THIRD EDITION

PART B

GARNER AND KLINTWORTH'S

PATHOBIOLOGY OF OCULAR DISEASE

Edited by

Gordon K. Klintworth
Duke University, Durham, North Carolina, USA

Alec Garner
Institute of Ophthalmology, Moorfields Eye Hospital, London, UK

Associate Editors

J. Godfrey Heathcote
Dalhousie University, Halifax, Nova Scotia, Canada

J. Douglas Cameron
Mayo Clinic, Rochester, Minnesota, USA

Victor M. Elner
Kellogg Eye Institute, University of Michigan, Ann Arbor, Michigan, USA

Narsing A. Rao
Doheny Eye Institute, Keck School of Medicine, University of Southern California, Los Angeles, California, USA

informa
healthcare

New York London

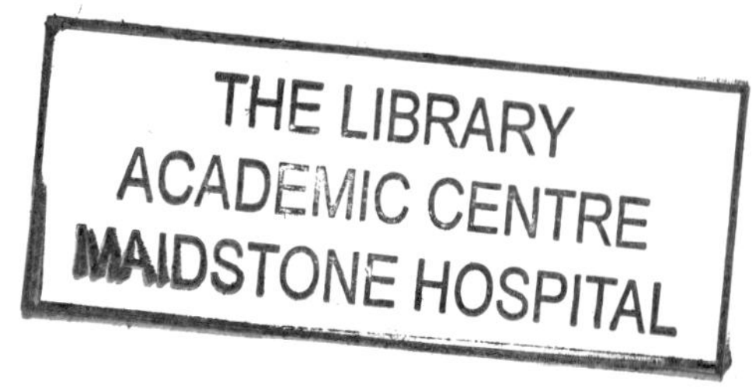

Informa Healthcare USA, Inc.
52 Vanderbilt Avenue
New York, NY 10017

Printed in the United States of America on acid-free paper
10 9 8 7 6 5 4 3 2 1

International Standard Book Number-10: 0-8493-9816-9 (Hardcover)
International Standard Book Number-13: 978-0-8493-9816-2 (Hardcover)
Part A: ISBN-10: 1-4200-7975-1; ISBN-13: 978-1-4200-7975-3
Part B: ISBN-10: 1-4200-7976-X; ISBN-13: 978-1-4200-7976-0

Library of Congress Cataloging-in-Publication Data

Garner and Klintworth's pathobiology of ocular disease/edited by Gordon K. Klintworth, Alec Garner.—3rd ed.
p. ; cm.
Rev. ed. of: Pathobiology of ocular disease/edited by Alec Garner, Gordon K. Klintworth. 2nd ed. c1994.
Includes bibliographical references and index.
ISBN-13: 978-0-8493-9816-2 (hardcover: alk. paper)
ISBN-10: 0-8493-9816-9 (hardcover: alk. paper)
1. Eye—Pathophysiology. 2. Eye—Diseases—Pathophysiology. I. Klintworth, Gordon K. II. Garner, Alec. III. Pathobiology of ocular disease. IV. Title: Pathobiology of ocular disease.
[DNLM: 1. Eye Diseases—pathology. 2. Eye Diseases—physiopathology. 3. Eye Diseases—etiology. WW 140 G234 2007]
RE67.P38 2007
617.7′1—dc22 2007030661

For Corporate Sales and Reprint Permissions call 212-520-2700 or write to: Sales Department, 52 Vanderbilt Avenue, 16th floor, New York, NY 10017.

Visit the Informa Web site at www.informa.com

and the Informa Healthcare Web site at www.informahealthcare.com

GARNER AND KLINTWORTH'S

PATHOBIOLOGY OF OCULAR DISEASE

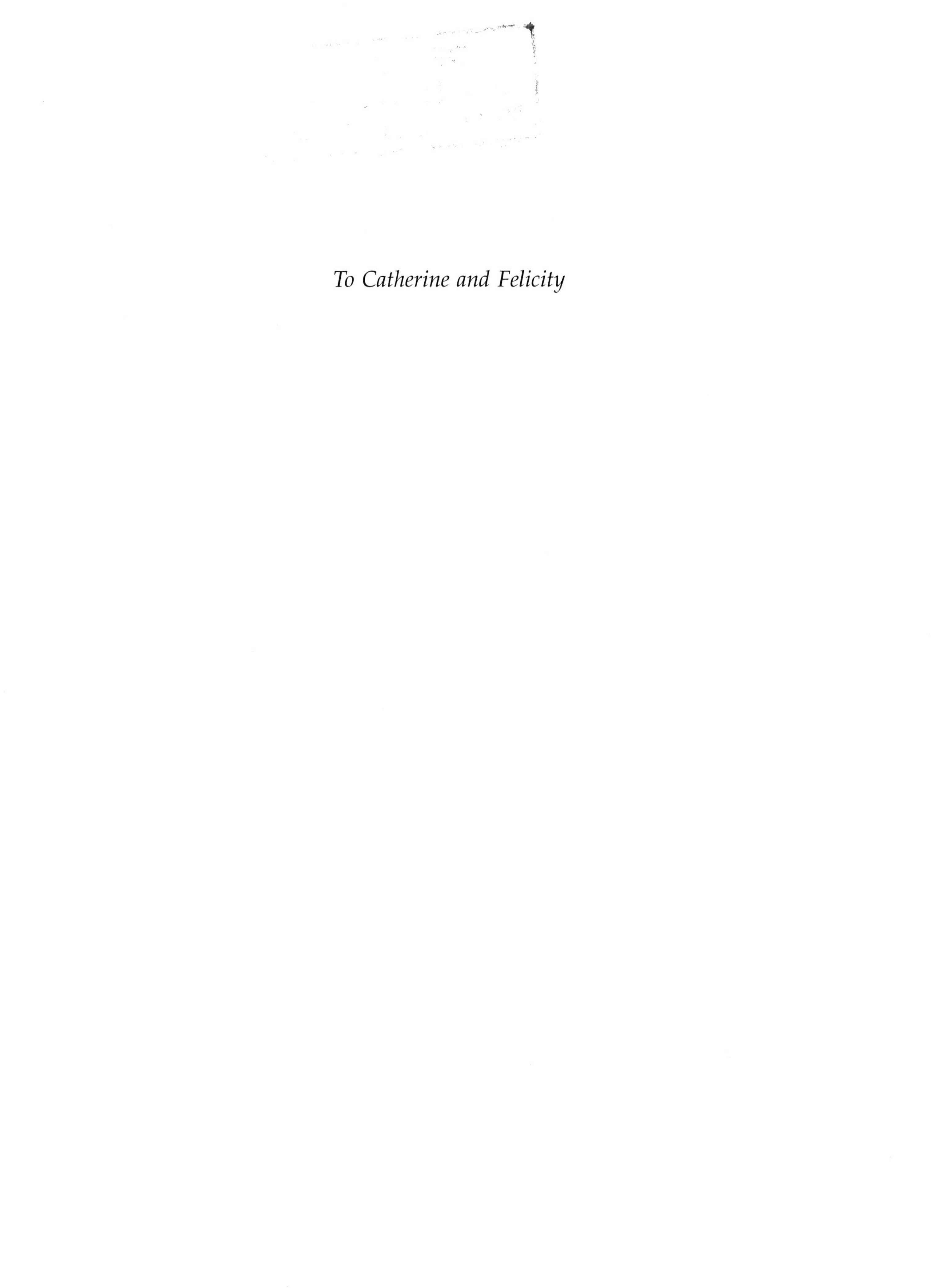

To Catherine and Felicity

Foreword to the Third Edition

A quarter of a century has passed since the first edition of *Pathobiology of Ocular Disease: A Dynamic Approach* was published. This successful, unique text, which is edited by two of the very few pathologists who have devoted major portions of their careers to ophthalmic pathology, has now gone into a third edition after a lapse of more than a decade. Unlike most books on ophthalmic pathology, this one devotes a large amount of space to a consideration of the etiology and pathogenesis of the diseases that afflict the tissues of the eye and its adnexa, as well as the visual pathways within the central nervous system. The current status of knowledge about the common blinding diseases of cataract, glaucoma, age-related maculopathy, and diabetic retinopathy is reviewed, but the vast numbers of infectious, immunologic, metabolic, toxic, degenerative, neoplastic, vascular, traumatic, and genetic diseases are also considered. By covering the embryologic development of the eye, the nature of ocular developmental anomalies can be appreciated.

Because this ambitious undertaking is multidisciplinary, the chapters were prepared by almost one hundred contributors with variable backgrounds from different parts of the world.

An understanding of the causes, variable behavior, and mechanisms underlying specific diseases is essential to their rational therapy. Although the editors decided not to cover therapy because of space restrictions and uncertainties about the ideal treatment of diseases, the text provides a background for the development of rational therapeutic approaches.

The third edition is vastly different from the second edition because of the amazing amount of new information that has emerged as a result of the combined research efforts of numerous individuals, involving, in particular, molecular genetic techniques. The Human Genome Project, completed in 2003 after thirteen years, was a major factor in the exponential increase in information, and it is not surprising that the current edition contains so much new information about mutated genes and the newly discovered metabolic pathways, such as those involved in programmed cell death (apoptosis). This body of information has necessitated an increase in the number of chapters from 54 to 72.

I congratulate the editors in bringing together this group of respected contributors to provide a comprehensive overview of the current status of knowledge about the diseases that affect the eye and vision. The book will undoubtedly be a valuable asset to those desiring information about the enormous array of ophthalmic disorders.

Lorenz E. Zimmerman, MD
Emeritus Chairman,
Department of Ophthalmic Pathology
Armed Forces Institute of Pathology,
Walter Reed Army Medical Center
Washington, DC, U.S.A.

Foreword from the Second Edition

Over a decade has passed since I contributed a foreword to the first edition of this scholarly work, and in that short time biomedical research has advanced further than could have been imagined. This second edition is accordingly expanded, and the fifty-four chapters, covering a wide range of disciplines, illustrate in a striking way the influence of this progress in the field of ophthalmology. The advances derive in the main from highly sophisticated developments in research technology, providing new concepts rather than etiological revelations. Thus, many blinding diseases, as from cataract, glaucoma, diabetes, and age-related maculopathy, still await definitive explanations of their cause, but our increasing appreciation of the many factors apparently playing a role in their pathogenesis, so well expounded here, provide a sure foundation for tomorrow's achievements in rational therapy.

Whether the authors are clinicians, pathologists, or other scientists, they are all authorities in their subjects and together present, to a standard equal to the best in medical literature, our latest knowledge of eye disease, within the context of cognate progress in general pathology. It is a most impressive work and surely unequalled in its particular approach to diseases of the eye, not as an organ sequestered in the orbit, but as one vulnerable to diseases of the body as a whole.

In congratulating the authors I express my hope that this second edition will continue to provide both pleasure and profit to the wide readership it will undoubtedly attract.

Norman Ashton, CBE, FRS
Emeritus Professor of Pathology
University of London and
The Royal College of Surgeons of England

Foreword from the First Edition

No systematized presentation of the pathology of the eye existed in any language until 1808 when James Wardrop, a Scotsman then aged 26, published his first edition of *Essays on the Morbid Anatomy of the Human Eye,* followed the next year by *Fungus Haemotodes or Soft Cancer* which established retino-blastoma as a recognized entity. Although these books were not the first to describe or illustrate specimens or ocular disease, and in fact contained little morbid anatomy as now defined, they introduced, by dissections and macroscopical studies, an area of investigation eventually to become the specialty of ophthalmic pathology.

The subsequent development of microscopy in the late nineteenth century and early twentieth century and its wider use throughout all aspects of laboratory science led to an immense and still expanding increase in knowledge. The revelations of histology and histopathology had as dramatic an impact as those of electron microscopy in modern times, and ophthalmic pathology in its turn became largely concerned with the documentation of macroscopical and microscopical features of diseased ocular tissues. There followed many textbooks dealing exclusively or predominantly with these aspects; the most widely admired are beautifully illustrated first with superb paintings and drawings and later by photographic reproductions, which in the last two decades reached the highest quality. These remain classic textbooks in ophthalmology and are of inestimable value, but curiously ophthalmic pathology continued to be confined to morbid anatomy long after pathology itself had branched out to found the present main disciplines of histopathology, chemical pathology, hematology, medical microbiology, and immunopathology. Even today ophthalmic pathology is usually equated with histopathology of the eye; that is certainly the main interest of American, Canadian, and European ophthalmic pathology societies. This has been at least partly due to the fact that for many years ophthalmic pathology was a part-time pursuit of ophthalmologists engaged in exacting clinical practice, and perhaps it would be as reasonable to expect them to have had the time to become conversant with the many developments in pathology as it would be to expect a general pathologist to be skilled, for instance, in the latest methods of cataract extraction or the management of glaucoma. Thus while freely acknowledging that the present sum of knowledge in ophthalmic pathology is much indebted to them, I have always been convinced that future progress must be more widely based. In 1957, I wrote …

"If in the future, eye pathology is to be taught and practised in the traditional way, as an elaborate recording of histologic minutiae, then the subject is not too demanding and may well be undertaken as a part-time pursuit, and probably best by the ophthalmologist who is most able to extract the greatest clinical value from the findings. But if the study of ocular pathology is to have its full meaning, the eye must be regarded as a unit of an entire organism, and its behavior in disease must as far as possible be related to that of the whole. Research in this field, in common with the general tendency, should concern itself with disease mechanisms rather than with disease patterns, and for this purpose the widest possible knowledge of pathologic processes is desirable and the whole armamentarium of modern scientific method should be available. To establish ocular pathology on this broad basis will demand the full and concentrated attention of workers trained and experienced in the appropriate disciplines."*

Nearly a quarter of a century later I have nothing to add to these convictions and I warmly welcome this monumental work in two volumes planned and executed on the lines I had so hopefully visualized, and I am proud that such a notable work should have been assembled by Professor Alec Garner, my successor as director of the Department of Pathology at the Institute of Ophthalmology in London, and Professor Gordon Klintworth, some-time visiting professor there. With their able collaborators they present in these comprehensive volumes exactly the approach to ocular disease that is essential both for its immediate elucidation and for the whole future development of the subject, not in isolation but within the context of pathology as a whole.

With this conviction I warmly commend this book to everyone interested and involved in this fascinating field of learning, and wish all those concerned in its production the success so richly deserved.

Norman Ashton, CBE, FRS
Emeritus Professor of Pathology
University of London and
The Royal College of Surgeons of England

* Am. J. Ophthalmol. 44:5-6, 1957.

Preface to the Third Edition

Pathology at the clinical level is principally concerned with diagnosis, and rightly so. But it has an even deeper significance, which stems from its very definition. Pathology is the study of disease. In other words, it is fundamentally concerned with the processes underlying the clinical manifestations of disease. This is the principle we have tried to uphold in putting the present compilation together.

What is unique about this book? Before providing an answer, let us consider other books on ophthalmic pathology. Several are designed for the trainee in clinical ophthalmology and focus on clinically relevant information that examiners require of persons taking professional examinations. Such books are valuable to persons intent on persuading their examiners that they know enough pathology to be allowed to practice clinical ophthalmology. Other books provide a manual of diagnostic ophthalmic pathology and concentrate on descriptive morphology and are often extensively illustrated. *Garner and Klintworth's Pathobiology of Ocular Disease, Third Edition*, contains some elements of both of these types of books, but it goes far beyond material necessary to pass examinations or diagnose disorders based on morphologic criteria. Morphology continues to be the bedrock in defining the pathology of any disorder and, where appropriate, our contributors have not shied away from spelling out the clinical and histological aspects of the conditions they describe. But because pathology goes far beyond morbid anatomy, they have sought, where possible, to use these definitions as a basis for describing the underlying cellular events at a molecular level.

Back in the 1960s, when the editors were learning the trade, knowledge about eye diseases was proving elusive, largely from lack of appropriate methods of investigation. But since then the introduction of such techniques as electron microscopy, precise histochemical stains, and tissue and cell culture revolutionized the functional appreciation of a multitude of diseases. The revolution has continued unabated with the application of extremely sophisticated molecular biology techniques able to exploit an ever-expanding understanding of cytogenetics and immunology.

In the preface to the first edition of a much-valued textbook on pathology that was current when the editors of this book were medical students (1), we were reminded that, "Pathology is the elucidation of the vital processes which underlie the end-results studied by the morbid anatomist. It is the study of disease from the physiological point of view." Indeed, this has always been the real goal of the pathologist, a point purportedly made more than a hundred years ago by the distinguished surgeon, scientist, and one-time professor of pathology, Sir Victor Horsley (1857–1916), who was intent on pushing back the limitations of clinical practice when he wrote, "What is currently thought of as pathology is nothing of the sort—it is morbid anatomy. The pathologist should be a student of disordered function." It is to this understanding of ophthalmic pathology that we and our contributors have been committed in this multi-disciplinary book purposely titled, *Pathobiology of Ocular Disease*.

As with the two earlier editions, the book was designed with the ophthalmic practitioner in mind to provide, as far as is possible, an appreciation of the processes responsible for producing the disorders observed in hospital clinics and consulting rooms. While therapy is not considered because of space restrictions and the fact that it is often empirical, the information provided about the cause and basic mechanisms of specific diseases provides insight into potential therapeutic approaches. The effective rational therapy of any disease must be derived from a sound understanding of the underlying basic mechanisms.

In the decade that has intervened since the last edition, major advances have been made, particularly in the realms of molecular biology, cytogenetics, computerized databases, and, more recently, in molecular genetics. The ability to amplify DNA with the polymerized chain reaction, to sequence the human genome, and to identify specific proteins in different tissues with the highly sensitive matrix-assisted laser desorption ionization–time of flight mass spectrometry has played an important role in furthering knowledge. The study of ocular disease has shared in this advance, and the findings have impinged on the etiology and pathogenesis of many ocular diseases. This knowledge has expanded exponentially, largely as a result of research by scientists with a wide variety of techniques and the rapid dissemination of information on the Internet.

Such has been the increase in knowledge that several chapters were completely revamped and several new chapters added. The vast increase in knowledge about the genetics of many ocular diseases spawned specific chapters dealing with molecular genetic aspects of glaucoma and cataracts, as well as corneal, retinal, and optic nerve disease. Other new chapters focus on the molecular pathways of apoptosis, wound healing, the vasculitides, aging, age-related maculopathy, the aging lens, myopia, and amblyopia.

In the first edition we diligently avoided abbreviations, despite their emerging popularity in biomedical publications. By the second edition, abbreviations were unavoidable, and in this new edition the number increased immensely, largely due to the use of acronyms and conventions that have arisen regarding the nomenclature of the vast number of identified genes and their encoded proteins. When possible, we used accepted abbreviations that have come into common usage among experts who are furthering knowledge about diseases. For example, for consistency we used italicized uppercase letters for human genes and non-italicized letters for the protein products. Mouse genes that are involved in many animal models of ocular diseases are designated according to the accepted format of lowercase italicized letters. For readers not familiar with abbreviations, we have insisted that they be defined the first time that they are used in each chapter, and for the ease of finding the definition, the separate section on abbreviations has been retained. Hopefully, the large number of abbreviations in some chapters is not a chaotic alphabet soup.

So many human genetic diseases are now recognized that each has a Mendelian Inheritance in Man (MIM) number (2). Information about these diseases is freely available on the Internet, with links to information about the involved genes and their protein products. To facilitate the reader's access to this material, the Mendelian Inheritance in Man number for specific inherited diseases that are discussed in the book is provided when possible.

Another significant editorial change in the book is the rejection of the possessive form of eponyms for diseases, syndromes, anatomic structures, and other eponymous terms. This was done for multiple reasons, as outlined elsewhere (3), and the trend is gradually gaining momentum in medical writings.

We are fortunate to have been able to enlist the services of some of the most highly qualified investigators in their respective fields who provide authoritative accounts of the current understanding of the enormous spectrum of ocular diseases. To assist us in the critical evaluation of the text and the editing process we also recruited four highly respected ophthalmic pathologists as associate editors (Drs. J. Godfrey Heathcote, J. Douglas Cameron, Victor M. Elner, and Narsing A. Rao). We are most grateful to these individuals, who have expertise in different areas of the subject, for their constructive comments and editorial suggestions. We would also like to acknowledge several other individuals who helped bring this book to fruition: Mr. Geoffrey Greenwood, who convinced us to embark on a third edition, and Ms. Sandra Beberman, Ms. Dana Bigelow, Ms. Beth Campbell, Ms. Mary Drabot, and Mr. Christopher DiBiase of Informa Healthcare, as well as Ms. Paula Garber, Ms. Joanne Jay, and Mr. Peter Compitello of The Egerton Group Ltd., who were most helpful in bringing this book to fruition. As with the previous two editions, we wish to acknowledge the support and encouragement provided by our wives, Felicity and Catherine, and have great pleasure in dedicating this third edition to them.

The preparation of each edition of this book has aptly confirmed the impression of the great British soldier, statesman, author, and first honorary citizen of the United States, Sir Winston Churchill (1874–1965), who stated, "Writing a book is an adventure. To begin with it is a toy, then an amusement. Then it [becomes] a mistress, and then it becomes a master, and then it becomes a tyrant and, in the last stage, just as you are about to be reconciled to your servitude, you kill the monster and fling him to the public" (Grosvenor House, London, November 2, 1949) (4).

Gordon K. Klintworth
Alec Garner

REFERENCES

1. Boyd W. A Textbook of Pathology: An Introduction to Medicine. 1st ed. Philadelphia: Lea and Febiger, 1932.
2. http://www.ncbi.nlm.nih.gov/entrez/query.fcgi?db=OMIM
3. Iverson C, Flanagin A, Fontanarosa PB, et al. American Medical Association Manual of Style: A Guide for Authors and Editors. 9th ed. Baltimore: Williams and Wilkins, 1998.
4. The words from the original speaking notes for Churchill's address after receiving the Times Literary Award. Churchill Archives Centre Cambridge, CHUR 5/28A, paragraph 4, page 2.

Preface from the Second Edition

A knowledge of pathology is the basis of sound medicine, and the thinking ophthalmologist is keen to understand, as well as may be, the forces responsible for the clinical manifestations of eye disease. Only then can management be pursued in a rational manner. The descriptive elements of ophthalmic pathology are fundamental and need to be precisely defined in the interests of accurate diagnosis. But beyond that utilitarian function is their importance as building blocks in comprehending the nature of the disease processes per se, and it is to this second objective in particular that the present text is directed. Correspondingly, we have not sought to provide a detailed manual of diagnostic pathology—there are now a number of excellent texts and atlases available that achieve this purpose far better than we could ever have hoped to do. Instead, where possible, we have tried to interpret the facts and to provide a feeling for the dynamic aspects of ophthalmic pathology.

As noted in the preface to the first edition, laudable though such a purpose may be, it is difficult to succeed. Firstly, depending on the particular disease state under consideration, it requires a sound knowledge of a range of complementary disciplines such as molecular biology, biochemistry, immunology, and genetics. In this regard, we have been fortunate in having the services of many recognized experts in these various fields capable of writing with authority. Secondly, not all the necessary building blocks are yet identified, let alone in position. Nevertheless, an incredible body of new information has accrued in almost every field in the twelve years since the first edition, especially in the understanding of disease at the molecular level, and an update of our text had become imperative if it was to remain relevant. We were encouraged to take up the challenge by the favorable reception of the first edition and because, despite the welcome increase in textbooks related to the pathology of eye disease, ours remains the only reasonably comprehensive attempt to address the functional aspects of the subject.

As with the first edition, this has been a daunting task, and we are more than grateful to our contributors, who have responded to their briefs quite magnificently. For one reason or another, we have had to enlist the help of a number of new authors, and such has been the enormous volume of new material to be covered that even existing authors have had to engage in extensive revision of their chapters, amounting in some cases to a complete rewrite.

Again, we very much hope that the attraction of the book will extend beyond the precious but small number of practicing ophthalmic pathologists to pathologists working in other fields, because study of the eye has relevance far beyond its own orbit. Clinical ophthalmologists too will, we trust, find much to assist them in the evaluation and treatment of their patients. We hope that others outside the medical community—those employed in related disciplines of biology, immunology, and genetics—will also discover something of value.

We are very conscious of and more than happy to acknowledge the enormous assistance provided by our secretaries, Pat Goodwin, Carmen Quarrie, Wanda Dietze, Elizabeth Barnard, Karen Alliume, and Kristina Boewe. We are also indebted to Allan T. Summers for his painstaking role in verifying and completing countless references. Finally, as before, we want to thank our wives, Catherine and Felicity, who have been most supportive, and we hope they will find pleasure in the outcome which we take great delight in dedicating to them.

Alec Garner
Gordon K. Klintworth

Preface from the First Edition

Such is the volume of ophthalmologic and pathological writing that only by stepping aside completely from one's commitment to engage actively in these disciplines would it be possible to absorb all that might profitably be read. It would be irresponsible of any potential author or editor to unleash on the busy student yet more reading matter should it not fill a real need. There are in existence already several excellent treatises relating to the pathological anatomy of the eye, and it would have been redundant for us to seek to emulate them; rather we have sought to direct attention to dynamic considerations and disease mechanisms, and so complement the emphasis on descriptive pathology to be found in other writings on the subject. Hence the title *Pathobiology of Ocular Disease: A Dynamic Approach*.

It is our belief that knowing the appearance of a lesion and being able to recognize it is only the beginning of the story. If appropriate and rational treatment is to be instituted, it is also necessary to understand what is happening and, where possible, why. For instance, from the practicing clinician's standpoint, more important than to recognize granulomatous inflammation when seen in a microscopical preparation is to have some idea of what that means in terms of causative factors and likely behavior. That is not to say we decry descriptive pathology—far from it, for morphology and function are but the two sides of the same coin and are patently interdependent. But the job of the pathologist is both to identify disease processes and to interpret them in behavioral terms. It was with this dual role of pathology in mind that we invited the various contributors to compose their chapters.

However, success is an elusive goal when the brief is so demanding. To state what and where is one thing; to ask how and why is quite another. Nevertheless, as editors, we feel that our contributors have responded magnificently and it is our fervent hope that the result will meet the needs of serious students of ophthalmology, be they trainees or more experienced practitioners, who are keen to understand the nature of the disorders they are called on to treat. The emphasis on dynamic disease processes inevitably encompasses the whole gamut of pathological disciplines—microbiology, immunology, and biochemistry, as well as histopathology, and this all-embracing interpretation of pathology serves further to distinguish our book from existing texts.

For a variety of reasons, which need not be spelt out here, ophthalmic pathology is commonly viewed with suspicion by other pathologists. Trained as general pathologists ourselves, we as editors hope that, by relating the specific matters of ocular pathology to the basic and more general aspects of disease processes, we will have gone some way towards persuading our colleagues that study of the eye is both fascinating and rewarding.

Inevitably, to assemble a multiauthor compendium of the sort we have compiled, such that there is not too much diversity of approach, has involved a great deal of effort, not only for the editors, but also for the gallant contributors who have had to contend with a seemingly endless stream of queries and comments. We want to thank them for their cooperation and forbearance.

Other people whose assistance has been invaluable are acknowledged elsewhere but we would also put on record our appreciation of the unstinting advice and practical help provided by the staff of our publisher, Marcel Dekker, Inc., and of the colossal support we have received from our secretaries, Catherine Thornton, Pat Goodwin, Louise Hart, Frances Slocum, Candiss Weaver, Pat Burks, Bonnie Lynch, Diane Evans, Linda Brogan, Marge Penny, and Virginia Hotelling. Lastly, if for no other reason than that they are the ones who at the end of the day have had to bear with us when the task of preparing the book weighed overheavily on our shoulders, we want to thank our wives and children for their tolerance and encouragement.

This book would not have been possible without the assistance of many individuals. Aside from the vital role of the authors and the editorial staff of Marcel Dekker, Inc., numerous individuals provided critical reviews of chapters. In this regard, we wish to thank the following:

Mathea R. Allansmith
Douglas R. Anderson
Norman Ashton
Elaine R. Berman
Stanley Braverman
Robert P. Burns
R. Jean Campbell
Leo T. Chylack
David G. Cogan
Byron P. Croker, Jr.
Anthony J. Dark
D. Doniach
Roberta Meyers Elliot
Bernard F. Fetter
Ben S. Fine
Ramon L. Font

Robert Y. Foos
Doyle G. Graham
Donald B. Hackel
Hal K. Hawkins
Hannah Kinney
Jin H. Kinoshita
John F. R. Kuck, Jr.
Robert Machemer
Kenneth S. McCarty, Jr.
Don Minckler
Ralph Muller
G. Richard O'Connor
M. Bruce Shields
James Tiedeman
Robert Trelstad
F. Stephen Vogel
Lorenz E. Zimmerman

Allan Summers, Susan Feinglos, Ginger Reeves, Betty Adams, Mary Ann Brown, and Janet Shields were most helpful in checking and completing the innumerable references.

The following assisted authors with specific chapters: Nancy L. Robinson, Glenn P. Kimball, and Karen A. Pelletier (Chapter 49), David Andrews (Chapter 48), Joseph Hackett (Chapter 40).

Alec Garner
Gordon K. Klintworth

Contents of Part B

NORMAL AND ABNORMAL DEVELOPMENT

TUMORS

BLOOD VESSELS IN OCULAR DISEASE

OCULAR INVOLVEMENT IN DISORDERS OF NERVOUS AND MUSCULAR SYSTEMS

Contents of Part A

DISORDERS OF THE VITREOUS

DISORDERS OF THE ANTERIOR SEGMENT

METABOLIC AND GENETIC DISORDERS

Contributors

Anthony P. Adamis Eyetech Pharmaceuticals, New York, New York, U.S.A.

D. Cory Adamson Departments of Neurosurgery and Neurobiology, Duke University, Durham, North Carolina, U.S.A.

Daniel M. Albert Department of Ophthalmology and Visual Sciences, University of Wisconsin, Madison, Wisconsin, U.S.A.

Thomas Albini Bascom Palmer Eye Institute, Miller School of Medicine, University of Miami, Miami, Florida, U.S.A.

R. Rand Allingham Department of Ophthalmology, Duke University, Durham, North Carolina, U.S.A.

Fahd Anzaar Massachusetts Eye Research and Surgery Institute and Harvard University, Boston, Massachusetts, U.S.A.

Pelin Atmaca-Sönmez Kellogg Eye Institute, University of Michigan, Ann Arbor, Michigan, U.S.A.

William Robert Bell Wilmer Eye Institute, Johns Hopkins University, Baltimore, Maryland, U.S.A.

Elaine R. Berman (deceased) Hadassah-Hebrew University Medical School, Jerusalem, Israel

Paul N. Bishop Faculty of Medical and Human Sciences and Wellcome Trust Centre for Cell-Matrix Research, University of Manchester, Manchester, U.K.

Zita F. H. M. Boonman Department of Ophthalmology, Leiden University Medical Center, Leiden, The Netherlands

Ray P. Boot-Handford Faculty of Life Sciences, Wellcome Trust Centre for Cell Matrix Research, University of Manchester, Manchester, U.K.

Edward H. Bossen Department of Pathology, Duke University, Durham, North Carolina, U.S.A.

Rose-Mary Boustany Departments of Pediatrics and Neurobiology, Duke University, Durham, North Carolina, U.S.A. and Abu-Haidan Neuroscience Institute, American University of Beirut, Beirut, Lebanon

Harry H. Brown Harvey and Bernice Jones Eye Institute, University of Arkansas for Medical Sciences, Little Rock, Arkansas, U.S.A.

Matthew J. Burton International Centre for Eye Health, London School of Hygiene and Tropical Medicine, London, U.K.

J. Douglas Cameron Department of Ophthalmology, Mayo Clinic, Rochester, Minnesota, U.S.A.

George M. Cherian Departments of Pathology, Pharmacology, and Toxicology, University of Western Ontario, London, Ontario, Canada

Chung-Jung Chiu Department of Ophthalmology and the Jean Mayer USDA Human Nutrition Research Center on Aging, Tufts University, Boston, Massachusetts, U.S.A.

M. Joseph Costello Department of Cell and Developmental Biology, University of North Carolina, Chapel Hill, North Carolina, U.S.A.

J. Oscar Croxatto Departments of Teaching and Research and Laboratory of Ophthalmic Pathology, Fundación Oftalmológica Argentina Jorge Malbran, Buenos Aires, Argentina

Thomas J. Cummings Departments of Pathology and Ophthalmology, Duke University, Durham, North Carolina, U.S.A.

Karim F. Damji University of Ottawa Eye Institute, Ottawa, Ontario, Canada

Hakan Demirci Kellogg Eye Institute, University of Michigan, Ann Arbor, Michigan, U.S.A.

Erin Demo Divison of Genetics and Metabolism, University of North Carolina, Chapel Hill, North Carolina, U.S.A.

Susan G. Elner Kellogg Eye Institute, University of Michigan, Ann Arbor, Michigan, U.S.A.

Victor M. Elner Kellogg Eye Institute, University of Michigan, Ann Arbor, Michigan, U.S.A.

Geoffrey G. Emerson Casey Eye Institute, Oregon Health and Science University, Portland, Oregon, U.S.A.

Jan J. Enghild Department of Molecular Biology, University of Aarhus, Aarhus, Denmark

Andrew Flint Department of Pathology, University of Michigan, Ann Arbor, Michigan, U.S.A.

C. Stephen Foster Massachusetts Eye Research and Surgery Institute and Harvard University, Boston, Massachusetts, U.S.A.

Peter J. Francis Casey Eye Institute, Oregon Health and Science University, Portland, Oregon, U.S.A.

Anne B. Fulton Department of Ophthalmology, Children's Hospital, Boston, Massachusetts, U.S.A.

David M. Gamm Department of Ophthalmology and Visual Sciences, University of Wisconsin, Madison, Wisconsin, U.S.A.

Alec Garner Institute of Ophthalmology, Moorfields Eye Hospital, London, U.K.

Devin M. Gattey Casey Eye Institute, Oregon Health and Science University, Portland, Oregon, U.S.A.

Jennifer B. Green Division of Endocrinology, Department of Medicine, Duke University, Durham, North Carolina, U.S.A.

W. Richard Green Wilmer Eye Institute, Johns Hopkins University, Baltimore, Maryland, U.S.A.

Ian Grierson Unit of Ophthalmology, School of Clinical Sciences, University of Liverpool, Liverpool, U.K.

Hans E. Grossniklaus Departments of Ophthalmology and Pathology, Emory University, Atlanta, Georgia, U.S.A.

Duane L. Guernsey Departments of Pathology, Ophthalmology and Visual Sciences, Surgery, Physiology, and Biophysics, Dalhousie University, Halifax, Nova Scotia, Canada

Avinash Gurbaxani Kings College Hospital, London, U.K.

Robyn H. Guymer Centre for Eye Research Australia, University of Melbourne, East Melbourne, Victoria, Australia

John R. Guyton Department of Medicine, Duke University, Durham, North Carolina, U.S.A.

Sarah Hale University Hospital of Wales, Cardiff, U.K.

John J. Harding Nuffield Laboratory of Ophthalmology, University of Oxford, Oxford, U.K.

J. Godfrey Heathcote Departments of Pathology and Ophthalmology and Visual Sciences, Dalhousie University, Halifax, Nova Scotia, Canada

John R. Heckenlively Kellogg Eye Institute, University of Michigan, Ann Arbor, Michigan, U.S.A.

Mitchell T. Heflin Center for Aging and Human Development, Duke University, Durham, North Carolina, U.S.A.

Paul Hiscott Unit of Ophthalmology, School of Clinical Sciences, University of Liverpool, Liverpool, U.K.

David N. Howell Department of Pathology, Duke University and Durham Veterans Administration Medical Center, Durham, North Carolina, U.S.A.

Martine J. Jager Department of Ophthalmology, Leiden University Medical Center, Leiden, The Netherlands

Henrik Karring Department of Experimental Medical Science, Lund University, Lund, Sweden

Cay M. Kielty Faculty of Life Sciences, Wellcome Trust Centre for Cell Matrix Research, University of Manchester, Manchester, U.K.

Priya S. Kishnani Division of Medical Genetics, Duke University, Durham, North Carolina, U.S.A.

Mary K. Klassen-Fischer Armed Forces Institute of Pathology, Washington, D.C., U.S.A.

Gordon K. Klintworth Departments of Pathology and Ophthalmology, Duke University, Durham, North Carolina, U.S.A.

Dwight D. Koeberl Division of Medical Genetics, Duke University, Durham, North Carolina, U.S.A.

Amol D. Kulkarni Department of Ophthalmology and Visual Sciences, University of Wisconsin, Madison, Wisconsin, U.S.A.

Jerome R. Kuszak Department of Ophthalmology, Rush University Medical Center, Chicago, Illinois, U.S.A.

Anand Shreeram Lagoo Department of Pathology, Duke University, Durham, North Carolina, U.S.A.

Susan Lightman Department of Clinical Ophthalmology, Moorfields Eye Hospital, London, U.K.

Lyndell L. Lim Centre for Eye Research Australia, University of Melbourne, East Melbourne, Victoria, Australia

Ming Lu Vantage Eye Center, Monterey, California, U.S.A.

Helen Lum Durham Veterans Administration Medical Center, Durham, North Carolina, U.S.A.

Curtis E. Margo University of South Florida, Tampa, Florida, U.S.A.

Suzanne P. McKee Smith-Kettlewell Eye Research Institute, San Francisco, California, U.S.A.

Stuart J. McKinnon Departments of Ophthalmology and Neurobiology, Duke University, Durham, North Carolina, U.S.A.

Janine D. Mendola Center for Advanced Imaging, West Virginia University School of Medicine, Morgantown, West Virginia, U.S.A.

Ravikanth Metlapally Duke Center for Human Genetics and Duke Eye Center, Duke University, Durham, North Carolina, U.S.A.

Sara E. Miller Department of Pathology, Duke University, Durham, North Carolina, U.S.A.

David Millington Division of Medical Genetics, Duke University, Durham, North Carolina, U.S.A.

Torben Møller-Pedersen Department of Molecular Biology, University of Aarhus, Aarhus, Denmark

Anne Moskowitz Department of Ophthalmology, Children's Hospital, Boston, Massachusetts, U.S.A.

Ronald C. Neafie Armed Forces Institute of Pathology, Washington, D.C., U.S.A.

Thomas T. Norton Department of Vision Sciences, University of Alabama at Birmingham, Birmingham, Alabama, U.S.A.

Terrence P. O'Brien Bascom Palmer Eye Institute of the Palm Beaches, Palm Beach Gardens, Florida, U.S.A.

Alan D. Proia Department of Pathology, Duke University, Durham, North Carolina, U.S.A.

Narsing A. Rao Doheny Eye Institute, Keck School of Medicine, University of Southern California, Los Angeles, California, U.S.A.

Johane M. Robitaille Departments of Ophthalmology and Visual Sciences and Pathology, Dalhousie University, Halifax, Nova Scotia, Canada

Diva R. Salomão Department of Pathology, Mayo Clinic, Mayo Foundation, and Mayo Medical School, Rochester, Minnesota, U.S.A.

Ursula Schlötzer-Schrehardt University of Erlangen-Nürnberg, Erlangen, Germany

Bryan J. Schwent Department of Ophthalmology, Emory University, Atlanta, Georgia, U.S.A.

Alan Shiels Department of Ophthalmology and Visual Sciences, Washington University School of Medicine, St. Louis, Missouri, U.S.A.

Brian S. F. Shine Department of Clinical Biochemistry, John Radcliffe Hospital, and Oxford Centre for Diabetes, Endocrinology, and Metabolism, Oxford, U.K.

Barbara A. W. Streeten State University of New York Upstate Medical University, Syracuse, New York, U.S.A.

Allen Taylor Department of Ophthalmology and the Jean Mayer USDA Human Nutrition Research Center for Aging, Tufts University, Boston, Masssachusetts, U.S.A.

René E. M. Toes Department of Rheumatology, Leiden University Medical Center, Leiden, The Netherlands

Julie H. Tsai University of South Carolina School of Medicine, Columbia, South Carolina, U.S.A.

Richard Vander Heide Wayne State University Medical School and John D. Dingell Veterans Administration Medical Center, Detroit, Michigan, U.S.A.

Bret M. Wehrli Department of Pathology, University of Western Ontario, London, Ontario, Canada

Janey L. Wiggs Department of Ophthalmology, Harvard Medical School, and Massachusetts Eye and Ear Infirmary, Boston, Massachusetts, U.S.A.

David J. Wilson Casey Eye Institute, Oregon Health and Science University, Portland, Oregon, U.S.A.

Carolyn S. Wu Department of Ophthalmology, Children's Hospital, Boston, Massachusetts, U.S.A.

Hai Yan Department of Pathology, Duke University, Durham, North Carolina, U.S.A.

Sarah Young Division of Medical Genetics, Duke University, Durham, North Carolina, U.S.A.

Terri L. Young Duke Eye Center and Duke Center for Human Genetics, Duke University, Durham, North Carolina, U.S.A.

36

Ocular Proteins and Proteomics

Henrik Karring
Department of Experimental Medical Science, Lund University, Lund, Sweden

Torben Møller-Pedersen and Jan J. Enghild
Department of Molecular Biology, University of Aarhus, Aarhus, Denmark

Gordon K. Klintworth
Departments of Pathology and Ophthalmology, Duke University, Durham, North Carolina U.S.A.

INTRODUCTION

The eye is a complex organ with a vast number of different proteins. Each ocular tissue and cell type has distinct protein expression profiles reflecting the function and condition of the cell/tissue. Thus, to better understand the molecular processes of the eye in health and disease a determination of proteins in the different compartments of the eye is important. In addition, many differentially expressed proteins in ophthalmic diseases are potential targets for therapeutic agents or suggest what processes are distorted in the disease (356). Previously, protein characterization involved only one or a few proteins at a time. However, recent technological developments now enable the simultaneous analysis of all the proteins in a system and the evaluation of changes in the protein expression as a consequence of disease and external factors.

In the first part of this chapter we describe the synthesis and modification of proteins, methods to analyze and characterize individual proteins and complex protein mixtures, and provide an overall classification of proteins according to function and structure. In the second part of the chapter we review proteome research on various healthy and diseased ocular tissues and the role of specific proteins in different ocular diseases.

PROTEOME AND PROTEOMICS

The human genome is estimated to contain 20,000 to 25,000 protein-encoding genes (168,219,385), but considerably more proteins are suspected due to alternative splicing of mRNA and post-translational modifications (PTMs) which result in different structures and functions of the mature protein. While the genome is static and identical in all cells the protein expression profile is cell- and tissue-specific and dynamically changes over time and with the conditions. The term *proteome* embraces the entire complement of proteins in a given organism or biological system at a given time and under specific conditions, i.e., the protein products of the genome (397,403,404). Therefore, analyzing biological systems at a protein rather than mRNA level has enormous advantages since proteins are the functional molecules. In addition, mRNA analyses may not truly reflect protein quantity (16) and analyses of nucleic acids do not predict the nature or position of PTMs that often regulate protein activity. More than 200 different types of PTMs are estimated to exist, dramatically increasing the complexity (257). Thus, gene-processing and PTMs could easily bring the number of different proteins in the human proteome to more than one million (223,260). Furthermore, genomics often does not predict the existence or the function of proteins emphasizing the need for direct protein analysis. The term *proteomics* describes the large-scale systematic study of proteins including their identification, characterization, quantification, structure, intermolecular protein–protein interactions, and functions (159,290). Proteomics therefore presents a powerful way to identify the constellation of proteins and protein modifications leading to biological perturbations and disease. To study the proteome of organs, tissues, or cells it is essential to use techniques that permit the simultaneous separation of thousands of different proteins and high throughput methodology for protein identification and characterization.

PROTEIN SYNTHESIS AND PTMs

When a gene is expressed its genetic information is first converted into RNA in the transcription process. The resulting primary transcript, the precursor messenger RNA (pre-mRNA), is processed and undergoes splicing in the nucleus to generate the mature mRNA that is exported to the cytosol. In the cytosol, the mRNA serves as template for protein synthesis carried out by the ribosome in a process termed translation (277). In addition to the mRNA and ribosome, transfer RNAs (tRNAs) and protein translation factors, are required in the protein expression machinery. Eukaryotic protein synthesis can be divided into initiation, elongation, and termination phases (182), which are controlled by specific factors. The initial amino acid in protein synthesis is methionine and in the initiation phase, ribosome subunits, mRNA, and Met-$tRNA_i^{Met}$ assemble to form an initiation complex (80S) that is ready for the elongation phase (304). In this complex the anticodon of $tRNA_i^{Met}$ interacts with the start codon of the mRNA. The peptide becomes elongated as amino acids carried by tRNAs are added one at a time to the C-terminus of the growing polypeptide chain. Translation termination is encoded by a stop codon of the mRNA. After the protein is synthesized the complete protein is released from the ribosome and the ribosome complex disassembles and becomes recycled ensuring that the ribosomal subunits are available for new initiations of protein synthesis.

Once synthesized, proteins are subjects to a multitude of PTMs (392), which may alter and regulate their function, stability, and solubility. They are cleaved (thus eliminating signal sequences, transit or pro-peptides, and initiator methionines); amino acids can be chemically modified (e.g., deamidation of glutamine and asparagine); many simple chemical groups, such as acetyl, methyl, phosphate, can be covalently attached to them. More complex molecules, such as sugars, lipids, and even other proteins or peptides can also become connected and finally, proteins can be internally or externally cross-linked by disulfide bridges (a bond between two cysteine residues). Thus, many secretory proteins have disulfide bridges due to the oxidative redox milieu in the extracellular matrix (ECM). In addition, many extracellular proteins including those in the circulation are glycoproteins in which carbohydrates are attached covalently to asparagine (N-glycans) or serine/threonine residues (O-glycans).

One of the main PTMs is ubiquitination, designed to signal rapid degradation of misfolded and damaged proteins. In this process the abnormal protein becomes attached to a unique protein called ubiquitin (76 amino acids) through an isopeptide bond, which tags it for degradation by a proteolytic digestion complex known as the proteasome. The proteasome is localized in the cytoplasm and nucleus and composed of a cylindrical core particle (20S proteasome) containing 28 subunits (two copies of 14 different proteins), and two identical regulatory particles (19S caps) formed by 14 different proteins. The complete proteasome is termed the 26S proteasome. This ubiquitin-mediated degradation of proteins is known as the ubiquitin-proteasome system (UPS) (129,323). Thus, since genomic information does not predict most PTMs, these protein modifications can only be identified by characterizing the proteins.

PROTEIN SEPARATION AND IDENTIFICATION

A precise identification of specific proteins requires their separation by techniques, such as two-dimensional (2D) gel electrophoresis (Appendix 1) (Fig. 1) and their identification, which is best performed by amino terminal protein sequencing (Edman degradation) or mass spectrometry using Matrix-Assisted Laser Desorption Ionization-Time of Flight Mass Spectrometry (MALDI-TOF MS) and peptide mass fingerprinting or electrospray ionization liquid chromatography tandem mass spectrometry (ESI-LC-MS/MS) (Appendix 1).

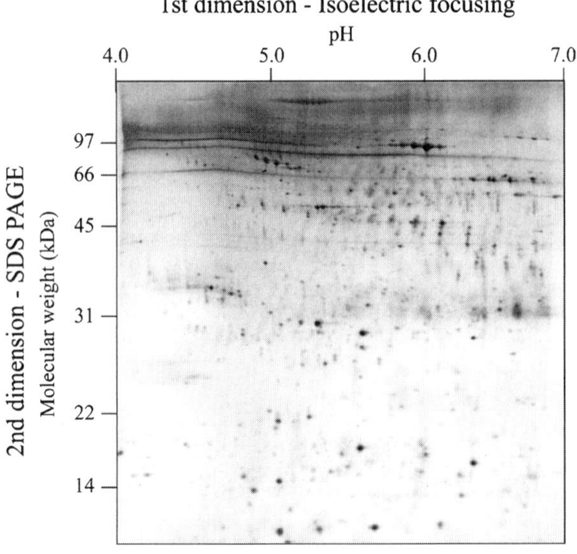

Figure 1 Two-dimensional polyacrylamide gel electrophoresis (2D PAGE) of the human cornea proteome. Proteins from the human cornea were extracted and analyzed by 2D PAGE. The depicted 2D gel (size: 18×23.4 cm) was developed with IEF (first dimension) using pH gradient 4.0 to 7.0. In the second dimension the proteins are separated according to their size. The molecular weight standards are indicated on the left. The separated proteins were visualized by silver staining. Each spot contains one protein. *Source*: The 2D gel is from Ref. 183.

PURIFICATION OF PROTEINS AND PEPTIDES

After a protein has been identified it is often important to characterize its function and determine the three-dimensional (3D) structure which require native and pure protein in significant amounts. Due to the lack of authentic sources (donor organs, tissue, or cells) or the low abundance of a protein in vivo, recombinant protein expression systems (cell-free systems, bacteria, yeast, insect cells, mammalian cells) are often used for functional and structural studies. Thus, the protein of interest can be synthesized by the organism/system after the insertion of the foreign gene into such systems (126). These so-called recombinant organisms can normally be grown easily at low cost and studies of the recombinant genes and proteins have extended our knowledge about many ocular proteins, such as those of the lens (38,40), retina (66,376), and cornea (69,70). The choice of recombinant expression system normally depends on potential PTMs and their ability to correctly fold the protein. Thus, certain expression systems may not provide the correct modifications to the protein or may be unable to assist in folding the protein.

Several chromatographic techniques are available for the purification of proteins under native conditions in which the structure and function of the target protein is maintained. After extraction of the soluble protein from the tissue or expression system, the proteins can be separated based on their physical characteristics (e.g., charge, size, hydrophobicity) (Appendix 1, Chromatographic Purification of Proteins and Peptides).

CLASSIFICATION OF PROTEINS

Proteins can be water-soluble (globular proteins) or insoluble (membrane proteins, fibrous proteins) and can be classified according to their subcellular localization, sequence and structural similarity, or their biological function. Basically, all proteins can be classified into three main groups based on their main subcellular localization; intracellular, extracellular (secreted), or plasma membrane-bound. The intracellular proteins can further be grouped in reference to their localization in the cell; cytosol, cytoskeleton, nucleus, or other organelles (e.g., mitochondria, endoplasmic reticulum, Golgi apparatus, vacuoles, vesicles, ribosomes). In addition, proteins can be classified into groups with similar sequence and/or fold (3D structure). Thus, by comparing multiple sequences and structural folds of proteins using advanced sequence alignment algorithms and bioinformatic tools, closely related proteins can be recognized (18,270,391). If a protein has been functionally annotated it can also be classified into a group reflecting its biological functionality. Important functional classes of proteins related to ocular health and disease are as follows:

A. **Structural cytoplasmic proteins**. Most structural proteins are fibrous and insoluble. The cytoplasmic structural proteins include tubulins, actins, and intermediate filaments such as cytokeratins and vimentin. The crystallins (α-, β- and γ-crystallins) are structural non-fibrous proteins giving the lens its optical properties.
B. **Structural extracellular matrix proteins**. The ECM contains structural proteins such as collagens (see Chapter 44), elastin, fibrin, and proteoglycans (PGs). PGs are not fibrous but provide structural integrity to tissues (see Chapter 40).
C. **Enzymes**. Enzymes such as proteases, ligases, kinases, lyases, isomerases, hydrolases, transferases catalyze a wide range of different reactions and are essential in metabolism and catabolism.
D. **Enzyme inhibitors**. Known inhibitors of enzymes include protease inhibitors, protein kinase inhibitors, and protein phosphatase inhibitors.
E. **Cell–cell and cell–extracellular adhesive proteins**. Proteins that are involved in cell–cell and cell–ECM adhesion include fibronectin, laminin, integrin, and transforming growth factor beta induced protein (TGFBIp) (discussed in the section titled Adhesion Proteins) and help cells to attach to the ECM.
F. **Membrane proteins**. Proteins found in cellular and intracellular membranes include receptors, ion channels, water channels, ion carriers, and other transport proteins. They can be integral membrane proteins or peripheral membrane proteins and are essential in transport of various molecules and ions across membranes (e.g., aquaporins, glucose transporter, Na^+-K^+-ATPase pump) and in signal transduction cascades for movement of signals from outside to the inside of the cell (e.g., receptor tyrosine kinases, G-protein-coupled receptors like rhodopsin).
G. **Blood/plasma carrier proteins**. The blood contains albumin, apolipoproteins, transferrin, hemoglobin, and many other water-soluble and globular proteins that transport particular substances/nutrients (e.g., vitamins, fatty acids/lipids, hormones, minerals, other proteins) in the circulation.
H. **Heat shock proteins (stress proteins) and chaperones**. After being exposed to unfavorable environmental conditions, such as heat stress and adverse chemical agents, eukaryotes synthesize specific proteins known as heat shock proteins (HSPs) (234,336,365). These proteins include Hsp27, Hsp70, Hsp90, and α-crystallins. They are molecular chaperones and assist in protein folding, prevent protein aggregation, and transport misfolded protein to the proteasome for degradation.
I. **Nucleoproteins**. The protein component conjugated with DNA and RNA can be histones, transcription factors, RNA and DNA polymerases, spliceosome proteins, ribosomal proteins, and some translation factors.
J. **Immune defense proteins**. Immune defense proteins are part of the adoptive immune defense system [e.g., immunoglobulins, major histocompatibility complex (MHC)], or the innate immune defense system (such as lysozyme, antimicrobial peptides, proteins of the complement system).
K. **Redox and oxidative stress-defense proteins**. Proteins, which regulate the redox potential in cells include glutathione S-transferases, thioredoxins, and peroxiredoxins. Redox proteins are important as antioxidative and regulatory components in many molecular processes. Proteins that somehow prevent/reduce the formation or scavenge reactive oxygen species (ROS) protect against oxidative damages.
L. **Growth factors and cytokines**. Growth factors and cytokines are signaling molecules that bind to specific receptors and stimulate specific responses. Growth factors, such as epidermal growth factor (EGF), transforming growth factor-β (TGFβ), and fibroblast growth factors (FGFs) activate cellular proliferation and/or differentiation, while cytokines [e.g., chemokines, interleukins, lymphokines, tumor necrosis factors (TNFs), interferons (IFNs)] stimulate immune responses.
M. **Peptide/protein hormones**. The numerous peptide/protein hormones include insulin, vasopressin, angiotensins, and oxytocin. They are signaling molecules secreted into the bloodstream and move by circulation to the target organs/cells, where they bind and regulate specific cellular mechanisms such as metabolism, muscle contraction, and immune defense.
N. **Intracellular signaling proteins**. Various groups of signaling proteins regulate intracellular processes such as DNA replication, cell cycle progression, differentiation, cell growth, and motility. For example various cyclins are important in replication and division and appear during the S phase (cyclin A), G1 phase (C, D, and E cyclins), or G2 phase (B1 and B2 cyclins), while members of the Ca^{2+}-binding S100 proteins are able to relocate in the cell through specific calcium-dependent signal transduction pathways.

O. **Proteins of unknown function**. The molecular functions of many proteins remain unknown. However, their potential roles can often be partially predicted by sequence similarities with other proteins with known function.

P. **Hypothetical proteins**. Hypothetical proteins are predicted translation products of predicted protein-encoding genes with no significant sequence similarity to characterized proteins and for which there is no experimental evidence that they are expressed in vivo.

OCULAR PROTEOMICS IN HEALTH AND DISEASE

The protein content in some parts of the eye differs partly as a consequence of the blood-aqueous and blood-retina barriers.

Several studies have characterized the proteome of healthy ocular cells/tissues and compared the protein expression profiles of healthy and diseased tissues to identify differential expressed proteins associated with ocular disorders. In this section we review proteomic studies on some ocular tissues and cells and describe some proteins important for the specific tissue or cell-type in ocular health and disease. A full discussion of all proteins relevant to normal and diseased ocular tissues are beyond the scope of this chapter. The interested reader should refer elsewhere for details (7,30,303,327).

The Cornea

Apart from those cellular proteins that are common to all cells (house-keeping proteins) and the ECM, such as PGs (see Chapter 40), collagens (see Chapter 44), and laminin and fibronectin (discussed elsewhere in this chapter), a number of other proteins are highly expressed in the cornea. As mentioned in Chapter 44 numerous collagen types are expressed in the cornea (132,201,240,281,331,401).

In a comprehensive proteome analysis of the normal intact avascular human cornea, 141 distinct proteins as well as several different protein isoforms were identified by peptide mass fingerprinting and LC-MS/MS (183). A significant number of traditional blood/plasma proteins have been identified in the cornea. A comparison of the identified corneal proteins with gene expression data strongly indicated that most of the common plasma proteins (including albumin, haptoglobin, hemopexin, amyloid P-component, transferrin, transthyretin, and immunoglobulin chains) are not synthesized in the cornea but originate from the surrounding pericorneal tissue (185). In another study, of an in vitro model of wound-healing keratocytes, the water-soluble fraction from serum-cultured human keratocytes disclosed 118 distinct proteins (184).

By comparative proteomics the protein expression profile of the rat cornea during angiogenesis induced by silver/potassium nitrate cauterization has been analyzed at various stages of blood vessel formation (369). This study identified more than 100 differentially expressed proteins including blood/plasma proteins that were upregulated during the first days of angiogenesis reflecting an increased vascular permeability and the development of new blood vessels.

Furthermore, to learn more about the nature of the abnormal protein deposits that accumulate within the cornea in corneal disorders, such as chronic actinic keratopathy (see Chapter 30) investigators are trying to isolate and determine the identity of the accumulated corneal proteins.

Due to its abundance in the cornea, aldehyde dehydrogenase family 3 subfamily A member 1 (ALDH3A1) and other enzymes such as transketolase (TKT) and α-enolase (2,74,386) have been termed corneal enzyme-crystallins, defined as proteins present at a concentration exceeding 5% of the total water-soluble protein content of cornea cells (306). However, ALDH3A1-deficient mice (273) and haplodeficient transketolase ($TKT^{+/-}$) mice have normal transparent corneas indicating that the enzyme-crystallins are not required for ocular transparency (413). Rabbit expresses ALDH1A1 rather than ALDH3A1 (discussed later).

The Sclera

Like in the cornea, collagen type I is the major extracellular structural protein in sclera (188). In addition, collagen types III, V, VI, XII, and XIII have been detected in the sclera (292,331,398,401). The organization of the collagens is likely to be assisted by the small leucine-rich PGs such as decorin, biglycan, lumican, and aggrecan (23,255,313). No comprehensive proteome analysis of the sclera is available, but characterization of the gene expression profile provides a useful list of genes/proteins for elucidating the molecular mechanism of such conditions as myopia (124,418). However, in a recent study using a proteomic approach, apolipoprotein A-I was identified as a "STOP" signal for myopia both in the retina and sclera in a chicken ocular growth model (37).

Lamina Cribrosa. Based on immunohistochemical studies, the ECM of lamina cribrosa contains elastin, laminin, collagen types I, III, IV, VI, fibronectin, and PGs (154,265,266,267,334). A comparison of the protein expression of various human ocular cells and tissues including the trabecular meshwork and lamina cribrosa using 1D and 2D PAGE of radiolabelled proteins indicate that trabecular meshwork cells and lamina cribrosa, which are both compromised in primary open-angle glaucoma, have similar protein expressions (358). This result suggests that in addition to morphological similarities, the lamina cribrosa and the trabecular meshwork share functional properties and imply that glaucoma may have a common causal origin in the two tissues.

Corneoscleral Limbus. The soluble proteins secreted by limbal fibroblasts have been compared with those of corneal and conjunctival fibroblasts to identify proteins selectively secreted by limbal fibroblasts (347). "Secreted protein, acidic, cysteine-rich" (SPARC or osteonectin) (58), vimentin, serine protease, collagen alpha2 (I) chain, tissue inhibitor of metalloproteinase 2 (TIMP2), and 5,10-methlenetetrahydrofolate reductase (MTHFR) were preferentially detected in the supernatant of limbal fibroblasts. It is suggested that SPARC secreted by limbal fibroblasts may inhibit adhesion of basal limbal epithelial cells.

Trabecular Meshwork. Research on glaucoma has spawned an interest in the protein composition of the trabecular meshwork. Collagen types I, III, IV, V, VI, VIII, XIII, and XVIII, fibronectin, laminin, elastin, and different integrins important for the cell adhesion are found in the trabecular meshwork or synthesized by trabecular meshwork cells (112,281,331,419,420,424). A proteomic study identified 368 proteins in normal and glaucomatous trabecular meshwork tissue (44). In addition to cochlin (discussed later), 51 proteins were detected only in glaucomatous tissue.

To better understand the pathophysiology of glaucoma, researchers have also analyzed the proteome of a transformed/immortalized trabecular meshwork cell strain (GTM3) (357) that apparently has a protein expression with many similarities to primary and normal cultured trabecular meshwork cells (291). In the proteomic investigation, 87 distinct proteins and different protein isoforms were identified in GTM3 cells. In addition, changes in the gene and protein expression in normal trabecular meshwork cells after treatment with TGFβ1 and TGFβ2 have been characterized (421). The TGFβ treatment caused alterations in cytoskeletal proteins, metabolic enzymes, and proteins involved in redox regulation, protein synthesis, and secretion.

Crystalline Lens

The crystalline lens proteome is the most thoroughly determined of all ocular tissue. The lens capsule is mainly composed of collagen types I, III, IV, and XVIII (189,240,281,335). Because the lens is dominated by a few abundant water-soluble proteins (α-, β-, and γ-crystallins) its proteome is relatively less complex than other tissues (50,305). Furthermore, studies have shown that PTMs, such as oxidation and deamidation of the crystallins, which comprise about 90% of the total protein mass in the vertebrate crystalline lens, accumulate with age and play vital roles in the development of cataract characterized by the aggregation of crystallins (51) (see Chapter 24). Studies on lens proteomics have been performed on the whole lens and specific regions of healthy and diseased lenses (lens cortex, nucleus, epithelial cells, and fiber cells) (160). The lens proteome has been analyzed especially by 2D PAGE, which has generated maps of the lenticular proteins and their modifications from various species, including human (77,119), mouse (161,180,381), rat (218), and chicken (407). Efforts have been made to produce complete 2D gel maps and datasets of human lenticular proteins (52,216, 217,239,241), which are useful for comparing protein expression profiles and have revealed the abundance of both cleavage and PTMs of crystallins. In more detailed studies, a large number of specific crystallin modifications in normal and cataractous lenses have been identified (140,160,241) (see Chapter 24). Recently, the largest sets of PTMs in human lens proteins including 155 age-related crystallin PTM sites have been identified (380,406) using advanced search algorithms on MS/MS data from cataractous lenses (344). Together these studies suggest that N- and C-terminal truncations, deamidation, oxidation, cysteine methylation, phosphorylation, disulfide bonding, acetylation, and glycation are among the major modifications of lens crystallins and that they accumulate with lenticular development and aging (259,381). Eventually, the damaging modifications lead to conformational changes, unfolding, subunit disassembly, and aggregation of crystallins, a condition know as age-related cataract (51,144). ROS, e.g., H_2O_2, ·OH, and O_2^-, damage tissues as they can irreversibly oxidize proteins and give rise to various chemical modifications of amino acid side chains, protein–protein cross-links, and fragmentations (35). Thus, oxidative stress conditions where ROS levels are elevated and/or the concentration of glutathione is reduced are known to be key factors in the development of lenticular opacifications (237,377). To study the protein response of human lens epithelial (HLE) cells, which is probably the first site of damage during oxidative stress conditions (354), a comparative 2D PAGE analysis of intracellular proteins from H_2O_2-treated and untreated cultured HLE cells has been performed (300). In this study, seven proteins with altered expression and two with elevated oxidation damages in response to the H_2O_2 exposure were identified. The proteomes of freshly isolated HLE cells (undifferentiated and partially differentiated), cultured immortalized HLE-B3 cells, and fully differentiated human fiber cells have also been investigated and compared by 2D PAGE (393). While undifferentiated and partially differentiated cells had similar protein expression profiles, transformed and cultured HLE cells had an altered protein expression profile including a marked decrease in the levels of crystallins.

Altogether, characterization of lens proteins using a proteomic approach has revealed important changes in the protein expression profile and PTM pattern associated with lenticular development, homeostasis, aging, and cataract formation.

Sensory Retina and Retinal Pigment Epithelium

Most proteomic retina research has been done on tissue containing retinal pigment epithelium (RPE) and photoreceptor cells, which are affected in age-related macular degeneration (AMD) and retinitis pigmentosa (see Chapter 35) (138,191). Thorough proteomic studies on RPE have been performed. In one study, the proteome of normal human RPE was fractionated, applied to 1D and 2D gel analysis, and 278 distinct proteins were identified using LC-MS/MS and peptide mass fingerprinting (400). Besides recognizing many "housekeeping proteins," several of the identified proteins are involved in retinoid metabolism and the visual cycle, protein degradation, and oxidative stress defense reflecting the RPE cell's function in retinoid-based systems (recycling of visual pigments) and phagocytosis of rod and cone outer segments. The proteins identified from freshly isolated human RPE were different from those identified in a cultured rat immortalized RPE cell line thus verifying previous proteomic results (399) and suggesting that the rat RPE cell line is not an appropriate in vitro model system for studies of the visual cycle pathway. In another study the protein expression profile of native differentiated and cultured dedifferentiated human RPE have been analyzed and compared by 2D PAGE (11). This proteomic comparison revealed that proteins such as cellular retinaldehyde- and retinol-binding proteins (CRALBP and CRBP), which are associated with the visual pigment regeneration, are not expressed by dedifferentiated cultured RPE, while proteins associated with phagocytosis and exocytosis are maintained. Furthermore, differentially expressed cytosolic proteins between dividing (pre-confluent culture) and resting (post-confluent culture) RPE have been identified and quantified using metabolic labeling of cells by the SILAC (Stable Isotope Labeling with Amino acids in Cell culture) approach followed by accurate measurements of protein ratios by mass spectrometry (146). To better understand the molecular processes of visual pigment transport and regeneration, 283 proteins were identified from isolated mouse RPE microvilli (55,56). Proteomic analyses of diseased retinal tissue and cells have also been performed. In a recent study researchers compared the RPE protein expression profile at four different progressive stages of AMD, and identified proteins that exhibited altered expression at early and late stages of the disease (279). In the early stages of obvious disease, altered expression of proteins involved in protection of protein unfolding and aggregation, mitochondrial trafficking, and regulation of apoptosis was observed, while proteins CRALBP and CRABP associated with the visual cycle changed expression in the later stages of the disease. Thus, in accordance with previous reports (228) these results may indicate that oxidative damage, mitochondrial dysfunction, and RPE apoptosis are important factors contributing to the development of AMD. Using a similar proteomic approach, the proteomes of the macular and peripheral region of the neurosensory retina from different stages of AMD were compared (98). Proteins exhibiting significant and exclusively region-specific altered expression at early disease stages, with AMD progression, or late disease stages were identified. This suggests that both regions are affected at the molecular level but differently during AMD development. In accordance with the study of the changes in the RPE during AMD (279), the levels of chaperone and stress-related proteins decreased in the early stages of AMD in both neurosensory retina regions. In contrast, decreased levels of proteins involved in microtubule formation and regulation were observed in the neurosensory retina suggesting that the microtubule pathway is only affected in the central and peripheral retina during AMD progression. The appearance of soft drusen, which are extracellular lipoproteinaceous deposits observed between the RPE and Bruch membrane in the macula, correlates significantly with the early-stage development of AMD. Consequently, to study the molecular changes associated with the early stages of AMD, Crabb et al. (72) analyzed the protein composition of drusen and detected 129 proteins in drusen preparations from eyes with and without AMD. Moreover, they found that tissue inhibitor of metalloproteinase 3 (TIMP3), clusterin, vitronectin, and albumin were the most common proteins in non-age-related drusen, but several crystallins were more common in AMD eyes. The study revealed that modifications caused by oxidative damage of proteins were more abundant in AMD, suggesting that oxidative protein modifications are important in drusen development. Hopefully, the characterization of drusen composition will lead to new insights into drusen formation and the molecular mechanisms of AMD (54,328).

Lipofuscin, which accumulates in RPE (101) is composed of proteins and lipids. It is abundant in several retinal diseases including AMD, Stargardt disease (MIM #248200, #600110, %603786), and Best macular dystrophy (MIM #153700). Almost 100 distinct proteins including several photoreceptor specific proteins, such as rhodopsin, have been identified in isolated granules (342,343,394). These analyses suggest that the granules are partly composed of oxidatively damaged and undegradable proteins derived from phagocytosed photoreceptor outer segments.

Several oxidative modifications of retinal proteins have been identified in a chronic pressure-induced rat model of glaucoma supporting the notion that retinal oxidative damage occurs in glaucoma (368).

Cultured retinal Müller cells have also revealed dramatic changes in proteins using a proteomic approach (147). The changes in the protein expression profile suggest that the cells acquire a fibroblastic phenotype under in vitro conditions.

Aqueous Humor

Aqueous humor contains a small amount of protein, derived largely from the blood, but the concentration is about 500 times less than in plasma (36). The plasma protein content in some animals varies with the circadian rhythm (425), but apparently not in humans (287). Elevations in aqueous humor protein content account for the flare that is clinically evident as in ocular inflammatory disorders. In a proteomic comparison no significant differences in the protein profile of aqueous humor from different pathological eyes (cataract, cataract plus glaucoma, and cataract plus pseudoexfoliation syndrome) were observed (322). Furthermore, surface-enhanced laser desorption ionization time-of-flight (SELDI-TOF) mass spectrometry has been used on aqueous humor as a diagnostic tool to search for tumor markers in uveal melanoma (262).

Vitreous

The major structural macromolecules of the vitreous gel are hyaluronan and collagen type II. Other structural-associated proteins in vitreous include collagen types V/XI, VI, and IX (see Chapter 29), various PGs, and fibrillin (46,57). In addition, numerous non-structural proteins have been identified in vitreous from eyes with diabetic retinopathy and macular holes (207,271,415). In the proteome investigation by Yamane et al. (415), 18 distinct proteins in vitreous from eyes with idiopathic macular holes and 38 proteins from subjects with proliferative diabetic retinopathy were identified. A comparison of the protein profiles of vitreous and serum from the patients revealed a high similarity but proteins differentially present in vitreous from both diseases as well as proteins only present in vitreous from eyes with proliferative diabetic retinopathy were also recognized. In another study, seven proteins with altered abundance associated with diabetic macular edema were identified in vitreous from eyes with preproliferative diabetic retinopathy (288). Furthermore, changes in the vitreous proteome following cataract extraction (272) and in endotoxin-induced uveitis (27) have been characterized. A number of glycoproteins associate with the surface of vitreous collagen fibrils including vitrin and opticin (248,315). Vitrin is a member of a superfamily of proteins that includes cochlin (discussed under the section entitled Proteins of Unknown Function). The chick vitreous contains abundant tenascin (411), but this molecule is rare in the mammalian vitreous (318).

Uvea

Collagen types I and IV have been identified as components of the uvea (236), but few studies on uveal proteins have been reported. Zuidervaart et al. (427) have used a proteomic approach to identify markers of potential dissemination of uveal malignant melanomas. They identified 24 proteins in metastatic cell lines of uveal melanomas that were not present in a cell line of the primary tumor. Together with a gene expression analysis this disclosed potential markers to discriminate between uveal melanomas of different prognostic significance (428).

Tears

The tear proteome has been extensively characterized and numerous proteins and protein isoforms have been identified (25,79,116,226,422,423). Among the most abundant proteins in the tear fluid are lysozyme, lactoferrin, secretory immunoglobulin A (109), tear lipocalin (316), lipophilin, proline-rich proteins, and plasma proteins (e.g., albumin, apolipoprotein, transferrin, β2-microglobulin). The tear fluid proteins originate from the lacrimal glands (127), the ocular surface epithelium, blood vessels in the conjunctiva, or the meibomian glands (378). Many of the tear proteins are antimicrobial factors, immune defense components, proteases, protease inhibitors, oxidative stress-defense proteins, and lipid-binding proteins, all important factors for the protection of the ocular surface and maintenance of the optical properties of the eye. Clinical diagnosis of ocular diseases based on changes of tear proteins is of significant interest partly due to the accessibility of tears (non-invasive test). Thus, mass spectrometric analyses have been applied to tear proteomes to elucidate disease pathogenesis and discover novel protein markers of ocular disorders and conditions such as blepharitis (204), Sjögren syndrome (373), allergic conjunctival disease (156), and ocular rosacea (14).

PROTEINS IN OCULAR DISEASES

General Remarks

Because proteins are the product of DNA transcription all genetically determined disorders basically result from the synthesis of abnormal proteins or from the failure of certain essential proteins to be produced (see Chapter 31). Some proteins are antigens that play an important role in immunological reactions and autoimmune diseases (see Chapters 4–6), while in other diseases proteins are altered by oxidative damage as in the lens (see Chapter 24) and retina (see Chapter 18).

Intracytoplasmic Protein Storage Diseases

Examples of protein storage diseases include α-1 antitrypsin deficiency, an inherited defect that results in accumulation of a mutated protein that can lead to cirrhosis of the liver. Protein aggregates of α-synuclein account for the Lewy body of Parkinson disease and the neurofibrillary tangles within neurons in Alzheimer disease result from the abnormal hyperphosphorylated microtubule-associated protein tau (see Chapter 70). In several disorders eosinophilic fibers (Rosenthal fibers) accumulate especially in the white matter of the central nervous system (CNS), including Alexander disease (MIM #203450) caused by a mutation in the *GFAP* gene (see Chapter 70) and astrocytomas of the optic nerve (see Chapter 63). By transmission electron microscopy (TEM) these structures are composed of condensations of microfilaments (128,139) and immunohistochemical methods have disclosed that they stain positively for the degradation-signaling protein ubiquitin (238). Examination of purified Rosenthal fibers has indicated that they consist of aggregates of αB-crystallin with glial fibrillary acidic protein (GFAP) and ubiquitin (372). For other examples of abnormal protein accumulations, the reader is referred to a general pathology textbook.

Extracellular Protein Accumulation

In some inherited and acquired diseases proteins accumulate within ocular tissues. These disorders include hypergammaglobulinemia, the amyloidoses (see Chapter 37), chronic actinic keratopathy (see Chapter 30), and inherited corneal disorders caused by mutations in the *TGFBI* gene (see Chapter 32). The precise identification of the particular protein in question is crucial to the understanding of these disorders.

Destruction of ECM

The matrix metalloproteases (MMPs) play an important role in many ocular diseases by cleaving the ECM. This occurs for example during angiogenesis when they are believed to cleave the ECM ahead of the newly forming blood vessels so that the barrier obstructing the new blood vessels can be removed. MMP-2 and MMP-9 appear to be proangiogenic, but MMP-7 seems to inhibit blood vessel growth.

SPECIFIC PROTEINS IN OCULAR HEALTH AND DISEASE

Structural Cytoplasmic Proteins

Tubulin

The globular polypeptide tubulin consists of a dimer composed of two closely related polypeptides (α-tubulin and β-tubulin). Polymers of tubulin molecules become assembled to form microtubules and within cilia these microtubules are precisely organized by specific proteins (dynein and nexin) which retain this configuration by forming links between adjacent doublets (nexin) and the side arms (dynein).

Actin

Actin filaments (F-actin) (microfilaments) consist of globular subunits (G-actin) arranged into two helical fibrils. The globular molecules are stabilized by tightly bound calcium ions and are covalently bound to adenosine 5′-triphosphate (ATP). Hydrolysis of the terminal phosphate of the bound ATP causes G-actin to polymerize into the actin filaments.

Actin is a constituent of virtually all cells and in cells with the zonula adherens type of cell junctions they converge on this intermediate cell junction. Mammals express at least six actin genes (*ACTA1, ACTA2, ACTB, ACTC, ACTG1, ACTG2*) and some of them are restricted to specific cell types [two sarcomeric actins (α-cardiac and α-skeletal actins), two smooth muscle actins (α-vascular smooth muscle actin and γ non-vascular smooth muscle actin), and two non-muscle actins (α and γ; cytoplasmic actins)] (7,339,340). The practical value of this information has already emerged. For example, analyses of the actin isoforms in leiomyosarcomas support the assumption that these smooth muscle tumors are heterogeneous in nature (339,340). Also, the immunohistochemical demonstration of sarcomeric α-skeletal actin in tumor cells is useful in establishing the diagnosis of rhabdomyosarcoma (64).

Intermediate Filaments

The intermediate filaments (10 nm in diameter and 21 nm axial periodicity) form a filamentous intracytoplasmic system in eukaryotic cells. These filaments, which are morphologically similar in all cell types, can be divided into six distinct classes by biochemical and immunological methods: cytokeratins (68,111,220, 221,263,371), GFAP, vimentin, desmin (123), neurofilaments, and nestin (370). All have sequence similarities and form a complex multigene family (123).

Immunocytochemical studies using monoclonal antibodies that recognize specific intermediate filaments can help classify tumors derived from mesenchymal, muscle, epithelial, glial, or neural cells and are useful in confirming histopathologic diagnoses, and in differentiating between different diagnostic possibilities (64,285,339,366).

Cytokeratins (tonofilaments), the most complex and highly developed of the various classes of intermediate filaments, are the major structural protein of all epithelial cells and they anchor into desmosomes. In the human, 19 different keratin species are recognized each of which is encoded by a specific gene. The keratins have been classified into the smaller acidic keratins (# 10–19) (keratin type I) (pI 4.5–5.3; M_r 40–56.5 kDa) and the larger basic keratins (# 1–8) (keratin type II) (pI 5.5–7.5; M_r 52–67 kDa). Each cytokeratin filament is composed of the products of two distinct gene families (111).

Most epithelia express several cytokeratins. The type of cytokeratin expressed varies with the species, tissue epithelium, and the cell's state of differentiation and keratinization.

The cornea contains specific cytokeratins (cytokeratins 3 and 12) that can be detected with particular monoclonal antibodies (320). When one of these cytokeratins is abnormal due to mutations in the *KRT3* or *KRT12* genes an inherited disorder of the corneal epithelium mutated results (Meesmann corneal dystrophy) (MIM # 122100) (see Chapter 32).

Structural ECM Proteins

ECM is a complex structure containing collagens, laminins, fibronectins, PGs, growth factors, and integrins. A considerable body of information related to proteins in the ECM has accumulated since the recognition by early histologists of different types of fibrous and structural components in tissue. This chapter considers some of them. Other chapters discuss disorders of collagen (see Chapter 44), disorders of PGs (see Chapter 40), and the amyloidoses (see Chapter 37).

Reticulin

The designation reticulin was originally introduced for the argyrophilic fibrous structure that forms a delicate network (reticulum) around some cells. Reticulin is not present in all tissues. Current evidence suggests that it consists of collagen fibers of a finer diameter than usual and that it varies in different tissues. Some reticulin fibers contain laminin and collagen type III (186,187), others seem to consist of only collagen type III (32,122,383), which retains its aminopropeptide (186). In other situations the composition seems to be collagen types I and III (103,166,203,249). Reticular fibers are interwoven in delicate networks rather than in coarse bundles, and with silver impregnation techniques stain more intensely than typical collagen. When viewed by TEM reticulin possesses the periodic ultrastructure that typifies collagen, and fibers with the properties of reticulin precede typical collagenous fibers, which gradually replace them in the differentiation of mesenchyme into loose connective tissue. Reticular fibers persist, however, around certain cells, such as adipose cells and the endothelium of capillaries. Past analyses of the protein portion of reticulin suggested collagen with more carbohydrate (4.25% against 0.55%) and 10% bound fatty acids (63).

From the standpoint of ocular disease abundant reticulin often surrounds neoplastic melanoma cells in the choroid. Indeed, at one time its presence was thought to be of prognostic significance—a view that is no longer accepted. In neoplasms of capillaries, the location of the reticulin can aid in the differentiation between hemangioendotheliomas and hemangiopericytomas. Reticulin is also conspicous around capillaries in diabetic retinopathy.

Proteins in Elastic and Related Fibers

Mature elastic fibers possess two distinct components: elastin and elastic fiber microfibrillary protein. These constituents are discernible in different tissues by TEM as a central homogeneous component (elastin) enveloped by tubular microfibrils (Fig. 2). Elastic

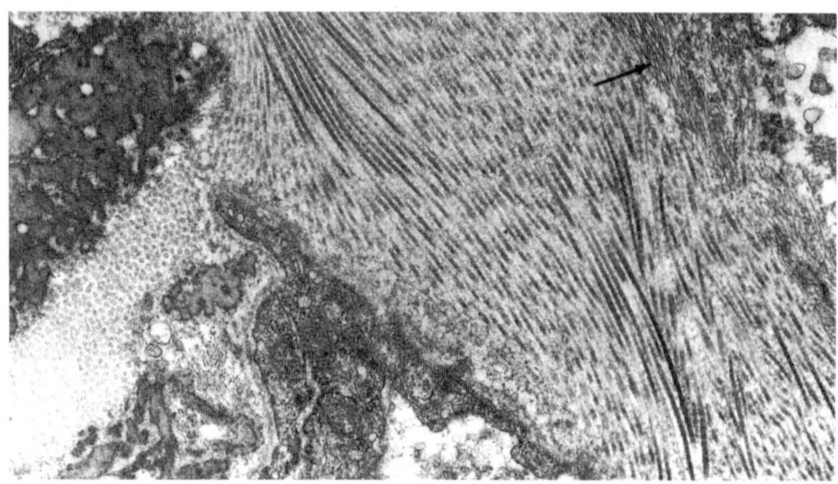

Figure 2 At the top left are homogeneous amorphous masses of typical elastic fibers. Just below these are cross-sections of normal collagen fibers, which are readily visible in longitudinal section in the middle of the field. These exhibit typical 55–64 nm macroperidicity characteristic of mature collagen. At the far right (*arrow*), strands of procollagen are visible (×22,600). *Source*: Courtesy of Dr. John D. Shelburne.

fibers occur in close proximity to collagen, PGs, glycoproteins, and other constituents of the ECM in most tissues, but vary considerably in amount. This structural component of connective tissue can be demonstrated with a variety of stains, including orcein, aldehyde fuschsin, Weigert resorcin fuchsin, Verhoeff iron hematoxylin stain, orcinol-new fuchsin (orcinol-new fuchsin has a high degree of specificity for elastic fibers, while some dyes such as aldehyde fuchsin, also react with other substances) (115). Elastic microfibrils possess an affinity for cationic substances such as lead or uranyl acetate, while anionic stains like phosphotungstic acid have an affinity for the non-filamentous component (325,326).

Each elastic fiber microfibril measures approximately 11 nm in diameter and a glycoprotein is associated with the microfibrillary protein in the elastic fibers (325). The microfibrillar protein in elastic tissue differs from both elastin and collagen in being rich in cystine, aspartic acid, glutamic acid and glycine, relatively poor in neutral and basic amino acids and containing no hydroxyproline, hydroxylysine, desmosine, or isodesmosine (326).

From the standpoint of the eye, elastic fibers are present in Bruch membrane, the sclera, conjunctiva and in the walls of some blood vessels, but are curiously absent from the normal cornea. An extensively studied, but incompletely understood disease involving elastic tissue is the pseudoexfoliation syndrome (PEX) (see Chapter 25).

Elastase, which possesses general proteolytic as well as elastolytic activity, degrades the elastin component of elastic fibers more than the microfibrils (326), but in contrast to elastin the elastic fiber microfibrils, are digested by trypsin, chymotrypsin, and pepsin (326). All other mammalian proteases either do not act on elastin or their activity is very slow. However, several non-mammalian proteases (papain, pronase, ficin, bromelin, nagarase) possess marked elastolytic activity.

Elastin and Tropoelastin

Elastin surrounds elastic tissue microfibrils. Pure elastin is rich in glycine, proline, alanine, and valine and these uncharged hydrophobic residues render the molecule insoluble in water. Elastin contains multiple cross-links between the polypeptide chains of the molecule that impart rubber-like properties on elastic tissue. Lysine plays a significant role in the formation of these cross linkages and this is achieved in part by lysine or leucine and the two amino acid isomers, desmosine, and isodesmosine (greek, *desmos*=band). Elastin, the most insoluble of all connective tissue elements can apparently be solubilized only after cleavage of peptide bonds either by chemical or enzymatic procedures.

Genes for elastin have been mapped to the long arm of chromosome 2 (95) and to chromosome 7 (7q11.2) (*ELN*) (253). The initial translational product of the *ELN* gene is known as tropoelastin (molecular mass 72 kDa). This soluble precursor of elastin, is a linear polymer of about 800 amino acids (molecular mass about 67 kDa) (329,330). It is highly hydrophobic and has a similar, but not identical amino acid composition to mature elastin. Tropoelastin has a higher content of lysine than elastin, but lacks the desmosine, isodesmosine, and lysine or leucine components known to participate in cross-links or to be precursors of cross-links.

Pseudoxanthoma elasticum (MIM #264800) and the Buschke-Ollendorff syndrome (MIM #166700) are suspected of being genetic defects of elastin (324). In Menkes disease (MIM #219100) (see Chapter 48) the synthesis of elastin is defective as a consequence of deficient cross-linking of elastin secondary to a deficiency of the enzyme lysyl oxidase, which needs both copper and pyridoxal as cofactors (76).

Pseudoxanthoma elasticum is a rare progressive inherited disorder of elastic tissue with prominent clinically significant manifestations in the skin, eye, and cardiovascular system. The elastic tissue fibers become fragmented and calcify. The disorder derives its name from small yellow cutaneous macules, papules and plaques that form especially in the flexural areas. Angioid streaks are common (see Chapter 27). Considerable heterogeneity exists in pseudoxanthoma elasticum and several forms are recognized (310,387). The disorder usually has an autosomal recessive mode of inheritance, but rarely it is autosomal dominant (309). Both varieties are due to mutations in the *ABCC6* gene on chromosome 16 (16p13.1). Two types of autosomal dominant pseudoxanthoma elasticum are recognized: type I (associated with "severe choroiditis") and type II (has myopia and blue sclera).

Cataracts are common in the Buschke-Ollendorff (osteopoikilosis) syndrome (317), a rare autosomal dominant disorder characterized by asymptomatic circumscribed areas of bony sclerosis and multiple skin lesions with abnormal elastic fibers (disseminated dermatofibrosis). In contrast to pseudoxanthoma elasticum elastic fiber fragmentation or calcification are not features of this disorder, which is caused by a heterozygous loss of function mutations in the *LEMND3* gene on chromosome 12 (12q14).

Fibrillin

A component of the elastin-associated microfibrils is a glycoprotein known as fibrillin. Three human genes encode for it. One has been mapped to the long arm of chromosome 15 (15q21.1) (*FBN1*) (82), another involves a locus on human chromosome 5 (5q23–q31)

(*FBN2*) (225), and a third one is on chromosome 19 (19p13.3–p13.2) (*FBN3*) (71). Fibrillin is the major widely distributed component of ECM. It is found in connective tissue microfibrils throughout the body and surrounds the amorphous cores of elastic fibers.

Marfan syndrome, one of the commonest connective tissue disorders has an autosomal dominant mode of inheritance, but almost 15% of cases occur sporadically (252). Two distinct types are recognized: Marfan syndrome type I (MIM # 154700) and Marfan syndrome type II (MIM # 154705). Cardinal features of the Marfan syndrome type I involve the eye as well as the cardiovascular and skeletal systems. Affected persons tend to be tall with elongated scrawny limbs, and long slender spidery fingers and toes (arachnodactyly). A shortened life time of persons with the Marfan syndrome is attributed to the cardiovascular manifestations that include: (*i*) an enfeebling aortic media that occasionally culminates in a lethal dissecting aneurysm, most frequently in the ascending aorta; (*ii*) pulmonary artery and aortic ring dilatation and a stretching of the aortic cusps that may result in marked aortic regurgitation. Skeletal anomalies include kyphoscoliosis, a prominent sternum and/or an undue depression in the sternum (pectus excavatum). The joints are often hypermobile with redundant ligaments and capsules.

A characteristic ocular abnormality in Marfan syndrome type I is ectopia lentis, which occurs in approximately 50–80% of affected persons (73,252,311) (Fig. 3). Slit lamp biomicroscopy discloses thin, redundant, and occasionally severed zonules. The crystalline lens tends to dislocate upward, perhaps because of particularly weak zonular attachments between the inferior portion of the lens and the ciliary body. Unlike homocystinuria (73), the lens rarely becomes displaced into the anterior chamber. The reason for this probably rests in the clinical observation that the pupil is nearly always miotic and generally unresponsive to mydriatics. As a consequence of the lens dislocation, the unsupported iris trembles with ocular movement (iridodonesis).

Individuals with the Marfan syndrome often have a myopic refractive error for which two potential reasons exist: an enlarged globe and microphakia (389). The markedly elongated globe, which sometimes enlarges under normal intraocular pressure, perhaps reflects involvement of scleral elastic tissue. Surgical treatment may become necessary for a resultant staphyloma (130). The elongated myopic eye that forms in persons with the Marfan syndrome probably predisposes these individuals to retinal detachment, especially after lens extraction (252). The sclera of persons with the Marfan syndrome is thinner than normal and this causes an apparent blue color of this tissue in some cases (48). The pathologic state may also affect the cornea and cause keratoconus (24).

Individuals with Marfan syndrome type II lack ocular abnormalities, but otherwise exhibit similar cardiovascular and skeletal abnormalities to Marfan syndrome type I.

After immunohistochemical studies pointed to a defect in fibrillin in the Marfan syndrome a metabolic abnormality of fibrillin was identified in many patients with Marfan syndrome (225). Mutations in the fibrillin-1 gene (*FBN1*) on chromosome 15 (15q21.1) account for Marfan syndrome type 1, which may be familial or sporadic (82). Marfan syndrome type 2 is caused by mutations in the *TGFBR2* gene on chromosome 3 (3p22) which encodes for the TGF beta receptor 2 (83). A condition with phenotypic similarities to Marfan syndrome has been linked to the fibrillin gene on chromosome 5 (225).

Fibulins

A family of proteins known as fibulins (fibulins 1–6) are involved in the organization and stability of extracellular proteins, including elastin, which is a major component of Bruch membrane.

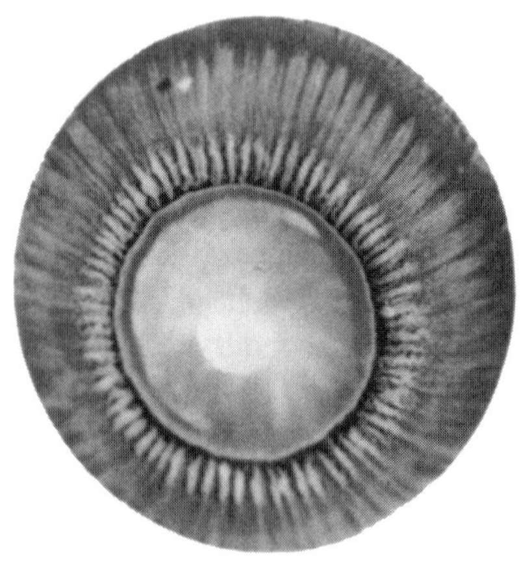

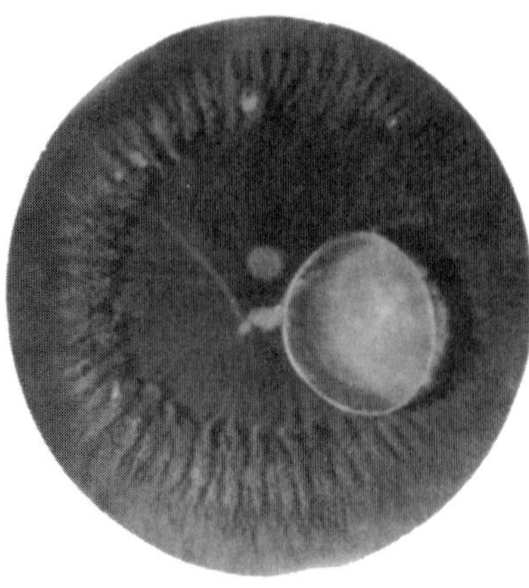

Figure 3 Crystalline lens, ciliary body, and iris viewed from behind. In contrast to the normal eye (*left*), the lens in the Marfan syndrome (*right*) is small, spherical, and displaced. The pupil of the abnormal eye is miotic. *Source*: From Klintworth GK, Landers MB III. The Eye: Structure and Function in Disease. Baltimore, MD: Williams & Wilkins, 1976.

Fibulin 3 encoded by the *FBLN3* (*EFEMP1*) gene accumulates within the RPE and underlying drusen found in malattia levantinese (Doyne honeycomb retinal dystrophy) (246) presumably because the misfolded mutant protein impairs its secretion from RPE. Genes encoding for fibulin 5 (*FBLN5*) and fibulin 6 (*FBLN6*) have been implicated in age-related maculopathy (338,363) (see Chapter 18). Fibulin 5 is involved in the binding and organization of elastin fibers (179) and missense mutations in the encoding gene (*FBLN5*) is associated with a systemic disease cutis laxa (MIM #219100), a connective tissue disease characterized by loose skin known as cutis laxa (235,258).

Oxytalan

In 1958, Fullmer and Lillie (114) discovered by serendipity a connective tissue fiber with some attributes of elastic tissue. The fibers were more resistant to acid hydrolysis than collagen and were hence designated oxytalan (greek, *oxys*=acid; *talas*=enduring). Such structures become apparent in tissue with certain stains for elastic tissue (aldehyde fuchsin, orcein, and Weigert resorcin fuchsin) after a prior exposure of tissue to a strong oxidizing agent, such as peracetic acid, performic acid, or potassium peroxymonosulfate but not otherwise (114). The grouping with which orcein-new fuchsin and the Verhoeff stain reacts is absent in oxytalan both before and after oxidation with peracetic acid. That oxidation is required for fiber staining suggests that it may contain a reduced form of some component of elastic fibers. Elastase is only able to digest formalin-fixed oxytalan fibers after oxidation with peracetic acid or other appropriate oxidizing agents (114). Oxytalan is also susceptible to β-glucuronidase after oxidation (but not before it). The precise composition of oxytalan remains unknown, however, although the fibers do not contain cystien, arginine, tryptophan, tyrosine, or disulfide reactive sites in amounts detectable by histochemical procedures (114,115). Oxytalan fibers appear to have a protein portion and a stainable component digestible with β-glucuronidase after oxidation (115). TEM has disclosed that oxytalan fibers consist of fibrils (approximately 10–15 nm in diameter) (115), which resemble the fibrotubular component of elastic fibers, and like elastic fibers they are sometimes associated with variable amounts of a homogeneous material.

Oxytalan has been identified in several tissues (114), including the cornea, a tissue normally devoid of elastic tissue.

Oxytalan has been identified beneath the epithelium of the cornea in keratoconus (9) and in post-inflammatory or post-traumatic scarring, but not in normal corneas (Fig. 4) (8,9,120). Oxytalan has also been demonstrated in the excrescences on Descemet membrane in Fuchs corneal dystrophy (120). The nature of oxytalan has not been established with certainty but it seems to be a component of elastic microfibrils.

Extracellular Matrix Protein 1

A mutation in the *ECMI* gene that encodes ECM protein 1 causes lipoid proteinosis (Urbach–Wiethe Syndrome) (MIM #247100) (137). This rare multisystem autosomal recessive disorder is characterized by an accumulation of hyaline material in the skin, mucous membranes, various organs, and at other sites, with hoarseness, stiffening and thickening of the lips and tongue, and blotchy cutaneous lesions. Neurological involvement, particularly psychomotor epilepsy and rage attacks, may stem from calcified

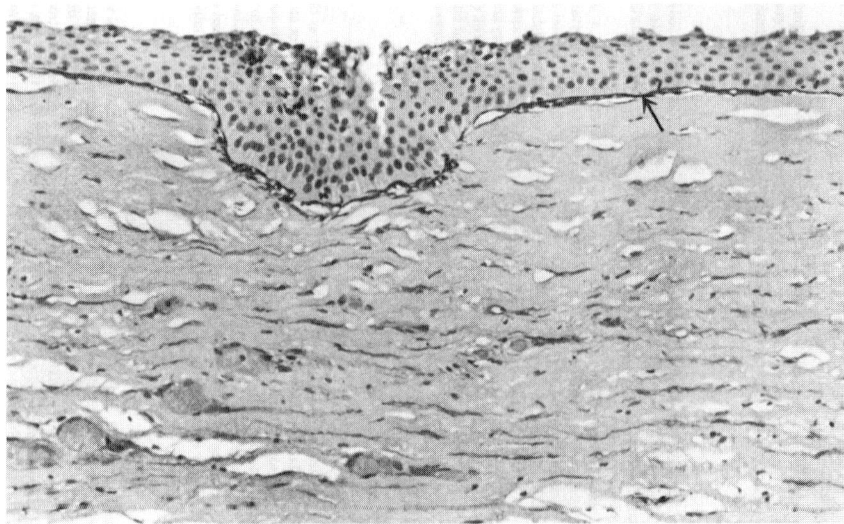

Figure 4 Oxytalan fibers in cornea (peracetic acid/orcein, ×170). *Source*: From Alexander RA, Garner A. Oxytalan fibre formation in the cornea: a light and electron microscopical study. Histopathology 1977; 1:189–99.

intracerebral lesions (276). Although sometimes present in infancy or early childhood, this chronic disorder has a generally benign course with low direct mortality except when severe laryngeal obstruction is not controlled. The periocular tissues are characteristically involved, with numerous waxy nodules forming in the eyelid margins in more than 60% of cases, together with loss of eyelashes (107). Infiltration less commonly involves the cornea, conjunctiva, and Bruch membrane.

Histologically, the characteristic lesion is an extracellular accumulation of hyaline material (268). The basal lamina of small blood vessels in the dermis are multilaminated from a neighboring deposition of fibrillar material, giving an onionskin appearance (104). The hyaline material is diastase resistant and reacts positively with the periodic acid Schiff stain and with lipophilic stains, such as Sudan red and oil red O (107,175). There is extensive evidence of disordered production of collagen subunits and of excess production of normal associated non-collagenous proteins (104,143, 148,284).

Enzymes

Plasminogen

Plasminogen is a normal constituent of the plasma and this zymogen is activated to plasmin by urokinase, which cleaves an Arg-Val bond between residues 560–561. A major function of plasmin is to digest fibrin in blood clots.

In the rare chronic pseudomembranous variety of conjunctivitis known as ligneous conjunctivitis, the conjunctiva acquires a hard woody character due to the accumulation of an amorphous acellular eosinophilic hyaline material that has been shown by histochemical and immunohistochemical stains, as well as TEM to contain fibrin (90,157,163,250), but immunofluorescence studies have also disclosed that immunoglobulins (especially IgG) are a prominent component of the hyaline material (157,163). The disorder is caused by homozygous or compound heterozygous mutations in the *PLG* gene that encodes for plasminogen (341). Hence an absent or inactive enzyme results in a protein accumulation particularly of fibrin.

Aldehyde Dehydrogenase

Aldehyde dehydrogenase (ALDH) (molecular mass about 54 kDa), the major soluble protein of the mammalian cornea (70), accounts for 30% of the soluble corneal proteins (2,10,202,211,348,384,386). ALDH converts and removes toxic aldehydes generated by lipid peroxidation (297,298), but it has also been suggested that it serves a structural role and thereby contributes to the transparency of the corneal cells (176). The precise cellular localization of ALDH is uncertain. One study found it concentrated just above the nuclei in the basal corneal epithelium in a pattern corresponding to the cell membranes (99); in isolated bovine and human corneal epithelial cells in another study ALDH was almost exclusively localized on the inner surface of the plasma membrane when determined by immunofluorescence microscopy using rabbit anti-ALDH antibodies, but not on the cell surface (202). The finding that rabbit anti-bovine ALDH reacts with corneas of many species, including rabbit, suggests that the antigen is not only conserved in many species but normally sequestered within corneal cells.

Immunofluorescence microscopy has disclosed ALDH in the rat corneal and conjunctival epithelium, but also in the fibroblasts and extracellular matrix of the corneal stroma, the corneal endothelium, the lens epithelium, and ciliary body, but not in other parts of the eye (99). In the human cornea, ALDH3A1 is expressed in epithelial cells and keratocytes, but not endothelial cells (298).

Soluble corneal proteins, such as ALDH, may be important antigens involved in immunologically mediated diseases. Using the indirect immunofluorescence assay on whole corneal sections and an ELISA test for ALDH antibodies, circulating antibodies to ALDH and other corneal proteins have been detected in a high percentage of patients with anterior uveitis without apparent corneal disease [including Fuchs heterochromic iridocyclitis (FHI)], in almost one quarter (26%) of patients with various corneal diseases, but in only 4% of controls (99,151,176,210,211,213,297,298,348,384). Despite the presence of anti-corneal antibodies in 88% of patients with FHI, humoral immunity to ALDH was detected in only about half the patients and in 17% of individuals with posterior uveitis (384) indicating that some anti-corneal antibodies detected in these patients are directed at antigens other than ALDH. Antibody production to corneal epithelium can be triggered after corneal damage (210). Lymphocytes in patients with uveitis have an increased responsiveness to ALDH (384), and the incidence of positive responses has been highest in patients with FHI (20 of 28 patients) compared to individuals with posterior uveitis (2 of 14 patients). Only one healthy control had a positive reaction (384). The significance of the immune response to ALDH in these conditions remains to be clarified. Perhaps, ALDH functions as an autoantigen in the initiation and development of immunopathologic processes in uveitis and some chronic keratopathies following its leakage from injured corneas. Although antibody production to corneal epithelial antigens is easily triggered, these antibodies do not bind to the corneal epithelium in rats following the intravenous injection of rabbit ALDH antiserum (99). Instead immunoglobulins deposit weakly in the corneal stroma and sclera, but do not enter the corneal epithelium (99).

Protein Kinase C

Mutations in the *PRKCG* gene that encodes for the protein kinase C in retina causes retinitis pigmentosa type 11 (MIM #600138) (388).

Enzyme Inhibitors

Known enzyme inhibitors include the tissue inhibitors of metalloproteinases (TIMPs). A mutation in the gene that encodes TIMP3 (*TIMP3*) causes Sorsby fundus dystrophy (MIM #126900) (see Chapter 35) (231,242).

Adhesion Proteins

Cell–cell and cell–extracellular adhesive proteins play an important role in mediating fundamental interactions between cells and the ECM. Such interactions are vital in normal and pathologic processes, including the control of cellular growth and neoplasia, migration and differentiation, cell-to-cell inflammatory and immunologic reactions, as well as angiogenesis.

TGFβ-Induced Protein

TGFβ-induced protein (TGFBIp) (also known by several other names) is one of the most abundant extracellular proteins in the cornea. It is encoded by the *TGFBI* gene (formerly designated *BIGH3*) which was first discovered in a lung adenocarcinoma cell line exposed to TGFβ (352). The precursor protein is composed of 683 residues including a 23 amino acid signal peptide and according to alignment analyses the protein contains four fasciclin domains, which were first identified in fasciclin 1, a cell adhesion protein from insects (426). Mature TGFBIp contains an integrin-binding RGD motif (residues Arg619-Gly620-Asp621) that interacts with different integrins (26,193,194,195,282), fibronectin (45), and collagen types I, II, IV, and VI (141,145) and stimulates cell migration. Thus, the interaction of TGFBIp with these ligands suggests that TGFBIp plays a role in cell adhesion but its specific physiological role remains unclear. The *TGFBI* gene is expressed in many tissues but TGFBIp is especially abundant in the cornea (97,199). Biochemical studies of TGFBIp purified from human and porcine corneas revealed that most corneal TGFBIp has a mature molecular mass of 68 kDa and is truncated in the C-terminus immediately after the RGD sequence (15). In addition, the authentic corneal TGFBIp most likely lacks PTMs. Furthermore, about 60% of the corneal TGFBIp is covalently associated with insoluble components, likely collagen. Mutations in the *TGFBI* gene are associated with an accumulation of mutant TGFBIp in several inherited corneal disorders that lead to impaired vision (see Chapter 32) (149,197,269).

Membrane Proteins

Rhodopsin

Much is known about the biosynthesis and basic composition of rhodopsin, the light-sensitive pigment composed of the protein opsin attached to retinal. This predominant protein within membranes of retinal rod outer segments is synthesized within the inner segments of these photoreceptors and is then inserted into the membranes of their outer segments (293) in such a manner that it is oriented across the membrane of the rod outer segments with its C-terminal region being on the cytoplasmic surface of the disc bilayer (142). Autoradiographic and immunocytochemical studies of opsin indicate that after its synthesis on ribosomes of the rough endoplasmic reticulum (RER) the apoprotein of rhodopsin passes through the Golgi apparatus (295,296) probably on water-insoluble membranes of its inner segment (294). Oligosaccharides of known structure are attached to two asparagine residues (Asn2 and Asn15) on rhodopsin (113,227).

One variety of autosomal dominant retinitis pigmentosa (adRP) is caused by a mutation in the rhodopsin gene (*RHO*) (see Chapter 35) (254). A point mutation resulting in a proline-to-histidine substitution has been observed in exon 1 at codon 23 of the *RHO* gene, in about 12% of American patients with adRP, but this mutation was not found in 91 European pedigrees with adRP (100) stressing the heterogeneity of adRP.

Peripherin

Retinal perpherin (molecular mass 39 kDa, also termed retinal degeneration slow protein or tetraspanin-22) is a glycoprotein localized to the rim of the photoreceptor-cell disc membrane and is encoded by the *RDS* (retinal degeneration slow) gene (66).

Mice homozygous for the mutant *RDS* gene fail to develop the outer segment of photoreceptors. The *RDS* mutation is caused by a 10 kb insertion of exogenous sequence into the protein coding exon of the gene (376). Some human cases of adRP have a mutated retinal peripherin gene (see Chapter 35).

Blood/Plasma Carrier Proteins

Ocular tissues may be affected adversely by abnormalities of hemoglobin and the circulating plasma immunoglobulins (see the section entitled Immune Defense Proteins). Several normal constituents of the blood (serum protein AA, β2-microglobulin, transthyretin, and apolipoprotein A1) are related to various forms of amyloidosis (see Chapter 37).

Hemoglobin

Human hemoglobin consists of two pairs of dissimilar polypeptide chains (containing 574 amino acid residues), with a heme group (ferro protoporphyrin IX) linked covalently to a specific site in each globin polypeptide chain. Five structurally different globin polypeptide chains, designated as α, β, γ, δ, and ε are synthesized. Alpha chains contain 141 amino acids in linear sequence, while β, δ, and γ chains have 146 residues. In adult erythrocytes HbA ($\alpha_2\beta_2$) comprises over 90% of the total hemoglobin, while about 2.5% is A2 ($\alpha_2\delta_2$). During fetal development, fetal hemoglobin (HbF) ($\alpha_2\gamma_2$) is produced while the ε-globin chains are only detected during the first 3 months of gestation.

More than 500 hemoglobins have been characterized with potential for an enormous number of hemoglobinopathies. From the standpoint of ocular pathobiology an understanding of hemoglobin is particularly important in sickle-cell disease (MIM #603903) and because of the concepts that the hemoglobinopathies provide about other inherited disorders. The defect in most known abnormal hemoglobins is in the α or β chains. Many of them are rare and not of ophthalmic importance. The hemoglobinopathies represent the prototype of genetic abnormalities that can occur at a mutant site. The amino acid composition of the polypeptide chains of the globin fraction of hemoglobin is altered in the hemoglobinopathies, and in these genetically determined disorders there is usually a substitution of a single amino acid.

One of the most widespread and well known genetic diseases is sickle cell anemia. In this disorder, a simple base change in the nucleic acid alters the mRNA triplet coding for glutamic acid (GAG) in the sixth position from the N-terminal of the β polypeptide chain to a triplet coding for valine (GUG) (Fig. 5). This single amino acid change causes deoxygenated

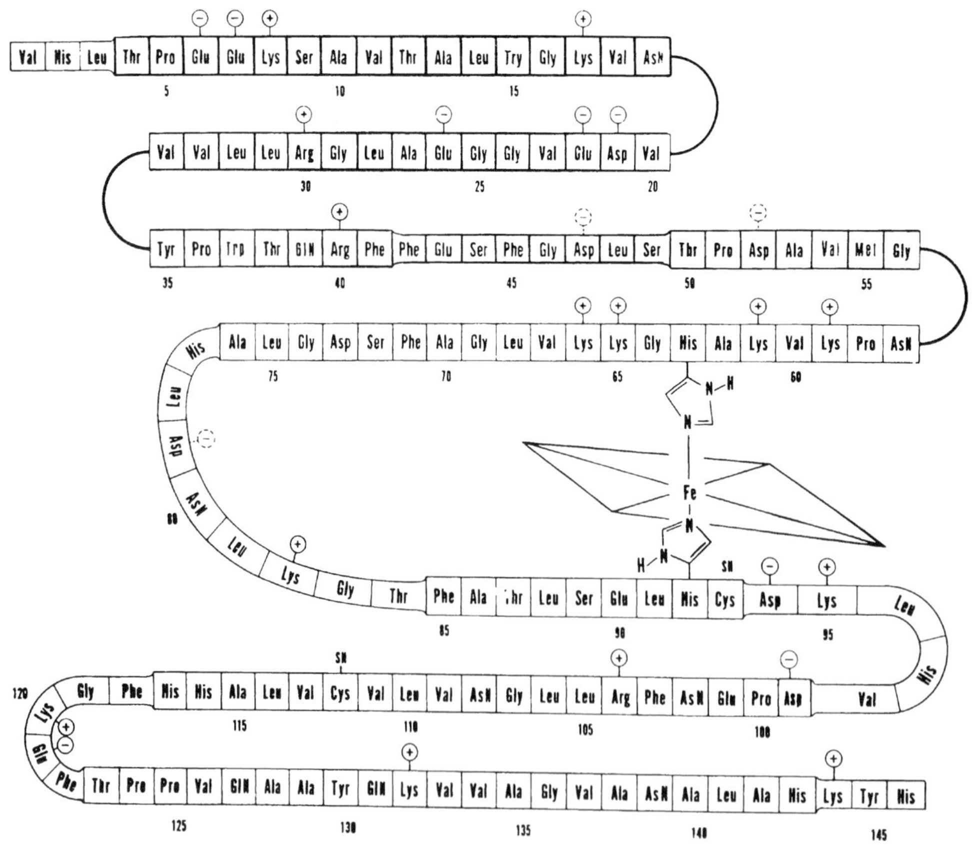

Figure 5 Amino acid sequence of hemoglobin. Beta chain contains 146 of the amino acid links in the massive hemoglobin molecule. *Source*: From Murayama M. Molecular mechanism of human red cell (with HbS) sickling. In: Nalbandian RM, ed. Molecular Aspects of Sickle Cell Hemoglobin, Clinical Application. Springfield, Illinois: C.C. Thomas, 1971.

hemoglobin S (HbS) to associate into long fibers which distort the erythrocytes into a characteristic sickle shape. Up to 20% of the population in parts of Central and West Africa have the gene for sickle cell disease. Hypoxic states, such as respiratory infections or high altitude flying, reduce HbS to relatively insoluble long rods. The eye is commonly affected in sickle cell disease because of occlusive vascular disease (see Chapter 67).

In hemoglobin C (HbC), the second hemoglobinopathy to be discovered, lysine is substituted for glutamic acid in the sixth position of the β polypeptide chain. HbC occurs most frequently in West Africa in the vicinity of North Ghana where from 17% to 28% of the population possess this hemoglobin (91) while 2–3% of the black population in the United States have HbC (337). Individuals who are heterozygous for both HbA and HbC (HbC trait) are asymptomatic, but a moderate chronic hemolytic anemia with splenomegaly occurs in individuals homozygous for HbC disease (HbCC disease) and HbSC disease. In hemoglobin SC disease there is a high incidence of vaso-occlusive disorders and the retina is significantly affected (see Chapter 67).

Fibrinogen and Fibrinoid Material

In several disorders including malignant hypertension, systemic lupus erythematosus, rheumatoid arthritis, rheumatic fever, polyarteritis nodosa, and the endotoxin-induced Schwartzman phenomenon an acellular, eosinophilic proteinaceous material, with staining attributes of fibrin accumulates in the walls of the ocular blood vessels or in the connective tissue. The term fibrinoid stems from the resemblance of this material to precipitated fibrin. Its composition, however, is variable and depends on the circumstances in which it is deposited. Both immunofluorescent microscopy and TEM indicate that fibrin is usually, if not always an important component. Fibrin has a characteristic ultrastructure with an axial periodicity of about 25 nm (less than half the periodicity of collagen) (Figs. 6 and 7). Fibrinoid material probably results from the insudation or exudation of several plasma proteins, including immunoglobulins, complement, and fibrinogen. Fibrin accumulation also occurs with excessive formation or defective fibrinolysis.

Amyloid-Related Blood Proteins

Apart from immunoglobulins, several other normally constituents of the blood (serum protein AA, β2-microglobulin, transthyretin, and apolipoprotein A1) are related to various forms of amyloid (see Chapter 37).

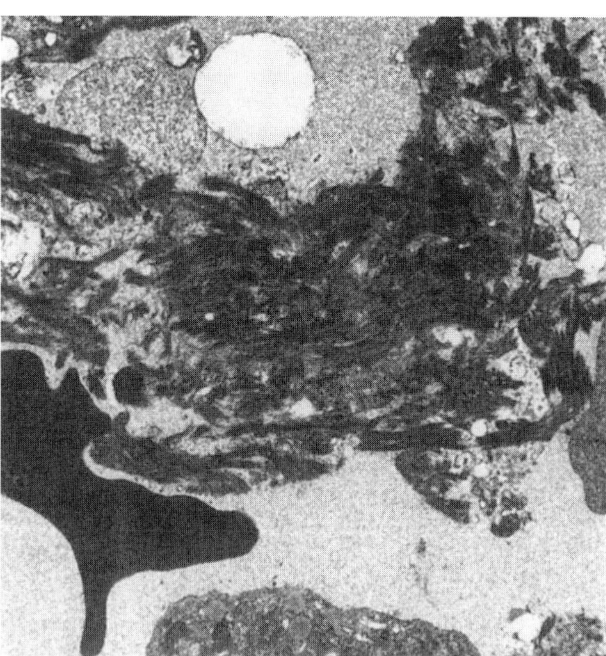

Figure 6 Typical low-magnification appearance of masses of fibrin. At higher magnification no periodicity (see Fig. 7) was visible (×8,200). *Source*: Courtesy of Dr. John D. Shelburne.

Heat Shock Proteins (Stress Proteins) and Chaperones

α-Crystallins

The α-crystallins are among the most abundant proteins in the crystalline lens of all vertebrates (409) and consist of both α-crystallin subunits (αA and αB). Both of which have considerable amino acid sequence similarity with sHSPs (167) and these genes (*CRYAA* and *CRYAB*) are regulated by stress (167,196,408). The αB subunit of the α-crystallins resides in many nonlenticular tissues (39,89,170,172,173). A diffuse reactivity with antibodies to αB-crystallin has been detected in several characteristic lesions of tuberous sclerosis (see Chapter 53) (171,174).

Heat Shock Protein 70 (Hsp70)

Hsp70 has been identified by immunohistochemistry in the atrophic corneal epithelium of rats with an inherited retinal degeneration (Royal College of Surgeon dystrophic rats) perhaps as a response to products of degenerating rod outer segments (414).

Nucleoproteins

Examples of mutated nucleoproteins that cause ocular disease that have been identified include TCF8 and FOXE3.

TCF8

Mutations in the *TCF8* gene causes posterior polymorphous corneal dystrophy (MIM #122000) (see

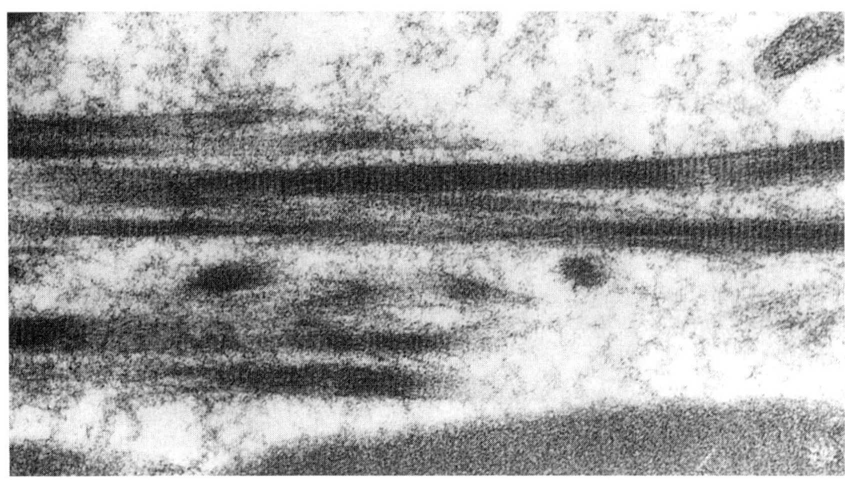

Figure 7 The typical 22 nm periodicity of fibrin is easily visible in this transmission electron micrograph of human blood (×34,000). *Source*: Courtesy of Dr. John D. Shelburne.

Chapter 32) and an ectopic expression of COL4A3 by corneal endothelial cells (208). TGF8 has a binding site in the promoter of the *COL4A3* gene.

FOXE3

The *FOXE3* gene, which encodes the forkhead transcription factor is expressed in the anterior lens epithelium and it is mutated in some patients with anterior segment ocular dysgenesis and cataracts as well as in mice with small cataractic lenses and anterior segment anomalies (345). The predicted translation of *FOXE3* exhibits an 80% homology to the mouse protein with 100% identity within the DNA-binding forkhead domain.

Immune Defense Proteins

Immunoglobulin

Immunoglobulins are synthesized by lymphocytes and plasma cells and variable amounts of these constituents of the plasma exist in the normal ocular tissues (see Chapter 3). Several abnormalities of the immunoglobulins affect the ocular tissues.

Plasma cell neoplasms, such as multiple myeloma, extramedullary plasmacytoma, solitary osseous plasmacytoma, Waldenström macroglobulinemia, heavy chain disease, plasma cell leukemia, monoclonal gammopathy of undetermined significance, synthesize and secrete into the serum electrophoretically homogeneous immunoglobulins ('M-components'). Various designations have been applied to conditions with an excessive proliferation of a single clone of immunoglobulin producing cells but the designation of plasma cells dyscrasias has much to commend it.

Several manifestations of plasma cell dyscrasias (including a predisposition to infections, hemorrhages, cold sensitivity, and the hyperviscosity syndrome) result from physiochemical properties of the excessive immunoglobulins that accumulate, such as an intrinsic high viscosity, the ability to form complexes with coagulation factors and other serum proteins, and a cold insolubility (cryoglobulins) (Fig. 8).

Macroglobulinemia

An excessive proliferation of plasma cells and lymphocytes that synthesize IgM globulins results in the syndrome of macroglobulinemia, first recognized

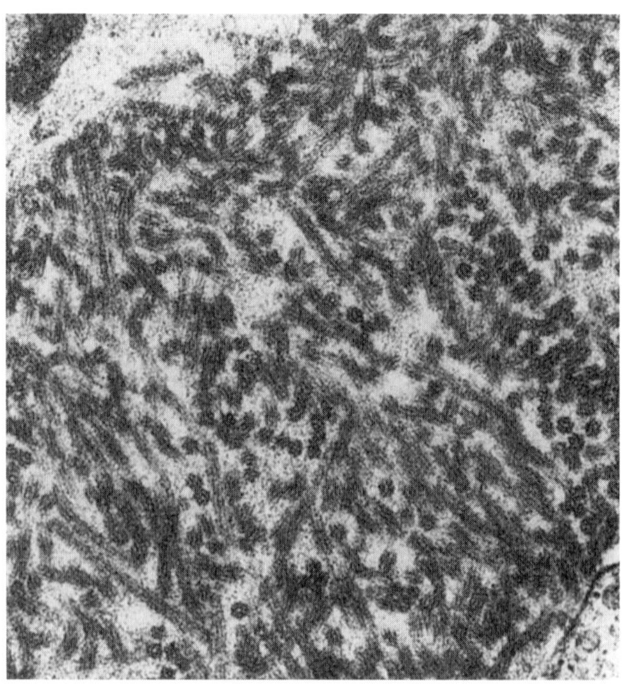

Figure 8 Typical cryoglobulin precipitate in a dermal capillary lumen. Note the clustered small tubular arrays (×40,300). *Source*: Courtesy of Dr. John D. Shelburne.

by Waldenström in 1944 (390). Bleeding manifestations and anemia are accompanied by symptoms related to the presence of excessive quantities of monoclonal (M-type) IgM globulins (macroglobulins) in the plasma.

Ocular Manifestations of Hypergammaglobulinemia

Hypergammaglobulinemia is relatively common and not usually associated with ocular disease. Immunofluorescence microscopy has disclosed several immunoglobulins (IgA, IgD, IgE, IgG) in the epithelium and stroma of the normal human cornea, but only occasionally trace amounts of IgM (12). However, rarely in hyperglobulinemia intra- and extracellular deposits accumulate in the cornea, conjunctiva, and other tissues in patients with multiple myeloma (20,31,33,49,59,102,106,108,162,198,360), rheumatoid arthritis (121,261,289), lymphoproliferative diseases (Hodgkin and non-Hodgkin lymphomas) (31,121,261), "reticulohistiocytosis" (280) or monoclonal gammopathies of undetermined significance (61,62,94,102,209,212,214,230,278,286,307,321, 355), probable monoclonal gammopathy of undetermined significance (256), chronic lymphocytic leukemia (118) and indeed may be the first indication of the systemic disorder (198).

The corneal opacities are bilateral and their clinical appearance varies considerably from case-to-case (355). The opacities may form a superficial gray crystalline thin ring concentric to the corneoscleral limbus, spongy fissures in the posterior corneal layers, or gray-brown homogenous spots (106). Frequently iridescent, polychromatic, or yellow-white punctate or linear delicate scintillating crystals appear within the cornea (Fig. 9), bulbar conjunctiva or lens, but corneal non-crystalline deposits with other appearances also occur. A diffuse corneal opacification due to deep hyaline-like corneal deposits has been reported in a patient with 38% plasma cells in the sternal marrow, but who surprisingly did not manifest hypergammaglobulinemia or other confirmatory evidence of multiple myeloma (108). Corneal immunoglobulin deposits may account for the clinical entity designated "deep filiform corneal dystrophy" (417), and may simulate end stage lattice corneal dystrophy (355).

The location of the corneal immunoglobulin deposits varies considerably from case-to-case. They may involve the central (198,417), peripheral (94), or midperipheral (321) cornea or may be diffusely dispersed throughout the tissue. Some deposits occupy the epithelium (Figs. 10 and 12) (198,360), Bowman layer and superficial stroma (61,94,289), the entire corneal stroma (31,261), posterior stroma (280), and in the stroma immediately anterior to Descemet membrane (162,321,417). They have also been observed within keratocytes (31,61,286,360,417) (Fig. 13) as well as extracellularly (94,198,261, 321,417). Small deposits of apparently similar material has been noted in the ciliary body (including the ciliary processes) and choroid (261).

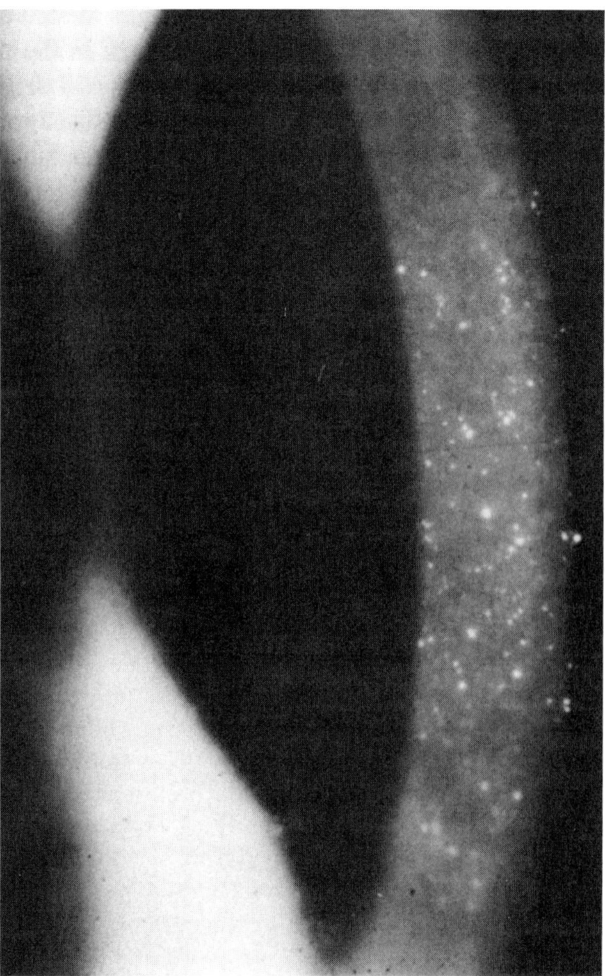

Figure 9 Slit lamp photograph of cornea in patient with multiple myeloma showing numerous crystals. *Source*: From Klintworth GK, Bredehoeff SJ, Reed JW. Analysis of corneal crystalline deposits in multiple myeloma. Am J Ophthalmol 1978; 86:303–13.

Some investigators once thought that the crystals of plasma cell dyscrasias were composed of cholesterol (20) or cholesteryl stearate, but the nature of the crystals became apparent only after their recognition in tissue sections. That they could be identified in tissue which had passed through lipid solvents indicated that lipid was not a significant component (165,198,307,321). Like many other proteins, the crystals are eosinophilic, but difficult to recognize in hematoxylin and eosin-stained preparations. They appear a brilliant red with the commonly used modified Masson trichrome stain (containing the red dyes Ponceau 2R, acid fuchsin, and azophloxine)

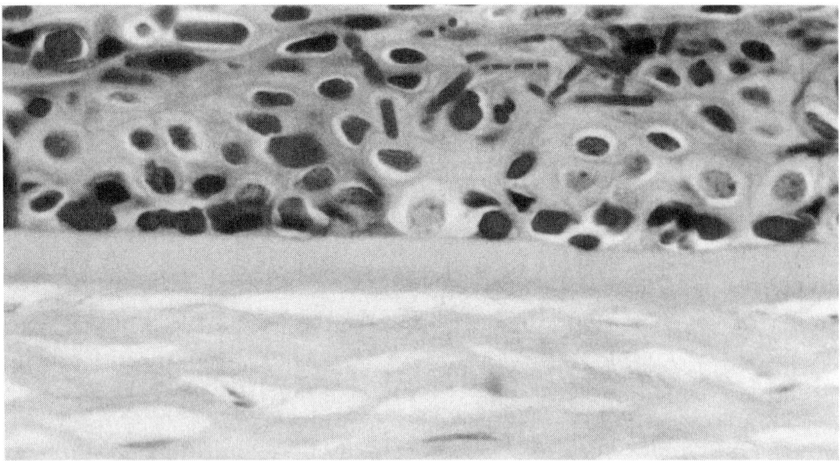

Figure 10 Crystalline deposits sectioned at variable depths in the corneal epithelium (Masson trichrome, ×680). *Source*: From Klintworth GK, Bredehoeff SJ, Reed JW. Analysis of corneal crystalline deposits in multiple myeloma. Am J Ophthalmol 1978; 86:303–13.

(198,261) and are also readily seen after staining with Movat pentachrome technique (red), the Warthin-Starry method (black), and the Danielli reaction for tyrosine-rich proteins (red) (31).

TEM has disclosed elongated crystals of variable length (up to 32.5 mm) and width (up to 7.5 mm) within the corneal epithelium (Figs. 11 and 12). In non-ocular tissue similar intracellular crystals have been identified within the cisternae of the RER (Fig. 14) as well as extracisternally (181). The crystals form in the renal tubular epithelium and extracellularly in multiple myeloma (169,181), as well as intracytoplasmically within neoplastic or reactive plasma cells. Such crystals are hexagonal in cross-section and possess parallel sides when cut longitudinally (198). The crystals have an internal periodicity of approximately 10–11 nm (31,121,198,321).

Several lines of evidence indicate that the crystals are composed of immunoglobulin (198,321). They react positively with antisera against immunoglobulins (121,198,355,360) and closely resemble crystallized immunoglobulins (81). Crystals of isolated IgG are elongated and range in length (up to 180 mm) and in width (to about 10 mm) (81).

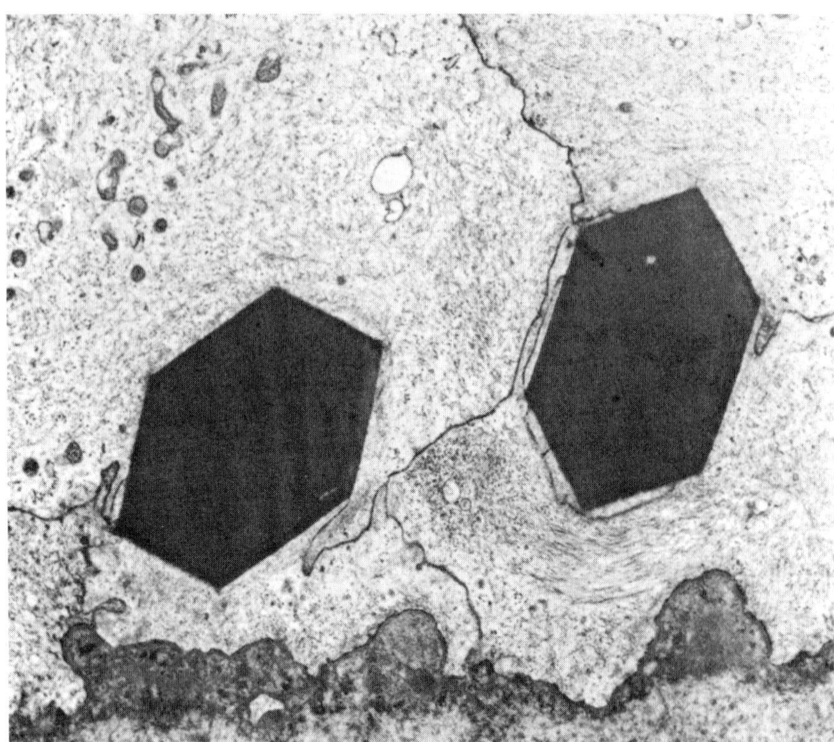

Figure 11 Hexagonal profiles of immunoglobulin crystals in basal portion of corneal epithelium of patient with multiple myeloma (×8,600). *Source*: From Klintworth GK, Bredehoeff SJ, Reed JW. Analysis of corneal crystalline deposits in multiple myeloma. Am J Ophthalmol 1978; 86:303–13.

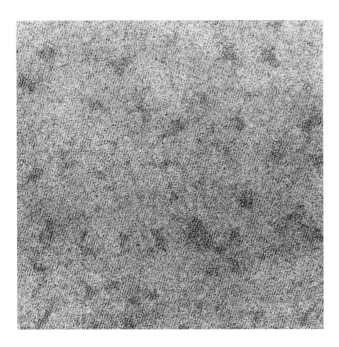

Figure 12 Higher magnification of electron dense immunoglobulin crystal in cornea showing a periodic inner structure (×52,400). *Source*: From Klintworth GK, Bredehoeff SJ, Reed JW. Analysis of corneal crystalline deposits in multiple myeloma. Am J Ophthalmol 1978; 86:303–13.

In multiple myeloma ($IgG_{2\kappa}$) spontaneously crystallizing cryoglobulin microtubules are hexagonal in cross-section, and possess internal and external diameters of about 10 and 20 nm, respectively. Such tubules have been observed within plasma cells, extracellularly in tissue (181), as well as in serum (53) and apparently aggregate into larger structures composed of tightly packed parallel nonbranching subunits. Crystals of this nature vary in length and appear hexagonal when cut perpendicular to their long axis. In cross-sectional profile the crystals have a fine honeycomb-lattice pattern consisting of alternating electron dense and electron lucent lines with a periodicity of about 6–9 nm (average 7.5 nm) (169). In multiple myeloma the periodicity of longitudinal sections of crystals in the serum is about 11 nm (229). The ultrastructural pattern of immunoglobulin crystals varies with the type of immunoglobulin. For example, the appearance of human cryoglobulins varies with the nature of the involved immunoglobulin. Monoclonal IgG_{κ} and cryoglobulins with antibody activity form crystalline rods and annuli (22 nm diameter) (362). Polyclonal cryoglobulins form filaments (6 nm wide) and cryoprecipitates of mixed IgG and IgM appear as cylindrical and annular bodies (12 nm internal diameter; 62 nm total diameter) (362). When IgM predominates over IgG globular condensations result (30 nm diameter) (362). Fingerprint-like periodic condensations occur with mixtures in which IgG is more abundant than IgM (362). On the other hand corneal extracellular microtubular deposits of IgG_{κ} immunoglobulin form hollow rods with a diameter of about 30–40 nm (150,361). Morphologically similar structures as well as others derived from immunoglobulins occasionally accumulate in renal tissue, where the entity is designated immunotactoid glomerulopathy (fibrillary glomerulonephritis) because of the composition (immunoglobulin) and polymeric morphology (tactoid) (205). The term immmunotactoid keratopathy has been proposed for the corneal lesions (118) and this has merit in bringing the nomenclature of different subspecialties of pathology together when the basic pathologic processes are identical.

The spontaneous crystallization of extracellular immunoglobulin in the absence of a tissue infiltration by cells with cytoplasmic crystals accounts for virtually all corneal immunoglobulin deposits (165,198,321), but the corneal crystals have been associated with intracytoplasmic crystals or granular accumulations of conjunctival plasma cells (162,307).

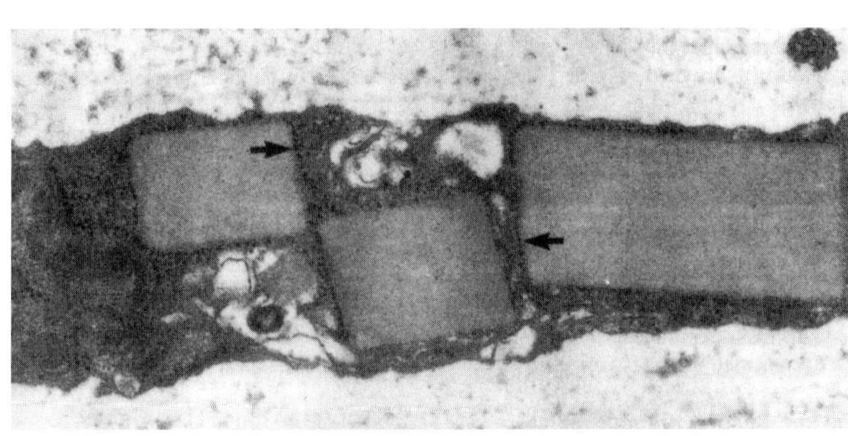

Figure 13 Monoclonal gammopathy. Crystals lined by ribosomes (*arrows*) are present within the cytoplasm of a keratocyte (×21,700). *Source*: From Barr CC, Gelender H, Font RL. Corneal crystalline deposits associated with dysproteinemia: report of two case reviews of the literature. Arch Ophthalmol 1980; 98:884–9.

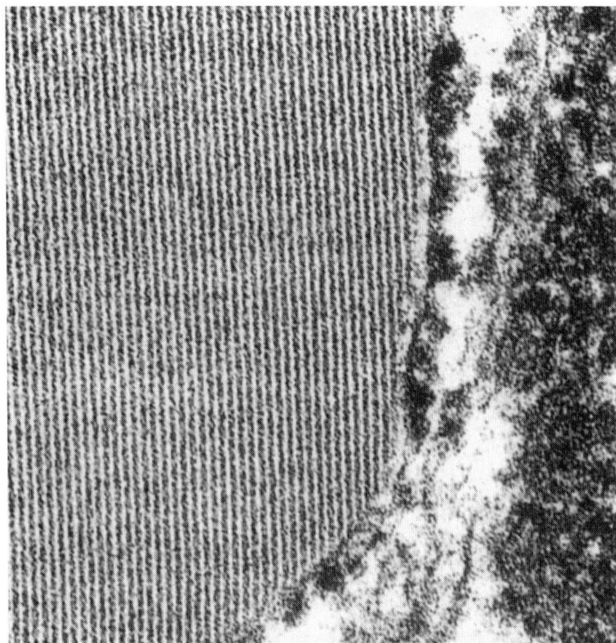

Figure 14 This plasma cell from a region of chronic inflammation exhibits crystallized protein within the cisterna of the RER. This high magnification view of a small portion of one such crystal shows its definite periodicity (×162,000). *Source*: Courtesy of Dr. John D. Shelburne.

Some hypergammaglobulinemic patients with corneal crystals have had crystalline inclusions within plasma cells of the bone marrow (20,214,307). Tears, aqueous humor, and the extravascular interstitial fluid contain immunoglobulins derived from plasma and neighboring plasma cells and in hypergammaglobulinemia increased quantities of immunoglobulins presumably reach the cornea from these sites. Immunoglobulin may diffuse into the conjunctiva and corneal stroma after passing through the conjunctival microcirculation. Alternatively, plasma cells in the conjunctiva and other ocular tissues can produce immunoglobulins, and it is noteworthy that corneal crystals are sometimes preceded by episodes of conjunctivitis or anterior uveitis, which perhaps provide an increased number of crystalline containing plasma cells. The possibility that immunoglobulin accumulation within the cornea may follow its local synthesis, by corneal fibroblasts has been raised (417), but this view is contrary to the prevailing belief that immuno globulins are products only of plasma cells and their precursor B-lymphocytes. However, crystals that react immunochemically with antibodies to immunoglobulins and with a comparable structure to those in plasma cell dyscrasias have been observed in the absence of detectable serum immunoglobulin abnormalities using standard methods (417).

Crystals have not been identified in tissue sections of the lens in hypergammaglobulinemia, but have been observed clinically within the lens in multiple myeloma (198). As cells do not invade the intact lens capsule, immunoglobulins presumably can diffuse into the lens and crystallize there. In multiple myeloma the corneal (162) and lenticular crystals (198) may diminish in number while on chemotherapy, suggesting that crystallized immunoglobulins can resolubilize in the patient.

Why immunoglobulins should crystallize so rarely in individuals with hypergammaglobulinemia remains an enigma. The deposits do not appear to reflect a specific immunoglobulin as they have been associated with IgG_{κ} (31,61,121,162,214,286,355,360), IgG_{λ} (102,158,417) and IgA_{κ} (278). In some instances non-ocular crystals have been associated with spontaneously crystallizing cryoglobulin in the plasma (181). An understanding of the crystallization of immunoglobulin in the cornea clearly would have broad biological importance, as γ-globulin crystallizes spontaneously so uncommonly (67) and the induction of crystals by purified immunoglobulin is difficult in the laboratory (78). Some patients with corneal crystals have had a relatively benign outcome even before the advent of therapy (198), but because of the extremely variable clinical course in patients with multiple myeloma the question of whether corneal deposits are a favorable prognostic indicator remains unanswered.

The precipitation from serum of IgA, IgG, or IgM at temperatures below 37°C (cryoglobulins) are common in multiple myeloma, plasma cell dyscrasias, and a variety of systemic diseases (including rheumatoid arthritis). Seeing that cryoglobulins precipitate below the normal body temperature, one might anticipate that in affected patients this phenomenon would occur spontaneously in the cornea where the temperature is normally about 35°C. Indeed, corneal opacities have accompanied cryoglobulinemia on rare occasions (209,256,280,289). But, if temperature is important, deposition should be maximal at the interpalpebral level which is the coolest region in the cornea. Experience does not confirm that this is so.

Cysts of the Ciliary Body

Multiple cysts of the ciliary body develop in individuals with hypergammaglobulinemia due to multiple myeloma, plasma cell dyscrasias, systemic lupus erythematosus, a variety of liver diseases and other conditions (21,29,177,178,332,333,353). The cysts are lined on their inner surface by the non-pigmented epithelium of the ciliary body and externally by this tissue's pigmented epithelium. They most often involve the pars plicata, but can also affect the corona ciliaris and orbiculus ciliaris of the ciliary body (29). In all likelihood an elevated serum gammaglobulin reaches the ciliary body by way of the circulation, passes through its pigmented epithelium and becomes entrapped in the potential space separating the pigmented and non-pigmented epithelia of the ciliary body. The cysts vary considerably in size and may reach a sufficient dimension to partially sublux the lens and displace it and the iris anteriorly (29). One reported patient with multiple myeloma and unilateral angle closure glaucoma was associated with such displacements and recurrent iridocyclitis (29). The cysts contain immunoglobulins and other proteins, and in multiple myeloma they have been shown by immunoelectrophoresis to contain the M-protein that is elevated in the serum (178). When observed clinically the ciliary cysts are translucent (29), and they remain so until the eye is placed in a fixative which precipitates the protein making the cyst milky white (Fig. 15) (29,178). Similar cysts sometimes develop in the choroid plexuses of the brain in individuals with hypergammaglobulinemia. Why ciliary body cysts do not occur in all individuals with hypergammaglobulinemia remains unknown, but the presence or absence of cysts, and their size is not related to the serum gammaglobulin level at the time of death (177).

Hyperviscosity Manifestations

The hyperviscosity of the plasma that occurs especially in primary macroglobulinemia (IgM globulins) and in certain cases of multiple myeloma and other plasma cell dyscrasias with monoclonal IgG results in a microcirculatory stasis. This accounts for a variety of retinal vascular lesions (dilated veins, retinal hemorrhages, microaneurysms, and exudates) (3,22,60,65,75,86,164).

Increased Susceptibility to Infection

In multiple myeloma, and to a lesser extent in macroglobulinemia, an increased susceptibility to infection results partly from an impaired capacity for antibody formation. This is reflected by a decreased serum concentration of normal IgA, IgG, and IgM (402). A metastatic bacterial endophthalmitis has been documented (29).

Hemorrhagic Manifestations

Hemorrhages can follow thrombocytopenia or coagulation defects in patients with multiple myeloma. Some of the latter may be related to the formation of a complex between the specific M-type globulins and coagulation factors (including platelets, fibrinogen, factors V, VII, VIII, and prothrombin) (402).

Amyloidosis

Amyloid may deposit in the ocular tissues in multiple myeloma (see Chapter 37).

Hypogammaglobulinemia

In numerous congenital and acquired conditions the serum level of one or more immunoglobulins is diminished or absent. Diseases that cause a lack of B-lymphocytes result in hypogammaglobulinemia. The resulting low level of immunoglobulins in the blood predispose to recurrent infections by specific viruses, bacteria, and fungi (see Chapters 8, 9, and 11).

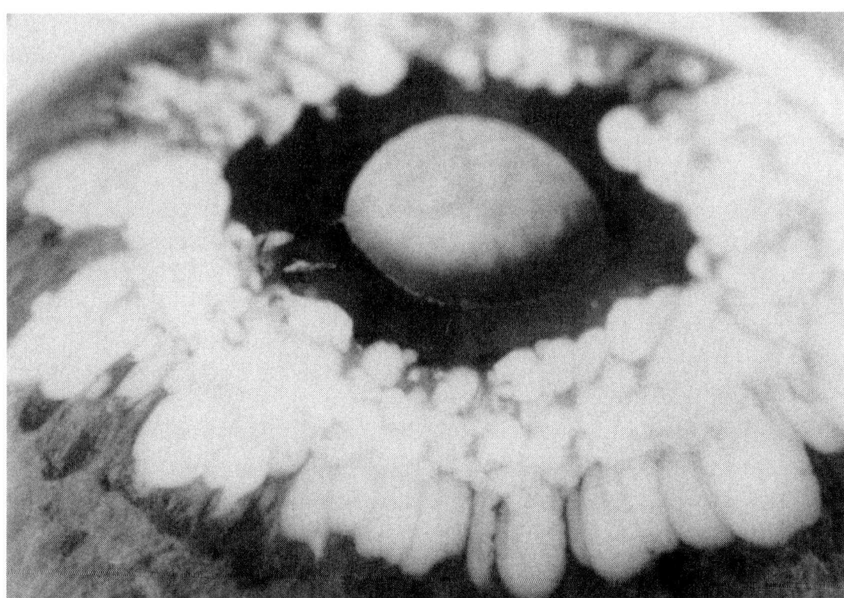

Figure 15 Milky white cysts of ciliary body in formalin fixed eye from individual with multiple myeloma. *Source*: From Baker TR, Spencer WH. Ocular findings in multiple myeloma: a report of two cases. Arch Ophthalmol 1974; 91:110–3.

Light Chain and Light and Heavy Chain Deposition Disease

On rare occasions monoclonal plasma cell populations, especially malignant plasma cell proliferations, only produce abundant quantities of immunoglobulin light chains. Under such circumstances the immunoglobulin light chains deposit in the kidney and various other tissues (117,251,314). A retinal vasculopathy has been documented in light chain disease, but without histopathologic confirmation (96).

Oxidative Stress-Defense Proteins

Lactoferrin

Lactoferrin is an iron-binding protein that is absent in the normal cornea, but is present in tears where it may protect the corneal epithelium from UV-induced generation of damaging ROS (28). Lactoferrin was identified in subepithelial deposits of amyloid in two cases of familial subepithelial corneal amyloidosis (gelatinous drop-like dystrophy of the cornea) (see Chapter 32) by amino terminal protein sequencing (200) and subsequently in corneas with amyloidosis associated with trichiasis (17,19,283). A Glu561Asp polymorphism in the *LTF* gene may facilitate the amyloid deposition in trichiasis (19).

Growth Factors and Cytokines

Growth factors and cytokines are involved in the inflammation and wound healing and many immunologic processes and tumors that affect the ocular tissues.

Intracellular Signaling Proteins

Calgranulin C

Calgranulin C (S100A12) is a Ca^{2+}-binding inflammatory mediator belonging to the large family of S100 proteins, which are localized in the cytoplasm and/or nucleus, where they regulate intracellular processes through calcium-dependent signal transduction pathways. Calgranulin C is constitutively expressed in PMNs (80) and is suspected of being the cornea-associated antigen responsible for Mooren ulcer (see Chapter 5) (135,136). The protein is inherently present in the cornea, and is upregulated in corneal fibroblasts by proinflammatory cytokines (134).

Recoverin

Recoverin is a calcium-sensitive protein that is apparently unique to the human and bovine retina (also known as p26) (84,215,375). Similar, and perhaps functionally equivalent, proteins have been isolated from the retina of chicken (visinin) and frogs (sensitivity-modulating protein or S-modulin). This modulator protein stimulates guanylate cyclase to resynthesize cGMP when calcium concentrations are low inducing a reopening of the sodium-calcium-ion channels in the retinal photoreceptors. This allows the rods and cones to react to further photons of light that traverse the retina even in the absence of calcium. The serum of a certain subset of patients with malignant neoplasms that have not invaded the retina or nervous system, but who develop a cancer-associated retinopathy (see Chapter 27) contain antibodies to this protein (308).

Arrestin

Arrestin (previously known as retinal S-antigen or "48K protein"), a well-characterized soluble protein present in the photoreceptor layer of the retina and in the pineal gland, is highly immunogenic and causes severe cell-mediated autoimmune uveitis and pinealitis in previously sensitized rats (see Chapter 4) (87,88). Immunization with several small synthetic peptides corresponding to certain amino acid sequences in bovine arrestin induce the same reaction as the native protein suggesting that multiple uveitopathogenic sites may be present in the molecule (349,350). An analysis of purified arrestin from the retina in several species, as well as from the pineal gland, has disclosed a considerable amount of sequence identity among species and between arrestin in the retina and pineal gland. Such studies have also revealed the presence of the same consensus phosphoryl-binding site that characterizes many GTP/GDP-binding proteins and a homologous sequence found in the C-terminus of α-transducin. These sequences may play a role in the action of arrestin in transmembrane signal transduction (1,379). Arrestin is implicated in the negative control of visual transduction. It binds to phosphorylated rhodopsin and interferes with the interaction of rhodopsin and transducin (206).

Proteins of Unknown Function

Cochlin

Cochlin, which is a product of the coagulation factor C homology gene (*COCH*), is a major non-collagen component of the ECM of the inner ear. Its function remains unclear. Cochlin accumulation is suspected of being a potential causal factor in primary open angle glaucoma through altered interactions with the ECM. Cochlin and GAG-cochlin deposits have been found in the trabecular meshwork around Schlemm channel of human eyes with glaucoma and in a DBA/2J mouse model of glaucoma prior to the appearance of an elevated intraocular pressure (IOP) (41–44).

Myocilin

Myocilin is a 66 kDa protein of unknown function. The gene that encodes it is mutated in some cases of glaucoma (see Chapter 34) (364). Myocilin interacts with Huntington, RAB8, and transcription factor IIIA and is implicated in the TNF_{α} pathway. It is expressed in the trabecular meshwork, non-pigmented ciliary epithelium, retina, brain, and kidney and is induced in mesangioproliferative glomerulonephritis (131).

WRD-36

An unusual ECM protein belonging to the small leucine repeat PG/protein family has been designated WD-repeat-containing protein 36 (WRD-36). It is present throughout the vitreous, but is concentrated in the internal limiting membrane (ILM) where it colocalizes with collagen type XVIII. This protein is mutated in a form of primary open angle glaucoma (264).

Other Proteins

Optineurin

Optineurin the product of the *OPTN* gene interacts with huntingtin (a protein that is mutated in Huntington disease), transcription factor IIA, and a Ras-associated protein (RAB8A). It is mutated in some cases of primary open angle glaucoma (see Chapter 34) (319).

Opticin

Opticin is member of a leucine-rich repeat (LRR) family of extracellular matrix proteins that was discovered in the retina, but which is also present in the vitreous humor and other parts of the eye. A mutation in the encoding gene has been detected in patient with severe neovascular age-related maculopathy (110).

Hyalin-Like Proteins

On purely morphologic grounds the designation hyalin has been applied to homogeneous, structureless eosinophilic material occurring in the epithelium or connective tissue, but hyalin is not an entity and the term embraces several different substances. From the standpoint of ocular tissues this pigeonhole is applicable to the excrescences that occur on the periphery of Descemet membrane in the cornea with aging (Hassall–Henle bodies), and to the almost identical nodules (corneal guttae) that extend across the entire cornea in Fuchs corneal dystrophy, macular corneal dystrophy (see Chapter 32), and interstitial keratitis (395). In the latter situations, collagen is a major constituent of the hyalin, but other substances such as glycoproteins are probably involved as well. Thick bands of amorphous eosinophilic material occur in the walls of arterioles and medium-sized arteries in diabetes mellitus and hypertension of long standing. It, like the hyaline material in the walls of arterioles with arteriolosclerosis, is believed to be derived from an insudation of plasma proteins, as well as by local production. The hyalin present in connective tissue in certain diseases appears to consist of excessive amounts of glycoprotein deposited between the collagen fibrils and other constituents of the extracellular matrix. Hyalin is commonly observed in connective tissue with aging, and in the conjunctiva in chronic conjunctivitis, notably trachoma, but the exact mechanism of its production in these situations is not clear.

The extracellular eosinophilic deposits in the cornea in granular corneal dystrophy were referred to as hyalin in the past, but these the deposits contain mutated TGFBIp (see Chapter 32).

ACKNOWLEDGMENT

Henrik Karring was supported by a post doctoral stipend from the Carlsberg Foundation to work at the University of Aarhus, Denmark. This work was accomplished while Henrik Karring was employed at the University of Aarhus.

REFERENCES

1. Abe T, Yamaki K, Tsuda M, et al. Rat pineal S-antigen: sequence analysis reveals presence of alpha-transducin homologous sequence. FEBS Lett 1989; 247:307–11.
2. Abedinia M, Pain T, Algar EM, Holmes RS. Bovine corneal aldehyde dehydrogenase: the major soluble corneal protein with a possible dual protective role for the eye. Exp Eye Res 1990; 51:419–26.
3. Ackerman AL. The ocular manifestations of Waldenström's macroglobulinemia and its treatment. Arch Ophthalmol 1962; 67:701–7.
4. Aebersold R, Goodlett DR. Mass spectrometry in proteomics. Chem Rev 2001; 101:269–95.
5. Aebersold R, Mann M. Mass spectrometry-based proteomics. Nature 2003; 422:198–207.
6. Alban A, David SO, Bjorkesten L, et al. A novel experimental design for comparative two-dimensional gel analysis: two-dimensional difference gel electrophoresis incorporating a pooled internal standard. Proteomics 2003; 3:36–44.
7. Alberts B, Bray D, Lewis J, et al. Molecular Biology of the Cell, 2nd ed. New York: Gartland Publishing, Inc, 1989.
8. Alexander RA, Clayton DC, Howes RC, Garner A. Effect of oxidation upon demonstration of oxytalan fibres: a light and electron microscopical study. Med Lab Sci 1981; 38:91–101.
9. Alexander RA, Garner A. Oxytalan fibre formation in the cornea: a light and electron microscopical study. Histopathology 1977; 1:189–99.
10. Alexander RJ, Silverman B, Henley WL. Isolation and characterization of BCP54, the major soluble protein of bovine cornea. Exp Eye Res 1981; 32:205–16.

11. Alge CS, Suppmann S, Priglinger SG, et al. Comparative proteome analysis of native differentiated and cultured dedifferentiated human RPE cells. Invest Ophthalmol Vis Sci 2003; 44:3629–41.
12. Allansmith MR, Whitney CR, McClellan BH, Newsome LP. Immunoglobulins in the human eye. Arch Ophthalmol 1973; 89:36–45.
13. Allen G. Determination of peptide sequences (Chapter 6). In: Burdon RH, van Knippenberg PH, eds. Laboratory Techniques in Biochemistry and Molecular Biology. Sequencing of Proteins and Peptides, 2nd revised ed. Amsterdam: Elsevier, 1989;207–91.
14. An HJ, Ninonuevo M, Aguilan J, et al. Glycomics analyses of tear fluid for the diagnostic detection of ocular rosacea. J Proteome Res 2005; 4:1981–7.
15. Andersen RB, Karring H, Moller-Pedersen T, et al. Purification and structural characterization of transforming growth factor beta induced protein (TGFBIp) from porcine and human corneas. Biochemistry 2004; 43:16374–84.
16. Anderson L, Seilhamer J. A comparison of selected mRNA and protein abundances in human liver. Electrophoresis 1997; 18:533–7.
17. Ando Y, Nakamura M, Kai H, et al. A novel localized amyloidosis associated with lactoferrin in the cornea. Lab Invest 2002; 82:757–66.
18. Andreeva A, Howorth D, Brenner SE, et al. SCOP database in 2004: refinements integrate structure and sequence family data. Nucleic Acids Res 2004; 32: D226–9.
19. Araki-Sasaki K, Ando Y, Nakamura M. et al. Lactoferrin Glu561Asp facilitates secondary amyloidosis in the cornea. Br J Ophthalmol 2005; 89:684–8.
20. Aronson SB II, Shaw R. Corneal crystals in multiple myeloma. Arch Ophthalmol 1959; 61:541–6.
21. Ashton N. Ocular changes in multiple myelomatosis. Arch Ophthalmol 1965; 73:487–94.
22. Ashton N, Kok DA, Foulds WS. Ocular pathology in macroglobulinaemia. J Path Bact 1963; 86:453–61.
23. Austin BA, Coulon C, Liu C-Y, et al. Altered collagen fibril formation in the sclera of lumican-deficient mice. Invest Ophthalmol Vis Sci 2002; 43:1695–1701.
24. Austin MG, Schaefer RF. Marfan's syndrome with unusual blood vessel manifestations: primary medionecrosis dissection of right innominate, right carotid, and left carotid arteries. Arch Pathol 1957; 64:205–9.
25. Azzarolo AM, Brew K, Kota S, et al. Presence of tear lipocalin and other major proteins in lacrimal fluid of rabbits. Comp Biochem Physiol B Biochem Mol Biol 2004; 138:111–7.
26. Bae JS, Lee SH, Kim JE, Choi JY, et al. Betaig-h3 supports keratinocyte adhesion, migration, and proliferation through alpha3beta1 integrin. Biochem Biophys Res Commun 2002; 294:940–8.
27. Bahk SC, Lee SH, Jang JU, et al. Identification of crystallin family proteins in vitreous body in rat endotoxin-induced uveitis: involvement of crystallin truncation in uveitis pathogenesis. Proteomics 2006; 6:3436–44.
28. Baker EN, Anderson BF, Baker HM, et al. Three-dimensional structure of lactoferrin. Implications for function, including comparisons with transferrin. Adv Exp Med Biol 1998; 443:1–14.
29. Baker TR, Spencer WH. Ocular findings in multiple myeloma: a report of two cases. Arch Ophthalmol 1974; 91:110–3.
30. Balazs EA, ed. Chemistry and Molecular Biology of the Intercellular Matrix (3 vols.). New York: Academic Press, 1970.
31. Barr CC, Gelender H, Font RL. Corneal crystalline deposits associated with dysproteinemia: report of two case and review of the literature. Arch Ophthalmol 1980; 98:884–9.
32. Becker U, Nowack H, Gay S, Timpl R. Production and specificity of antibodies against the aminoterminal region in type III collagen. Immunology 1976; 31:57–65.
33. Beebe WE, Webster RG Jr. Spencer WB. Atypical corneal manifestations of multiple myeloma: a clinical and immunohistochemical report. Cornea 1989; 8:274–80.
34. Berggren K, Chernokalskaya E, Steinberg TH et al. Background-free, high sensitivity staining of proteins in one- and two-dimensional sodium dodecyl sulfate-polyacrylamide gels using a luminescent ruthenium complex. Electrophoresis 2000; 21:2509–21.
35. Berlett BS, Stadtman ER. Protein oxidation in aging, disease, and oxidative stress. J Biol Chem 1997; 272: 20313–16.
36. Berman ER. Biochemistry of the Eye. Plenum Press, 1991.
37. Bertrand E, Fritsch C, Diether S, et al. Identification of apolipoprotein A-I as a 'STOP' signal for myopia. Mol Cell Proteomics 2006; 5:2158–66.
38. Bhat SP, Jones RE, Sullivan MA, Piatigorsky P. Chicken lens crystallin DNA sequences show at least two α-crystallin genes. Nature 1980; 284:234–8.
39. Bhat SP, Nagineni CN. αB subunit of lens-specific protein α-crystallin is present in other ocular and non-ocular tissues. Biochem Biophys Res Commun 1989; 158:319–25.
40. Bhat SP, Piatigorsky J. Molecular cloning and partial characterization of α-crystallin cDNA sequences in a bacterial plasmid. Proc Natl Acad Sci U S A 1979; 76: 3299–303.
41. Bhattacharya SK. Focus on molecules: cochlin. Exp Eye Res 2006; 82:355–6.
42. Bhattacharya SK, Annangudi SP, Salomon RG, et al. Cochlin deposits in the trabecular meshwork of the glaucomatous DBA/2J mouse. Exp Eye Res 2005; 80: 741–4.
43. Bhattacharya SK, Peachey NS, Crabb JW. Cochlin and glaucoma: a mini-review. Vis Neurosci 2005; 22:605–13.
44. Bhattacharya SK, Rockwood EJ, Smith SD, et al. Proteomics reveal Cochlin deposits associated with glaucomatous trabecular meshwork. J Biol Chem 2005; 280:6080–4.
45. Billings PC, Whitbeck JC, Adams CS, et al. The transforming growth factor-beta-inducible matrix protein (beta)ig-h3 interacts with fibronectin. J Biol Chem 2002; 277:28003–9.
46. Bishop PN. Structural macromolecules and supramolecular organisation of the vitreous gel. Prog Retin Eye Res 2000; 19:323–44.
47. Bjellqvist B, Ek K, Righetti PG, et al. Isoelectric focusing in immobilized pH gradients: principle, methodology and some applications. J Biochem Biophys Methods 1982; 6:317–39.
48. Black HH, Landay LH. Marfan's syndrome: report of five cases in one family. Am J Dis Child 1955; 89:414–20.
49. Blobner F. Kristallinsche degeneration der Bindehaut und Hornhaut. Klin Mbl Augenheilkd 1938; 100:588–93.
50. Bloemendal H, ed. Molecular and Cellular Biology of the Ocular Lens. New York: Wiley and Sons, 1981.
51. Bloemendal H, de Jong W, Jaenicke R, et al. Ageing and vision: structure, stability and function of lens crystallins. Prog Biophys Mol Biol 2004; 86:407–85.
52. Bloemendal H, van de gaer K, Benedetti EL, et al. Towards a human crystallin map. Two-dimensional gel electrophoresis and computer analysis of water-soluble

crystallins from normal and cataractous human lenses. Ophthalmic Res 1997; 29:177–90.
53. Bogaars HA, Kaldenon AE, Cummings FJ, et al. Human IgG cryoglobulin with tubular crystal structure. Nature New Biol 1973; 245:117–8.
54. Bok D. New insights and new approaches toward the study of age-related macular degeneration. Proc Natl Acad Sci USA 2002; 99:14619–21.
55. Bonilha VL, Bhattacharya SK, West KA, et al. Proteomic characterization of isolated retinal pigment epithelium microvilli. Mol Cell Proteomics 2004; 3:1119–27.
56. Bonilha VL, Bhattacharya SK, West KA, et al. Support for a proposed retinoid-processing protein complex in apical retinal pigment epithelium. Exp Eye Res 2004; 79:419–22.
57. Bos KJ, Holmes DF, Meadows RS, et al. Collagen fibril organisation in mammalian vitreous by freeze etch/ rotary shadowing electron microscopy. Micron 2001; 32: 301–6.
58. Brekken RA, Sage EH. SPARC, a matricellular protein: at the crossroads of cell-matrix communication. Matrix Biol 2001; 19:816–27.
59. Burk EV. Über Hornhautveränderungen bei einem Fall von multiplem Myeloma (Plasmocytom). Ophthalmologia 135: 565–72.
60. Carr R, Henkind P. Retinal findings associated with serum hyperviscosity. Am J Ophthalmol 1963; 56:23–31.
61. Cherry PMH, Kraft S, McGowan H, et al. Corneal and conjunctival deposits in monoclonal gammopathy. Can J Ophthalmol 1983; 18:142–9.
62. Cherry PMH, Scott JG. Corneal and conjunctival deposits in monoclonal gammopathy: addendum and correction (letter). Can J Ophthalmol 1983; 18:256.
63. Chvapil ML. Physiology of Connective Tissue. London: Butterworth, 1967;229–33.
64. Cintorino M, Vindigni C, Del Vecchio MT, et al. Expression of actin isoforms and intermediate filament proteins in childhood orbital rhabdomyosarcomas. J Submicrosc Cytol Pathol 1989; 21:409–19.
65. Clarke E. Ophthalmological complications of multiple myelomatosis. Br J Ophthalmol 1955; 39:233–6.
66. Connell G, Bascom R, Molday L, et al. Photoreceptor peripherin is the normal product of the gene responsible for retinal degeneration in the (rds) mouse. Proc Natl Acad Sci USA 1991; 88:723–6.
67. Connell GE, Freedman MH, Nyburg SC, et al. A human IgG myeloma protein crystallizing with rhombohedral symmetry. Can J Biochem 1973; 51:1137–41.
68. Cooper D, Schermer A, Sun T-T. Biology of disease: classification of human epithelia and their neoplasms using antibodies to keratins: strategies, applications, and limitations. Lab Invest 1985; 52:243–56.
69. Cooper DL, Baptist EW, Enghild J, et al. Partial amino acid sequence determination of bovine corneal protein 54K (BCP54). Curr Eye Res 1990; 9:781–6.
70. Cooper DL, Baptist EW, Enghild JJ, et al. Bovine corneal protein 54K (BCP54) is a homologue of the tumor-associated (class 3) rat aldehyde dehydrogenase (RATALD). Gene 1991; 98:201–7.
71. Corson GM, Charbonneneau NL, Keene DR, Sakai LY. Differential expression of fibrillin-3 adds to microfibril variety in human and avian, but not rodent, connective tissues. Genomics 2004; 83:461–72.
72. Crabb JW, Miyagi M, Gu X, et al. Drusen proteome analysis: an approach to the etiology of age-related macular degeneration. Proc Natl Acad Sci USA 2002; 99: 14682–7.
73. Cross HE, Jensen AD. Ocular manifestations in the Marfan syndrome and homocystinuria. Am J Ophthalmol 1973; 75: 405–20.
74. Cuthbertson RA, Tomarev SI, Piatigorsky J. Taxon-specific recruitment of enzymes as major soluble proteins in the corneal epithelium of three mammals, chicken, and squid. Proc Natl Acad Sci USA 1992; 89: 4004–8.
75. Danis P, Brauman S, Coppez P. Lesions of the fundus of the eye found in certain hyperproteinemias, particularly those of myelomatous origin. Acta Ophthalmol 1955; 33: 33–52.
76. Danks D.M. Disorders of copper transport. In: Scriver CR, Beaudet AL, Sly WS, Valle D, eds. The Metabolic Basis of Inherited Disease, 6th ed., Vol. 1, Chapter New York: McGraw-Hill, 1989;1411–31.
77. Datiles MB, Schumer DJ, Zigler JS Jr, et al. Two-dimensional gel electrophoretic analysis of human lens proteins. Curr Eye Res 1992; 11:669–77.
78. Davies DR, Padlan EA, Segal DM. Three-dimensional structure of immunoglobulins. Ann Rev Biochem 1975; 44:639–67.
79. de Souza GA, Godoy LM, Mann M. Identification of 491 proteins in the tear fluid proteome reveals a large number of proteases and protease inhibitors. Genome Biol 2006; 7: R72.1–11.
80. Dellangelica EC, Schleicher CH, Santome JA. Primary structure and binding properties of calgranulin C, a novel S100-like calcium-binding protein from pig granulocytes. J Biol Chem 1994; 269:28929–36.
81. Deutsch HF, Suzuki T. A crystallin G1 human monoclonal protein with an excessive H chain deletion. Ann NY Acad Sci 1971; 190:472–86.
82. Dietz HC, Cutting GR, Pyeritz RE, et al. Marfan's syndrome caused by a recurrent de novo missense mutation in the fibrillin gene (see comments). Nature 1991; 352:337–9.
83. Disbella E, Grasso M, Marziliano N, et al. Two novel and one known mutation of the TGFBR2 gene in Marfan syndrome not associated with *FBNI* gene defects. Eur J Hum Genet 2006; 14:34–8.
84. Dizhoor AM, Ray S, Kumar S, et al. Recoverin: a calcium sensitive activator of retinal rod guanylate cyclase. Science 1991; 251:915–8.
85. Domon B, Aebersold R. Mass spectrometry and protein analysis. Science 2006; 312:212–7.
86. Donnelly EJ. Ocular complications of multiple myelomatosis. Am J Ophthalmol 1959; 47:211–4.
87. Dua HS, Liversidge J, Forrester JV. Immunomodulation of experimental autoimmune uveitis using a rat antiretinal S-antigen specific monoclonal antibody: evidence for a species difference. Eye 1989; 3:69–78.
88. Dua HS, Sewell HF, Forrester JV. The effect of retinal S-antigen-specific monoclonal antibody therapy on experimental autoimmune uveoretinitis (EAU) and experimental autoimmune pinealitis (EAP). Clin Exp Immunol 1989; 75:100–5.
89. Dubin RA, Wawrousek EF, Piatigorsky J. Expression of the murine αB-crystallin gene is not restricted to the lens. Mol Cell Biol 1989; 9:1083–91, 1989.
90. Eagle RC Jr, Brooks JSJ, Katowitz JA, et al. Fibrin as a major constituent of ligneous conjunctivitis. Am J Ophthalmol 1986; 101:493–4.
91. Eddington GN, Lehmann H. A case of sickle cell-hemoglobin C disease in a survey of hemoglobin incidence in West Africa. Trans World Soc Trop Med Hyg 1954; 48:332 6.

92. Edman P. Method for determination of the amino acid sequence in peptides. Acta Chem Scand 1950; 4:283–93.
93. Edman P, Begg G. A protein sequenator. Eur J Biochem 1967; 1:80–91.
94. Eiferman RA, Rodrigues MM. Unusual superficial stromal corneal deposits in IgGk monoclonal gammopathy. Arch Ophthalmol 1980; 98:78–81.
95. Emanuel BS, Cannizzarol L, Ornstein-Goldstein N, et al. Chromosomal localization of the human elastin gene. Am J Hum Genet 1985; 37:873–82.
96. Enzenauer RJ, Stock JG, Enzenauer RW, et al. Retinal vasculopathy associated with systemic light chain deposition disease. Retina 1990; 10:115–8.
97. Escribano J, Hernando N, Ghosh S, et al. cDNA from human ocular ciliary epithelium homologous to beta ig-h3 is preferentially expressed as an extracellular protein in the corneal epithelium. J Cell Physiol 1994; 160: 511–21.
98. Ethen CM, Reilly C, Feng X, et al. The proteome of central and peripheral retina with progression of age-related macular degeneration. Invest Ophthalmol Vis Sci 2006; 47:2280–90.
99. Eype AA, Kruit PJ, van der Gaag R, et al. Autoimmunity against corneal antigens. II. Accessibility of the 54 kD corneal antigen for circulating antibodies. Curr Eye Res 1987; 6:467–75.
100. Farrar GJ, Kenna P, Redmond R, et al. Autosomal dominant retinitis pigmentosa: absence of the rhodopsin proline-histidine substitution (codon 23) in pedigrees from Europe. Am J Hum Genet 47:1990; 941–5.
101. Feeney-Burns L, Hilderbrand ES, Eldridge S. Aging human RPE: morphometric analysis of macular, equatorial, and peripheral cells. Invest Ophthalmol Vis Sci 1984; 25:195–200.
102. Firkin FC, Lee N, Ramsay R, Robertson I. Visual loss caused by corneal crystals in myeloma: rapid improvement with plasma exchange and chemotherapy. Med J Aust 1979; 2:677–8.
103. Fleischmajer R, Jacobs L II, Perlish JS, et al. Immunochemical analysis of human kidney reticulin. Am J Pathol 1992; 140:1225–35.
104. Fleischmajer R, Krieg T, Dziadek M, et al. Ultrastructure and composition of connective tissue in hyalinosis cutis et mucosae skin. J Invest Dermatol 1984; 82:252–8.
105. Fodor IK, Nelson DO, Alegria-Hartman M, et al. Statistical challenges in the analysis of two-dimensional difference gel electrophoresis experiments using DeCyder. Bioinfor matics 2005; 21:3733–40.
106. Francois J. Paraproteinaemic thesaurismosis of the cornea in Kahler's multiple myelomatosis. Eye Ear Nose Throat Mon 1967; 46:857–60.
107. Francois J, Bacskulin J, Follmann P. Manifestations oculaires du syndrome d'Urbach-Wiethe. Hyalinosis cutis et mucosae. Ophthalmologica 1968; 155:433–48.
108. Francois J, Rabaey M. Dystrophie cornéene et paraproteinemie. Bull Soc Belge Ophthalmol 1960; 125:1007–17.
109. Franklin RM. The ocular secretory immune system: a review. Curr Eye Res 1989; 8:599–606.
110. Friedman JS, Faucher M, Hiscott P, et al. Protein localization in the human eye and genetic screen of opticin. Hum Mol Genet 2002; 11:1333–42.
111. Fuchs EV, Coppock SM, Green H, Cleveland DW. Two distinct classes of keratin genes and their evolutionary significance. Cell 1981; 27:75–84.
112. Fuchshofer R., Welge-Lussen U, Lutjen-Drecoll E, Birke M. Biochemical and morphological analysis of basement membrane component expression in corneoscleral and cribriform human trabecular meshwork cells. Invest Ophthalmol Vis Sci 2006; 47:794–801.
113. Fukuda MN, Papermaster DS, Hargrave PA. Rhodopsin carbohydrate: structure of small oligosaccharides attached at two sites near the NH2 terminus. J Biol Chem 1979; 254:8201–7.
114. Fullmer HM, Lillie RD. The oxytalan fiber: a previously undescribed connective tissue fiber. J Histochem Cytochem 1958; 6:425–30.
115. Fullmer HM, Sheetz JH, Narkates AJ. Oxytalan connective tissue fibers: a review. J Oral Pathol 1974; 3:291–316.
116. Fung KY, Morris C, Sathe S, et al. Characterization of the in vivo forms of lacrimal-specific proline-rich proteins in human tear fluid. Proteomics 2004; 4:3953–9.
117. Ganeval D, Noel LH, Preud'homme JL, Droz D, Grünfeld JP. Light-chain deposition disease: its relation with A1-type amyloidosis. Editorial review. Kidney Int 1984; 26:1–9.
118. Garibaldi DC, Gottsh HJ, de la Cruz Z, Mark H, Green WR. Immunotactoid keratopathy: a clinicopathologic case report and a review of corneal involvement in the systemic paraproteinemias. Surv Ophtahlmol 2005; 50: 61–80.
119. Garland DL, Duglas-Tabor Y, Jimenez-Asensio J, et al. The nucleus of the human lens: demonstration of a highly characteristic protein pattern by two-dimensional electrophoresis and introduction of a new method of lens dissection. Exp Eye Res 1996; 62:285–91.
120. Garner A, Alexander RA. Pre-elastic (oxytalan) fibres in corneal pathology. Proc VIth Congr Eur Soc Ophthalmol: London, Academic Press and Royal Society of Medicine, 1980;213–6.
121. Garner A, Kirkness CM. Corneal gammopathy. Cornea 1988; 7:44–9.
122. Gay S, Fletzek PP, Remberger K, et al. Liver cirrhosis: immunofluorescence and biochemical studies demonstrate two types of collagen. Klin Wochenschr 1975; 53: 205–8.
123. Geisler N, Weber K. The amino acid sequence of chicken muscle desmin provides a common structural model for intermediate filament proteins. EMBO J 1982; 1:1649–56.
124. Gentle A, Liu Y, Martin JE, et al. Collagen gene expression and the altered accumulation of scleral collagen during the development of high myopia. J Biol Chem 2003; 278: 16587–94.
125. Gharahdaghi F, Weinberg CR, Meagher DA, et al. Mass spectrometric identification of proteins from silver-stained polyacrylamide gel: a method for the removal of silver ions to enhance sensitivity. Electrophoresis 1999; 20:601–5.
126. Gilbert W, Villa-Komaroff L. Useful proteins from recombinant bacteria. Sci Am 1980; 242:74–94.
127. Glasgow BJ. Tissue expression of lipocalins in human lacrimal and von Ebner's glands: colocalization with lysozyme. Graefes Arch Clin Exp Ophthalmol 1995; 233: 513–22.
128. Gluszcz A, Giernat L, Habryka K, et al. Rosenthal fibers, birefringent gliofibrillary changes and intracellular homogenous conglomerates in tissue cultures of gliomas. Acta Neuropathol 1971; 17:54–67.
129. Goldberg AL. Protein degradation and protection against misfolded or damaged proteins. Nature 2003; 426:895–9.
130. Goldberg MF, Ryan SJ. Intercalary staphyloma in Marfan's syndrome. Am J Ophthalmol 1969; 67:329–35.
131. Goldwich A, Baulmann DC, Ohlmann A, et al. Myocilin is expressed in the glomerulus of the kidney and induced in mesangioproliferative glomerulonephritis. Kidney Int 2005; 67:140–51.

132. Gordon MK, Fitch JM, Foley JW, et al. Type XVII collagen (BP 180) in the developing avian cornea. Invest Ophthalmol Vis Sci 1997; 38:153–66.
133. Görg A, Obermaier C, Boguth G, et al. The current state of two-dimensional electrophoresis with immobilized pH gradients. Electrophoresis 2000; 21:1037–53.
134. Gottsch JD, Li Q, Ashraf F, et al. Cytokine-induced calgranulin C expression in keratocytes. Clin Immunol 1999; 91:34–40.
135. Gottsch JD, Liu SH. Cloning and expression of human corneal calgranulin C (CO-Ag). Curr Eye Res 1998; 17: 870–4.
136. Gottsch JD, Liu SH, Minkovitz JB, et al. Autoimmunity to a cornea-associated stromal antigen in patients with Moorens ulcer. Invest Ophthalmol Vis. Sci. 1995; 36: 1541–7.
137. Hamada T, Wessagowit V, South AP, et al. Extracellular matrix protein 1 gene (ECM1) mutations in lipoid proteinosis and genotype-phenotype correlation. J Invest Dermatol 2003; 120:345–50.
138. Hamdi HK, Kenney C. Age-related macular degeneration: a new viewpoint. Front Biosci 2003; 8:e305–14.
139. Hamilton AM, Garner A, Tripathi RC, Sanders MD. Malignant optic nerve glioma: report of a case with electron microscope study. Br J Ophthalmol 1973; 57: 253–64.
140. Hanson SR, Hasan A, Smith DL, Smith JB. The major in vivo modifications of the human water-insoluble lens crystallins are disulfide bonds, deamidation, methionine oxidation and backbone cleavage. Exp Eye Res 2000; 71: 195–207.
141. Hanssen E, Reinboth B, Gibson MA. Covalent and non-covalent interactions of betaig-h3 with collagen VI. Beta ig-h3 is covalently attached to the amino-terminal region of collagen VI in tissue microfibrils. J Biol Chem 2003; 278:24334–41.
142. Hargrave PA, Fong SL. The amino- and carboxyl-terminal sequence of bovine rhodopsin. J Supramol Struct 1977; 6:559–70.
143. Harper JL, Duance VC, Sims TJ, Light ND. Lipoid proteinosis: an inherited disorder of collagen metabolism? Br J Dermatol 1985; 113:145–51.
144. Harrington V, McCall S, Huynh S, et al. Crystallins in water soluble-high molecular weight protein fractions and water insoluble protein fractions in aging and cataractous human lenses. Mol Vis 2004; 10:476–89.
145. Hashimoto K, Noshiro M, Ohno S, Kawamoto T, et al. Characterization of a cartilage-derived 66-kDa protein (RGD-CAP/beta ig-h3) that binds to collagen. Biochim Biophys Acta 1997; 1355:303–14.
146. Hathout Y, Flippin J, Fan C, et al. Metabolic labeling of human primary retinal pigment epithelial cells for accurate comparative proteomics. J Proteome Res 2005; 4:620–7.
147. Hauck SM, Suppmann S, Ueffing M. Proteomic profiling of primary retinal Muller glia cells reveals a shift in expression patterns upon adaptation to in vitro conditions. Glia 2003; 44:251–63.
148. Hausser I, Blitz S, Rauterberg E, Frosch PJ, Anton-Lamprecht I. Hyalinosis cutis et mucosae (Morbus Urbach-Wiethe). Ultrastrukturelle und immunologische Merkmale. Hautarzt 1991; 42:28–33.
149. Hedegaard CJ, Thogersen IB, Enghild JJ, et al. Transforming growth factor beta induced protein accumulation in granular corneal dystrophy type III (Reis-Bucklers dystrophy). Identification by mass spectrometry in 15 year old two-dimensional protein gels. Mol Vis 2003; 9:355–9.
150. Henderson DW, Stirlng JW, Lipsett J, et al. Paraproteinemic crystalloidal keratopathy: an ultrastructural study of two cases, including immunoelectron microscopy. Ultrastruct Pathol 1993; 17:643–68.
151. Henley WL, Kong S. Antibody to corneal proteins in uveitis. Pediatr Res 1986; 20(Suppl.):294A.
152. Henzel WJ, Billeci TM, Stults JT, et al. Identifying proteins from two-dimensional gels by molecular mass searching of peptide fragments in protein sequence databases. Proc Natl Acad Sci USA 1993; 90:5011–5.
153. Herbert B. Advances in protein solubilisation for two-dimensional electrophoresis. Electrophoresis 1999; 20: 660–3.
154. Hernandez MR, Luo XX, Igoe F, Neufeld AH. Extracellular matrix of the human lamina cribrosa. Am J Ophthalmol 1987; 104:567–76.
155. Heukeshoven J, Dernick R. Improved silver staining procedure for fast staining in PhastSystem Development Unit. I. Staining of sodium dodecyl sulfate gels. Electrophoresis 1988; 9:28–32.
156. Hida RY, Ohashi Y, Takano Y, et al. Elevated levels of human alpha-defensin in tears of patients with allergic conjunctival disease complicated by corneal lesions: detection by SELDI ProteinChip system and quantification. Curr Eye Res 2005; 30:723–30.
157. Hidayat AA, Riddle PJ. Ligneous conjunctivitis: a clinicopathologic study of 17 cases. Ophthalmology 1987; 94:949–59.
158. Hill JC, Mulligan GP. Subepithelial corneal deposits in IgG lambda myeloma. Br J Ophthalmol 1989; 73:552–4.
159. Hochstrasser DF, Sanchez JC, Appel RD. Proteomics and its trends facing nature's complexity. Proteomics 2002; 2: 807–12.
160. Hoehenwarter W, Klose J, Jungblut PR. Eye lens proteomics. Amino Acids 2006.
161. Hoehenwarter W, Kumar NM, Wacker M, et al. Eye lens proteomics: from global approach to detailed information about phakinin and gamma E and F crystallin genes. Proteomics 2005; 5:245–57.
162. Hoisen H, Ringvold A, Kildahl-Anderson O. Corneal crystalline deposits in multiple myeloma: a case report. Acta Ophthalmol 1983; 61:493–500.
163. Holland EJ, Chan C-C, Kuwabara T, et al. Immmunologic findings and results of treatment with cyclosporine in ligneous conjunctivitis. Am J Ophthalmol 1989; 107: 160–6.
164. Holt JM, Gordon-Smith EC. Retinal abnormalities in diseases of the blood. Br J Ophthalmol 1969; 53:145–60.
165. Horácèk J. Kristallinische Augendegeneration als erstes Anzeichen der plasmozytären Myeloms. Zentral Allg Pathol Anat 1963; 104:264–7.
166. Huang TW. Chemical and histochemical studies of human alveolar collagen fibers. Am J Pathol 1977; 86:81–97.
167. Ingolia TD, Craig EA. Four small Drosophila heat shock proteins are related to each other and to mammalian α-crystallin. Proc Natl Acad Sci USA 1982; 79:2360–4.
168. International Human Genome Sequencing Consortium. Finishing the euchromatic sequence of the human genome. Nature 2004; 431:931–45.
169. Ito S, Goshima K, Niiomi M, et al. Electron microscopic studies of the crystalline inclusions in the myeloma cells and kidney of κ-Bence-Jones protein type myeloma. Acta Haem Jpn 1970; 33:598–617.
170. Iwaki A, Iwaki T, Goldman JE, Liem RKH. Multiple mRNAs of rat brain α-crystallin B chain result from alternative transcriptional initiation. J Biol Chem 1990; 265:22197–203.

171. Iwaki T, Iwaki A, Miyazono M, Goldman JE. Preferential expression of αB-crystallin in astrocytic elements of neuroectodermal tumors. Cancer 1991; 68:2230–40.
172. Iwaki T, Kume-Iwaki A, Goldman JE. Cellular distribution of αB-crystallin in non-lenticular tissues. J Histochem Cytochem 1990; 38:31–9.
173. Iwaki T, Kume-Iwaki A, Liem RKH, Goldman JE. αB-crystallin is expressed in non-lenticular tissues and accumulates in Alexander's disease brain. Cell 1989; 57: 71–8.
174. Iwaki T, Takeishi J. Immunohistochemical demonstration of αB-crystallin in hamartomas of tuberous sclerosis. Am J Pathol 1991; 139:1303–8.
175. Jensen AD, Khodadoust AA, Emery JM. Lipid proteinosis: report of a case with electron microscopic findings. Arch Ophthalmol 1972; 88:273–7.
176. Jester JV, Moller-Pedersen T, Huang J, et al. The cellular basis of corneal transparency: evidence for 'corneal crystallins'. J Cell Sci 1999; 112(Pt 5):613–22.
177. Johnson BL. Proteinaceous cysts of the ciliary epithelium. II. Their occurrence in non-myelomatous hypergammaglobulinemic conditions. Arch Ophthalmol 1970; 84: 171–5.
178. Johnson BL, Storey JD. Proteinaceous cysts of the ciliary body. I. Their clear nature and immunoelectrophoretic analysis in a case of multiple myeloma. Arch Ophthalmol 1970; 84:166–70.
179. Johnson LV, Anderson DH. Age-related macular degeneration and the extracellular matrix. N Engl J Med 2004; 351:320–22.
180. Jungblut PR, Otto A, Favor J, et al. Identification of mouse crystallins in 2D protein patterns by sequencing and mass spectrometry. Application to cataract mutants. FEBS Lett 1998; 435:131–7.
181. Kalderon AE, Bogaars HA, Diamond I, et al. Ultrastructure of myeloma cells in a case with crystal cryoglobulinemia. Cancer 1977; 39:1475–81.
182. Kapp LD, Lorsch JR. The molecular mechanics of eukaryotic translation. Annu Rev Biochem 2004; 73: 657–704.
183. Karring H, Thogersen IB, Klintworth GK, et al. A dataset of human cornea proteins identified by peptide mass fingerprinting and tandem mass spectrometry. Mol Cell Proteomics 2005; 4:1406–8.
184. Karring H, Thogersen IB, Klintworth GK, et al. Proteomic analysis of the soluble fraction from human corneal fibroblasts with reference to ocular transparency. Mol Cell Proteomics 2004; 3:660–74.
185. Karring H, Thogersen IB, Klintworth GK, et al. The human cornea proteome: bioinformatic analyses indicate import of plasma proteins into the cornea. Mol Vis 2006; 12:451–60.
186. Karttunen T, Alavaikko M, Apaja-Sarkkinen M, Autio-Harmainen H. An immunohistochemical study of laminin, type IV collagen and type III pN-collagen with relation to reticular fibres in Hodgkin's disease. Int J Cancer 1988; 41:52–8.
187. Karttunen T, Sormunen R, Risteli L, et al. Immunoelectron microscopic localization of laminin, type IV collagen and type III pN-collagen in reticular fibres of human lymph nodes. J Histochem Cytochem 1988; 37: 279–86.
188. Keeley FW, Morin JD, Vesely S. Characterisation of type I collagen from normal human sclera. Exp Eye Res 1984; 39:663–72.
189. Kelley PB, Sado Y, Duncan MK. Collagen IV in the developing lens capsule. Matrix Biol 2002; 21:415–23.
190. Kemper C, Berggren K, Diwu Z, Patton WF. An improved, luminescent europium-based stain for detection of electroblotted proteins on nitrocellulose or polyvinylidene difluoride membranes. Electrophoresis 2001; 22:881–9.
191. Kennan A, Aherne A, Humphries P. Light in retinitis pigmentosa. Trends Genet 2005; 21:103–110.
192. Kerenyi L, Gallyas F. A highly sensitive method for demonstrating proteins in electrophoretic, immunoelectrophoretic and immunodiffusion preparations. Clin Chim Acta 1972; 38:465–7.
193. Kim JE, Jeong HW, Nam JO, et al. Identification of motifs in the fasciclin domains of the transforming growth factor-beta-induced matrix protein betaig-h3 that interact with the alphavbeta5 integrin. J Biol Chem 2002; 277: 46159–65.
194. Kim JE, Kim SJ, Lee BH, et al. Identification of motifs for cell adhesion within the repeated domains of transforming growth factor-beta-induced gene, betaig-h3. J Biol Chem 2000; 275:30907–15.
195. Kim MO, Yun SJ, Kim IS, Sohn et al. Transforming growth factor-beta-inducible gene-h3 (beta(ig)-h3) promotes cell adhesion of human astrocytoma cells in vitro: implication of alpha6beta4 integrin. Neurosci Lett 2003; 336:93–6.
196. Klemenz R, Fröhli E, Steiger RH, et al. αB-crystallin is a small heat shock protein. Proc Natl Acad Sci USA 1991; 88:3652–6.
197. Klintworth GK. The molecular genetics of the corneal dystrophies—current status. Front Biosci 2003; 8: d687–713.
198. Klintworth GK, Bredehoeft SJ, Reed JW. Analysis of corneal crystals in multiple myeloma. Am J Ophthalmol 1978; 86:303–13.
199. Klintworth GK, Enghild JJ, Valnickova Z. Discovery of a novel protein (big-h3) in normal human cornea. Invest Ophthalmol Vis Sci 1994; 35(Suppl.):1938.
200. Klintworth GK, Valnickova Z, Kielar RA, et al. Familial subepithelial corneal amyloidosis–a lactoferrin-related amyloidosis. Invest Ophthalmol Vis Sci 1997; 38: 2756–63.
201. Koch M, Laub F, Zhou P, et al. Collagen XXIV, a vertebrate fibrillar collagen with structural features of invertebrate collagens: selective expression in developing cornea and bone. J Biol Chem 2003; 278:43236–44.
202. Kong SA, Henley WL, Luntz MH. Immunochemical localization of corneal protein BCP 54 in epithelial cells. Invest Ophthalmol Vis Sci 1989; 30(Suppl.):519.
203. Konomi H, Sano J, Nagai Y. Immunohistochemical localization of type I-III and IV (basement membrane) collagens in the lymph node: codistribution of types I and III collagens in the reticular fibers. Biomed Res 1981; 2: 536–45.
204. Koo BS, Lee DY, Ha HS, et al. Comparative analysis of the tear protein expression in blepharitis patients using two-dimensional electrophoresis. J Proteome Res 2005; 4: 719–24.
205. Korbet SM, Schwartz MM, Lewis EJ. Immunotactoid glomerulopathy (fibrillary glomerulonephritis). Clin J Am Soc Nephrol 2006; 1:1351–6.
206. Kotake S, Hey P, Mirmira RG, Copeland RA. Physicochemical characterization of bovine retinal arrestin. Arch Biochem Biophys 1991; 285:126–33.
207. Koyama R, Nakanishi T, Ikeda T, Shimizu A. Catalogue of soluble proteins in human vitreous humor by one-dimensional sodium dodecyl sulfate-polyacrylamide gel electrophoresis and electrospray ionization mass spectrometry including seven angiogenesis-regulating factors.

J Chromatogr B Analyt Technol Biomed Life Sci 2003; 792: 5–21.
208. Krafchak CM, Pawar H, Moroi SE, Sugar A. Mutations in TCF8 cause posterior polymorphous corneal dystrophy and ectopic expression of COL4A3 by corneal endothelial cells. Am J Hum Genet 2005; 77:694–708.
209. Kremer I, Wright P, Merin S, et al. Corneal subepithelial monoclonal kappa IgG deposits in essential cryoglobulinaemia. Br J Ophthalmol 1989; 73:669–73.
210. Kruit PJ, Broersma L, van der Gaag R, Kijlstra A. Clinical and experimental studies concerning circulating antibodies to corneal epithelium antigens. Doc Ophthalmol 1986; 64:43–51.
211. Kruit PJ, van der Gaag R, Broersma L, Kijlstra A. Autoimmunity against corneal antigens. I. isolation of a soluble 54 kD corneal epithelium antigen. Curr Eye Res 1986; 5:313–20.
212. Kyle RA, Greipp PR. Monoclonal gammopathies of undetermined significance. In: Wiernik PH, Canellos GP, Kyle RA, Schiffer CA, eds. Neoplastic Disesases of the Blood, Vol. 2. New York: Churchill Livingstone, 1985;653–76.
213. La Hey E, Baarsma GS, Rothova A, et al. High incidence of corneal epithelium antibodies in Fuch's heterochromic cyclitis. Br J Ophthalmol 1988; 72:921–5.
214. Laibson PR, Damiano VV. X-ray and electron diffraction of ocular and bone marrow crystals in paraproteinemia. Science 1969; 163:581–3.
215. Lambrecht H-G, Koch K-W. A 26 kD calcium binding protein from bovine rod outer segments as modulator of photoreceptor guanylate cyclase. EMBO J 1991; 10:793–8.
216. Lampi KJ, Ma Z, Hanson SR, et al. Age-related changes in human lens crystallins identified by two-dimensional electrophoresis and mass spectrometry. Exp Eye Res 1998; 67:31–43.
217. Lampi KJ, Ma Z, Shih M, et al. Sequence analysis of betaA3, betaB3, and betaA4 crystallins completes the identification of the major proteins in young human lens. J Biol Chem 1997; 272:2268–75.
218. Lampi KJ, Shih M, Ueda Y, et al. Lens proteomics: analysis of rat crystallin sequences and two-dimensional electrophoresis map. Invest Ophthalmol Vis Sci 2002; 43: 216–24.
219. Lander ES, Linton LM, Birren B, et al. Initial sequencing and analysis of the human genome. Nature 2001; 409: 860–921.
220. Lane EB. Monoclonal antibodies provide specific intramolecular markers for the study of epithelial tonofilament organization. J Cell Biol 1982; 92:665–73.
221. Lane EB, Bartek J, Purkis PE, Leigh IM. Keratin antigens in differentiating skin. Ann. NY Acad Sci 1985; 455: 241–58.
222. Lauber WM, Carroll JA, Dufield DR, et al. Mass spectrometry compatibility of two-dimensional gel protein stains. Electrophoresis 2001; 22:906–18.
223. Laurell T, Marko-Varga G. Miniaturisation is mandatory unravelling the human proteome. Proteomics 2002; 2: 345–51.
224. Laursen RA. Solid-phase Edman degradation. An automatic peptide sequencer. Eur J Biochem 1971; 20:89–102.
225. Lee B, Godfrey M, Vitale E, et al. Linkage of Marfan syndrome and a phenotypically related disorder to two different fibrillin genes (see comments). Nature 1991; 353: 330–4.
226. Li N, Wang N, Zheng J, et al. Characterization of human tear proteome using multiple proteomic analysis techniques. J Proteome Res 2005; 4:2052–61.
227. Liang CJ, Yamashita K, Muellenberg CG, et al. Structure of the carbohydrate moieties of bovine rhodopsin. J Biol Chem 1979; 254:6414–8.
228. Liang FQ, Godley BF. Oxidative stress-induced mitochondrial DNA damage in human retinal pigment epithelial cells: a possible mechanism for RPE aging and age-related macular degeneration. Exp Eye Res 2003; 76:397–403.
229. Lièvre JA, Camus JP, Lèvy R, et al. Myéloma a globulin cristallisable: étude physiocochemique et microscopie electronique. Nouv Rev Fr Hematol 1961; 1:23–35.
230. Lightman MA. Essential and secondary monoclonal gammopathies. In: Williams WJ, Beutler E, Erslev AJ, Lichtman MA, eds., Hematology, 4th. ed. New York: McGraw Hill, 1990;1109–14.
231. Lin RJ, Blumenkranz MS, Binkley J, et al. A novel His158Arg mutation in TIMP3 causes a late-onset form of Sorsby fundus dystrophy. Am J Ophthalmol 2006; 142: 839–48.
232. Link AJ, ed. 2-D Proteome Analysis Protocols. Totowa, NJ: Humana Press, 1998;1–608.
233. Link AJ, Eng J, Schieltz DM, et al. Direct analysis of protein complexes using mass spectrometry. Nat Biotechnol 1999; 17:676–82.
234. Linquist S. The heat-shock response. Ann Rev Biochem 1986; 55:1151–91.
235. Loeys B, Van Maldergem L, Mortier G, et al. Homozygosity for a missense mutation in fibulin-5 (FBLN5) results in a severe form of cutis laxa. Hum Mol Genet 2002; 11:2113–8.
236. Los LI, van der Worp RJ, van Luyn MJ, Hooymans JM. Presence of collagen IV in the ciliary zonules of the human eye: an immunohistochemical study by LM and TEM. J Histochem Cytochem 2004; 52:789–95.
237. Lou MF. Redox regulation in the lens. Prog Retin Eye Res 2003; 22:657–82.
238. Lowe J, Mayer RJ. Ubiquitin, cell stress and diseases of the nervous system. Neuropathol Appl Neurobiol 1990; 16:281–91.
239. Ma Z, Hanson SR, Lampi KJ, et al. Age-related changes in human lens crystallins identified by HPLC and mass spectrometry. Exp Eye Res 1998; 67:21–30.
240. Maatta M, Heljasvaara R, Sormunen R, et al. Differential expression of collagen types XVIII/endostatin and XV in normal, keratoconus, and scarred human corneas. Cornea 2006; 25:341–9.
241. MacCoss MJ, McDonald WH, Saraf A, et al. Shotgun identification of protein modifications from protein complexes and lens tissue. Proc Natl Acad Sci USA 2002; 99:7900–5.
242. Majid MA, Smith VA, Easty DL, et al. Sorsby's fundus dystrophy mutant tissue inhibitors of metalloproteinase-3 induce apoptosis of retinal pigment epithelial and MCF-7 cells. FEBS Lett 2002; 529:281–5.
243. Malone JP, Radabaugh MR, Leimgruber RM, Gerstenecker GS. Practical aspects of fluorescent staining for proteomic applications. Electrophoresis 2001; 22:919–32.
244. Mann M, Hojrup P, Roepstorff P. Use of mass spectrometric molecular weight information to identify proteins in sequence databases. Biol Mass Spectrom 1993; 22: 338–45.
245. Mann M, Jensen ON. Proteomic analysis of post-translational modifications. Nat Biotechnol 2003; 21:255–61.
246. Marmorstein LY, Munier FL, Arsenijevic Y, et al. Aberrant accumulation of EFEMP1 underlies drusen formation in Malattia Leventinese and age-related macular degeneration. Proc Natl Acad Sci USA 2002; 99:13067–72.

247. Marouga R, David S, Hawkins E. The development of the DIGE system: 2D fluorescence difference gel analysis technology. Anal Bioanal Chem 2005; 382:669–78.
248. Mayne R, Ren ZX, Liu J, et al. VIT-1: the second member of a new branch of the von Willebrand factor A domain superfamily. Biochem Soc Trans 1999; 27:832–5.
249. McCurley TL, Gay RE, Gay S, et al. The extracellular protein in 'sclerosing' follicular center cell lymphomas. Hum Pathol 1986; 17:930–8.
250. McGrand JC, Rees DM, Harry J. Ligneous conjunctivitis. Br J Ophthalmol 1969; 53:373–81.
251. McKay K, Striker L, D'Amico G, Striker G. Dysproteinemias and paraproteinemias. In: Tisher CC, Brenner BM, eds. Renal Pathology. Philadelphia: Lippincott, 1989;1363–416.
252. McKusick VA. Heritable Disorders of Connective Tissue, 4th ed. St Louis, MO: C.V. Mosby, 1972.
253. McKusick VA. Mendelian Inheritance in Man. Catalogs of Autosomal Dominant, Autosomal Recessive and X-linked Phenotypes, 10th ed. Baltimore: Johns Hopkins University Press, 1992.
254. McWilliam P, Farrar GJ, Kenna P, et al. Autosomal dominant retinitis pigmentosa (ADRP): localization of an ADRP gene to the long arm of chromosome 3. Genomics 1989; 5:619–22, 1989.
255. Meek KM, Fullwood NJ. Corneal and scleral collagens—a microscopist's perspective. Micron 2001; 32:261–72.
256. Meesmann A. Über eine eigenartige Hornhaut degeneration. (Ablagerung der Bence-Jonesschen Einweiss korper in der Hornhaut). Ber Dtsch Ophthalmol 1934; 50:311–5.
257. Meri S, Baumann M. Proteomics: posttranslational modifications, immune responses and current analytical tools. Biomol Eng 2001; 18:213–20.
258. Midwood KS, Schwarzbauer JE. Elastic fibers: building bridges between cells and their matrix. Curr Biol 2002; 12: R279–81.
259. Miesbauer LR, Zhou X, Yang Z, et al. Post-translational modifications of water-soluble human lens crystallins from young adults. J Biol Chem 1994; 269:12494–502.
260. Miklos GL, Maleszka R. Protein functions and biological contexts. Proteomics 2001; 1:169–78.
261. Miller KH, Green WR, Stark WJ, et al. Immunoprotein deposition in the cornea. Ophthalmology 1980; 87:944–50.
262. Missotten GS, Beijnen JH, Keunen JE, Bonfrer JM. Proteomics in uveal melanoma. Melanoma Res 2003; 13: 627–9.
263. Moll R, Franke WW, Schiller DL, et al. The catalog of human cytokeratins: patterns of expression in normal epithelia, tumors and cultured cells. Cell 1982; 31:11–24.
264. Monemi S, Spaeth G, DaSilva A, et al. Identification of a novel adult-onset primary open-angle glaucoma (POAG) gene on 5q22.1. Hum Mol Genet 2005; 14:725–33.
265. Morrison JC, Dorman-Pease ME, Dunkelberger GR, Quigley HA. Optic nerve head extracellular matrix in primary optic atrophy and experimental glaucoma. Arch Ophthalmol 1990; 108:1020–4.
266. Morrison JC, Jerdan JA, L'Hernault NL, Quigley HA. The extracellular matrix composition of the monkey optic nerve head. Invest Ophthalmol Vis Sci 1988; 29:1141–50.
267. Morrison JC, Rask P, Johnson EC, Deppmeier L. Chondroitin sulfate proteoglycan distribution in the primate optic nerve head. Invest Ophthalmol Vis Sci 1994; 35:838–45.
268. Moy LS, Moy RL, Matsuoka LY, Ohta A, Uitto J. Lipoid proteinosis: ultrastructural and biochemical studies. J Am Acad Dermatol 1987; 16:1193–201.
269. Munier FL, Korvatska E, Djemai A, et al. Kerato-epithelin mutations in four 5q31-linked corneal dystrophies. Nat Genet 1997; 15:247–51.
270. Murzin AG, Brenner SE, Hubbard T, Chothia C. SCOP: a structural classification of proteins database for the investigation of sequences and structures. J Mol Biol 1995; 247:536–40.
271. Nakanishi T, Koyama R, Ikeda T, Shimizu A. Catalogue of soluble proteins in the human vitreous humor: comparison between diabetic retinopathy and macular hole. J Chromatogr B Analyst Technol Biomed Life Sci 2002; 776: 89–100.
272. Neal RE, Bettelheim FA, Lin C, et al. Alterations in human vitreous humour following cataract extraction. Exp Eye Res 2005; 80:337–47.
273. Nees DW, Wawrousek EF, Robison WG Jr, Piatigorsky J. Structurally normal corneas in aldehyde dehydrogenase 3a1-deficient mice. Mol Cell Biol 2002; 22:849–55.
274. Neuhoff V, Arold N, Taube D, Ehrhardt W. Improved staining of proteins in polyacrylamide gels including isoelectric focusing gels with clear background at nanogram sensitivity using Coomassie Brilliant Blue G-250 and R-250. Electrophoresis 1988; 9:255–62.
275. Neuhoff V, Stamm R, Pardowitz I, et al. Essential problems in quantification of proteins following colloidal staining with coomassie brilliant blue dyes in polyacrylamide gels, and their solution. Electrophoresis 1990; 11: 101–17.
276. Newton FH, Rosenberg RN, Lampert PW, O'Brien JS. Neurological involvement in Urbach-Wiethe's disease (lipoid proteinosis): a clinical, ultrastructural, and chemical study. Neurology 1971; 21:1205–13.
277. Nierhaus KH, Wilson DN, eds. Protein Synthesis and Ribosome Structure: Translating the Genome, New York: Wiley-VCH, 2004; 1–579.
278. Nik NA, Martin WF, Berler DK. Corneal crystalline deposits and drusenosin associated with IgA-kappa chain monoclonal gammopathy. Ann Ophthalmol 1985; 17:303–7.
279. Nordgaard CL, Berg KM, Kapphahn RJ, et al. Proteomics of the retinal pigment epithelium reveals altered protein expression at progressive stages of age-related macular degeneration. Invest Ophthalmol Vis Sci 2006; 47:815–22.
280. Oglesby RB. Corneal opacities in a patient with cryoglobulinemia and reticulohistiocytosis. Arch Ophthalmol 1961; 65:63–6.
281. Ohlmann AV, Ohlmann A, Welge-Lussen U, May CA. Localization of collagen XVIII and endostatin in the human eye. Curr Eye Res 2005; 30:27–34.
282. Ohno S, Noshiro M, Makihira S, et al. RGD-CAP ((beta) ig-h3) enhances the spreading of chondrocytes and fibroblasts via integrin alpha(1)beta(1). Biochim Biophys Acta 1999; 1451:196–205.
283. Okuda T, Matsumoto K, Ando Y, et al. A case of corneal lactoferrin amyloidosis secondray to trichiasis. Nippon Ganka Gakkai Zasshi 2003; 107:105–8.
284. Olsen DR, Chu ML, Uitto J. Expression of basement zone genes coding for type IV procollagen and laminin by human skin fibroblasts in vitro: elevated alpha 1(IV) collagen mRNA levels in lipoid proteinosis. J Invest Dermatol 1988; 900:734–8.
285. Orcutt JC, Reeh MJ, Gown AM, Lindquist TD. Diagnosis of orbital and periorbital tumors: use of monoclonal antibodies to cytoplasmic antigens (intermediate filaments). Ophthal Plast Reconstruct Surg 1987; 3:159–78.

286. Ormerod LD, Collin HB, Dohlman CH, et al. Paraproteinemic crystalline keratopathy. Ophthalmology 1988; 95:202–12.
287. Oshika T, Sakurai M, Araie M. A study on diurnal fluctuation of blood-aqueous barrier permeability of plasma proteins. Exp Eye Res 1993; 56:129–33.
288. Ouchi M, West K, Crabb JW, Kinoshita S, et al. Proteomic analysis of vitreous from diabetic macular edema. Exp Eye Res 2005; 81:176–82.
289. Palm E. A case of crystal deposits in the cornea: precipitation of a spontaneously crystallizing plasma globulin. Acta Ophthalmol 1947; 25:165–74.
290. Pandey A, Mann M. Proteomics to study genes and genomes. Nature 2000; 405:837–46.
291. Pang IH, Shade DL, Clark AE, et al. Preliminary characterization of a transformed cell strain derived from human trabecular meshwork. Curr Eye Res 1994; 13:51–63.
292. Panjwani N. Cornea and sclera. In: Harding JJ, ed. Biochemistry of the Eye, 1st ed. London: Chapman & Hall, 1997; 16–51.
293. Papermaster DS, Burstein Y, Schecter I. Opsin mRNA isolation from bovine retina and partial sequence of the in vitro translation product. Ann NY Acad Sci 1980; 343: 347–55.
294. Papermaster DS, Converse CA, Siu J. Membrane biosynthesis in the frog retina: opsin transport in the photoreceptor cell. Biochemistry 1975; 14:1343–52.
295. Papermaster DS, Schneider BG, Zorn MA, Kraehenbuhl JP. Immunocytochemical localization of opsin in outer segments and Golgi zones of frog photoreceptor cells: an electron microscope analysis of cross-linked albumin-embedded retinas. J Cell Biol 1978; 77:196–210.
296. Papermaster DS, Schneider BG, Zorn MA, Kraehenbuhl JP. Immunocytochemical localization of a large intrinsic membrane protein to the incisures and margins of frog rod outer segment disks. J Cell Biol 1978; 78: 415–25.
297. Pappa A, Chen C, Koutalos Y, et al. Aldh3a1 protects human corneal epithelial cells from ultraviolet- and 4-hydroxy-2-nonenal-induced oxidative damage. Free Radic Biol Med 2003; 34:1178–89.
298. Pappa A, Estey T, Manzer R, et al. Human aldehyde dehydrogenase 3A1 (ALDH3A1): biochemical characterization and immunohistochemical localization in the cornea. Biochem J 2003; 376:615–23.
299. Pappin DJ, Hojrup P, Bleasby AJ. Rapid identification of proteins by peptide-mass fingerprinting. Curr Biol 1993; 3:327–32.
300. Paron I, D'Elia A, D'Ambrosio C, et al. A proteomic approach to identify early molecular targets of oxidative stress in human epithelial lens cells. Biochem J 2004; 378: 929–37.
301. Patterson SD, Aebersold R. Mass spectrometric approaches for the identification of gel-separated proteins. Electrophoresis 1995; 16:1791–814.
302. Patton WF. A thousand points of light: the application of fluorescence detection technologies to two-dimensional gel electrophoresis and proteomics. Electrophoresis 2000; 21:1123–44.
303. Pérez-Tamayo R, Rojkind M, eds. Molecular Pathology of Connective Tissues. New York: Marcel Dekker, 1973.
304. Pestova TV, Kolupaeva VG, Lomakin IB, et al. Molecular mechanisms of translation initiation in eukaryotes. Proc Natl Acad Sci U S A 2001; 98:7029–36.
305. Piatigorsky J. Lens differentiation in vertebrates. A review of cellular and molecular features. Differentiation 1981; 19: 134–53.
306. Piatigorsky, J. Gene sharing in lens and cornea: facts and implications. Prog Retin Eye Res 1998; 17:145–74.
307. Pinkerton RMH, Robertson DM. Corneal and conjunctival changes in dysproteinemia. Invest Ophthalmol 1969; 8:357–64.
308. Polans AS, Buczylko J, Crabb J, Palczewski K. A photoreceptor calcium binding protein is recognized by autoantibodies obtained from patients with cancer-associated retinopathy. J Cell Biol 1991; 112:981–9.
309. Pope FM. Autosomal dominant pseudoxanthoma elasticum. J Med Genet 1974; 11:152–7.
310. Pope FM. Historical evidence for the genetic heterogeneity of pseudoxanthoma elasticum. Br J Dermatol 1975; 92: 493–509.
311. Pyreritz RE, McKusick VA. The Marfan syndrome: diagnosis and management. N Engl J Med 1979; 300:772–7.
312. Rabilloud T, Vuillard L, Gilly C, Lawrence JJ. Silver-staining of proteins in polyacrylamide gels: a general overview. Cell Mol Biol (Noisy-le-grand) 1994; 40:57–75.
313. Rada JA, Achen VR, Perry CA, Fox PW. Proteoglycans in the human sclera. Evidence for the presence of aggrecan. Invest Ophthalmol Vis Sci 1997; 38:1740–51.
314. Randall RE, Williamson WC, Mullinax F, Tung MY, Still WJ. Manifestations of systemic light chain deposition. Am J Med 1976; 60:293–9.
315. Reardon AJ, Le Goff M, Briggs MD, et al. Identification in vitreous and molecular cloning of opticin, a novel member of the family of leucine-rich repeat proteins of the extracellular matrix. J Biol Chem 2000; 275:2123–9.
316. Redl B. Human tear lipocalin. Biochim Biophys Acta 2000; 1482:241–8.
317. Reinhart LA, Rountree CB, Wilkin JK. Buschke-Ollendorff syndrome. Cutis 1983; 31:94–6.
318. Ren ZX, Brewton RG, Mayne R. An analysis by rotary shadowing of the structure of the mammalian vitreous and zonular apparatus. J Ultrastruct Biol 1991; 106: 57–63.
319. Rezaie T, Child A, Hitchings R, et al. Adult-onset primary open-angle glaucoma caused by mutations in optineurin. Science 2002; 295:1077–9.
320. Rodrigues M, Ben-Zvi A, Krachmer J, et al. Suprabasal expression of a 64-kilodalton keratin (no.3) in developing human corneal epithelium. Differentiation 1987; 34:60–7.
321. Rodrigues MM, Krachmer JH, Miller SD, Newsome DA. Posterior corneal crystalline deposits in benign monoclonal gammopathy: a clinicopathologic case report. Arch Ophthalmol 1979; 97:124–8.
322. Rohde E, Tomlinson AJ, Johnson DH, Naylor S. Comparison of protein mixtures in aqueous humor by membrane preconcentration–capillary electrophoresis–mass spectrometry. Electrophoresis 1998; 19:2361–70.
323. Roos-Mattjus P, Sistonen L. The ubiquitin-proteasome pathway. Ann Med 2004; 36:285–95.
324. Rosenbloom J. Elastin: relation of protein and gene structure to disease. Lab Invest 1984; 51:605–23.
325. Ross R, Bornstein P. The elastic fiber. I. The separation and partial characterization of its macromolecular components. J Cell Biol 1969; 40:366–81.
326. Ross R, Bornstein P. Studies of the components of the elastic fiber. In: Balazs EA, ed. Chemistry and Molecular Biology of Intercellular Matrix, Vol. 1. New York: Academic Press, 1970; 641–55.
327. Ruoslahti E. Structure and biology of proteoglycans. Ann Rev Cell Biol 1988; 4:229–55.
328. Sakaguchi H, Miyagi M, Shadrach KG, et al. Clusterin is present in drusen in age-related macular degeneration. Exp Eye Res 2002; 74:547–9.

329. Sandberg LB, Hackett TN Jr, Carnes WH. The solubilization of an elastin-like protein from copper deficient porcine aorta. Biochim Biophys Acta 1969; 181:201–7.
330. Sandberg LB, Weissman N, Smith DW. The purification and partial characterization of a soluble elastin-like protein from copper deficient procine aorta. Biochemistry 1969; 8:2940–5.
331. Sandberg-Lall M, Hagg PO, Wahlstrom I, Pihlajaniemi T. Type XIII collagen is widely expressed in the adult and developing human eye and accentuated in the ciliary muscle, the optic nerve and the neural retina. Exp Eye Res 2000; 70:401–10.
332. Sanders TE, Podos S. Pars plana cysts in multiple myeloma. Trans Am Acad Ophthalmol Otolaryng 1966; 70:951–8.
333. Sanders TE, Podos SM, Rosenbaum LJ. Intraocular manifestations of multiple myeloma. Arch Ophthalmol 1967; 77:789–94.
334. Sawaguchi S, Yue BY, Fukuchi T, et al. Age-related changes of sulfated proteoglycans in the human lamina cribrosa. Curr Eye Res 1993; 12:685–92.
335. Sawhney RS. Immunological identification of types I and III collagen in bovine lens epithelium and its anterior lens capsule. Cell Biol Int 2005; 29:133–7.
336. Schesinger MJ. Heat shock proteins: the search for function. J Cell Biol 1986; 103:321–5.
337. Schneider RG. Incidence of hemoglobin C trait in 505 normal negroes: a family with homozygous hemoglobin C and sickle-cell trait union. J Lab Clin Med 1954; 44: 133–44.
338. Schultz DW, Klein ML, Humpert AJ, et al. Analysis of the ARMD1 locus: evidence that a mutation in HEMICENTIN-1 is associated with age-related macular degeneration in a large family. Hum Mol Genet 2003; 12: 3315–23.
339. Schürch W, Skalli O, Lagace R, et al. Intermediate filament proteins and actin isoforms as markers for soft tissue tumor differentiation and origin. III. Hemangio pericytomas and glomus tumors. Am J Pathol 1990; 136: 771–86.
340. Schürch W, Skalli O, Seemayer TA, Gabbiani G. Intermediate filament proteins and actin isoforms as markers for soft tissue tumor differentiation and origin. I. Smooth muscle tumors. Am J Pathol 1987; 128:91–103.
341. Schuster V, Seidenspinner S, Zeitler P, et al, Compound-heterozygous mutations in the plasminogen gene predispose to the development of ligneous conjunctivitis. Blood 1999; 93:3457–66.
342. Schutt F, Bergmann M, Holz FG, Kopitz J. Proteins modified by malondialdehyde, 4-hydroxynonenal, or advanced glycation end products in lipofuscin of human retinal pigment epithelium. Invest Ophthalmol Vis Sci 2003; 44:3663–8.
343. Schutt F, Ueberle B, Schnolzer M, et al. Proteome analysis of lipofuscin in human retinal pigment epithelial cells. FEBS Lett 2002; 528:217–21.
344. Searle BC, Dasari S, Wilmarth PA, et al. Identification of protein modifications using MS/MS de novo sequencing and the OpenSea alignment algorithm. J Proteome Res 2005; 4:546–54.
345. Semina EV, Brownell I, Mintz-Hittner HA, Murray JC, Mutations in the human forkhead transcription factor FOXE3 associated with anterior segment ocular dysgenesis and cataracts. Hum Mol Genet 2001; 10:231–6.
346. Shevchenko A, Wilm M, Vorm O, Mann M. Mass spectrometric sequencing of proteins silver-stained polyacrylamide gels. Anal Chem 1996; 68:850–8.
347. Shimmura S, Miyashita H, Higa K, et al. Proteomic analysis of soluble factors secreted by limbal fibroblasts. Mol Vis 2006; 12:478–84.
348. Silverman B, Alexander RJ, Henley WL. Tissue and species specificity of BCP 54, the major soluble protein of the bovine cornea. Exp Eye Res 1981; 33:19–29.
349. Singh VK, Nussenblatt RB, Donoso LA, et al. Identification of a uveitopathogenic and lymphocyte proliferation site in bovine S-antigen. Cell Immunol 1988; 115:413–9.
350. Singh VK, Yamaki K, Donoso LA, Shinohara T. S-antigen: experimental autoimmune uveitis induced in guinea pigs with two synthetic peptides. Curr Eye Res 1988; 7:87–92.
351. Siuzdak G. Mass Spectrometry for Biotechnology. San Diego, CA: Academic Press, 1996; 1–161.
352. Skonier J, Neubauer M, Madisen L, et al. cDNA cloning and sequence analysis of beta ig-h3, a novel gene induced in a human adenocarcinoma cell line after treatment with transforming growth factor-beta. DNA Cell Biol 1992; 11: 511–22.
353. Slansky HH, Bronstein M, Gartner S. Ciliary body cysts in multiple myeloma: their relation to urethane, hyperproteinemia, and duration of the disease. Arch Ophthalmol 1966; 76:686–9.
354. Spector A, Wang GM, Wang RR, et al. The prevention of cataract caused by oxidative stress in cultured rat lenses. I. H_2O_2 and photochemically induced cataract. Curr Eye Res 1993; 12:163–79.
355. Spiegel P, Grossniklaus HE, Reinhart WJ, Thomas RH. Unusual presentation of paraproteinemic corneal infiltrates. Cornea 1990; 9:81–5.
356. Steely HT Jr, Clark AF. The use of proteomics in ophthalmic research. Pharmacogenomics 2000; 1:267–80.
357. Steely HT, Dillow GW, Bian L, et al. Protein expression in a transformed trabecular meshwork cell line: proteome analysis. Mol Vis 2006; 12:372–83.
358. Steely HT Jr, English-Wright SL, Clark AF. The similarity of protein expression in trabecular meshwork and lamina cribrosa: implications for glaucoma. Exp Eye Res 2000; 70: 17–30.
359. Steinberg TH, Jones LJ, Haugland RP, Singer VL. SYPRO orange and SYPRO red protein gel stains: one-step fluorescent staining of denaturing gels for detection of nanogram levels of protein. Anal Biochem 1996; 239: 223–37.
360. Steuhl K-P, Knorr M, Rohrbach JM, et al. Paraproteinemic corneal deposits in plasma cell myeloma. Am J Ophthalmol 1991; 111:312–8.
361. Stirling JW, Henderson DW, Rozenbilds MA, et al. Crystalloidal paraprotein deposits in the cornea: an ultrastructural study of two new cases with tubular crystalloids that contain IgG kappa light chains and IgG gamma heavy chains. Ultrastruct Pathol 1997; 21:337–44.
362. Stoebner P, Renversez JC, Groulade J, et al. Ultrastructural study of human IgG and IgG–IgM crystalcryoglobulins. Am J Clin Pathol 1979; 71:404–10.
363. Stone EM, Braun TA, Russell SR, et al. Missense variations in the fibulin 5 gene and age-related macular degeneration. N Engl J Med 2004; 351:346–53.
364. Stone EM, Fingert JH, Alward WL, et al. Identification of a gene that causes primary open angle glaucoma. Science 1997; 275:668–70.
365. Subjeck JR, Shyy T-T. Stress protein systems of mammalian cells. Am J Physiol 1986; 250:C1–17.
366. Sun XL, Zheng BH, Li B, et al. Orbital rhabdomyosarcoma: immunohistochemical studies of seven cases. Chin Med J Peking 1990; 103:485–8.

367. Switzer RC III, Merril CR, Shifrin S. A highly sensitive silver stain for detecting proteins and peptides in polyacrylamide gels. Anal Biochem 1979; 98:231–7.
368. Tezel G, Yang X, Cai J. Proteomic identification of oxidatively modified retinal proteins in a chronic pressure-induced rat model of glaucoma. Invest Ophthalmol Vis Sci 2005; 46:3177–87.
369. Thompson LJ, Wang F, Proia AD, et al. Proteome analysis of the rat cornea during angiogenesis. Proteomics 2003; 3: 2258–66.
370. Tohyama T, Lee VM, Rorke LB, et al. Nestin expression in embryonic human neuroepithelium and in human neuroepithelial tumor cells. Lab Invest 1992; 66:303–13.
371. Tölle H-G, Weber K, Osborn M. Microinjection of monoclonal antibodies specific for one intermediate filament protein in cells containing multiple keratins allow insight into the composition of particular 10 nm filaments. Eur J Cell Biol 1985; 38:234–44.
372. Tomokane K, Iwaki T, Tateishi J, et al. Rosenthal fibers share epitopes with αB crystallin, glial fibrillary acidic protein, and ubiquitin, but not vimentin: immunoelectron microscropy with colloidal gold. Am J Pathol 1991; 138: 875–85.
373. Tomosugi N, Kitagawa K, Takahashi N, et al. Diagnostic potential of tear proteomic patterns in Sjögren's syndrome. J Proteome Res 2005; 4:820–5.
374. Tonge R, Shaw J, Middleton B, et al. Validation and development of fluorescence two-dimensional differential gel electrophoresis proteomics technology. Proteomics 2001; 1:377–96.
375. Touchette N. Recoverin illuminates mechanisms of visual adaptation. J NIH Res 1991; 3:58–64.
376. Travis GH, Sutcliffe JG, Bok D. The retinal degeneration slow (rds) gene product is a photoreceptor disc membrane-associated glycoprotein. Neuron 1991; 6:61–70.
377. Truscott RJ. Age-related nuclear cataract-oxidation is the key. Exp Eye Res 2005; 80:709–25.
378. Tsai PS, Evans JE, Green KM, et al. Proteomic analysis of human meibomian gland secretions. Br J Ophthalmol 2006; 90:372–7.
379. Tsuda M, Syed M, Bugra K, et al. Structural analysis of mouse S-antigen. Gene 1988; 73:11–20.
380. Tsur D, Tanner S, Zandi E, et al. Identification of post-translational modifications by blind search of mass spectra. Nat Biotechnol 2005; 23:1562–7.
381. Ueda Y, Duncan MK, David LL. Lens proteomics: the accumulation of crystallin modifications in the mouse lens with age. Invest Ophthalmol Vis Sci 2002; 43:205–15.
382. Unlu M, Morgan ME, Minden JS. Difference gel electrophoresis: a single gel method for detecting changes in protein extracts. Electrophoresis 1997; 18:2071–7.
383. Unsworth DJ, Scott DL, Almond TJ, et al. Studies on reticulin I: serological and immunohistological investigation of the occurrence of collagen type III, fibronectin and the non-collagenous glycoprotein of PRAS and GLYNN in reticulin. Br J Exp Pathol 1982; 63:154–66.
384. van der Gaag R, Broersma L, Rothova A, et al. Immunity to a corneal antigen in Fuchs' heterochromic cyclitis patients. Invest Ophthalmol Vis Sci 1989; 30:443–8.
385. Venter JC, Adams MD, Myers EW, et al. The sequence of the human genome. Science 2001; 291:1304–51.
386. Verhagen C, Hoekzema R, Verjans GM, Kijlstra A. Identification of bovine corneal protein 54 (BCP 54) as an aldehyde dehydrogenase. Exp Eye Res 1991; 53:283–4.
387. Viljoen DL, Pope FM, Beighton P. Heterogeneity of pseudoxanthoma elasticum: delineation of a new form? Clin Genet 1987; 32:100–5.
388. Vithana EN, Abu-Safieh L, Allen MJ, et al. A human homolog of yeast pre-mRNA splicing gene, PRP31, underlies autosomal dominant retinitis pigmentosa on chromosome 19q13.4 (RP11). Mol Cell 2001; 8:375–81.
389. Wachtel JG. The ocular pathology of Marfan's syndrome: including a clinico-pathological correlation and an explanation of ectopia lentis. Arch Ophthalmol 1966; 76: 512–22.
390. Waldenström J. Incipient myelomatosis or 'essential' hyperglobulinemia with fibrinogenopenia—a new syndrome? Acta Med Scand 1944; 117:216–47.
391. Wallace IM, Blackshields G, Higgins DG. Multiple sequence alignments. Curr Opin Struct Biol 2005; 15:261–6.
392. Walsh CT, Garneau-Tsodikova S, Gatto GJ Jr. Protein posttranslational modifications: the chemistry of proteome diversifications. Angew Chem Int Ed Engl 2005; 44:7342–72.
393. Wang-Su ST, McCormack AL, Yang S, et al. Proteome analysis of lens epithelia, fibers, and the HLE B-3 cell line. Invest Ophthalmol Vis Sci 2003; 44:4829–36.
394. Warburton S, Southwick K, Hardman RM, et al. Examining the proteins of functional retinal lipofuscin using proteomic analysis as a guide for understanding its origin. Mol Vis 2005; 11:1122–34.
395. Waring GO, Font RL, Rodrigues MM, Mulberger RD. Alterations of Descemet's membrane in intersitial keratitis. Am J Ophthalmol 1976; 81:773–85.
396. Washburn MP, Wolters D, Yates JR III. Large-scale analysis of the yeast proteome by multidimensional protein identification technology. Nat Biotechnol 2001; 19: 242–7.
397. Wasinger VC, Cordwell SJ, Cerpa-Poljak A, et al. Progress with gene-product mapping of the Mollicutes: *Mycoplasma genitalium*. Electrophoresis 1995; 16:1090–4.
398. Wessel H, Anderson S, Fite D, et al. Type XII collagen contributes to diversities in human corneal and limbal extracellular matrices. Invest Ophthalmol Vis Sci 1997; 38: 2408–22.
399. West KA, Yan L, Miyagi M, et al. Proteome survey of proliferating and differentiating rat RPE-J cells. Exp Eye Res 2001; 73:479–91.
400. West KA, Yan L, Shadrach K, Sun J, et al. Protein database, human retinal pigment epithelium. Mol Cell Proteomics 2003; 2:37–49.
401. White J, Werkmeister JA, Ramshaw JA, Birk DE. Organization of fibrillar collagen in the human and bovine cornea: collagen types V and III. Connect Tissue Res 1997; 36:165–74.
402. Whitt JW, Wood BC, Sharma JN, Crouch TT. Adult polycystic kidney disease and lattice corneal dystrophy: occurrence in a single family. Arch Intern Med 1978; 138: 1167–8.
403. Wilkins MR, Pasquali C, Appel RD, et al. From proteins to proteomes: large scale protein identification by two-dimensional electrophoresis and amino acid analysis. Biotechnology (NY) 1996; 14:61–5.
404. Williams KL, Hochstrasser DF. Introduction to the proteome. In: Wilkins MR, Williams KL, Appel RD, Hochstrasser DF, eds., Proteome Research: New Frontiers in Functional Genomics, 1st ed. Berlin Heidelberg: Springer Verlag, 1997;1–12.
405. Wilm M, Shevchenko A, Houthaeve T, et al. Femtomole sequencing of proteins from polyacrylamide gels by nano-electrospray mass spectrometry. Nature 1996; 379: 466–9.
406. Wilmarth PA, Tanner S, Dasari S, et al. Age-related changes in human crystallins determined from

comparative analysis of post-translational modifications in young and aged lens: does deamidation contribute to crystallin insolubility? J Proteome Res 2006; 5:2554–66.
407. Wilmarth PA, Taube JR, Riviere MA, et al. Proteomic and sequence analysis of chicken lens crystallins reveals alternate splicing and translational forms of beta B2 and beta A2 crystallins. Invest Ophthalmol Vis Sci 2004; 45: 2705–15.
408. Wistow G. Evolution of a protein superfamily: relationships between vertebrate lens crystallins and microrganism dormancy proteins. J Mol Evol 1990; 30:140–5.
409. Wistow GJ, Piatigorsky J. Lens crystallins: the evolution and expression of proteins for a highly specialized tissue. Annu Rev Biochem. 57:479–504, 1988.
410. Wolters DA, Washburn MP, Yates JR III. An automated multidimensional protein identification technology for shotgun proteomics. Anal Chem 2001; 73:5683–90.
411. Wright D, Mayne R. Vitreous humor of chicken contains two fibrillar systems: an analysis of their structure. J Ultrastruct Mol Struct Res 1988; 100:224–34.
412. Wu CC, Yates JR III. The application of mass spectrometry to membrane proteomics. Nat Biotechnol 2003; 21:262–7.
413. Xu ZP, Wawrousek EF, Piatigorsky J. Transketolase haploinsufficiency reduces adipose tissue and female fertility in mice. Mol Cell Biol 2002; 22:6142–7.
414. Yamaguchi K, Yamaguchi K, Sheedlo HJ, Turner JE. Expression of heat shock protein in the atrophic corneal epithelium of the royal college of surgeon dystrophic rat. Cornea 1991; 10:161–5.
415. Yamane K, Minamoto A, Yamashita H, et al. Proteome analysis of human vitreous proteins. Mol Cell Proteomics 2003; 2:1177–87.
416. Yan JX, Harry RA, Spibey C, Dunn MJ. Postelectrophoretic staining of proteins separated by two-dimensional gel electrophoresis using SYPRO dyes. Electrophoresis 2000; 21:3657–65.
417. Yassa NH, Font RL, Fine BS, Koffler BH. Corneal immunoglobulin deposition in the posterior stroma: a case report including immunohistochemical and ultrastructural observations. Arch Ophthalmol 1987; 105: 99–103.
418. Young TL, Scavello GS, Paluru PC, et al. Microarray analysis of gene expression in human donor sclera. Mol Vis 2004; 10:163–76.
419. Yue BY. The extracellular matrix and its modulation in the trabecular meshwork. Surv Ophthalmol 1996; 40:379–90.
420. Yun AJ, Murphy CG, Polansky JR, et al. Proteins secreted by human trabecular cells. Glucocorticoid and other effects. Invest Ophthalmol Vis Sci 1989; 30:2012–22.
421. Zhao X, Ramsey KE, Stephan DA, Russell P. Gene and protein expression changes in human trabecular meshwork cells treated with transforming growth factor-beta. Invest Ophthalmol Vis Sci 2004; 45:4023–4.
422. Zhou L, Beuerman RW, Barathi A, Tan D. Analysis of rabbit tear proteins by high-pressure liquid chromatography/electrospray ionization mass spectrometry. Rapid Commun Mass Spectrom 2003; 17:401–12.
423. Zhou L, Beuerman RW, Foo Y, et al. Characterisation of human tear proteins using high-resolution mass spectrometry. Ann Acad Med Singapore 2006; 35:400–7.
424. Zhou L, Zhang SR, Yue BY. Adhesion of human trabecular meshwork cells to extracellular matrix proteins. Roles and distribution of integrin receptors. Invest Ophthalmol Vis Sci 1996; 37:104–13.
425. Zhou LX, Liu JHK. Circadian variation of mouse aqueous humor protein. Mol Vis 2006; 12:639–43.
426. Zinn K, McAllister L, Goodman CS. Sequence analysis and neuronal expression of fasciclin I in grasshopper and *Drosophila*. Cell 1988; 53:577–87.
427. Zuidervaart W, Hensbergen PJ, Wong MC, et al. Proteomic analysis of uveal melanoma reveals novel potential markers involved in tumor progression. Invest Ophthalmol Vis Sci 2006; 47:786–93.
428. Zuidervaart W, van der Velden PA, Hurks, MH, et al. Gene expression profiling identifies tumour markers potentially playing a role in uveal melanoma development. Br J Cancer 2003; 89:1914–9.

APPENDIX

PROTEIN SEPARATION AND IDENTIFICATION

Two-Dimensional Gel Electrophoresis

The global analysis of the proteins expressed in a system has been challenging. Improvements in the technique of 2D PAGE (47) mean that it is now a cardinal method in proteome analysis (133,153,232). 2D PAGE has the capacity to separate proteins by two characteristics; charge and molecular mass (M_r). The charged amino acid residues confer a specific protein with an overall charge and thus an isoelectric point (pI), the pH value where the net-charge of the protein is zero. Thus, in the first dimension of 2D PAGE the proteins are separated by isoelectric focusing (IEF) according to their charge in an immobilized pH gradient applied with an electric field. In the second dimension the proteins are separated by size using sodium dodecyl sulphate–polyacrylamide gel electrophoresis (SDS–PAGE). Due to the high separation capacity 2D PAGE can resolve protein isoforms generated by post-translational additions or proteolytic processing. Thus, the same protein may be identified in two or more different spots in the gel due to the addition of a charged modification (alteration of the pI in the first dimension) or by protein cleavage resulting in a reduced molecular mass (fast migration in the second dimension). However, not all proteins in a complex mixture can be separated by classical 2D PAGE. Thus, proteins with abnormal pI values and insoluble proteins such as membrane proteins containing hydrophobic transmembrane domains are not resolved in the pH gradients of the first dimension. In addition, very small and large proteins are not resolved in the second dimension. Thus, analysis and characterization of these proteins require other techniques such as traditional 1D SDS–PAGE, chromatographic methods, and LC-MS/MS (see Appendix section, Electrospray Ionization Liquid Chromatography Tandem Mass Spectrometry).

Differences detected in protein maps derived from 2D PAGE of diverse proteomes frequently uncover differences in protein expression furthering knowledge about biological changes at the protein level. Due to the complexity of the topic, the analysis and comparison of protein expression profiles require sophisticated methods and computer programs. The technique termed 2D difference gel electrophoresis (2D DIGE) allows multiple samples to be co-separated and visualized on one 2D gel with high sensitivity and accurate quantification (382) (see Appendix section, Protein Visualization).

Protein Visualization

Colorimetric Protein Staining

Proteins separated by 1D or 2D PAGE are often visualized by colorimetric staining with dyes having an electrostatic affinity for proteins. The Coomassie brilliant blue dyes are normally used in staining procedures giving low background staining and higher sensitivity (274). The procedure is simple to use and has a protein detection limit of about 10–50 ng. Furthermore, Coomassie brilliant blue staining has a linear dynamic range extending over three orders of magnitude, which makes it useful for quantitative protein studies (275,302). Since Coomassie brilliant blue staining does not modify the proteins it is compatible with subsequent protein identification by amino-terminal protein sequencing or mass spectrometry (see Appendix section, Protein Identification).

Protein Silver Staining

Another common method for visualization of electrophoretically separated proteins is silver staining in which Ag^+ is first bound to the proteins and then reduced to metallic silver ($Ag_{(s)}$) by which the proteins are colored brown (Fig. 1) (192,312). Silver staining methods are at least 10 times more sensitive than Coomassie brilliant blue staining and therefore the method of choice when low amounts of protein (1–10 ng) have to be detected on electrophoresis gels (155,367). Silver staining techniques are, however, more complex to use and are not universally applicable. They only have a narrow linear dynamic range within two orders of magnitude, which makes it less suitable for quantification and comparison of protein levels in different samples. Classical protein silver staining methods are not suitable for amino-terminal protein sequencing and mass spectrometry-based protein identification as they contain compounds (glutaraldehyde and formaldehyde) that chemically modify the proteins and procedures that inhibit trypsin, the protease normally used for in-gel digestion (see Appendix section, Mass Spectrometry-Based Protein Identification). However, improved silver staining protocols compatible for mass spectrometry are available (125,346).

Fluorescent Protein Staining

Fluorescent detection of proteins in 1D and 2D gels has several advantages over colorimetric and silver staining including a greater sensitivity and broader linear dynamic range. The different fluorophores available for protein detection are either bound non-covalently or covalently to the proteins and either before or after the electrophoretic separation. Thus, one group of fluorescent dyes [e.g., the SYPRO™ dyes Red, Orange, and Tangerine, 8-anilino-l-naphthalene-sulfonate (ANS), and Nile Red] become fluorescent upon non-covalent binding with SDS-protein complexes and are therefore used for the detection of proteins after SDS–PAGE (359,416). Other fluorescent dyes (SYPRO™ Ruby and SYPRO™ Rose) with electrostatic affinity for proteins are termed "luminescent transition metal chelate dyes" (34,190). In general, these fluorophores have protein detection sensitivities between 0.2 and 10 ng, high linear dynamic ranges (three orders of magnitude), and are compatible with mass spectrometry identification techniques, which make them suitable for quantitative proteomic studies (222,243,302).

Different fluorophores [e.g., monobromobimane, 2-methoxy-2,4-diphenyl-3(2H)-furanone (MDPF), cyanine dyes] are available for covalent derivatization of cysteine residues and primary amines (N-terminus and lysine residues) of proteins prior to SDS–PAGE (302). The fluorescent cyanine dyes Cy2, Cy3, and Cy5 (CyDye DIGE Fluors GE Healthcare Life Science) label lysine residues and have been optimized for detection of differential expressed proteins using 2D DIGE and with a linear dynamic range of three to five orders of magnitude (382). By pre-labeling two different proteome preparations (e.g., healthy and diseased) with two distinct CyDye DIGE Fluors and analyzing them simultaneously on the same 2D gel together with an internal standard (reference sample) (6) labeled with the third fluor, no gel-to-gel variation is obtained and the relative abundance of the individual proteins can be determined with high accuracy in all samples (105,247). The most established 2D DIGE procedure uses minimal labeling of the proteins in which only about 3% of the lysine residues are labeled. The sensitivity of the minimal labeling 2D DIGE technique is about 0.1 ng, thus more than 10 times more sensitive than silver staining. In addition, the minimal labeling ensures that most of the proteins are not covalently modified which makes the technique compatible with subsequent Edman degradation or mass spectrometry analysis (374) (see Appendix section, Protein Identification).

Visualization of protein in gels can also be performed with other methods such as zymographic assays and radiolabeling.

Protein Identification

Comparison of proteomes derived from normal and diseased cells/tissues/organs followed by identification of differentially expressed proteins may provide new insights to disease mechanisms and thus new avenues for therapeutic intervention. Thus, it is essential to determine identities of the proteins of interest. Proteins differ in size (molecular mass), amino acid sequence, electric charge, hydrophobicity, and tertiary structure. Hence, most proteins are indistinguishable using traditional histochemical dyes that only demonstrate functional groups in amino acids. For example, eosin is an acid dye that effectively binds positively charged arginine, histidine, and lysine residues, which are shared by many different proteins. Furthermore, immunohistochemical and immunocytochemical methods where specific proteins can be stained suffer from the inherent weakness that antibodies may react with portions of molecules that are basically dissimilar, which is known as cross-reactivity or non-specific binding. Thus, the limitations of the numerous histochemical techniques are the identification of novel proteins, low specificity, and risk of false-positives. These indirect methods of protein identification, which are dependent on molecular recognition and binding of the dyes/reporters, are therefore less reliable than direct methods such as enzymatic activity assays, amino acid sequencing, and mass spectrometry. Enzyme histochemistry and zymography are useful techniques for directly detecting specific enzyme activities within a tissue section (e.g., staining for ATPase or acid phosphatase activities) or electrophoretic gel (e.g., proteases or lipases), respectively. However, identification of an enzyme by measuring enzymatic activity requires that the reaction is specifically catalyzed by only that enzyme. Thus, these techniques do not distinguish between isoenzymes (also known as isozymes).

Amino-terminal Protein Sequencing by Edman Degradation

Edman degradation is a chemical method for determining the amino acid sequence from the amino-terminus of proteins (or peptides) (92). After the protein has been purified by electrophoresis or liquid chromatography (13), the amino-terminal residue of the protein is coupled with phenylisothiocyanate (PITC) under alkaline conditions to form a phenylthiocarbamoyl (PTC) derivative that subsequently can be cleaved under acidic conditions. The released thiazolinone amino acid is then converted to a more stable derivative [phenylthiohydantoin (PTH)-amino acid]. The amino acid derivative is then analyzed by liquid chromatography to determine its identity. Thus, by repeating this procedure several times the sequence from the amino-terminal of the protein/peptide can be determined. By using an advanced automated protein sequencer (93) based on solid phase Edman chemistry (224) and with the latest technology, as little as 5 pmol of protein (nanogram level) can be sequenced. However, the Edman degradation reaction is not completely efficient and, therefore, no more than about 50 residues can be sequenced. Normally, this is normally more than enough to identify the protein by a computer-assisted database search. However, if the amino-terminus is blocked by a PTM, the Edman chemistry is not usable. Likewise, glycosylated and phosphorylated amino acids may result in blank cycles.

Mass Spectrometry-Based Protein Identification

Due to technical advances mass spectrometry has essentially replaced Edman degradation for protein identification and primary structure characterization (5,351) including analyses of PTMs (245). Different types of mass spectrometers have been developed for protein analysis but there are basically two approaches to determine protein identify (5,85). The proteins or peptides are volatilized and ionized either by MALDI or electrospray ionization (ESI). After the ionized molecules have entered the gas phase and introduced into the mass spectrometer their mass-to-charge ratio (m/z where m is the mass and z is the charge) is measured with high accuracy. Using the identified masses to search databases several hundred proteins can be identified from 1D and 2D gels (301) or even from non-separated complex protein mixtures.

Mass spectrometry-based protein identification and characterization is much faster and more sensitive than Edman degradation. Thus, ESI-MS offers reliable sensitivity and MS/MS sequencing of a few femtomoles (picogram) (4,405).

MALDI-TOF MS and Peptide Mass Fingerprinting

Intact proteins separated by electrophoresis (1D or 2D PAGE) or chromatographic techniques (ion-exchange, reverse phase, gel-filtration, or affinity) (see Appendix section, Purification of Proteins and Peptides) are often easily identified by "peptide mass fingerprinting" using MALDI-TOF MS. In this method the protein of interest is digested with a specific protease (e.g., trypsin which cleaves exclusively at the carboxyl side of arginine and lysine residues) and the accurate masses (m/z ratio) of the resulting peptides are then determined by MALDI-TOF MS (152,244,299). Before being subjected to enzymatic digestion the protein must be reduced to break potential disulfide bridges. Since it is difficult to extract intact proteins from the polyacrylamide gel, individual proteins from excised 1D or 2D gel spots are in-gel digested. The generated peptides are usually small enough (<3 kDa) to diffuse out of the gel from where they are collected for MALDI-TOF MS analysis. The isolated peptides are then mixed with a MALDI matrix (e.g., α-cyano-4-hydroxycinnamic acid) and spotted onto a solid MALDI target plate where the peptides co-crystallize with the matrix. By firing a pulsed laser onto the sample the peptides volatize and become ionized by the addition of a proton to generate positive single-charged peptides, which can be analyzed in the mass spectrometer. The list of experimentally determined peptide masses, the "peptide mass fingerprint" of the protein, is then subjected to database searches and compared to the theoretical peptide masses generated in silico from each of all the genes in the human genome. The accurate masses of a few peptides (<5) from a protein normally provide sufficient information for successful identification.

Peptide mass fingerprinting is a rapid protein identification method but requires that the proteins have been separated and purified. Thus, only a single or a few different proteins must be present in the sample which makes the technique powerful in combination with 1D and 2D PAGE, where each band and spot represents individual proteins. However, contamination of the sample with environmental keratin can be a major problem. Proteins with low molecular mass give rise to fewer peptides and, therefore, are in general more difficult to identify than larger proteins.

Electrospray Ionization Liquid Chromatography Tandem Mass Spectrometry

Individual proteins can also be identified by the technique ESI-LC-MS/MS where the peptides in solution are separated by reverse phase liquid chromatography before being introduced directly into the mass spectrometer. At the end of the reverse phase column the peptides become protonated and are transferred into the gas phase by electrospray ionization to generate positive multiple-charged peptides (+1, +2, +3, etc.). In the mass spectrometer the masses (m/z ratio) of the peptides are determined and subsequently, the individual peptides are selected and fragmented (in the peptide bond) into smaller peptides to generate a fragmentation spectrum. The complete collection of determined peptide masses and fragment mass data is subjected to database searches and the peptides (the protein) are identified based on a so-called "sequence tag," which is a short string of consecutive amino acid residues that are recognized based on mass differences in the fragmentation spectrum. Normally, MS/MS analysis of a single peptide is sufficient to identify a protein, which makes ESI-LC-MS/MS a highly efficient method in proteomics. Since MS/MS data in contrast to peptide mass fingerprinting bear sequence information of individual peptides, multiple proteins can be identified by ESI-LC-MS/MS in an unpurified sample.

The design of "high performance" mass spectrometers has enabled the development of "shotgun" techniques to identify a large number of proteins in complex proteins mixtures with high detection efficiency and sensitivity. Thus, "Multidimensional Protein Identification Technology" (MudPIT) is a high-throughput proteomic approach to identify proteins from very complex mixtures such as cell or tissue extracts without separating the intact proteins prior to the MS analysis. The crude protein extract is immediately digested with a specific protease such as trypsin and the peptide mixture is separated by multidimensional liquid chromatography (e.g., strong cation exchange followed by reversed phase chromatography). The peptides are progressively eluted into the mass spectrometer and identified by MS/MS (233,396,410). Since MudPIT does not involve a separation of intact proteins it facilitate the identification of insoluble membrane bound proteins (412) and insoluble structural proteins in connective tissues such as the cornea (183,185). In this approach the insoluble proteins are first converted into soluble peptides by chemical digestion using e.g., cyanogen bromide making them suitable for analysis by mass spectrometry. In addition, proteins too large/small or too acidic/basic to be separated by traditional 2D PAGE can be identified by this technique.

Because the amount of data generated by LC-MS/MS and MudPIT analysis is enormous, this protein identification method requires advanced software programs for the database searches. Thus, bioinformatics is an essential part of mass spectrometry-based proteomics.

CHROMATOGRAPHIC PURIFICATION OF PROTEINS AND PEPTIDES

Different chromatographic techniques are used for the purification of native proteins. By ion-exchange liquid chromatography, the proteins are separated according to their charge distribution. Thus, negatively charged proteins will bind to a column of positively charged beads (anion exchange chromatography), while positively charged proteins will bind to negatively charged beads (cation exchange chromatography). The bound proteins can then be eluted and separated by increasing the concentration of a salt. The charged salt ions will compete with the protein for the binding to the column. The native proteins can also be separated according to their size by gel filtration chromatography. In a column containing porous beads, larger proteins will move mainly in the solution between the beads while smaller proteins can enter the beads. Thus, larger molecules have a shorter path through the column and will elute earlier. Affinity chromatography utilizes the affinity of some proteins for other molecules (e.g. glucose, antibodies, divalent cations). After the protein(s) with an affinity to the immobilized molecules on the column have bound, the unbound proteins are washed away with a buffer and the desired protein(s) can be eluted by adding the ligand-molecule in a solute form to the column. Alternatively, the interaction with the protein can be disrupted by changing the pH or salt concentration. Reverse phase chromatography is mostly used for the purification of peptides. The peptides are dissolved in water and applied to a column containing beads with hydrophobic chemical groups. The most hydrophobic peptides bind strongest to the column. By increasing the concentration of an organic solution the peptides can be separated and eluted.

37

Amyloidoses

Gordon K. Klintworth
Departments of Pathology and Ophthalmology, Duke University, Durham, North Carolina, U.S.A.

INTRODUCTION

The amyloidoses are a heterogeneous group of protein misfolding disorders that share common attributes. They all have extracellular eosinophilic deposits that stain with Congo red imparting a unique green birefringence and dichroism in such stained preparations when viewed in a polarizing microscope (160). This is in contrast to elastic tissue and some other components of connective tissue that also have an affinity for Congo red. Amyloid also stains metachromatically with certain triphenylmethane (crystal violet) and thiazine dyes (toluidine blue), most consistently when fresh unfixed tissue is examined. Amyloid is often autofluorescent or exhibits fluorescence after staining with thioflavin-T or thioflavin-S. In tissue, all types of amyloid appear by transmission electron microscopy (TEM) as fine nonbranching fibrils (approximately 10 nm in diameter) organized in random array. The diameter of isolated amyloid fibrils (7–7.5 nm) is thinner than those in tissue sections and a subunit of about 3.5 nm has also been identified.

PROTEIN CONFORMATIONAL DISORDERS

Cells synthesize numerous proteins and many normally fold to perform their function before eventually becoming degraded by the proteasome (see Chapter 36) (56). Glycosylation and deglycosylation reactions enable correctly folded proteins to be distinguished from misfolded proteins (148). In an increasing number of diseases known as protein conformational diseases certain proteins become misfolded and escape cellular surveillance and degradation by proteolytic enzymes (37,148,202). Specific proteins in these proteopathies escape proteolysis and this leads to the accumulation over time of these proteins because of aggregation, cross-linking, or posttranslational modifications. The misfolded proteins self-associate and form intracellular or extracellular protein aggregates by at least one of three mechanisms: cross-β spine, end-to-end stacking, and three-dimensional (3D) domain swapping (9). The cross-β spine mechanism accounts for the cross-β diffraction pattern of amyloid deposits.

The protein deposition diseases can be divided into the amyloidoses in which amyloid accumulates and those in which the deposits lack the attributes of amyloid. In some diseases, such as sickle cell anemia (hemoglobin S) (see Chapter 36), Huntington disease (huntingtin in the Huntington bodies), Parkinson disease (α-synuclein in the Lewy bodies) and Alzheimer disease (tau in the neurofibrillary tangles) (see Chapter 70), the protein accumulation is intracellular in contrast to amyloid, which is extracellular. Misfolded proteins known as prions are implicated in the spongiform encephalopathies [Creutzfelt–Jakob disease and its variants, kuru, Gerstmann–Sträussler–Scheinker disease, fatal familial insomnia, scrapie, and bovine spongiform encephalopathy ("mad cow disease")] (see Chapter 70) and they possess the remarkable property of being infectious.

AMYLOID

Historical Remarks

Rokitansky (169) is usually credited with the first description of what is currently known as amyloid, but he did not use the term and included the disease under the designation lardaceous disease. The word amyloid was created in 1839 from the Greek (*αμυλον*) and Latin (*amylum*) words for starch (223) and became used in botany. In 1854, Virchow (222) coined the word amyloid for the corpora amylacea in brain because they develop a violet hue after treatment with iodine and sulfuric acid as in starch (27). However, corpora amylacea, notwithstanding their high carbohydrate content, have no relationship to what is currently designated amyloid. Amyloid despite the origin of the word is largely protein and not predominantly carbohydrate in composition (27), but it contains glycosaminoglycans (GAGs).

Initially amyloid was a subject for pathologists and then also for physicians involved in its clinical diagnosis and treatment. Later biochemists, biophysicists, and molecular geneticists began unraveling the mysteries of amyloid and the amyloidoses yielding a considerable body of information about the subject. It has gradually become evident that the amyloidoses are disorders of protein misfolding, aggregation, and deposition. Indeed the journal *Amyloid* considers itself a journal of protein folding disorders. Several reviews provide additional information on the history of amyloid (112,120,187).

Nomenclature

Initially, the terminology of amyloid proteins was confusing because of the lack of a standardized nomenclature. A system for naming amyloid fibril proteins and related serum components recommended by an international committee has clarified the situation immensely (83,228). When possible the amyloid should be classified by the fibril protein that has been characterized by amino acid sequencing. The term protein precursor refers to the protein from which the amyloid fibril is believed to arise. For amyloid proteins derived from immunoglobulin the immunoglobulin chain nomenclature is used. In situations where new inadequately characterized amyloid proteins are detected in tissue the prefix A is followed by a provisional term to identify the particular protein. The Nomenclature Committee of the International Society for Amyloidosis has established a list of acceptable amyloid proteins and of their precursors (Table 1) (228). The term "amylog" has been suggested in preference to amyloid for fibrils that are created, sometimes after harsh nonphysiologic conditions, from synthetic peptides with properties of amyloid (21).

Over time confusion regarding the terminology of amyloid has emerged. Some authors have inappropriately categorized all disorders with intracellular fibrillar protein aggregates as amyloidoses, even though the inclusions do not bind to Congo red. In the absence of a typical reaction with Congo red, positive immunohistochemical reactions with antibodies to amyloid proteins have been misinterpreted as indicating amyloid despite the fact that they may only indicate the precursor protein. The precursor protein will usually react with antibodies to the smaller amyloid fragment. Such false conclusions are particularly true with regard to an alleged identification of intracellular amyloid, which has only been unequivocally recognized extracellularly.

Composition of Amyloid

Since variations occur in the staining attributes of amyloid in different situations amyloid has long been suspected of being chemically heterogeneous and this was confirmed after different purified amyloid fibrils were identified in various types of amyloidosis in humans and animals (8,27,43,53,87,88,188,211).

The composition of amyloid in some varieties of amyloidosis has not yet been established, but at least 23 distinct unrelated amyloid proteins derived from precursor proteins have been identified (158). Despite their diversity in the native state proteins convert at least partly to stacked beta sheets with main chain hydrogen bonds parallel to the fibril axis and side chains perpendicular to the fibril axis.

Most amyloid proteins in the systemic amyloidoses are derived from precursors that are constituents of plasma, such as immunoglobulin light chain (AL), immunoglobulin heavy chain (AH), serum protein AA (SAA), β_2-microglobulin, transthyretin,

Table 1 Amyloid Proteins and Their Precursors

Amyloid protein	Precursor protein	Gene	Associated diseases
AA	Apo serum AA	*SAA1*	Secondary amyloidosis in familial Mediterranean fever (MIM #249100), certain malignancies, and following persistent acute inflammation
AANF	Atrial natriuretic factor	*NPPA*	Isolated atrial amyloidosis
AApoAI	Apolipoprotein AI	*APOA1*	FAP, Iowa type
AApoAII	Apolipoprotein AII	*APOA2*	Familial amyloidosis
AApoAIV	Apolipoprotein AIV	*APOA4*	Sporadic age-related amyloidosis
Aβ	Aβ protein precursor	*APP*	Alzheimer disease (MIM #104300); Down syndrome; hereditary cerebral hemorrhage with amyloid, Dutch type; aging
Aβ_2M	β_2-microglobulin	*B2M*	Hemodialysis-related amyloidosis
ACal	(Pro)calcitonin	*CALCA*	C-cell thyroid tumors
ACys	Cystatin C	*CST3*	Amyloidosis VI (cerebroarterial amyloidosis, Icelandic type) (MIM #105150)
AFib	Fibrinogen α-chain	*FGA*	Hereditary renal amyloidosis (amyloidosis VIII) (MIM #105200)
AGel	Gelsolin	GSN	Amyloidosis V (amyloidosis, Finnish type) (MIM #105120)
AH	Gamma immunoglobulin heavy chain	*IGHG1*	Waldenström macroglobulinemia
AIAPP	Islet amyloid polypeptide	*IAPP*	Insulinomas, diabetes mellitus
AIMP2B	Integral membrane protein 2B	*IMP2B*	Familial dementia, British (MIM #176500), familial dementia, Danish (MIM #117300)
AIns	Insulin	*INS*	Diabetic iatrogenic amyloidosis
AKer	Keratoepithelin	*TGFBI*	*TGFBI* gene-related corneal amyloidoses (see Chapter 32)
AL	Immunoglobulin κ or λ light chain	*IGLJ*	Primary amyloidosis, multiple myeloma and plasma cell dyscrasia-associated amyloid
ALac	Lactoferrin	*LTF*	GDCD, trichiasis-associated corneal amyloid
ALys	Lysozyme	*LYZ*	Amyloidosis VIII (familial visceral amyloidosis) (MIM #105200)
AMed	Lactadherin	*MFGE8*	Age-related amyloidosis of the aorta
APro	Prolactin	*PRL*	Pituitary age-related amyloidosis
APrP	Prion protein	*PRNP*	Spongioform encephalopathies
ATTR	Transthyretin	TTR	FAP, age-related systemic amyloidosis

Abbreviations: GDCD, gelatinous droplike corneal dystrophy; FAP, familial amyloid polyneuropathy; MIM, mendelian inheritance in man.

cystatin C, fibrinogen, gelsolin, apolipoprotein AI, apolipoprotein AII, apolipoprotein AIV and presumably reach tissues from the blood.

The composition of amyloid in various situations differs not only in the protein of the amyloid fibrils, but in disparate associated proteoglycans (PGs), GAGs, collagen, fibrinogen, lipoproteins, complement components, and other macromolecules (99).

Native amyloid fibrils are poorly immunogenic, but antigenic determinants are liberated following its degradation with sodium hydroxide. Antiserum elaborated against such material is capable of reacting with native amyloid (44).

Aside from having a major amyloid protein component the various types of amyloidosis share constituents, including amyloid P component (AP) and GAGs.

AP is a pentagonal protein identical to, or derived from a normal circulating serum protein known as serum amyloid P (SAP) and encoded by the *APCS* gene, which is situated close to the *CRP* gene for C-reactive protein. AP and serum C-reactive protein possess a similar pentagonal structure and share an amino acid sequence similarity. AP has been detected by indirect immunofluorescence techniques in normal cultured human skin fibroblasts suggesting that it may be a product of such cells (197).

AP is abundant in partially purified tissue extracts of amyloid, but has not been recognized in tissue sections (190). It appears as rod or "doughnut"-shaped particles (measuring up to 8–10 nm in diameter). These structures, which represent a small constituent of amyloid, are composed of five small subunits each 2 to 2.5 nm in diameter, clustered around a clear central zone with stacks of the pentagonal structures sometimes forming regularly beaded rods. AP is associated with amyloid fibrils yet the serum SAP levels do not significantly vary with the presence of amyloidosis (189).

Amyloid fibrils from different sources share a structural similarity regardless of the nature of the precursor protein. This is evident by electron microscopy, solid state nuclear magnetic resonance (NMR), and electron spin resonance (ESR) (131,207). Moreover natural and synthetic amyloid fibrils give similar high-resolution synchrotron X-ray diffraction patterns (208). The latter are consistent with a helical array of β-sheets parallel to the fiber long axis with strands perpendicular to this axis.

How the polypeptides in the amyloid proteins become aligned to form amyloid fibrils remains incompletely understood, but interactions between aromatic amino acids may play an important role in the so-called π-stacking interaction (a nonbonded interaction between planar aromatic rings) known to be involved in molecular recognition and self-assembly in many areas of chemistry and biochemistry (46). Amyloid fibrils manifest a self-seeding characteristic and the peptide segments are bound to neighboring segments through stacks of both backbone and side-chain hydrogen bonds (149).

Topography of Deposits

Amyloidosis characteristically involves specific tissues, and even in the eye amyloid deposition occurs in different sites. Heller and colleagues (72) classified amyloidosis into perireticulin and pericollagen types depending upon the site of initial amyloid deposition. In primary and myeloma-associated amyloidosis, the heart, tongue, gastrointestinal tract, skin, and nerves are frequently affected and the amyloid tends to deposit in mesenchymal tissue where collagen fibrils prevail ("pericollagenous amyloid") (adventitia of arteries and veins, connective tissue, sarcolemma of muscle and neurolemma of nerves) (mesenchymal tissue distribution pattern I). In amyloidosis associated with an overt inflammatory disease or malignancy (secondary or reactive amyloidosis) on the other hand, the amyloid occurs especially in parenchymal locations rich in reticulin. With this so-called perireticulin pattern, the liver, spleen, kidneys, intestine, and adrenal glands are generally involved, but the heart and other organs may be affected too. Why amyloid is regularly distributed in some organs, but rarely in others is not clear, perhaps the initial binding is a physicochemical reaction.

Secondary Effects

Amyloid deposits were once regarded as inert and dysfunctions in affected tissue were considered to be due to the displacement of adjacent cells and extracellular constituents. Most clinical manifestations, including those in the eye, occur by virtue of the space that amyloid occupies. However, certain substances in the serum, such as the blood clotting factors IX and X bind to the polyanionic amyloid fibrils possibly resulting in other secondary effects such as a bleeding diathesis. Foreign body giant cells commonly surround amyloid in the ocular adnexa as in primary orbital amyloidosis (70,82), but as amyloid in most situations does not elicit an inflammatory response, the giant cells may be an independent reaction to an underlying disease process. In some varieties of amyloidosis soluble amyloid oligomers are suspected of being toxic to cells leading to cell death (50). In the brain prefibillary beta-amyloid may cause tau-dependent microtubule disassembly (98). Some mutations in the *TTR* gene that encodes transthyretin lead to amyloid accumulation in the vitreous, but this is not associated with retinal dysfunction as vision is readily restored after a vitrectomy.

Etiology and Pathogenesis of Amyloidosis

The disparate conditions included under the connotation "amyloidosis" do not represent a single disorder, but rather a group of diseases characterized by an abnormal deposition of an extracellular protein. The amyloidoses have common morphologic, structural, and staining attributes. In each instance the major protein component of the amyloid fibrils usually shares a beta-pleated configuration and the fibrils are composed of two or more protofibrils, each with a central spine of β strands running perpendicular to the fibril axis (cross-β spine). This attribute orientates the fibrils so that they stain with Congo red and produce birefringence under polarized light and manifest a cross-β diffraction pattern. By TEM amyloid fibrils appear as rigid nonbranching structures of variable length that measure about 6 to 13 nm in diameter. Amyloid deposition is an end product of a complex chain of reactions in which genetic (89) and antigenic determinants are important.

Secondary Reactive Amyloidosis

An excessive antigenic stimulation characterizes secondary reactive amyloidosis associated with persistent acute inflammation, familial Mediterranean fever and certain malignant neoplasms, autoimmune disorders, and other conditions that may lead to amyloid production. The immune response in these situations may manifest itself in a production of normal or abnormal immunoglobulins or immunoglobulin light chains. Amyloid formation may depend on the characteristics of the immunoglobulin light chain as some of them form amyloid fibrils more easily than others, and not all individuals with Bence–Jones proteins (light chain polypeptides of immunoglobulin) develop amyloidosis. Also, fibrils obtained from the cleavage of some, but not all, Bence–Jones proteins by peptic digestion manifest typical attributes of amyloid fibrils: characteristic green birefringence in the polarizing microscope after Congo red staining, a distinctive ultrastructure and a typical X-ray diffraction pattern (51).

Immunoamyloid

Plasma cells, which synthesize and secrete immunoglobulins, undoubtedly play a cardinal role in the genesis of amyloid light chain proteins in primary nonfamilial systemic amyloidosis, and in amyloidosis associated with multiple myeloma and other plasma cell dyscrasias. Plasma cells presumably produce light chains, which are both excreted in the urine as Bence–Jones proteins, and subjected to proteolytic breakdown or polymerization with the formation of amyloid.

In many tissues investigators have alluded to a cellular origin of amyloid. The implicated cells have included the plasma cell which is the source of the precursors for AH and AL. Macrophages and other phagocytic cells also seem to participate in the formation of amyloid. The fibroblast is suspected of playing a role in amyloidogenesis as well, and two normal serum proteins associated with amyloid (AP and AA) have been identified in fibroblasts, which may be the source of them (197).

Some localized deposits of amyloid in the conjunctiva and orbit are preceded by chronic inflammation and associated with a prominent infiltrate of lymphocytes and plasma cells (70,104), but in most instances this is not the case.

The deposition of at least some types of amyloid (AA, AL, Aβ, ATTR) require the presence of a specific amyloid-enhancing factor (AEF), which has been identified as the AA fiber itself (128).

TYPES OF AMYLOIDOSIS

Overview

Amyloid deposition occurs in numerous localized and systemic settings (10). One variety of systemic amyloidosis occurs in the absence of a positive family history without significant antecedent or coexistent disease (primary idiopathic nonfamilial systemic amyloidosis) (111). It is associated with a high incidence of serum and/or urine immunoglobulin abnormalities and a high percentage of such patients (92% of 50 patients) have Bence–Jones proteinuria and characteristic M proteins (88).

Another type of systemic amyloidosis known as reactive systemic amyloidosis (secondary systemic amyloidosis) follows chronic infections (tuberculosis, tertiary syphilis, chronically infected burns, leprosy, infections with paraplegia, Whipple disease), chronic inflammatory diseases (regional enteritis, Reiter syndrome, ulcerative colitis), autoimmune conditions (rheumatic carditis, rheumatoid arthritis, scleroderma, systemic lupus erythematosus, and other "collagen vascular diseases"), and certain malignant neoplasms (renal cell carcinoma, Hodgkin disease). Reactive systemic amyloidosis can be produced experimentally with powerful antigenic stimulants like casein and Freund adjuvant.

Nonspecific immunoglobulin abnormalities frequently occur in patients with reactive systemic amyloidosis, but rarely if ever is a myeloma or Bence–Jones protein detected in such individuals. In one series of 17 patients with secondary generalized amyloidosis 53% had characteristic M proteins (53).

The term "primary familial amyloidosis," widely used in the literature, lacks precision as several distinct heredofamilial types of amyloidosis exist (130,141,171) including (*i*) familial visceral amyloidosis (systemic nonneuropathic amyloidosis, Ostertag type amyloidosis) (MIM #105200) due to mutations in the *APOA1*, *FGA*, or *LYZ* genes, (*ii*) autosomal recessive familial Mediterranean fever (MIM #249100), and autosomal dominant familial Mediterranean fever (MIM #134610), which are both caused by mutations in the *MEFV* gene, (*iii*) urticaria–deafness–amyloidosis syndrome (Muckle–Wells syndrome, MIM #19100) and familial cold hypersensitivity (MIM #120100), which are both caused by mutations in the *CIAS1* gene, and (*iv*) the cardiac amyloidoses, and familial amyloid polyneuropathies (FAPs) due to mutations in transthyretin, gelsolin, and apolipoprotein A1 (Table 1). With the exception of autosomal recessive familial Mediterranean fever, all systemic primary heredofamilial varieties of amyloidoses have an autosomal dominant mode of inheritance.

Small deposits of amyloid are commonly seen postmortem in the central nervous system (CNS), aorta, pancreas, seminal vesicles, and several other organs in the elderly (amyloidosis of aging) (235).

Solitary or multiple small localized deposits of amyloid may occur in the skin, respiratory tract, bladder, urethra, and other tissues sometimes simulating neoplasms clinically. The cornea, conjunctiva, orbit, and eyelid may be involved (discussed elsewhere in this chapter). Localized forms of cutaneous amyloidosis may be associated with miscellaneous lesions of the skin (including basal cell carcinoma, calcifying epithelioma of Malherbe and psoriasis). Several types of familial cutaneous amyloidosis have been documented: a bullous type with an onset at about 10 to 13 years of age (33), a hyperpigmented papular variety (172), a localized amyloidosis of the skin associated with psoriasis (86), and familial lichen amyloidosis (154).

AMYLOID PROTEINS, PRECURSOR PROTEINS, AND TYPES OF AMYLOIDOSES

Overview

Amyloid-like fibrils can be formed from a variety of proteins with all classes of secondary structure (174) in vitro, and it has been suggested that any protein can form such fibrils under appropriate conditions (26). The type of amyloid can be identified in formalin-fixed tissue (92). There is a striking similarity in amyloid formation of different proteins (15,24).

Types of Amyloid and Different Varieties of Amyloidosis

Protein SAA-Derived Amyloid (AA)

Amyloid fibrils in human and animal amyloidosis that follows persistent acute inflammation, some malignant neoplasms and familial Mediterranean fever (secondary or reactive amyloidosis) contain a unique fibrillar protein (AA) (molecular mass 8–8.5 kDa) (8) that is derived from a larger precursor in the serum (SAA). The serum of normal individuals contains minute quantities of SAA (molecular mass about 80 kDa), which is the cleavage product of an acute-phase reactant protein (SAAL) that is formed in the liver. SAA is found in the lipoprotein fraction of plasma [mainly with the high-density lipoproteins (HDL)] (234). A cluster of four closely linked genes on chromosome 11 (11p15.1) gives rise to four different isotypes of SAA (SAA1, SAA2, SAA3, and SAA4) (185), which are present in human serum from the time of birth. SAA rises in acute inflammatory diseases (an acute-phase protein) as well as in pregnancy (189) and usually after 70 years of age without relation to specific age-related diseases. The SAA level is of no practical value in the diagnosis of different types of amyloidosis as it is elevated in primary, secondary, and multiple myeloma-associated amyloidosis (even in forms of amyloidosis in which amyloid fibrils are devoid of AA).

A polymorphism in the SAA1-alpha variant of SAA imparts a sevenfold increased risk for renal amyloidosis in familial Mediterranean fever (234).

Atrial Natriuric Peptide Amyloidosis (AANF)

Atrial natriuric peptide (ANP), which consists of multiple peptides of variable molecular weight, is encoded by the *NPPA* gene and synthesized as a larger precursor (atrial pronatriodilatin) (239). Amyloid derived from ANP has been identified within the atrium of individuals with atrial fibrillation (55,118).

Apolipoprotein AI-Derived Amyloid (AApoA1)

Apolipoprotein AI is the major apoprotein of HDL (see Chapter 46). It is encoded by the *APOA1* gene (25) and at least seven mutations (Gly26Arg, Trp50Arg, Leu60Arg, Leu90Pro, Arg173Pro, Leu174Ser, Ala175Pro) cause phenotypes with amyloidosis. The Gly26Arg mutation causes amyloid polyneuropathy—nephropathy, Iowa type (formerly amyloidosis IV) (MIM *107680) (150), which involves the nerves in all four extremities at the onset in this disorder. In contrast to the transthyretin forms of FAP vitreous opacities have not been reported (238). Peptic ulcers may be present and cataracts sometimes develop (138). An amyloid nephropathy causing the nephrotic syndrome is common and is the usual cause of death.

Apolipoprotein AII-Derived Amyloid (AApoAII)

Human mutations in the *AOPA2* gene for apolipoprotein AII (ApoA2) can also cause hereditary renal amyloidosis (12). Variants of apoA2 correlate with the susceptibility to senile amyloidosis in the SAMP1 stain of mouse. Amyloid deposits in the conjunctiva, in blood vessel walls near the anterior chamber angle and in the sheaths of the extraocular muscles, but not in the retina or choroid in these mice (186). Amyloid fibrils derived from apoA2 accelerate amyloid deposition in mice with senile amyloidosis (107).

Apolipoprotein AIV-Derived Amyloid (AApoAIV)

In a patient with systemic amyloidosis amyloid fibrils derived from both transthyretin and apolipoprotein A4 (apoA4) have been detected in different tissues (13,14). The AApoAIV amyloid fibrils were derived from the product of a nonmutated *APOA4* gene (14).

Beta-Amyloid (Aβ)

The senile plaques of Alzheimer disease have been known to stain with Congo red since 1927 (36), but this only became accepted as being due to amyloid many years later (133). The protein in the amyloid plaques of Alzheimer disease were purified by Glenner and Wong in 1984 and named beta-amyloid (52). The highly conserved *APP* gene encodes for β-amyloid (57) and mutations in it cause familial Alzheimer disease (MIM #104300), early onset Alzheimer disease with cerebral amyloid angiopathy (MIM #104300) and several types of hereditary cerebral amyloidosis (62). Soluble forms of β-amyloid elicit apoptosis (198) (see Chapter 2) and deceased synaptic plasticity (227). In brains with Alzheimer disease the senile plaques, but not the neurofibrillary tangles, contain amyloid (see Chapter 70) (25,232).

β_2-Microglobulin-Derived Amyloid ($A\beta_2M$)

β_2-Microglobulin, which is coded by the *B2M* gene (67), is a normal serum constituent with amino acid sequence similarities to the immunoglobulins. β_2-Microglobulin is present on the surface of all cells as the light chain of the human leukocyte antigen (HLA) complex and it is also a secretory product of plasma cells. After long-term hemodialysis for severe renal disease β_2-microglobulin deposits particularly in the synovium and bone of patients, where it takes on the fibrillary pattern of amyloid, causing an osteoarthropathic syndrome (carpal tunnel syndrome, arthropathy, and lytic bone lesions that are prone to spontaneous fractures) (hemodialysis-related amyloidosis) (47,137). β_2-Microglobulin has a β-pleated sheet structure and is associated with the major histocompatibility complex (MHC) class I heavy chains. Amyloid derived from it is coupled with a codeposition of calcium. This form of amyloid has not been identified within ocular tissues.

Calcitonin-Derived Amyloid (ACal)

Amyloid associated with medullary thyroid carcinoma is derived from calcitonin (97,192). This neoplasm occurs in the multiple endocrine neoplasia syndrome type IIB, which has several ophthalmic manifestations (see Chapter 55), which can lead to an early diagnosis of this malignant tumor.

Cystatin C-Derived Amyloid (ACys)

Cystatin C (cytostatin 3) is a serum protein produced by all nucleated cells. It is a potent inhibitor of lysosomal proteinases (65,123) and a marker of renal glomerular function. Cystatin is encoded by the *CST3* gene and is unrelated to the statins (pharmaceutical agents that lower plasma cholesterol levels).

Amyloid derived from cytostatin accumulates in amyloidosis type VI (cerebroarterial amyloidosis, Icelandic type) (MIM #105150). This autosomal dominant disease, which was first described in Iceland, is caused by a Leu68Gln mutation in the *CST3* gene (1). It has a predilection for cerebral arteries and arterioles and affected individuals die from cerebral hemorrhage before they reach 40 years of age (66). The disease has also been recognized among fishermen along the Dutch North Sea coast (129). Following its purification and analysis the amyloid in this condition was identified as cystatin C. It is noteworthy that the amyloid found in the clinically similar Dutch form of cerebroarterial amyloidosis (MIM #609065) is not caused by a mutation in the *CST3* gene that encodes cystatin C, but in the *APP* gene that is responsible for amyloid precursor protein (217). The different genes can cause these phenotypically identical forms of amyloidosis illustrates genetic heterogeneity. Although the ocular vasculature could conceivably be affected in cerebral amyloid angiopathy, amyloid deposits have thus far not been documented within the eye or its adnexal tissues in the cerebroarterial amyloidoses.

Fibrinogen-Derived Amyloid (AFib)

Some mutations in the *FGA* gene (Arg554Leu, Glu526Val,1bp-del, FS548Ter) that encode fibrinogen alpha chain cause autosomal dominant renal amyloidosis (6,11,113,214).

Gelsolin-Derived Amyloid (AGel)

Gelsolin, an actin-binding and actin-fragmenting protein, is a constituent of normal plasma and virtually all cells (110). The amyloid protein in Finnish patients with amyloidosis V (MIM #105120), which has lattice corneal dystrophy (LCD) type II as a manifestation (see Chapter 32) is a 71-amino acid long fragment (7–12 kDa) of gelsolin with an Asp187Asn mutation (48,68,77,122,134–136). The same mutation has also been found in an American family of Irish descent (59). Only one other mutation in *GSN* has been discovered in amyloidosis V (Asp187Tyr) (32). Postmortem examination of patients with amyloidosis V has disclosed amyloid in arterial walls of almost all organs, as well as in the heart, kidney (glomeruli), nerves, skin, and other tissues in addition to the cornea.

Islet Amyloid Polypeptide Amyloidosis (AIAPP)

A localized form of amyloidosis is found in the pancreatic islets of Langerhans in diabetes mellitus type II (see Chapter 45) as well as in insulinomas. This amyloid consists of a 37-amino acid polypeptide derived by proteolytic processing from an 89-amino acid precursor produced by beta cells in the islets of Langerhans (amylin) that is encoded by the *IAPP* gene (178). The extent of the amyloid deposition correlates with the severity of the diabetes. Studies in transgenic mice strongly suggest that the amyloid deposits are toxic to the beta cells and cause diabetes (219). The sequence Ala-Ile-Leu-Ser-Ser corresponding to positions 25 to 29 in human amylin is strongly amyloidogenic (229).

Integral Membrane Protein 2B Amyloid (AIMP2B)

Amyloid deposition associated with CNS degeneration occurs in two forms of dementia that differ from Alzheimer disease (see Chapter 25) [British familial dementia (presenile dementia with spastic ataxia, MIM #176500) and Danish familial dementia (cerebellar ataxia, cataract, deafness, and dementia or psychosis, MIM #117300)]. Both diseases are caused by mutations in the *ITM2B* gene, which encodes integral membrane protein 2B (221), which was formerly thought to be two different protein precursors (ABriPP and ADanPP). The Danish disease has a widespread amyloid angiopathy throughout the CNS and retinal blood vessels are involved. Posterior polar cataracts seem to be the initial manifestation in the Danish variant and appear between the ages of 20 to 30 years. Vidal et al. (220) identified the amyloid in the British variant as a unique 4-kDa protein subunit of a fragment of a longer than the usual integral membrane protein 2B, caused by a single base substitution at a stop codon in the mutated *ITM2B* gene.

Immunoamyloid (AH and AL)

More than five decades ago, Vazquez and Dixon (218) using immunofluorescence microscopy identified gamma globulin in amyloid deposits. Subsequently, it became recognized that the major component of amyloid fibril in primary nonfamilial systemic amyloidosis and in the amyloidosis associated with multiple myeloma and plasma cell dyscrasias is a fragment of immunoglobulin light chains (54,88,111,153,188,211).

Amyloidosis occurs in approximately 15% of cases of multiple myeloma and other plasma cell dyscrasias. This amyloid, now designated AL (53,87) is considered to consist of polymerized fragments of entire light chains (211) or in combination with fragments of κ or λ light chains, which probably consist of the variable portion, and part of the constant region portion of the light chain (54). These subunits consist of the first 30 residues of light chains. Human light chain-related amyloidosis can be induced experimentally by injecting Bence–Jones proteins obtained from patients with AL amyloid into mice (195). Under such circumstances amyloid deposits in the spleen, liver, and other organs. Mice do not develop amyloidosis after they are inoculated with nonamyloid-associated Bence–Jones proteins indicating that only some light chains and Bence–Jones proteins are amyloidogenic (195). Bone marrow cells from patients with AL amyloidosis, as well as from either light chain or light and heavy chain deposition disease, have invariably synthesized monoclonal light chains corresponding to the class found in the tissue deposits (22). AH amyloid, derived from the heavy chain of gamma globulin may be associated with Waldenström macroglobulinemia. Immunoamyloid is found in some localized forms of amyloid, such as a nodular localized form of amyloidosis in the lung (54).

Iatrogenic Amyloidosis (AIns)

Patients who receive a continuous local infusion of insulin for 6 weeks develop granulation tissue together with amyloid deposits around the tip of the catheter. This iatrogenically produced amyloid reacts with anti-insulin antibody (204).

Lactoferrin Amyloid (ALac)

Lactoferrin has been identified within amyloid deposits in cornea (3,5,103), seminal vesicles (213), and brain. Initially the role of lactoferrin in the amyloid was unclear as it may have coprecipitated with other components of amyloid. However, it is now recognized as an amyloid precursor protein (228). Nilsson and Dobson (152) have found that lactoferrin does not by itself form amyloid fibrils, but a particular sequence in lactoferrin (Asn-Ala-Gly-Asp-Val-Ala-Phe-Val) is highly amyloidogenic and lactoferrin-derived amyloid may follow damage to this protein as by proteolysis. Lactoferrin is found, together with beta amyloid, in the senile plaques of Alzheimer disease and Down syndrome (121). Within the brain lactoferrin has also been identified within the lesions of amyotrophic lateral sclerosis and Pick disease (121). A Glu561Asp polymorphism in the *LTF* gene that encodes lactoferrin is thought to facilitate amyloid deposition in corneas associated with trichiasis (5).

Lysozyme-Derived Amyloid (ALys)

A rare variety of nonneuropathic hereditary amyloidosis is caused by several mutations in the *LYZ* gene (Ile56Thr, Phe57Ile, Trp64Arg, Asp67His) that encodes lysozyme (63). Renal manifestations are often the most prominent feature but gastrointestinal symptoms and bleeding complications may be prominent. Keratoconjunctivitis sicca may be present (63).

Medin Amyloid (AMed)

Medin amyloid is thought to be the most common variety of amyloid. It is found in the medial layer of the aorta in almost all Caucasians >50 years old (115). Medin is a 5.5 kDa fragment of the cell adhesion protein lactadherin, which is a mammary epithelial cell expressed glycoprotein encoded by the *MFGE8* gene. A hexapeptide truncated portion of medin (Asn-Phe-Gly-Ser-Val-Gln) can form typical amyloid fibrils (164). Both medin and lactadherin bind to tropoelastin via the medin domain and the interaction elastic fibers may be important in medin amyloid formation (116).

Prion Amyloid (APrP)

A sialoglycoprotein designated prion protein is believed to be the causative agent of several spongioform encephalopathies, including Creutzfelt–Jakob disease and scrapie (see Chapter 70) (19). The scrapie isoform of this protein (PrP^{SC}) as well as the component that is found in the CNS of normal individuals (PrP^{C}) polymerizes into amyloid rods (prion amyloid).

Prolactin-Derived Amyloid (APro)

Spheroidal concentric localized deposits of amyloid derived from prolactin have been identified in the pituitary gland in association with prolactin-secreting adenomas (17,78). They have also been found associated with aging.

Transforming Growth Factor Beta-Induced Protein Amyloid (AKer)

Amyloid deposits in LCD type I and in other corneal amyloidoses caused by specific mutations in the *TGFBI* gene (see Chapter 32). The amyloid (AKer) represents fragments of transforming growth factor beta-induced protein (TGFBIp) (also known as keratoepithelin and other terms) (see Chapter 36). Takacs et al. (209) and Korvatska et al. (108) have provided evidence that the amyloid in LCD type I results from an accumulation of a 44 kDa N-terminal part of the mutated TGFBIp.

Transthyretin Amyloid (ATTR)

Transthyretin, a normal constituent of human plasma and cerebrospinal fluid (CSF), is encoded by the *TTR* gene. It is synthesized predominantly in the liver, but is also produced in the choroid plexus of the brain

(35), and by the retinal pigment epithelium (RPE) (31,74). This acidic protein has an affinity for thyroxine and retinol-binding protein and partakes in their plasma transportation. On electrophoresis it migrates in front of albumin, hence its older designation of prealbumin. Transthyretin is made up of four identical subunits, each consisting of 127 amino acids about half of which form a β-pleated sheet.

Transthyretin is the precursor of the amyloid protein known as ATTR and all forms of transthyretin amyloidosis have autosomal dominant modes of transmission and a striking feature of these disorders is the varied tissue distribution of the amyloid caused by the different mutations in the *TTR* gene. To date almost 50 distinct mutations in the *TTR* gene have been identified mostly with systemic deposits of amyloid (Table 2) (84). Some amino acid substitutions are polymorphisms without pathologic consequences. An acidic transthyretin may also result (His90Asn). Most *TTR* mutations cause a FAP. Other mutations affect predominantly the heart, often with other tissues, and the cardiomyopathy may be fatal (84). Leptomeningeal amyloidosis results from certain *TTR* mutations and in such cases the eye is commonly affected (16,58,159,215,216). It is noteworthy that the substitution of alanine for threonine in position 60 results in FAP with major deposits in the heart (unlike the other mutations). The eye is only known to be affected in some mutations, but the reason remains to be determined. Some investigators have found amyloid fibrils of senile systemic amyloidosis to be derived from normal transthyretin (230); others have found an age-related deposition of amyloid in the heart, lungs, liver, and other tissues (senile systemic amyloidosis) with mutated *TTR* (61). With some mutations the amyloid deposition may not have a striking predominant tissue predisposition. Aside from amyloidosis another clinical manifestation of some *TTR* mutations is euthyroid hyperthyroxinemia resulting from increased binding of thyroxine to the mutated transthyretin (146,165,179).

A carpal tunnel syndrome is sometimes the initial manifestation of a transthyretin amyloidosis and with some *TTR* mutations (Tyr114His) it may be the sole clinical abnormality. Vitreous deposits of amyloid are features of some mutations in transthyretin (Table 2) (95,105,147).

Amyloid polyneuropathy (Andrade or Portuguese type) (MIM +176300) is an example of a phenotype caused by a specific *TTR* mutation (Val30Met) (180). This form of amyloidosis was first described by Andrade in 1952 (4) in patients from a small area of northwestern Portugal. Subsequently it was identified in persons of Portuguese, Japanese, Swedish, Greek, and other origins (138,210). The disorder starts in the lower extremities with thermal, superficial pain, touch, and position sense loss in that order. In this disease early impotence in the male, perforating ulcers of the feet, diarrhea, sphincter disturbances, and weight loss are common. Amyloid deposits in blood vessels throughout the body and in almost all organs, but clinically significant renal disease is conspicuously absent. The pupils become irregular in contour, unequal in size, and dilated with absent or sluggish reactions to light and accommodation. The pupil develops a characteristic scalloped appearance. Ocular signs and symptoms may result from the neuropathy, vascular fragility, or vitreous opacification.

Amyloid polyneuropathy (Indiana type) (MIM +176300) is caused by a Ile84Ser mutation in the *TTR* gene. It starts later in life and progresses more slowly than the Andrade type of FAP and the hands are affected with the carpal tunnel syndrome (130). Ecchymoses of the eyelids, extraocular muscle weakness, internal ophthalmoplegia, and anisocoria may occur (41). In a postmortem study of an eye from a patient with this variety of amyloidosis extensive deposits of amyloid have been found in blood vessels, ciliary nerves, and extraocular muscles, but not in the iris sphincter muscle or cornea (156). The amyloid in this condition is a variant of transthyretin with a serine substitution for isoleucine at position 84 (225). Amyloid polyneuropathy (Maryland type) (MIM +176300) resembles the Indiana type of amyloid neuropathy clinically, but the *TTR* mutation differs (Leu58His) (151). Another variant of amyloid polyneuropathy (German–American type) discovered in a patient of German descent with peripheral neuropathy and bowel dysfunction results from a Ser77Tyr *TTR* mutation (226).

Yet to Be Identified Amyloidoses

Aside from the aforementioned types of amyloid derived from specific proteins numerous other proteins are suspected of being amyloidogenic, but have not yet been identified. Cells that arise from the neural crest and secrete polypeptide hormones have been designated amine precursor uptake and decarboxylation (APUD) cells. Neoplasms derived from these cells (apudomas) (pheochromocytomas, medullary carcinomas of the thyroid gland, gastrinomas and insulinomas) produce a variety of localized forms of amyloid (apudamyloid) (157). As discussed above with insulinomas the amyloid is AIAPP, and with medullary carcinoma the amyloid is ACal, but in the other apudomas the amyloid awaits identification. However, it may be derived from the nonhormone residue of the relevant prohormone or a polypeptide produced concomitantly with the hormone itself. Apudamyloid differs from immunoamyloid in not demonstrating yellow autofluorescence when examined under UV light, and in lacking tryptophan and tyrosine.

Table 2 Mutations in the *TTR* Gene Encoding Transthyretin

Phenotype	Mutations	MIM#	Remarks
Amyloid polyneuropathy	Cys10Arg	+17630	
Amyloid polyneuropathy, Andrade type	Val30Met	+17630	Vitreous involved
Amyloid polyneuropathy	Val30Ala	+17630	
Amyloid polyneuropathy	Val30Leu	+17630	
Amyloid polyneuropathy, Jewish type	Phe33Ile	+17630	
Amyloid polyneuropathy, Polish-American type	Phe33Leu	+17630	
Amyloid polyneuropathy	Ala36Pro	+17630	
Amyloid polyneuropathy	Glu42Gly	+17630	
Amyloid polyneuropathy	Phe44Ser	+17630	
Amyloid polyneuropathy	Gly47Arg	+17630	
Amyloid polyneuropathy	Gly47Ala	+17630	
Amyloid polyneuropathy	Ser50Arg	+17630	
Amyloid polyneuropathy, Maryland type	Leu58His	+17630	
Amyloid polyneuropathy	Leu58Arg	+17630	
Amyloid polyneuropathy, Appalachian type	Thr60Ala	+17630	
Amyloid polyneuropathy	Glu61Lys	+17630	
Amyloid polyneuropathy	Phe64Leu	+17630	
Amyloid polyneuropathy	Lys70Asn	+17630	
Amyloid polyneuropathy	Val71Ala	+17630	
Amyloid polyneuropathy, German–American type	Ser77Tyr	+17630	
Amyloid polyneuropathy, Indiana type	Ile84Ser	+17630	
Amyloid polyneuropathy	His90Asn	+17630	Vitreous involved
Amyloid polyneuropathy	Ala97Gly	+17630	
Amyloid polyneuropathy	Arg104His	+17630	Vitreous involved
Amyloid polyneuropathy	Ile107Val	+17630	
Amyloid polyneuropathy	Tyr114Cys	+17630	Vitreous involved
Amyloid polyneuropathy	Val122Del	+17630	

(*Continued*)

Table 2 Mutations in the *TTR* Gene Encoding Transthyretin (*Continued*)

Phenotype	Mutations	MIM#	Remarks
Age-related systemic amyloidosis	Val122Ile	+17630	Amyloid in heart, lungs, liver and other tissues
Amyloid cardiopathy	Val20Ile	+17630	
Amyloid cardiopathy	Ala45Thr	+17630	
Amyloid cardiopathy	Ser50Ile	+17630	
Amyloid cardiopathy	Thr60Ala	+17630	
Amyloid cardiopathy	Ile68Leu	+17630	
Amyloid cardiopathy, Denmark type	Leu111Met	+17630	
Leptomeningeal amyloidosis	Asp18Gly	#105210	
Leptomeningeal amyloidosis	Val30Gly	#105210	
Leptomeningeal amyloidosis	Gly53Glu	#105210	
Leptomeningeal amyloidosis	Phe64Ser	#105210	
Leptomeningeal amyloidosis	Tyr69His	#105210	
Oculoleptomeningeal amyloidosis	Phe64Ser	#105210	
Familial carpal tunnel syndrome	Tyr114His	+17630	
Euthyroid hyperthyroxinemia	Ala109Thr	+17630	
Euthyroid hyperthyroxinemia	Ala109Val	+17630	
Euthyroid hyperthyroxinemia	Thr119Met	+17630	
Nonpathologic polymorphism	Gly6Ser	+17630	
Nonpathologic polymorphism	Tyr116Val	+17630	
Familial amyloidosis	Leu12Pro	+17630	Amyloidosis without predominant tissue distribution
Familial amyloidosis	Thr49Ala	+17630	
Familial amyloidosis	Leu55Pro	+17630	
Familial amyloidosis	Glu89Gln	+17630	

OCULAR AMYLOIDOSES

Cornea

Lattice Corneal Dystrophy Type I and Related Amyloidoses

Certain *TGFBI* mutations are responsible for LCD type I (MIM #12200) and other conditions with corneal amyloid deposition (see Chapter 32) (Fig. 1) (101,184,194,196). In these cases the amyloid is AKer. Available evidence indicates that the amyloid deposits in LCD type I are restricted to the cornea and that clinical systemic disease is not associated. Amyloid has not been observed in surgically excised tissue from several sites (skin, lymph nodes, cartilage, nerve,

Table 3 A Comparison Between Some Familial Amyloid Polyneuropathies

Characteristic	Type I (Andrade, Portuguese type)	Type II (Rukavina, Indiana, Swiss type), type IIB (Mahloudji, Maryland type)	Type III (Van Allen, Iowa type)	Type IV (Meretoja, Finnish type)
Usual age at onset	Third decade	Fifth decade	Fourth decade	Third decade
Site of onset	Feet	Hands	Feet and hands	Cornea
Gastrointestinal complaints	Common	Rare	Common	Rare
Impotence and sphincter disturbances	Common	Rare	Common	Rare
Trophic ulcers	Common	Rare	Rare	Rare
Average duration of illness	4–12 years	14–40+ years	12 years	69 years
Nephropathy	Rare	Absent	Invariable	Common, usually mild
Eye	Abnormal pupils	Vitreal amyloid	Cataracts (sometimes)	Lattice corneal dystrophy
Type of amyloid	Transthyretin	Transthyretin	Apolipoprotein Aj	Gelsolin

Source: Modified from Ref. 130.

muscle, and the wall of a Baker cyst) in subjects with LCD type I (101). Following keratoplasty for LCD type I amyloid deposits may recur in the grafted donor tissue some 2 to 14 years later (102,114). Prior to the discovery that mutations in the *TGFBI* gene cause LCD type I several investigators came to incorrect conclusions about the identification of the amyloid (18,127,145,231) demonstrating the shortcoming of immunohistochemistry when trying to identify an unknown protein in amyloid deposits.

Evidence that fibroblasts play a role in amyloid production elsewhere together with an intimate association of some corneal fibroblasts (keratocytes) with amyloid and the prominent rough endoplasmic reticulum disclosed by TEM within such cells (81,101,236) in LCD type I supports the possibility that the amyloid may be a product of corneal fibroblasts. However, another potential source is the corneal epithelium.

Lattice Corneal Dystrophy Type II

The cornea is also accompanied by amyloid deposition in persons with a systemic form of amyloidosis (amyloidosis V) (MIM #105120) caused by two mutations in the *GSN* gene (Asp187Tyr and Asp187Asn). These individuals have LCD type II (see Chapter 32), which is the only form of amyloidosis in which corneal and noncorneal tissues are affected. In eyes examined at necropsy with LCD type II amyloid has been identified predominantly in the corneal stroma (142,143). Surgically excised corneal tissue has occasionally been examined following a superficial keratectomy or penetrating keratoplasty (161,201). A neurotrophic persistent epithelial defect complicated the postoperative course in one of these cases (201). The corneal amyloid in LCD type II reacts with antibodies against amyloid P component (201) and the gelsolin mutant protein (60), but not with AP or transthyretin antibodies (201).

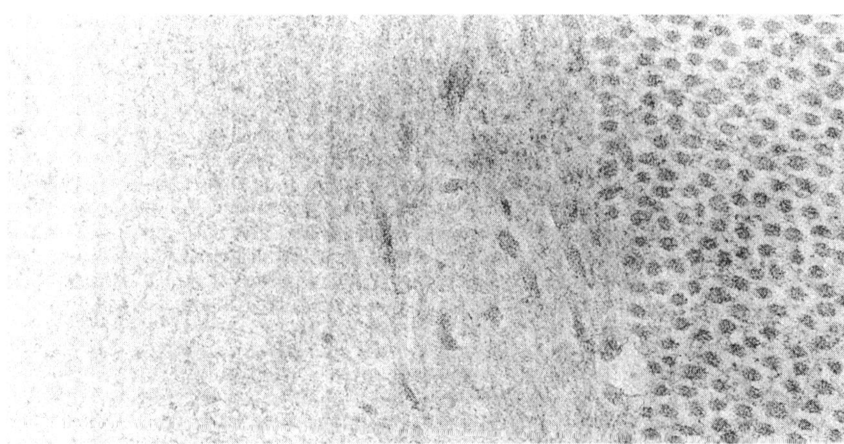

Figure 1 Transmission electron micrograph of amyloid deposit in corneal stroma of lattice corneal dystrophy type I. The amyloid fibrils are adjacent to wider collagen fibers (*right side*) (×58,400).

Possibly relevant to the pathogenesis of LCD type II, is the yet unconfirmed observation from Finland, which the corneal changes in LCD type II are preceded by acute episodes reminiscent of iritis or scleritis, during which crystals are evident in the cornea, bulbar conjunctiva, and aqueous (96).

Gelatinous Droplike Corneal Dystrophy

Another inherited corneal disease with subepithelial deposits of amyloid is the autosomal recessive disorder gelatinous droplike corneal dystrophy (Fig. 2) (familial subepithelial corneal amyloidosis) (MIM 204870) (see Chapter 32) (103). Most cases of this disorder result from mutations in the *TACSTD2* gene, but there is evidence for genetic heterogeneity. The encoded product of *TACSTD2* affects the permeability of the bulbar surface epithelial, but it is not the precursor of the amyloid. Instead the major component of the subepithelial amyloid is ALac (a derivative of lactoferrin), which is also a component of other corneas with amyloidosis (3,5), including those associated with trichiasis (5).

The unfortunate designation of "gelatinous droplike dystrophy of the cornea," is one of the synonyms for chronic actinic keratopathy (see Chapter 30). In an immunofluorescent study of this form of corneal amyloidosis (144) the amyloid deposits have been noted to react with antibodies to AP, but not with antibodies to AA, immunoglobulins, light chains, or transthyretin.

Other Forms of Primary Corneal Amyloidosis

Partington and colleagues (155) reported a family in which 2 males and 7 females had brown pigmentation of the skin with the pigmentation mimicking incontinentia pigmenti in the females. In both sexes the skin was slightly hyperkeratotic with melanin in its basal layer. Amyloid was present in the papillary dermis. Both males did not survive infancy and one was almost blind with amyloid deposits in the cornea.

Secondary Corneal Amyloidosis

Amyloid deposits in the cornea without conjunctival involvement in numerous apparently unrelated chronic nonspecific disorders, such as the retinopathy of prematurity (retrolental fibroplasia) (140,199), trauma (28,45,140), keratoconus (139,140,203), phlyctenular keratoconjunctivitis (140), congenital glaucoma (34,100), glaucoma secondary to uveitis (40), endothelial decompensation (79,100), sympathetic ophthalmia (140), trachoma (34,75), trichiasis (5,71), syphilitic interstitial keratitis (39,76), Schnyder crystalline corneal dystrophy (40), and lipid keratopathy (140). In such instances the amyloid often occurs most conspicuously immediately beneath the corneal epithelium, but it may be scattered among the collagen fibers in the substantia propria. Spontaneous nonfamilial deposits of amyloid have also been described under the designation *polymorphic amyloid degeneration* of the cornea (109,132). Loeffler and colleagues (127) reported a positive reaction of monoclonal antibodies to gelsolin with the amyloid of *polymorphic amyloid degeneration*, but others have found no reactivity with antibodies to mutant gelsolin (59). The literature contains a noteworthy single example of bilateral corneal amyloidosis coupled with hypergammaglobulinemia (106).

Conjunctiva and Eyelid

The first documented example of ocular amyloidosis appears to involve the conjunctiva (73). Conjunctival amyloidosis usually affects both eyes in individuals between 20 and 30 years of age. As a rule it begins at the fornix and eventually extends into the bulbar and palpebral conjunctiva. Chronic conjunctivitis (especially trachoma), repeated pyogenic conjunctivitis, and chronic idiopathic conjunctivitis may lead to

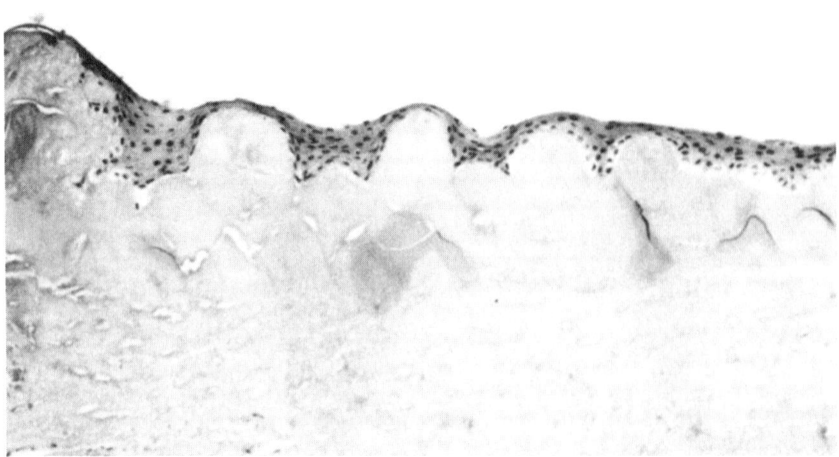

Figure 2 Nodular deposits of amyloid in the superficial cornea in gelatinous droplike dystrophy of the cornea (hematoxylin and eosin, ×100).

localized deposits of amyloid in the eyelid and conjunctiva, but sometimes amyloid accumulates in the absence of a known antecedent disorder, as a painless swelling of the eyelid (7,193,200).

Vitreous

Opaque vitreal deposits were first reported in 1953 by Kantarjian and de Jong (91). Vitreal amyloidosis occurs in several types of FAP related to amino acid substitutions in transthyretin (see also Chapter 29) (41,80,85,91,94,95,156,175), yet not in FAP type IIA (transthyretin Leu58His), or with some other mutations in *TTR* (Table 2). Clinically the amyloid appears as bilateral vitreous opacities or floaters. In some forms of amyloidosis it can severely impair vision and it is often the first clinical manifestation of the systemic disease. In FAP type II vitreal involvement is most conspicuous. Rarely amyloid has been observed in the vitreous in the absence of a positive family history or overt systemic manifestations (42,80,176,183,191). In one such case that was thoroughly studied a *TTR* mutation was detected (191). In another family with a different TTR mutation (Ala36Pro) vitreous amyloidosis was isolated and not accompanied by a FAP (173).

Clinical and histopathological observations suggest that the amyloid reaches the vitreous from the retinal blood vessels. In the retina prominent perivascular sheathing is often a prominent early clinical manifestation of vitreal amyloidosis. Tissue sections of eyes with FAP (69,117,233) have disclosed an extension of amyloid from the walls of retinal blood vessels into the vitreous and when amyloid does not deposit in the walls of retinal blood vessels vitreal amyloidosis does not seem to occur. Although transthyretin reaches the eye from the circulation another potential source is the RPE, which has been shown to synthesize transthyretin (31).

Vitreous amyloid is frequently mistaken clinically for old hemorrhage and its presence is often not appreciated until cytological evaluation of a vitrectomy specimen (64). Pars plana vitrectomy offers an opportunity for not only diagnosing the nature of the vitreal opacities, but it is also a sole beneficial therapy for removing the amyloid (93,95). Such treatment can improve vision markedly but the amyloid gradually reaccumulates over weeks to years (38,80,93,181).

The only type of amyloid that has been identified in the vitreous is ATTR (176,177,191). Amyloid fibrils (Fig. 3) composed of AH or AL have not been detected in the vitreous. It is also noteworthy that the amyloid deposition has not been documented in either the retinal vessels or vitreous in amyloid polyneuropathy–nephropathy, Iowa type (MIM *107680) or amyloidosis V (MIM #105120), and that amyloid may be absent from the vitreous and retinal blood vessels despite other extensive ocular deposits in both multiple myeloma and primary idiopathic systemic amyloidosis (29,212).

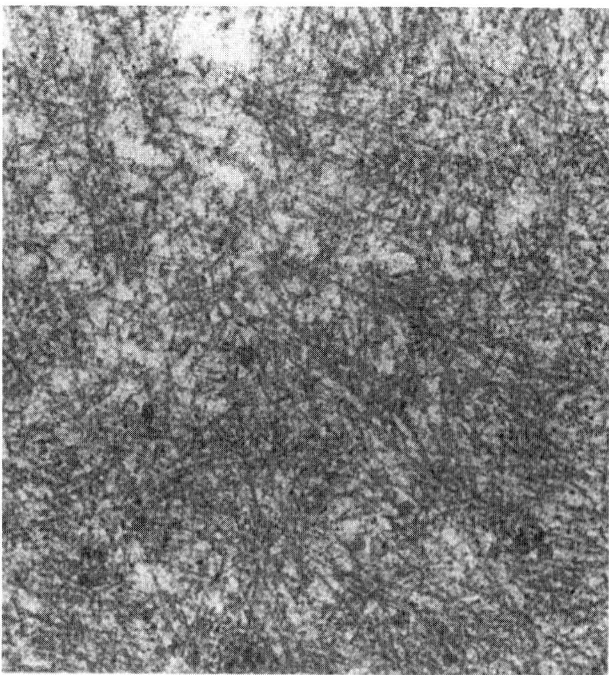

Figure 3 A high magnification view of densely matted amyloid fibrils (×50,900). *Source*: Courtesy of John D. Shelburne.

Orbit

Orbital amyloidosis is uncommon and generally not preceded by overt local disease (70,82,104,182). It may cause proptosis, but diplopia and loss of visual acuity are not prominent clinical manifestations. Ptosis may be a presenting feature of localized amyloidosis of the eyelid and orbit and several cases have simulated myasthenia gravis (182). Exophthalmos may occur in FAP types I (Andrade or Portuguese type) (91) or FAP type II (Rukavina or Indiana type) (41) suggesting that amyloid deposits in the orbit in these varieties of amyloidosis, but this has not been confirmed by tissue examination at either biopsy or autopsy. Ophthalmoplegia is sometimes associated with amyloid infiltrations of the extraocular muscles in multiple myeloma (162). The types of amyloid found in the orbit include AL (multiple myeloma) (162), AA (chronic inflammation) (59), and ATRR (59).

Iris

In 1975, Lessell et al. (119) drew attention to a "scalloping" of the pupils in two patients with an autosomal dominant type of FAP. This pupillary abnormality is a feature of the Andrade type of FAP due to a *TTR* mutation (MIM +176300). The pupils may be small, irregular, of different size and react poorly to light and accommodation like the Argyl–Robertson pupils of neurosyphilis (4). The pathogenesis of the scalloped pupils, which may also be a feature of other types of FAP (119,170), remains to be determined.

Other

In 1973, Ringvold and Husby (167) drew attention to features of amyloid in the exfoliated material of the pseudoexfoliation syndrome (PEX) (see Chapter 25). Unlike most forms of amyloid, however, the fibers in PEX rarely exhibit dichoism after staining with Congo red. PEX material reacts with antibodies to AP and a variety of basement membrane and elastic fiber system proteins (2,124,125,206,224) including a reaction with a crude AA antiserum (167), probably due to contamination with AP. Monoclonal antibodies against AA, AB, transthyretin, or immunoglobulin light chains have yielded negative results (30,166,205). One of the downregulated genes in PEX tissues is *SAA1*, which encodes for SAA1. β-Amyloid the precursor for Aβ in Alzheimer disease is found in the aqueous humor of PEX patients (90). Amyloid-associated proteins, which are not part of the fibrils, include AP, GAGs, extracellular matrix components, complement proteins, apolipoproteins, and cytokines, which also occur in association with PEX fibrils. Polymorphisms of apolipoprotein E (ApoE), which promotes the aggregation of amyloidogenic proteins into the beta-pleated sheet conformation in many amyloidoses, is associated with PEX (237). Although PEX is not an amyloidosis according to the current definition it is probably a protein conformational disorder, like the amyloidoses, with an accumulation of an altered structural protein (see Chapter 36).

Ocular Involvement in the Systemic Amyloidoses

The incidence of ocular involvement in the systemic amyloidoses is not known, but in a retrospective clinical review of a heterogeneous group of 154 published patients with primary systemic amyloidoses (171) an overall incidence of ocular involvement was found in 8.4% of the cases. This biased sample included many cases of transthyretin amyloidosis, which has a high incidence of vitreal amyloidosis.

With the exception of the transthyretin and gelsolin amyloidoses clinically significant ocular amyloid deposits usually indicate a localized disease. Amyloid in the vitreous is the hallmark of a systemic disorder and amyloidosis of the eyelids is virtually pathognomonic of systemic amyloidosis (20,162). Although orbital amyloidosis is usually a localized disorder it may be a manifestation of multiple myeloma (162). Deposits of amyloid may apparently be localized to the palpebral conjunctiva, but may also be a component of systemic amyloidosis (200), including multiple myeloma-associated amyloid (162).

Glaucoma can accompany vitreal amyloidosis (126,156), and amyloid has been noted in the trabecular meshwork of an eye with secondary open angle glaucoma (156), but has not been documented in this part of the eye in patients with normal intraocular pressure. A hemorrhagic diathesis is common in systemic forms of amyloidosis apparently due to a deficiency of clotting factor X, which seems to bind nonspecifically to amyloid fibrils. Ecchymoses of the eyelids and retinal hemorrhages can develop in such cases.

Histopathologic studies of ocular tissues in patients with the systemic amyloidoses have disclosed variable amounts of amyloid in ocular and adnexal tissues, and particularly in the choroidal blood vessels. The vascular deposition of amyloid does not appear to interfere with the transport of nutrients across blood vessels as marked choroidal amyloidosis with occlusion of the choriocapillaris in a fatal case of multiple myeloma still had a morphologically normal overlying retina (212).

The vascular walls in the conjunctiva, retina, choroid, and extraocular muscles may contain amyloid in idiopathic primary systemic amyloidosis, as well as in some inherited varieties of amyloidosis mentioned above. In several histopathologic studies the uveal blood vessels, particularly those of the choroid, have contained variable amounts of amyloid.

Rarely small clinically insignificant deposits of amyloid have been documented in the eyelid, sclera, conjunctiva, uvea, optic nerve, extraocular muscles, and other orbital tissues in systemic secondary amyloidosis (49,163,168). In lepromatous leprosy with secondary amyloidosis, amyloid has been noted in the vascular walls of the choriocapillaris, and in larger choroidal blood vessels as well as in Bruch membrane (168), in the iris of a patient with leprosy (163). Amyloid deposits have not been documented in the retina and vitreous in secondary amyloidosis.

REFERENCES

1. Abrahamson M, Grubb A. Increased body-temperature accelerates aggregation of the Leu-68-Gln mutant cystatin-C, the amyloid-forming protein in hereditary cystatin-C amyloid angiopathy. Proc Natl Acad Sci USA 1994; 91: 1416–20.
2. Amari F, Umihira J, Nohara M. Electron microscopic immunohistochemistry of ocular and extraocular pseudoexfoliative material. Exp Eye Res 1997; 65:51–6.
3. Ando Y, Nakamura M, Kai H, et al. A novel localized amyloidosis associated with lactoferrin in the cornea. Lab Invest 2002; 82:757–65.
4. Andrade C. A peculiar form of peripheral neuropathy: familiar a typical generalized amyloidosis with special involvement of the peripheral nerves. Brain 1952; 75: 408–27.

5. Araki-Sasaki K, Ando Y, Nakamura M, et al. Lactoferrin Glu561Asp facilitates secondary amyloidosis in the cornea. Br J Ophthalmol 2005; 89:684–8.
6. Asl LH, Liepnicks JJ, Uemichi T, et al. Renal amyloidosis with a frame shift mutation in fibrinogen A (alpha)-chain gene producing a novel amyloid protein. Blood 1997; 90: 4799–805.
7. Behal ML. Secondary amyloid infiltration around the limbus. Br J Ophthalmol 1964; 48:622–3.
8. Benditt EP, Eriksen N. Chemical classes of amyloid substance. Am J Pathol 1971; 65:231–49.
9. Bennett MJ, Sawaya MR, Eisenberg D. Deposition diseases and 3D domain swapping. Structure 2006; 14: 811–24.
10. Benson MD. Amyloidosis. In: Scriver CR, Beaudet AL, Sly WS, Valle D, eds. The Metabolic Basis of Inherited Disease, vol 4, 8th ed. New York, NY: McGraw-Hill, 2001:5345–78 [chap. 209].
11. Benson MD, Liepnieks J, Uemichi T, et al. Hereditary renal amyloidosis associated with a mutant fibrinogen alpha-chain. Nature Genet 1993; 3:252–5.
12. Benson MD, Liepnieks JJ, Yazaki M, et al. A new human hereditary amyloidosis: the result of a stop-codon mutation in the apolipoprotein AII gene. Genomics 2001; 72:272–7.
13. Bergstrom J, Murphy C, Eulitz M, et al. Codeposition of apolipoprotein A-IV and transthyretin in senile systemic (ATTR) amyloidosis. Biochem Biophys Res Commun 2001; 285:903–8.
14. Bergstrom J, Murphy CL, Weiss DT, et al. Two different types of amyloid deposits—apolipoprotein A-IV and transthyretin—in a patient with systemic amyloidosis. Lab Invest 2004; 84:981–8.
15. Bitan G, Kirkitadze MD, Lomakin A, et al. Amyloid beta-protein (A beta) assembly: a beta 40 and A beta 42 oligomerize through distinct pathways. Proc Natl Acad Sci USA 2003; 100:330–5.
16. Blevins G, Macaulay R, Harder S, et al. Oculoleptomeningeal amyloidosis in a large kindred with a new transthyretin variant Tyr69His. Neurology 2003; 60:1625–30.
17. Bononi PL, Martinez AJ, Nelson PB, et al. Amyloid deposits in a prolactin-producing pituitary-adenoma. J Endocrinol Invest 1993; 16:339–43.
18. Bowen RA, Hassard DTR, Wong VG, et al. Lattice dystrophy of the cornea as a variety of amyloidosis. Am J Ophthalmol 1970; 70:822–5.
19. Brown P, Goldfarb LG, Gajdusek DC. The new biology of spongiform encephalopathy: infectious amyloidosis with genetic twist. Lancet 1991; 337:1019–22.
20. Brownstein MH, Elliot R, Helwig EB. Ophthalmologic aspects of amyloidosis. Am J Ophthalmol 1970; 69:423–30.
21. Buxbaum JN. Diseases of protein conformation: what do in vitro experiments tell us about in vivo diseases? Trends Biochem Sci 2003; 28:585–92.
22. Buxbaum J, Caron D, Gallo G. AL amyloid, L-chain and L and H-chain deposition diseases: comparison of Ig synthesis and tissue deposition. In: Natvig JB, Førre O, Husby G, Husebekk A, Skogen B, Sletten K, Westermark P, eds. Amyloid and Amyloidosis. Dordrecht: Kluwer Academic Publishers, 1991:197–200.
23. Castano EM, Frangione B. Human amyloidosis, Alzheimer's disease and related disorders. Lab Invest 1988; 58:122–32.
24. Caughey B, Lansbury PT. Protofibrils, pores, fibrils, and neurodegeneration: separating the responsible protein aggregates from the innocent bystanders. Ann Rev Neurosci 2003; 26:267–98.
25. Cheung P, Kao, F-T, Law ML, et al. Localization of the structural gene for human apolipoprotein A-1 on the long arm of human chromosome 11. Proc Natl Acad Sci USA 1984; 81:508–11.
26. Chiti F, Webster P, Taddei N, et al. Designing conditions for in vitro formation of amyloid protofilaments and fibrils. Proc Natl Acad Sci USA 1999; 96:3590–4.
27. Cohen AS, Cathcart ES, Skinner M. Amyloidosis: current trends in its investigation. Arth Rheum 1978; 21:153–60.
28. Collyer RT. Amyloidosis of the cornea. Can J Ophthalmol 1968; 3:35–8.
29. Crawford JB. Cotton wool exudates in systemic amyloidosis. Arch Ophthalmol 1967; 78:214–6.
30. Dark AJ, Streeten BW, Cornwall CC. Pseudoexfoliative disease of the lens: a study in electron microscopy and histochemistry. Br J Ophthalmol 1977; 61:462–72.
31. Defoe DM, Martone RL, Caldwell RB, et al. Transthyretin secretion by cultured rat retinal pigment epithelium. Invest Ophthalmol Vis Sci 1992; 33(Suppl.):911.
32. de la Chapelle A, Tolvanen R, Boysen G, et al. Gelsolin-derived familial amyloidosis caused by asparagine or tyrosine substitution for aspartic acid at residue 187. Nat Genet 1992; 2:157–60.
33. De Souza AR. Amiloidose cutanea bulhosa familial observacao de 4 casos. Rev Hosp Clin Fac Med S Paulo 1963; 18:413–7.
34. Dhermy P, Pouliquen Y, Salvodelli M. Amylose secondaire localisée de la cornée. Arch Ophtalmol (Paris) 1973; 33:501–23.
35. Dickson PW, Schreiber G. High levels of messenger RNA for transthyretin (prealbumin) in human choroid plexus. Neurosci Lett 1986; 66:311–5.
36. Divry P. Etude histo-chimique des plaques séniles. J Neurol Psychiat 1927; 27:643–7.
37. Dobson CM. Principles of protein folding, misfolding and aggregation. Semin Cell Develop Biol 2004; 15:3–16.
38. Doft DH, Machemer R, Skinner M, et al. Pars plana vitrectomy for vitreous amyloidosis. Ophthalmology 1987; 94:607–11.
39. Dutts S, Elner VM, Soong HK, et al. Secondary localized amyloidosis in interstitial keratitis: clinicopathologic findings. Ophthalmology 1992; 99:817–23.
40. Eiferman RA, Rodrigues MM, Laibson PR, Arentsen JJ. Schnyder's crystalline dystrophy associated with amyloid deposition. Metab Pediatr Ophthalmol 1979; 3: 15–20.
41. Falls HF, Jackson J, Carey JH, et al. Ocular manifestations of hereditary primary systemic amyloidosis. Arch Ophthalmol 1955; 54:660–4.
42. Ferry AP, Leiberman TW. Bilateral amyloidosis of the vitreous body: report of a case without systemic and familial involvement. Arch Ophthalmol 1976; 94:982–91.
43. Franklin EC, Pras M. Immunologic studies of water-soluble human amyloid fibrils: comparative studies of eight amyloid preparations. J Exp Med 1969; 130:797–808.
44. Franklin EC, Rosenthal CJ, Pras M, Levin M. Recent progress in amyloid. In: Beers RF, Basset EG, eds. The Role of Immunological Factors in Infectious, Allergic, and Autoimmune Processes. New York, NY: Raven Press, 1976:163–74.
45. Garner A. Amyloidosis of the cornea. Br J Ophthalmol 1969; 53:73–81.
46. Gazit E. A possible role for π-stacking in the self-assembly of amyloid fibrils. FASEB J 2002; 16:77–83.
47. Gejyo F, Maruyama S, Maruyama N, et al. β_2-Microglobulin-derived amyloid and calcium in long-term dialysis patients. In: Natvig JB, Forre O, Husby G,

Husebekk A, Skogen B, Sletten K, Westermark P, eds. Amyloid and Amyloidosis. Dordrecht: Kluwer Academic Publishers, 1991:377–80.
48. Ghiso J, Haltia M, Prelli F, et al. Gelsolin variant (ASN-187) in familial amyloidosis, Finnish type. Biochem J 1990; 272:827–30.
49. Giarelli L, Bonito L, Di Melato M. Dans quelle mesure les tissue orbitaires (intra-et extra-ocularies) sont concernés dans l'amyloidose-Lignes de comportement déduites sur la base de 10 observations. Arch Ophtalmol (Paris) 1973; 33:757–62.
50. Glabe CG, Kayed R. Common structure and toxic function of amyloid oligomers implies a common mechanism of pathogenesis. Neurology 2006; 66:S74–8.
51. Glenner GG, Ein D, Eanes ED, et al. Creation of amyloid fibrils from Bence–Jones proteins in vitro. Science 1971; 174:712–4.
52. Glenner GG, Wong CW. Alzheimers-disease—initial report of the purification and characterization of a novel cerebrovascular amyloid protein. Biochem Biophys Res Commun 1984; 120:885–90.
53. Glenner GG, Terry W, Harada M, et al. Amyloid fibril proteins: proof of homology with immunoglobulin light chains by sequence analysis. Science 1971; 172: 1150–1.
54. Glenner GG, Terry WD, Isersky C. Amyloidosis: its nature and pathogenesis. Semin Hematol 1973; 10:65–86.
55. Goette A, Rocken C. Atrial amyloidosis and atrial fibrillation: a gender-dependent "arrhythmogenic substrate"? Eur Heart J 2004; 25:1185–6.
56. Goldberg AL. Protein degradation and protection against misfolded or damaged proteins. Nature 2003; 426: 895–9.
57. Goldgaber D, Lerman MI, McBride OW, et al. Characterization and chromosomal localization of a cDNA encoding brain amyloid of Alzheimer's disease. Science 1987; 235:877–80.
58. Goren H, Steinberg MC, Farboody GH. Familial oculoleptomeningeal amyloidosis. Brain 1980; 103: 473–95.
59. Gorevic PD, Munoz PC, Gorgone G, et al. Amyloidosis due to a mutation of the gelsolin gene in an American family with lattice corneal dystrophy type II. N Engl J Med 1991; 325:1780–5.
60. Gorevic PD, Munoz PC, Rodrigues M, et al. Shared gelsolin antigenicity between familial amyloidosis Finnish type (FAF) and one form of familial lattice corneal dystrophy (LCD) with polyneuropathy from the United States. In: Natvig JB, Forre O, Husby G, Husebekk A, Skogen B, Sletten K, Westermark P, eds. Amyloid and Amyloidosis. Dordrecht: Kluwer Academic Publishers, 1991:423–35.
61. Gorevic PD, Prelli FC, Wright J, et al. Systemic senile amyloidosis. Identification of a new prealbumin (transthyretin) variant in cardiac tissue: immunologic and biochemical similarity to one form of familial amyloidotic polyneuropathy. J Clin Invest 1989; 83:836–43.
62. Grabowski TJ, Cho HS, Vonsattel JPG, et al. Novel amyloid precursor protein mutation in an Iowa family with dementia and severe cerebral amyloid angiopathy. Ann Neurol 2001; 49:697–705.
63. Granel B, Valleix S, Serratrice J, et al. Lysozyme amyloidosis—report of 4 cases and a review of the literature. Medicine 2006; 85:66–73.
64. Green WR. Diagnostic cytopathology of ocular fluid specimens. Ophthalmology 1984; 91:726–49.
65. Grubb A, Jensson O, Gudmundsson G, et al. Abnormal metabolism of gamma-trace alkaline microprotein: the basic defect in hereditary cerebral hemorrhage with amyloidosis. N Engl J Med 1984; 311:1547–9.
66. Gundmundsson G, Hallgrimsson J, Jonasson TA, Bjarnason O. Hereditary cerebral haemorrhage with amyloidosis. Brain 1972; 95:387–404.
67. Gussow D, Rein R, Ginjaar I, et al. The human beta-2-microglobulin gene—primary structure and definition of the transcriptional unit. J Immunol 1987; 139:3132–8.
68. Haltia M, Prelli F, Ghiso J, et al. Amyloid protein in familial amyloidosis (Finnish type) is homologous to gelsolin, an actin-binding protein. Biochem Biophys Res Commun 1990; 167:927–32.
69. Hamburg A. Unusual cause of vitreous opacities: primary familial amyloidosis. Ophthalmologica 1971; 162:173–7.
70. Handousa A. Localized intra-orbital amyloid disease. Br J Ophthalmol 1954; 38:510–1.
71. Hayasaka S, Setogawa T, Ohmura M. Secondary localized amyloidosis of the cornea caused by trichiasis. Ophthalmologica 1987; 194:77–81.
72. Heller H, Missmahl H-P, Sohar E, Gafni J. Amyloidosis: its differentiation into peri-reticulin and peri-collagen types. J Path Bact 1964; 88:15–34.
73. Herbert H. Colloid degeneration of the conjunctiva. Trans Ophthalmol Soc UK 1902; 22:261–6.
74. Herbert J, Mizuno R, Cavallaro T. Transthyretin gene expression in the developing rat retinal pigment epithelium (RPE). Invest Ophthalmol Vis Sci 1991; 32(Suppl.): 1011.
75. Hidayat AA, Risco JM. Amyloidosis of the corneal stroma in patients with trachoma: a clinicopathologic study of 62 cases. Ophthalmology 1989; 8:1203–11.
76. Hill JC, Maske R, Bowen RM. Secondary localized amyloidosis of the cornea associated with tertiary syphilis. Cornea 1990; 9:98–101.
77. Hiltunen T, Kiuru S, Hongell T, et al. Finnish type of familial amyloidosis: cosegregation of ASP_{187}?ASN mutation of gelsolin with the disease in three large families. Am J Genet 1991; 49:522–8.
78. Hinton DR, Polk RK, Linse KD, et al. Characterization of spherical amyloid protein from a prolactin-producing pituitary adenoma. Acta Neuropathol 1997; 93:43–9.
79. Hinzpeter EN, Naumann G. Zur sekundären Amyloidose der Hornhaut. Albrecht Graefes Arch Clin Exp Ophthalmol 1974; 192:19–25.
80. Hitchings RA, Tripathi RC. Vitreous opacities in primary amyloid disease: a clinical, histochemical, and ultrastructural report. Br J Ophthalmol 1976; 60:41–54.
81. Hogan MJ, Alvarado J. Ultrastructure of lattice dystrophy of the cornea: a case report. Am J Ophthalmol 1967; 64: 656–60.
82. Howard GM. Amyloid tumours of the orbit. Br J Ophthalmol 1966; 50:421–5.
83. Husby G, Araki S, Benditt EP, et al. The 1990 guidelines for nomenclature and classification of amyloid and amyloidosis. In: Natvig JB, Forre O, Husby G, Husebekk A, Skogen B, Sletten K, Westermark P, eds. Amyloid and Amyloidosis. Dordrecht: Kluwer Academic Publishers, 1991:7–11.
84. Husby G, Ranlov PJ, Sletten K, Marhaug G. Prealbumin nature of the amyloid in familial amyloid cardiomyopathy of Danish origin. In: Glenner GG, Osserman EF, Benditt EP, Calkins E, Cohen AS, Zucker-Franklin D, eds. Amyloidosis. New York, NY: Plenum, 1986:391–9.

85. Inouye H, Domingues FS, Damas AM, et al. Analysis of x-ray diffraction patterns from amyloid of biopsied vitreous humor and kidney of transthyretin (TTR) Met30 familial amyloidotic polyneuropathy (FAP) patients: axially arrayed TTR monomers constitute the protofilament. Amyloid-International J Exp Clin Invest 1998; 5:163–74.
86. Isaak L. Localized amyloidosis cutis associated with psoriasis in siblings. Arch Dermatol Syph 1950; 61: 859–62.
87. Isersky C, Ein D, Page EL, et al. Immunochemical cross-reactions of human amyloid proteins with human immunoglobulin light polypeptide chains. J Immunol 1972; 108:486–93.
88. Isobe T, Osserman EF. Patterns of amyloidosis and their association with plasma cell dyscrasia, monoclonal immunoglobulins and Bence–Jones protein. N Engl J Med 1974; 290:473–7.
89. Jacobson DR, Buxbaum JN. Genetic aspects of amyloidosis. Adv Hum Genet 1991; 20:69–123.
90. Janciauskiene S, Krakau T. Alzheimer's peptide: a possible link between glaucoma, exfoliation syndrome and Alzheimer's disease. Acta Ophthalmol Scand 2001; 79:328–9.
91. Kantarjian AD, de Jong RN. Familial primary amyloidosis with nervous system involvement. Neurology 1953; 3: 399–409.
92. Kaplan B, Martin BM, Livneh A, et al. Biochemical subtyping of amyloid in formalin-fixed tissue samples confirms and supplements immunohistologic data. Am J Clin Pathol 2004; 121:794–800.
93. Kasner D, Miller G, Taylor WH, et al. Surgical treatment of amyloidosis of the vitreous. Trans Am Acad Ophthalmol Otolaryngol 1968; 72:410–21.
94. Kaufman HE. Primary familial amyloidosis. Arch Ophthalmol 1958; 60:1036–43.
95. Kaufman HE, Thomas LB. Vitreous opacities diagnostic of familial primary amyloidosis. N Engl J Med 1959; 261: 1267–71.
96. Kaunisto N. Lattice dystrophy of the cornea: its connection with preceding episodes of crystals and with subsequent amyloidosis. Acta Ophthalmol 1973; 51: 335–52.
97. Khurana R, Agarwal A, Bajpai VK, et al. Unraveling the amyloid associated with human medullary thyroid carcinoma. Endocrinol 2004; 145:5465–70.
98. King ME, Kan HM, Baas PW, et al. Tau-dependent microtubule disassembly initiated by prefibrillar beta-amyloid. J Cell Biol 2006; 175:541–6.
99. Kisilevsky R, Fraser P. Proteoglycans and amyloid fibrillogenesis. In: Bock GR, Goode JA, eds. The Nature and Origin of Amyloid Fibrils, Ciba Foundation Symposium 199, New York, NY: John Wiley & Sons, 1996:58–72.
100. Klemen UM, Kulnig W, Radda TM. Secondary corneal amyloidosis: clinical and pathological examinations. Albrecht Graefes Arch Klin Exp Ophthalmol 1983; 220: 130–8.
101. Klintworth GK. Lattice corneal dystrophy: an inherited variety of amyloidosis restricted to the cornea. Am J Pathol 1967; 50:371–99.
102. Klintworth GK, Ferry AP, Sugar A, Reed J. Recurrence of lattice corneal dystrophy type 1 in the corneal grafts of two siblings. Am J Ophthalmol 1982; 94:540–6.
103. Klintworth GK, Valnickova Z, Kielar RA, et al. Familial subepithelial corneal amyloidosis—a lactoferrin-related amyloidosis. Invest Ophthalmol Vis Sci 1997; 38: 2756–63.
104. Knowles DM, Jakobiec FA, Rosen M, Howard G. Amyloidosis of the orbit and adnexae. Surv Ophthalmol 1975; 19:367–84.
105. Koga T, Ando E, Hirata A, et al. Vitreous opacities and outcome of vitreous surgery in patients with familial amyloidotic polyneuropathy. Am J Ophthalmol 2003; 135: 188–93.
106. König B, Pur S. Amyloidoza rohovky. Cesk Oftal 1966; 22: 187–91.
107. Korenaga T, Yan JM, Sawashita J, et al. Transmission of amyloidosis in offspring of mice with AApoAII amyloidosis. Am J Pathol 2006; 168:898–906.
108. Korvatska E, Henry H, Mashima Y, et al. Amyloid and non-amyloid forms of 5q31-linked corneal dystrophy resulting from kerato-epithelin mutations at Arg-124 are associated with abnormal turnover of the protein. J Biol Chem 2000; 275:11465–9.
109. Krachmer JH, Dubord PJ, Rodrigues MM, Mannis MJ. Corneal posterior crocodile shagreen and polymorphic amyloid degeneration. Arch Ophthalmol 1983; 101: 54–9.
110. Kwiatkowski DJ, Stossel TP, Orkin SH, et al. Plasma and cytoplasmic gelsolins are encoded by a single gene and contain a duplicated actin-binding domain. Nature 1986; 323:455–8.
111. Kyle RA. Primary systemic amyloidosis (AL) in 1990. In: Natvig JB, Forre O, Husby G, Husebekk A, Skogen B, Sletten K, Westermark P, eds. Amyloid and Amyloidosis. Dordrecht: Kluwer Academic Publishers, 1991:147–52.
112. Kyle RA. Amyloidosis: a convoluted story. Br J Haem 2001; 114:529–38.
113. Lachman HJ, Chir B, Booth DR, et al. Misdiagnosis of hereditary amyloidosis as AL (primary) amyloidosis. New Eng J Med 2002; 346:1786–91.
114. Lanier JD, Fine M, Togni B. Lattice corneal dystrophy. Arch Ophthalmol 1976; 94:921–4.
115. Larsson A, Peng SW, Persson H, et al. Lactadherin binds to elastin—a starting point for medin amyloid formation? Amyloid 2006; 13:78–85.
116. Lee S, Eisenberg D. Seeded conversion of recombinant prion protein to a disulfide-bonded oligomer by a reduction-oxidation process. Nat Struct Biol 2003; 10: 725–30.
117. Legrand J, Guenel J, Dubigeon P. Glaucome et opacification du vitré par amylose. Bull Soc Ophthalmol Fr 1968; 68:13–20.
118. Leone O, Boriani G, Chiappini B, et al. Amyloid deposition as a cause of a trial remodelling in persistent valvular atrial fibrillation. Eur Heart J 2004; 25: 1237–41.
119. Lessell S, Wolf PA, Benson MD, Cohen AS. Scalloped pupils in familial amyloidosis. N Engl J Med 1975; 293: 914–5.
120. Letterer E. History and development of amyloid research. In: Mandema E, Ruinen L, Scholten JH, Cohen AS, eds. Amyloidosis, Proceedings of the Symposium on Amyloidosis, University of Groningen, the Netherlands, September 24–28, 1967. Amsterdam, Excerpta Medica, 1968:3–9.
121. Leveugle B, Spik G, Perl DP, et al. The iron-binding protein lactotransferrin is present in pathologic lesions in a variety of neurodegenerative disorders: a comparative immunohistochemical analysis. Brain Res 1994; 650: 20–31.

122. Levy E, Haltia M, Fernandz-Madrid I, et al. Mutation in gelsolin gene in Finnish hereditary amyloidosis. J Exp Med 1990; 172:1865–7.
123. Levy E, Lopez-Otin C, Ghiso J, et al. Stroke in Icelandic patients with hereditary amyloid angiopathy is related to a mutation in the cystatin C gene, an inhibitor of cysteine proteases. J Exp Med 1989; 169:1771–8.
124. Li Z-Y, Streeten, BW, Wallace RN. Association of elastin with pseudoexfoliative material. An immunoelectron microscopic study. Curr Eye Res 1988; 7:1163–72.
125. Li Z-Y, Streeten BW, Yohai N. Amyloid P protein in pseudoexfoliative fibrillopathy. Curr Eye Res 1989; 8: 217–27.
126. Limon S, Rousselie F, Joseph E. A propos d'une observation familiale d'amylose vitrénne héréditaire associée à un glaucome. Arch Ophtalmol (Paris) 1973; 33:525–8.
127. Loeffler KU, Edward DP, Tso MOM. An immunohistochemical study of gelsolin immunoreactivity in corneal amyloidosis. Am J Ophthalmol 1992; 113:546–54.
128. Lundmark K, Westermark GT, Nystrom S, et al. Transmissibility of systemic amyloidosis by a prion-like mechanism. Proc Natl Acad Sci USA 2002; 99: 6979–84.
129. Luyendiijk W, Bots GTAM. Hereditary cerebral haemorrhage (letter). Scand J Clin Lab Invest 1986; 46:391.
130. Mahloudji M, Teasdall RD, Adamkiewicz JJ, et al. The genetic amyloidoses with particular reference to hereditary neuropathic amyloidosis, type II (Indiana or Rukavina type). Medicine 1969; 48:1–37.
131. Makin OS, Serpell LC. Structures for amyloid fibrils. FEBS J 2005; 272:5950–61.
132. Mannis MJ, Krachmer JH, Rodrigues MM, Pardos GJ. Polymorphic amyloid degeneration of the cornea. Arch Ophthalmol 1981; 99:1217–23.
133. Margolis G. Senile cerebral disease—a critical survey of traditional concepts based upon observations with newer techniques. Lab Invest 1959; 8:335–70.
134. Maury CPJ. Isolation and characterization of cardiac amyloid in familial amyloid polyneuropathy type IV (Finnish): relation of amyloid protein to variant gelsolin. Biochem Biophys Acta 1990; 1096:84–6.
135. Maury CPJ, Alli K, Baumann M. Finnish hereditary amyloidosis: amino acid sequence homology between the amyloid fibril protein and human plasma gelsoline. FEBS Lett 1990; 260:85–7.
136. Maury CPJ, Alli K, Baumann M. Complete primary structure of amyloid protein in Finnish hereditary amyloidosis. Identification of a new type of amyloid protein derived from variant (Asn-187) gelsolin. In: Natvig JB, Forre O, Husby G, Husebekk A, Skogen B, Sletten K, Westermark P, eds. Amyloid and Amyloidosis. Dordrecht: Kluwer Academic Publishers, 1991:405–8.
137. McClure J, Bartley CJ, Ackrill P. Carpal tunnel syndrome caused by amyloid containing beta-2-microglobulin: a new amyloid and a complication of long term haemodialysis. Ann Rheum Dis 1986; 45:1007–11.
138. McKusick VA. Mendelian Inheritance in Man: a Catalog of Human Genes and Genetic Disorders. 12th ed. Baltimore: Johns Hopkins University Press, 1998.
139. McPherson SD Jr., Kiffney GT Jr. Some histologic findings in keratoconus. Arch Ophthalmol 1968; 79: 669–73.
140. McPherson SD Jr., Kiffney GT Jr., Freed CC. Corneal amyloidosis. Trans Am Ophthalmol Soc 1966; 64:148–62 (also in Am J Ophthalmol 1966; 62:1024–33.)
141. Meretoja J. Familial systemic paramyloidosis with lattice dystrophy of the cornea, progressive cranial neuropathy, skin changes and various internal symptoms. I. A previously unrecognized heritable syndrome. Ann Clin Res 1969; 1:314–24.
142. Meretoja J. Comparative histopathological and clinical findings in eyes with lattice corneal dystrophy of two different types. Ophthalmologica 1972; 165:15–37.
143. Meretoja J, Teppo L. Histopathological findings of familial amyloidosis with cranial neuropathy as principal manifestation. Acta Path Microbiol Scand (A) 1971; 79: 432–40.
144. Mondino BJ, Rabb MF, Sugar J, et al. Primary familial amyloidosis of the cornea. Am J Ophthalmol 1981; 92: 732–6.
145. Mondino BJ, Sundar Raj CV, Skinner M, et al. Protein AA and lattice corneal dystrophy. Am J Ophthalmol 1980; 89: 377–80.
146. Moses AC, Lawlor J, Haddow J, Jackson IM. Familial euthyroid hyperthyroxinemia resulting from increased thyroxine binding to thyroxine-binding pre-albumin. New Engl J Med 1982; 306:966–9.
147. Murakami A, Fujiki K, Hasegawa S, et al. Transthyretin Ser-44 mutation in a case with vitreous amyloidosis. Am J Ophthalmol 2002; 133:272–3.
148. Nayeem MS, Khan RH. Misfolded proteins and human diseases. Protein Peptide Lett 2004; 11:593–600.
149. Nelson R, Sawaya MR, Balbirnie M, et al. Structure of the cross-beta spine of amyloid-like fibrils. Nature 2005; 435: 773–8.
150. Nichols WC, Dwulet FE, Liepnieks J, Benson MD. Variant apolipoprotein A1 as a major constituent of a human hereditary amyloid. Biochem Biophys Res Commun 1988; 156:762–8.
151. Nichols WC, Liepnieks JJ, McKusick VA, Benson MD. Direct sequencing of the gene for Maryland/German familial amyloidotic polyneuropathy type II and genotyping by allele-specific enzymatic amplification. Genomics 1989; 5:535–40.
152. Nilsson MR, Dobson CM. In vitro characterization of lactoferrin aggregation and amyloid formation. Biochemistry 2003; 42:375–82.
153. Osserman EF. Analysis of amyloid-related Bence–Jones proteins (TEW BJκ and MCG BJλ) and the "non-immunoglobulin" amyloid protein AA: hypervariable region homologies and their possible significance. In: Wegelius O, Pasternack A, eds. Amyloidosis, Proceedings of the Fifth Sigrid Jusélius Foundation Symposium. New York, NY: Academic Press, 1976:223–31.
154. Ozaki M. Familial lichen amyloidosis. Int J Dermatol 1984; 23:190–3.
155. Partington MW, Marriott PJ, Prentice RSA, et al. Familial cutaneous amyloidosis with systemic manifestations in males. Am J Med Genet 1981; 10:65–75.
156. Paton D, Duke JR. Primary familial amyloidosis: ocular manifestations with histopathologic observations. Am J Ophthalmol 1966; 61:736–47.
157. Pearse AGE, Ewen SWB, Polak JM. The genesis of apudamyloid in endocrine polypeptide tumours: histochemical distinction from immunoamyloid. Virchows Arch Abt B Zellpath 1972; 10:93–107.
158. Pepys MB. Amyloidosis. Ann Rev Med 2006; 57: 223–41.
159. Petersen RB, Goren H, Cohen M, et al. Transthyretin amyloidosis: a new mutation associated with dementia. Ann Neurol 1997; 41:307–13.

160. Puchtler H, Sweat F, Levine M. On binding of Congo red by amyloid. J Histochem Cytochem 1962; 10: 355–64.
161. Purcell JJ Jr., Rodrigues MM, Chishti MI, et al. Lattice corneal dystrophy associated with familial systemic amyloidosis (Meretoja's syndrome). Ophthalmology 1983; 90:1512–7.
162. Raflo GT, Farrell TA, Siossat RS. Complete ophthalmoplegia secondary to amyloidosis associated with multiple myeloma. Am J Ophthalmol 1981; 92:221–4.
163. Ratnakar KS, Mohan M. Amyloidosis of the iris. Can J Ophthalmol 1976; 11:256–7.
164. Reches M, Gazit E. Amyloidogenic hexapeptide fragment of medin: homology to functional islet amyloid polypeptide fragments. Amyloid 2004; 11:81–9.
165. Refetoff S, Marinov VSZ, Tunca H, et al. A new family with hyperthyroxinemia caused by transthyretin Val (109) misdiagnosed as thyrotoxicosis and resistance to thyroid hormone—a clinical research center study. J Clin Endocrinol Metab 1996; 81:3335–40.
166. Ringvold A. Update on etiology and pathogenesis of the pseudoexfoliation syndrome. New Trends Ophthalmol 1993; 8:177–80.
167. Ringvold A, Husby G. Pseudoexfoliation material: an amyloid-like substance. Exp Eye Res 1973; 17:289–99.
168. Rodrigues M, Zimmerman LE. Secondary amyloidosis in ocular leprosy. Arch Ophthalmol 1971; 85:277–9.
169. Rokitansky K. Handbuch der Pathologischen Anatomie, Vol. 3. Vienna: Bramüller und Seidel, 1842–1846:311–2.
170. Rubinow A, Cohen AS. Scalloped pupils in familial amyloid polyneuropathy. Arth Rheumat 1986; 29:445–7.
171. Rukavina JG, Block WD, Jackson CE, et al. Primary systemic amyloidosis: a review and an experimental, genetic and clinical study of 29 cases with particular emphasis on the familial form. Medicine 1956; 35: 239–334.
172. Sagher F, Shanon J. Amyloidosis cutis: familial occurrence in three generations. Arch Dermatol 1963; 87: 171–5.
173. Salvi G, Salvi F, Mencucci R, et al. Transthyretin-related (TTR) hereditary amyloidosis of the vitreous body: clinical and molecular characterization in two Italian families. Communication to IX Meeting of the International Society for Genetic Eye Disease and VI International Symposium on Retinoblastoma, Siena, Italy, June 1–3, 1992.
174. Sambashivan S, Liu YS, Sawaya MR, et al. Amyloid-like fibrils of ribonuclease A with three-dimensional domain-swapped and native-like structure. Nature 2005; 437: 266–9.
175. Sandgren O, Holmgren G, Lundgren E. Vitreous amyloidosis associated with homozygosity for the transthretin methionine-30 gene. Arch Ophthalmol 1990; 108:1584–6.
176. Sandgren O, Holmgren G, Lundgren E, Steen L. Restriction fragment length polymorphism analysis of mutated transthyretin in vitreous amyloidosis. Arch Ophthalmol 1988; 106:790–2.
177. Sandgren O, Westermark P, Stenkula S. Relation of vitreous amyloidosis to prealbumin. Ophthalmic Res 1986; 18:98–103.
178. Sanke T, Bell GI, Sample C, et al. An islet amyloid peptide is derived from an 89-amino acid precursor by proteolytic processing. J Biol Chem 1988; 263:17243–6.
179. Saraiva MJM. Transthyretin mutations in hyperthyroxinemia and amyloid diseases. Hum Mutat 2001; 17: 493–503.
180. Saraiva MJM, Costa PP, Goodman DS. Biochemical marker in familial amyloidotic polyneuropathy, Portuguese type: family studies on the transthyretin (prealbumin)-methionine-30 variant. J Clin Invest 1985; 76:2171–7.
181. Savage DJ, Mango CA, Streeten BW. Amyloidosis of the vitreous: fluorescein angiographic findings and association with neovascularization. Arch Ophthalmol 1982; 100: 1776–9.
182. Savino PJ, Schatz NJ, Rodrigues MM. Orbital amyloidosis. Can J Ophthalmol 1976; 11:252–5.
183. Schwartz MF, Green WR, Michels RG, et al. An unusual case of ocular involvement in primary systemic nonfamilial amyloidosis. Ophthalmology 1982; 89: 394–401.
184. Seitelberger F, Nemetz UR. Beitrag zur Frage der gittrigen Hornhaut-dystrophie. Albrecht von Graefes Arch Ophthalmol 1961; 164:102–11.
185. Sellar GC, Oghene K, Boyle S, et al. Organization of the region encompassing the human serum amyloid-A (Saa) gene family on chromosome-11p15.1. Genomics 1994; 23: 492–5.
186. Shoji M, Matsushita T, Higuchi K, et al. Senile ocular amyloidosis in SAM and BALB/c strains of mice. Mech Ageing Develop 2000; 120:87–94.
187. Sipe JD, Cohen AS. Review: history of the amyloid fibril. J Struc Biol 2000; 130:88–98.
188. Skinner M, Benson MD, Cohen AS. Amyloid fibril protein related to immunoglobulin λ-chains. J Immunol 1975; 114: 1433–5.
189. Skinner M, Cohen AS, Benson MD. Serum amyloid p-component (SAP) levels in normals, amyloidotic patients and in malignancy. Fed Proc 1978; 37:753.
190. Skinner M, Cohen AS, Shirahama T, Cathcart ES. P-component (pentagonal unit) of amyloid: isolation, characterization and sequence analysis. J Lab Clin Med 1974; 84:604–14.
191. Skinner M, Harding J, Skare J, et al. A new transthyretin mutation associated with amyloidotic vitreous opacities: asparagine for isoleucine at position 84. Ophthalmology 1992; 99:503–8.
192. Sletten K, Westermark P, Natvig JB. Characterization of amyloid fibril proteins from medullary carcinoma of thyroid. J Exp Med 1976; 143:993–8.
193. Smith ME, Zimmerman LE. Amyloidosis of the eyelid and conjunctiva. Arch Ophthalmol 1966; 75: 42–50.
194. Smith ME, Zimmerman LE. Amyloid in corneal dystrophies: differentiation of lattice from granular and macular dystrophies. Arch Ophthalmol 1968; 79:407–12.
195. Solomon A, Weiss DT. Experimental production of human amyloidosis AL. In: Natvig JB, Forre O, Husby G, Husebekk A, Skogen B, Sletten K, Westermark P, eds. Amyloid and Amyloidosis. Dordrecht: Kluwer Academic Publishers, 1991:193–6.
196. Souza Queiroz L, de Brick M. Degenerançāo reticular familial da cornea apresentaçāe de 10 casos e etudo histopathologico. Arg Inst Penido Burnier, Sao Paulo 1961; 18:94–106.
197. Spark EC, Shirahama T, Skinner M, Cohen AS. Identification of amyloid p-component (protein AP) in normal cultured human fibroblasts. Lab Invest 1978; 38: 556–9.
198. Sponne I, Fifre A, Drouet A, et al. Apoptotic neuronal cell death induced by the non-fibrillar amyloid-beta peptide proceeds through an early reactive oxygen

species-dependent cytoskeleton perturbation. J Biol Chem 2003; 278:3437–45.
199. Stafford WR, Fine BS. Amyloidosis of the cornea: report of a case without conjunctival involvement. Arch Ophthalmol 1966; 75:53–6.
200. Stansbury JR. Conjunctival amyloidosis in association with systemic amyloid disease. Am J Ophthalmol 1965; 59:24–9.
201. Starck T, Kenyon KR, Hanninen LA, et al. Clinical and histopathologic studies of two families with lattice corneal dystrophy and familial systemic amyloidosis (Meretoja syndrome). Ophthalmology 1991; 98:1197–206.
202. Stefani M, Dobson CM. Protein aggregation and aggregate toxicity: new insights into protein folding, misfolding diseases and biological evolution. J Mol Med 2003; 81: 678–99.
203. Stern GA, Knapp A, Hood CI. Corneal amyloidosis associated with keratoconus. Ophthalmology 1988; 95: 52–5.
204. Storkel S, Schneider HM, Muntefering H, Kashiwagi S. Iatrogenic, insulin-dependent, local amyloidosis. Lab Invest 1983; 48:108–11.
205. Streeten BW. Aberrant synthesis and aggregation of elastic tissue components in pseudoexfoliative fibrillopathy: a unifying concept. New Trends Ophthalmol 1993; 8:187–96.
206. Streeten BW, Gibson SA, Dark AJ. Pseudoexfoliative material contains an elastic microfibrillar-associated glycoprotein. Trans. Am Ophthalmol Soc 1986; 84:304–20.
207. Sunde M, Blake C. The structure of amyloid fibrils by electron microscopy and X-ray diffraction. Adv Protein Chem 1997; 50:123–59.
208. Sunde M, Serpell LC, Bartlam M, et al. Common core structure of amyloid fibrils by synchrotron X-ray diffraction. J Mol Biol 1997; 273:729–39.
209. Takacs L, Boross P, Tozser J, et al. Transforming growth factor-beta induced protein, betaIG-H3, is present in degraded form and altered localization in lattice corneal dystrophy type I. Exp Eye Res 1998; 66:739–45.
210. Tawara S, Nakazato M, Kangawa K, et al. Identification of amyloid prealbumin variant in familial amyloidotic polyneuropathy (Japanese type). Biochem Biophys Res Commun 1983; 116:880–8.
211. Terry WD, Page DL, Kimura S, et al. Structural identity of Bence–Jones and amyloid fibril proteins in a patient with plasma cell dyscrasia and amyloidosis. J Clin Invest 1973; 52:1276–81.
212. Ts'o MOM, Bettman JW. Occlusion of choriocapillaris in primary nonfamilial amyloidosis. Arch Ophthalmol 1971; 86:281–6.
213. Tsutsumi Y, Serizawa A, Hori S. Localized amyloidosis of the seminal vesicle: identification of lactoferrin immunoreactivity in the amyloid material. Pathol Int 1996; 46: 491–7.
214. Uemichi T, Liepnieks JJ, Yamada T, et al. A frame shift mutation in the fibrinogen A-alpha chain gene in a kindred with renal amyloidosis. Blood 1996; 87:4197–203.
215. Uemichi T, Uitti RJ, Koeppen AH, et al. Oculoleptomeningeal amyloidosis associated with a new transthyretin variant Ser64. Arch Neurol 1999; 56:1152–5.
216. Uitti RJ, Donat JR, Rozdilsky B, et al. Familial oculoleptomeningeal amyloidosis—report of a new family with unusual features. Arch Neurol 1988; 45:1118–22.
217. Van Duinen SG, Castano EM, Prelli F, et al. Hereditary cerebral hemorrhage with amyloidosis in patients of Dutch origin is related to Alzheimer's disease. Proc Natl Acad Sci USA 1987; 84:5991–4.
218. Vazquez JJ, Dixon FJ. Immunohistochemical analysis of amyloid by the fluorescence technique. J Exp Med 1956; 104:727–36.
219. Verchere CB, Dalessio DA, Palmiter RD, et al. Islet amyloid formation associated with hyperglycemia in transgenic mice with pancreatic beta cell expression of human islet amyloid polypeptide. Proc Natl Acad Sci USA 1996; 93:3492–6.
220. Vidal R, Frangione B, Rostagno A, et al. A stop-codon mutation in the BRI gene associated with familial British dementia. Nature 1999; 399:776–81.
221. Vidal R, Revesz T, Rostagno A, et al. A decamer duplication in the 3′ region of the BRI gene originates an amyloid peptide that is associated with dementia in a Danish kindred. Proc Natl Acad Sci USA 2000; 97:4920–5.
222. Virchow R. Ueber eine im Gehirn und Ruckenmark des Menschen aufgefunde Substaz mit der chemischen Reaction der Cellulose. Virchows Arch Path Anat 1854; 6:135–8.
223. Vogel and Scheiden Ann Phys Chem XLVI 327, 1839 cited in The Oxford English Dictionary, second edition, vol 1, Simpson JA, Weiner ESC, editors. Oxford, England: Clarendon Press, 1989:323.
224. Vogiatzis A, Marshall GE, Konstas AG, Lee WR. Immunogold study of non-collagenous matrix components in normal and exfoliative iris. Br J Ophthalmol 1994; 78:850–8.
225. Wallace MR, Dwulet FE, Conneally PM, Benson MD. Biochemical and molecular genetic characterization of a new variant prealbumin associated with hereditary amyloidosis. J Clin Invest 1986; 78:6–12.
226. Wallace MR, Dwulet FE, Williams EC, et al. Identification of a new prealbumin variant, Tyr-77 and detection of the gene by DNA analysis. J Clin Invest 1988; 81:189–93.
227. Walsh DM, Klyubin I, Fadeeva JV, et al. Naturally secreted oligomers of amyloid beta protein potently inhibit hippocampal long-term potentiation in vivo. Nature 2002; 416:535–9.
228. Westermark P, Benson MD, Buxbaum JN, et al. Amyloid: toward terminology clarification—report from the Nomenclature Committee of the International Society of Amyloidosis. Amyloid-J Protein Fold Disorder 2005; 12:1–4.
229. Westermark P, Engstrom U, Johnson KH, et al. Islet amyloid polypeptide—pinpointing amino-acid-residues linked to amyloid fibril formation. Proc Natl Acad Sci USA 1990; 87:5036–40.
230. Westermark P, Sletten K, Johansson B, Cornwell GG III. Fibril in senile systemic amyloidosis is derived from normal transthyretin. Proc Natl Acad Sci USA 1990; 87: 2843–5.
231. Wheeler GE, Eiferman RA. Immmunohistochemical identification of the AA protein in lattice dystrophy. Invest Ophthalmol Vis Sci 1981; 20(Suppl.):115.
232. Wisniewski HM, Terry RD. Reexamination of the pathogenesis of the senile plaque. In: Zimmerman HM, ed. Progress in Neuropathology, vol. 2, New York, NY: Grune and Stratton, 1973:1–26.
233. Wong VG, McFarlin DE. Primary familial amyloidosis. Arch Ophthalmol 1967; 78:208–13.
234. Woo P, Betts J, Edbrooke M. The human serum amyloid A genes and their regulation by inflammatory cytokines. In: Natvig JB, Forre O, Husby G, Husebekk A, Skogen B, Sletten K, Westermark P, eds. Amyloid and Amyloidosis, Dordrecht: Kluwer Academic Publishers, 1991:13–9.
235. Wright JR, Calkins E, Breen WJ, et al. Relationship of amyloid to aging: review of the literature and systematic

study of 83 patients derived from a general hospital population. Medicine 1969; 48:39–60.
236. Yanoff M, Fine BS, Colosi NJ, Katowitz JA. Lattice corneal dystrophy: report of an unusual case. Arch Ophthalmol 1977; 95:651–5.
237. Yilmaz A, Tamer L, Ates NA, et al. Effects of apolipoprotein E genotypes on the development of exfoliation syndrome. Exp Eye Res 2005; 80:871–5.
238. Zalin AM, Jones S, Fitch NJ, Ramsden DB. Familial nephropathic non-neuropathic amyloidosis: clinical features, immunohistochemistry and chemistry. Quart J Med 1991; 81:945–56.
239. Zivin RA, Condra JH, Dixon RAF, et al. Molecular-cloning and characterization of DNA-sequences encoding rat and human atrial natriuretic factors. Proc Natl Acad Sci USA Biol Sci 1984; 81:6325–9.

38

Lysosomal Storage and Transport Disorders

Erin Demo
Divison of Genetics and Metabolism, University of North Carolina, Chapel Hill, North Carolina, U.S.A.

Dwight D. Koeberl and Priya S. Kishnani
Division of Medical Genetics, Duke University, Durham, North Carolina, U.S.A.

INTRODUCTION

Lysosomes were discovered in 1959 through a series of brilliant investigations by de Duve and coworkers (14,15). These cytoplasmic organelles, ubiquitous in distribution in living cells, show great diversity in form, origin, and function. Varying in diameter from approximately 0.25 to 0.5 μm, they are easily recognizable by their characteristic biochemical and morphological properties. Lysosomes are a component of a system of intracellular organelles known as the endosomal–lysosomal system (16). This system consists of three parts: the early endosome, the late endosome and the lysosome (primary and secondary) which together are responsible for trafficking and digestion of endocytosed molecules and also for recycling and sorting of materials within the cellular matrix (51). Lysosomes are the sole site of digestive activity in living cells.

ENDOLYSOSOMAL PATHWAY

Endosomes

Endosomes are the first organelles along the endolysosomal pathway. The early endosome is a major sorting station. The early endosome is responsible for dissociating certain lipoproteins from their receptors, at which point the receptors are recycled and the ligands are trafficked via the endosome carrier vesicle to the late endosome (43). The late endosome contains lysosomal hydrolases and lysosome-associated proteins. Late endososmes and lysosomes are believed to be in dynamic equilibrium.

Lysosomes

Lysosomes are membrane-bound vacuoles. A modern definition of the lysosome is that it is the terminal organelle in the endocytic pathway devoid of recycling receptors (27). Lysosomes contain a broad spectrum of hydrolytic enzymes (acid hydrolases) that degrade polymers into their monomeric subunits. In the past, it was thought that these acid hydrolases were only present in lysosomes; however, it is now known that they are also present in early and late endosomes, phagosomes and autophagosomes (42).

When considering a morphological definition of lysosomes, two major groups of organelles are distinguishable (Fig. 1). *Primary lysosomes* are small membrane-limited granules or vesicles containing a full complement of acid hydrolases. They are defined by two highly specific characteristics: (*i*) They have not yet acquired substrates for digestion, and (*ii*) they contain mannose 6-phosphate receptors (see following discussion) that transport newly synthesized hydrolases from the Golgi apparatus to endosomes which are in the process of being transformed into lysosomes (44). *Secondary lysosomes* which are defined as vesicles that have acquired degradable substrates through endocytosis or autophagy and have lost their mannose-6-phosphate (Man-6-P) markers.

Both primary and secondary lysosomes are membrane-limited structures, and under normal conditions, the acid hydrolases within them are not in contact with the rest of the cell. The lipoprotein membrane surrounding the lysosome serves as a protective barrier against the indiscriminate destruction of cellular components. Lysosome-associated membrane proteins are two distinct but highly homologous proteins which comprise close to 50% of the total integral membrane proteins in purified preparations of lysosomes. All of them have single hydrophobic membrane-spanning segments and short cytoplasmic tails. They are extensively glycosylated, and their high-content of sialic acid accounts for the low-isoelectric points (pH 2–4). It is thought that this composition of complex oligosaccharides rich in sialic acid located on the internal surface of the lysosomal membrane protect the membrane from attack by intralysosomal acid hydrolases (44,53). Most importantly, these membrane proteins are neither phosphorylated, nor do they contain Man-6-P recognition markers demonstrating that the mode of synthesis of lysosomal membrane proteins is distinctly different from that of soluble acid hydrolases.

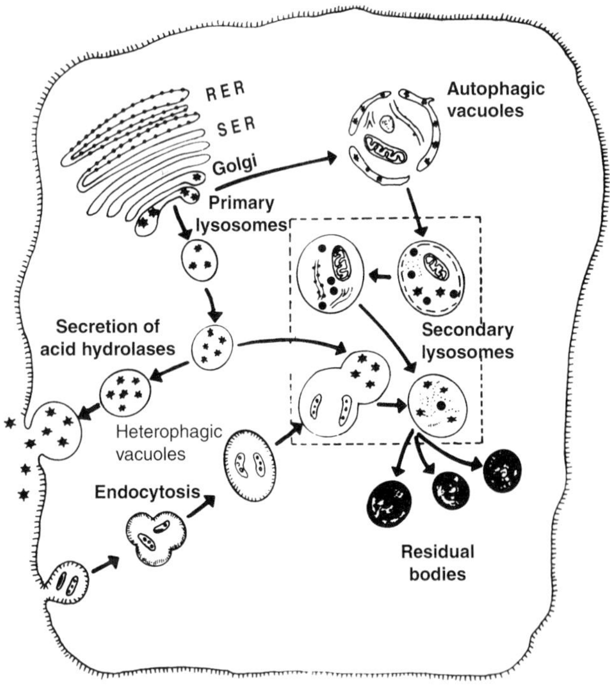

Figure 1 Various aspects of lysosomal digestion. *Abbreviations*: RER, rough endoplasmic reticulum; SER, smooth endoplasmic reticulum.

Lysosomal Enzymes

Acid hydrolases in the lysosomes include esterases, proteases, peptidases, glycosidases, nucleases, phospholipases, phosphatases, and sulfatases. Acid hydrolases are synthesized in the rough endoplasmic reticulum (ER), they then migrate to the lumen of the ER, where they lose their signal sequence by *N*-glycosylation. The majority of lysosomal enzymes acquire a Man-6-P ligand which is a required step for appropriate targeting into the lysosomes (51). Proteolysis, folding and aggregation are the final steps for the mature form of the enzyme. If these steps do not occur, the enzymes cannot enter the lysosome and substrate breakdown cannot occur. Alterations to this pathway is one of the major mechanisms for lysosomal storage diseases (LSDs) (36).

The optimum activity of lysosomal enzymes is at an acid pH. The acidic environment of the lysosomes is maintained at 4.8–5.0 by hydrogen ion (proton) pumps located in the lysosomal membrane. They are inactive at the neutral pH values of the intracellular cytosol and extracellular fluids.

The digestive action of lysosomes is directed toward substances deriving from sources which must first gain access to the interior of the lysosome by either phagocytosis/endocytosis or via autophagy for material from the cytosol.

Endocytosis

Extracellular substances, soluble materials as well as solid particles, are taken up by receptor-mediated endocytosis. In this process, the cell surface receptors bind specific substances (such as hormones, growth factors, and lipoproteins) in concentrated regions or invaginations of the plasma membrane known as coated pits. A specific protein termed clathrin covers the surface of the coated pit. These vesicles are then pinched off or invaginated into the cytoplasm, resulting in the formation of coated vesicles that are still surrounded by clathrin. In the next step, the clathrin coat is quickly lost from the coated vesicles as they fuse with the endosomes. At this stage, the material adsorbed on the cell surface and carried in the coated vesicles is transferred to the endosomes.

Phagocytosis

Phagocytosis is another mechanism used by the lysosome to transport extracellular materials into the internal portion of the organelle. The process involves many steps, the first of which is the stimulation of receptors on the lysosomal cell surface that causes the plasma membrane to create pseudopods that will make a phagosome. This phagosome then fuses with the lysosome and once this occurs the phagosome dissolves, leaving the particle of interest inside of the lysosome. This process is regulated tightly by antigens and enzymes to ensure that it occurs correctly (6).

Autophagy

Endogenous substances originating within the cell itself are handled differently. In this case, the primary lysosome in the form of a Golgi cistern may enclose any type of cellular structure, including mitochondria, ER, microbodies, and particulate glycogen. Some of the steps in this process resemble the receptor-mediated endocytosis just described, but a full description is beyond the scope of the present discussion. The organelles resulting from fusion of intracellular structures with primary lysosomes are known as autophagosomes or autophagic vacuoles.

Once taken up by the lysosomes, the battery of lysosomal enzymes allow the near complete degradation of a variety of soluble macromolecules, as well as membranous biological structures. Most proteins are degraded to peptides and amino acids, complex carbohydrates (glycoproteins, proteoglycans, and glycolipids) to monosaccharides and other small molecules, nucleic acids to nucleosides and phosphates, and complex lipids to free fatty acids and other components. Not all hydrolytic enzymes are present in all cell types; moreover, the activities of those present vary considerably from one tissue to the next.

Despite the highly effective battery of hydrolytic enzymes, not all substances, either particulate or soluble, are completely degraded by lysosomal digestion. After heterophagic and autophagic vacuoles fuse with lysosomes, the enclosed enzymes degrade the contents to substances of low-molecular weight, most of which traverse the lysosomal membrane and enter the cytoplasmic ground substance. Indigestible residues of lysosomal acid hydrolase activity form electron-dense bodies termed residual bodies (Fig. 1). Under some circumstances they may be extruded from the cell by exocytosis. However, in most cell types these residual bodies accumulate and are ultimately recognized by their characteristic autofluorescence. These organelles are abundant in many tissues, such as brain, liver, and heart; in ocular tissues they have been most extensively investigated in the retinal pigment epithelium (RPE), where they form part of the phagolysosomal system of the cell (22). These residual bodies are thought to play a role in the pathogenesis of Batten disease (neuronal ceroid lipofuscinosis), as discussed in Chapter 41.

BIOGENESIS OF SOLUBLE LYSOSOMAL ACID HYDROLASES

The biogenesis of lysosomal enzymes, that is, the synthesis, transport, and packaging of hydrolytic enzymes into primary lysosomes, is an exceedingly complex process; its elucidation during the past decade represents an important breakthrough in cellular biology and biochemistry. Several excellent reviews describe in great detail the individual steps involved in the targeting of lysosomal enzymes from their site of synthesis in the rough ER to their final destination in primary lysosomes (12,35,40, 42,51).

The first steps in the biogenesis of lysosomal enzymes consists of their synthesis on ribosomes, acquisition of cleavable terminal peptide signals, translocation into the lumen of the ER, cleavage of the N-terminal region, and acquisition of N-linked high-mannose oligosaccharides through a dolichol pyrophosphate intermediate. These events are similar to the early stages in the biosynthesis of secretory glycoproteins. Subsequent steps are markedly different; however, in that proteins destined to become lysosomal hydrolases are specifically modified by the addition of a unique marker, Man-6-P. This occurs in the cis-Golgi apparatus through the concerted action of two enzymes, *N*-acetylglucosoaminyl phosphotransferase and α-*N*-acetylglucosaminidase. The first (the phosphotransferase) catalyzes the transfer of phosphate from an *N*-acetylglucosaminyl-1-phosphate residue, through UDP-*N*-acetylglucosamine, to the C-6 hydroxy group of the high-mannose oligosaccharide of the hydrolase. This results in the formation of a phosphodiester intermediate linking the mannose to the *N*-acetylglucosamine. The second enzymatic step releases the *N*-acetylglucosamine and exposes the Man-6-P marker. It is the first enzyme that is defective in I-cell disease (mucolipidosis II) and pseudo-Hurler polydystrophy (mucolipidosis III), two disorders of lysosomal enzyme biosynthesis in which nonphosphorylated lysosomal hydrolases are secreted extracellularly and are not taken up by the cell owing to the lack of the Man-6-P marker (see Chapter 42).

The function of the Man-6-P marker is to mediate the binding of prelysosomal hydrolases to specific receptors in the Golgi membranes; two such receptors are known, a 275 kDa cation independent MPR and a 46 kDa cation dependent (calcium or other) MPR. These receptors play a central role in the targeting of hydrolases to lysosomes. These receptors have different affinities for the soluble precursors, depending on their carbohydrate structure and they are able to sort the various soluble precursors for targeting to the endolysosomal system. The cation independent MPR not only recognizes the Man-6-P residues of prelysosomal hydrolases but also serves as an insulin-like growth factor II receptor (42). Cloning of the cDNA for the two receptors has shown that both contribute to the targeting of newly synthesized enzymes, but in different ways. It is thought that the calcium-independent receptor not only plays a role in the direct intracellular route of acid hydrolase biosynthesis but also mediates endocytosis of lysosomal enzymes from the extracellular environment. The latter is now considered a minor pathway (12,35,51).

Binding of the acid hydrolase to one (or both) of the Man-6-P receptors results in the formation of a unique, albeit unstable, type of complex; which is transported to the endosome. Here, a rise in pH causes dissociation of the complex. The Man-6-P receptors are recycled to the trans-Golgi apparatus to mediate further rounds of transport; the hydrolases enter the lysosomes, where they undergo what is known as trimming, that is, loss or modification of some of their oligosaccharide chains by deglycosylation. The final step(s) in maturation of the acid hydrolases consist of proteolytic cleavage, which is thought to take place in the lysosome itself. A unique feature of the acid hydrolases is the ability to self-regulate, without the need for intra-lysosomal inhibitors.

At one time it was thought that the endocytic pathway from the cell surface to the lysosomes was a major route of delivery of newly synthesized acid hydrolases to these organelles. It is now clear, however, that in most cell types the majority of acid hydrolase enzymes are targeted to lysosomes through the intracellular Man-6-P-dependent pathway in the Golgi apparatus (6,35).

CARRIER-MEDIATED TRANSPORT SYSTEMS

The foregoing discussion is centered on the biogenesis of soluble lysosomal acid hydrolases. Carrier-mediated transport systems specific for cystine, neutral and cationic amino acids, monosaccharides, and other low-molecular-weight solutes have been identified in lysosomal membranes (44). Monosaccharides appear to be transported across the lysosomal membrane by facilitated diffusion. Ion flux and control of pH are mediated by an ATP-dependent proton pump that maintains an acid environment within the lysosomal lumen.

Two lysosomal disorders, cystinosis and sialic acid storage disease(s), are now known to be caused by defects in the carrier-mediated transport of cystine and sialic acid, respectively, across the lysosomal membrane (24,46). Cystinosis (MIM #219800) is caused by a mutation in the *CTNS* gene located on chromosome 17 (17p), which causes the cystine transporter to be defective, leading to a buildup of cystine in the lysosome. Sialic acid storage disease(s) (MIM #269920, MIM #604369) are caused by mutations in the *SLC1745* gene on chromosome 6 that results in abnormal metabolism and transport of sialic acid into the lysosome (46).

INHERITED LYSOSOMAL STORAGE DISORDERS

General Remarks

Tay-Sachs disease (MIM #272800), first described in 1881, was the first description of a LSD (51). The concept of inborn LSDs stemmed from the elegant transmission electron microscopic (TEM) studies of Baudhuin and coworkers (1), who were the first to show that the glycogen-engorged cytoplasmic granules in the liver of a patient with Pompe disease (glycogen storage disease type II; MIM #232300) are abnormally distended lysosomes. The concomitant deficiency of lysosomal acid α-glucosidase in this disorder led to the proposal that glycogen storage disease type II was caused by a failure in the intralysosomal enzymatic hydrolysis of glycogen, resulting in the accumulation of undegraded polysaccharide within the organelle. Following this initial observation, many more lysosomal diseases were delineated by both biochemical and morphological criteria, all of them having one distinguishing feature in common: The intracellular accumulation of enlarged lysosomes filled with storage substances not normally found in the cells. The bizarre alterations in ultrastructure of the abnormal lysosomes has become the morphological hallmark of this group of inborn errors of metabolism, of which nearly 40 are now known. Over the years, the biochemical and enzymatic defects have been elucidated in nearly all (Table 1), and more recently, the molecular basis of these disorders has been established by cloning of the cDNA as well as the genes encoding both normal and aberrant lysosomal enzymes.

Inborn LSDs have been defined as pathological conditions resulting from a defect of a lysosomal enzyme. In some instances two lysosomal enzymes may be involved, as in galactosialidosis, indicating the existence of combined deficiencies, in this case β-galactosidase and neuraminidase (47). Nevertheless, most known LSDs involve deficiency of a single acid hydrolase.

Table 1 Lysosomal Storage and Transport Disorders and Associated Enzyme or Protein Deficiencies

Disorder	MIM #	Gene	Gene location	Enzyme or protein deficiency
Cholesterol ester and triglyceride-degradation				
Wolman disease	+278000	*LIPA*	10q24–q25	Acid lipase
Glycogen degradation				
Pompe disease (glycogenosis type II)	#232300	*GAA*	17q25.2–q25.3	Acid α-glucosidase
Glycoprotein degradation				
Aspartylglycosaminuria	+208400	*AGA*	4q32–q33	Aspartylglycosaminidase
Fucosidosis	+230000	*FUCA1*	1p34	α-L-Fucosidase
Galactosialidosis	+256540	*PPGB*	20q13.1	Cathepsin protective protein (neuraminidase and β-galactosidase)
α-Mannosidosis	+248500	*MAN2B1*	19cen–q12	α-Mannosidase
β-Mannosidosis	+248510	*MANBA*	4q22–q25	β-Mannosidase
Sialidosis	# 256550	*NEU1*	6p21.3	Neuraminidases (sialidase)
Glycosaminoglycan degradation (mucopolysaccharidoses)				
Hurler syndrome (MPS IH)	# 607014	*IDUA*	4p16.3	α-L-Iduronidase
Scheie syndrome (MPS IS)	# 607016	*IDUA*	4p16.3	
Hunter syndrome (MPS II)	+309900	*IDS*	Xq28	Iduronate-2-sulfatase
Sanfillipo syndrome (MPS III)				
Sanfillipo syndrome type A (MPS IIIA)	# 252900	*SGSH*	17q25.3	Heparan *N*-sulfatase (sulphamidase)
Sanfillipo syndrome type B (MPS IIIB)	# 252920	*NAGLU*	17q21	α-*N*-Acetylglucosaminidase
Sanfillipo syndrome type C (MPS IIIC)	# 252930	*HGSNAT*	8p11.1	Acetyl-CoA-glucosamine *N*-acetyltransferase
Sanfillipo syndrome type D (MPS IIID)	# 252940	*GNA*	*12q14*	*N*-Acetylglucosamine 6-sulfatase
Morquio syndrome (MPS IV)				
Morquio syndrome type A (MPS IVA)	+253000	*GALNS*	16q24.3	Galactose 6-sulfatase
Morquio syndrome type B (MPS IVB)	# 230500	*GLB1*	3p21.33	β-Galactosidase sulfatase
Maroteaux–Lamy syndrome (MPS VI)	+253200	*ARSB*	5q11–q13	Arylsulfatase B
Sly syndrome (MPS VII)	+253220	*GUSB*	7q21.11	β-D-glucuronidase
Natowicz disease (MPS IX)	# 601492	*HYAL1*	3p21.3–p21.2	Hyaluronidase
Lysosomal enzyme biosynthesis				
I-cell disease	# 252500	*GNPTAB*	12q23.3	N-acetylglucosamine 1-phosphotransferase
Pseudo–Hurler polydystrophy	# 252600	*GNPTAB*	12q23.3	N-acetylglucosamine 1-phosphotransferase
Lysosomal membrane transport				
Cystinosis	# 219800	*VTNS*	17p13	Cystine transport
Sialic acid storage disorders[a]				Sialic acid transport
Salla disease	# 604369	*SLC17A5*	6q14–q15	Sialic acid transport
Infantile sialic acid storage disease (ISSD)	# 269920	*SLC17A5*	6q14–q15	Sialic acid transport
Sphingolipid degradation				
Fabry disease	+301500	*GLA*	Xq22	α-Galactosidase A
Farber disease	+228000	*ASAH*	8p22–p21.3	Ceramidase
Gaucher disease type I	# 230800	*GBA*	1q21	Glucocerebrosidase
Gaucher disease type II	# 230900	*GBA*	1q21	
Gaucher disease type III	323100	*GBA*	1q21	
GM_1 gangliosidosis	+230500	*GLB1*	3p21.33	β-Galactosidase
GM_2 gangliosidoses				
Activator deficiency				GM_2 ganglioside activator
Sandhoff disease	# 268800	*HEXB*	5q13	β-Hexosaminidase (β subunit)
Tay–Sachs disease	# 272800	*HEXA*	15q23–q24	β-Hexosaminidase (α subunit)
Krabbe disease	# 245200	*GALC*	14q31	Galactosylceramidase
Metachromatic leukodystrophy				
Activator-deficient type	# 249900	*PSAP*	10q22.1	Saposin sulfatide activator
Enzyme-deficient type	# 250100	*ARSA*	22q13.31	Arylsulfatase A
Mucolipidosis type IV	# 252650	*MCOLN1*	19p13.3–qter	Ganglioside sialidase[a]
Multiple sulfatase deficiency	# 272200	*SUMF1*	3p26	All sulfatase substrates
Niemann–Pick disease type A	# 257200	*SMPD1*	11p15.4–p15.1	Sphingomyelinase
Niemann–Pick disease type B	# 607616	*SMPD1*	11p15.4–p15.1	Sphingomyelinase
Niemann–Pick disease type C and D	# 25722	*NPC1*	18q11–q12	A lipid trafficking protein
Schindler disease	# 609241	*NAGA*	22q11	α-*N*-Acetylgalactosaminidase

[a] Probably a secondary enzyme deficiency (46).

The enzymatic deficiency of a single acid hydrolase causes a metabolic block in the catabolism of one or more macromolecules that require the specific enzyme for their degradation. In some cases, as in Gaucher disease (MIM #230800), a single undegraded metabolite, glucocerebroside, accumulates as a result of the defective lysosomal acid hydrolase, glucocerebrosidase. The gene for this enzyme has been isolated and characterized, and several mutations have been identified (2). In other LSDs, the chemical pathology is far more complex, since a variety of seemingly unrelated substances are stored. For example, in generalized GM_1 gangliosidosis, the metabolic block leads to the accumulation of both lipids (GM_1 gangliosides) and carbohydrates [glycosaminoglycans (GAGs) or glycoproteins] (8). The mutant enzyme is unable to cleave terminal β-galactose residues from naturally occurring substrates; hence, the mutation giving rise to the inactive β-galactosidase leads to the storage of a large variety of macromolecules, all having one structural feature in common, a terminal β-galactose unit. Although the enzyme is inactive, immunoreactive β-galactosidase (GLB1) has been detected in most GM_1 gangliosidosis patients (47). Patients with GM_1 gangliosidosis have various phenotypes (infantile, late infantile, juvenile and adult) which correlate to the degree of clinical severity, age of onset and the residual enzyme activity of GLB1 (8).

Molecular cloning techniques are being increasingly applied to study normal and aberrant lysosomal enzymes, and many sequence homologies have been established in a variety of species (49). These studies have been helpful in elucidating the biochemical defect in several more LSDs. Additionally, these studies have been able to identify the genotypes of many of the LSDs. The specific mutations in genes encoding arylsulfatase A (in metachromatic leukodystrophy), α-L-fucosidase (in infantile fucosidosis), glucocerebrosidase (in Gaucher disease), β-hexosaminidase (in Tay–Sachs disease and Sandhoff disease) amongst others have been characterized and are discussed in detail in Chapter 41. These studies have identified both the type and the location of the mutation, information that provides an understanding of the molecular basis of catalytically inactive enzymes and also in some instances a genotype–phenotype correlation.

In addition to mutations affecting the active site of lysosomal enzymes, other mechanisms for inherited LSDs are now well established. For example, two disorders, I-cell disease and pseudo-Hurler polydystrophy, are caused by a failure of the enzyme phosphotransferase to synthesize acid hydrolases with Man-6-P markers. As a result, these enzymes are mislocated; they are found predominantly in extracellular fluids, such as serum, but are essentially undetectable intracellulary (36). Another important type of lysosomal malfunction involves carrier-mediated transport across the membranes (39). Only two disorders in this category are known at present, cystinosis and sialic acid storage disease(s) (46). Mutations implicated in these disease processes have been identified and are providing researchers new information about the function of lysosomal trafficking as well as the opportunity for carrier testing (39).

The majority of LSDs have ocular effects (Table 2), many of which are important in the clinical diagnosis of certain disorders, for example the cherry-red spot in the GM_2 gangliosidoses and other LSDs (Table 3). That the eye is affected in such a variety of systemic inherited disorders should come as no surprise. The cornea and retina, for example, are specialized examples of connective tissue (extracellular matrix) and neural tissue, respectively; hence, generalized disorders that affect either or both of these tissues systemically are likely to affect their ocular counterparts as well. There is a wide variation among these conditions which can cause difficulty in the diagnosis and early treatment for these disorders. Additionally, many of these disorders present with similar symptoms, making a clinical diagnosis impossible.

Diagnosis of Inherited Lysosomal Storage Diseases

For several LSDs a number of mutations have been delineated across the gene, several private and some recurring mutations. There is genetic heterogeneity as well as allelic heterogenity in many of the LSDs. Due to overlapping symptoms, and the number of mutations for a particular disorder, mutation analysis, is not practical for diagnosing a patient initially presenting to a clinician (52). A more definitive way to diagnose new patients is via enzymatic testing and or identification of the storage products. Easily accessible cells, such as leukocytes, cultured skin fibroblasts, or serum, can be assayed for enzyme activity, thus circumventing the need for biopsies of liver, brain, or other tissues, which either carry much risk and discomfort to the patient or are impractical.

A majority of the LSDs can be diagnosed with enzymatic testing on leukocytes or plasma; however, there are some such as Niemann Pick type C, sialidosis, and Farber disease that require skin fibroblasts for a definitive diagnosis (52). Urine samples may also be sent for storage material such as urine GAGs for the mucopolysaccharidoses and oligosaccharides such as, Hex_4 for Pompe disease. The limitation for the latter is that if present, they provide a clue but are not diagnostic for a specific LSD. Another limitation is the high-rate of false negatives and false positives, which makes the use of storage material in urine an adjunct to

Table 2 Inherited Lysosomal Disorders Affecting the Eye

Disorder	Ocular signs
Glycogen degradation	
Pompe disease (glycogenosis type II)	Abnormal deposits in smooth and striated muscles
Glycoprotein degradation	
Fucosidosis	Vascular tortuosities in retina and conjunctiva
Galactosialidosis	Macular cherry-red spots
α-Mannosidosis	Lens opacities
Sialidosis[a]	Macular cherry-red spots; punctate corneal opacities
Glycosaminoglycan degradation (mucopoly-saccharidoses)	
Hurler and Scheie syndromes (MPS IH and MPS IS)	Corneal clouding, pigmentary retinopathy, optic atrophy
Hunter syndrome (MPS II)	Pigmentary retinopathy, late corneal clouding (atypical finding)
Sanfilippo syndrome (MPS III) types A–D	Pigmentary retinopathy, no corneal clouding
Morquio syndrome (MPS IV) types A and B	Corneal clouding, pigmentary retinopathy
Maroteaux–Lamy syndrome (MPS VI)	Corneal clouding, optic atrophy pigmentary retinopathy
Sly syndrome (MPS VII)	Mild corneal clouding, pigmentary retinopathy
Lysosomal enzyme biosynthesis	
I-cell disease	Mild corneal opacities
Pseudo-Hurler polydystrophy	Fine corneal stromal opacities
Lysomal membrane transport	
Cystinosis	Corneal crystals, pigmentary retinopathy
Sialic acid storage disorders[b]	
Salla disease	Myopia, divergent strabismus
Infantile sialic acid storage disease (ISSD)	Divergent strabismus
Sphingolipid degradation	
Fabry disease	Corneal verticillata, cataract, crystalline posterior capsule linear deposits, retinal vessel tortuisity, conjunctival vessel microaneurysm
Farber disease	Macular cherry-red spots
Gaucher disease-neuronopathic (types II and III)	Pingueculae, squint, horizontal saccades, saccadic slowing
GM_1 gangliosidosis	Macular cherry-red spots, optic atrophy
GM_2 gangliosidoses	
Tay-Sachs disease (GM_2 type I)	Cherry red spot
Sandhoff disease (GM_2 type II)	Cherry red spot
GM_2 activator deficiency	
Infantile forms	Macular cherry-red spots, optic atrophy

(*Continued*)

Table 2 Inherited Lysosomal Disorders Affecting the Eye (*Continued*)

Disorder	Ocular signs
GM_2 activator deficiency	
Juvenile forms	Optic atrophy, pigmentary retinopathy
Adult-onset forms	Visual disturbances[c]
Krabbe disease	Optic atrophy
Metachromatic leukodystrophy	Macular cherry-red spot
Activator-deficient type	
Enzyme-deficient type	
Late infantile form	Optic atrophy, grayish discoloration of macula nystagmus
Juvenile and adult forms	Visual disturbances[c]
Mucolipidosis IV	Early corneal clouding, later pigmentary retinopathy
Niemann–Pick disease type A	Macular degeneration, cherry-red spots
Niemann–Pick disease type B	Type B macular halo, macular cherry-red spots in 1/3
Schindler disease	Strabismus, optic atrophy, cortical blindness

[a] Formerly called mucolipidosis I; two or three types are known. Enzyme defects include either α-neuraminidase or β-galactosidase, or both, resulting in accumulations of sialoconjugates (19,24).
[b] Accumulation of free sialic acid resulting from defect in lysosomal transport of sialic acid (24).
[c] Not clearly defined owing to uncertainties in clinical diagnoses.

enzymatic/genotyping in making a definitive diagnosis. Additionally, some LSDs, such as galactosialidosis, are not definitively diagnosed when there is the presence of a low-value for one enzyme (52).

Recent advances have facilitated lysosomal enzymatic testing on dried blood spots (DBS) (37). New methods have been developed that assay lysosomal enzyme activity in DBS extracts. Isolation of the respective enzymes from DBS extracts by immunocapture or competitive inhibition has been used or are in development for several LSDs (37). These technology platforms will facilitate early diagnosis and also their use in newborn screening programs.

Conjunctiva and Tears in the Diagnosis of Lysosomal Storage Disorders

Of special historic interest to the ophthalmologist is that conjunctiva and tear fluid, can provide a convenient and a reliable source material for the diagnosis of LSDs. The ultrastructural abnormalities found in the conjunctival fibroblasts, epithelial cells, capillary endothelium, or Schwann cells are indistinguishable from those present in neural and visceral tissues of affected individuals. Tear fluid contains lysosomal enzymes at concentrations 5 to 10 times greater than those found in plasma. Both conjunctiva and tear fluid are readily available, noninvasive sources of material that have been used for the

Table 3 Differential Diagnosis of the Cherry-Red Spot at the Macula

Disorder	Deficient enzyme	Other features	Refs.
GM_1 gangliosidosis	β-Galactosidase		50
Tay–Sachs disease	Hexosaminidase A		11,25
Sialidosis type 1	Marked reduction in neuraminidase	Seizures	28
Sandhoff disease		Bilateral optic atrophy	54

ultrastructural and enzymatic diagnosis, respectively, of many LSDs (50).

Conjunctival Biopsy

Abnormal storage vacuoles in subepithelial conjunctival tissue were first noted by Kenyon and Sensenbrenner (34) in a biopsy specimen from a patient with I-cell disease (mucolipidosis type II). Studies of conjunctival ultrastructure were subsequently extended to include other LSDs, of which nearly 20 have been examined (32). Sufficient evidence has now accumulated to warrant the following generalizations.

In all the mucopolysaccharidoses, except MPS IV (Morquio syndrome), both the epithelial cells and the fibroblasts are engorged with single-membrane-limited vacuoles containing fibrillogranular material (33). The Schwann cells in some cases have membranous lamellar storage bodies, but the capillary endothelium is not affected.

The ultrastructural changes in the mucolipidoses reflect metabolic abnormalities in both lipid and carbohydrate metabolism (33). The storage vacuoles usually consist of two types: single-membrane-limited vacuoles in the epithelial cells and fibroblasts similar to those found in the mucopolysaccharidoses, and dense lamellar bodies or opaque globules representing intralysosomal deposits of lipid. Abnormal inclusion bodies are also found in the endothelial cells of the capillary endothelium in some of the mucolipidoses, although this is not a constant finding.

Ultrastructural changes in the sphingolipidoses are less uniform than those in the mucopolysaccharidoses. Thus, single-membrane-limited vacuoles in the epithelial cells and in fibroblasts are especially prominent in GM_1 gangliosidoses, GM_2 gangliosidosis type II, Niemann–Pick disease type A, and Fabry disease and are either less prominent or totally absent in TSD, metachromatic leukodystrophy, and Krabbe disease. Nearly all the sphingolipidoses, except Niemann–Pick disease types B and C, contain membranous cytoplasmic bodies and other abnormal lipid-storing organelles in the Schwann cells. Ultrastructural lesions are prominent in the endothelial cells of capillaries in all the sphingolipidoses except Tay–Sachs disease, metachromatic leukodystrophy, and Krabbe disease.

Tear Fluid

Tay–Sachs and Fabry diseases were the first storage diseases to be diagnosed by analyzing lysosomal enzymes in tear fluid (9,27,38). The enzymes originate in the secretory cells of the lacrimal gland and pass directly through the duct into the tear fluid, thus they reflect a true tissue source. Moreover, because they are concentrated in a small volume with a relatively low-protein content, the specific activity of the enzymes is very high. Tear fluid is easy to obtain on strips of Whatman fllter paper. After collection, the strip is dried and in this form can be mailed to laboratories for processing (11). The enzymes are stable, especially if stored at –30°C. For analysis, the dried tear fluid is simply extracted into buffer and the enzyme assayed with no further processing. At least 11 LSDs have been correctly diagnosed by analyses of tear fluid (Table 3) (25).

Therapeutic Approaches Based on Fundamental Knowledge

Enzyme Replacement Therapy, Bone Marrow/Cord Blood Transplantation, and Substrate Reduction Therapy

Therapy for LSDs has been possible due to the principle of cross-correction of lysosomal enzyme deficiencies. Cross-correction depends upon the Man-6-P receptor-mediated uptake of lysosomal enzymes (37). Enzyme replacement therapy (ERT) and bone marrow transplantation were initiated based upon the principle that receptor-mediated uptake could correct the deficiency of the spectrum of tissues affected by various LSDs.

The first success of ERT in Gaucher disease established a paradigm for later attempts in other LSDs. The confluence of purification of mannosylated glucocerebrosidase, the passage of the Orphan Drug Act, and widespread success of Gaucher disease patients on treatment assured the success of ERT for this disorder (2). ERT for Gaucher disease corrects anemia, thrombocytopenia, and hepatosplenomegaly reliably. The paradigm of receptor-mediated uptake was confirmed, when efficacy was achieved with glucocerebrosidase that was modified to expose terminal mannose residues. The relevance of the blood–brain barrier to ERT was illustrated by the resistance of neuronopathic Gaucher disease to ERT (5).

An alternative, cell-based approach through bone marrow transplantation has ameliorated the progression of neurologic involvement, at least in MPS IH (Hurler disease), X-linked adrenoleukodystropy, and Krabbe disease, if accomplished prior to the onset of neurologic involvement (3). The prevention of developmental regression was possible in Hurler disease patients, if successful bone marrow transplantation occurred in the first several years of life. Hepatosplenomegaly resolved, although the response of less vascularized tissues such as bone and heart valves has been mixed. Recently cord blood transplantation has demonstrated remarkable efficacy in neonatal onset Krabbe disease; however, transplantation in the first weeks of life prior to the onset of symptoms was most efficacious (21). Bone marrow or cord blood transplantation hinges upon the presence of an HLA-matched donor, which is more likely in the context of a large cord blood or bone marrow repository.

Further confirmation of the peripheral response to ERT has been confirmed in Fabry disease, Pompe disease, MPS IH (Hurler syndrome), MPS II (Hunter syndrome) and MPS VI (Maroteaux-Lamy syndrome). The attenuated forms of LSDs with no neurological or minimal neurological involvement are the ones with maximum benefit from ERT. Under development are ERT for Niemann–Pick type B disease and others (Table 4) (4).

Another therapeutic strategy for LSDs with neurologic involvement consists of substrate reduction therapy (SRT). SRT inhibits the synthesis of storage materials upstream of the deficient enzyme. For instance, SRT with *N*-butyldeoxynojirimycin has reduced the accumulation of glucocerebroside in the blood of Gaucher disease patients. Consequently, SRT has been approved for Gaucher patients ineligible for or unresponsive to ERT. SRT would only be effective for those lysosomal storage disorders in which there is residual enzyme and where glycosphingolipids, accumulate. The efficacy of SRT was initially demonstrated in preclinical studies with Sandhoff disease mice based upon prolongation of survival (31). A potential advantage of SRT lies in the permeability of the blood–brain barrier to these agents, in contrast to ERT with lysosomal enzymes that do not as a rule cross into the brain from the vasculature. SRT thus has a potential role in LSDs with a neurologic component (18). Additional studies are needed to demonstrate if there is a CNS effect and long-term safety.

Chaperone therapy is another treatment approach for lysosomal diseases that result from protein misfolding and/or mistrafficking. In this approach chaperones are used to rescue the misfolded protein thereby enhancing protein function and amelioration of symptoms. Its potential advantages are ability to cross the blood–brain barrier and reversible binding to the protein, allowing for its dissociation once targeted to the lysosome. It is currently in development for LSDs such as Fabry disease, Gaucher disease, and Pompe disease.

Preclinical Experimental Therapeutic Studies

New therapies under development include gene therapy strategies with viral vectors. The viral vectors depend upon replacement of the defective gene with a therapeutic transgene delivered by a replication-deficient viral vector. Currently favored viral vectors include adeno-associated virus (AAV) vectors, lentiviral vectors, and murine retroviral vectors, although adenoviral vectors have been established proof of

Table 4 Lysosomal Storage Diseases and Associated Enzyme Deficiencies

Disorder	Deficient enzyme	Refs.
Sphingolipidoses		
GM_1 gangliosidosis	B-Galactosidase	48
GM_2 gangliosidosis		
Tay–Sachs disease	Hexosaminidase A	11,25
Sandhoff disease	Hexosaminidase A and B	25
Fabry disease	α-Galactosidase A	17,38
Metachromatic leukodystrophy	Arylsulfatase A	50
Mucopolysaccharidoses		
Hurler (MPS IH) and Scheie (MPS IS) syndromes	α-L-Iduronidase	50
Mucolipidoses		
Fucosidosis	α-L-Fucosidase	50
Mannosidosis	α-D-Mannosidase	25
I-cell disease	Multiple lysosomal enzymes	50
Glycogen storage disorders		
Glycogenosis type II	Acid α-glucosidase	50

Table 5 Lyosomal Storage Disease and Available Therapies

Disorder	Enzyme or substrate treatment	Stage of approval for therapy
Hunter syndrome (MPS II)	Enzyme replacement therapy	FDA approved
Pompe disease (glycogenosis type II)	Enzyme replacement therapy	FDA approved
Gaucher disease	Enzyme replacement therapy/substrate reduction therapy	FDA approved
Fabry disease	Enzyme replacement therapy	FDA approved
Hurler and Scheie disease (MPS IH and MPS IS)	Enzyme replacement therapy	FDA approved
Maroteaux–Lamy disease (MPS VI)	Enzyme replacement therapy	FDA approved
Niemann–Pick disease	Enzyme replacement therapy	Phase I/II trials

Abbreviation: FDA, Food and Drug Administration.

principle for gene therapy in several animal models for LSDs. Mouse models for many LSDs have become available through knock-out technology, while large animal models have been bred from naturally occurring mutations among pet and farm animal breeding programs. The availability of viral vectors for moderately efficient gene delivery has spawned a number of successful preclinical studies in the last several years (Table 5).

The principal successes of gene therapy in LSDs have been through neonatal delivery or intracerebral injection to correct the brain (45). Neonatal delivery of AAV vectors corrected the tissues of MPS VII (Sly disease) mice generally, including the brain, apparently related to permeability of the vasculature to the vector in newborn mice (13). Similarly, murine retroviral vectors had marked efficacy in the canine models for MPS IH (Hurler disease) and MPS VII (Sly disease) if administered in the newborn animals (44). Intracerebral injection of AAV or adenoviral vectors corrected the enzyme deficiency and storage material accumulation distal to the injection site in MPS VII (Sly disease) mice (23). Injection of deep cerebral nuclei with newer AAV vectors, cross-packaged with alternative serotypes featuring enhanced tissue tropism, has corrected both the storage material accumulation and behavioral deficits in Niemann–Pick type A mice (20).

Retinal function was improved in the MPS VII and Batten disease mouse models following intraocular administration of AAV vectors (26,29). Very intriguingly, injection of an AAV vector into the vitreal space corrected both the optic tract and adjacent regions of the brain in MPS VII mice, presumably related to retrograde transport of the α-gluconidase enzyme from retinal ganglion cells (28). These latter results emphasize the role of the retina as an extension of the central nervous system that could serve as a portal of entry for therapeutic gene delivery.

The chief hurdles to implementation of gene therapy include safety and efficacy concerns. The safety of retroviral vectors has been questioned, especially in light of the high-frequency of leukemia related to retroviral gene therapy in a clinical trial for X-linked severe combined immune deficiency (SCID). The unique prevalence of leukemia in SCID stems from a strong selective pressure for corrected lymphocytes that drives clonal expansion of cells with an activated oncogene secondary to retroviral vector insertion (7). Prevention of oncogene activation could be possible through disabling the enhancer in retroviral vectors or replacing it with a tissue-specific promoter that is inactive in hematologic cells. Nonetheless, new clinical trials proposing to use integrating retroviral vectors will face additional scrutiny. The difficulty of translating efficacy in animal models of genetic disease to clinical trials was illustrated by the clinical trials for hemophilia B, because patients expressed subtherapeutic levels of coagulation factor IX and mounted unanticipated immune responses to the AAV vector at higher particle number doses (30). Therefore, clinical trials in lysosomal storage disorders will be feasible only in those disorders with high, early mortality and an acceptably risk to benefit ratio.

ACKNOWLEDGMENT

This chapter is a modification of the one originally prepared for the first two editions by the late Dr. Elaine Berman.

REFERENCES

1. Baudhuin P, Hers HG, Loeb H. An electron microscopic and biochemical study of type II glycogenosis. Lab Invest 1964; 13:1139–52.
2. Beutler E. Lysosomal storage diseases: Natural natural history and ethical and economic aspects. Mol Genet Metab 2006; 88:208–15.
3. Boelens JJ. Trends in haematopoietic cell transplantation for inborn errors of metabolism. J Inherit Metab Dis 2006; 29:413–20.
4. Brady RO. Emerging strategies for the treatment of hereditary metabolic storage disorders. Rejuvenation Res 2006; 9:237–44.
5. Brady RO. Enzyme replacement for lysosomal diseases. Annu Rev Med 2006; 57:283–96.
6. Braun V, Niedergang F. Linking exocytosis and endocytosis during phagocytosis. Biol Cell 2006; 98: 195–201.

7. Buckley RH. Gene therapy for SCID—a complication after remarkable progress. Lancet 2002; 360:1185–6.
8. Caciotti A, Donati MA, Bardelli T, et al. Primary and secondary elastin-binding protein defect leads to impaired elastogenesis in fibroblasts from GM1-gangliosidosis patients. Am J Pathol 2005; 167:1689–98.
9. Carmody PJ, Rattazzi MC, Davidson RG. Tay-Sachs disease – the use of tears for the detection of heterozygotes. N Engl J Med 1973; 289:1072–4.
10. Chinchurreta-Capote A, Beltran-Urena FJ, Espana-Contreras M. [Sialidosis type I. Two cases in a family]. Arch Soc Esp Oftalmo 2005; 80:537–40.
11. Cotlier E, Kivlin J, Del Monte, MA. Mail screening for inborn errors of metabolism with tears. Birth Defects Orig Artic Ser 1976; 12:105–14.
12. Dahms NM, Lobel P, Kornfeld S. Mannose 6-phosphate receptors and lysosomal enzyme targeting. J Biol Chem 1989; 264:12115–8.
13. Daly TM, Vogler C, Levy B, et al. Neonatal gene transfer leads to widespread correction of pathology in a murine model of lysosomal storage disease. Proc Natl Acad Sci USA 1999; 96:2296–300.
14. de Duve C. Lysosomes, a new group of cytoplasmic particles. In: Hayashi T, ed. Subcellular Particles Particles. New York: Ronald Press, 1959:128–59.
15. de Duve C, Pressman BC, Gianetto R, et al. Tissue fractionation studies. 6. Intracellular distribution patterns of enzymes in rat-liver tissue. Biochem J 1955; 60: 604–17.
16. De Duve, C, Wattiaux R. Functions of lysosomes. Annu Rev Physiol 1966; 28:435–92.
17. Del Monte, MA, Johnson, DL, Cotlier, E, Desnick RJ. Diagnosis of inherited enzymatic deficiencies with tears: Fabry disease. Birth Defects Orig Artic Ser 1976; 12:209–19.
18. Desnick RJ. Enzyme replacement and enhancement therapies for lysosomal diseases. J Inherit Metab Dis 2004; 27: 385–410.
19. Deutsch JA, Asbell PA. Sialidosis and galactosialidosis. In: *The Eye in Systemic Disease*, DH Gold DH and, TA Weingeist TA, (Eds), The Eye in Systemic Disease (pp. 376–77). JB Lippincott, Philadelphia: JB Lippincott, pp. 376–7 1990:376–7.
20. Dodge JC, Clarke J, Song A, et al. Gene transfer of human acid sphingomyelinase corrects neuropathology and motor deficits in a mouse model of Niemann-Pick type A disease. Proc Natl Acad Sci USA 2005; 102:17822–7.
21. Escolar ML, Poe MD, Provenzale JM, et al. Transplantation of umbilical-cord blood in babies with infantile Krabbe's disease. N Engl J Med 2005; 352:2069–81.
22. Feeney-Burns L, Berman ER, Rothman H Lipofuscin of human retinal pigment epithelium. Am J Ophthalmol 1980; 90:783–91.
23. Frisella WA, O'Connor LH, Vogler CA, et al. Intracranial injection of recombinant adeno-associated virus improves cognitive function in a murine model of mucopolysaccharidosis type VII. Mol Ther 2001; 3:351–8.
24. Gahl WA, Schneider J, Thoene JG Lysosomal transport disorders: Ccystinosis and sialic acid storage disorders. In: CR Scriver CR, AL Beaudet AL, WS Sly WS, & D. Valle D, (Eds)., The metabolic Metabolic basis Basis of inherited Inherited disease Disease, (8th ed., (pp. 5085–108). New York: McGraw-Hill, 2001:5085–108.
25. Goldberg JD, Truex JH, Desnick RJ. Tay-Sachs disease: an improved, fully-automated method for heterozygote identification by tear beta-hexosaminidase assay. Clin Chim Acta 1977; 77:43–52.
26. Griffey M, Macauley SL, Ogilvie JM, Sands MS. AAV2-mediated ocular gene therapy for infantile neuronal ceroid lipofuscinosis. Mol Ther 2005; 12:413–21.
27. Griffiths GM. Secretory lysosomes—a special mechanism of regulated secretion in haemopoietic cells. Trends Cell Biol 1996; 6:329–32.
28. Hennig AK, Levy B, Ogilvie JM, et al. Intravitreal gene therapy reduces lysosomal storage in specific areas of the CNS in mucopolysaccharidosis VII mice. J Neurosci 2003; 23:3302–7.
29. Hennig AK, Ogilvie JM, Ohlemiller KK, et al. AAV-mediated intravitreal gene therapy reduces lysosomal storage in the retinal pigmented epithelium and improves retinal function in adult MPS VII mice. Mol Ther 2004; 10:106–16.
30. High KA, Manno CS, Sabatino DE. Immune reseponses to AAV and to factor IX in a phase 1 study of AAV-mediated, liver-directed gene transfer for hemophilia B. Blood 2003; 102:154A–5A.
31. Jeyakumar M, Butters TD, Cortina-Borja M, et al. Delayed symptom onset and increased life expectancy in Sandhoff disease mice treated with *N*-butyldeoxynojirimycin. Proc Natl Acad Sci U S A 1999; 96:6388–93.
32. Kenyon KR. Ocular manifestations and pathology of systemic mucopolysaccharidoses. In: MF. Goldberg MF, (Ed), In genetic Genetic and Metabolic Eye Disease. Boston: Brown, 1974.
33. Kenyon KR. Ocular manifestations and pathology of systemic mucopolysaccharidoses. Birth Defects Orig Artic Ser. 1976; 12:133–53.
34. Kenyon KR, Sensenbrenner JA. Mucolipidosis II (I-cell disease): ultrastructural observations of conjunctiva and skin. Invest Ophthalmol 1971; 10:555–67.
35. Kornfeld S, Mellman I. The biogenesis of lysosomes. Annu Rev Cell Biol 1989; 5:483–525.
36. Kudo M, Brem MS, Canfield WM. Mucolipidosis II (I-cell disease) and mucolipidosis IIIA (classical pseudo-hurler polydystrophy) are caused by mutations in the GlcNAc-phosphotransferase alpha/beta-subunits precursor gene. Am J Hum Genet. 2006; 78:451–63.
37. Li Y, Scott CR, Chamoles NA, et al. Direct multiplex assay of lysosomal enzymes in dried blood spots for newborn screening. Clin Chem, 2004; 50:1785–96.
38. Libert J, Tondeur M, Van Hoof F. The use of conjunctival biopsy and enzyme analysis in tears for the diagnosis of homozygotes and heterozygotes with Fabry disease. Birth Defects Orig Artic Ser 1976; 12:221–39.
39. Mancini GM, Havelaar AC, Verheijen FW. Lysosomal transport disorders. J Inherit Metab Dis 2000; 23: 278–92.
40. Neufeld EF. Lysosomal storage diseases. Annu Rev Biochem, 1991; 60:257–80.
41. Neufeld EF, Fratantoni JC. Inborn errors of mucopolysaccharide metabolism. Science 1970; 169:141–6.
42. Pillay CS, Elliott E, Dennison C. Endolysosomal proteolysis and its regulation. Biochem J 2002; 363: 417–29.
43. Ponder KP, Melniczek JR, Xu L, et al. Therapeutic neonatal hepatic gene therapy in mucopolysaccharidosis VII dogs. Proc Natl Acad Sci U S A 2002; 99:13102–7.
44. Sabatini DD, Adesnik MB. The biogenesis of membranes and organelles. In: Scriver CR, Beaudet AL, Sly WS, and Valle D, Eds. The metabolic Metabolic basis Basis of inherited Inherited diseases Diseases. (8th ed, New York: McGraw-Hill, 2001:433–7.
45. Sands MS, Davidson BL. Gene therapy for lysosomal storage diseases. Mol Ther 2006; 13:839–49.

46. Scriver CR, Beaudet AL, Sly WS, Valle D. (Eds.) The Metabolic and Molecular Bases of Inherited Disease (8th ed.) New York: McGraw-Hill, 2001.
47. Suzuki Y, Oshima A, Nanba E. Beta-galactosidase deficiency (GM1-gangliosidosis, galactosialidosis, and Morquio syndrome type B). In: CR Scriver CR, AL Beaudet AL, WS. Sly WS, Valle D. (Eds). The Metabolic Basis of Inherited Disease (8th ed.) New York: McGraw-Hill; 2001:3775–801.
48. Tsuboyama A, Miki F, Yoshida M, et al. The use of tears for diagnosis of GM1 gangliosidosis. Clin Chim Acta 1977; 80: 237–42.
49. Vallance H, Ford J. Carrier testing for autosomal-recessive disorders. Crit Rev Clin Lab Sci. 2003; 40:473–97.
50. van Hoof, F, Libert J, Aubert-Tulkens G, Serra MV. The assay of lacrimal enzymes and the ultrastructural analysis of conjunctival biopsies: New techniques for the study of inborn lysosomal diseases. Metab. Ophthalmol 1977; 1: 165–71.
51. Vellodi A. Lysosomal storage disorders. Br J Haematol 2005; 128:413–31.
52. Wenger DA, Coppola S, Liu SL. Lysosomal storage disorders: diagnostic dilemmas and prospects for therapy. Genet Med 2002; 4:412-4–19.
53. Winchester B. Lysosomal metabolism of glycoproteins. Glycobiology 2005; 15:1R–15R.
54. Yun YM, Lee SN. A case report of Sandhoff disease. Korean J Ophthalmol, 2005; 19:68–72.

39

Glycogen Storage Diseases

Alan D. Proia
Department of Pathology, Duke University, Durham, North Carolina, U.S.A.

INTRODUCTION

Glycogen is the storage form of glucose in virtually all animal cells, but it is most abundant in liver and muscle (7,15,31). Glycogen is a highly branched polymer with a treelike structure that can accommodate up to 60,000 glucose units in a single globular molecule with a molecular mass of approximately 10,000 kDa (2,7,31). Because of this unique structure, 7% to 10% of the glucose residues are terminal and thus easily accessible to the action of both biosynthetic and degradative enzymes. When viewed by transmission electron microscopy (TEM), glycogen molecules are easily recognized as spherical electron-dense particles approximately 30 nm in diameter. These spherules are called β particles. In the liver, where the concentration of glycogen is considerably higher than in other tissues, β particles form large rosette-shaped aggregates ranging in size from 110 to 150 nm and reaching molecular weights as high as 100,000 kDa (7,31). These structures are called α particles.

The concentration of liver glycogen varies from as little as 0.1% during fasting to approximately 5% under normal nutritional conditions. Glycogen concentration may reach values as high as 14% in livers of fasted, re-fed rats (18). The regulation of such large changes in concentration is exceedingly complex; it is carried out through controlled interactions between a dozen or more enzymes and several hormones, including glucagon and insulin (2,7,15,31).

Glycogen storage diseases (GSDs) (also termed "glycogenoses") are inherited disorders of glycogen metabolism that result from defects in the enzymes involved in synthesis or degradation of glycogen (7,11,38). The glycogen in these disorders may be abnormal in quality, quantity, or both. Defects in almost all of the synthetic and degradative enzymes of glycogen metabolism have been discovered to cause GSD and the disorders have been assigned numbers based on the chronological order in which their enzymatic defects were identified (7). Over 20 forms of GSD are known at present, and 18 of them have been reasonably well characterized (Table 1) (7,11,38). With the exception of GSD type IXa (which has X-linked inheritance), all are inherited as autosomal recessive traits. Liver (38) and skeletal muscle (11), which normally contain abundant glycogen, are the most commonly and seriously affected tissues in the GSDs. Hepatic GSDs are usually associated with hepatomegaly and hypoglycemia (7,38). Muscle GSDs are manifested as episodic, recurrent exercise intolerance with muscle cramps, myalgia, and myoglobinuria, or as continuous, often progressive weakness (11). As shown in Table 1, only GSD type I (von Gierke disease, MIM +232200) and GSD type II (Pompe disease, MIM #232300) have ocular changes; these are for the most part mild in nature and, moreover, are not documented in all cases.

The other GSDs are not lysosomal disorders; instead, the defective enzymes are localized in other cell organelles.

GLYCOGEN STORAGE DISEASE TYPE I

Glycogen storage disease type I represents two genetically determined autosomal recessive disorders resulting from defects in the glucose-6-phosphatase complex (7,9,10,27,30). Numerous mutations in the *G6PC* gene encoding for glucose-6-phosphatase are responsible for GSD type Ia, while mutations in the *G6PT1* gene encoding microsomal glucose-6-phosphate translocase (glucose-6-phosphate transporter) cause GSD type Ib (7,9,10,27,30). Von Gierke first described the clinical features of GSD type I in 1929, while Cori and Cori in 1952 demonstrated that it was an absence of glucose-6-phosphatase activity that caused the disorder (7,9). The estimated frequency of GSD type I is 1 in 100,000 newborns (30). A strict correlation does not exist between location of the mutation and phenotype for either GSD type Ia (10) or GSD type Ib (27).

Defects in the glucose-6-phosphatase complex cause deranged glucose homeostasis and inadequate hepatic production of glucose, since this enzyme complex catalyzes the hydrolysis of glucose-6-phosphate to glucose and phosphate in the terminal steps of gluconeogenesis and glycogenolysis (10). Glycogen accumulates primarily in the liver and kidney in both GSD type Ia and GSD type Ib, resulting in hepatomegaly and nephromegaly (10). Hyperuricemia results from both decreased renal tubular secretion of uric acid and increased uric acid production by the liver and other tissues. The latter may be a consequence of diminished levels of inorganic phosphate and adenosine triphosphate in the tissues, which secondarily leads to an enhanced breakdown of adenine nucleotides (10). Hyperlipidemia results from increased lipolysis, overproduction of substrates and cofactors for lipid biosynthesis, and a diminished capacity of the liver to synthesize apolipoproteins (10).

The major clinical features of GSD type Ia are massive hepatomegaly, growth retardation, enlarged kidneys, hypoglycemia, hyperuricemia, hyperlipidemia, and lactic acidemia (7,9). The clinical features of GSD type Ib are similar to those of GSD type Ia, with the addition of neutropenia and neutrophil dysfunction (27), which predispose GSD type Ib patients to severe infections and inflammatory bowel disease (27). Progressive renal disease and complications from liver adenomas are likely to be the major causes of morbidity and mortality in children treated with dietary therapy, although new complications may be uncovered as more children survive to adulthood (30).

Only rare reports exist concerning ophthalmological abnormalities in GSD type I (1,6,12,20). Fine et al. (12) noted multiple bilateral, symmetrical, yellowish, nonelevated, discrete paramacular lesions in three of five patients with GSD type I, ranging in age from 13 to 17 years. Vision was not impaired. Fine et al. (12) and Hockman (20) speculate that the lesions are a result of the patients' hyperlipidemia. A faint brown cloudy infiltration invading the cornea from the periphery was reported in one case by Bron and Tripathi (6). In one report, a 40-year-old woman with GSD type Ia had a gradual attenuation of the b-wave on electroretinographic examination, while a 15-year-old girl with GSD type Ib had a delayed appearance of the choroidal flush on fluorescein angiography, a subnormal Arden ratio (the ratio of light peak to dark trough) on electrooculography, and atrophy of the retinal pigment epithelium (RPE) and choriocapillaris (1).

GLYCOGEN STORAGE DISEASE TYPE II

Glycogen storage disease type II (also termed Pompe disease, glycogenosis type II, acid α-glucosidase deficiency, or acid maltase deficiency) results from defects in the activity of lysosomal acid α-glucosidase, an enzyme essential for the degradation of glycogen (19,29). The disease was first described by Pompe in 1932 (19,29), and its enzymatic defect and the subcellular localization of the enzyme were identified by Hers et al. in the early 1960s (3,19). GSD type II is the prototype of an inherited lysosomal storage disease, a concept first introduced by Hers in 1965 (17,19) (see Chapter 38). Whereas in normal liver and other cells glycogen is dispersed throughout the cytoplasm, in GSD type II the greatest concentration is found in giant single-membrane-limited vacuoles, which Baudhuin et al. (3) identified as abnormally distended lysosomes. Following these early

Table 1 Glycogen Storage Diseases

Disorder	Eponym	MIM #	Tissues affected	Enzyme deficiency	Mode of transmission	Gene	Gene locus	Ocular signs
GSD type 0		#240600	Liver	Glycogen synthase	AR	*GYS2*	12p12.3	ND
GSD type Ia	von Gierke disease	+232200	Liver, kidney, intestine	Glucose-6-phosphatase	AR	*G6PC*	17q21	Yellowish paramacular lesions; attenuated b-wave on electroretinography
GSD type 1b		#232220	Liver	Glucose-6-phosphate transporter	AR	*G6PT1*	11q23	Delayed choroidal flush on fluorescein angiography; subnormal Arden ratio on electrooculography; atrophy of RPE and choriocapillaris
GSD type II	Pompe disease	#232300	All	Lysosomal acid α-glucosidase	AR	*GAA*	17q25.2–q25.3	Extraocular muscle weakness
GSD type IIIa	Cori disease or Forbes disease	+232400	Liver, muscle, heart	Glycogen debranching enzyme	AR	*AGL*	1p21	ND
GSD type IIIb		+232400.0002	Liver	Glycogen debranching enzyme	AR	*AGL*	1p21	ND
GSD type IV	Andersen disease	#232500	Generalized	Glycogen branching enzyme	AR	*GBE1*	3p12	ND
GSD type V	McArdle disease	#232600	Skeletal muscle	Muscle phosphorylase	AR	*PYGM*	11q13	ND
GSD type VI	Hers disease	+232700	Liver	Liver phosphorylase	AR	*PYGL*	14q21–q22	ND
GSD type VII	Tarui disease	+232800	Skeletal muscle, erythrocytes	Muscle phosphofructokinase	AR	*PFKM*	12q13.3	ND
GSD type VIII[a]		+30600						
GSD type IXa		+306000	Liver, erythrocytes, leukocytes	Liver isoform of α subunit of phosphorylase kinase	XR	*PHKA2*	Xp22.2–p22.1	ND
GSD type IXb		#261750	Liver, muscle, erythrocytes, leukocytes	β-subunit of liver and muscle phosphorylase kinase	AR	*PHKB*	16q12–q13	ND
GSD type IXc		604549	Liver	Testis/liver isoform of γ subunit of phosphorylase kinase	AR	*PHKG2*	16q11–p12	ND
GSD type IXd		*311870	Skeletal muscle	Muscle isoform of α subunit of phosphorylase kinase	AR	*PHKA1*	Xq13	ND
GSD type X		+261670	Skeletal muscle	Muscle phosphoglycerate mutase	AR	*PGAM2*	7p13–p12.3	ND
GSD type XI		+150000	Skeletal muscle	Lactate dehydrogenase M-subunit	AR	*LDHA*	11p15.4	ND
GSD type XII		+103850	Skeletal muscle, erythrocytes	Fructose 1,6-bisphosphate aldolase A	AR	*ALDOA*	16q22–q24	ND
GSD type XIII		+131370	Skeletal muscle	β-enolase (also called enolase 3)	AR	*ENO3*	17pter–p12	ND

[a] GSD type VIII is currently classified as GSD type IX (1).
Abbreviations: AR, autosomal recessive; GSD, glycogen storage disease; ND, not described; XR, X-linked recessive.

observations, many additional lysosomal storage disorders have been delineated.

Three forms of GSD type II (infantile, childhood/juvenile and adult onset) are traditionally recognized based on age of onset of symptoms and the severity of the disease, which is related to the degree of enzyme deficiency (22,29). All of these forms are inherited as autosomal recessive traits (19). More than seventy mutations have been identified in the *GAA* gene that encodes acid α-glucosidase (29), but the location of the mutation in the gene is not always predictive of clinical severity (29).

Classic infantile-onset GSD type II presents at a mean age of 1.6 to 2.0 months, usually with feeding difficulties and/or a failure to thrive, motor abnormalities such as muscular weakness, motor retardation, or paucity of movements, or respiratory problems like airway infections and respiratory difficulty (21,34). Less common, the first symptoms are malaise, sweating, fatigue, irritability, a weak cry, constipation, vomiting, regurgitation, spasm, tremor, and questionable mental retardation (34). The most common findings on physical examination at presentation are cardiomegaly, hypotonia, tachypnea, dyspnea, pallor or cyanosis, an enlarged tongue, cardiac murmurs, and moderate hepatomegaly (21,34). Infants with classic infantile-onset GSD type II have a rapidly progressive cardiac hypertrophy, impaired motor development, and decreased body weight for age even when receiving nasogastric tube feeding (34). The median age at death is 6 to 9 months (21,34). Death is from cardiac and/or respiratory failure (19,21,34). This form of GSD type II has a complete or near complete deficiency of acid α-glucosidase. The incidence of classic infantile-onset GSD type II varies in different ethnic groups and ranges from 1/14,000 in African Americans to 1/100,000 to 1/200,000 in the Caucasian population (19,21).

Autopsy of children with classic infantile-onset GSD type II reveals marked glycogen accumulation in the heart and skeletal muscle (about 10 times normal) and an approximately threefold increase in glycogen in the liver (19). Glycogen accumulation is predominantly within lysosomes, but is also within the cytoplasmic cytosol (26). The latter glycogen accumulation may result from glycogen release from lysosomes or possibly because the pathway to the lysosome is saturated (29). In addition to the heart, skeletal muscle, and liver, virtually every organ that has been examined accumulates glycogen. Widespread intralysosomal glycogen storage has been noted in smooth muscle, vascular endothelial cells, kidney, lymphocytes, skin, and the nervous system (19). Nervous system involvement is more marked in the spinal cord and brain stem than in the cerebral cortex (19). Prominent glycogen buildup is reported in Schwann cells, anterior horn cells of the spinal cord, motor nuclei of the brain stem, spinal ganglia, myenteric plexus, astrocytes, and oligodendroglia, as well as in pericytes (13,19).

The second form of GSD type II is termed childhood, juvenile, or muscular variant GSD type II (19). Approximately one-half of these individuals have an age of onset of symptoms at less than 2 years of age, while the other one-half present from 2 to 15 years of age (19). Muscle weakness is the dominant feature of childhood/juvenile-onset GSD type II, and cardiomegaly is absent (19,36). Muscle weakness in childhood/juvenile GSD type II progresses more slowly than in classic infantile-onset GSD type II, but death ensues from respiratory failure usually before the end of the third decade (19,36).

At the other end of the age spectrum from the classic infantile-onset GSD type II is an adult-onset form of the disease that presents as a slowly progressive myopathy beginning in the third to sixth decade of life (16,29,34). Muscle weakness is proximal with greater involvement of the lower extremities than the upper extremities, and truncal involvement is ubiquitous (16,19,29). Approximately 30% of patients with adult-onset GSD type II present with symptoms such as somnolence, morning headache, orthopnea, or exertional dyspnea (19,29). Cardiomegaly is absent in adult-onset GSD type II, and death results from respiratory failure (19,29,36). Minimal or no specific abnormalities are usually found in tissues other than skeletal muscle at autopsy (19), although cases with vacuolar myopathy of smooth muscle (35) and cerebral vascular involvement are documented (19,23).

Ophthalmological abnormalities in GSD type II have been reported rarely, and only in the infantile-onset form of the disease (16,36). The only clinical manifestation of infantile-onset GSD type II that has been reported is extraocular muscle weakness (14,32). Smith and Reinecke reported a 3-year-old boy with clinical signs of childhood GSD type II who had surgical correction of his esotropia (32). TEM of the left inferior oblique muscle demonstrated abundant glycogen within myocytes, as well as in capillary endothelium and pericytes in the connective tissue (32). Toussaint and Danis reported the ocular histopathological findings in a 5-month-old girl with classic infantile-onset GSD type II (33). Using light microscopy, they noted vacuolization and excess glycogen in the extraocular striated muscles, smooth muscle of the ciliary body and iris, corneal endothelial cells, and in the retina (ganglion cells, Müller cells, and pericytes of retinal capillaries) (33). Ultrastructural examination of eyes from two aborted fetuses with GSD type II revealed extensive deposits of lysosomal glycogen in virtually all ocular tissues (24,28). Libert et al. examined a 22-week-old female fetus and found lysosomal glycogen accumulation in conjunctiva and corneal epithelial cells, keratocytes, corneal endothelial cells, fibroblasts of the conjunctiva, iris, choroid and sclera, capillary endothelial cells of the conjunctiva, uvea, and retina, ganglion cells, Müller cells, and photoreceptors of the retina, and glial cells of the optic nerve (24). Only the RPE was noted to be unaffected (24). Pokorny et al. had virtually identical findings in a 16-week-old fetus; only the iris and RPE were spared from glycogen accumulation (28). The only report of an ocular examination from an older child with classic infantile-onset GSD type II was by Goebel et al., who documented a 9-month-old boy with strabismus, but visual impairment and funduscopic abnormalities were not recorded (14). Goebel et al. focused their studies on the retina, and noted lysosomal glycogen accumulation in ganglion cells, cells of the inner nuclear layer, and the inner segments of photoreceptors (14). The RPE lacked glycogen within lysosomes (14).

Several years ago, this author examined both eyes from an approximately 1-year-old girl with infantile-onset GSD type II who had been treated for 4 months with recombinant human acid α-glucosidase (4,37). She died 2 days following an episode of aspiration, and the eyes were removed approximately 2 hours after death. Light microscopy of tissue sections stained with hematoxylin and eosin revealed that both eyes had a vacuolar myopathy of smooth muscle in the iris, ciliary body, and scleral blood vessels, lacy vacuolization of the iris pigment epithelium, prominent vacuolization of lens epithelial cells, and vacuolar myopathy of the superior rectus and inferior oblique muscles (Fig. 1). The periodic acid Schiff (PAS) reagent disclosed glycogen accumulation within the corneal epithelium and endothelium, the sphincter pupillae, iris pigment epithelium, ciliary smooth muscle cells, lens epithelium, retinal ganglion cells, the inner plexiform layer of the retina along with approximately 20% of the cells in the inner nuclear layer, smooth muscle within the walls of scleral and orbital arteries and arterioles, glial cells within the optic nerve, and skeletal muscle fibers of the inferior oblique muscle. TEM revealed lysosomes engorged with glycogen in several cell types: conjunctival epithelium, scleral fibroblasts, non-pigmented ciliary epithelium, smooth muscle of the ciliary body, retinal ganglion cells (Fig. 2), cells of the inner nuclear layer of the retina, retinal capillary pericytes, an occasional photoreceptor, and the inferior oblique muscle. In the inner nuclear layer of the retina, glycogen accumulation was prominent in bipolar cells and Müller cells, and it was less in the amacrine and horizontal cells. Some of the inferior oblique muscle fibers contained massive amounts of glycogen, which was both within lysosomes and free in the cytoplasm (Fig. 3). Lysosomes containing glycogen were not observed in the pigmented ciliary epithelium or the RPE.

Ocular histopathological studies in adult-onset GSD type II have apparently not been reported. However, this author recently examined the eyes from an approximately 60-year-old woman who died

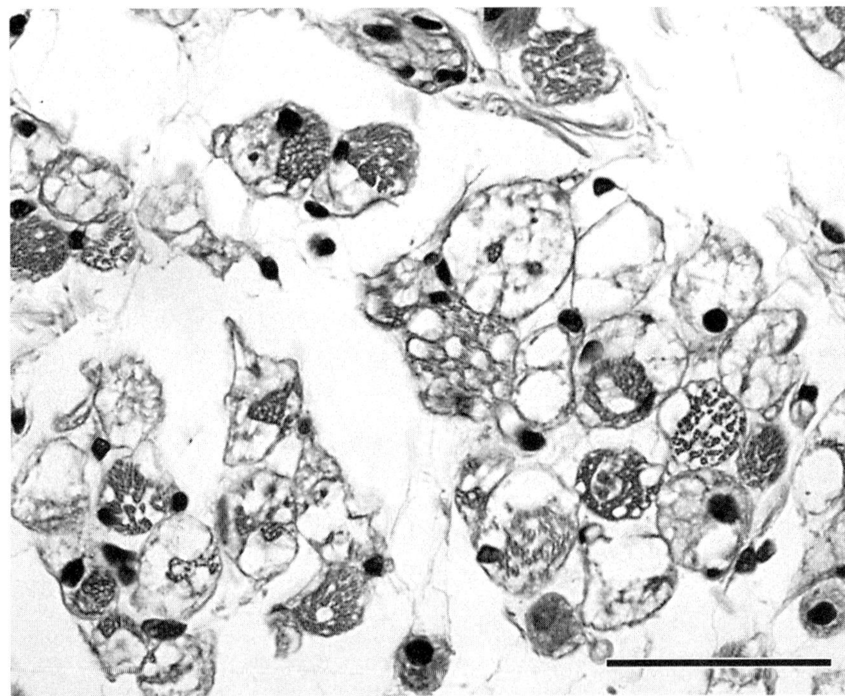

Figure 1 Inferior oblique muscle from a child with infantile-onset glycogen storage disease type II. Light microscopy shows typical vacuolar change ("vacuolar myopathy") due to distension of the skeletal muscle fibers by glycogen (hematoxylin and eosin; bar = 1μm).

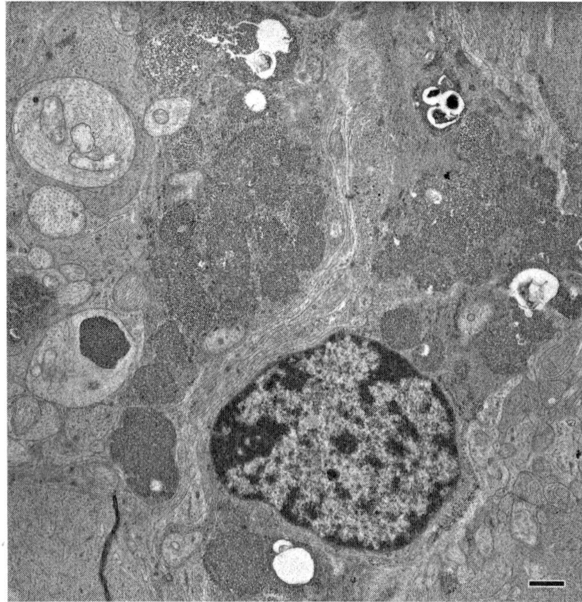

Figure 2 Transmission electron microscopy of the retina from a child with infantile-onset glycogen storage disease type II showing prominent accumulation of glycogen within lysosomes of the retinal ganglion cells (bar = 1μm).

with this disorder. Light microscopy of sections stained with hematoxylin and eosin did not disclose any pathological changes within the eyes or extraocular muscles, and glycogen accumulation was not detected using the PAS reagent.

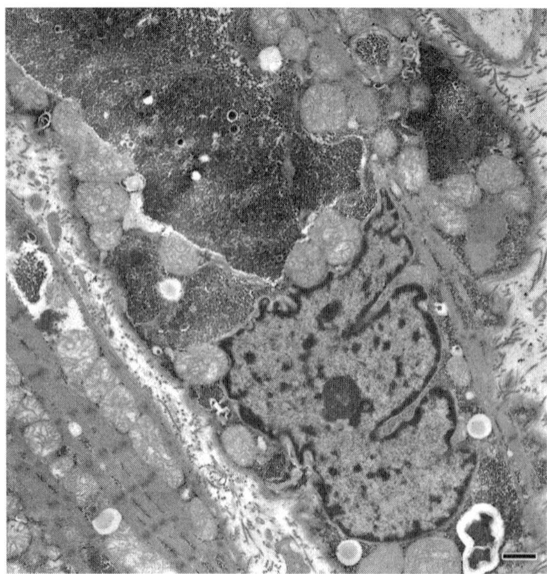

Figure 3 Transmission electron microscopy of the inferior oblique muscle from a child with glycogen storage disease type II discloses abundant free glycogen deposits, probably originating from disrupted lysosomes, and lysosomes (membrane-bound vacuoles) distended with glycogen (bar = 1μm).

The presence of lysosomal glycogen accumulation within the ocular tissues of children with infantile-onset GSD type II indicates that more detailed ophthalmological evaluations are warranted in children receiving enzyme replacement therapy or gene therapy (8,25). The prominent glycogen accumulation in the lens epithelium has the potential to cause early cataract formation, while that in the retina may cause aberrant visual function. Specialized techniques such as pattern electroretinograms and visual evoked potentials may be particularly useful for assessing subtle retinal derangement as the children age (5).

REFERENCES

1. Abe T, Tamai M. Ocular changes of glycogen storage disease type I. Ophthalmologica 1995; 209:92–5.
2. Alonso MD, Lomako J, Lomako WM, Whelan WJ. A new look at the biogenesis of glycogen. FASEB J 1995; 9: 1126–37.
3. Baudhuin P, Hers HG, Loeb H. An electron microscopic and biochemical study of type II glycogenosis. Lab Invest 1964; 13:1139–52.
4. Brady RO. Enzyme replacement for lysosomal diseases. Annu Rev Med 2006; 57:283–96.
5. Brecelj J, Strucl M, Zidar I, Tekavcic-Pompe M. Pattern ERG and VEP maturation in schoolchildren. Clin Neurophysiol 2002; 113:1764–70.
6. Bron AJ, Tripathi RC. Corneal disorders. In: Goldberg MF, ed. Genetic and Metabolic Eye Disease. Boston: Litlte Brown, 1974:281–323.
7. Chen YT. Glycogen storage diseases. In: CR Scriver, AL Beaudet, WS Sly, D Valle, B Childs, KW Kinzler, B Vogelstein, eds. The Metabolic & Molecular Bases of Inherited Disease. 8th ed. New York: McGraw-Hill, 2001: 1521–51.
8. Chen YT, Amalfitano A. Towards a molecular therapy for glycogen storage disease type II (Pompe disease). Mol Med Today 2000; 6:245–51.
9. Chou JY. The molecular basis of type 1 glycogen storage diseases. Curr Mol Med 2001; 1:25–44.
10. Chou JY, Matern D, Mansfield BC, Chen YT. Type I glycogen storage diseases: disorders of the glucose-6-phosphatase complex. Curr Mol Med 2002; 2:121–43.
11. DiMauro S, Lamperti C. Muscle glycogenoses. Muscle Nerve 2001; 24:984–99.
12. Fine RN, Wilson WA, Donnell GN. Retinal changes in glycogen storage disease type I. Am J Dis Child 1968; 115: 328–31.
13. Gambetti P, DiMauro S, Baker L. Nervous system in Pompe's disease. Ultrastructure and biochemistry. J Neuropathol Exp Neurol 1971; 30:412–30.
14. Goebel HH, Kohlschutter A, Pilz H. Ultrastructural observations on the retina in type II glycogenosis (Pompe's disease). Ophthalmologica 1978; 176:61–8.
15. Greenberg CC, Jurczak MJ, Danos AM, Brady MJ. Glycogen branches out: new perspectives on the role of glycogen metabolism in the integration of metabolic pathways. Am J Physiol Endocrinol Metab 2006; 291:E1–8.
16. Hagemans ML, Winkel LP, Van Doorn PA, et al. Clinical manifestation and natural course of late-onset Pompe's disease in 54 Dutch patients. Brain 2005; 128:671–7.

17. Hers HG. Inborn lysosomal diseases. Gastroenterology 1965; 48:625–33.
18. Hers HG, van Hoof F, de Barsy T. Glycogen storage diseases. In: CR Scriver, AL Beaudet, WS Sly, D Valle, eds. The Metabolic Basis of Inherited Disease. 6th ed. New York: McGraw-Hill, 1989:425–52.
19. Hirschhorn R, Reuser AJJ. Glycogen storage disease type II: acid α-glucosidase (acid maltase) deficiency. In: Scriver CR, Beaudet AL, Sly WS, Valle D, Childs B, Kinzler KW, Vogelstein B, eds. The Metabolic & Molecular Bases of Inherited Disease. 8th ed. New York: McGraw-Hill, 2001: 3389–420.
20. Hockman IH. Glycogen storage disease: type I. Am J Dis Child 1969; 117:736.
21. Kishnani PS, Hwu WL, Mandel H, et al. A retrospective, multinational, multicenter study on the natural history of infantile-onset Pompe disease. J Pediatr 2006; 148: 671–6.
22. Kishnani PS, Steiner RD, Bali D, et al. Pompe disease diagnosis and management guideline. Genet Med 2006; 8: 267–88.
23. Kretzschmar HA, Wagner H, Hubner G, et al. Aneurysms and vacuolar degeneration of cerebral arteries in late-onset acid maltase deficiency. J Neurol Sci 1990; 98: 169–83.
24. Libert J, Martin JJ, Ceuterick C, Danis P. Ocular ultrastructural study in a fetus with type II glycogenosis. Br J Ophthalmol 1977; 61:476–82.
25. Mah C, Cresawn KO, Fraites TJ Jr, et al. Sustained correction of glycogen storage disease type II using adeno-associated virus serotype 1 vectors. Gene Ther 2005; 12:1405–9.
26. Martin JJ, De Barsy T, De S, Leroy JG, Palladini G. Acid maltase deficiency (type II glycogenosis). Morphological and biochemical study of a childhood phenotype. J Neurol Sci 1976; 30:155–66.
27. Melis D, Fulceri R, Parenti G, et al. Genotype/phenotype correlation in glycogen storage disease type 1b: a multicentre study and review of the literature. Eur J Pediatr 2005; 164:501–8.
28. Pokorny KS, Ritch R, Friedman AH, Desnick RJ. Ultrastructure of the eye in fetal type II glycogenosis (Pompe's disease). Invest Ophthalmol Vis Sci 1982; 22: 25–31.
29. Raben N, Plotz P, Byrne BJ. Acid alpha-glucosidase deficiency (glycogenosis type II, Pompe disease). Curr Mol Med 2002; 2:145–66.
30. Rake JP, Visser G, Labrune P, et al. Glycogen storage disease type I: diagnosis, management, clinical course and outcome. Results of the European Study on Glycogen Storage Disease Type I (ESGSD I). Eur J Pediatr 2002; 161 (Suppl. 1):S20–34.
31. Roach PJ. Glycogen and its metabolism. Curr Mol Med 2002; 2:101–20.
32. Smith RS, Reinecke RD. Electron microscopy of ocular muscle in type II glycogenosis (Pompe's disease). Am J Ophthalmol 1972; 73:965–70.
33. Toussaint D, Danis P. Ocular histopathology in generalized glycogenosis (Pompe's disease). Arch Ophthalmol 1965; 73:342–9.
34. van den Hout HM, Hop W, van Diggelen OP, et al. The natural course of infantile Pompe's disease: 20 original cases compared with 133 cases from the literature. Pediatrics 2003; 112:332–40.
35. van der Walt JD, Swash M, Leake J, Cox EL. The pattern of involvement of adult-onset acid maltase deficiency at autopsy. Muscle Nerve 1987; 10:272–81.
36. Winkel LP, Hagemans ML, van Doorn PA, et al. The natural course of non-classic Pompe's disease; a review of 225 published cases. J Neurol 2005; 252:875–84.
37. Winkel LP, Kamphoven JH, van den Hout HJ, et al. Morphological changes in muscle tissue of patients with infantile Pompe's disease receiving enzyme replacement therapy. Muscle Nerve 2003; 27:743–51.
38. Wolfsdorf JI, Weinstein DA. Glycogen storage diseases. Rev Endocr Metab Disord 2003; 4:95–102.

40

Disorders of Glycosaminoglycans (Mucopolysaccharides) and Proteoglycans

Gordon K. Klintworth
Departments of Pathology and Ophthalmology, Duke University, Durham, North Carolina, U.S.A.

INTRODUCTION

A significant component of all tissues is the complex polysaccharides known as glycosaminoglycans (GAGs). In the past the term "acid mucopolysaccharide" was used to designate these extracellular macromolecules containing a preponderance of carbohydrate. As this nomenclature was confusing and lacked precision, the GAGs became the preferred designation (117). A vast body of information about GAGs now exists, and an understanding of the mucopolysaccharidoses (MPSs) requires an appreciation of the basic structure of the GAGs and proteoglycans (PGs).

GLYCOSAMINOGLYCANS

Overview

Several GAGs are recognized and they differ in their sugar composition: hyaluronic acid (hyaluronan) (HA), heparin (H), heparan sulfate (HS), dermatan sulfate (DS), chondroitin sulfates (chondroitin-4-sulfate [C4S], chondroitin-6-sulfate [C6S]), keratan sulfate(s) (KS). Each of these macromolecules is a polysaccharide polymer comprising unbranched disaccharide repeating units composed of alternating hexosaminic (*N*-acetylglucosamine, *N*-acetylgalactosamine) and uronic acid (D-glucuronic acid, L-iduronic acid—an epimer of D-glucuronic acid) moieties. The nature of the predominant repeating unit is typical for each GAG. Complex modification patterns are present in the GAGs and there is some chemical microheterogeneity in the hexosamine and uronic acid portion of each polysaccharide polymer. Modifications in the sugar residues of the GAGs create a tremendous molecular diversity and this is suspected of influencing interactions between GAGs/PGs and different molecules (33,251). A sulfate group is attached to oxygen or nitrogen in various positions in all GAGs except in the nonsulfated HA. Both oxygen esters R–O–SO_3– ("*O*-sulfates") and derivates of sulfamic acid (R–NH–SO_3 "*N*-sulfates") exist. With the exception of

H and HS, all sulfated GAGs are *O*-sulfated. The site of the sulfate esters varies in the different GAGs. With DS and HS, which are hybrid molecules containing nonidentical disaccharide or tetrasaccharide regions, the iduronic acid and hexosamine is variably sulfated, but the glucuronic acid is not.

KS differs from the other GAGs by containing galactose instead of uronic acid and it has a great degree of variability (163). Moreover, KS-containing proteins resemble glycoproteins rather than PGs in chemical composition.

KS was once thought to be present only in cartilage and the cornea, where it accounts for approximately 45% to 60% of the total sulfated GAGs. However, studies employing molecular biological techniques have disclosed KS containing PGs in other sites including aorta (79,200), tendon (14), and even sclera (14).

Two main types of KS are recognized: corneal KS (KS-I) and cartilaginous KS (KS-II) (133). Skeletal KS (KS-II) is subclassified into two groups: KS-IIA and KS-IIB (175). KS chains from articular and intervertebral disc cartilage (KS-IIA) contain α-(1,3)-fucose and α-(2,6)-linked *N*-acetyl-neuraminic acid residues, that are absent from KS from tracheal or nasal-septum cartilage (KS-IIB) (174). Serum levels of KS are elevated in patients with generalized osteoarthritis, reflecting an elevated rate of cartilage PG catabolism in these individuals (241).

Corneal Glycosaminoglycans

Corneal thickness varies considerably among species and alcian blue staining at a critical electrolyte concentration, suggestive of KS, increases as corneas thicken (214). Differences in KS content, especially its oversulfated terminal domain, which is absent from mouse cornea, account in part for the species variation in corneal thickness (214). The KS content increases with corneal thickness, whereas DS increases in thin corneas (214). Scott and Haigh (215) have suggested that the oxygen tension, which varies with corneal thickness may influence the CS/KS ratio. This view finds support in the observation that the amount of radioactivity incorporated into corneal KS increases markedly with decreased oxygen tension or an increased lactate concentration, whereas the biosynthesis of other GAGs decreases concomitantly (19).

Also, corneal thickness relates to the water content of the cornea and this correlates with the distribution of PGs and their water sorptive and retentive capacity (37). Of the GAGs, KS plays a particularly important part in this regard. The bound (nonfreezable) water content within the cornea decreases in progressing from epithelium to endothelium, while the total and free (freezable) water content increases from the epithelium to endothelium (37). In this regard it is noteworthy that the anterior part of the rabbit cornea synthesizes mostly a KS rich GAG fraction, while the posterior part produces mostly CS and DS (47).

The peripheral cornea has less acidic GAGs and KS than the central cornea, where chondroitin is replaced by CS (26). In contrast to the cornea, sclera contains DS and hyaluronate (26).

With the exception of HA other GAGs are covalently linked to a protein core at a site containing monosaccharides. The connecting link for CS, DS, H, and HS consists of glucuronic acid-galactose-galactose-xylose-serine, whereas KS is linked to serine/threonine or asparagine (104).

PROTEOGLYCANS

Overview

The PGs are anionic polymers with a polypeptide core and GAG side chains and they are abundant in the extracellular matrix (ECM), basement membranes, and at cell surfaces. Branched oligosaccharide side chains are also attached to the core protein.

Recombinant DNA methodology has led to considerable advances in our understanding of the structure, function, and metabolism of PGs. Most well-defined PGs have poetic names related to their structure or presumed function. The core proteins of PGs contain structural motifs, such as transmembrane domains, cysteine-rich regions, and globular segments, but no structural domain is common to all PGs (62,104).

A vast body of information is available about the PGs, and about corneal PGs (lumican, decorin, keratocan, mimecan) (17,45,62,94,106,107,146,164,221) and a detailed discussion about them is beyond the scope of this chapter. For additional information on PGs and their role in development the reader should refer to various reviews (33,62,64,87,104,114,139,158,206,242).

The PGs can be classified according to the predominant GAG that attaches to the core protein and according to major families based on similarities in their structure (Table 1). The main families are small interstitial PGs with leucine-rich repeat (LRR) regions, cell surface HS PGs, HA-binding PGs, perlecan, and secretory granule PGs.

Small Interstitial Leucine-Rich Proteoglycans

A superfamily of small PGs containing tandem arrays of leucine-rich repeats (SLRRs) includes nyctalopin, which is apparently only expressed in the kidney and retina (photoreceptors, bipolar interneurons, amacrine cells, and ganglion cells) (20). Several small interstitial PGs (lumican, decorin, biglycan, fibromodulin, and epiphycan) share similar primary structures.

A cluster of genes for some SLRRs [asporin (*ASPN*), ECM protein 2 (*ECM2*) osteomodulin (*OMD*), and osteoglycin (*OGN*)] is located on chromosome 9 (9q21.3–q22).

Table 1 Representative Proteoglycan Core Proteins

Core protein	Human gene	Gene location	Attached GAGs	References
Small interstitail proteins with leucine-rich repeats (SLRRs)				
Asporin (periodontal ligament-associated protein 1)	*ASPN*	9q21.3–q22	CS/DS	149
Biglycan (proteoglycan I)	*BGN*	Xq28	CS/DS	211,245
Decorin (proteoglycan II)	*DCN*	12q13.2	CS/DS	29,49
Epiphycan (PG-Lb9, dermatan sulfate proteoglycan 3)	*DSPG3*	12q21	CS/DS	52
Extracellular matrix protein 2	*ECM2*	9q22.3	Not known	176
Fibromodulin	*FMOD*	1q32.1	KS	233
Keratocan	*KERA*	12q22	KS	185,237
Lumican (keratan sulfate proteoglycan)	*LUM*	12q21.3–q22	KS	38
Osteomodulin (osteoadherin)	*OMD*	9q22	KS	181
Osteoglycin (mimecan)	*OGN*	9q22.3	KS	238
Nyctalopin	*NYX*	Xp11.4	KS	20,193,272
Opticin/oculoglycan	*OPTC*	Unknown	KS	73
PRELP (proline arginine-rich end leucine rich repeat)	*PRELP*	1q32	KS	96
CS/DS				
Chondroitin sulfate proteoglycan 1 (aggrecan)	*AGC1*	15q26.1	CS/DS	86
Chondroitin sulfate proteoglycan 2 (versican)	*CSPG2*	5q12–q14	CS/DS	115,165
Chondroitin sulfate proteoglycan 3 (neuroan)	*NCAN*	19p12	CS/DS	190,278
Chondroitin sulfate proteoglycan 4 (NG2, Mel-CSPG)	*CSPG4*	Chromosome 15	CS/DS	225
Neuroglycan C/CALEB (chondroitin sulfate proteoglycan 5)	*CSPG5*	3p21.3	CS/DS	274
Bamacan (chondroitin sulfate proteoglycan 6)	*CSPG6*	10q25	CS/DS	83
Brevican (chondroitin sulfate proteoglycan 7)		Mouse chromosome 3	CS/DS	273
Tenascin C (cytotactin, hexabrachion)	*TNC*	9q33	CS/DS	263
Tenascin R (restrictin)	*TNR*	1q24	CS/DS	207
HS core proteins				
Perlecan (heparan sulfate proteoglycan of basement membrane)	*HSPG2*	1p36.1	HS	15,56,230
Collagen type XVIII	*COL18A1*	21q22.3	HS	75
Agrin	*AGRN*	1pter–p32	HS	22
Transmembrane cell surface proteoglycans				
Syndecan-like integral membrane proteoglycans (SLIPS)				
Syndecan 1 (syndecan, CD138 antigen)	*SDC1*	2p24.1	HS	6
Syndecan 2 (fibroglycan, heparan sulfate glycoprotein)	*SDC2*	8q22–q24	HS	25
Syndecan 3 (N-syndecan)	*SDC3*	1p32	HS	21,44
Syndecan 4 (amphiglycan, ryudocan)	*SDC4*	20q12–q13	HS	25,50
Glypican-related integral membrane glycoproteins (GRIPS)				
Glypican 1	*GPC1*	2q35–q37	HS	127,254
Glypican 2 (cerebroglycan)	*GPC2*	7q22.1	HS	116
Glypican 3	*CPC3*	Xq26	HS	188,256
Glypican 4	*GPC4*	Xq26	HS	258
Glypican 5	*GPC5*	13q32	HS	257
Glypican 6	*GPC6*	13q32	HS	184,255
Secretory granule proteoglycans				
Serglycin (proteoglycan 1)	*PRG1*	10q22.1	CS/HS/H	111

Abbreviations: CS, chondroitin sulfate; DS, dermatan sulfate; GAG, glycosaminoglycans, H, heparin; HS, heparin sulfate; KS, keratan sulfate.

Asporin

ASPN, which has similarities to decorin, derives its name from its unique aspartate-rich N-terminus, but it is probably not a traditional PG because it lacks the serine-glycine dipeptide needed for an *O*-linked GAG attachment.

Biglycan

Biglycan is a small cellular or pericellular PG that is expressed at high levels in the growing skeleton and in human skin at the cell surface of differentiating keratinocytes. The core protein consists predominantly of a series of 11 tandem repeats apparently for protein–protein, protein–cell, or cell–cell interactions (65). Biglycan binds transforming growth factor beta (TGFβ) in vitro.

Decorin

Decorin (galactosaminoglycan PG) is involved in the regulation of extracellular matrix (ECM) formation and cell proliferation. This PG, which occurs in the cornea, contains protein, oligosaccharides, CS, DS, and in some tissues some KS. Decorin interacts with collagen via the CS chains (221).

Extracellular Matrix Protein 2

ECM protein 2 (ECM2) has about one-third amino acid identity with both keratocan and decorin.

Fibromodulin

Fibromodulin from sclera and other tissues contains *N*-glycosidically linked oligosaccharides, some of which are extended to KS chains (14). Fibromodulin produced by scleral and other fibroblasts in culture contains tyrosine sulfate residues (14).

Lumican

Lumican is the main corneal KS-containing PG (24) (Fig. 1). Vertebrate corneas contain multiple lumican core protein isoforms that may arise as products of separate mRNAs (122). The corneal fibroblasts are the only cells that continuously produce KS and lumican under physiological conditions and in the chick this synthesis begins after neural crest derived cells arrive in the primitive corneal stroma (76).

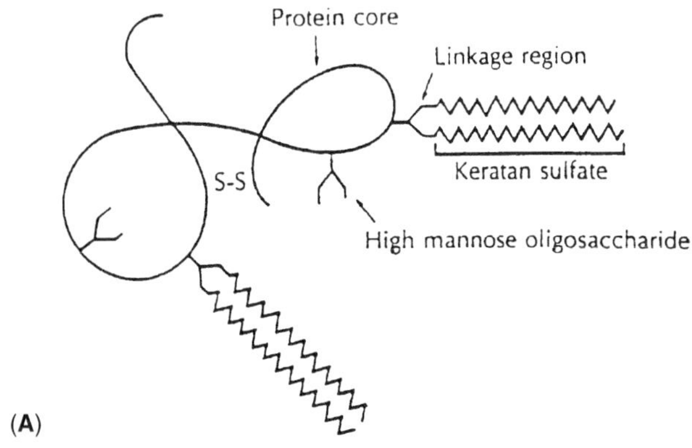

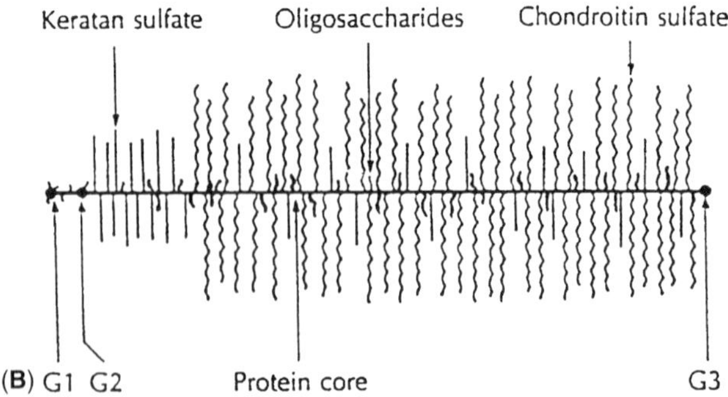

Figure 1 (**A**) Model of corneal keratan sulfate proteoglycan. Note that the keratan sulfate molecule is the only type of glycosaminoglycan attached to the protein core. *Source*: Hassell J, Hascall VC, Ledbetter S, et al. Corneal proteoglycan biosynthesis and macular corneal dystrophy. In: Heredity and Visual Development. Sheffield JB, Hifner SR, eds. New York: Springer-Verlag, 1985. (**B**) Model of cartilage proteoglycan containing chondroitin sulfate, keratan sulfate, and oilgosaccharide chains covalently linked to a common protein core. The protein core contains three globular domains: the binding region (G1), which contains a specific hyaluronate binding site, a second globular domain (G2), and a C-terminal domain (G3). *Source*: Modified from Hardingham TE, Beardmore-Gray M, Dunham DG, et al. Cartilage proteoglycans. In: Functions of Proteoglycans. Evered D, Whelan J, eds. Ciba Foundation Symposium, 1986; 124:30–46.

Originally thought to only be a constituent of cornea, lumican is now known to be present in several tissues. For example, chick lumican is present in muscle and intestine in addition to cornea and lumican core protein and mRNA are synthesized by these tissues (24). The abundance of low sulfate lumican in many tissues indicates that this protein occurs predominantly as a glycoprotein rather than as highly sulfated corneal PG (79). A glycoprotein containing unsulfated lactosaminoglycan chains with similarities to corneal lumican has been isolated from bovine aorta (79) as well as atherosclerotic pigeon aorta (200). The expression of lumican in tissues other than cornea suggests that its physiological role is broader than a function solely in corneal transparency (24), but it also illustrates the weakness in using presumed functional attributes in coining terms for PGs.

Osteoglucin

Osteoglucin (mimecan), a major KS-containing corneal PG, induces bone formation with TGFβ1 and TGFβ2.

Osteomodulin

Osteomodulin, a PG expressed by osteoblasts, is encoded by the *OMD* gene and plays a role in the pathogenesis of some aneurysmal bone cysts (see Chapter 65) (181).

Hyaluronate-Binding Proteoglycans

Although hyaluronan is not one of the GAGs linked directly to the core protein of the PGs it binds strongly to certain PGs [aggregan, versican, Hermes antigen (CD44)].

Aggrecan

Aggrecan is a large aggregating chondroitin sulfate (CS) PG (13,57). The human sequence contains two regions of highly conserved repeats of a hexameric sequence in the KS attachment domain, Glu-Glu-Pro-(Ser,Phe)-Pro-Ser; and a 19 amino acid sequence reiterated 19 times, in the CS-1 portion of the serine-glycine-containing region (57).

Versican

A large connective tissue CS PG expressed by fibroblasts was designated versican from *versatile* and *proteoglycan* (278). It has a 2389 amino acid long core protein and a 20-residue signal peptide and has potential hyaluronan-binding and GAG attachment sites. The carboxy-terminal region of versican contains the same structural motifs (EGF-like repeats, a lectin-like sequence and a complement regulatory protein-like domain) as in the cell adhesion molecules termed LEC-CAMS (selectins). Versican may function in cell recognition by connecting ECM components and cell surface glycoproteins (278). Versican is present in vitreous and probably binds to the HA in an interaction stabilized by a link protein (see Chapter 29) (199).

Heparan Sulfate Proteoglycans of Basement Membrane

Perlecan

The name perlecan was coined for a HS PG with a structure consisting of a series of globules separated by rods, or "beads on a string" (178). It consists of three HS side chains linked to a large core protein of approximately 400 kDa (178). Human perlecan contains 507 amino acid residues. The major protein core of human perlecan without the signal peptide of 21 amino acids, has a Mr of 466,564 and contains five different domains most of which contain internal repeats (166,178): domain I, near the amino terminus, contains a typical signal transfer sequence, a unique segment of 172 amino acids and three Ser-Gly-Asp sequences that are probable sites for HS attachment (166,178). Domain II contains four conserved cysteine- and acidic amino acid-rich repeats that are similar to those found in the low-density lipoprotein receptor (166,177). Domain III shares homology to the short arm of laminin A chain and consists of four cysteine-rich repeats intercalated among three globular regions (178). Domain IV, the largest part with more than 2000 residues, contains 14 to 21 repeats of the immunoglobulin superfamily that are similar to the immunoglobulin-like repeats in the neural cell adhesion molecule (N-CAM) (166,178). The variety of domains in perlecan suggest multiple interactions with other molecules (178).

Perlecan is a constituent of all basement membranes studied to date, including those in the cornea, crystalline lens, and retinal capillaries (107,108,146). It is found in all vascularized, and some other connective tissues. Perlecan is synthesized by basement membrane-producing cells as well as several cell types, including fibroblasts (178).

Cell Surface Heparan Sulfate Proteoglycans

The cell surface PGs are composed of an integral transmembrane protein or are anchored to the cell membrane by a phosphoinositol linkage and almost all are HS PGs (104). They are divided into two families: (*i*) the syndecan-like integral membrane PGs (SLIPS) and (*ii*) the glypican-related integral membrane PGs (GRIPS). A retinal HS containing PG interacts with a N-CAM (42).

Syndecan-Like Integral Membrane Proteoglycans

The SLIPS are characterized by a core protein that spans the cytoplasmic membrane. They include syndecan 1 (180,209), syndecan 2 (fibroglycan) (187), syndecan 3 (*N*-syndecan) (36,93), syndecan 4 (amphiglycan, ryudocan) (50,138) and a cell surface PG known as 48K5 (154,159). These integral cell-surface HS PGs are encoded by different genes and occur in many diverse tissues and cells. They possess highly similar, but unique cytoplasmic and transmembrane domains, including the conservation of four tyrosine residues and the most proximal and most distal cytoplasmic sequences. The core protein of the syndecans have three domains: a matrix-interacting extracellular domain containing several clustered putative GAG attachment sites that may be occupied by HS, a hydrophobic membrane-spanning domain, and a relatively short cytoplasmic tail.

Syndecan 1 acts as a receptor for several ECM components, including basic fibroblast growth factor (bFGF) thus promoting bFGF association with its high-affinity receptor (131). It binds via HS chains to collagen types I, II, and V, fibronectin, tenascin, and thrombospondin (104). This highly conserved PG (104,154,209) is predominantly expressed on epithelial cells and the expression undergoes striking spatial and temporal changes during embryonic development (232).

Syndecan 2 with properties similar to other syndecans is encoded by the *SCD2* gene, which is located in the region of the *MYC* gene.

A prominent feature of syndecan 3 (*N*-syndecan) is an extensive threonine, serine, and proline-rich domain with close similarities to comparable regions in mucin-like proteins in which *O*-linked oligosaccharides are bound to the threonine and serine residues (93). Multiple functional domains of syndecan 3 provide potential sites for mediating adhesive cell–matrix interactions and cytoskeletal reorganization (93). It contains three potential GAG attachment sites, as well as a threonine- and proline-rich region (36).

Syndecan 4, also known as ryudocan (from *ryûdousei* a Japanese word for fluidity) and amphiglycan. The alternative designation amphiglycan stems from the extension of its domain structure on both sides of the plasma membrane, and to its localization around cells of both epithelial and fibroblastic origin (50). The core protein is 198 amino acids long and except for the sequences that represent putative HS chain attachment sites, the extracellular domain of this protein has a unique structure (50). Syndecan 4 is an anticoagulantly active HS PG, which was thought to play a major role in the maintenance of blood fluidity (138). Syndecan 4 exhibits only three potential GAG attachment sites within the extracellular region, in contrast to syndecan's five GAG attachment sites within the same domain (138).

Glypican-Related Integral Membrane Glycoproteins

The GRIPS are a family of cell surface HS PGs in which the core protein is anchored to the cytoplasmic membrane by glycosyl phoshatidylinositol. To date six distinct members of the GRIPS family have been identified: glypican 1, glypican 2, glypican 3, glypican 4, glypican 5, and glypican 6. The GRIPS are thought to play important roles in cell signaling related to growth and division. For example, there is evidence that glypican 3 may modulate the action of insulin-like growth factor 2 (ILGF2) (188).

Secretory Granule Proteoglycans

Another PG, serglycin (111), is a secretory granule which contains a series of serine-glycine repeats (104). It is stored in many hematopoietic cells and contains several *O*-linked GAGs (HS, DS, H).

Other Proteoglycans

The cytokine TGFβ induces the expression of *TGFBI* gene (see Chapter 32) and mediates multiple cellular processes under its control by an interaction with several receptors on the surface of cells. One of these receptors, TGFβ receptor type III (betaglycan), is a polymorphic membrane-anchored PG with high affinity for TGFβ. Its core protein has an extracellular domain with clustered sites for potential attachment of GAG chains (148). The transmembrane region and the short cytoplasmic tail of betaglycan are similar to these regions in an endothelial cell membrane glycoprotein involved in intercellular recognition (endoglin). The ectodomain of betaglycan can be released as a soluble PG; a potential cleavage site near the transmembrane region is identical to the highly regulated cleavage site of the membrane-anchored TGFβ precursor. The unique features of betaglycan suggest important roles in cell interaction with TGFβ.

DEGRADATION OF PROTEOGLYCANS AND GLYCOSAMINOGLYCANS

A variety of proteases can hydrolyze the protein part of the PGs, while the carbohydrate component is catabolized intracellularly by a series of lysosomal acid hydrolases. Exoglycosidases (such as α-L-iduronidase, or β-*N*-acetylhexosaminidase) sequentially cleave the terminal glycosyl units from the linear polysaccharide chains. Should the terminal sugar not be removed due to a deficiency of the appropriate enzyme the chain is not further degraded by other exoglycosidases. However, endoglycosidases such as hyaluronidase can degrade some GAGs to variable sized fragments (147). Sulfatases with a remarkably high degree of specificity toward the sugar moiety of the substrate molecule are involved in the hydrolysis of particular sulfate esters.

As some GAGs share specific glycoside linkages with each other and with glycoproteins and glycolipids, hydrolases capable of cleaving such bonds sometimes act on several different macromolecules. As expected, deficiencies of such glycosidases result in the accumulation of more than one type of carbohydrate-containing substance. Indeed decreased levels of GM_1- and GM_2-gangliosides and ceramide lactoside have been identified within the brain in MPSs with neuronal storage (27,91,120,141,235,236). Also, several enzymes participate in the degradation of specific GAGs. For example α-L-iduronidase, sulfoiduronate sulfatase, and β-glucuronidase degrade DS and HS. These two compounds accumulate when α-L-iduronidase (MPS I) or sulfoiduronate sulfatase (MPS II), or β-glucuronidase (MPS VII) are deficient.

The defective genes and enzymes have been identified in all well-defined MPSs (Table 2). When these specific lysosomal enzymes are deficient, proteases and endoglycosidases degrade some of these molecules partially, so that variable-sized fragments of GAGs accumulate in the tissues or become excreted in the urine as products of incomplete degradation (68,137).

DISORDERS OF GLYCOSAMINOGLYCANS

Overview

A perspective of some historical highlights in our understanding of the MPSs will be provided as these diseases have taught much despite their rarity. In retrospect, others probably recognized patients with these disorders before Hunter (112), but his report in 1917 was the first definitive one. Two years later Hurler (113) documented two infants with a similar grotesque phenotype but with corneal clouding, a gibbus, and mental retardation. By 1938 it was well established that a wide variety of cells in patients with the Hunter–Hurler syndrome were distended with abnormal material (141). Particularly important from the ocular standpoint was an article by Njå (177) who not only recognized forms of gargoylism with X-linked recessive and autosomal recessive modes of inheritance, but stressed that corneal clouding was absent in the X-linked cases [now known as MPS type II (MPS II)]. In 1952, Brante (27) introduced the term MPS after demonstrating an accumulation of substances composed of hexosamine, glucuronic acid, and sulfur in the liver of two patients of what was still designated gargoylism. Several years later, Brown (31) isolated HS from the liver of an affected individual.

The next breakthrough occurred from chemical analyses of urine, when Dorfman and Lorincz (59)

Table 2 Mucopolysaccharidoses

Disorder	MIM #	Gene	Gene location	Enzyme or protein deficiency
Muopolysaccharidosis type IH (Hurler syndrome) (MPS IH)	#607014	*IDUA*	4p16.3	α-L-Iduronidase
Muopolysaccharidosis type IS (Scheie syndrome) (MPS IS)	#607016	*IDUA*	4p16.3	α-L-Iduronidase
Muopolysaccharidosis type II (Hunter syndrome) (MPS II)	+309900	*IDS*	Xq28	Iduronate-2-sulfatase
Muopolysaccharidosis type IIIA (Sanfillipo syndrome type A) (MPS IIIA)	#252900	*SGSH*	17q25.3	Heparan *N*-sulfatase (sulphamidase)
Muopolysaccharidosis type IIIB (Sanfillipo syndrome type B) (MPS IIIB)	#252920	*NAGLU*	17q21	α-*N*-acetylglucosaminidase
Muopolysaccharidosis type IIIC (Sanfillipo syndrome type C) (MPS IIIC)	#252930	*HGSNAT*	8p11.1	Acetyl-CoA-α glucosamine *N*-acetyltransferase
Muopolysaccharidosis type IIID (Sanfillipo syndrome type D) (MPS IIID)	#252940	*GNA*	*12q14*	*N*-acetylglucosamine 6-sulfatase
Muopolysaccharidosis type IVA (Morquio syndrome type A) (MPS IVA)	+253000	*GALNS*	16q24.3	Galactose 6-sulfatase
Muopolysaccharidosis type IVB (Morquio syndromes type B) (MPS IVB)	#230500	*GLB1*	3p21.33	β-Galactosidase
Muopolysaccharidosis type V (Scheie syndrome) (MPS V) now called MPS IS				
Muopolysaccharidosis type VI (Maroteaux–Lamy syndrome) (MPS VI)	+253200	*ARSB*	5q11–q13	Arylsulfatase B
Muopolysaccharidosis type VII (Sly syndrome (MPS VII)	+253220	*GUSB*	7q21.11	β-D-glucuronidase
Muopolysaccharidosis type VIII (MPS VIII) No longer an excepted entity				
Muopolysaccharidosis type IX (Natowicz disease) (MPS IX)	#601492	*HYAL1*	3p21.3–p21.2	Hyaluronidase

Abbreviations: CS, chondroitin sulfate; DS, dermatan sulfate; H, heparin; KS, keratan sulfate.

discovered excessive amounts of DS and HS in the urine of a patient with Hurler syndrome (MPS IH). They postulated, before the concept of lysosomal storage diseases (LSDs), that the basic defect was an overproduction of GAGs (designated mucopolysaccharides at that time). A chemical basis for distinguishing certain MPSs became recognized when Harris (98) found that an excessive urinary excretion of HS alone typified a specific clinical entity (now known as MPS III) (98,208). The possibility of the MPSs being LSDs (see Chapter 38) due to a faulty degradation of GAGs was first raised by Van Hoof and Hers (253) because of transmission electron microscopic (TEM) observations on cells distended with a storage product. Knowledge of the MPSs increased immensely with studies on isolated fibroblasts cultured from skin biopsies. Matalon and Dorfman (161) found that large amounts of DS accumulate in such cultured fibroblasts. Radioactive kinetic studies in cultured fibroblasts provided a major breakthrough in elucidating the enzymatic defects in the MPSs. Utilizing ^{35}S-sulfate, Frantantoni and colleagues (69) established the fundamental disorder to be in the degradation of sulfated GAGs. Subsequently, Neufeld and her collaborators discovered that the abnormal accumulation in cultured cells with the Hurler syndrome (MPS IH) and Hunter syndrome (MPS II) could be prevented by growing the mutant cells with others that were either normal or from individuals with the other MPSs (70,71). Subsequently, it became established that fibroblasts derived from each of the MPSs were deficient in specific enzymes. Corrective factors for specific MPSs were isolated and purified from various tissues and the urine (35,71,140,169,170). Enzymes secreted by normal fibroblasts in culture are taken up by defective fibroblasts permitting them to complete the degradation of the stored GAGs. With some diseases, such as MPS IH and MPS IS, mutual correction by cocultured fibroblasts was not observed (266), whereas fibroblasts from certain patients with the phenotypical Sanfilippo syndrome (MPS III) cross-reacted with each other suggesting that it consisted of more than one entity, each presumably lacking a different enzyme required for HS degradation (170).

Mucopolysaccharidoses

Several distinct MPSs are recognized each with its own characteristic clinicopathologic features and a vast literature pertaining to them is reviewed elsewhere (171,222,265). Most MPSs are characterized by a gargoyle-like facies, skeletal abnormalities, variable degrees of mental retardation, abnormal mucopolysacchariduria, and a visceral storage of GAGs. Almost all recognized MPSs have an autosomal recessive mode of inheritance, the only exception being MPS II (Hunter syndrome), which has the mutant gene located on the long arm of the X-chromosome (Xq28.1) (151).

Basically, the MPSs are progressive LSDs caused by an inherited deficiency of specific exoglycosidases or sulfatases. A deficiency of one of these enzymes, necessary for the degradation of GAGs, results in an accumulation of the corresponding macromolecule within numerous tissues and their increased excretion in the urine. As with other LSDs, undegraded material accumulates in single membrane delimited intracellular vacuoles.

The widely accepted classification of the MPSs, as accomplished by McKusick (265) is based on a combination of clinical features and enzymatic defects (Table 2). Not only do the specific MPSs differ from each other, but within the recognized types, the age of onset and the clinical severity vary. Poorly understood regulatory mechanisms and the existence of some enzymes as multiple isozymes may contribute to this clinical variability.

A fascinating aspect of the MPSs is the manner in which a deficiency of a particular enzyme can cause striking phenotypic differences. This point is illustrated by the marked differences between MPS IH and MPS IS, both of which are expressions of a deficiency of α-L-iduronidase. In MPS IH mental deficiency is the rule and corneal opacification is severe before the second year of life. This sharply contrasts with MPS IS, in which individuals are of normal or superior intelligence and lack corneal opacities until after the age of 4 years.

Affected tissues in all of the MPSs have a similar ultrastructure. Membrane-bound cytoplasmic vacuoles contain flocculent, fibrillogranular and/or lamellar bodies, often with transverse striations ("zebra bodies"). The latter type of inclusion is typical of the stored intraneuronal material in the brain (7,61,91,252,261) and retina (243) and corresponds to a storage of gangliosides (53). Nonneural tissues such as the liver contain electron-lucent vacuoles (due to the solubility of the stored material in solutions used for the processing of the tissue) or accumulate fibrillogranular material.

Spontaneous animal models have been found for several MPSs [MPS I (cat) (99,227), (dog) (43,218); MPS VI (cat) (3,101,259); MPS VII (dog) (100,103,229,270), (mouse) (23,260)] and these offer opportunities for further studies on the pathobiology of the MPSs.

Mucopolysaccharidosis Type I (Hurler Syndrome, Scheie Syndrome)

Located within the *IDUA* gene encoding for α-L-iduronidase (151) are mutations that account for two entities that manifest a deficiency of this enzyme. These conditions vary in severity with MPS IH (Hurler syndrome) being the most serious, and MPS IS (Scheie syndrome) the least severe. Separate genetic mutations are responsible for these two disorders and only one clinical phenotype develops in affected families.

Striking physical abnormalities characterize the phenotype of MPS IH. These include a grotesque facies with a prominent brow, an oversized tongue, a large saddle-shaped nose with broad nostrils, and a short neck associated with dwarfism, limitations in the mobility of joints, a protuberant abdomen with hepatosplenomegaly, umbilical and/or inguinal hernias, cardiac abnormalities, deafness, and mental retardation. Skeletal abnormalities of the vertebrae are accompanied by a large shallow sella turcica, and broad stubby fingers due to hyperplastic terminal pharyngeal bones.

Infants with MPS IH may appear normal at birth, but have inguinal or umbilical hernias. Corneal clouding and the other characteristic physical findings of MPS IH are seldom recognized until 6 to 24 months after birth. Yet an abnormal accumulation of GAGs within the tissue has been confirmed in fetuses with MPS IH aborted at 20 weeks gestation (46). Excessive DS and HS are excreted in the urine and, it is noteworthy the disease affects cartilage, bone and the cornea, tissues that do not normally contain detectable amounts of these GAGs. In MPS IH, death usually ensues before the reproductive age is reached.

Patients with MPS IS manifest deformities of the hands and feet, coarse facies, and hirsutism (212). Intellect is not impaired and some affected individuals have been of more than normal intelligence. Their life span is normal, but most patients have aortic regurgitation due to aortic valve disease. The frequent deformities of the hand result from compression of the median nerve as it passes through the wrist ("carpal tunnel syndrome"). Despite the clinical differences between MPS IH and MPS IS, both conditions resemble each other biochemically (266).

Because the mutations responsible for MPS IH and MPS IS are allelic (i.e., at the same locus on a chromosome 4), one would expect a rare individual to inherit one gene for each of these diseases and to manifest a phenotype intermediate between MPS IH and MPS IS and indeed, such individuals designated MPS IH/S (Hurler–Scheie syndrome) have been identified. More than two decades ago, McKusick and colleagues (152) hypothesized that the genetic mutations responsible for MPS IH and MPS IS involved allelic mutations at the α-L-iduronidase locus and that individuals with the "Hurler–Scheie compound" inherited a Hurler gene from one parent and the Scheie gene from the other. Others, however, suggested that a single different mutation might be responsible (48,118,124,145), and support for this view was the inbred family reported by Jensen and colleagues (118) that was thought to be more likely to be homozygous at one locus than heterozygous at two loci.

Ocular Manifestations

A diffuse cloudy luster occurs, particularly in the central cornea in MPS IH due to an abnormal accumulation of GAGs in the cornea demonstrable with histochemical methods. A pigmentary retinopathy and optic atrophy are common; rarely, papilledema follows increased intracranial pressure.

By light microscopy the epithelium, fibroblasts (keratocytes) (especially beneath the epithelium) and endothelium of the cornea contain stored material. When examined by TEM the affected corneal cells contain fibrillogranular or amorphous material and occasional myelin figures, within numerous small, round, or oval membrane-bound vacuoles (54,132,162,189,203,249). Long-spacing collagen (see Chapter 44) is sometimes evident in the stroma (249). The lesions in canine MPS I are virtually identical to those in humans, but in contrast to humans with MPS IH the corneal epithelium of affected dogs has been unremarkable (43). Corneal clouding has cleared in humans (95,110) and dogs (43) with MPS IH following bone marrow transplantation. The ocular manifestations of MPS IS include corneal clouding, a pigmentary retinopathy, bilateral narrow or closed angle glaucoma, and chronic papilledema with optic atrophy (197,212,265). By light microscopy the keratocytes as well as the basal epithelial cells in the cornea are vacuolated and stain with reagents that demonstrate GAGs (212). In some cases of MPS IS, Bowman layer has been markedly attenuated (192,212,247,276), but this has not been an invariable finding (205).

Histologically, the lesions in MPS IS are indistinguishable from those in MPS IH. Multiple single membrane-delimited vacuoles containing fibrillogranular material appear in fibroblasts and the epithelium of the conjunctiva in MPS IS (195).

Cornea clouding invariably occurs in MPS IH/S and some patients have had corneal grafts that have remained clear for 2, 4, and 8 years (124,125). Corneal specimens from patients with MPS IH/S have disclosed numerous vacuoles containing a predominance of fibrillogranular and multimembranous materials within corneal epithelial cells, histiocytes, keratocytes, and endothelial cells (125).

Aside from corneal opacification visual impairment may be due retinal degeneration. The ERG is sometimes extinguished (39,118,125) and a pigmentary retinopathy with "bone spicule" shaped areas of pigmentation may be present (118,123). Papilledema has also been reported (226,269).

In MPS I the tears can be used to evaluate the efficiency of bone marrow transplantation (264).

Mucopolysaccharidosis Type II (Hunter Syndrome)

The X-chromosome linked recessive MPS II resembles MPS IH clinically, but the condition is less severe with some cases surviving to adulthood. Mental retardation may not be a feature and the cornea is usually clear, but a slight haze sometimes develops in older patients and may only be evident on slit-lamp biomicroscopy. As in MPS IH and MPS IS excessive amounts of HS and DS are excreted in the urine, although a slightly greater proportion of HS is excreted in MPS II. Severe (MPS IIA) and mild (MPS IIB) phenotypes are recognized with such differences being explained by different allelic mutations (265). The defective enzyme in MPS II is sulfoiduronate sulfatase (18). This MPS is caused by a mutation in the *IDS* gene on the X-chromosome (Xq28) (151).

Ocular Manifestations

The ocular lesions in MPS II have been studied by light microscopy and TEM (88,150,243). In a cornea lacking macroscopic corneal clouding (but having a slight posterior stromal haze on slit-lamp examination) minimal abnormalities were apparent by TEM. Intracellular clear fibrillogranular and homogeneous vacuoles occur in the epithelia of the cornea and ciliary body and in fibroblasts of the cornea, choroid, and sclera (Fig. 2). Vacuoles containing membranous lamellar bodies are prominent in both the ganglion and pigment epithelial cells, which have migrated into the retina, as well as in corneal, scleral and choroidal fibroblasts, and the ciliary epithelium. The iris pigment epithelium and the nonpigmented epithelium of the ciliary body are thickened and contain accumulations consistent with GAGs by histochemical techniques. A pigmentary retinopathy with loss of photoreceptors and pigment epithelial migration into the retina occurs (Fig. 3). The sclera may be thickened (88), but this is not a constant feature of MPS II. Descemet membrane is unremarkable (88) and in contrast to human MPS IH the corneal epithelium is spared.

Mucopolysaccharidosis Type III (Sanfilippo Syndrome)

Sanfilippo syndrome (MPS III) is characterized by severe progressive mental retardation, hepatosplenomegaly, and other clinical features that resemble

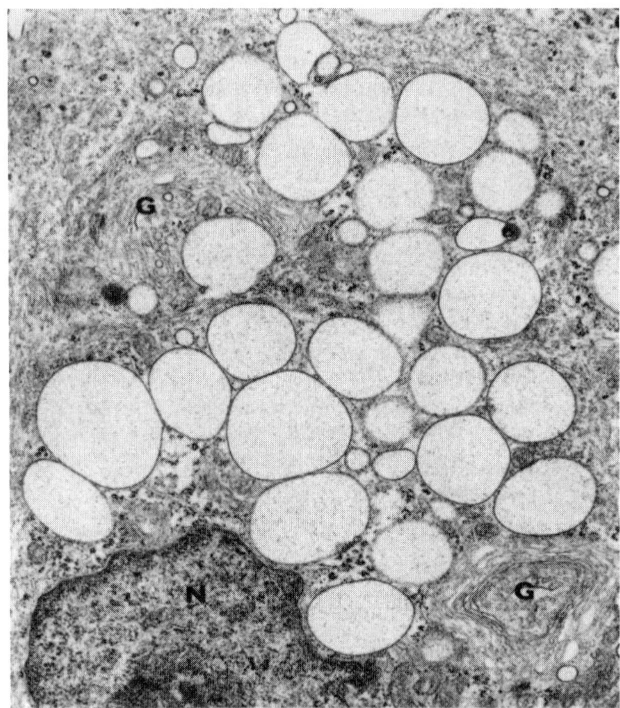

Figure 2 Conjunctiva in mucopolysaccharidosis type II, showing numerous cytoplasmic vacuoles with fibrillogranular material. *Abbreviations*: G, Golgi apparatus; N, nucleus. *Source*: Reproduced from Kenyon KR. Ocular ultrastructure of inherited metabolic disease. In: Goldberg MF, ed. Genetic and Metabolic Eye Disease. Boston: Little Brown, 1974.

MPS 1H and MPS II (except with less dwarfing) and an excessive urinary excretion of HS but not DS. Although phenotypically indistinguishable, four forms of Sanfilippo syndrome are recognized: MPS IIIA, MPS IIIB, MPS IIIC, and MPS IIID. They are due to mutations if different genes that lead to deficiencies of heparan-*N*-sulfatase (*SGSH*), α-*N*-acetylglucosaminidase (*NAGLU*), acetyl-CoA: α-glucosaminide-*N*-acetyltransferase (*HGSNAT*), and *N*-acetylglucosamine-6-sulfatase (*GNA*), respectively. In contrast to MPS IH and MPS IS the different forms of MPS III are due to nonallelic mutations. MPS IIIC is a LSD in which the defective enzyme is not an acid hydrolase.

Ocular Manifestations

A pigmentary retinopathy may occur in MPS III, and like other such retinopathies, it is associated with abnormal visual receptors and retinal pigment epithelium (RPE). In one of the very few eyes with MPS IIIA to be examined microscopically, the outer nuclear layer was thin, with a virtual absence of photoreceptors, and the retinal ganglion cells contained a foamy vacuolated cytoplasm. The RPE had hypopigmentated and hyperplastic areas and also contained fibrillogranular inclusions in addition to the lipofuscin (residual bodies) that normally occurs in the RPE (128).

The study of an eye with MPS IIIB has disclosed fibrillogranular material in single membrane-bound intracytoplasmic vacuoles within the endothelium of the trabecular meshwork, iris stroma, iris pigment epithelium, nonpigmented and pigmented epithelium of the ciliary body, lens epithelium, retinal ganglion cells, as well as in the corneal, choroidal, and scleral fibroblasts (144). The neuroepithelial pigment layers of the iris, ciliary body, and retina were hypopigmented and photoreceptor degeneration was similar to that found in retinitis pigmentosa (144).

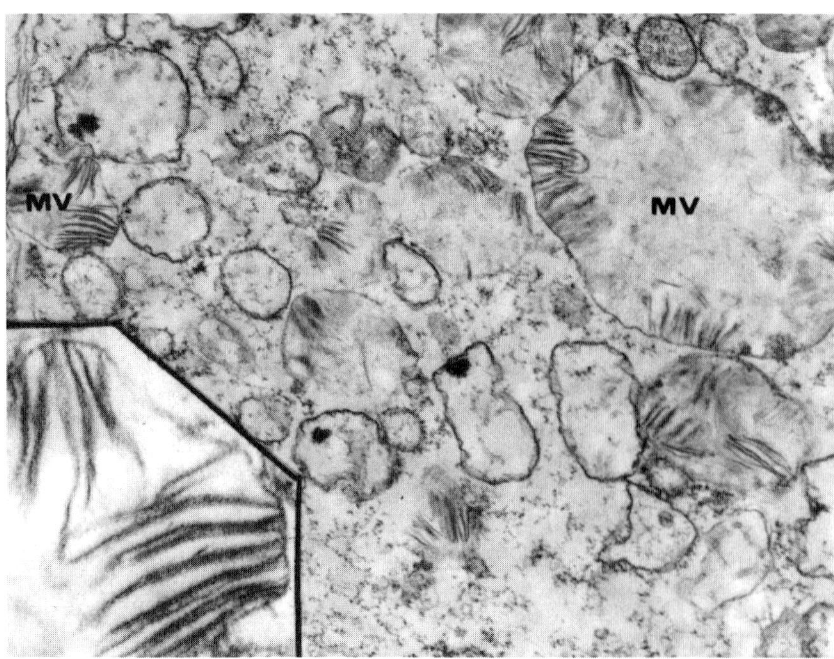

Figure 3 Retina in mucopolysaccharidosis type II. The cytoplasm contains numerous vacuoles with membranous lamellar bodies. *Abbreviation*: MV, membranous lamellar vacuoles. *Source*: From Ref. 243.

Mucopolysaccharidosis Type IV (Morquio Syndrome)

Individuals with the Morquio syndrome (MPS IV) are dwarfs with short trunks and skeletal abnormalities (spondyloepiphyseal dysplasia) distinct from patients with other MPSs. Affected persons are of normal intelligence and excrete an increased amount of KS and CS in their urine. In contrast to other MPSs cultured fibroblasts in this disorder do not accumulate sulfated GAGs, because skin fibroblasts do not synthesize KS in culture (134). However, skin fibroblasts are deficient in their ability to release $^{35}SO_4$ from labeled C6S (160). Two enzyme deficiencies result in MPS IV. In MPS IVA *N*-acetylgalactosamine-6-sulfatase (galactose-6-sulfatase), which removes sulfate from the sulfated carbon-6 linkage of the galactose moiety in KS is defective (55,109). The defect of MPS IVB involves β-galactosidase and the responsible mutation is in the *GLB1* gene on chromosome 3 (3p21–p14.2) (151,216). Different mutations in the same gene are responsible for GM_1-gangliosidosis (see Chapter 41).

Ocular Manifestations

In MPS IV fine corneal opacities are detectable early in life by slit-lamp examination, but do not become obvious until after 8 to 10 years of life, when they may become severe. Ghosh and McCulloch (84) reported a light microscopic and TEM study of corneal biopsies from two patients with MPS IV. The epithelium and its basement membrane as well as Bowman layer were normal, but vacuoles containing fibrillogranular and lamellar material were evident particularly by TEM within the corneal fibroblasts. Long-spaced collagen was also noted in the corneal stroma. However, the diagnosis in these cases is questionable, as they did not excrete excessive amounts of KS and CS in the urine, in contrast to the usual patients with MPS IV.

Mucopolysaccharidosis Type VI (Maroteaux–Lamy Syndrome)

Maroteaux–Lamy syndrome (MPS VI) resembles MPS II clinically, but marked corneal clouding is present (157). Mild, intermediate, and severe phenotypes occur. Unlike MPS IH, affected individuals survive longer and have a normal intelligence. There is an excessive urinary excretion and tissue storage of DS. A deficiency of arylsulfatase B was reported in the viscera (252), and in cultured fibroblasts (67) using a synthetic substrate, but using a more specific substrate the enzymatic defect has been identified as *N*-acetylgalactosamine-4-sulfatase (179). MPS VI results from a mutation in the *ASRB* gene.

Ocular Manifestations

Marked corneal clouding is a striking feature of MPS VI and corresponds to the storage of GAGs within keratocytes, the epithelium (Fig. 4) and the endothelium, and probable histiocytes within Bowman zone as well as between the collagen lamellae (196). In both the mild and severe phenotypes of MPS VI the basal epithelial cells and fibroblasts of the cornea contain numerous single-limited vacuoles with finely granular and membranous lamellar material as in several other MPSs (130,196). The corneal fibroblasts are less involved in the mild cases than in the severe ones (196). In arylsulfatase B-deficient cats DS and CS accumulates in the RPE (228).

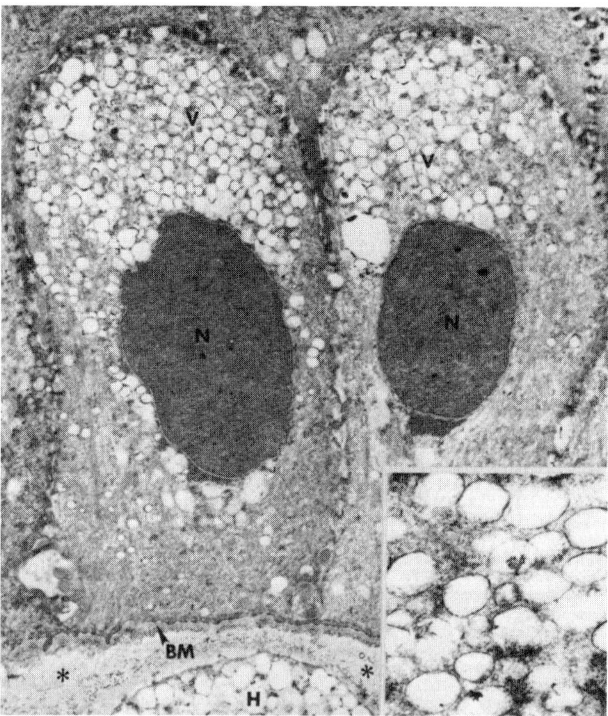

Figure 4 Vacuolated cells in corneal epithelium in mucopolysaccharidosis type VI (Maroteaux-Lamy). *Abbreviations*: N, nucleus; BM, basement membrane; H, vacuolated histiocytes; v, intracytoplasmic vacuoles; *, abnormal extracellular material. *Source*: From Ref. 130.

Despite an expectation that the cornea would thicken due to the concomitant intracytoplasmic storage of GAGs, nonprogressive stromal thinning is a feature of the corneal involvement in MPS VI in cats (3,4). The reason for this remains to be determined, but an impaired synthesis of collagen and other ECM components is possible (2).

In humans with MPS VI significant corneal clearing has not followed bone marrow transplantation (142), but clearing of the recipient cornea adjacent to the graft has been described (168). Initial accounts in cats with MPS VI that underwent corneal grafts drew attention to a similar situation (82,262), but these were not confirmed by follow-up studies (102). In a study in cats involving "normal to MPS VI" and "MPS

VI to normal" corneal grafts, Aguirre and colleagues failed to detect any clearing of MPS VI graft or host beds over a 14- to 30-month period by clinical observations or by light microscopy or TEM (2).

Unlike several other MPSs, a pigmentary retinopathy has not been reported in MPS VI. In a postmortem study of two siblings Kenyon and colleagues (130) observed marked thickening of the posterior sclera, especially at the posterior pole temporally, where it was approximately two- and one-half times normal thickness. The parafoveal region also contained fewer ganglion cells than normal. Cells in numerous sites (corneal stroma, Bowman zone, trabecular meshwork, sclera, corneal epithelium, nonpigmented epithelium of ciliary body) contained granular fibrillary material within membrane bound vacuoles. Optic atrophy is common (130) and may be secondary to papilledema, which follows a communicating hydrocephalus (89).

Mucopolysaccharidosis Type VII (Sly Syndrome)

The clinical features of MPS VII are suggestive of MPS IH and include coarse facies, growth and mental retardation, hepatosplenomegaly, and skeletal deformities. However, CS, rather than DS and HS, are excreted in excessive amounts in the urine (97,220).

The corneas were clear in infants with this rare condition (220,223), but ocular observations have not been documented beyond the age of 30 months (220) and human ocular tissue has not been examined by light microscopy or TEM. Canine (100,103,229,270) and murine (23,260) models of MPS VII are recognized. Although corneas appear clear in murine MPS VII the corneal fibroblasts are vacuolated due to the accumulation of GAGs (260).

MPS VII results from a mutation in the *GUSB* gene, which causes a complete deficiency of the lysosomal enzyme β-D-glucuronidase and DS, HS and CS accumulate within lysosomes (74,151). The mutation causing murine MPS VII has been mapped to the homologous region of the mouse chromosome 5 within 3.7 centimorgans of the structural gene for β-glucuronidase (23).

Mucopolysacchaidosis Type VIII (MPS VIII) (Di Ferrante Syndrome)

The entity once designated MPS VIII is no longer regarded as a specific entity (171) and may be the product of scientific misconduct. It had features of MPS IIID and was alleged to be associated with a deficiency of *N*-acetyl-glucosamine-6-sulfatase (55,85), but the impaired degradation and urinary excretion of GAGs involved KS in addition to HS.

Mucopolysaccharidosis Type IX (MPS IX) (Natowitz Disease)

MPS type IX is a LSD of HA caused by a mutation in the *HYAL1* gene. It is characterized by a deficiency hylauronidase and multiple periarticular soft-tissue masses in children of short stature (248). The plasma HA is markedly elevated and plasma hyaluronidase activity is absent.

Miscellaneous Unclassified and Suspected Mucopolysaccharidoses

Aside from the aforementioned clearly defined entities, several other MPSs may exist. Corneal opacification associated with excessive KS in the urine has been reported in two patients with a short trunk type of dwarfism, skeletal abnormalities of dysostosis multiplex, and an extrapyramidal disorder (34,156). A few patients with variable clinical phenotypes, but with corneal opacification, excrete excessive urinary CS (72,186,224,240). Morphologic studies of the tissue in these disorders of CS have not been documented. Edmison and colleagues (60) in a light microscopic and TEM study of the cornea from a patient with an atypical MPS with only a minimal increase in the urinary GAGs found Descemet membrane, the corneal endothelium and the epithelium to be unremarkable, while extracellular vacuoles were evident.

Winchester syndrome (MIM #277950), which is characterized by coarse facial features associated with progressive grotesque deformities of the trunk and limbs, was categorized as a possible MPS in the past. This entity, first recognized in the offspring of a consanguineous marriage, resembles rheumatoid arthritis clinically and roentgenographically. Peripheral corneal opacities become apparent by the age of 2 years and progress centrally, but unlike recognized systemic MPSs, the peripheral cornea becomes thin and vascularized. A biopsy from the peripheral cornea of one affected child was found to have morphologically abnormal basal epithelial cells and keratocytes (32), but unlike the abnormalities in established MPSs. An excessive urinary excretion of GAGs was not observed, but cultured cutaneous fibroblasts manifest increased metachromasia (an unreliable indicator of a MPS) (32,267). Increased amounts of uronic acid were stated to be present using nonspecific histochemical methods (267). It is now established that Winchester syndrome is an inherited osteolysis syndrome caused by a mutation in the *MMP2* gene that encodes for matrix metalloproteinase-2 (MMP-2) (204,277).

Furthermore, the precise diagnosis of some reports on the ocular manifestations of MPSs is questionable. For example, Klika and Kloucek (132) reported a presumed case of MPS IH, but without conclusive supporting clinical and biochemical data. Also, unlike most patients with MPS IH the patients described by Rosen and colleagues (202) had a normal intellect at ages of 13 and 15 years. Furthermore, the diagnosis of the case reported by Tremblay and colleagues as MPS IS (247) is doubtful as only trace amounts of HS were present in a 24 h urine specimen.

Ocular Abnormalities in the Mucopolysaccharidoses

Overview

Seeing that GAGs are a noteworthy component of the ocular tissues, it is not surprising that most systemic MPSs have clinically significant lesions of the eye, with the cornea and retina being most conspicuously involved.

Cornea

Corneal clouding occurs in almost all MPSs typically with diffuse fine punctate opacities. In some of these diseases (MPS IH, MPS IS, and MPS VI) it is a significant and clinical feature, while in MPS II it is a late manifestation. Although clinically detectable corneal abnormalities have not been described in MPS III, MPS VII, and MPS IX, the corneal fibroblasts are abnormal and manifest a slight intracellular accumulation of finely granular material in MPS III (128) and MPS VII (260).

Tissue examinations of clouded corneas in the MPSs have revealed similar morphologic alterations in the various disorders (54,130,132,173,189,196,203,212). When reviewed by TEM, several different types of corneal cells (epithelium, fibroblasts, endothelium, and subepithelial "histiocytes") contain numerous membrane-bound vacuoles, sometimes enclosing delicate fibrillogranular material. In MPS IH (132,203,249), MPS VI (130,196), and a questionable MPS IV (84) involvement of the basal epithelial cells and corneal fibroblasts has been conspicuous. Broad-banded collagen has been observed in the corneal stroma in MPS IH (249), MPS IS (205,234,276), and MPS IV (84) and is not specific for MPS IS as suggested by some authors (205,276).

In contrast to macular corneal dystrophy (MCD), which was once thought to be a MPS localized to the cornea (see Chapter 32) (136), Descemet membrane is normal in the MPSs. Also, although an extracellular accumulation of GAGs occurs in the MPSs (234,244) it is not a prominent feature. As the cornea becomes opaque (90) when the collagenous stromal lamellae are separated by distances exceeding 200 nm, the loss of corneal transparency in the MPSs is readily explained by light scattering caused by distended corneal fibroblasts and the associated extracellular pools of GAGs. But why significant corneal opacification only develops in some MPSs and not in others is an unanswered question of fundamental importance. For instance, HS and DS, which are not normally found in the cornea, accumulate throughout the body and are excreted in excess in MPS IH, MPS IS, and MPS II, yet the cornea in MPS II remains clear until late in life. These observations perhaps indicate that there are α-L-iduronate, but not sulfoiduronate, linkages in the corneal GAGs.

Conjunctiva

Clinically detectable abnormalities are not manifest in the conjunctiva, but biopsies of this accessible part of the eye have disclosed basal epithelial and subconjunctival connective tissue cells distended with intracytoplasmic vesicles containing material with cytochemical attributes of GAGs (128,129,212). When viewed in the TEM, most affected cells contain fibrillogranular accumulates similar to those within lysosomes elsewhere in these diseases. However, concentric membranous inclusions, like those in the brain and retina, occur in Schwann cells (128).

Retina

A pigmentary retinopathy occurs frequently in MPS IH, MPS IS, MPS II, MPS IIIA, and MPS IIIB, but has not been documented in MPS IV or MPS VI. In MPS IV, however, diminished ganglion cells has been observed in the parafoveal region in tissue sections (130).

Optic Nerve

In MPS IH, MPS II, and MPS VIA, optic atrophy may be a sequel to the diseased ganglion cells in the retina, papilledema, or glaucoma (130,153). In some of the MPSs (MPS IH, MPS II, and MPS IV) (89,172) papilledema follows increased intracranial pressure due to hydrocephalus related to obstruction to the CSF pathways caused by thickened leptomeninges, the latter often being associated with cyst formation (Fig. 5).

Other Ocular Manifestations

Glaucoma can occur in MPS IS (197,212,265) and MPS IV (51), but the mechanism whereby the intraocular pressure becomes elevated has not been established. Marked thickening of the posterior sclera has been noted in some patients with MPS II (88) and MPS IV (130), but this is not a constant feature in MPS II.

After a partial refurbishment of the lacking enzyme by bone marrow transplantation, several reports have documented a partial clearing of the cornea in some human patients and animals with certain MPSs [MPS I (human) (95,110,231) and (dogs) (30,43,217,219), MPS II (human) (95), MPS IIIB (human) (95), MPS IV (human) (95), MPS VI (human) (95), (cats) (82)].

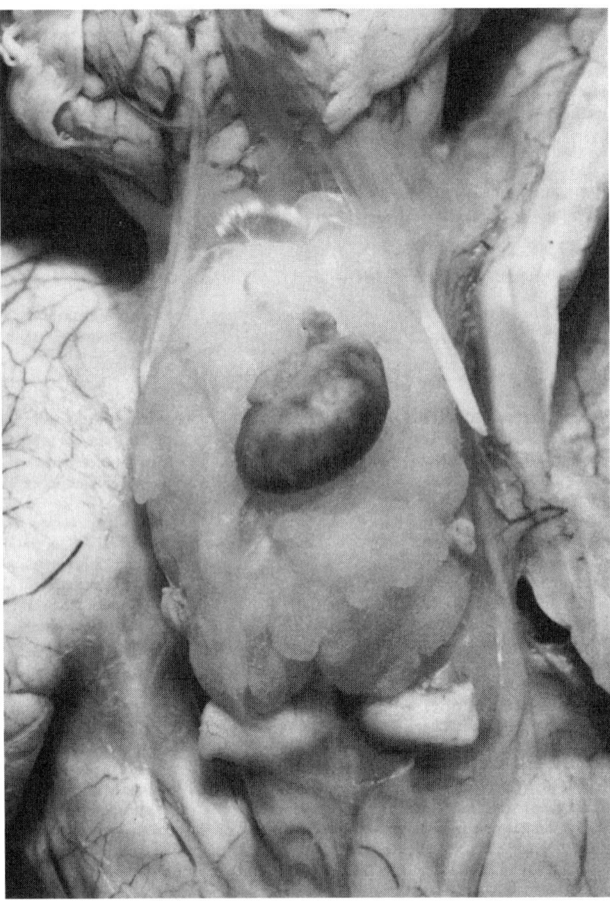

Figure 5 Thickening of leptomeninges and cyst in subarachnoid space of patient with systemic mucopolysaccharidosis. *Source*: From Ref. 172.

GENETIC DISORDERS OF PROTEOGLYCANS

Mutations have been detected in several of the core proteins in PGs and some of them result in abnormalities that affect the eye and vision.

Decorin

Mutations in the *DCN* gene of the decorin core protein account for congenital stromal corneal dystrophy (MIM #610048) (see Chapter 32) (28) and expression of this gene is deficient in skin fibroblasts of some cases of Marfan syndrome (192).

Glypican

An epicanthus may be part of the coarse facies in the X-linked recessive Simpson–Golabi–Behmel syndrome (MIM #312870) (201). Cortical blindness may be a sequel to degenerative changes in the brain in this overgrowth disorder with multiple developmental disorders (182).

Keratocan

The *KERA* gene that encodes the core protein of keratocan is mutated in autosomal recessive cornea plana (MIM #217300) (see Chapter 32) (185).

Lumican

Although no human disease has been found that affects the core protein of lumican the KS component of the attached GAGs is affected in MCD (see Chapter 32). In MCD mutations in the *CHST6* gene impair the sulfotransferase that adds sulfate moieties to KS (5,135). Lumican interacts with collagen and collagen fibril formation in lumican deficient mice is altered in the sclera (16). Mice deficient in this major corneal PG manifest some features of Ehlers–Danlos syndrome (MIM #130000) (119).

Nyctalopin

Mutations in the *NYX* gene have been found in complete congenital stationary night blindness (MIM #310500) (see Chapter 35) (20,193,272).

Perlecan

Mutations in the *HSPG2* gene have been detected in the Schwartz–Jampel syndrome (MIM #255800) (15), a disorder characterized by blepharophimosis, dwarfism, skeletal and facial anomalies, and myotonia (see Chapter 72). Other ophthalmic manifestations that have been documented in this disorder of perlecan include orbital hypertelorism and myopia (1,15). Arthrogryposis multiplex congenita (MIM #108110) and the Schwartz–Jampel syndrome (MIM #255800) may be present in the same patient (66).

Versican

The inherited vitreoretinopathy known as Wagner syndrome (MIM #143200) is caused by mutations in the *CSPG2* gene that encodes for the core protein of versican (see Chapter 29) (165).

MISCELLANEOUS OCULAR DISORDERS

The finding of disordered GAG metabolism in association with a pathologic state does not necessarily indicate that the affiliation is causal one or even a related one. This point is underscored by an unrelated genetic mutation that causes β-glucuronidase deficiency in C_3H mice developing a retinal degeneration (183).

Corneal Disorders

Keratoconus

Inconstant abnormalities in the GAG and PG composition of keratoconus (KC) corneas have been documented by numerous investigators (see Chapter 30) (80,81,191,210,264,275). At least some of the reported abnormalities are probably secondary to scarring. The staining intensity of GAGs is weaker than normal in many KC corneas and biochemical and histochemical studies have disclosed a reduction of highly sulfated KS epitopes in KC corneas (80).

The periphery of some KC corneas stain normally for KS, but the coloring intensity decreases in the thinned central stroma apparently not only in scarred tissue (80). KC corneas contain only about half as much KS as normal corneas when assayed with anti-KS monoclonal antibody (81). The amount of lumican core protein in KC and normal corneal extracts do not differ significantly (81), but the lumican in KC corneas has fewer KS side chains than normal or structurally modified KS (81).

Decorin and lumican, as well as their core proteins, isolated from KC corneas are of the same size as those from healthy corneas, but the decorin/lumican ratio is increased in KC cornea and the KS chains of two lumicans from KC cornea were considerably shorter (Mr 44 and 33 kDa) than normal (271).

Cornea Edema

Alterations in the composition of stromal GAGs and PGs occur in opaque swollen corneas (191), including those with experimentally induced edema (8). Corneal edema produced in the rabbit by perfusion of the anterior chamber with a calcium-free balanced salt solution is associated with the loss of biochemically detectable stromal GAGs, including KS (126). TEM and X-ray diffraction studies of cuprolinic blue stained edematous corneas have confirmed a loss of stromal PGs normally associated with collagen and reduced levels of antigenic KS, while biochemical techniques revealed constant CS levels in the same corneas (194).

Corneal Wound Healing and Scars

The GAG composition of corneal wounds and scars differ from normal corneas and the PGs in corneal wounds and scars have been localized at an ultrastructural level after cuprolinic blue staining with and without prior specific enzymatic digestion (40).

Both glucosaminoglycans and galactosaminoglycans decrease in the healing area of perforating corneal wounds (12). In wound healing KS is reduced, while C4S synthesis increases (11). ^{3}H-glucosamine incorporation by the cornea diminishes markedly following injury to the corneal epithelium and/or endothelium and removal of both layers decreases the incorporation drastically (47). Injury to the anterior part of the cornea increases CS and DS synthesis but decreases KS production, while injury to the posterior cornea has the opposite effect (47). Especially during the peak of fibroblastic activity (1–3 weeks after corneal wounding) ^{35}S-sulfate becomes incorporated mainly into galactosaminoglycans rather than into glucosaminoglycans (58).

The GAGs within the first 8 weeks of corneal wound healing resemble those in normal developing cornea, but by the second year of healing they change to those of the normal adult (40). In 1-week-old corneal wounds in the rabbit KS is evident, but not in the anterior stroma adjacent to the wound (40). KS and CS are present in 1-week-old wounds and the adjacent stroma.

PG synthesis decreases with wound age and the quantity of PGs in scar and adjacent tissue increases with healing time, but scarred corneas synthesize PGs with lower sulfation than adjacent normal corneal tissue. The principal GAG of scar tissue is CS (12). Opaque scars lack lumican but contain HA (105). The lumican/decorin ratio in scars and the adjacent tissue is lower than normal, but especially in the scar (40). CS is abundant in 2-week-old scars, which contain primarily newly synthesized low-sulfated KS (40). KS is absent in the 2-week-old posterior scar (40). By week 8 of healing, KS is present throughout most of the scar, except along the posterior margin (40). Radioactive labeled PGs in normal stroma adjacent to the wound moves into scar tissue during healing (40).

Wounding markedly decreases the incorporation of labeled precursors into rabbit corneal PGs 1 and 2 weeks after partial-thickness radial scalpel incisions (77). The labeled PGs are more readily extracted after wounding. Labeled PGs from wounded corneas are larger than those from control corneas, a result of an increased amount of KS in the large molecular size fractions (77). After wounding the relative amounts of HS and KS increases (77) and the HS/DS ratio increases, while DS decreases (77). Scar tissue from perforating corneal wounds has less PG than normal and the KS sulfation is reduced, whereas a highly sulfated high-iduronic acid DS accumulates (77).

Two-week-old scars from experimental penetrating corneal wounds in rabbits contain less lumican than normal corneal tissue and this lumican is altered antigenically (78). PGs extracted from 2-, 4-, and 8-week-old scars synthesize PGs with lower sulfation than those of adjacent corneal tissue (40). Although PG synthesis in scars decreases with wound age, the synthesis in adjacent cornea remains the same. The quantity of PGs in scar and adjacent cornea increases with healing time (40). The ratios of lumican to decorin in normal cornea, scar, and adjacent cornea has been found to be 2.3, 0.6, and 1.5, respectively (40). The PGs from adjacent corneal tissue has a higher charge density than those from scar (40). The predominant adjacent cornea DS PG had a higher charge density than that in normal cornea (40). Cornea adjacent to the healing wound synthesizes PGs measurably different from those in scar and normal cornea (40).

Anterior Keratectomy

Sulfated KS is not detected immuohistochemically in the newly synthesized collagen stroma of the monkey cornea following excimer laser or mechanical anterior keratectomy (155).

An immunohistochemical analysis of healing penetrating nonperforating linear corneal incisions in rabbit with monoclonal antibodies against KS has disclosed that even after 6 months, the concentration of the sulfated epitopes of KSs in the regenerated stromal matrix are less than in the surrounding nonwounded regions (92).

Other Corneal Disorders

After penetrating keratoplasty the GAG content of the cornea decreases, perhaps because of postoperative edema, but returns to normal with successful transparent grafts (9). Nontransparent grafts contain DS, while the content of other GAGs, especially the KS, decrease further (71).

DS is also found in the cornea in certain other pathologic states including viral keratitis (10).

Anterior Chamber Angle Disorders

Histochemical and immunohistochemical studies of the juxtacanalicular meshwork in the ocular anterior chamber angle have shown the presence of GAGs. Because of their hydrophilicity they probably contribute to the resistance of aqueous outflow and are hence important in some forms of glaucoma (see Chapter 20) (63). The GAGs synthesized by human trabecular meshwork in perfusion organ culture anterior segments of human eyes after 7 and 14 days have similar incorporation profiles as fresh eyes (250).

Retinal Disorders

Murine retinal neurons produce a CS containing PG in culture and probably synthesize at least part of this PG that is found in the interphotoreceptor matrix (IPM). The photoreceptors may be critically involved in the maintenance of the IPM as these PGs disappear in mice with retinal degenerations, such as retinal degeneration slow (*rds* mouse) (239). Histochemical and immunocytochemical studies suggest that the distribution of PGs, especially those in the IPM, are altered in murine models of retinal degeneration (167).

Bruch membrane contains PGs, which may provide a selective filtration barrier for nutrients coming from the choriocapillaris to the outer retina. In human eyes the GAGs within Bruch membrane normally consist of approximately 75% CS/DS and 25% HS, but an increased proportion of HS has been observed in the presence of retinal disease (143).

Other

Two elderly patients with diffuse corneal stromal deposits of what appears to be GAGs, but without evidence of systemic disease were reported by Winterbotham and colleagues (268). Similar accumulations were found within the sclera in one case, but not in other ocular or extraocular tissues.

REFERENCES

1. Aberfeld DC, Hinderbuchner LP, Schneider M. Myotonia, dwarfism, diffuse bone disease and unusual ocular and facial abnormalities (a new syndrome). Brain 1965; 88: 313–22.
2. Aguirre G, Raber I, Yanoff M, Haskins M. Reciprocal corneal transplantation fails to correct mucopolysaccharidosis VI corneal storage. Invest Ophthalmol Vis Sci 1992; 33:2702–13.
3. Aguirre G, Stramm L, Haskins M. Feline mucopolysaccharidosis VI: General ocular and pigment epithelial pathology. Invest Ophthalmol Vis Sci 1983; 24: 991–1007.
4. Aguirre G, Stramm L, Haskins M, Jezyk P. Animal Models of Metabolic Eye Diseases. In: Renie WA, ed. Goldberg's Genetic and Metabolic Eye Disease. Boston, MA: Little, Brown and Company, 1986:139–67.
5. Akama TO, Nishida K, Nakayama J, et al. Macular corneal dystrophy type I and type II are caused by distinct mutations in a new sulphotransferase gene. Nat Genet 2000; 26:237–41.
6. Ala-Kapee M, Nevanlinna H, Mali M, et al. Localization of gene for human syndecan, an integral membrane proteoglycan and a matrix receptor, to chromosome 2. Somat Cell Molec Genet 1990; 16:501–5.
7. Aleu F, Terry RD, Zellweger H. Electron microscopy of two cerebral biopsies in gargoylism. J Neuropath Exp Neurol 1965; 24:304–17.
8. Anseth A. Studies on corneal polysaccharides. V. Changes in corneal glycosaminoglycans in transient stromal edema. Exp. Eye Res. 1969; 8:297–301.
9. Anseth A. Studies on corneal polysaccharides. VII Changes in the glycosaminoglycans in penetrating corneal grafts. Exp Eye Res 1969; 8:310–4.
10. Anseth A. Studies on corneal polysaccharides. VIII Changes in the glycosaminoglycans in some human corneal disorders. Exp Eye Res 1969; 8:438–41.
11. Anseth A, Fransson LA. Studies on corneal polysaccharides. VI. Isolation of dermatan sulfate from corneal scar tissue. Exp Eye Res 1969; 8:302–9.
12. Anseth A, Laurent TC. Polysaccharides in normal and pathologic corneas. Invest Ophthalmol 1962; 1: 195–201.
13. Antonsson P, Heinegard D, Oldberg A. The keratan sulfate-enriched region of bovine cartilage proteoglycan consists of a consecutively repeated hexapeptide motif. J Biol Chem 1989; 264:16170–3.
14. Antonsson P, Heinegard D, Oldberg A. Posttranslational modifications of fibromodulin. J Biol Chem 1991; 266: 16859–61.
15. Arikawa-Hirasawa E, Le AH, Nishino I, et al. Structural and functional mutations of the perlecan gene cause Schwartz–Jampel syndrome, with myotonic myopathy and chondrodysplasia. Am J Hum Genet 2002; 70 1368–75.

16. Austin BA, Coulon C, Liu CY, et al. Altered collagen fibril formation in the sclera of lumican-deficient mice. Invest Ophthalmol Vis Sci 2002; 43:1695–701.
17. Axelsson I, Heinegard D. Characterization of chondroitin sulfate-rich proteoglycans from bovine corneal stroma. Exp Eye Res 1980; 31:57–66.
18. Bach G, Eisenberg F Jr, Cantz M, Neufeld EF. The defect in the Hunter syndrome: deficiency of sulfoiduronate sulfatase. Proc Natl Acad Sci USA 1973; 70:2134–8.
19. Balduini, C, De Luca, G, Passi, A, et al. Effect of oxygen tension and lactate concentration on keratan sulphate and chondroitin sulphate biosynthesis in bovine cornea. Biochim Biophys Acta 1992; 1115:187–91.
20. Bech-Hansen NT, Naylor MJ, Maybaum TA, et al. Mutations in NYX, encoding the leucine rich proteoglycan nyctalopin, cause X-linked complete congenital stationary night blindness. Nature Genet 2000; 26:319–23.
21. Berndt C, Casaroli-Marano RP, Vilaro S, Reina M. Cloning and characterization of human syndecan-3. J Cell Biol 2001; 82:246–59.
22. Bezakova G, Ruegg MA New insights into the roles of agrin. Nat Rev Mol Cell Biol 2003; 4:295–308.
23. Birkenmeier E.H, Davisson MT, Beamer WG, et al. Murine mucopolyssacharidosis type VII: characterization of a mouse with β-glucuronidase deficiency. J Clin Invest 1989; 83:1258–66.
24. Blochberger TC, Vergnes J-P, Hempel J, Hassell JR. cDNA to chick lumican (corneal keratan sulfate proteoglycan) reveals homology to the small interstitial proteoglycan gene family and expression in muscle and intestine. J Biol Chem 1992; 267:347–52.
25. Bobardt MD, Saphire ACS, Hung H-C, et al. Syndecan captures, protects, and transmits HIV to T lymphocytes. Immunity 2003; 18:27–39.
26. Borcherding MS, Blacik LJ, Sittig RA, et al. Proteoglycans and collagen fibre organization in human corneoscleral tissue Exp Eye Res 1975; 21:59–70.
27. Brante G. Gargoylism: a mucopolysaccharidosis. Scand J Clin Lab Invest 1952; 4:43–6.
28. Bredrup C, Knappskog P M, Majewski J, et al. Congenital stromal dystrophy of the cornea caused by a mutation in the decorin gene. Invest Ophthal Vis Sci 2005; 46:420–6.
29. Bredrup C, Knappskog PM, Majweski J, et al. Congenital stromal dystrophy of the cornea caused by a mutation in the decorin gene. Invest Ophthamol Vis Sci 2005; 46: 420–6.
30. Breider MA, Shull RM, Constantopoulos G. Long-term effects of bone marrow transplantation in dogs with mucopolysaccharidosis I. Am J Pathol 1989; 134:677–92.
31. Brown DH. Tissue storage of mucopolysaccharides in Hurler–Pfaundler's disease. Proc Natl Acad Sci USA 1957; 43:783–90.
32. Brown SI, Kuwabara T. Peripheral corneal opacification and skeletal deformities: a newly recognized acid mucopolysaccharidosis simulating rheumatoid arthritis. Arch Ophthalmol 1970; 83:667–77.
33. Bülow, H.E., Hobert, O. The molecular diversity of glycoaminoglycans shapes animal development. Annu. Rev. Cell Dev. Biol. 2006; 22:375–-407, 2006.
34. Buscaino GA. Difficile inquadramento di una forma clinica di osteochondrodistrofia associata a disturbi neurologici di tipo extrapiramidale. Studio clinicobiochimico in 4 fratelli. Acta Neurol 1968; (Napoli) 23:34–60.
35. Cantz AM, Chrambach A, Neufeld EF. Characterization of the factor deficient in the Hunter syndrome by polyacrylamide gel electrophoresis. Biochem Biophys Res Commun 1970; 39:936–42.
36. Carey DJ, Evans DM, Stahl RC, et al. Molecular cloning and characterization of N-syndecan, a novel transmembrane heparan sulfate proteoglycan. J Cell Biol 1992; 117: 191–201.
37. Castoro, JA, Bettelheim, AA, Bettelheim, FA. Water gradients across bovine cornea. Invest Ophthalmol Vis Sci 1988; 29:963–8.
38. Chakravarti S, Stallings RL Sundar Raj N, et al. Primary structure of human lumican (keratan sulfate proteoglycan) and localization of the gene (LUM) to chromosome 12q21.3-q22. Genomics 1995; 27:481–8.
39. Chijiiwa T, Inomata H, Yamana Y, Kaibara N. Ocular manifestations of Hurler/Scheie phenotype in two sibs. Jap J Ophthalmol 1983; 27:54–62.
40. Cintron C, Covington HI, Kublin CL. Morphologic analyses of proteoglycans in rabbit corneal scars. Invest Ophthalmol Vis Sci 1990; 31:1789–98.
41. Cintron C, Gregory JD, Damle SP, Kublin CL. Biochemical analyses of proteoglycans in rabbit corneal scars. Invest Ophthalmol Vis Sci 1990; 31:1975–81.
42. Cole GJ, Burg M. Characterization of a heparan sulfate proteoglycan that copurifies with the neural cell adhesion molecule. Exp Cell Res 1989; 182:44–60.
43. Constantopoulos G, Scott JA, Shull RM. Corneal opacity in canine MPS I Invest Ophthalmol Vis Sci 1989; 30: 1802–7.
44. Cornelison DDW, Wilcox-Adelman SA, Goetinck PF, et al. Essential and separable roles for syndecan-3 and syndecan-4 in skeletal muscle development and regeneration. Genes Dev 2004; 18:2231–6.
45. Cornet PK, Blochberger TC, Hassel JR. Molecular polymorphism of lumican during corneal development. Invest Ophthalmol Vis Sci 1994; 35:870–7.
46. Crawford M. d'A, Dean MF, Hunt DM, et al. Early prenatal diagnosis of Hurler's syndrome with termination of pregnancy and confirmatory findings on the fetus. J Med Genet 1973; 10:144–53.
47. Dahl IMS, Laurent TC. Synthesis of glycosaminoglycans in corneal organ cultures. Exp Eye Res 1982; 34:83–98.
48. Danes BS. Variant of iduronidase deficient mucopolysaccharidoses: further evidence for genetic heterogeneity. J Med Genet 1977; 14:346–51.
49. Danielson KG, Fazzio A, Cohen I, et al. The human decorin gene: intron–exon organization, discovery of two alternatively spliced exons in the 5-prime untranslated region, and mapping of the gene to chromosome 12q23. Genomics 1993; 15:146–60.
50. David G, van der Schueren B, Marynen P, et al. Molecular cloning of amphiglycan, a novel integral membrane heparan sulfate proteoglycan expressed by epithelial and fibroblastic cells. J Cell Biol 1992; 118:961–9.
51. Davis DB, Currier FP. Morquio's disease: report of two cases. J Am Med Assoc 1934; 102:2173–6.
52. Deere M, Johnson J, Garza S, et al. Characterization of human DSPG3, a small dermatan sulfate proteoglycan. Genomics 1996; 38:399–04.
53. Dekaban AS, Patton VM. Hurler's and Sanfilippo's variants of mucopolysaccharidosis: cerebral pathology and lipid chemistry. Arch Pathol 1971; 91:434–43.
54. Desvignes P, Pouliquen Y, Legras M, Guyot JD. Aspect clinique, examen histologique et structural d'une cornée dystrophique de maladie de Hurler. Bull Mem Soc Fr Ophtalmol 1967; 80:43–8.
55. Di Ferrante N, Ginsberg LC, Donnelly PV, et al. Deficiencies of glucosamine-6-sulfate or galactosamine-6-sulfate sulfatases are responsible for different mucopolysaccharidoses. 1978, Science 199:79–81.

56. Dodge GR, Kovalszky I, Chu M-T, et al. Heparan sulfate proteoglycan and human colon: partial molecular cloning, cellular expression and mapping of the gene (HSPG2) to the short arm of human chromosome 1. Genomics 1991; 10:673–80.
57. Doege KJ, Sasaki M, Kimura T, Yamada Y. Complete coding sequence and deduced primary structure of the human cartilage large aggregating proteoglycan, aggrecan. Human-specific repeats, and additional alternatively spliced forms. J Biol Chem 1991; 266:894–902.
58. Dohlman CH, Praus R. The mucopolysaccharides in corneal wound healing. In: Dardenne MU, Nordmann J, eds. Biochemistry of the Eye. Basel, S. Karger, 1968: 120–7.
59. Dorfman A, Lorincz AE. Occurrence of urinary acid mucopolysaccharides in the Hurler syndrome. Proc Natl Acad Sci USA 1957; 43:443–6.
60. Edmison DR, Robertson DM, Rosen DA. Corneal mucopolysaccharidosis: light and electron microscopic study of an atypical case after keratoplasty. Can J Ophthalmol 1972; 7:271–6.
61. Escourolle R, Berger B, Poirier J. Biopsie cérébrale d'un cas de mucopolysaccharidose H.S. (oligophrénie polydystrophique ou maladie de Sanfilippo). Étude histochimique et ultrastructurale. Presse Med 1966; 74: 2869–74.
62. Esko JD. Genetic analysis of proteoglycan structure, function and metabolism. Curr Opin Cell Biol 1991; 3: 805–16.
63. Ethier CR, Kamm RD, Palaszewski BA, et al. Calculations of flow resistance in the juxtacanalicular meshwork. Invest Ophthalmol Vis Sci 1986; 27:1741–50.
64. Filmus J. Mini Review. Glypicans in growth control and cancer. Glycobiology 2001; 11:19R–23R.
65. Fisher LW, Heegaard AM, Vetter U, et al. Human biglycan gene. Putative promoter, intron-exon junctions, and chromosomal localization. J Biol Chem 1991; 266: 14371–7.
66. Fitch N, Karpati G, Pinsky L. Congenital blepharophimosis, joint contractures, and muscular hypotonia. Neurology 1971 21: 1214–20.
67. Fluharty AL, Stevens RL, Sanders DL, Kihara H. Arylsulfatase B deficiency in Maroteaux-Lamy syndrome cultured fibroblasts. Biochem Biophys Res Commun 1974; 59:455–61.
68. Fransson L-A, Sjöberg I, Dorfman A, Matalon R. Chemistry of dermatan sulphate accumulated intracellularly in Hunter's disease. In: Holton JB, Ireland JT, eds. Inborn Errors of Skin Hair and Connective Tissue. Baltimore, University Park Press, 1975:179–96.
69. Frantantoni JC, Hall CW, Neufeld EF. The defect in Hurler's and Hunter's syndromes: faulty degradation of mucopolysaccharides. Proc Natl Acad Sci USA 1968; 60: 699–706.
70. Frantantoni JC, Hall CW, Neufeld EF. Hurler and Hunter syndromes: mutual correction of defect in cultured fibroblasts. Science 1968; 162:570–2.
71. Frantantoni JC, Hall CW, Neufeld EF. The defect in Hurler and Hunter syndromes. II. Deficiency of specific factors involved in mucopolysaccharide degradation. Proc Natl Acad Sci USA 1969; 64:360–6.
72. Freitag F, Kuchemann K, Schuster W, Spranger J. Hepatic ultrastructure in chondroitin-4-sulfate mucopolysaccharidosis. Virchows Arch Abt B Zellpathol 1971; 8:1–15.
73. Friedman JS, Faucher M, Hiscott P, et al. Protein localization in the human eye and genetic screen of opticin. Hum Molec Genet 2002; 11:1333–42.
74. Frydman M, Steinberger J, Shabtai F, Steinherz R. Interstitial 7q deletion (46, XY, del(7)(pter cen::q112qtr)) in a retarded quadriplegic boy with normal betaglucuronidase. Am J Med Genet 1986; 25:245–9.
75. Fukai N, Eklund L, Marneros AG, et al. Lack of collagen XVIII/endostatin results in eye abnormalities. EMBO J 2002; 21:1535–44.
76. Funderburgh JL, Caterson B, Conrad GW. Keratan sulfate proteoglycan during embryonic development of the chicken cornea. Dev Biol 1986; 116:267–77.
77. Funderburgh JL, Chandler JW. Proteoglycans of rabbit corneas with nonperforating wounds. Invest Ophthalmol Vis Sci 1989; 30:435–42.
78. Funderburgh JL, Cintron C, Covington HI, Conrad GW. Immunoanalysis of keratan sulfate proteoglycan from corneal scars. Invest Ophthalmol Vis Sci 1988; 29:1116–24.
79. Funderburgh JL, Funderburgh ML, Mann MM, Conrad GW. Arterial lumican: properties of a corneal-type keratan sulfate proteoglycan from bovine aorta. J Biol Chem 1991; 266:24773–7.
80. Funderburgh JL, Funderburgh ML, Rodrigues MM, et al. Altered antigenicity of keratan sulfate proteoglycan in selected corneal diseases. Invest Ophthalmol Vis Sci 1990; 31:419–28.
81. Funderburgh JL, Panjwani N, Conrad GW, Baum J. Altered keratan sulfate epitopes in keratoconus. Invest Ophthalmol Vis Sci 1989; 30:2278–81.
82. Gasper PW, Thrall MA, Wenger DA, et al. Correction of feline arylsulfatase B deficiency (mucopolysaccharidosis VI) by bone marrow transplantation. Nature 1984; 312: 467–9.
83. Ghiselli G, Iozzo RV. Overexpression of bamacan/SMC3 cusese transformation. J Biol Chem 2000; 275:20235–8.
84. Ghosh M, McCulloch C. The Morquio syndrome: light and electron microscopic findings from two corneas. Can J Ophthalmol 1974; 9:445–52.
85. Ginsberg LC, Donnelly PV, Di Ferrante DT, et al. N-acetylglucosamine-6-sulfate sulfatase in man: deficiency of the enzyme in a new mucopolysaccharidosis. Pediatr Res 1978; 12:805–9.
86. Gleghorn L, Ramesar R, Beighton P, Wallis G. A mutation in the variable repeat region of the aggrecan gene (AGC1) causes a form of spondyloepihyseal dysplasia associated with severe, premature osteoarthritis. Am J Hum Genet 2005; 77:484–90.
87. Goetinck PF. Proteoglycans in development. Curr Topics Develop Biol 1991; 25:111–31.
88. Goldberg MF, Duke JR. Ocular histopathology in Hunter's syndrome: systemic mucopolysaccharidosis type II. Arch Ophthalmol 1967; 77:503–12.
89. Goldberg, MF, Scott CI, McKusick VA. Hydrocephalus and papilledema in the Maroteaux-Lamy syndrome (mucopolysaccharidosis type VI). Am J Ophthalmol 1970; 69:969–75.
90. Goldman JN, Benedek GB, Dohlman CH, Kravitt B. Structural alterations affecting transparency in swollen human corneas. Invest Ophthalmol 1968; 7:501–19.
91. Gonatas NK, Gonatas J. Ultrastructural and biochemical observations on a case of systemic late infantile lipidosis and its relationship to Tay-Sachs disease and gargoylismus. J Neuropath Exp Neurol 1965; 24:318–40.
92. Goodman WM, SundarRaj N, Garone M, et al. Unique parameters in the healing of linear partial thickness penetrating corneal incisions in rabbit: immunohistochemical evaluation. Curr Eye Res 1989; 8:305–16.
93. Gould SE, Upholt WB, Kosher RA. Syndecan 3: a member of the syndecan family of membrane-intercalated

proteoglycans that is expressed in high amounts at the onset of chicken limb cartilage differentiation. Proc Natl Acad Sci USA 1992; 89:3271–5.

94. Gregory JD, Coster L, Damle SP. Proteoglycans of rabbit corneal stroma: isolation and characterization. J Biol Chem 1982; 257:6965–70.
95. Groth C, Ringden O. Transplantation in relation to the treatment of inherited disease. Transplantation 1984; 38: 319–27.
96. Grover J, Chen X-N, Korenberg JR, et al. The gene organization, chromosome location, and expression of a 55-kDa matrix protein (PRELP) of human articular cartilage. Genomics 1996; 38:109–17.
97. Hall CW, Cantz M, Neufeld EF. A β-glucuronidase deficiency mucopolysaccharidosis: studies in cultured fibroblasts. Arch Biochem Biophys 1973; 155:32–8.
98. Harris RC. Mucopolysaccharide disorder: a possible new genotype of Hurler's syndrome. Am J Dis Child 1961; 102:741–2.
99. Haskins M, Aguirre G, Jezyk P, et al. The pathology of the feline model of mucopolysaccharidosis I Am J Pathol 1983; 112:27–36.
100. Haskins ME, Aguirre GD, Jezyk PF, et al. Animal model of human disease. Mucopolysaccharidosis type VII (Sly syndrome): beta-glucuronidase-deficient mucopolysaccharidosis in the dog. Am J Path 1991; 138: 1553–5.
101. Haskins ME, Aguirre GD, Jezyk P, Patterson DF. The pathology of the feline model of mucopolysaccharidosis VI. Am J Pathol 1980; 101:657–74.
102. Haskins M, Baker H, Birkenmeier E, et al. Transplantation in animal model systems. In: Desnick R, ed. Therapy of Genetic Disease. New York, NY: Churchill Livingston, 1992:183–201.
103. Haskins ME, Desnick RJ, DiFerrante N, et al. Beta-glucuronidase deficiency in a dog: a model for human mucopolysaccharidosis VII. Pediatr Res 1984; 10:980–4.
104. Hassell JR, Blochberger TC, Rada JA, et al. Proteoglycan gene families. In: Kleinman H, ed. Advances in Molecular and Cell Biology, vol. 7. Greenwich, CT: The Extracellular Matrix, JAI Press, 1993.
105. Hassell JR, Cintron C, Kublin C, Newsome DA. Proteoglycan changes during restoration of transparency in corneal scars. Arch Biochem Biophys 1983; 222: 362–9.
106. Hassell JR, Newsome DA, Hascall VC. Characterization and biosynthesis of proteoglycans of corneal stroma from rhesus monkey. J Biol Chem 1979; 254:12346–54.
107. Hassell J, Robey PG, Barrach HJ, et al. Isolation of a heparan sulfate-containing proteoglycan from basement membrane. Proc Natl Acad Sci USA 1980; 77:4494–8.
108. Heathcote JG, Bruns RR, Orkin RW. Biosynthesis of sulphated macromolecules by rabbit lens epithelium. II. Relationship to basement membrane formation. J Cell Biol 1984; 99:861–9.
109. Horwitz AL, Dorfman A. The enzymic defect in Morquio's disease: the specificity of N-acetyl- hexosamine sulfatases. Biochem Biophys Res Comm 1978; 80:819–25.
110. Hugh-Jones K, Hobbs J, Chambers D, et al. Bone marrow transplantation in mycopolysaccharidosis. In: Barranger JA, Brady, RO, eds. Molecular Basis of Lysosomal Storage Disorders. New York, NY: Academic Press, 1984:411–28.
111. Humphries DE, Nicodemus CF, Schiller V, Stevens RL. The human serglycin gene: nucleotide sequence and methylation pattern in human promyelocytic leukemia HL-60 cells and T-lymphoblast Molt-4 cells. J Biol Chem 1992; 267:13558–63.
112. Hunter C. A rare disease in two brothers. Proc R Soc Med 1917; 10:104–16.
113. Hurler G. Über einen Type multipler Abartungen, vorwiegend am Skellettsystem. Z Kinderheilkd 1919; 24:220–34.
114. Iozzo RV. Proteoglycans: structure, function, and role in neoplasia. Lab Invest 1985; 53:373–96.
115. Iozzo RV, Naso MF, Cannizzaro LA, et al. Mapping of the versican proteoglycan gene (CSPG2) to the long arm of human chromosome 5 (5q12-5q14). Genomics 1992; 14: 845–51.
116. Ivins JK, Litwack ED, Kumbasar A, et al. Cerebroglycan, a developmentally regulated cell-surface heparan sulfate proteoglycan, is expressed on developing axons and growth cones. Dev Biol 1997; 184:320–32.
117. Jeanloz RW. The nomenclature of acid mucopolysaccharides. Arthritis Rheum 1960; 3:323–7.
118. Jensen OA, Pederson C, Schwartz M, et al. Hurler/Scheie phenotype: report of an inbred sibship with tapeto-retinal degeneration and electron-microscopic examination of the conjunctiva. Ophthalmologica 1978; 176:194–204.
119. Jepsen KJ, Wu F, Peragallo JH, et al. A syndrome of joint laxity and impaired tendon integrity in lumican- and fibromodulin-deficient mice. J Biol Chem 2002; 277: 35532–40.
120. Jervis GA. Familial mental deficiency akin to amaurotic idiocy and gargoylism: an apparently new type. Arch Neurol Psychiatr 1942; 47:943–61.
121. Jones ST, Zimmerman LE. Histopathologic differentiation of granular, macular and lattice dystrophies of the cornea. Am J Ophthalmol 1961; 51:394–410.
122. Jost CJ, Funderburgh JL, Mann M, et al. Cell-free translation and characterization of corneal keratan sulfate proteoglycan core proteins. J Biol Chem 1991; 266: 13336–41.
123. Kaibara N, Eguchi M, Shibata K, Takugishi K. Hurler-Scheie phenotype: a report of two pairs of inbred sibs. Hum Genet 1979; 53:37–41.
124. Kajii T, Matsuda I, Ohsawa T, et al. Hurler/Scheie genetic compound (mucopolysaccharidosis IH/IS) in Japanese brothers. Clin Genet 1974; 6:394–400.
125. Kameen A, Jr, Maumenee IH, Green WR. Light and electron microscopic studies of the cornea in systemic mucopolysaccharidosis, type I-HS. Cornea 1986; 5:107–114.
126. Kangas TA, Edelhauser HF, Twining SS, O'Brien WJ. Loss of stromal glycosaminoglycans during corneal edema. Invest Ophthalmol Vis Sci 1990; 31:1994–2002.
127. Karumanchi SA, Jha V, Ramchandran R, et al. Cell surface glypicans are low-affinity endostatin receptors. Molec Cell 2001; 7:811–22.
128. Kenyon KR. Ocular manifestations and pathology of systemic mucopolysaccharidoses. Birth Defects 1976; 12: 133–53.
129. Kenyon KR, Quigley HA, Hussels IE, Wyllie RG. The systemic mucopolysaccharidoses: ultrastructural and histochemical studies of conjunctiva and skin. Am J Ophthalmol 1972; 73:811–33.
130. Kenyon KR, Topping TM, Green WR, Maumenee AE. Ocular pathology of the Maroteaux-Lamy syndrome (systemic mucopolysaccharidosis type VI): histologic and ultrastructural report of two cases. Am J Ophthalmol 1972; 73:718–41.
131. Kiefer MC, Ishihara M, Swiedler SJ, et al. The molecular biology of heparan sulfate fibroblast growth factor receptors. Ann NY Acad Sci 1991; 638:167–76.
132. Klika E, Kloucek F. L'histochimie et l'ultrastructure de la cornée dans un cas de gargoylisme. Ophthalmologica 1966; 151:568–79.

133. Klintworth GK. The cornea-structure and macromolecules in health and disease: a review. Am J Pathol 1977; 89:719–808.
134. Klintworth GK, Smith CF. Difference between glycosaminoglycans synthesized by corneal and cutaneous fibroblasts in culture. Lab Invest 1981; 44:553–9.
135. Klintworth GK, Smith CF, Bowling BL: CHST6 mutations in North American subjects with macular corneal dystrophy: a comprehensive molecular genetic review. Molec Vis 2006; 12:159–76.
136. Klintworth GK, Vogel FS. Macular corneal dystrophy: an inherited acid mucopolysaccharide storage disease of the corneal fibroblast. Am J Pathol 1964; 45:565–86.
137. Knecht J, Cifonelli JA, Dorfman A. Structural studies on heparitin sulfate of normal and Hurler tissues. J Biol Chem 1967; 242:4652–61.
138. Kojima T, Shworak NW, Rosenberg RD. Molecular cloning and expression of two distinct cDNA-encoding heparan sulfate proteoglycan core proteins from a rat endothelial cell line. J Biol Chem 1992; 267:4870–7.
139. Kornblihtt AR, Gutman A. Molecular biology of the extracellular matrix proteins. Biol Reviews Cambridge Phil Soc 1988; 63:465–507.
140. Kresse H, Neufeld EF. The Sanfilippo A corrective factor: purification and mode of action. J Biol Chem 1972; 247: 2164–70.
141. Kressler RJ, Aegerter EE. Hurler's syndrome (gargoylism): a summary of literature and report of case with autopsy findings. J Pediatr 1938; 12:579–91.
142. Krivit W, Pierpoint ME, Ayaz K, et al. Bone-marrow transplantation in the Maroteaux-Lamy syndrome (mucopolysaccharidosis type VI). N Eng J Med 1984; 311: 1606–11.
143. Landers RA, Tawara A., Varner HH, Hollyfield JG. Proteoglycans in the mouse interphotoreceptor matrix. IV Retinal synthesis of chondroitin sulfate proteoglycan. Exp Eye Res 1991; 52:65–74.
144. Lavery MA, Green WR, Jabs EW, et al. Ocular histopathology and ultrastructure of Sanfilippo's syndrome, type III B. Arch Ophthalmol 1983; 101:1263–74.
145. Leisti J, Rimoin DL, Kaback MM, et al. Phenotypic variation in alpha-L-iduronidase deficiency, letter to the editor. Lancet 1975; 1:1344.
146. Li W, Vergnes JP, Cornuet PK, Hassell JR. cDNA clone to chick corneal chondroitin/dermatan sulfate proteoglycan reveals identity to decorin. Arch. Biochem. Biophys. 1992; 296:190–7.
147. Lie SO, Schofield BH, Taylor HA Jr, Doty SB. Structure and function of the lysosomes of human fibroblasts in culture: dependence on medium pH. Pediatr Res 1973; 7: 13–9.
148. Lopez-Casillas F, Cheifetz S, Doody J, et al. Structure and expression of the membrane proteoglycan betaglycan, a component of the TGF-beta receptor system. Cell 1991; 67: 785–95.
149. Lorenzo P, Aspberg A, Onnerfjord P, et al. Identification and characterization of asporin: a novel member of the leucine-rich repeat protein family closely related to decorin and biglycan. J Biol Chem 2001; 276:12201–11.
150. McDonnell JM, Green WR, Maumenee IH. Ocular histopathology of systemic mucopolysaccharidosis, type II-A (Hunter syndrome, severe). Ophthalmology 1985; 92: 1772–9.
151. McKusick VA. Mendelian Inheritance in Man. Catalogs of Autosomal Dominant, Autosomal Recessive and X-linked Phenotypes, 10th ed. Baltimore, MD: Johns Hopkins University Press, 1992.
152. McKusick VA, Howell RR, Hussels IE, et al. Allelism, non-allelism, and genetic compounds among the mucopolysaccharidoses. Lancet 1972; 1:993–6.
153. Mailer C. Gargoylism associated with optic atrophy. Can J Ophthalmol 1969; 4:266–71.
154. Mali M, Jaakkola P, Arvilommi AM, Jalkanen M. Sequence of human syndecan indicates a novel gene family of integral. J Biol Chem 1990; 265:6884–9.
155. Malley DS, Steinert RF, Puliafito CA, Dobi ET. Immunofluorescence study of corneal wound healing after excimer laser anterior keratectomy in the monkey eye. Arch Ophthalmol 1990; 108:1316–22.
156. Maroteaux P. Un nouveau type de mucopolysaccharidose avec athétose et elimination urinaire de kératin-sulfate. Presse Med 1973; 81:975–9.
157. Maroteaux P, Lévêque B, Marie J, Lamy M. Une nouvelle dysotose avec élimination urinaire de chondroitine-sulfate B. Presse Med 1963; 71:1849–52.
158. Martin GR, Timpl R. Laminin and other basement membrane components. Annul Rev Cell Bio 1987; 3: 57–85.
159. Marynen P, Zhang J, Cassiman J, et al. Partial primary structure of the 48- and 90-kilodalton core proteins of the cell surface-associated heparan sulfate proteoglycans of lung fibroblasts: prediction of an integral membrane domain and evidence for multiple distinct core proteins at the cell surface of human lung fibroblasts. J Biol Chem 1989; 264:7017–24.
160. Matalon R, Arbogast B, Justice P, et al. Morquio's syndrome: deficiency of a chondroitin sulfate N-acetylhexosamine sulfate sulfatase. Biochem Biophys Res Commun 1974; 61:709–15.
161. Matalon R, Dorfman A. Hurler's syndrome: biosynthesis of acid mucopolysaccharides in tissue culture. Proc Natl Acad Sci USA 1966; 56:1310–6.
162. Matsuda H, Satake Y, Katsumata H. Ultrastructural observations of the cornea of Hurler's syndrome. Acta Soc Ophthalmol Jap 1970; 74:47–56.
163. Meyer K. Biochemistry and biology of mucopolysaccharides. Am J Med 1969; 47:664–72.
164. Midura, RJ, Hascall, VC. Analysis of the proteoglycans synthesized by corneal explants from embryonic chicken. II. Structural characterization of the keratan sulfate and dermatan sulfate proteoglycans from corneal stroma. J Biol Chem 1989; 264:1423–30.
165. Miyamoto T, Inoue H, Sakamoto Y, et al. Identification of a novel spice site mutation of the CSPG2 gene in a Japanese family with Wagner syndrome. Invest Ophthalmol Vis Sci 2005; 46:2726–35.
166. Murdoch AD, Dodge GR, Cohen I, et al. Primary structure of the human heparan sulfate proteoglycan from basement membrane (HSPG2/perlecan). A chimeric molecule with multiple domains homologous to the low density lipoprotein receptor, laminin, neural cell adhesion molecules, and epidermal growth factor. J Biol Chem 1992; 267:8544–57.
167. Murillo-Lopez F, Politi L, Adler R, Hewitt AT. Proteoglycan synthesis in cultures of murine retinal neurons and photoreceptors. Cell Mol Neurobiol 1991; 11:579–91.
168. Naumann G. Clearing of cornea after perforating keratoplasty in mucopolysaccharidosis type VI (Maroteaux-Lamy syndrome) (letter). N Engl J Med 1985; 312:995.
169. Neufeld EF. Replacement of genotype-specific proteins in mucopolysaccharidoses. In: Bergsma D, Desnick RJ, Berlohr RW, Krivit W, eds. Enzyme Therapy in Genetic Diseases. Baltimore, MD: Williams & Wilkins, 1973:27–30.

170. Neufeld EF, Cantz MJ. Corrective factors for inborn errors of mucopolysaccharide metabolism. Ann NY Acad Sci 1971; 179:580–7.
171. Neufeld EF, Muenzer J. The mucopolysaccharidoses. In: Scriver CR, Beudet AL, Sly WS, Valle D, eds. The Metabolic Basis of Inherited Disease, vol. 2. New York, NY: McGraw-Hill, 1989:1565–87.
172. Neuhauser EBD, Griscom NT, Gilles FH, Crocker AC. Arachnoid cysts in the Hurler-Hunter syndrome. Ann Radiol 1968; 11:453–69.
173. Newell FW, Koistinen A. Lipochondrodystrophy (gargoylism): pathologic findings in five eyes of three patients. Arch Ophthalmol 1955; 53:45–62.
174. Nieduszynski IA., Huckerby TN, Dickenson JM, et al. Structural aspects of skeletal keratan sulphates. Biochem Soc Trans 1990; 18:792–3.
175. Nieduszynski IA, Huckerby TN, Dickenson JM, et al. There are two major types of skeletal keratan sulphates. Biochem J 1990; 271:243–5.
176. Nishiu J, Tanaka T, Nakamura Y. Identification of a novel gene (ECM2) encoding a putative extracellular matrix protein expressed predominantly in adipose and female-specific tissues and its chromosomal localization to 9q22.3. Genomics 1998; 52:378–81.
177. Njå A. A sex-linked type of gargoylism. Acta Pediatr. 1946; 33:267–86.
178. Noonan DM, Fulle A, Valente P, et al. The complete sequence of perlecan, a basement membrane heparan sulfate proteoglycan, reveals extensive similarity with laminin A chain, low density lipoprotein-receptor, and the neural cell adhesion molecule. J Biol Chem 1991; 266: 22939–47.
179. O'Brien JF, Cantz M, Spranger J. Maroteaux-Lamy disease (mucopolysaccharidosis VI), subtype A: deficiency of a N-acetyl-galactosamine-4-sulfatase. Biochem Biophys Res Commun 1974; 60:1170–7.
180. Oettinger HF, Streeter H, Lose E, et al. Chromosome mapping of the murine syndecan gene. Genomics 1991; 11:334–8.
181. Oliveira AM, Perez AR, Cin PD, et al. Aneurysmal bone cyst variant translocations upregulate USP6 transcription by promoter swapping with the ZNF9, COL1A1, TRAP150, and OMD genes. Oncogene 2005; 24:3419–26.
182. Opitz JM. The Golabi–Rosen syndrome: report of a second family. Am J Med Genet 1984; 17:359–66.
183. Paigen K, Noell WK. Two linked genes showing a similar timing of expression in mice. Nature 1961; 190: 148–50.
184. Paine-Saunders S, Viviano BL, Sauders S. GPC6, a novel member of the glypican gene family, encodes a product structurally related to GPC4 and is colocalized with GPC5 on human chromosome 13. Genomics 1999; 57:455–8.
185. Pellegata NS, Dieguez-Lucena JL, Joensuu T, et al. Mutations in KERA, encoding keratacan, cause cornea plana. Nature Genet 2000; 25:91–5.
186. Philippart M, Sugarman GI. Chondroitin-4-sulfate mucopolysaccharidosis: a new variant of Hunter's syndrome. Lancet 1969; 2:854.
187. Pierce A, Lyon M, Hampson IN, et al. Molecular cloning of the major cell surface heparan sulfate proteoglycan from rat liver. J Biol Chem 1992; 267:3894–900.
188. Pilia G, Hughes-Benzie RM, MacKenzie A, et al. Mutations in GPC3, a glypican gene, cause the Simpson-Golabi-Behmel overgrowth syndrome. Nature Genet 1996; 12:241–7.
189. Pouliquen Y, Faure JP, Bisson J, Desvignes P. Ultrastructure de la cornée dans un cas de polydystrophie de Hurler. Arch Ophtalmol (Paris) 1967; 27:495–512.
190. Prange CK, Pennacchio LA, Lieuallen K, et al. Characterization of the human neurocan gene, CSPG3. Gene 1998; 221:199–205.
191. Praus R, Goldman JN. Glucosaminoglycans in human corneal buttons removed at keratoplasty. Ophthalmic Res 1971; 2:223–30.
192. Pulkkinen L, Alitalo T, Krusius T, Peltonen L. Expression of decorin in human tissues and cell lines and defined chromosomal assignment of the gene locus (DCN). Cytogenet. Cell Genet. 1992; 60:107–11.
193. Pusch CM, Zeitz C, Brandau O, et al. The complete form of X-linked congenital stationary night blindness is caused by mutations in a gene encoding a leucine-rich protein. Nature Gene 2000; 26:324–7.
194. Quantock AJ, Meek KM, Brittain P, et al. Alteration of the stromal architecture and depletion of keratan sulphate proteoglycans in oedematous human corneas: histological, immunochemical and X-ray diffraction evidence. Tissue Cell 1991; 23:593–606.
195. Quigley HA, Goldberg MF. Scheie syndrome and macular corneal dystrophy: an ultrastructural comparison of conjunctiva and skin. Arch Ophthalmol 1971; 85: 553–64.
196. Quigley HA, Kenyon KR. Ultrastructural and histochemical studies of a newly recognized form of systemic mucopolysaccharidosis (Maroteaux-Lamy syndrome, mild phenotype). Am J Ophthalmol 1974; 77:809–18.
197. Quigley AH, Maumenee AE, Stark WJ. Acute glaucoma in systemic mucopolysaccharidosis I-S. Am J Ophthalmol 1975; 80:70–2.
198. Rasteiro A. Nota anatomica-clinica: sindroma de Scheie. Exp Ophthalmol 1977; 3:62–4.
199. Reardon A, Heinegard D, McLeod D. The large chondroitin sulphate proteoglycan versican in mammalian vitreous. Matrix Biol 1998; 17:325–33.
200. Robbins RA, Wagner WD, Register TC, Caterson B. Demonstration of a keratan sulfate-containing proteoglycan in atherosclerotic aorta. Arterioscler Thromb 1992; 12: 83–91.
201. Rodriquez-Criado G, Mangano L, Segovia M, et al. Clinical and molecular studies on two further families with Simpson-Golabi-Behmel syndrome. Am J Med Genet 2005; 138A:272–7.
202. Rosen DA, Edmison DR, Robertson DM. Five year maintenance of corneal graft normality in systemic mucopolysaccharidosis. Can J Ophthalmol 1972; 7: 445–53.
203. Rosen DA, Haust MD, Yamashita T, Bryans AM. Keratoplasty and electron microscopy of the cornea in systemic mucopolysaccharidosis (Hurler's disease). Can J Ophthalmol 1968; 3:218–30.
204. Rouzier C, Vanatka R, Bannwarth S, et al. A novel homozygous MMP2 mutation in a family with Winchester syndrome. Clin Genet 2006; 69:271–6.
205. Rummelt V, Meyer HJ, Naumann GOH. Light and electron microscopy of the cornea in systemic mucopolysaccharidosis type I-S (Scheie's syndrome). Cornea 1992; 11:86–92.
206. Ruoslahti E. Structure and biology of proteoglycans. Ann Rev Cell Biol 1988; 4:229–55.
207. Saghatelyan A, de Chevigny A, Schachner M, Lledo P-M. Tenascin-R mediates activity-dependent recruitment of neuroblasts in the adult mouse forebrain. Nature Neurosci 2004; 7:37–356.

208. Sanfilippo SJ, Podosin R, Langer LO, Good RA. Mental retardation associated with acid mucopolysacchariduria (heparitin sulfate type). Pediatr 1963; 63:837–8.
209. Saunders S, Jalkanen M, O'Farrell S, Bernfield M. Molecular cloning of syndecan, an integral membrane proteoglycan. J Cell Biol 1989; 108:1547–56.
210. Sawaguchi S, Yue BYJT, Chang I, et al. Proteoglycan molecules in keratoconus corneas. Invest Ophthalmol Vis Sci 1991; 32:1846–53.
211. Schaefer L, Babelova A, Kiss E, et al. The matrix component biglycan is proinflammatory and signals through Toll-like receptors 4 and 2 in macrophages. J Clin Invest 2005; 115:2223–33.
212. Scheie HG, Hambrick GW Jr, Barness LA. A newly recognized forme fruste of Hurler's disease (gargoylism). Am J Ophthalmol 1962; 53:753–69.
213. Schrecengost PK, Blochberger TC, Hassell JR. Identification of chick corneal keratan sulfate proteoglycan precursor protein in whole corneas and in cultured corneal fibroblasts. Arch Biochem Biophys 1992; 292:54–61.
214. Scott, JE, Bosworth, TR. The comparative chemical morphology of the mammalian cornea. Basic Appl Histochem 1990; 34:35–42.
215. Scott, JE, Haigh, M. Keratan sulphate and the ultrastructure of cornea and cartilage: a 'stand-in' for chondroitin in conditions of oxygen lack? J Anat 1988; 158:95–108.
216. Shows TB, Scrafford-Wolf LR, Brown JA, Meisler M. Assignment of β galactosidase gene (β-Galα) to chromosome 3 in man. Cytogenet Cell Genet 1978; 22:219–222.
217. Shull RM, Hastings NE, Selcer RR, et al. Bone marrow transplantation in canine mucopolysaccharidosis I: Effects within the central nervous system. J Clin Invest 1987; 79:435–43.
218. Shull R, Helman R, Spellacy E, Constantopoulos G. Morphologic and biochemical studies of canine mucopolysaccharidosis I Am J Pathol 1984; 114:487–95.
219. Shull RM, Munger RJ, Spellacy E, et al. Canine α-L-iduronidase deficiency. Am J Pathol 1982; 109:244–8.
220. Sly WS, Quinton BA, McAlister WH, Rimoin DL. Beta glucuronidase deficiency: report of clinical, radiologic and biochemical features of a new mucopolysaccharidosis. 1973; J Pediatr. 82:249–57.
221. Speizale P, Bardoni A, Balduini C. Interactions between bovine cornea proteoglycans and collagen. Biochem J 1980; 187:655–9.
222. Spranger J. The systemic mucopolysaccharidoses. Ergeb Inn Med Kinderheilkd 1972; 32:165–265.
223. Spranger J. Morphological aspects of the mucopolysaccharidoses. In: Holton JB, Ireland JT, eds. Inborn Errors of Skin, Hair and Connective Tissues. Baltimore, MD: University Park Press, 1975:39–65.
224. Spranger J, Schuster W. Chondroitin-4-sulphate mucopolysaccharidosis. Helv Pediatr Acta 1971; 26:387–96.
225. Staub E, Hinzmann B, Rosenthal A. A novel repeat in the melanoma-associated chondroitin sulfate proteoglycan defies a new protein family. FEBS Lett. 2002; 527: 114-–118, 2002.
226. Stevenson RE, Howell RR, McKusick VA, et al. The iduronidase deficient mucopolysaccharidoses: clinical and roentgenographic features. Pediatrics 1976; 57: 111–22.
227. Stramm LE, Haskins ME, Aguirre G. Retinal pigment epithelial glycosaminoglycan metabolism: intracellular vs extracellular pathways. Invest Ophthalmol Vis Sci 1989; 30:2118–31.
228. Stramm L, Li W, Haskins M, Aguirre G. Glycosaminoglycan and collagen metabolism in arylsulfatase B-deficient retinal pigment epithelium in vitro. Invest Ophthalmol Vis Sci 1991; 32:2035–41.
229. Stramm L, Wolfe J, Schuchman E, et al. β-Glucuronidase mediated pathway essential for retinal pigment epithelial degradation of glycosaminoglycans. Disease expression and in vitro disease correction using retroviral mediated cDNA transfer. Exp Eye Res 1990; 50:521–32.
230. Stum M, Davoine C-S, Vicart S, et al. Spectrum of HSPG2 (perlecan) mutations in patents with Schwartz-Jampel syndrome. Hum Mutat 2006; 27:1082–91.
231. Summers CG, Purple RL, Krivit W, et al. Ocular changes in the mucopolysaccharidoses after bone marrow transplantation: a preliminary report. Ophthalmology 1989; 96:977–85.
232. Sutherland AE, Sanderson RD, Mayes M, et al. Expression of syndecan, a putative low affinity fibroblast growth factor receptor, in the early mouse embryo. Development 1991; 113:339–51.
233. Sztrovics R, Chen X-N, Grover J, et al. Localization of the human fibromodulin gene (FMOD) to chromosome 1q32 and completion of the cDNA sequence. Genomics 1994; 23:715–7.
234. Tabone E, Grimaud J-A, Peyrol S, et al. Ultrastructural aspects of corneal fibrous tissue in the Scheie syndrome. Virchows Arch [B] 1978; 27:63–7.
235. Taghavy A, Salsman K, Ledeen R. An abnormal ganglioside pattern from a gargoyle brain. Fed Proc 1964; 23:163.
236. Taketomi T, Yamakawa T. Glycolipids of the brain in gargoylism. Jap J Exp Med 1967; 37:11–21.
237. Tasheva ES, Pettanati M, von Kap-Her C, Conrad GW. Assignment of keratocan gene (KERA) to human chromosome band 12q22 by in situ hybridization. Cytogenet Cell Genet 2000; 88:244–5.
238. Tasheva ES, Pettenati M, von Kap-Her C, Conrad GW Assignment of mimecan gene (OGN) to human chromosome band 9q22 by in situ hybridization. Cytogenet Cell Genet 2000; 88:326–7.
239. Tawara A, Hollyfield JG. Proteoglycans in the mouse interphotoreceptor matrix. III Changes during photoreceptor development and degeneration in the rds mutant. Exp Eye Res 1990; 51:301–15.
240. Thompson GR, Nelson NA, Castor CW, Grobelny SL. A mucopolysaccharidosis with increased urinary excretion of chondroitin-4-sulphate. Ann Intern Med 1971; 75: 421–6.
241. Thonar EJ, Manicourt DM, Williams J, et al. Circulating keratan sulfate: marker of cartilage proteoglycan catabolism in osteoarthritis. J Rheumatol Suppl 1991; 27:24–6.
242. Threlked A, Adler R, Hewitt AT. Proteoglycan biosynthesis by chick embryo retina glial-like cells. Dev Biol 1989; 132:559–68.
243. Topping TM, Kenyon KR, Goldberg MF, Maumenee AE. Ultrastructural ocular pathology of Hunter's syndrome, systemic mucopolysaccharidosis type II. Arch Ophthalmol 1971; 86:164–77.
244. Toselli C, Volpi U, Pirodda A. Contributo alla conoscenza della distrofia maculata del parenchima corneale (dystrophie mouchetée di François e Neetens). Ann Ottalmol 1966; 92:770–7.
245. Traupe H, van den Ouweland AM, van Oost BA, et al. Fine mapping of the human biglycan (BGN) gene within the Xq28 region employing a hybrid cell panel. Genomics 1992; 13:481–3.
246. Tremblay M, Dubé I. Macular dystrophy of the cornea: ultrastructure of two cases. Can J Ophthalmol 1973; 8: 47–53.
247. Tremblay M, Dube I, Gagne R. Altérations de la cornée dans the maladie de Scheie (mucopolysaccharidose type

1-S). Etude ultrastructurale. J Fr Ophthalmol 1979; 2: 193–7.
248. Triggs-Raine B, Salo TJ, Zhang H, et al. Mutations in HYAL1, a member of a trandemly distributed multigene family encoding disparate hyaluronidase activities, cause a newly described lyosomal disorder, mucopolysaccharidosis IX. Proc Natl Acad Sci USA 1999; 96:6296–300.
249. Tripathi RC, Ashton N. Application of electron microscopy to the study of errors of metabolism. Birth Defects 1976; 12:69–104.
250. Tschumper RC, Johnson DH, Bradley JM, Acott TS. Glycosaminoglycans of human trabecular meshwork in perfusion organ culture. Curr Eye Res 1990; 9:363–9.
251. Turnbull J, Powell A, Guimond S. Heparan sulfate: decoding a dynamic multifunctional cell regulator. Trends Cell Biol 2001; 11:75–82.
252. Uchimura Y, Toshima Y, Sekiya T. Zur elektonmikroskopischen Pathomorphologie der Hirnrinde bei Gargoylismus. Acta Neuropathol 1965; 4:476–90.
253. van Hoof F, Hers HG. The abnormalities of lysosomal enzymes in mucopolysaccharidoses. Eur J Biochem 1968; 7:34–44.
254. Vermeesch JR, Mertens G, David G, Marynen P. Assignment of the human glypican gene (GPC1) to 2q35-q37 by fluorescence in situ hybridization. Genomics 1995; 25:327–9.
255. Veugelers M, De Cat B, Ceulemans H, et al. Glypican-6, a new member of the glycipan family of cell surface heparan sulfate proteoglycans. J Biol Chem 1999; 274: 26968–77
256. Veugelers M, De Cat B, Muyldermans SY, et al. Mutational analysis of the GPC3/GPC4 glypican gene cluster on Xq26 in patients with Simpson-Golabi-Behmel syndrome: identification of loss-of-function mutations in the GPC3 gene. Hum Molec Genet 2000; 9:1321–8.
257. Veugelers M, Vermeesch J, Reekmans G, et al. Characterization of glypican-5 and chromosomal localization of human GPC5, a new member of the glypican family. Genomics 1997; 40:24–30.
258. Veugelers M, Vermeesch J, Watanabe K, et al. GPC4, the gene for human K-glypican, flanks GPC3 on Xq26: deletion of the GPC3-GPC4 gene cluster in one family with Simpson-Golabi-Behmel syndrome. Genomics 1998; 53:1–11.
259. Vine D, McGovern M, Schuchman E, et al. Enhancement of residual arylsulfatase B activity in feline mucopolysaccharidosis VI by thiol-induced subunit association. J Clin Invest 1982; 69:294–302.
260. Vogler C, Birkenmeier EH, Sly WS, et al. A murine model of mucopolysaccharidosis VII: gross and microscopic findings in beta-glucuronidase-deficient mice. Am J Path 1990; 136:207–17.
261. Wallace BJ, Kaplan D, Adachi M, et al. Mucopolysaccharidosis type III: morphologic and biochemical studies of two siblings with Sanfilippo syndrome. Arch Pathol 1966; 82:462–73.
262. Wenger D, Gasper P, Thrall M, et al. Bone marrow transplantation in the feline model of arylsulfatase B deficiency. In: Krivit W, Paul N, eds. Bone Marrow Transplantation for Treatment of Lysosomal Storage Diseases. New York, NY: Alan R. Liss, 1986:177–86.
263. White DM, Mikol DD, Espinosa R, et al. Structure and chromosomal localization of the human gene for a brain form of prostaglandin D-2 synthase. J Biol Chem 1992; 267:23202–8.
264. Whitley C, Ramsey N, Kersey J, Krivit W. Bone Marrow Transplantation for Hurler Syndrome: Assessment of Metabolic Correction. In: Krivit W, Paul N, eds. Bone Marrow Transplantation for Treatment of Lysosomal Storage Diseases. New York, NY: Alan R. Liss, 1986: 7–24.
265. Whiteley CB. The mucopolysaccharidoses, In: Beighton P, ed. McKusick's Heritable Disorders of Connective Tissue. 5th ed. St. Louis, MO: CV Mosby, 1993:367–945.
266. Wiesmann U, Neufeld EF. Scheie and Hurler syndromes: apparent identity of the biochemical defect. Science 1970; 169:72–4.
267. Winchester P, Grossman H, Lim WN, Danes BS. A new mucopolysaccharidosis with skeletal deformities simulating rheumatoid arthritis. Am J Roentgenol 1969; 106: 121–8.
268. Winterbotham CTC, Torczynski E, Horwitz AL, et al. Unusual mucopolysaccharide disorder with corneal and scleral involvement. Am J Ophthalmol 1990; 109: 544–55.
269. Winters PR, Harrod MJ, Molenich-Heetred SA, et al. Alpha-L-iduronidase deficiency and possible Hurler-Scheie genetic compound. Neurology 1976; 26:1003–7.
270. Wolfe J, Schuchman E, Stramm L, et al. Restoration of normal lysosomal function in mucopolysaccharidosis type VII cells by gene transfer. Proc Natl Acad Sci USA 1990; 87:2877–81.
271. Wollensak J, Buddecke E. Biochemical studies on human corneal proteoglycans: a comparison of normal and keratoconic eyes. Graefes Arch Clin Exp Ophthalmol 228:517–23.
272. Xiao X, Jia X, Guo X, et al. CSNB1 in Chinese families associated with novel mutations in NYX. J Hum Genet 2006; 51:634–40.
273. Yamada, H, Watanabe K, Shimonaka M, Tamaguchi, Y Molecular cloning of brevican, a novel brain proteoglycan of the aggregan/verican family. J. Biol. Chem. 1994; 269: 10119–10126.
274. Yasuda Y, Tokita Y, Aono S, et al. Clong and chromosomal mapping of the human gene of neuroglycan C (NGC). A neural transmembrane chondrotin sulfate proteoglycan with an EGF module. Neurosci Res 1998; 32:313–22.
275. Yue BYJT, Baum JL, Silbert JE. The synthesis of glycosaminoglycans by cultures of corneal stromal cells from patients with keratoconus. J Clin Invest 1979; 63: 545–51.
276. Zabel RW, MacDonald IM, Mintsioulis G, Addison DJ. Scheie's syndrome: an ultrastructural analysis of the cornea. Ophthalmology 1989; 96:1631–8.
277. Zankl A, Bonafe L, Calcaterra V, et al. Winchester syndrome caused by a homozygous mutation affecting the active site of matrix metalloproteinase 2. Clin Genet 2005; 67:261–6.
278. Zimmerman DR, Ruoslahti E. Multiple domains of the large fibroblast proteoglycan versican. EMBO J 1989; 8: 2975–81.

41

Sphingolipidoses and the Neuronal Ceroid Lipofuscinoses

Rose-Mary Boustany
Departments of Pediatrics and Neurobiology, Duke University, Durham, North Carolina, U.S.A. and Abu-Haidan Neuroscience Institute, American University of Beirut, Beirut, Lebanon

INTRODUCTION

The sphingolipidoses are a group of inborn errors of metabolism caused by enzyme defects that involve the sphingolipids, which derive their name from sphingosine, an 18-carbon amino alcohol (Table 1; Fig. 1). The sphingolipidoses include Fabry disease, Farber disease, Gaucher disease (GD), GM_1-gangliosidoses, GM_2-gangliosidoses, Krabbe disease, metachromatic leukodystrophy (MLD), and Niemann–Pick disease (NPD) (Fig. 2). The neuronal ceroid lipofuscinoses (NCLs) (Batten disease) are a genetically heterogenous group of severe neurodegenerative disorders grouped together because of the constellation of clinical findings of seizures, blindness, motor, and cognitive decline and the presence of autofluorescent inclusions with a characteristic ultrastructural appearance within the cytoplasm of neurons and other cells.

Ocular findings are considered hallmarks in most of the sphingolipidoses and the NCLs. More often than not, these ocular manifestations lead to the correct diagnosis of these disorders. Considerable progress has been made in understanding the molecular pathobiology of the sphingolipidoses and the various NCLs over the past 15 years. Of note in this regard is the first description in Amish infantile epilepsy syndrome of a loss of function mutation of a key synthetic enzyme for gangliosides, GM_3-synthase, in humans (180). Also, several genes for the NCLs have been identified.

Basic knowledge about the pathobiology of the sphingolipidoses and NCLs has provided opportunities for therapy. Enzyme replacement for GD and Fabry disease is now available. Substrate reduction therapy (SRT) is being considered for GD, the gangliosidoses, and Fabry disease (100,138). Chaperone therapy with enzyme inhibitors at suboptimal concentrations to rapidly escort undegraded mutant enzymes through the secretory pathway, subsequently raising residual enzyme activity, is possible for few mutations (94). Presymptomatic bone marrow

Table 1 Sphingolipidoses

Disorder	MIM #	Gene	Enzyme or protein deficiency
GM_1-gangliosidoses			
GM_1-gangliosidosis type I	+230500	*GLB1*	Acid β-galactosidase
GM_1-gangliosidosis type II			
GM_1-gangliosidosis type III			
GM_2-gangliosidoses			
GM_2-gangliosidosis type I (Tay–Sachs disease)	#272800	*HEXA*	α-subunit of β-hexosaminidase A
GM_2-gangliosidosis type II (Sandhoff disease)	#268800	*HEXB*	β-subunit of β-hexosaminidase A
Sphingolipidoses			
Niemann–Pick disease		*GM2A*	GM_2-activator protein
Niemann–Pick disease type A	#257200	*SMPD1*	Acid sphingomyelinase
Niemann–Pick disease type B	#607616	*SMPD1*	Acid sphingomyelinase
Niemann–Pick disease type C1	#257220	*NPC1*	
Niemann–Pick disease type C2	#607625	*NPC2*	Epididymal secretory protein
Niemann–Pick disease type D			
Farber disease	+228000	*ASAH*	Ceramidase
Fabry disease	+301500	*GLA*	α-galactosidase
Gaucher disease type I	#230800	*GBA*	Acid beta-glucosidase
Gaucher disease type II	#230900	*GBA*	Acid beta-glucosidase
Gaucher disease type III	#231000	*GBA*	Acid beta-glucosidase
Gaucher disease, atypical		*PSAP*	Prosaposin
Krabbe disease	#245200	*GALC*	Galactosylceramidase
Metachromatic leukodystrophy	#250100	*ARSA*	Arylsulfatase A
Muopolysaccharidosis type IVA (Morquio syndromes type B) (MPS IVB)	#230500	*GLB1*	Acid β-galactosidase

replacement is recommended for early Krabbe disease, and patients with juvenile MLD. Oral drugs affecting biochemical processes, such as phosphocysteamine to break the thioester linkage in infantile NCL (INCL), are in trials. The antiapoptotic drug flupirtine is being tried as therapy for several NCLs (50). Virally mediated gene therapies are under study in animal models. Stem cell therapies are approved for safety trials in late INCL.

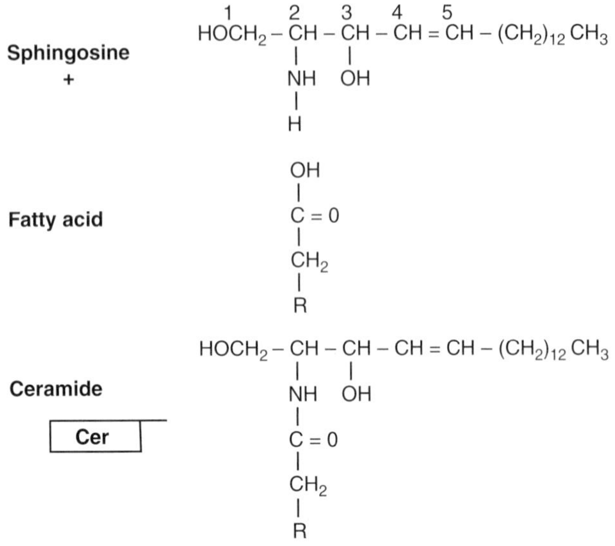

```
                 1       2     3      4      5
Sphingosine      HOCH2 – CH – CH – CH = CH – (CH2)12 CH3
    +                    |     |
                         NH    OH
                         |
                         H

                         OH
                         |
Fatty acid               C = 0
                         |
                         CH2
                         |
                         R

                 HOCH2 – CH – CH – CH = CH – (CH2)12 CH3
                         |     |
Ceramide                 NH    OH
                         |
   [ Cer ]               C = 0
                         |
                         CH2
                         |
                         R
```

Figure 1 Chemical structures of sphingosine and ceramide. The major fatty acids are palmitate and stearate, containing 16 and 18 carbon atoms, respectively. Small amounts of longer chain fatty acids, saturated or unsaturated, are also present. The overall fatty acid composition varies with the tissue source and the individual sphingolipid.

GANGLIOSIDOSES

GM_1-Gangliosidoses (β-Galactosidosis)

Overview

The GM_1-gangliosidoses are autosomal recessive lysosomal storage diseases (LSDs) (see Chapter 38), characterized by the storage of GM_1-ganglioside, oligosaccharides, and keratan sulfate (KS) (188). Decreased activity of the acid β-galactosidase can result in one of two diseases: GM_1-gangliosidosis (MIM +230500), or mucopolysaccharidosis type IVB (Morquio disease type B) (MPS IVB) (MIM #230500) (see Chapter 40) because allelic mutations in the *GLB1* gene that encodes for acid β-galactosidase cause Morquio disease type B. Patients with MPS IVB have no central nervous system (CNS) involvement, but manifest dysostosis multiplex and corneal opacities.

Clinical Presentation

There are three clinical types of GM_1-gangliosidosis: GM_1-gangliosidosis type I (the classic infantile type), GM_1-gangliosidosis type II (juvenile form), and GM_1-gangliosidosis type III (adult form).

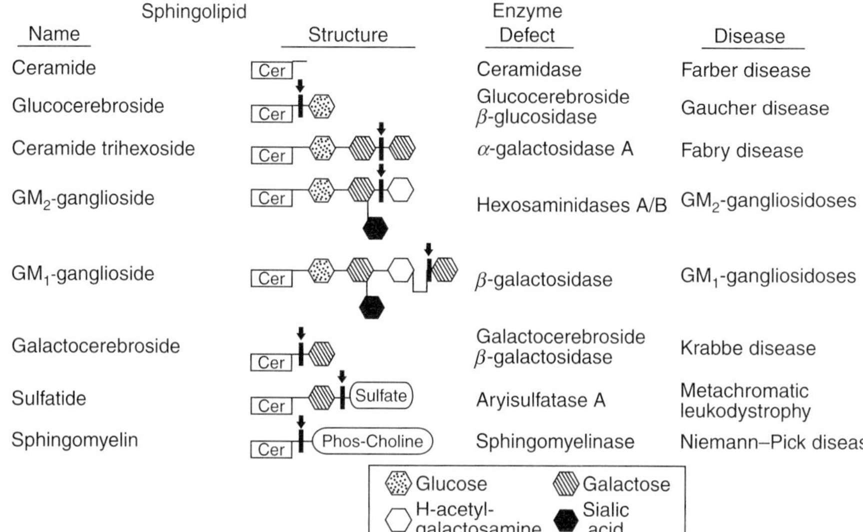

Figure 2 Structural formulas of the sphingolipids stored in the eight known groups of sphingolipidoses, with enzyme defects and the location of the metabolic blocks shown for each disorder.

GM_1-gangliosidosis type I is manifest by 5 to 6 months of age. Neuronal death and macular cherry red spots, and hepatosplenomegaly, cardiomegaly, and mild dysostosis multiplex, are common, with an initial presentation of failure to thrive. Gum hypertrophy, macroglossia, corneal clouding, a protuberant abdomen (165), flexion contractures, kyphoscoliosis, frontal bossing, coarse fascies, and hypertelorism also occur. These patients are retarded and floppy, have an exaggerated startle response, and develop generalized seizures. Death due to pneumonia and cardiopulmonary failure or arrest follows at the age of 2 years. GM_1-gangliosidosis type II is diagnosed before the age of 2 years with psychomotor retardation. Ataxia, dystonia, and spasticity of increasing severity follow, with death usually by the end of the second decade. Organomegaly, skeletal abnormalities, and cherry red spots are rare (193). GM_1-gangliosidosis type III appears later in childhood or adolescence with dementia, Parkinsonism and dystonia, and visceral, macular, and bony involvements are unusual. Age at the time of death is variable (223).

Diagnostic Testing

Low β-galactosidase activity in leukocytes is diagnostic, but is not a good screening method for carriers (2). Vacuolation of lymphocytes and histiocytes is present and histiocytosis is found in the liver and spleen. Lipid accumulates in bone marrow cells, neurons, and rectal ganglion cells. Dysostosis multiplex is evident on plain roentgenograms. There is hypoplasia and anterior beaking of vertebrae in the thoracolumbar region. Bone development is delayed. Computed tomography (CT) and magnetic resonance imaging (MRI) are notable for atrophy, demyelination, and occasionally basal ganglia changes, as well as a dilated ventricular system. CT may show increased density of the thalami and reduced intensity of basal ganglia. MRI also shows thalamic and basal ganglia hyperintensities on T2-weighted images and low densities on T1-weighted sections, suggesting a delay in myelination. Findings are similar in GM_1-gangliosidosis types I and II (95). The putamen may show increased intensity on T2-weighted scans in the adult variant. Cerebral fluorine-18 labeled 2-fluoro-2-deoxyglucose positron emission tomography (PET) is notable for decreased uptake regions (3). Electroretinography (ERG) is normal, but visual evoked responses (VER) demonstrate delays in peak latencies. Electroencephalography (EEG) frequently uncovers epileptogenic foci and slowing.

Histopathology

In GM_1-gangliosidosis, GM_1-ganglioside is stored in neurons. Coarse facial features, hepatosplenomegaly, and skeletal changes are only seen in GM_1-gangliosidosis type I (51). Neuronal cell death and connective tissue and skeletal abnormalities are caused by the intra- and extracellular storage of oligosaccharides with a terminal galactose. Neurons are filled with membranous cytoplasmic bodies (MCBs) and there is cortical brain atrophy in patients with early onset GM_1-gangliosidosis. Demyelination in GM_1-gangliosidosis type I results from defective axoplasmic transport, most likely secondary to neuronal storage of GM_1-ganglioside (200). Inflammation may play a role in the pathogenesis of GM_1-gangliosidoses and GM_2-gangliosidosis with evidence of microglia/macrophage activation in the brain (92). Histiocytes with the cytoplasm chock full of a fine granular material are observed in the liver, spleen, lymph nodes, and thymus (50). The connective tissue abnormalities in GM_1-gangliosidosis type I are probably due to defective elastic fiber assembly by fibroblasts (81).

Ocular Findings

Ocular changes are varied and are not always present. Mild corneal clouding, esotropia, and nystagmus have all been reported. Cherry red spots surrounded by a creamy macula are seen in 50% of GM_1-gangliosidosis type I cases, but have not been documented with later onset variants. Optic atrophy has been described in a juvenile case, and occasionally retinal hemorrhages are seen. The infantile cases become blind early in life. The juvenile cases develop blindness much later. Mild corneal clouding has also been reported. Ultrastructurally, retinal ganglion cells are filled with MCBs (Figs. 3 and 4). Corneal epithelial cells contain single-membrane-bound vesicles stuffed with finely granular material. Two fetuses with GM_1-gangliosidosis have had their eyes examined at 20 to 21 weeks of fetal age: storage inclusions were present in neuroectoderm, surface ectoderm, and mesoderm. By transmission electron microscopy (TEM) pleiomorphic, osmiophilic inclusions were seen in retinal neurons and to a lesser degree in other cell types, but electrolucent vacuoles were only observed in epithelial and mesenchymal cells (179).

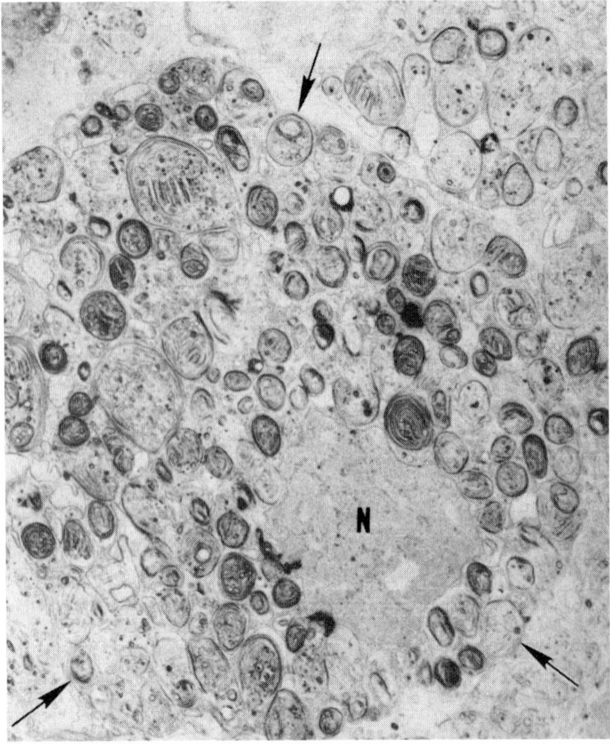

Figure 3 Retinal ganglion cell in GM_1-gangliosidosis type II contains scattered storage vesicles surrounded by single membranes (*arrows*). Some of the cytosomes have prominent lamellar membranes; others have vesicles only (× 8,500). *Source*: Reproduced from Goebel HH, Fix ID, Zeman W. Retinal pathology in GM_2-gangliosidosis, type II. Am J Ophthalmol 1973; 75:434–41.

Biochemistry

All forms of GM_1-gangliosidosis result from a deficiency in β-galactosidase activity. This enzyme is a glycoprotein containing ~9% carbohydrate. The terminal galactose of sphingolipids is usually cleaved by β-galactosidase, except for galactosylceramide (GalCer) and galactosylsphinganine. Acid β-galactosidase is a lysosomal hydrolase, which cleaves terminal beta-linked galactose from GM_1-ganglioside, generating GM_2-ganglioside. Patients therefore store excess GM_1-ganglioside, KS, asialo-GM_1, lyso-GM_1, and oligosaccharides in their tissues. β-galactosidase exists as a monomer, dimer, and/or in a multiprotein complex with neuraminidase (sialidase) and a protective glycoprotein. The latter associates with β-galactosidase and neuraminidase, stabilizing the former and activating neuraminidase (207). Differences in synthesis, posttranslational modification, or degradation of β-galactosidase can result in different clinical phenotypes such as MPS IVB or GM_1-gangliosidosis. GM_1-ganglioside is fourfold higher in the cortex of patients. Asialo-GM_1 is 20 times what it normally is. In GM_1-gangliosidosis type III, lipid accumulation is restricted to the caudate and putamen. Only a small amount of GM_1-ganglioside accumulates in the liver, but KS levels are 50 times higher than normal.

Genetics

The *GLBI* gene is responsible for GM_1-gangliosidoses. The mode of inheritance is autosomal recessive. Heterogeneous gene mutations in all clinical forms of GM_1-gangliosidosis with no clear genotype/phenotype correlation evident have been described. Cardiac abnormalities are correlated with specific gene defects, with some patients homozygous for certain mutations. A common mutation in Japan, Arg201Cys, affects interaction with the protective protein and results in a juvenile or adult variant (227). An Italian mutation affects synthesis (Arg482His), and a North American and Puerto Rican mutation (Arg208Cys) also impacts synthesis (27).

Experimental Models

Naturally occurring animal models of GM_1-gangliosidosis exist in cats, dogs (167), sheep (2), and calves. A GM_1-gangliosidosis mouse model has been created following targeted disruption of the murine

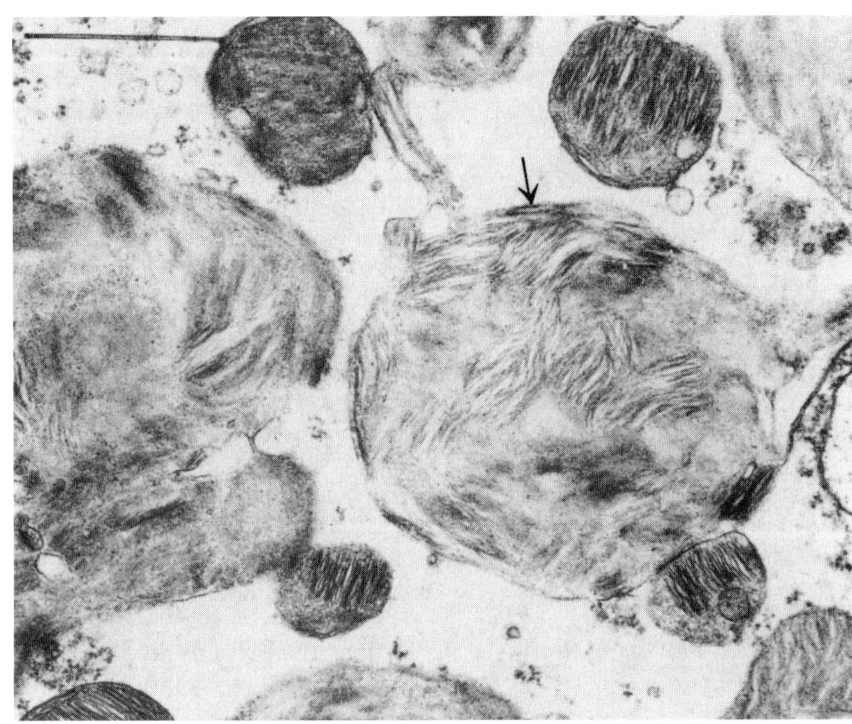

Figure 4 Membranous cytoplasmic bodies (*arrow*) in the ganglion cell layer of the retina in GM_1-gangliosidosis, type II. The abnormal storage bodies contain lamellar membranes that are embedded in an amorphous matrix (×27,000). *Source*: Courtesy of H.H. Goebel.

Glb1 gene (117). The imino sugar *N*-butyl-deoxygalactonojirimycin, a competitive inhibitor of ceramide glucosyltransferase, has been effective in lowering neonatal brain ganglioside levels in a mouse model of GM_1-gangliosidosis and acts as a means for substrate reduction (100). *N*-octyl-4-epi-beta-valienamine and *N*-octyl-beta-valienamine lead to a correction of enzyme activity in cultured fibroblasts from patients with GM_1-gangliosidosis (138).

GM_2-Gangliosidoses

Overview

The GM_2-gangliosidoses are lipid storage diseases resulting from mutations in one of three recessive genes, *HEXA*, *HEXB*, and *GM2A* (the gene for GM_2-activator protein). These gene defects cause an accumulation of GM_2-ganglioside. Three different proteins are needed for degradation of GM_2-ganglioside. These proteins are HEXA (α-subunit of β-hexosaminidase A), HEXB (β-subunit of β-hexosaminidase A), and the GM_2-activator protein. A defect in any of these proteins can lead to accumulation of GM_2-ganglioside, and to GM_2-gangliosidosis and clinical disease (96).

Clinical Presentation

Infantile Acute GM_2-Gangliosidosis

Clinical phenotypes of the infantile forms of the GM_2-gangliosidoses are very similar. These are infantile Tay–Sachs disease (TSD) (defects in the HEXA protein), Sandhoff disease (defects in HEXB protein), and the ABO variant due to defects in the GM_2-activator protein. Infants are normal at birth. An early sign is mild motor weakness at ~2 months of age, with slowing of growth and muted responses to stimuli. Hyperacusis, an exaggerated startle response to noise, is an early sign. Regression with loss of milestones occurs. Progressive weakness, hypotonia with loss of gross motor skills sets in before the age of 10 months. Seizures start a few months later. Fundoscopic examination reveals macular cherry red spots, which may fade with age. Progression of the disease is fast and the infant becomes less responsive to parents. Hyperacusis, blindness, and frequent seizures set in by 10 to 12 months of age (71,142). The EEG is abnormal and continues to deteriorate until death (142). The ERG is normal, but VER are often abnormal. Macrocephaly is evident by 16 to 18 months of age. Ultimately, decerebrate rigidity, problems with deglutition, increasing convulsions, and a vegetative state develop. Death is frequently caused by pneumonia before the age of 5 years. Low density in the thalami and basal ganglia are visualized on CT and high signal intensity on T2-weighted images by MRI. The caudate nuclei appear larger as the disease progresses. Cortical atrophy becomes prominent toward the end (58).

Late Onset Forms of GM_2-Gangliosidosis

Disease onset is anywhere from late infancy to adulthood. Deeper brain structures and the cerebral cortex are less involved compared to the massive gray matter involvement in the infantile variant. Dystonia, ataxia, spinocerebellar degeneration, and lower motor neuron disease are prominent. In the adult variant of TSD, an amyotrophic lateral sclerosis-like motor neuron involvement, and psychosis develop (137,219). Late onset forms of GM_2-gangliosidosis are either variant forms of TSD or Sandhoff disease. GM_2-activator deficiency only causes an infantile form of GM_2-gangliosidosis, almost identical to infantile TSD or Sandhoff disease (113).

Subacute GM_2-Gangliosidosis

Ataxia appears between the ages of 2 to 10 years. Motor regression and dementia are leading symptoms. Progressive deterioration, increasing spasticity, and epilepsy develop before the age of 10 years (113). Optic atrophy and retinitis pigmentosa (RP) appear late in the course, and are the reasons for blindness. A vegetative state and decerebrate rigidity are common by 10 to 15 years of age, soon followed by death, usually due to pneumonia. The disease may accelerate quickly, with death occurring before the age of 5 years (79).

Chronic GM_2-Gangliosidosis

The disease can begin anytime in childhood or adulthood (30). There is great variation in clinical manifestations and course. TSD variants are more commonly described than Sandhoff disease variants. Dystonia and extrapyramidal signs are common, with a clinical phenotype reminiscent of Friedreich ataxia. Cerebellar signs are often the major presenting symptoms (161,219). Prominence of cerebellar symptoms, spasticity and muscle wasting, often evoke an atypical form of Friedreich ataxia with increased deep tendon reflexes (91). Some older individuals have muscle wasting and weakness with fasciculation that is indistinguishable from late onset spinal muscular atrophy (Kugelberg–Welander disease) (see Chapter 72) (55). Others evoke the diagnosis of amyotrophic lateral sclerosis. The electromyogram (EMG) reveals chronic-active denervation with reinervation and normal nerve conduction velocities, and evidence for denervation atrophy on muscle biopsy. EEG is unremarkable. Rectal biopsy shows the MCBs. Neuroimaging studies reveal severe cerebellar atrophy and some mild cerebral atrophy (55). Psychiatric manifestations of depression and schizophrenia affect 40% of patients with the disease.

Ocular Findings

The hallmark of the GM_2-gangliosidoses is the cherry red spot, which tends to fade with age, as retinal ganglion cells are progressively lost (101). Ultrastructurally, the retina and optic nerve disclose abundant pleomorphic storage cytosomes in all neurons of the retina, including the inner segments of photoreceptor cells, and in the glial cells of the optic nerve (Figs. 5 and 6). TEM of the cornea from an infantile case with Sandhoff disease showed distended clear lysosomes that contained fibrogranular material and an occasional collection of lamellae within keratinocytes (31). Abnormal cytoplasmic membrane inclusions were also found in the retinal ganglion cells of a 20-week-old fetus with TSD (40).

Histopathology

Brain weight and volume increase during the second year of life due to gliosis. Cystic degeneration of the cerebral white matter and atrophy of the cerebellum is often present. Neuronal numbers are low and remaining neurons are ballooned due to the storage material. Glial cells are also ballooned. Spinal anterior horn cells are also involved explaining the low tone, diminished reflexes and weakness. Lipid-laden lysosomes appear throughout the cytoplasm of neurons by TEM. Macrophages engorged with lipid are found in liver, spleen, and lung. In late onset GM_2-gangliosidosis, storage is limited to thalamus, substantia nigra, cerebellum, and brainstem nuclei. GM_2-ganglioside accumulation in lysosomes gives rise to MCBs, which also contain cholesterol and sphingolipid. There is apoptosis of neurons, and phagocytic activation leads to chronic inflammation and elevated cytokine production and reactive oxygen species. A disturbed blood–brain barrier aggravates the inflammatory process, promoting oxidative stress, apoptosis, and neurodegeneration. Microglial/macrophage activation appears to contribute to the pathological process in mouse models for GM_1-gangliosidoses and GM_2-gangliosidoses (94).

Biochemistry

The defect in GM_2-gangliosidoses is due to an inability of mutant β-hexosaminidase to hydrolyze the terminal amino sugar from GM_2-ganglioside. Disease severity correlates inversely with the relative residual enzyme activity. This enzyme is one of two major isoenzymes, HEXA and HEXB. HEXA (αβ) is a thermolabile protein composed of a dimeric structure of α- and β-subunits. HEXB (ββ) is a heat-stable dimeric structure composed of two β chains (Fig. 7). The GM_2-activator protein is necessary for hydrolysis of GM_2-ganglioside. HEXA and HEXB hydrolyze *N*-acetyl hexosamine from glycoproteins, glycolipids, glycosaminoglycans (GAGS), and oligosaccharides. HEXA metabolizes GM_2-ganglioside. HEXB metabolizes all the compounds listed above, as well as globoside. In humans, GM_2 is degraded by β-hexosaminidase A, which removes the *N*-acetylgalactosaminyl group. The water-soluble enzyme

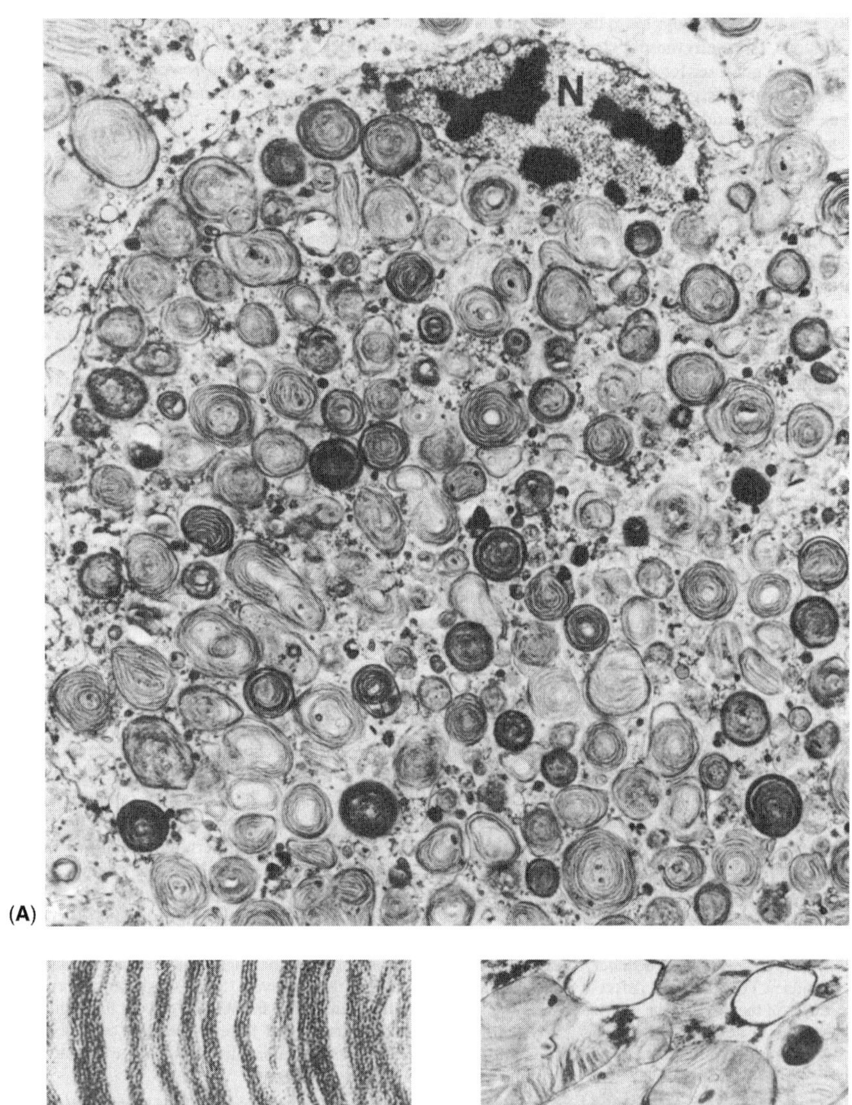

Figure 5 (**A**) Retinal ganglion cell in Tay–Sachs disease filled with membranous cytoplasmic inclusion bodies. The accumulation of round- or oval-shaped lamellar bodies has caused displacement of the nucleus peripherally (× 7,210). (**B**) Mem-branous lamellae at higher magnification (× 142,000). (**C**) Cytoplasmic lamellar inclusions in the inner nuclear layer of the retina in Tay–Sachs disease (× 18,700). *Source*: Reproduced from Tripathi RC, Aston N. Application of electron microscopy to the study of ocular inborn errors of metabolism. Birth Defects 1976; 12:69–104.

cannot hydrolyze the membrane-bound GM_2-ganglioside due to steric hindrance at the membrane surface. The GM_2-activator protein is essential, as its role is to make accessible to the water-soluble enzyme the GM_2-ganglioside lipid for terminal sugar hydrolysis. Both HEXA and HEXB and GM_2-activator protein are glycoproteins that are synthesized in the endoplasmic reticulum (ER), but are processed in the Golgi apparatus, and transported via the mannose-6-phosphate (Man-6-P) receptor to the lysosome. Both α- and β-subunits harbor an active site, yet dimer formation, as HEXA (α–β), HEXB (β–β), and HEXS (α–α), is usually required for catalytic activity. The α- and β-subunits exhibit different substrate specificities. The β-subunit preferentially hydrolyses neutral water-soluble substrates, and the α-subunit also hydrolyses negatively charged substrates such as GM_2-ganglioside, dermatan sulfate (DS), and chondroitin sulfate (CS). The primary amino acid sequences of α and β chains demonstrate a significant degree of primary structure homology. Also, gene structures of *HEXA* and *HEXB* are similar with respect to the number and arrangement of intron/exon junctions (71,153). Twelve of the 13 introns are located at corresponding positions. The GM_2-activator gene contains four exons. α-Subunit defects cause HEXA deficiency (TSD and juvenile and adult onset GM_2-gangliosidosis); β-subunit defects impact HEXA and HEXB (Sandhoff disease), and mutated GM_2-activator protein results in normal HEXA and HEXB activity with accumulation of GM_2-ganglioside (the ABO variant). In the B1 variant described in Portuguese patients the defect is in the α-catalytic site. Enzyme activity loss in this variant can only be demonstrated

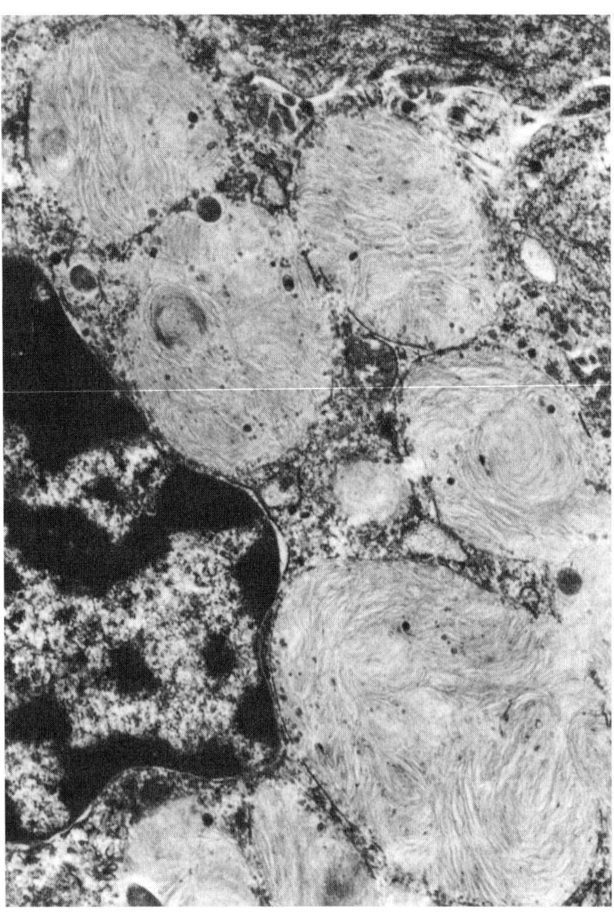

Figure 6 Retinal ganglion cell in Sandhoff disease filled with pleomorphic membranous cytoplasmic bodies varying in size from 0.5 to 6 μm in diameter. Some of the smaller bodies appear to be fused (× 18,400). *Source*: Reproduced from Garner A. Ocular pathology of GM_2-gangliosidosis, type II (Sandhoff disease). Br J Ophthalmol 1973; 57:514–20.

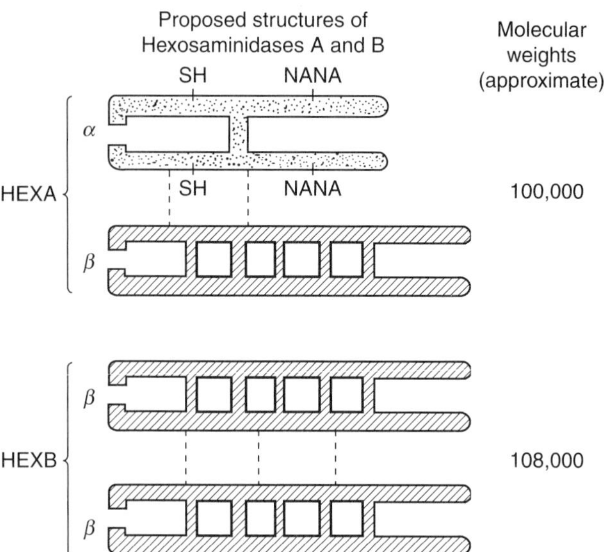

Figure 7 Hypothetical structural models pf hexosaminidase A (one α and one β chain, HEXA) and hexosaminidase B (two β chains, HEXB). Cross-linking is probably by S-S linkage. The chains contain sulfhydryl groups (SH) and sialic acid (NANA, N-acetylneuraminic acid).

when a sulfated artificial substrate is used to assay enzyme activity. Loading studies of fibroblasts using radiolabeled gangliosides can identify all variants, but is predominantly used for diagnosing the B1 and ABO variants (165). In GM_2-gangliosidosis, GM_2-ganglioside is elevated in the CNS, accounting for ~90% of neutral tissue gangliosides. Asialo and lyso forms of GM_2-ganglioside are also increased in brain tissue. GM_2-ganglioside is also stored in the liver and spleen. Lyso-compounds are cytotoxic, and are found in brains of MLD, Krabbe disease, and GD patients. The acute forms of GM_2-gangliosidosis are associated with complete HEXA deficiency and early death. Enzyme activity levels of ~5% are present in the juvenile and adult forms. Some individuals have only 10% enzyme activity compared to normal controls, but are normal themselves. Conzelmann and Sandhoff have postulated that 5% to 10% of normal HEXA activity levels constitutes a "critical threshold" below which clinical disease becomes apparent (42).

Genetics

Most mutations described result in infantile onset disease. The B1 subtype includes mutations in the catalytic α-subunit domain. They do not interfere with the synthesis and activity of the HEXA heterodimer, but the mutant protein does not hydrolyze the sulfated artificial fluorescent substrate used to determine enzyme activity, 4-methylumbelliferyl-*N*-acetylglucosamine-6-sulfate (4MUGS), as well as the natural substrate, GM_2-ganglioside. Mutations causing chronic disease clinical variants produce unstable α-protein that cannot associate with the β-subunit, or its processing is otherwise incomplete. HEXA pseudodeficiency is caused by a point mutation resulting in a mutant HEXA with lower activity toward the artificial substrate, but with sufficient GM_2-ganglioside hydrolyzing activity to escape storage of GM_2-ganglioside and clinical disease. Mutant TSD genes are more commonly carried by Ashkenazi Jews, French Canadians from eastern Quebec, Cajuns from Louisiana, and Pennsylvania Dutch. About 1 in 3600 Ashkenazi Jews are at risk for TSD, yet TSD is not restricted to these groups, but can occur in all ethnic groups. Juvenile TSD has no ethnic predominance. Inheritance is autosomal recessive. TSD is genetically heterogeneous, with numerous allelic mutations described. One ethnic group can harbor multiple mutations. Seventy mutations or more affect the gene for the α-subunit. Mutations can result in wide fluctuations in residual enzyme activity, distribution and level of GM_2-ganglioside in the brain and spinal cord, and tremendous diversity in clinical presentation. An exhaustive and complete online database cataloging alleles, mutations, phenotypes, and authors are available. Only four mutations have been described that affect the GM_2-activator protein A.

Diagnostic Tests

With the development of enzymatic and molecular diagnostic techniques, accurate ascertainment of carriers and affected patients is now feasible using tissues or body fluids (serum, tears), chorionic villi, skin fibroblasts, leukocytes, or buccal mucosa. In a family with a known mutation, prenatal and postnatal diagnosis of heterozygous, homozygotes, or compound heterozygotes, can be made by DNA analysis. The availability of rapid and inexpensive methods for identification of carriers has led to programs for screening of populations at risk. DNA-based diagnostics allows distinction between infantile, subacute, and chronic disease mutations, as well as pseudodeficiency alleles that do not result in disease. Carrier frequencie are 0.006 for *HEXA* mutations and 0.0036 for *HEXB* mutations. In Ashkenazi Jews, the carrier frequency for *HEXA* mutations is high at 0.033. Screening programs aimed at Ashkenazi Jewish groups have resulted in an impressive reduction in the incidence by almost 90%. The adult onset form has primarily been described in those of Ashkenazi Jewish descent. They carry the common Ashkenazi mutation on one allele, and a milder mutation on the other.

Experimental Models

GM_2-gangliosidosis occurs naturally in dogs (135), cats, and in pigs. They exhibit neuronal storage. Visceral storage is only described in the feline model. Gene therapy experiments have involved the production of a recombinant virus, either retrovirus or adenovirus containing the *HEXA* cDNA. Substrate deprivation therapy using oral administration of N-butyldeoxygalactonojirimycin (NB-DNJ), resulted in a 50% reduction in GM_2-ganglioside accumulation in TSD mice (6,100,162).

Amish Infantile Epilepsy Syndrome

Overview

The sphingolipidoses usually are caused by hydrolytic enzyme defects, but the Amish infantile epilepsy syndrome (GM_3-synthase deficiency) (MIM #609056) is caused by a defect in the synthetic pathway of gangliosides (185).

Clinical Description

Initial symptoms of irritability, poor feeding, and failure to thrive appear after 2 weeks of age and before 3 months. Generalized tonic-clonic seizures set in by 1 year. Many other types of seizures, including startle myoclonus, resistant to anticonvulsants are common. Developmental arrest followed by regression occurs. Patients become nonverbal and nonambulatory and develop random choreoathetoid movements. EEG is slow with superimposed epileptiform discharges. MRI demonstrates progressive cortical atrophy. Children are cortically blind with optic atrophy.

Biochemistry

The defective enzyme catalyzes the generation of GM_3-synthase from lactosylceramide. This is the first and key step in the formation of complex a- and b-series gangliosides. Patients lack GM_3-ganglioside and all its downstream derivatives, but accumulate the precursor, lactosylceramide with increased flux through the globoside/paragloboside pathways.

Genetics

Simpson et al. (185) reported GM_3-synthase deficiency in a large, older Amish pedigree, which is transmitted in an autosomal recessive manner. All described cases have a nonsense mutation in the *SIAT9* gene (Arg232stop), for GM_3-synthase.

Experimental Models

Mutant mice with a similar defect demonstrate a milder clinical symptomatology than humans with increased insulin resistance and no seizures.

SPHINGOLIPIDOSES

Niemann–Pick Disease

Overview

NPD encompasses a heterogeneous group of storage diseases with autosomal recessive inheritance. Four clinical forms are known that were initially grouped together because of pathologic similarities and the occurrence of sea-blue histiocytes in the reticuloendothelial system. NPD type A (MIM #257200) and NPD type B (MIM #607616) result from low acid sphingomyelinase (ASM) activity, and are characterized by accumulation of sphingomyelin and have defects in the same *SMPD1* gene (28). NPD type C1 (MIM #257220), described in a genetic isolate from Nova Scotia formerly known as NPD type D, accounts for 95% of all NPD type C patients. A second defect in the *NPC2* gene is now identified. NPD types C1 and C2 defects have a lipid trafficking abnormality of low-density lipoprotein (LDL)-derived cholesterol. The latter remains trapped in lysosomes. Concomitantly, sphingomyelin and other lipids are increased due to sequestration of cholesterol in lysosomes (146).

Niemann–Pick Disease, Types A and B

Clinical Presentation

In NPD type A (NP-A) (infantile or acute form), hepatosplenomegaly and moderate lymphadenopathy appear in the first few months of life. Most NP-A cases are of Ashkenazi Jewish descent. A moderate microcytic anemia, responsive to iron, and a decrease in platelet numbers are common. Neurologic signs of hypotonia, muscular weakness, and feeding difficulties appear. Recurrent vomiting and constipation are characteristic. Fifty percent of patients have macular cherry red spots. ERG amplitudes are diminished. EEG manifests nonspecific slowing and low voltage waves. Evoked brainstem responses are abnormal, and nerve conduction velocities can be reduced. Death follows by age 4 to 5 years. NP-B (chronic, non-neuronopathic forms) is the chronic, non-neuropathic form, with prolonged survival and no neurologic involvement. Hepatosplenomegaly is prominent in childhood. In most patients with NP-B, decreased pulmonary diffusion due to alveolar infiltration appears early and progresses. Patients can have significant pulmonary problems by 15 years of age with low oxygen tensions, dyspnea on exertion, life-threatening pneumonias and cor pulmonale. Liver involvement and cirrhosis may occur. NP-B patients have no neurologic involvement and are intellectually normal. Some NP-B patients have cherry red maculae or gray granular pigmentation around the fovea that gives a halo effect (39). Two adults with psychiatric and pulmonary symptoms as well as low ASM activity have been reported (108).

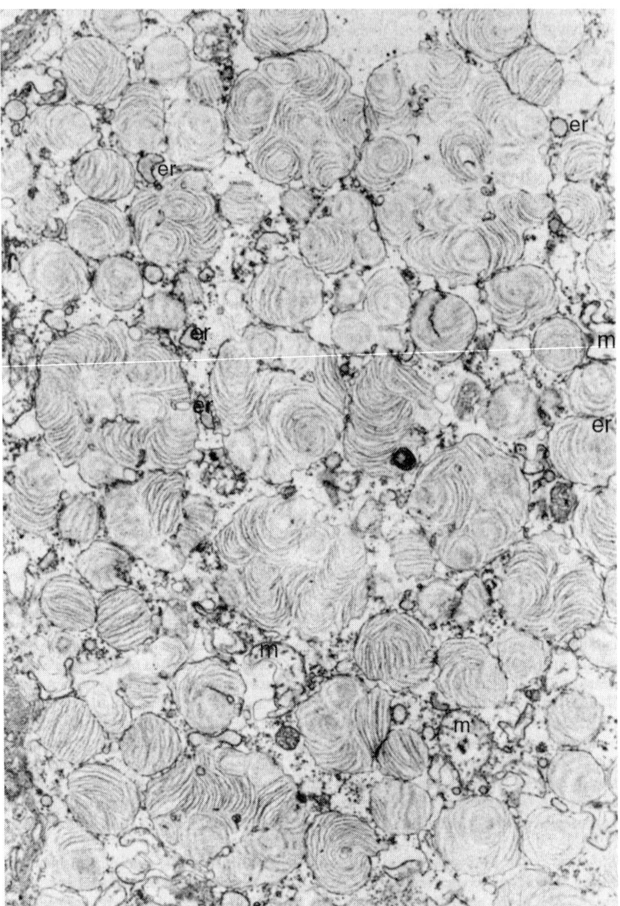

Figure 8 Retinal ganglion cell in Niemann–Pick disease type A, showing abundance of round inclusion bodies containing parallel or concentrically laminated membranes. Some appear to be compressed and in the process of fusing. Mitochondria (m) and endoplasmic reticulum (er) are also seen (×11,500). *Source*: Reproduced from Libett J, Touasaint D, Guiselings R. Ocular findings in Niemann–Pick disease. Am J Ophthalmol 1975; 80:991–1002.

Histopathology

Characteristic lipid-laden cells (foam cells) that appear as sea-blue histiocytes are seen in the bone marrow. These NPD cells are 30 to 70 μm in diameter and their cytoplasm is engorged with lipid droplets that have a mulberry-like morphology. NP-A brains are firm and have a reduced weight due to atrophy of the cerebellum and the cerebrum. Glial cells and foam cells stuffed with lipid are found close to blood vessels. Remaining neurons are swollen and there is demyelination. The spinal cord and deep nuclei are also affected. Peripheral nerves demonstrate loss of myelin and inclusion bodies in Schwann cells. The bone marrow and spleen are affected. The latter can be enlarged up to 10 times normal. Lymph nodes, liver, kidneys, and lungs are affected. In NP-B, lung involvement is severe with increased lung size and presence of invading foam cells in blood vessels and alveoli (102). The retinal ganglion cells contain characteristic inclusion bodies (Fig. 8) and so does the lens epithelium (Fig. 9). A 23-week fetus had lipid droplets in the inner plexiform layer of the retina, and membranous cytoplasmic bodies in corneal epithelium and keratocytes, lens epithelial cells, fibroblasts of choroid, and sclera and in muscles by TEM.

Biochemistry

ASM metabolizes sphingomyelin to ceramide and phosphorylcholine. NP-A and NP-B both manifest an accumulation of sphingomyelin in tissues due to ASM deficiency (206). Lipids stored in the reticuloendothelial system and visceral organs are similar. The profile of lipids in the brain differs with lysosphingomyelin elevated in the brain of two NP-A patients, but normal in the brain of one NP-B patient (168). Lysosphingolipids are toxic metabolites found in brains of patients with sphingolipid disorders. They are implicated in the pathogenesis of NPD as well as Krabbe disease. NP-A patients have levels of sphingomyelin up to 50-fold normal values, representing

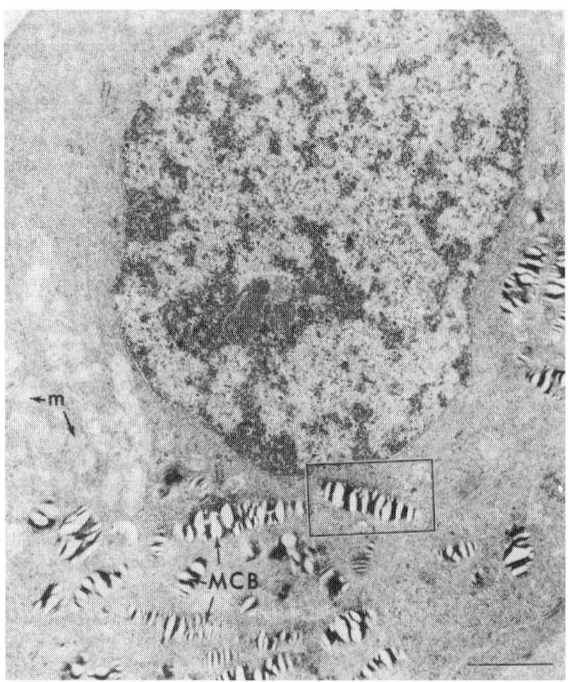

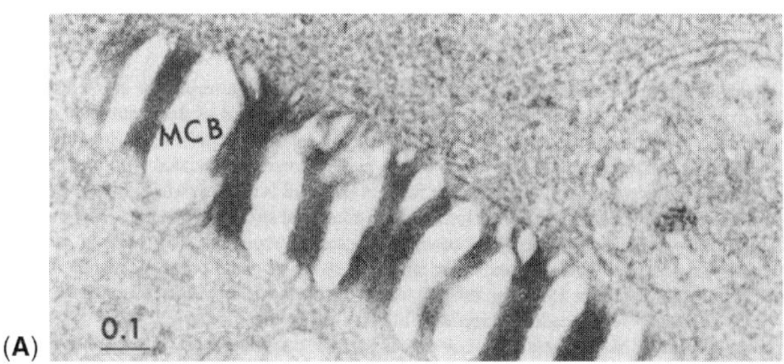

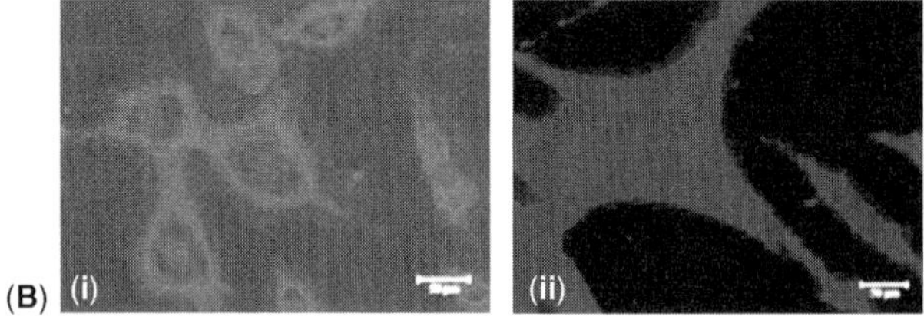

Figure 9 (**A**) (*Upper panel*) Lens epithelium in type A Niemann–Pick disease, showing single-membrane-bound cytoplasmic bodies with predominantly lamellar architecture. They are round or oval in shape, are surrounded by a single trilamellar membrane, and contain alternating osmiophilic and osmiophobic strands with periodicities of 5.5–6 nm. They contrast sharply with the mitochondria (m) (×11,800). (*Lower panel*) The structural details of the membrane-bound cytoplasmic bodies (MCB) enclosed in the rectangular area of the upper panel are shown in greater detail at higher magnification (× 50,000). *Source*: Reproduced from Robb RM, Kuwabara T. The ocular pathology of type A Niemann–Pick disease. Invest Ophthalmol 1973; 12:366–77. (**B**) Niemann–Pick type C fibroblasts store excess cholesterol (*i*) after Filipin staining, compared to (*ii*) normal fibroblasts.

2% to 5% of total body weight (99). Bis-monoacylglycero-phosphate is 100-fold normal and cholesterol is elevated. Glycolipids and glycosphingolipids (GSL) including glucocerebroside, GM_2-gangliosides and GM_3-gangliosides, lactocyl ceramide, globotriaosylceramide (GB3), and globotetraocylceramide accumulate in liver and spleen (34).

Patients with NP-A have nondetectable to 5% of normal ASM activity in cultured fibroblasts/leukocytes (61,152,206). ASM activity in cells or tissues from NP-B patients is more than that from NP-A patients and when determined in cultured cells, residual enzyme activities range between 2% and 10%. Measuring sphingomyelin hydrolysis with fluorescently labeled sphingomyelin loaded cells is useful and reveals a higher rate of sphingomyelin hydrolysis in cells from NP-B patients. This enzyme assay is not helpful in ascertaining carriers. For the detection of carriers it is best to analyze molecular DNA in families with known mutations. ASM activity, amniocyte cell loading studies, and/or DNA analysis are used in prenatal diagnosis.

Genetics

NP-A and NP-B have allelic defects in the *ASM* gene. Carrier frequency for NP-A in the Ashkenazi Jewish patient is 1:80 individuals. More than 50 mutations are known, three of which, Arg496Leu, Leu302Pro, fsPro330 (stop codon) account for 92% of mutant alleles in Ashkenazi Jews. NP-A has been described in non-Jewish patients. NP-B is unusual in the Ashkenazim. The Arg496Leu mutation appears in some NP-B Ashkenazi Jewish patients on one allele, and a second mutation on the other. One of these, the ΔArg608 mutation, is common to NP-B patients of Ashkenazi and North African background. This mutation accounts for 87% of NP-B alleles in the Maghreb (Algeria, Morocco, and Tunis). Cases with protracted neuronopathic disease are due to combinations of mutations that produce a greater deficiency in ASM than NP-B patients. NPD phenotype/genotype correlations hold for Ashkenazi Jewish mutations, yet identical alleles in other populations do not predict the same phenotype.

Experimental Models

Two mouse models of NP-A and NP-B disease have been generated. They are normal until 3 months, but manifest progressive ataxia and death at 7 months (86,171). Enzyme replacement has been successfully tried in mice with NP-B, but has not worked for NP-A due to an impenetrable blood–brain barrier. Stem cell-mediated gene therapy holds promise for treatment of NP-B, but not for NP-A, as trials in mice showed no improvement in the brain.

Niemann–Pick Disease, Types C and D

Clinical Presentation

Age of onset is anywhere from the newborn period to adulthood. Initial symptoms are neurologic, hepatic, or psychiatric. The clinical courses of systemic and neurologic disease are different. Liver involvement is present the first month of life and hepatosplenomegaly occurs in 85% of patients. The common type begins in childhood with ataxia, vertical supranuclear palsy, and psychomotor decline, dysarthria, dystonia, cataplexy, seizures, jaundice, and hepatosplenomegaly. Clinical presentation is variable with clinical signs appearing in the second to sixth decade. The subacute form of NP-C1 (formerly, NP-D) described in French-speaking Canadians of Acadian descent has a homogeneous phenotype. Most patients were traced to a common ancestor who immigrated to Nova Scotia from France and have the same genetic defect. There is an acute form with hydrops, an early neonatal form with congenital hepatitis, and a chronic form with progressive neurologic involvement and survival into adulthood. An early pulmonary lethal form of NP-C has been reported in three patients (98,225).

Histopathology

The cause of neurodegeneration in NP-C is unknown. NP-C1 or NP-C2 protein defects cause a "traffic jam" of lipids in the lysosome (110,111). Foam cells, called sea-blue histiocytes in bone marrow, are seen, are not specific, and may be absent in cases without organomegaly. Typical inclusions are seen in skin. Cytoplasmic ballooning of neurons and other cells by pleiomorphic, electron-dense inclusions are seen in the nervous system. Apoptotic Purkinje cells and other neurons are seen in the cerebellum, and meganeurites and axonal spheroids in the thalamus.

Biochemistry

The metabolic basis of NPD types C1 (NP-C1), C2 (NP-C2), and D (NP-D) was clarified recently. NP-D and NP-C1 are allelic variants with defects in the same gene, and are now classified as lipid-trafficking disorders (147,148). NP-D cases are a genetic isolate from Nova Scotia (60). ASM is elevated or normal in leukocytes and tissues of NP-C patients (17,205). Cultured fibroblasts may show a decrease in sphingomyelin degradation (105,206) and ASM activity. This is attributed to sequestration of cholesterol. GM_2-ganglioside also accumulates in lysosomes, even though hexosaminidase A activity is normal (226), and is due to impaired cellular transport of GM_2-ganglioside (172,211). There is elevation of free sphingoid bases in tissues and cells (168). The problem in NP-C is impaired transport of endocytosed cholesterol (110,148). The internalization, transport to endocytic vesicles, and hydrolysis of LDLs is normal, but transport of unesterified cholesterol is blocked, resulting in storage of unesterified cholesterol in the lysosomes and failure of inducing LDL-mediated homeostatic responses (205). In NP-C1, LDL cholesterol traffics to lysosomes via endosomes, and is entrapped, bypassing the plasma membrane (PM). NPC1 protein helps in LDL transport to PM (223) and in delivery of PM-derived cholesterol (217).

Genetics

NP-C is panethnic. Ninety-five percent of patients have mutations in the *NPC1* gene (56 kb, 25 exons). The remainder has defects in the *NPC2* gene (13.5 kb, 5 exons). *NPC1* encodes a 1278 amino acid membrane protein with 13 transmembrane domains, one cytoplasmic loop, three large luminal hydrophilic loops, a luminal amino terminus, and a cytoplasmic tail with a dileucine motif (47). There are over 133 disease-causing *NPC1* mutations known, 71% of which are missense mutations (60,98,125,198,205). These are distributed all over the *NPC1* gene and affect all functional domains, except for the leucine zipper motif (luminal amino terminus). Three common mutations described are: the Ile1061Thr, Pro1007Ala, and Gly992Trp. The Ile1061Thr mutation in patients of Western European origin accounts for 15% of U. S. alleles and 20% of alleles in France and the United Kingdom, and is prevalent in a Spanish American isolate in Southern Colorado and New Mexico. Pro1007Ala is the second most common European allele. Gly992Trp is typical of Nova Scotian patients and is rare elsewhere. Some mutations are prevalent in Japanese (Arg518Gln) (225) or Italian patients (Pro474Leu) (198). Molecular analysis of the *NPC1* gene is tedious due to the size of the gene, private mutations, and the existence of many polymorphisms. The *NPC2* (*HE1*) gene was discovered by a proteomic approach based on isolation of soluble lysosomal proteins (136). The 130-amino acid NP-C2 protein had been described (130) as a secretory protein of the mammalian epididymis that operates as a cholesterol transfer protein. Physiological functions of NP-C2 are preventing wrong sterol intercalation into lysosomal membranes, and presenting sterol to transporters like NP-C1. Only a few cases are described, all with nonsense or frameshift mutations. The Glu20Stop mutation accounts for 50% of reported alleles.

Diagnostic Tests

Diagnosis of NPC is based on Filipin staining of cultured fibroblasts grown in LDL medium. Filipin binds to excess unesterified cholesterol. This is visualized as birefringent cytoplasmic granules. Levels of impaired LDL-induced cholesterol esterification identifies 80% of cases, but Filipin staining is a more sensitive, cheaper, and easier test.

Experimental Models

A strain of BALB/C mice with characteristics of NPD has been identified (146). These mice have reduced

ASM activity and high levels of sphingomyelin and cholesterol. Another strain of C57BLKS/J mice has similar biochemical and clinical findings (130) and the murine *Asm* gene was normal in both strains (86) that are models for NP-C1.

Farber Disease

Overview

Farber disease (MIM +228000) is due to defects in acid ceramidase, the lysosomal enzyme that breaks down sphingomyelin-derived ceramide and ceramide storage in lysosomes, is rare. A triad of subcutaneous nodules over painful and arthritic extensor joints accompanied by hoarseness due to laryngeal involvement is typical. These nodules may involve eyelids, lips, and gums.

Clinical Description

Seven clinical variants are known, including a rare, fatal neonatal form presenting with hydrops fetalis, and a common classic variant is with presentation between 4 months and 4 years. Some cases have lung infiltrates, cherry red spots at the macula, organomegaly and neurologic deterioration involving CNS, anterior horn cell, and peripheral nerves. Most die after 1 to 2 years. Mild and intermediate forms exist with minimal neurologic involvement. A neurologically progressive form with no organomegaly or lung infiltration is described. An unusual case with both Farber and Sandhoff disease has been reported (106).

Histopathology

Macrophages, histiocytes, and foam cells are described, and sometimes multinucleated cells form around foam cells. Skin, joints, and larynx have granulomatous regions. The lungs and alveoli are infiltrated by macrophages. The aortic and mitral valve may be thickened with nodules. Storage material accumulates in the anterior horn cells, and in neurons of the brainstem nuclei, cerebellum, basal ganglia, cerebral cortex, and retinal ganglion cells. Tubular structures representing ceramide and zebra bodies because of ganglioside storage are seen by TEM.

Biochemistry

The ceramide content of subcutaneous nodules, liver, kidney, and brain can be very high. Some mild cases have normal levels. Glycolipids, particularly gangliosides, accumulate. PM and mitochondrial membrane ceramide have important bioregulatory roles impacting cell growth, apoptosis, and other stress responses. Ceramide accumulating in Farber disease due to ceramidase does not increase apoptosis of fibroblasts, unlike ceramide accumulation due to neutral and alkaline ceramidases that are distinct from acid ceramidase. Acid ceramidase is a heterodimer made up of a glycosylated β-subunit and a nonglycosylated α-subunit. Saposins (sphingolipid activator proteins) are soluble glycoproteins necessary for presentation of lipids like ceramide to lysosomal hydrolases for breakdown. Prosaposin is glycoprotein that is the precursor of saposin A (SAP-A), saposin B (SAP-B), saposin C (SAP-C), and saposin D (SAP-D). A deficiency of prosaposin and these four derivatives causes MLD, Farber disease, and atypical GD type II-like symptoms, including seizures, organomegaly, respiratory, and cardiac failure (81).

SAP-C and SAP-D present neutral ceramide for degradation into sphingosine and fatty acid by acid ceramidase in lysosomes. The water permeability barrier/intercellular lipid barrier of the stratum corneum consists of ceramide, cholesterol, and free fatty acids, with ceramide and proteins covalently bound at the skin surface (89).

Diagnostic Tests

Carrier diagnosis has been accomplished by enzyme assays and DNA analysis. Prenatal diagnosis is based on measurement of enzyme activity and/or cell loading studies of cultured amniocytes.

Genetics

Farber disease is rare, usually occurring in consanguineous marriages. No Jewish cases are known. Point or exon skipping mutations account for 12 of the defects, with less than 5% enzyme activity in leukocytes, fibroblasts, and tissues or chorionic villus.

Experimental Studies

Bone marrow transplantation (BMT) causes regression of nodules and organomegaly, but does not reverse neurologic deterioration. Experimental trials in cell model systems using viral gene delivery systems are in progress.

Gaucher Disease

Overview

GD, the most common lysosomal disorder, is due to defects in acid β glucosidase (19,29). It results in storage of glucosylceramide (GluCer) in phagocytes, causing hepatosplenomegaly and other symptoms (69). The three types of GD are: GD type I (nonneuronopathic GD), GD type II (acute neuronopathic GD), and GD type III (subacute neuronopathic GD).

Clinical Presentation

GD type I, the nonneuronopathic form of GD, accounts for most patients with GD in North America and Europe. The disease is panethnic, but prevalence is high in Ashkenazi Jews (1 in 850) compared to other groups (1 in 40,000). It can begin anywhere from birth to the eighth decade. Most patients present with hepatosplenomegaly, anemia, and thrombocytopenia, and bony abnormalities due to bone marrow space expansion. Mild cases are diagnosed late in life. Fatigability is common due to anemia and proinflammatory cytokines. Splenomegaly is present in 90% of cases and is often associated with splenic infarction, one of the most serious complications of GD. Liver failure, cirrhosis, and portal hypertension occur in <10% of cases (44). Early thrombocytopenia is due to splenic sequestration of platelets and responds to splenectomy, but it may be followed by bone marrow failure because of an extensive invasion by Gaucher cells. Lymphoproliferative disorders, amyloidosis, and gammopathies frequently occur in patients with GD type I. Skeletal involvement causes osteopenia and destructive lesions. Infarction of the bone marrow is common. Degenerative joint disease of the hips, thinning of cortical bone, and sacroiliac osteosclerosis are described. Pulmonary involvement occurs due to infiltration of alveoli, perivascular, peribronchial, and septal regions by Gaucher cells. Hepatosplenomegaly, kyphoscoliosis (127), and pulmonary hypertension can occur. Patients homozygous for the c.1226A>G mutation show minimal progression, but adult and pediatric heterozygotes with a different affected gene deteriorate. GD type II and variants of it manifest CNS involvement. Storage of GluCer occurs in neurons, but neuronal death best explains the symptoms in this type of GD, which is the most severe form due to early onset and rapid progression. Formerly known as the acute infantile GD, GD type II accounts for 1 case per 500,000 births. Bulbar signs, progressive spasticity, and choreoathetosis appear from 3 to 6 months of age, followed by neurological deterioration and seizures, with demise in the first 2 years of life. Gaucher cells infiltrate many organs, including the lung, liver, and spleen. GD type III appears at a later age, and is exemplified by a protracted course. Its incidence is less than 1 in 100,000 births. Early cases were reported from the Swedish region of Norbotten. A differentiation between GD type II and GD type III is based on the presence of bulbar signs, which only occur in GD type II (70). Involvement of organs outside of the nervous system is moderate in GD type III, but neurodegeneration with signs of dementia and ataxia is rapid. GD type III is subdivided into three variants: GD type IIIA (Norbotten form), GD type IIIB, and GD type IIIC. GD type IIIB occurs in early childhood with organ enlargement and death due to pulmonary and portal hypertension, and GD type IIIC [c.1342G>C (Asp409His)] has minor visceral signs and, typically, early appearing oculomotor paralysis. Homozygous GD type IIIC patients have cardiac disease with mitral and/or aortic valve lesions (66,126).

Cherry red spots at the macula are not seen, but in some cases perimacular grayness has been described.

Histopathology

Gliosis in the brain and progressive fibrosis of the viscera is common. Infarction, necrosis, and scarring are observed in bones and soft tissues, and there is neuronal death and loss. Visceral disease with its prominent storage material is explained by the wide distribution of macrophages filled with glycolipids derived from phagocytosed senescent leukocytes and erythrocytes (Gaucher cells). Why lipid storage results in disease in the neuronopathic forms of GD is obscure. Perhaps neuronal death follows an inhibition of protein kinase C by lysosphingolipids (78), but it may also be related to downregulation of bcl-2, a neuroprotective protein (84).

Adults with GD type I are stated to sometimes have brown, wedge-shaped pingueculae, but morphologic studies of the conjunctiva by light microscopy and TEM have not disclosed abnormalities. Lipid-laden macrophages have been reported in the ciliary body and in the inner layers of the retina.

Biochemistry

Human acid β-glucosidase is a homomeric glycoprotein or a dimeric protein (38,114). The existence of groups of mutant enzymes due to responses to different modifiers of acid β-glucosidase activity (1,145) and/or altered processing or stability is also possible. Two classes of mutant enzymes have been identified: (*i*) those with decreased stability, normal interaction with inhibitors, and decreased catalytic rate constants; and (*ii*) enzymes with normal stability but decreased affinity for site-directed inhibitors, and decreased catalytic rate constants. The first type of mutant enzymes explains non-Jewish patients with GD type I, II, and III patients; the second group of enzymes is found in Jewish cases.

Diagnostic Tests

Decreased acid β-glucosidase activity in leukocytes is diagnostic. Cultured fibroblasts also show decreased enzyme activity. Enzymatic activity does not distinguish the three types of GD, as there is no correlation between residual enzyme activity and the clinical type (23). Mutations accounting for cases of GD type I in Ashkenazi Jews can be diagnosed by analyzing five common alleles. The existence of numerous rare alleles in non-Jewish cases makes use of DNA diagnosis unwieldy, except in certain cases with known established molecular defects. Prenatal diagnosis by measuring acid β-glucosidase in chorionic villi at week 10 of gestation or in cultured amniotic cells at week 14 of pregnancy in fetuses at risk for GD type II or GD type III is possible.

Genetics

Mutations 84insG (84G>GC), c.1448T>C (Leu444Pro), and c.1226A>G (Asn370Ser) account for 8%, 20%, and 55% of the patient population with GD type I, respectively, although over 200 mutations are known. The (Asn370Ser) mutation is present in 6% of Ashkenazi Jews. Investigation of the above three mutations in Jewish patients permits diagnosis of 93% of alleles, and 95.5% if the IVS2+1G>A allele is also included. The first three mutations account for 70% of alleles in non-Jewish patients. Asn370Ser is described in patients from Portugal, Spain, Germany, and the Netherlands (5,23,43).

Deleterious alleles, or complex alleles (Rec*Nci*I and RecTL), occur in GD (43,230). They result from a gene–pseudogene crossover. Their presence implies disease severity (140). Novel mutations continue to be identified (126,140,183). Two cases of GD are known without defects in the *GBA* gene, but with mutations in the *PSAP* gene, which encodes the sphingolipid activator for SAP-C (81). The clinical phenotype ranges from an asymptomatic course to a very severe disease. The presence of an Asn370Sr allele implies absence of primary CNS disease, but carrying one or two Asn370Ser alleles predisposes to early onset and refractory Parkinson disease. In a sporadic cohort of Parkinsonian cases, 14% had low β-glucosidase enzyme levels.

Experimental Models

A glucocerebrosidase deficient mouse was generated using knockout strategies, but affected newborn mice died within 34 hr of birth and had extensive GluCer storage. Patients respond positively to enzyme replacement therapy (ERT) even if manifestations are severe (59,69,70,214). SRT relies on diminishing tissue GSL by inhibiting production of GluCer. The *N*-alkylated imino sugar analog, *N*-butyldeoxynojirimycin, is now approved for patients in whom ERT is not feasible (44). This oral drug traverses the blood–brain barrier. Pharmacological chaperones can expedite the trafficking of certain mutant forms of β-glucosidase (Asn370SEr) through the secretory pathway, preventing entrapment and degradation in the ER, which increases enzyme activity. The β-glucosidase inhibitor, *N*-nonyl-deoxynojirimycin, when added at suboptimal concentrations to cells, leads to a rise in enzyme levels. Reducing the secondary inflammatory response may also delay progression (138).

Krabbe Disease

Overview

Krabbe disease (galactosylceramide lipidosis, globoid cell leukodystrophy) (MIM #245200) results from low galactosylceramidase (galactocerebroside-β-galactosidase or GALC) activity that normally degrades GalCer. Krabbe (103) reported two infants with a familial and acute form of diffuse brain sclerosis in 1916, but there were other earlier reports of the same disease (32). Collier and Greenfield used the term globoid cells for multinucleated macrophages stuffed with GalCer (41) that are found in the brain and peripheral nervous system (PNS) of affected individuals. The symptoms are entirely neurologic. The infantile form presents in infants at 3 to 6 months of age with irritability, spasticity, and opisthotonic posturing. Krabbe babies are not comforted by touching or cuddling. They are blind by 2 years of ages and definitely by the time they expire. Late infantile, juvenile, and adult forms exist and are typified by variable spasticity, peripheral neuropathy, dementia, and blindness.

Clinical Presentation

After normal development, babies with infantile Krabbe disease become irritable, inconsolable, and opisthotonic with hands held in a claw-like position. Touching and holding provokes crying, because of hyperesthesias. Microcephaly is common. Optic atrophy appears early. Peripheral neuropathy is often described. Reflexes, initially hyperactive, diminish and are unobtainable towards the end. Epileptic fits appear late and children seldom survive beyond the age of 2 years. A Palestinian Muslim girl had neurologic deterioration noted at 3 months and progressed to death at 8 months. She had a mutation in the sphingolipid activator gene. The late infantile variant of Krabbe disease has an onset between 6 months and 3 years with psychomotor decline, irritability, ataxia, spasticity, blindness, peripheral neuropathy, and seizures. Affected children die within 2 years. Juvenile Krabbe disease is diagnosed between 3 and 8 years with spasticity, ataxia, hemiparesis, and peripheral neuropathy. Psychomotor decline occurs and then disease progression plateaus for many years, with some patients surviving to their late twenties (175,215). Patients with adult Krabbe disease always present diagnostic dilemmas. Although apparently neurologically normal in childhood, some cases give a history of fixed deficits like clubfeet, ataxia, tremor, or rigidity, which ultimately, worsens with age. A late dementia and a peripheral neuropathy are also described in some patients. A frequent presentation is one of familial spastic paraparesis (16,202).

Diagnostic Tests

Cerebrospinal fluid (CSF) protein is high in infantile and late infantile forms, and elevated lactate levels may raise suspicion for a mitochondrial disorder. MRI/CT helps in the differential diagnosis. High signal T2-weighted changes in thalami, corona radiata, cerebellum, internal capsule, and periventricular white matter and enhancement of cranial nerves or lumbosacral nerve roots appear in infantile Krabbe disease. Symmetric changes of pyramidal tracts and optic radiations were seen by fluid-attenuated inversion recovery MRI. Proton magnetic resonance spectroscopy (MRS) shows peaks of choline, lactate, and myoinositol with decreased N-acetyl aspartic acid (NAA) suggesting demyelination, and low NAA suggests a destructive neuronal and axonal disorder. Radial stripes by MRI correspond to perivenular globoid cell clusters filled with GalCer. EEGs are normal at the beginning but deteriorate later on. Nerve conduction velocities are slow in the early variants, and often in juvenile and adult patients. In the early Krabbe form, brainstem evoked responses (BAER) are abnormal in 88%, and flash visual evoked potentials (VEPs) are abnormal in 53% of cases. In later onset cases BAER were abnormal in 40%, but VEPs were normal in 100% of cases. The severity of findings correlates with abnormalities by MRI. Sixty-seven percent of symptomatic patients had abnormal VEPs, but presymptomatic children did not (11,115). Measuring galactocerebrosidase activity in leukocytes/fibroblasts, and/or using DNA diagnostics in specific ethnic groups, delivers the diagnosis. Prenatal diagnosis using amniotic fluid cells and chorionic villi from pregnancies at risk is reported. Obligate carriers should be tested simultaneously with affected family members. If enzyme activity and the gene sequence are normal, a defect in the activator, SAP-A, may be present. This diagnosis can only be made using natural substrate and cultured skin fibroblasts, or by determining the *PSAP* gene sequence. The finding of low GALC activity confirms the diagnosis of Krabbe disease.

Histopathology

Pathologic changes are limited to the PNS and CNS. The brain is shrunken and ventricles are wide. There is destruction of white matter, but the cortical layer is preserved. Three distinct findings are loss of myelin and oligodendroglia, presence of multinucleated globoid cells, and astrocytic gliosis. Demyelination is prominent in the centrum semiovale and cerebellum. Secondary axonal degeneration is present. Multinucleated giant globoid cells are phagocytic in origin and cluster around blood vessels. Globoid cells can be generated by injecting mouse brain with GalCer. Golgi preparations of large pyramidal neurons have preserved dendritic processes (103,218). Peripheral nerves are thick and demonstrate segmental demyelination. Endoneural fibrosis, fibroblast proliferation, presence of periodic acid Schiff (PAS)-positive macrophages and axonal degeneration are present. Schwann cells and globoid cells in the brain contain needle-like tubular inclusions by TEM (82,115,116).

Optic atrophy and slow pupillary reactions are common. Loss of vision appears early and may precede loss of the pupillary light reflex. TEM demonstrated tubular inclusions and globoid cells in a severely demyelinated nerve of an infantile Krabbe (Fig. 10).

Degeneration of the optic radiations and of the frontoparietal white matter with secondary degeneration of corticospinal tracts has been described in two siblings with late onset Krabbe disease. Peripheral

(A)

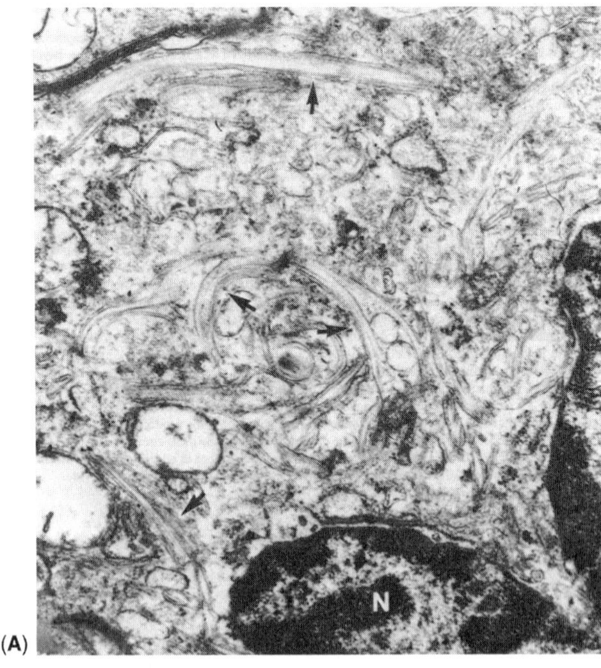

(B)

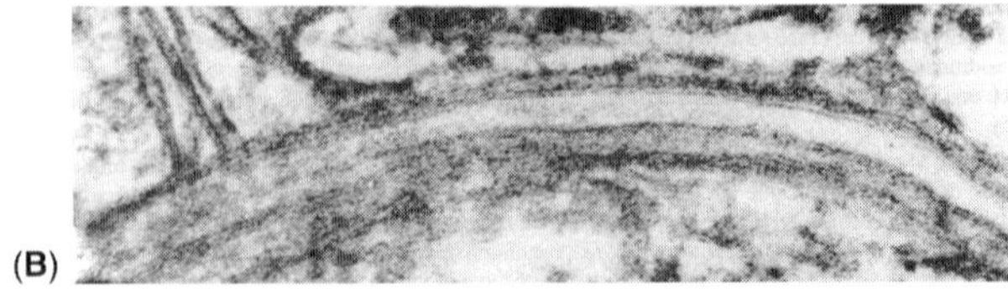

Figure 10 (**A**) Optic nerve in Krabbe disease, showing extensive demyelination. Globoid cells with indented nuclei (N) contain straight or gently curved paracrystalline filaments (*arrows*) similar to the helical tubules accumulating in neural tissue of Krabbe disease (×24,000). (**B**) The lamellar structure of the tubules at higher magnification (×102,900). *Source*: Reproduced from Tripathi RC, Ashton N. Application of electron microscopy to the study of ocular inborn errors of metabolism. Birth Defects: Original Article Series, 1976; 69–104.

nerves and Schwann cells with the typical needle-like inclusions have also been seen in nerve biopsies from older patients. In fetal Krabbe disease the spinal cord shows changes as early as 20 weeks gestation with globoid cells in the dorsal columns. The pons is also involved.

Biochemistry

GalCer and its sulfated form, sulfatide, are major components of normal myelin. Strangely, GalCer does not accumulate in the brains of Krabbe disease patients. There may be substrate specificity overlap between GALC and β-galactosidase, the enzyme defective in the GM_1-gangliosidoses and MPS IVB. The latter enzyme also degrades GalCer. Another substrate for GALC is psychosine, which is made up of galactose and sphingosine. The latter is not a substrate for β-galactosidase, and increases 100-fold in myelin.

Genetics

The human *GALC* gene contains 17 exons and 16 introns that code for a 669 amino acid protein. The precursor protein (80 kDa) is processed into a 50 to 52 kDa and a 30 kDa subunit, both important for the enzyme. Sixty mutations include the common 502T/del that accounts for 75% of Swedish cases and 50% of European cases. Two other mutations are reported: (*i*) in Palestinian Druze in Northern Israel, Thr1748Gly; and (*ii*) in a Palestinian Muslim group from a village next to Jerusalem, Gly1582Ala. The mutation consists of a 30 kb deletion beginning with a 502 C-to-T polymorphism in the middle of intron 10 and extends to the end. This eliminates all of the 30 kDa and 15% of the 50 to 52 kDa protein. Patients homozygous for this mutation have the infantile variant. A number of polymorphisms (Cys502Thr, Gly694Ala, Ala865Gly, Thr1637Cys) occur together, and may appear with disease-causing mutations in the same allele, and can contribute to disease severity.

Pathobiology

One hypothesis for Krabbe disease claims that accumulated psychosine kills oligodendrocytes via apoptosis and that rapidly vanishing oligodendrocytes prevent the normal formation and turnover of myelin, and preclude evidence for stored GalCer. Globoid cell formation is induced by GalCer, and the needle-like and tubular inclusions in Schwann cells and globoid cells resemble GalCer aggregates.

Experimental Models

Naturally occurring animal models for Krabbe disease exist include the Twitcher mouse (193,195). Crossing immunocompromised mice with Twitcher mice produces mice with mild disease. Estrogens present during pregnancy also result in mild forms of the illness in mice. Cross-breeding *Galc–/–* mice with a mouse heterozygous for GalCer synthase results in mice with mild disease, providing the rationale for SRT. Beneficial effects of BMT in Krabbe disease were first shown in Twitcher mice and have also been documented in presymptomatic infants or in late onset cases by BMT and cord blood transplants (35,54,121).

L-Cycloserine, a potent inhibitor of psychosine production, may be responsible for the beneficial effects of stem cell transplantation. The introduction into the brain of *GALC* in viruses or liposomes or stem cells, anti-inflammatory and antiapoptotic oral drugs, substrate reduction, or combinations of these methods are currently being investigated as treatment options for Krabbe disease.

Metachromatic Leukodystrophy

Overview

MLD (MIM #250100) results from lack of hydrolysis of sulfatide and other sulfated lipids of the PNS and CNS. MLD results from a deficiency in arylsulfatase A (ASA), the enzyme that desulfates 3-0-sulfogalactosyl-containing lipids. Sulfated glycolipids have a brown color in tissue sections stained with cresylviolet. The pathological feature is extensive demyelination in the CNS and the PNS. The first case of MLD may have been described by Alzheimer in 1906 (4). Excess sulfatides in tissues and defects in ASA enzyme were discovered in 1965. Mehl and Jazkewitz confirmed this fact, and discovered a heat-stable factor that increases enzyme activity known to be the activator saposin SAP-B (122). Defects in saposin SAP-B are responsible for cases of MLD with normal ASA activity (90). Another form of ASA deficiency with leukodystrophy, ichthyosis, and a mucopolysaccaridosis is known as multiple sulfatase deficiency (MSD) with seven deficient sulfatases reported (178,182). MLD families often include healthy individuals with normal ASA that harbor the "pseudodeficiency" or PD allele (65,163).

Clinical Presentation

The late infantile variant of MLD is usually diagnosed between 18 and 24 months of age and patients never outgrow the waddling gait stage. They have absent ankle jerks, due to nerve involvement, positive Babinski signs, and demyelination by MRI. Optic atrophy, a cognitive decline, and speech disturbances are present and patients become quadriparetic and die at the end of the first decade. Seizures develop late in the illness, and have elevated CSF protein. Papillomatosis of the gall bladder can present as acute cholecystitis or an abdominal mass due to a deposition of sulfatide in the gall bladder (9,75). Juvenile MLD appears before or after age 4 years, but before the age of 6 years. The late juvenile type has an age of onset between 6 and 16 years. Symptoms are an abnormal gait, ataxia, spasticity, peripheral neuropathy more prominent in early onset cases, and a slow cognitive decline. CSF protein is elevated, and optic atrophy may be present. Older onset cases may have a psychiatric presentation. Adult MLD almost always presents as a psychiatric disorder. Peripheral neuropathy may be present and the CSF protein is mildly elevated. A myelopathy with spasticity may develop. Ataxia, dystonia, bulbar signs, tremors, and optic atrophy may be present. The course can persist from a few years to several decades. At the end, patients develop quadriparesis, spasticity, hyperactive tendon reflexes, and, often seizures (73,164).

SAP-B deficiency MLD is extremely rare and the age of onset varies. It has a clinical picture resembling ASA deficiency, but ASA activity is normal. The presence of a progressive demyelinating illness and normal ASA levels leads to the diagnosis, which can be established by measurement of urine sulfatides, analysis of sulfatide metabolism in fibroblasts, or by sequencing the *ASA* gene (224).

Multiple Sulfatase Deficiency

A clinical phenotype reminiscent of late infantile MLD with white matter changes, and MPS-like features of coarse fascies, deafness, dysostosis multiplex, and visceromegaly, are consistent with MSD. The most common form is an infantile variant with mild MPS features, clear corneas, ichthyosis, optic atrophy, retinal degeneration, and, occasionally, a cherry red macula. Severe neonatal, and early infantile variants in patients less than 1 year of age are described with dwarfism, craniosynostosis, hydrocephalus and cervical cord strangulation, and an absence of ichthyosis or retinitis. MSD results from low activity of seven different sulfatases including ASA and this is a result of a change in posttranslational modification (178,182).

Diagnostic Tests

The diagnosis is based on low ASA levels, excessive urine sulfatide, slow sulfatide turnover in fibroblasts, and DNA sequence analysis. CSF protein is high in late infantile and early juvenile variants. Progressive loss of myelin in MLD has a typical appearance by CT and MRI. The centrum semiovale has low signal on T1-weighted images and bright signal on T2-weighted sections. There is involvement of frontal and parieto-occipital white matter with occipital regions being most affected. There is a tigroid pattern to the white matter. Proton MRS shows an elevation in myoinositol, a reduced *N*-acetylaspartate peak, and a lactate peak in myelin. The PET scan shows low metabolism in the thalami (139,164). The EEG is initially normal, but eventually becomes slow and abnormal. Some patients have epileptiform activity and many develop seizures late in the course (22). Nerve conduction velocities are diminished in the late infantile and early juvenile variants, and may be delayed in late juvenile and adult variants. Visual, brainstem, and somatosensory evoked responses may be slowed in all types, but more so in early onset types (196).

Histopathology

There is massive demyelination within deep gray structures, and metachromatic granules that stain brown with cresylviolet. These are observed in nerves and viscera as 15 μm spherical structures. Prismatic inclusions with a herringbone lattice appear to have a honeycomb pattern on cross-sections. Tuffstone-like inclusions are also observed in the thalami of adult cases. Demyelination of the brainstem and spinal cord is extensive, with reduction in the number of oligodendrocytes and a reactive gliosis in the late infantile form. The cerebellum is atrophied due to Purkinje cell and granule cell death and loss. Some Purkinje cells may have torpedo-like swellings. In the early onset severe forms of MLD there is segmental demyelination and metachromatic granules are present in macrophages and Schwann cells. In muscle type I, and fibers are atrophic (see Chapter 72) and myelin sheaths are thinned. Kidneys, gallbladder, and testis accumulate sulfated lipids and intrahepatic bile duct cells contain metachromatic granules in adult MLD.

Optic atrophy is often present and demyelination of the optic nerve is the most striking feature (Fig. 11). Optic atrophy results from retrograde degeneration and in adult MLD it is reported late in the disease. Foveal grayness has also been alluded too. Cherry red spots are not typical in MLD. TEM studies of the retina in an affected adult disclosed an extensive loss of ganglion cells. TEM of conjunctival biopsies in MLD reveals osmiophillic inclusions. Pigmentary retinal degeneration has also been observed.

Biochemistry

Sulfatide levels are elevated in myelin in persons with late infantile MLD. They are also high in the cerebellum, brainstem, and spinal cord of a 24-week fetus. Deacylated sulfatide also is high. Myelin sulfatide is not elevated in adult MLD, but gray matter sulfatide is. Sulfatides are stored in the gall bladder and the kidney. Other sulfated glycolipids including lactosylceramide-3-sulfate and seminolipid accumulate. Sulfatide is a sulfated ester of GalCer with the sulfate joined by an ester bond to the C-3

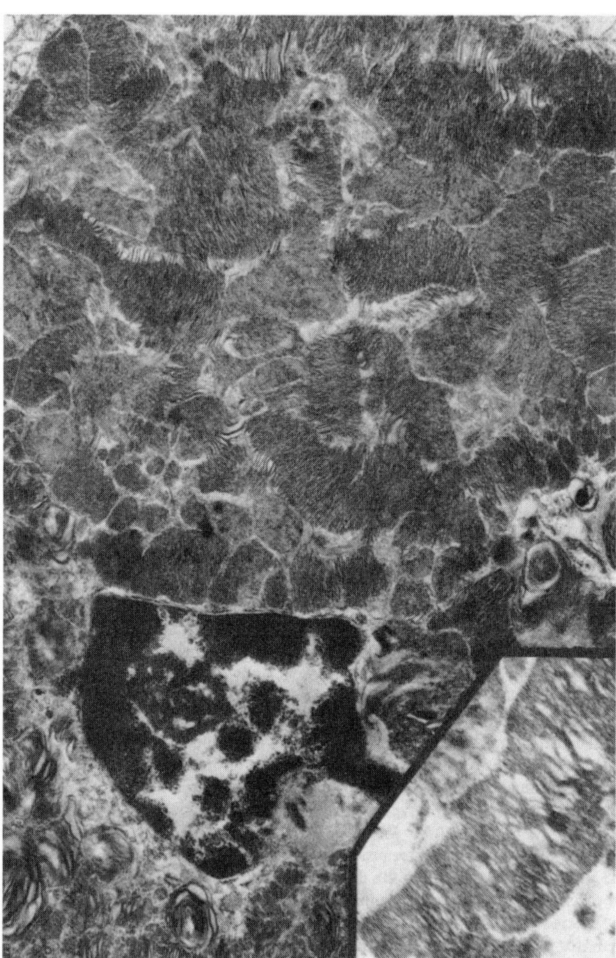

Figure 11 Optic nerve in adult-onset metachromatic leukodystrophy containing abnormal glial cells filled with single-membrane-limited lamellar inclusion bodies. The cells are larger than normal glia and are devoid of cellular processes (× 13,200). (*Inset*) Lamellar inclusion body at higher magnification (× 36,900). *Source*: Reproduced from Quigley HA, Green WR. Clinical and ultrastructural ocular histopathological studies of adult-onset metachromatic leukodystrophy. Am J Ophthalmol 1975; 82:472–9.

hydroxyl of galactose. GalCer, and its derivative sulfatide maintain insulator function, can undergo hydrophilic and hydrophobic reactions, are active in sodium transport, and are involved in binding of γ-amino butyric acid, opiates, gp120 of HIV, prionic protein and β-amyloid to the cell surface. Residual enzyme activity is present and sulfatide accumulates more slowly than in early MLD (24,80).

Genetics

All MLD variants, and cases with MSD, are inherited in an autosomal recessive manner because of allelic mutations in *ASA*. The defect in MSD is obscure and affects the serine at position 69 in *ASA*, which normally becomes formylglycine that is necessary for catalytic function of sulfatases. In Sweden, the incidence of the disease is 1 in 40,000 and is lower than that in other European countries. Habbanite Jews (231) living in Israel and originating from Yemen have an elevated incidence because of a high degree of consanguinity (231). Arabs from an area to the north of Nazareth have an incidence of 1 in 8000. The ASA PD allele results in low enzyme activity (5–10% of normal) but no clinical symptoms. The PD allele often exists in families who also carry a true MLD allele. The frequency of the PD allele in Europe ranges from 10% to 20%. The incidence for heterozygotes carrying a PD and an *ASA* allele simultaneously is 1 in 1500 individuals. A small proportion of them have neurologic symptoms unrelated to MLD. The PD allele has two polymorphisms. One causes loss of one glycosylation signal resulting in a short protein (Asn350Ser). The other polymorphism affects the polyadenylation signal, which precludes generation of long ASA transcripts. The *N*-glycosylation defect causes a drop of 50% in ASA activity. Presence of the second polymorphism results in ASA activity that is 10% of normal. More than 68 mutations in *ASA* are described in MLD. Three alleles cover most European cases. One of these 459+1A→G causes loss of a splice acceptor site and is the mutation in Arab cases. Seven of the MLD-causing mutations occur concomitantly with a PD allele as well. Residual enzyme activity determined with sulfatide loading correlates the most with disease severity. Patients with both a PD and an MLD allele have 5% to 10% enzyme activity and are normal. Adult MLD patients have 2% to 5% enzyme activity, and late infantile MLD activities range from 0% to 2% when determined in this manner. The Ile179Ser allele is found in those presenting with psychiatric symptoms. The sulfatide loading test also identifies saposin SAP-B–deficient cases. Urine sulfatide excretion can also distinguish between these variants. Awareness of mutations of obligate carriers in a family is helpful for determining carrier status, or for prenatal diagnosis. Determining if the parents carry a PD allele is also important. Sulfatide loading tests become very important in this case (163).

Experimental Models

A transgenic mouse is available and demonstrates sulfatide storage in brain, kidney, and other viscera. The neuropathologic lesion of astrogliosis is similar to that seen in humans. Mice have normal glia at 1 year of age. Glial activation is observed by 2 years. Strikingly though, mice do not show demyelination, and have very mild symptoms (64). Intravenous ASA enzyme replacement in transgenic mice given once a week for four weeks reduced sulfatide storage in organs, spinal cord, and the brain (20). Efficacy in humans has not been evaluated, but so far the mice data seems promising (118).

Fabry Disease

Overview

Fabry disease (MIM + 301500) is an X-linked recessive LSD with systemic deposition of neutral GSL, because of defects and low activity in the enzyme α-galactosidase (49). The disease was initially described by Anderson and Fabry in the 1800s.

Clinical Presentation

Clinical onset can be in childhood or adolescence, but can be delayed until the late thirties. Excruciating pain is incapacitating, and can be intermittent or steady and is known as acroparesthesias. Fever, exercise, fatigue, and stress trigger painful flare-ups. Patients experience hypohidrosis, anhydrosis, and fever. Another feature is the development, typically around puberty, of angiokeratomas (angiokeratoma corporis diffusum) in a bathing trunk distribution affecting buttocks and scrotum, hips, thighs, umbilicus, and mucosal surfaces (18). Cardiac involvement affects valves, sometimes resulting in mitral insufficiency or left ventricular enlargement, and affects the conduction system (15). Electrocardiograph changes result from GSL deposition in the myocardium. Some patients have a milder "cardiac variant" with only cardiac symptoms but without painful acroparesthesias or angiokeratomas. Cerebrovascular disease results from involvement of small blood vessels, which may lead to thrombosis, transient ischemic attacks, basilar artery aneurysm, seizures, aphasia, hemiplegia, and hemianesthesia. Decreased erythrocyte survival causes anemia. MRI and proton MRS are helpful in assessing cerebrovascular disease (133,199). GSL deposition in the kidney results in proteinuria and a deteriorating renal function, and uremia at midlife. Birefringent lipid globules or "maltese crosses" are observed in desquamated cells in the urinary sediment using polarization microscopy. MRI of kidneys is notable for loss of corticomedullary differentiation. Death often results from renal failure. Gastrointestinal disease arises from GSL storage in intestinal small vessels and in autonomic ganglia, causing diarrhea, abdominal and flank pain, nausea, and vomiting. Airflow obstruction and reduced oxygen diffusing capacity can cause chronic bronchitis, wheezing, and dyspnea. Minor changes are described in the EEG and EMG. Musculoskeletal involvement is described because of damage to the distal interphalangeal joints with joint limitations and avascular necrosis of the head of femur or talus, and involvement of metacarpal, metatarsal, and temporomandibular joints (48).

Ophthalmic Manifestations

A keratopathy and star-like opacities in the posterior region of the lens are hallmarks. Blood vessels of the conjunctiva and retina are prominent and appear tortuous with dilatations and aneurysms due to deposition of ceramide trihexoside (CTH). Central retinal artery occlusion with sudden loss of vision has been reported, as have partial segmental infarcts of the retina. Cornea verticillata is striking and occurs in all affected males. By examination this appears as spoke-like radiations from a central region in the epithelial and subepithelial layers. Heterozygote carrier females may or may not have all the above or some of those ocular findings. Whorl-like deposits are observed in a majority of carrier females. Retinal infarcts are common.

Histopathology

Deposition of crystalline glycosphingolipids in vascular endothelial cells of all areas of the body is observed. These lipids are birefringent and appear as characteristic "maltese crosses" under polarization microscopy. Deposition occurs in lysosomes of the endothelium, pericyte, and smooth muscle cells of blood vessels, and some in reticular and histiocytic cells. GSL accumulate in epithelial cells of the glomerulus and of the distal renal tubules, and lipid-laden tubular epithelial cells are dehisced with the urinary sediment. Renal blood vessels with arterial fibrinoid deposits are common. GSL deposition affects the liver sinus epithelial and Kupffer cells, but not hepatocytes. In the heart, deposition affects myocardial cells and valvular fibrocytes (56). Vascular ischemia and lipid deposition in the perineurium of peripheral nerves causes a painful peripheral neuropathy with conduction defects (184). Sweat glands blocked by lipid deposition result in an inability to sweat increasing body temperature during hot weather and exercise exacerbating a painful small myelinated fiber and unmyelinated fiber neuropathy. Immunohistochemical studies with an anti-globotriaosylceramide monoclonal antibody demonstrates selective neuronal involvement of spinal cord, ganglia, brainstem, amygdala, hypothalamus, and entorhinal cortex. The eyes, adrenal glands, gastrointestinal tract, prostate, testes, bladder, and thyroid gland show vessel smooth muscle and nerve involvement.

The cornea, lens, conjunctiva, and retina are affected (Fig. 12). Spoke-like opacities in the corneas and characteristic lenticular inclusions are often seen by slit-lamp biomicroscopy (57,188). Lamellar osmiophillic deposits are found in the lens and iris pigment epithelium, vascular endothelial cells and pericytes of ocular blood vessels, and smooth muscle cells of choroidal vessels. Conjunctival cells also contain these inclusions beyond the age of 7 years and provide a convenient source for diagnostic investigation. These changes often precede corneal and other clinical signs.

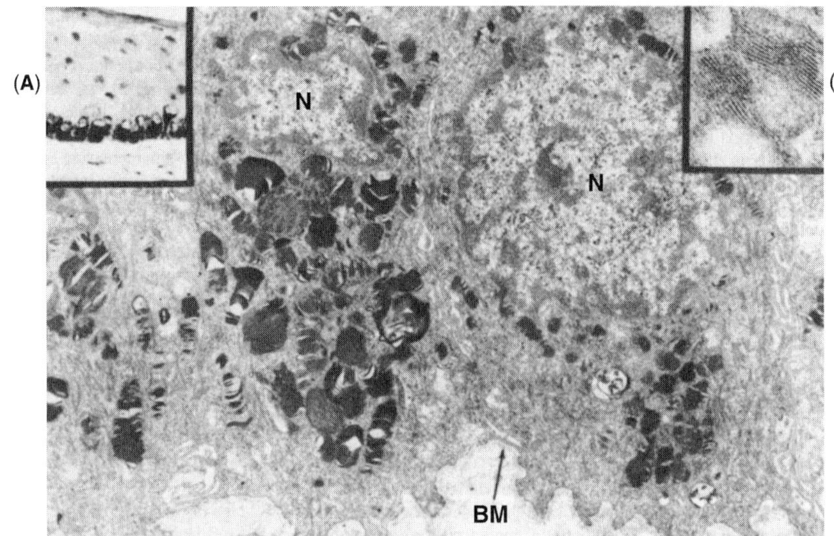

Figure 12 Lamellar inclusion bodies accumulating in the basal cells of the corneal epithelium in Fabry disease (× 5,600). *Inset* (**A**): The same region of the epithelium at lower magnification (× 220). Dense staining with Sudan black B and oil red O is observed mainly in the basal cells and rarely in the superficial cells. *Inset* (**B**): The lamellar deposits at high magnification (× 63,800). *Abbreviations*: N, nuclei; BM, basal membrane. *Source*: Reproduced from Font RL, Fine BS. Ocular pathology in Fabry's disease: histochemical and electron microscopic observations. Am J Ophthalmol 1972; 73:419–30.

Biochemistry

Low α-galactosidase A results in storage of neutral GSL with terminal α-galactosyl residues. Accumulation of GB3 or CTH in lysosomes of vascular endothelial and smooth muscle cells, and in epithelial and perithelial cells of most organs is severe. CTH levels in hemizygote males are 30 to 300 times higher than in normal controls (129,176). Galabiosylceramide levels are elevated in a tissue-specific manner affecting kidney, pancreas, right heart, lung, renal tubule cells, and spinal and sympathetic ganglia (88). Blood groups B and B1 GSL inhibitory to blood group B agglutination accumulate in those with blood groups B and AB. GSL are degraded in a stepwise fashion by specific exoglycosidases. These exoglycosidases are glycoproteins with optimal catalytic activity at acidic pH. α-Galactosidase A defects cause Fabry disease, and α-galactosaminidase B defects cause a type of neuroaxonal dystrophy (Schindler disease) (MIM #609241) (48,177). α-Galactosidase A is a 101 kDa protein. Affected males have normal plasma α-galactosidase A levels, but deficient peripheral leukocyte enzyme. Changes in urinary CTH are a sensitive and specific measure of tissue CTH burden (143).

Genetics

Fabry disease is panethnic. The α-galactosidase A protein is encoded by a 12 kb gene mapped to the long arm of the X chromosome, and is 7 exons long. In Fabry disease 57% of alleles are missense mutations, 18% partial gene deletions, 11% nonsense mutations, 6% insertions, and 6% RNA processing defects. Mutations have been found in all 7 exons (7). Most mutations are private and confined to a single Fabry pedigree yet several occur in unrelated families (143). Many of the latter occur at CpG islands or mutation hot spots because of deamination of methylcytosine to involve these hot spots. The majority of mutations are private; therefore, genotype/phenotype correlation is not feasible. Several mutations, Asn215S, Gln279Glu, Met296Val, and Arg301Gln, are in exons 5 or 6 and cause atypical, mild disease. The closely located missense mutation, Ser297Phe adjacent to Met296Val, results in severe disease. Patients from unrelated families with the Gly328Arg, Arg301Gln, and Arg112His have presented with classic disease in one family and mild disease in another (7). The diagnosis of Fabry disease should lead to counseling and screening of family members. Obligate female carriers may be symptomatic because of "nonrandom" X inactivation.

Diagnostic Tests

Low α-galactosidase A activity in leukocytes, or cultured fibroblasts is diagnostic. Enzyme activity does not distinguish affected hemizygous males from obligate carrier females. In an affected family carrier status should be determined by molecular DNA techniques if the defect is known or by linkage analysis if the defect is not known. Carrier detection can be established by amazing elevations in total glycolipids of CTH and digalactosylceramide in urine. The diagnosis can be made prenatally by measuring enzyme activity and/or determining the sex of the fetus, DNA analysis of chorioni villi, or cultured amniocytes.

Experimental Models

A mouse model for Fabry disease was generated by knocking out the *Gla* gene. Tissues from these mice lack α-galactosidase A activity (210) and have elevated levels of GB3. They were not clinically affected. They are, however, an excellent model for assessment of treatment modalities. In the 1980s, α-galactosidase A enzyme was shown to diminish circulating GB3. A patient with a cardiac variant of Fabry received galactose infusions, one of the first attempts at chaperone-mediated therapy. ERT should be given to all hemizygous males to slow down continued organ damage (151). Many patients require kidney transplantation and dialysis. Substrate depletion, gene therapy, and chemical chaperone therapy at subinhibitory doses to the enzyme all play a role in therapy.

NEURONAL CEROID LIPOFUSCINOSES

Overview

The NCLs (Batten disease) are pediatric neurodegenerative diseases caused by a number of gene and protein defects. Clinical features include seizures, blindness, intellectual, and motor decline resulting in early demise. The clinical variants include: (*i*) NCL type 1 (classical infantile NCL) (INCL/CLN1); (*ii*) NCL type 2 (classical late infantile NCL, Scottish juvenile NCL) (LINCL/CLN2); (*iii*) NCL type 3 (classical juvenile NCL)(JNCL/CLN3); (*iv*) NCL type 4 (CLN4); (*v*) NCL type 5 (variant late infantile Finnish NCL) (CLN5); (*vi*) NCL type 6 (variant late infantile NCL) (vLINCL/CLN6); (*vii*) NCL type 8 (includes what was formerly NCL type 7 and epilepsy with mental retardation) (EPMR/CLN8); and (*viii*) NCL type 9 (variant juvenile NCL (vJNCL/CLN9) (26,67). Six genes causing NCL have been identified: *CLN1*, *CLN2*, *CLN3*, *CLN5*, *CLN6*, and *CLN8* (Table 1).

Autofluorescent material is stored in neurons and affected cells. Most forms exhibit neuronal and photoreceptor cell death. Neuronal loss is visualized by CT and MRI as cerebral and cerebellar cortical atrophy. Apoptosis of photoreceptor cells translated into low amplitude a and b waves by ERG. Ultrastructural features include granular osmiophilic deposits or GRODS in INCL, curvilinear bodies in late infantile neuronal ceroid lipofuscinosis (LINCL), curvilinear and/or fingerprint-like inclusions in JNCL or different combinations of the above. These inclusions are found in many different cell types, including neurons, liver, muscle, and conjunctiva and the type of inclusion varies with the NCL (Table 2).

A mountain of information has emerged over the past decade pertinent to the genetics, molecular and cell biology, and proteins, but CLN1 and CLN2 are not LSDs. CLN6 and CLN8 are ER proteins, and CLN3 protein travels between Golgi apparatus, early recycling endosomes, and lipid rafts at the PM. CLN3, CLN6, and CLN8 are hydrophobic membrane proteins. CLN5 is reported to be a lysosomal membrane glycoprotein. Many animal models of NCLs exist. The *nclf* mouse and the New Zealand Southhampshire sheep represent models for the CLN6-deficient variant. Transgenic mouse models for CLN1-, CLN2-, CLN3-, and CLN6-deficient variant LINCL are available.

Diagnosis is suggested by clinical findings and telltale neuroradiologic and electrophysiologic

Table 2 Neuronal Ceroid Lipofuscinoses

Synonyms	MIM #	Gene	Protein product
Infantile neuronal ceroid lipofuscinosis (INCL), Haltia–Santavuori disease	#256730	*CLN1*	Palmitoyl-protein thioesterase 1 (PPT1)
Ceroid lipofuscinosis, neuronal type 2 (CLN2), late infantile neuronal ceroid lipofuscinosis (LINCL), Jansky–Bielchowski disease	#204500	*CLN2*	Tripeptidyl peptidase (TTP1)
Ceroid lipofuscinosis, neuronal type 3 (CLN3), juvenile neuronal ceroid lipofuscinosis (JNCL), Spielmeier–Vogt disease	#204200	*CLN3*	Some refer to it as Batterin
Ceroid lipofuscinosis, neuronal type 4 (CLN4), adult neuronal ceroid lipofuscinosis (ANCL), Kufs disease, dominant forms known as Parry disease (dominant forms of ANCL)	#204300	Unknown	Unknown
Ceroid lipofuscinosis, neuronal type 5 (CLN5), variant late infantile neuronal ceroid lipofuscinosis (vLINCL), Finnish late infantile neuronal ceroid lipofuscinosis	#256731	*CLN5*	
Ceroid lipofuscinosis, neuronal type 6 (CLN6), late infantile neuronal ceroid lipofuscinosis (vLINCL), Costa Rican, Portuguese, Indian neuronal ceroid lipofuscinosis	#601780	*CLN6*	Some refer to it as Linclin
Some cases similar to ceroid lipofuscinosis, neuronal type 8			
Ceroid lipofuscinosis, neuronal type 8 (CLN8), Turkish variant of late infantile neuronal ceroid lipofuscinosis (vLINCL Turkish) (CLN7), Northern epilepsy with mental retardation (EPMR)	#600143 #601780	*CLN8*	
Ceroid lipofuscinosis, neuronal type 9 (CLN9), variant juvenile neuronal lipofuscinosis (vJNCL)		CLN9	

Table 3 Comparison of the Neuronal Ceroid Lipofuscinoses

	Age of onset	Ethnic predilection or country of origin	Clinical hallmarks	TEM	Diagnosis and tests
INCL, Haltia–Santavuori	9–18 months	Primarily Finnish, described in others	Seizures, cognitive/motor decline, blindness, microcephaly	GRODS	PPT1 enzymatic assay, gene-based, skin biopsy, isoelectric EEG by age 3 years
LINCL, Jansky–Bielchowski	2.5–3.5 years	Panethnic	Seizures, ataxia, cognitive/motor decline, retinitis pigmentosa	Curvilinear	TTP1 enzymatic assay, gene-based test, giant occipital EEG spike, ERG
JNCL, Spielmeier–Vogt	4–8 years	Northern European, described in many others	Retinitis pigmentosa, seizures, echolalia, psychosis, dystonia, tremor, bradycardia	Fingerprint/ curvilinear	Gene-based test, ERG
ANCL, Kufs disease, dominant forms known as Parry disease	30 years		Early dementia, psychosis, type A myoclonic seizures, type B extrapyramidal signs, facial dyskinesias	Fingerprint, pigmented	Clinical, by pathology, exclude other dementias
vLINCL, Finnish late infantile	5–7 years	Finnish	Clumsiness, visual failure, cognitive and motor decline, seizures	Curvilinear/ fingerprint	Gene-based test
vLINCL, Costa Rican, Portuguese, Indian	4–6 years	Costa Rican, Portuguese, Indian, Pakistani	Loss of speech, seizures, retinitis, cognitive and motor decline	Fingerprint/ curvilinear, rectilinear, lipid drops	Gene-based test
vLINCL Turkish	5–7 years	Turkish		Fingerprint/ curvilinear	
EPMR or Northern Epilepsy with mental retardation	5–8 years	Finnish	Seizures ↑with puberty ↓with age, clumsy, dysarthria, ↓cognition agitation, ↓visual acuity	Curvilinear-like, fine GRODS lipid drops	Gene-based test, EEG
vLINCL Turkish (previously classified as CLN7)	5–7 years	Turkish	Loss of speech, seizures, retinitis, cognitive and motor decline	Curvilinear, fingerprint	Clinical, exclude CLN2, CLN5 CLN6
vJNCL	4–8 years	Serbian, German	Myoclonus, seizures, cognitive and motor decline	Fingerprint/ curvilinear/ GRODS	TEM, ↑cell growth, ↓cell adhesion, GeneChip

Notes: Rare cases of adolescent and adult forms of CLN1-deficiency have been described. Patients with CLN2-deficiency of later onset and survival into the 4th and 5th decade exist. *CLN4*, *CLN7*, and *CLN9* genes still unidentified. *Abbreviations*: ANCL, adult neuronal ceroid lipofuscinosis; EEG, electroencephalogram; TEM, transmission electron microscopy; EPMR, epilepsy with mental retardation; ERG, electroretinography; CLN, neuronal ceroid lipofuscinoses; GRODS, granular osmophilic deposits; INCL, infantile neuronal ceroid lipofuscinoses; JNCL, juvenile neuronal ceroid lipofuscinoses; LINCL, late infantile neuronal ceroid lipofuscinoses; PPT1, palmitoyl-protein thioesterase 1; TTP1, tripeptidyl peptidase 1; v, variant; ↑, increase(d); ↓, decrease(d).

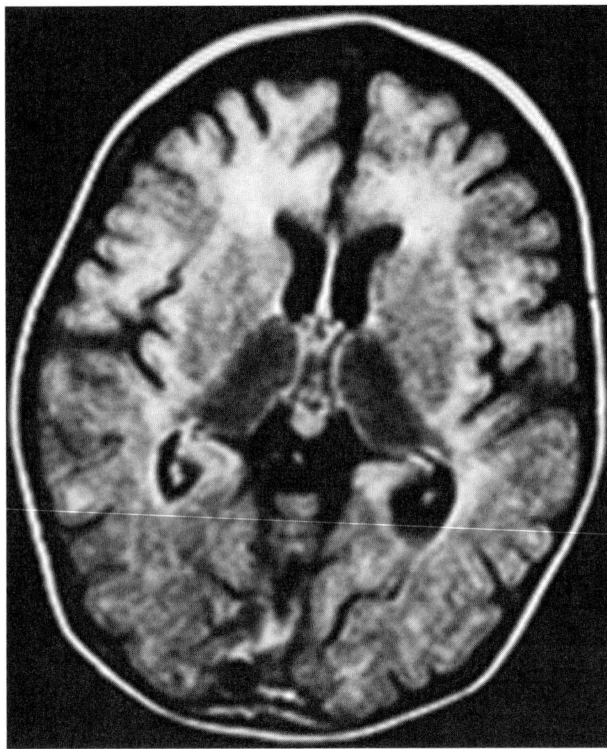

Figure 13 Magnetic resonance imaging of shrunken juvenile neuronal ceroid lipofuscinosis brain weighing 650 g with wide sulci, large ventricles, and abnormal signal in the white matter.

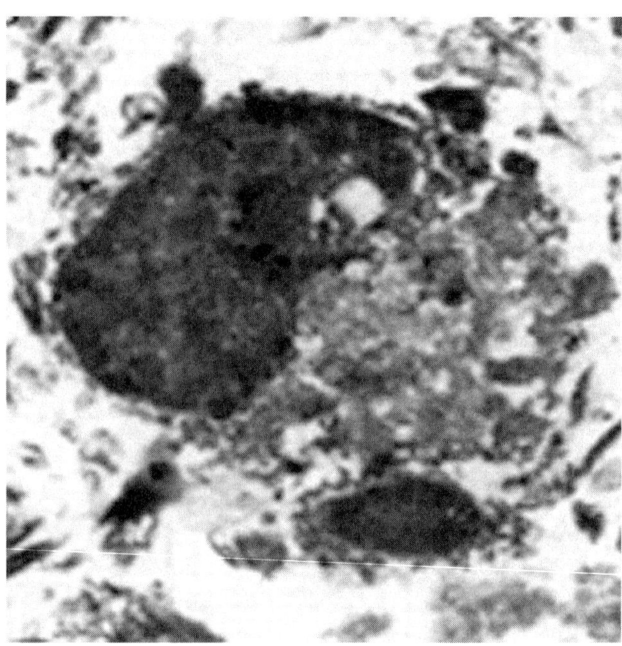

Figure 14 Apoptotic neuron with condensed and fractured chromatin from frontal cortex of a juvenile neuronal ceroid lipofuscinosis brain.

studies. It is established by an enzymatic (PPT1 or TTP1 activity in CLN1 and CLN2 deficiencies) or a DNA-based laboratory test. Ultrastructure of a punch skin biopsy remains an important diagnostic tool, particularly when delineation of novel variants with unknown gene defects are being described. A typical ultrastructure and a classical picture led to identification of the CLN1-, CLN5-, CLN8-, CLN6-, and CLN9-deficient forms.

Targeted therapies based on biochemical and cell biological processes include using cysteamine or Cystagon in INCL, and flupirtine in INCL-, LINCL-, JNCL-, CLN6-, and CLN9-deficient variants (13,50). Gene- and protein-based delivery systems for the classical late infantile and infantile types with defects in soluble proteins have been explored in generated mouse models, and for LINCL, in humans.

Stengel described the first JNCL cases in 1926, followed by descriptions attributed to Batten, Mayou, Spielmeyer, Vogt, and Sjögren (119,209). The CLN3 gene causing JNCL was identified in 1995 (107). The LINCL variant was initially reported by Jansky and Bielchowski in 1908 and 1913 (93). LINCL and JNCL were previously classified as Batten disease. Batten disease presently refers to all forms. The adult form (Kufs disease) consisting of an early onset dementia with seizures without visual findings was described in 1925 (51). Sporadic and familial reports of ANCL, with some families suggesting a dominant mode of inheritance, are also reported. The *CLN4* genes responsible for adult disease are not known. NCL was coined by Zeman and Dyken in 1969 to portray the autofluorescent, waxy, dusky lipid accumulation observed in endosomes (228). The infantile form or INCL was initially recognized by Hagberg, followed by detailed descriptions by Haltia and Santavuori in 1973 (74,170). The *CLN1* gene was cloned in 1995, and the *CLN2* gene for LINCL was discovered in 1997 (187). Numerous variant late infantile forms and early juvenile forms with defects in the CLN5, CLN6, and CLN8 genes are now described (174,216). A CLN9 form clinically similar to the juvenile form is now well-characterized, but the responsible gene remains to be identified (109,181).

The terminology of the NCLs is complex and impractical. Some terms, such as INCL, LINCL, JNCL, and ANCL, classify these diseases according to age of onset, but for many variants this is not valid. The discovery of additional genes and the ascertainment of atypical cases have rendered a classification based on the age of onset almost obsolete. Defects in one particular gene can present with a variable clinical course and multiple ages of onset. A reference to the specific gene defect may be best. The naming of the genes as ceroid lipofuscinosis neuronal (CLN) as opposed to NCL is unfortunate, as yeast cyclin genes

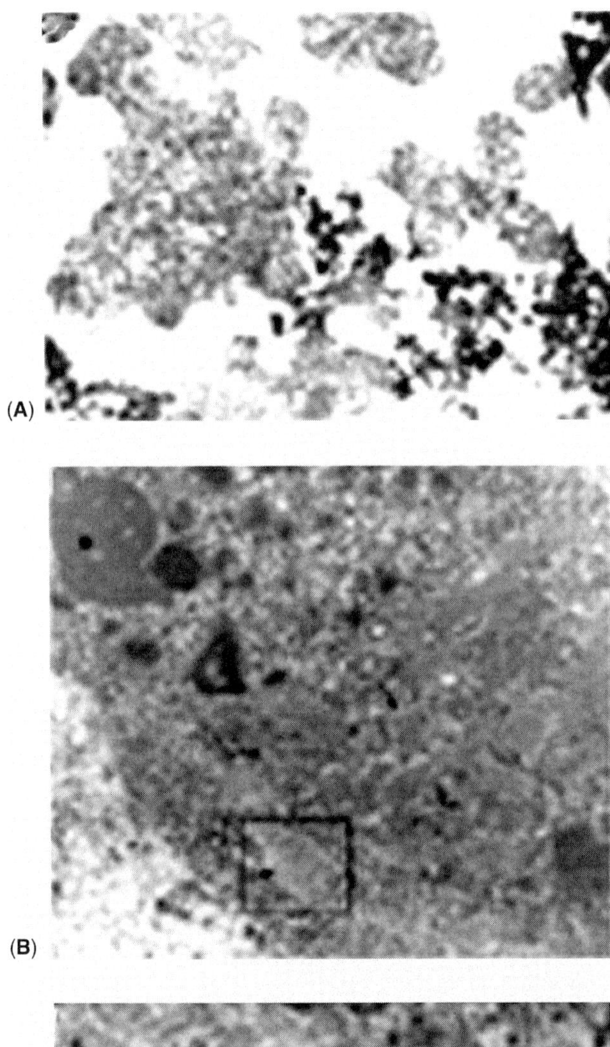

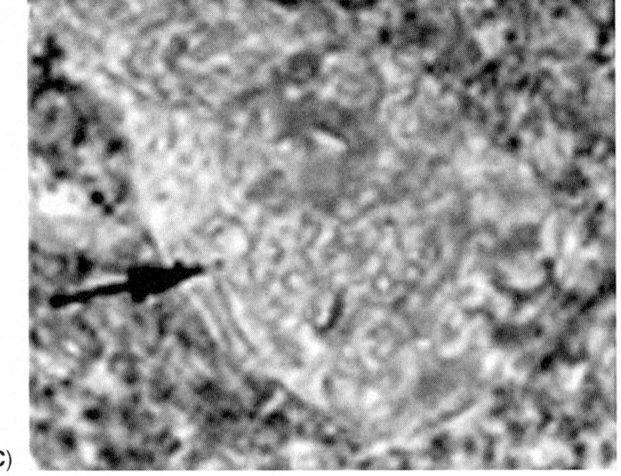

Figure 15 Curvilinear and granular osmophilic deposit-like inclusions from frontal cortex of a neuronal ceroid lipofuscinosis type 9-deficient brain biopsy.

are called *CLN* genes. Attempting a switch at this point in time will only muddy the waters. All variants are now referred to collectively as Batten disease. Although historically incorrect, it is a matter of practicality, ease of pronunciation, and convenience. Batten disease is the term now used by families, physicians, private foundations, and government agencies in the United States.

Infantile Ceroid Lipofuscinosis

Overview

Infantile ceroid lipofuscinosis (INCL, Haltia-Santavuori variant, *CLN1* defective, palmitoyl-protein thioesterase or PPT1-deficient) was initially described by Hagberg (74). A complete clinical and pathological description of this recessive disorder appeared later (76,170). The disorder arises because of a deficiency in PPT1.

Clinical Description

Early development is normal until 10 to 18 months of age. Head growth rate decelerates beginning at 5 months, with patients ultimately becoming microcephalic. Further developmental progress does not take place, and hypotonia and ataxia follow. Visual difficulties present at 1 year of age result in blindness at age 2 years. Myoclonic jerks and generalized seizures start at age 1 year. Some patients acquire Rett-like hand knitting movements that disappear by 2 years. At age 3 years, children are bedridden, irritable, hypotonic, and spastic. Flexion contractures, acne, hirsutism, and precocious puberty are common. Death occurs between 7 and 13 years. An adolescent onset form similar to the juvenile type occurs in affected individuals of Scottish descent (128). A single report describes two families with late adult onset and mild, indolent course.

Optic atrophy, thinned retinal vessels and a discolored brownish macula are present. Cones are affected before rods as reflected in an abnormal ERG. Pupillary reflexes are diminished by 24 months of age and there is optic atrophy with attenuated vessels. Occasionally, in older children a bony spicule-like retinopathy appears. By then the ERG is completely extinguished.

Diagnostic Tests

Low PPT1 enzyme activity in leukocytes is diagnostic (46). A dried blood spot on filter paper, ethylene diaminetetraacetic acid (EDTA) blood, or cultured fibroblasts are good sources of enzyme. Patients have <5% of normal enzyme activity in INCL. Diagnosis based on DNA analysis is also available. TEM examination reveals characteristic membrane-bound granular osmiophilic deposits or GRODS seen in the endothelium and pericytes of blood vessels in the skin, and nerve cells of the submucosal myenteric nerve plexus in the rectum. The EEG gradually worsens. Sleep spindles are absent as is the attenuation in amplitude observed with eye opening by 16 to

24 months. The EEG is isoelectric after the age of 3 years. ERG, VEPs, and SEPs are abnormal. CT and MRI reveal signal loss in the thalami, cerebral atrophy, and thinned periventricular rims early in the course. Postmortem MRI T2-weighted images expose hypointensity of gray matter with respect to white matter. Prenatal diagnosis using chorionic villus samples (CVS) at 11 weeks, and amniocytes at 16 to 18 weeks has been accomplished: TEM reveal GRODS, and low PPT1 activity and/or defects by DNA analysis are necessary to establish the diagnosis. TEM is most useful, particularly when enzyme analysis is not available, and the family DNA defect is unknown. Ideally, the three diagnostic modalities should be used. The diagnosis of a normal or carrier fetus should be rechecked at birth using cord blood.

Histopathology

Brain weight is only 250 to 400 g. Cortical neuronal loss sets in at 1 year of age, and there is a near total loss of neurons by age 4 years. Betz cells and neurons in the CA1 and CA4 sectors of the hippocampus are intact, with a prominence of reactive astrocytes. GRODS in neurons and macrophages appear early at 8 weeks of fetal life. Purkinje cells and granule cells disappear and are replaced by Bergman glia with extensive gliosis. The brainstem and basal ganglia are affected as well, and anterior horn cells manifest a prominent storage of ceroid and lipofuscin. Although storage granules are everywhere, there is evidence for cell loss only in brain and retina (68,221).

Biochemistry

The activity of PPT1, which detaches long-chain fatty acids attached in thioester linkage to proteins (180) is diminished. The fatty acylated cysteine residue containing proteins found at the inner PM leaflet are usually acylated and deacylated. Protein–protein and protein–lipid membrane interactions are affected if this capability is lost. *S*-acylated protein degradation is also impaired. What accumulates in the cell has no link to the actual defect. PPT1 is taken up via Man-6-P into lysosomes, but is active at neutral and basic pH, and must function in other parts of the cell. Normally, PPT1 colocalizes with synaptophysin to presynaptic vesicles in neurons. Sphingolipid activator proteins A and D are stored in cytosomes (203). Brain sphingomyelin and other phospholipids are low in brains with INCL. Apoptosis is accelerated in lymphocytes, cultured lymphoblasts, and skin fibroblasts, as well as in neurons lacking PPT1 (37). Defective deacylation of *S*-acylated proteins and the apoptosis of PPT1-deficient cells have given rise to specific therapies. Virally mediated *CLN1* gene therapy reduces storage material and clinical symptoms in a *Cln1-deficient* knockout mouse. Stem cell therapies and clinical trials with phosphocysteamine, an oral medication protein deacylater with antiapoptotic therapies, are ongoing.

Genetics

Finnish cases result from a missense mutation (Arg122Trp) in the *CLN1* gene that changes an arginine to a tryptophan, producing a mutant protein that is degraded in the ER (131). Carrier frequency is 1 in 70 and disease incidence is 1 in 2000. In the United States, INCL accounts for 20% of all cases of Batten disease. A threonine to proline substitution at amino acid 75 produces a juvenile variant of this disorder (128). This mutation and a premature stop codon at arginine 151 accounts for nearly all alleles in North America that occur in patients with Irish or Scottish ancestry. Forty mutations of the *CLN1* gene have been reported.

Late Infantile Neuronal Ceroid Lipofuscinosis

Overview

LINCL [late infantile Bassen disease, Jansky–Bielchowski disease, *CLN2* defective NCL, tripeptidyl peptidase (TTP1)-deficient NCL] arises from defects in the lysosomal *TTP1* gene (187). Initial reports were made by Jansky in 1908 and Bielchowski in 1913. European, Middle-Eastern, Chinese, Pakistani, and Indian patients are described. LINCL is common in the United States, although affected cases at any point in time do not number more than 500.

Clinical Description

Affected children present with a seizure and/or ataxia between 2.5 and 3.5 years of age. Within 4 to 6 months vision declines and motor and cognitive skills are lost, with blindness setting in at 4 years because of tapetoretinal degeneration. Children become nonambulatory and mute by 5 years, and require gavage feeding. Myoclonic jerks appear in the face and body. Hypotonia, ultimately followed by contractures, is prominent. Hypothalamic disease causes both hyper- and hypothermia. Copious secretions and shallow breathing end up causing lung infections. Infections and unmanageable seizures cause death at the end of the first decade or in the early teen years (26,229). Atypical cases with late onset and a milder disease are described.

Ocular Manifestations

The ERG shows reduced amplitudes preceding the appearance of thinned blood vessels and optic pallor, and is extinguished after a few months. Giant occipital polyspike discharges appear in response to a single flash of light and to low frequency repetitive stimulation on the EEG. These are an expression of an exaggerated VEP. VEP and somatosensory evoked response wave amplitudes are elevated.

Diagnostic Tests

Low TPP1 activity is the cornerstone of diagnosis. Values are <5% in leukocytes, skin fibroblasts, cultured amniocytes, and blood spotted on filter paper. Measurement of TPP1 enzyme activity is the most practical tool for diagnosis. Prenatal diagnosis relies on analyzing the ultrastructure of amniocytes, low enzyme activities, and molecular DNA analysis (220). DNA diagnostics are less practical, especially if the mutations are new. Ultrastructural studies of skin biopsies provide valuable diagnostic clues. Curvilinear bodies within single-membrane endosomes in endothelial cells, pericytes, and Schwann cells are typical. Fingerprint profiles may also be found. CT or MRI may be normal, but within 6 months both cerebral and cerebellar atrophy are visible. There is a 40% loss of cerebellar volume and an increase in lateral ventricle/hemisphere volume. The caudate nuclei and thalamus are diminished in size, and brainstem volume appears relatively preserved (25).

Histopathology

Brain weight is drastically reduced to 250 to 650 g, and the skull is thick. Sulci are wide. Cerebellar folia are prominent and ventricles are enlarged. Massive neuronal loss results in laminar necrosis with preservation of layer III, with the presence of meganeurites. Purkinje cells and granule cells are absent. Neuronal loss is also prominent in the putamina, subthalamic, and brainstem nuclei. The white matter manifests reactive astrocytosis and activation of microglia, but monocyte-derived macrophages are absent, which implies that neuronal loss is the initial event, with a secondary, reactive gliosis occurring later. Remaining neurons have engorged cell bodies and their granular cytoplasm stains positively with PAS, luxol fast blue, and Sudan black B. The white matter is intact. Condensed chromatin, increase in neuroprotective Bcl-2, and terminal deoxynucleotidyl transferase (TdT) mediated Z′-deoxyuridine 5′-triphosphate (dUTP) nick-end labelling (TUNEL) positivity substantiates apoptosis (154,155). Reactivity to subunit C of mitochondrial ATP synthase antibodies is robust (95). Mitopsis (engulfing of mitochondrial fragments by phagocytes), a form of apoptosis seen in neurodegenerative disease, may cause this. Neurons and other cells harbor curvilinear bodies (Figs. 16 and 17) sometimes admixed with fingerprint profiles. Smooth muscle cells, eccrine sweat glands, endothelial cells, and pericytes outside the brain also are involved.

Biochemistry

Defects in a pepstatin-insensitive lysosomal TTP1 cause LINCL. TPP1 is a 46 kDa protein. Subunit C or 9 of mitochondrial ATP synthase is the major protein stored in cytosomes. Other NCL disorders also accumulate subunit C. This may very well be a secondary process connected to the occurrence of apoptosis in CLN2, CLN3, CLN6, and CLN8 deficiencies.

Genetics

LINCL is a panethnic, autosomal recessive disease. There are no known African or Jewish cases described. It is the second most common form of Batten disease in the United States and accounts for a third of cases. Over 53 mutations are known. Two defects are responsible for 65% of the U.S. LINCL

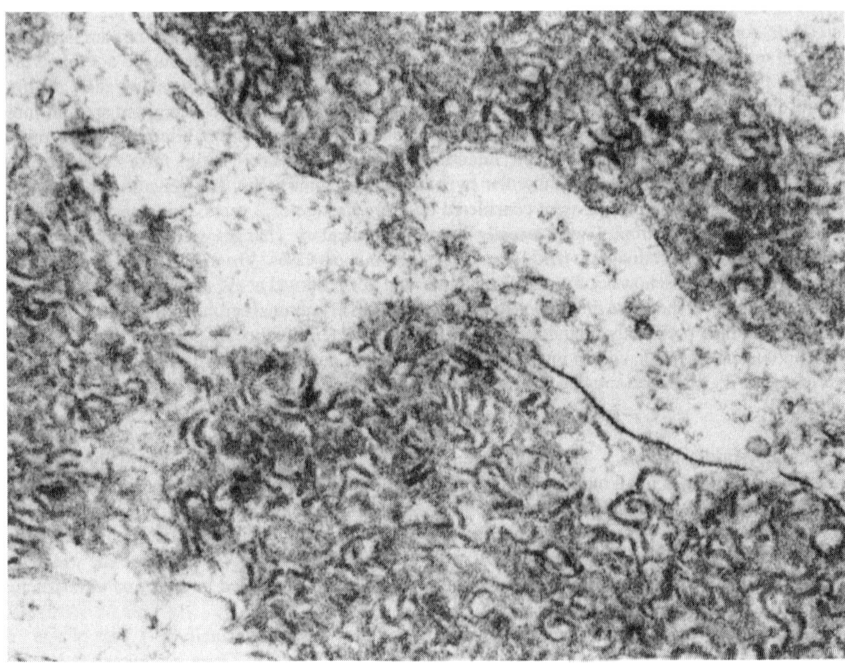

Figure 16 Ultrastructure of neural tissue in late infantile neuronal ceroid lipofuscinosis. The cell is filled with cytosomes containing curvilinear inclusion bodies (×83,600). *Source*: Courtesy of B.D. Lake.

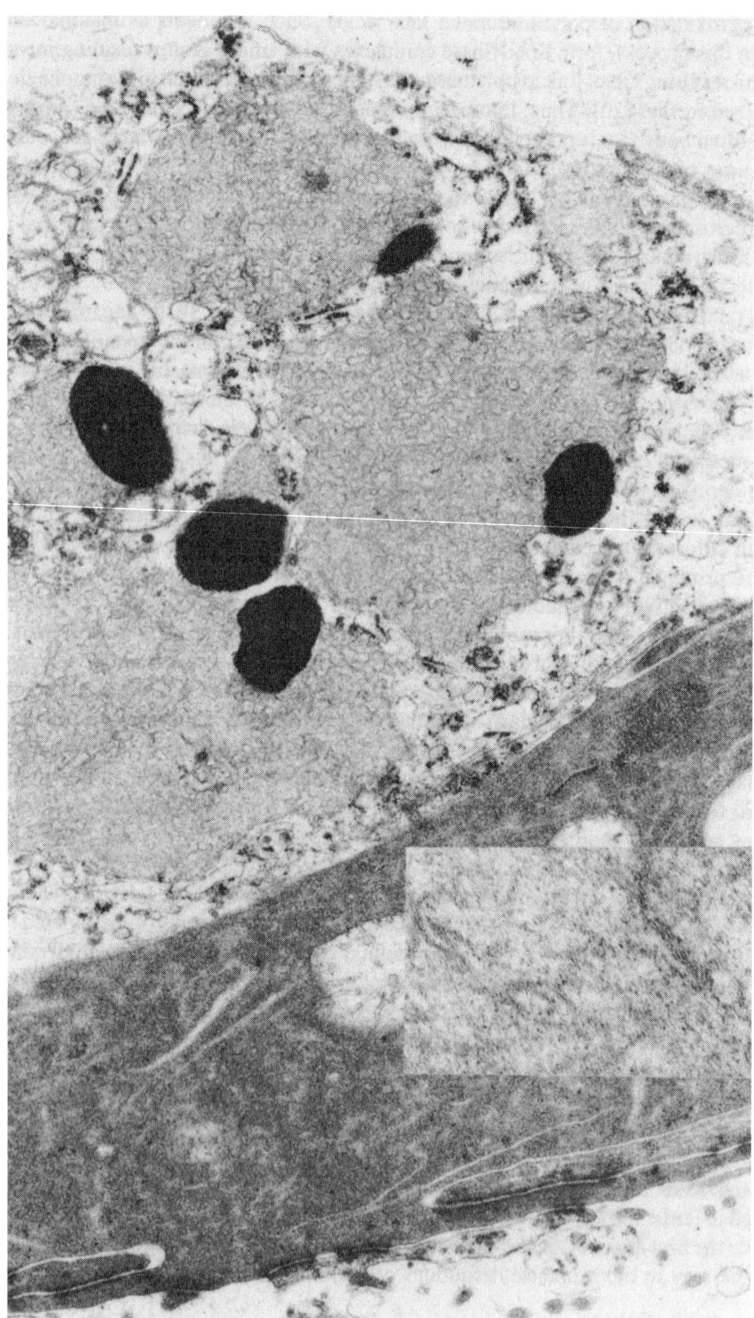

Figure 17 Equatorial region of the retina in late infantile neuronal ceroid lipofuscinosis. In the pigment epithelial cells, melanin granules are fused with curvilinear bodies (× 21,500). *Inset*: substructure of the curvilinear bodies at higher magnification, showing alternating dark and light unordered membranous sheets (× 109,500). *Source*: Reproduced from Goebel HH, Zeman W, Damaske E. An ultrastructural study of the retina in the Jansky–Bielschowsky type of neuronal ceroid-lipofuscinosis. Am J Ophthalmol 1977; 83:70–3.

cases: a nonsense mutation, Arg208Stop, and a splice junction site, IVS5-1G>C. A mild course with later onset implies one of these two mutations is on one allele, and an Arg447His on the second allele.

Experimental Models

A mouse model for this disease has been generated (186). Gene replacement via a number of strategically placed burr holes in children with advanced disease has been tried without any tangible benefit. Stem cell therapy is currently being explored. The antiapoptotic drug, flupirtine, may slow disease progression by numerous anecdotal reports. The wide safety margin for the oral drug, flupirtine, and its associated analgesic, antispasmodic, and antiepileptic properties makes its use attractive and feasible (50).

Variant Late Infantile Forms of Neuronal Ceroid Lipofuscinosis

Overview

Variant late infantile forms of NCL (vLINCL; Finnish: CLN5-deficient; Costa Rican/Portuguese/Lake-Cavanaugh form: CLN6-deficient; Northern epilepsy or epilepsy with mental retardation/EPMR, and Turkish vLINCL or tLINCL: CLN8-deficient) is a series of variant late infantile types with an age of onset spanning 5 to 8 years, and a clinical picture similar but milder than classic LINCL and a protracted course are known. Three genes have been discovered. The *CLN5* gene causes the Finnish type, a rare variant circumscribed in an area in Finland affecting 16 families. One Swedish and one Dutch case have been identified. The *CLN8* gene responsible for Northern epilepsy was discovered in Finnish patients from the Finnish North-East. Some of the Turkish variant LINCL patients have mutations in a different part of the *CLN8* gene. Variant LINCL Costa Rican/Portuguese that is CLN6-deficient was discovered in patients with Costa Rican, Venezuelan, Pakistani, and Indian heritage. A case from the United States has also been published. Early reports refer to this variant as the "early juvenile" or Lake-Cavanaugh type (62,174,216).

Clinical Description

Finnish Variant LINCL (CLN5-Deficient)

Individuals with *Finnish variant LINCL* (*CLN5-deficient*) typically have motor clumsiness at age 4.5 years, cognitive decline at age 6 years, and generalized and myoclonic epilepsy at age 8 years, with children becoming blind at 8 years, then losing the ability to walk by age 10 years, and dying between the age of 14 to 34 years.

Northern Epilepsy (Epilepsy with Mental Retardation) (EPMR) (CLN8-Deficient)

Presents with frequent and brief generalized tonic clonic convulsions and complex partial seizures, as well as a cognitive decline to a low average level after the age of 5 years, but before the onset of puberty (160). After puberty, the second stage, which is noted for slowness of movements and a plateauing effect for the rate of cognitive decline, sets in. In the final stages, seizures decrease in frequency, and mental dullness results in early dementia by age 40 years. Toward the end patients are characteristically clumsy, ataxic, and have impaired vision. They usually die anytime from the age of 17 years to late middle age.

Turkish vLINCL or tLINCL (CLN8-Deficient)

Turkish vLINCL has a clinical phenotype that is more severe than the Finnish cases with EPMR. Patients present between the ages of 2 and 5 years with seizures, loss of intellectual capabilities, blindness, and behavioral problems. The latter are prominent by the age of 8 to 9 years. Most patients are wheelchair-bound by 10 years of age.

Costa Rican/Portuguese vLINCL/ Lake-Cavanaugh Variant (CLN6-Deficient)

The initial symptoms in the Costa Rican/Portuguese vLINCL/Lake-Cavanaugh variant (CLN6-deficient) at the age of 4 years consists of ataxia, and problems with speech (200). Visual failure secondary to RP, myoclonic jerks, and other seizures and intellectual decline follow. Patients succumb to the disease by the mid-teens.

Diagnostic Tests

JNCL with atypical features suggestive of classical LINCL, normal TPP1 enzyme activity, absence of vacuolated lymphocytes and a normal *CLN3* gene, together with a skin biopsy TEM, country of origin, and mild and subtle characteristics for one of these variants suggests a variant LINCL type. Fingerprint and rectilinear structures suggest the Finnish variant; combined curvilinear and fingerprint bodies favors the Costa Rican/Portuguese variant; Finnish CLN8 TEM findings are noted for loose curvilinear-like structures; and the Turkish variant has dense fingerprint profiles as well as dark amorphous material. The confirmatory test is DNA-based, and should uncover a defect in one of three genes: *CLN5*, *CLN6* or *CLN8*. Costa Rican, Portuguese, and Venezuelan CLN6-deficient and Finnish vLINCL are reported to have severe cerebral and cerebellar cortical atrophy, low densities in the thalami/basal ganglia, and hyperintensities of the white matter by MRI, but the MRI of tLINCL is characterized by atrophy of the brainstem and cerebellar and cerebral atrophy. Giant amplitude occipital spikes in response to low frequency photic stimulation on the EEG are noted in all the variants.

Histopathology

Finnish Variant LINCL (CNL5-Deficient)

The brain weighs about 500 g and severe cerebellar atrophy is documented. Findings are otherwise very similar to classical LINCL. Strong immunoreactivity to subunit C or 9 of mitochondrial ATP synthase and weak immunoreactivity to the SAPs is reported. TEM of affected tissues is conspicuous for the presence of rectilinear profiles, and both curvilinear and fingerprint bodies (67,68,201,220).

Northern Epilepsy or Epilepsy with Mental Retardation (CLN8-Deficient)

The brain weight at autopsy can exceed 1000 g but is less than 1600 g. The brain may appear normal or mildly atrophic. Storage material is prominent in layer III of the cerebral cortex and neuronal loss is most conspicuous in cortex layer V. Deep gray matter structures and cerebellar Purkinje cells are relatively spared. There is strong reactivity with antibodies to β-amyloid, subunit C, and SAP-D. TEM of the storage bodies is characterized by curvilinear bodies and granular material.

Turkish vLINCL or tLINCL (CLN8-Deficient)
TEM of skin biopsies is characterized by curvilinear, rectilinear, and fingerprint profiles (201), but detailed reports on brain have not been documented.

Costa Rican/Portuguese vLINCL/Lake-Cavanaugh Variant (CLN6-Deficient)
The brain weight is between 600 and 900 g. Neuronal loss is pervasive and very prominent in neocortex layer V. Granule cells in the cerebellum are wiped out completely, but few Purkinje cells remain. There is strong immunoreactivity with subunit C in neuronal tissues, which is absent from peripheral organs. By TEM, fingerprint bodies and few rectilinear profiles are observed in the CNS. Rectilinear, fingerprint, and curvilinear bodies are also observed in peripheral viscera.

Genetics

Finnish Variant LINCL (CLN5-Deficient)
A 2 bp deletion in exon 4 (c.1175delAT) accounts for 94% of Finnish cases. A minor Finnish mutation, Asp279Asn, and two other mutations found in rare Dutch and Swedish cases, Trp75Stop and c669insC, are described.

Northern Epilepsy or Epilepsy with Mental Retardation (CLN8-Deficient) and Variant Turkish tLINCL
A single point mutation, Arg24Gly, accounts for all Northern Epilepsy patients. The four other mutations cause the clinically more severe Turkish tLINCL phenotype. Two missense mutations are reported in exon 3, Arg204Cys, and Trp263Cys, as well as two others, Leu16Met and Thr170Met. Arg204Cys occurs in the conserved TLC lipid-sensing domain and may predict a potential role for CLN8 in sphingolipid metabolism/trafficking.

Costa Rican/Portuguese vLINCL/Lake-Cavanaugh Variant (CLN6-Deficient)
Nineteen mutations are now recognized. The nonsense mutation reported in 20 Costa Rican families, c.214G>T is the most common, followed by the 3 bp deletion in six Portuguese families, I154del (200). Other mutations are described in patients with Venezuelan, Indian, Pakistani, Greek, American, and Trinidadian or East-Indian ancestry. The *nclf* mouse is a naturally occurring model for CLN8-deficient vLINCL (132).

Biochemistry

CLN6 and CLN8 proteins are transmembrane proteins that reside in the ER. The CLN5 protein is a secreted lysosomal glycoprotein. CLN5 coimmunoprecipitates with the CLN2 protein, and with CLN3 (208). This implies that there are potential interactions between these proteins, that they are found in more than one subcellular localization, and that they may be functionally related. This can have useful implications for therapy. CLN2 is soluble and amenable to protein and/or gene replacement therapy, whereas transmembrane proteins (e.g., CLN8) are not.

Experimental Models

The motor neuron degeneration or "mnd" mouse is a naturally occurring animal model for the CLN8-deficient variant (159).

Juvenile Neuronal Ceroid Lipofuscinosis

Overview

There is a preponderance of juvenile NCL (juvenile Batten disease, Spielmeier–Vogt–Batten–Mayou disease, CLN3-defective/deficient NCL) cases with Northern European ancestry (Finland, Iceland, Norway, Sweden, Denmark, Germany, and Holland), and a conspicuous and notable absence of African or Jewish cases. Japanese, Portuguese, Polish, British, Turkish, Moroccan, Lebanese cases have been reported and so have cases from many other countries. JNCL is the most prevalent type of NCL in the United States (26). The first Batten disease variant to be recognized was JNCL, and the gene responsible for it, *CLN3*, was also the first NCL gene to be cloned (107). The description of the first juvenile cases is credited to the Danish physician, Otto Christian Stengel, in 1826 (190). The four affected siblings of the described Norwegian family established the genetic nature of the illness.

Clinical Description

Early development is unremarkable and the first symptom is decreased vision due to RP at 4 to 6 years of age. Patients become completely blind at variable ages from 10 to 14 years. Complete blindness and a disturbed sleep–wake cycle and insomnia are common. A subset of affected children manifests difficult behavior between the ages of 7 to 9 years. By age 10 years, cognitive decline is apparent. Diagnosis is often first suspected by teachers for the blind who are familiar with this condition in the pediatric visually impaired population. Seizures appear at the age of 12 years or sooner, but may not declare themselves until the age of 14 years. Early onset seizures, particularly when difficult to control, often foretell a more rapidly declining course. Repetitive echolalic speech is universal to all cases. Perseveration of speech and motor actions is familiar to all cases. A cogwheel rigidity of the limbs and a stooped, shuffling gait is reminiscent of patients with Parkinson disease. Intention tremor may be present and is of variable severity. Patients stabilize for a few years in their mid-teens. Many become depressed and agitated, or aggressive and psychotic, requiring neuroleptics. There usually is a positive family history for unipolar or bipolar illness in this subset. Treatment unfortunately aggravates extrapyramidal signs and symptoms. Hallucinations are common, but are often of a pleasant, repetitive, and familiar nature. A number of patients have frequent conversations with imaginary friends that become part of who they are. Growth and physical maturity are normal, and sexual development eventually becomes a problem. Drooling, difficulty in swallowing, and weight loss are a nuisance late in the course. Temperature instability with hypothermia alternating with hyperthermia are caused by hypothalamic involvement. Seizures increase to 150 to 200 per day in spite of multiple drugs and are recalcitrant to treatment. Few patients develop a cardiomyopathy or sick sinus syndrome with bradycardia. Patients succumb in their early to mid-twenties to uncontrollable seizures or due to cardiopulmonary arrest. A small number of patients survive into the fourth decade.

Diagnostic Tests

DNA-based *CLN3* gene tests confirm the diagnosis. The EEG is abnormal from the age of 9 years due to large amplitude spike and slow wave complexes. CT and MRI, though initially normal, ultimately reveal cerebral atrophy with gaping sulci and enlarged ventricles (Fig. 13). Cerebellar atrophy is a prominent feature. Morphometric MRI measurements document loss of hemisphere, caudate, thalamic, and lenticular volumes (25). Low signal is documented in the white matter in T2-weighted images. PET scans confirm decreased glucose utilization in the calcarine area, which progresses to involve all gray matter structures. The techniques of morphometric volume analysis and PET are not routinely performed, but were means to better understand disease progression. The ERG is often abnormal before decreased vision becomes apparent. Visual evoked potentials show reduced amplitude potentials, and somatosensory evoked potentials are enhanced. TEM of a skin biopsy is often of assistance, particularly if the known and common mutations are not found in the patient's *CLN3* gene. Schwann cells, endothelial cells, pericytes, neurons, macrophages, and eccrine sweat glands contain typical inclusions. Fingerprint-like inclusions enclosed by a unit membrane are common, usually associated with curvilinear bodies. Vacuolated lymphocytes are a hallmark of JNCL, but their detection is impractical from a diagnostic standpoint because the sample has to be processesd swiftly and correctly, otherwise false positives are to be expected. Skin TEM is more robust and therefore more reliable.

Histopathology

Brain weight is between 450 and 1100 g. There is thinning of the cortical mantle with moderate neuronal loss, gliosis, and accumulation of autofluorescent material that stains with Sudan black B and is PAS-positive. Meganeurites are seen in the basolateral amygdaloid complex and in cortical layer V. Purkinje cell and granule cell loss are dramatic. Apoptotic neurons with dark, shrunken, and fragmented chromatin are seen in the cerebral cortex by TEM (Fig. 14). A number of neurons are TUNEL positive, confirming the existence of apoptotic neurons. Surviving neurons are immunoreactive with antibodies to Bcl-2 and subunit C or 9 of mitochondrial ATP synthase. Lipopigment accumulates in anterior horn cells of the spinal cord and the receptor cells of the organ of Corti. In neurons, fingerprint profiles are common, and in cells of peripheral organs and tissues, curvilinear inclusions prevail.

Biochemistry

Ceramide, the proapoptotic lipid second messenger, was elevated in JNCL brains (156). This correlated with the identification of apoptosis in JNCL brain and antiapoptotic residues and motifs stretches within the CLN3 protein (150). More recently it was determined that other GSL and sphingomyelin were also elevated, pointing to a general enhanced production of sphingolipids (149). The CLN3 RNA and protein were upregulated in human and mouse cancer cell lines, and solid colon cancer specimens, further supporting an antiapoptotic role for the CLN3 protein (169). The CLN3 protein localizes to the Golgi apparatus, early recycling endosomes, and lipid rafts in PMs. CLN3 protein has embedded in it a GalCer lipid raft binding domain. In CLN3-deficient cells, mutant CLN3 mislocalizes to late endosomes and lysosomes, and both mutant CLN3 protein and GalCer remain in the Golgi apparatus, and do not reach their final destination or lipid rafts. Restoring CLN3 to deficient cells reverses this insinuating CLN3 may function as a GalCer transporter. Apoptosis is initiated from lipid rafts in many instances, and the enhanced production of sphingolipids may be an attempt to compensate for the GalCer deficiency in lipid rafts.

Genetics

The prevalence of this autosomal recessive disease is 7 in 100,000 live births in Iceland, and 0.71 in 100,000 live births in Germany. The prevalence drops the further one travels from Scandinavian or Northern European countries. The gene has 15 exons, and the protein is 438 amino acids long. It is a hydrophobic protein with 5 to 7 potential transmembrane domains and is highly conserved across species. There are more than 36 documented mutations. A 1.02 kb deletion accounts for 85% of the U.S. cases.

Diagnostic Tests

DNA-based carrier testing is available, and is more straightforward if the specific family mutation is known. Prenatal diagnosis has been achieved by TEM and/or DNA-based methodologies as early as 11 weeks of gestation. It is advisable to confirm diagnosis by retesting umbilical cord blood at birth.

Experimental Models

There are multiple mouse models for JNCL. They provide hope for a better understanding of the cell biology and biochemistry of this disease and for the development of logical therapies.

CLN9 Deficient Juvenile-Like Variant of Neuronal Ceroid Lipofuscinoses

Overview

Two German brothers and two American sisters of Serbian descent diagnosed with the JNCL variant that were found to have an intact *CLN3* gene and enzyme assays and molecular tests for all known NCL variants were normal. However, analysis of cDNA from CLN3 deficient and other NCL variants, and cDNA from these cases using Affymetrix GeneChips, identified a distinct gene profile allowing their grouping together as a new variant (109,181).

Clinical Description

The clinical course in this variant of NCL is similar to that of JNCL with decreased vision at age 4 years, cognitive decline at age 6 years, and ataxia and rigidity by age 9 years. They became dysarthric, develop scanning speech, and become mute by age 12 years. One of the cases developed hallucinations and behavior problems. They all developed seizures in their early teens. A pigmentary retinopathy was documented in one brother. One of the German cases died at 15 years of age because of infection and the other at age 19 years following uncontrolled seizures. The two sisters are still alive. One is in her early twenties, though bedridden since the age of 14 years. She has well-controlled seizures and a feeding tube. The younger sister is 12 years old and is following a similar course.

Diagnostic Tests

ERG showed diminished wave amplitudes in one case. EEGs in all four patients were abnormal with slowing and frequent polyspike discharges. TEM of lymphocytes revealed membrane bound inclusions containing a mixture of electron-dense/fingerprint patterns. CT scans and MRIs documented cerebral and cerebellar cortical atrophy. Abnormal signal intensity in the periventricular white matter has been described. A diagnostic brain biopsy from one case showed neurons that contained granular osmiophilic inclusions and curvilinear bodies.

Histopathology

The brain weight of one of the brothers at the time of death was 1,140 g. Large neurons remaining in the cerebral cortex and the deep gray structures were ballooned with a fine granular material. The substantia nigra, thalamus, and spinal cord was characterized by an astrocytic gliosis, and autofluorescent storage material that stained with Sudan black. Neurons contained GRODS and curvilinear bodies by TEM. Also, neurons had increased reactivity to subunit C or 9 protein (this is a subunit of the F1Fo protein complex of mitochondrial ATP synthase) a feature common to many of the NCLs.

Genetics

The gene is yet to be discovered and candidate genes are thought to code for proteins that impact sphingolipid metabolic pathways. There is evidence that the *CLN9* gene could be an activator of dihydroceramide synthase.

Biochemistry

The biochemistry and cell biology of this variant are well delineated. CLN9-deficient cells have a distinctive morphology and biochemical phenotype. Cells are small and rounded and manifest a cell adhesion defect. A number of genes involved in cell adhesion and apoptosis are dysregulated by gene profiling (see www.dbsr.duke.edu/pub/cln9/). Gene expression of cyclins A2, B1, C, E2, G1, and T2 were increased, and expression of cyclin D1, a protooncogene involved in malignant transformation of breast tissue, was decreased; member 1A increased. Ceramide and sphingomyelin levels, lactosylceramide, CTH and globoside levels were 60% to 100% decreased compared to normal. The key regulating enzyme in the ceramide de novo synthetic pathway, serine palmitoyl transferase, was upregulated.

REFERENCES

1. Aerts JMFG, Donker-Koopman WE, Brul S, et al. Comparative study on glucocerebrosidase in spleens from patients with Gaucher disease. Biochem J 1990; 269:93–100.
2. Ahern-Rindell AJ, Murnane RD, Prieur DJ. B-Galactosidase activity in fibroblasts and tissues from sheep with a lysosomal storage disease. Biochem Genet 1988; 26:733–46.
3. Al-Essa MA, Bakheet SM, Patay ZJ, et al. Cerebral fluorine-18 labeled 2-fluoro-2-deoxyglucose positron emission tomography (FDG PET), MRI, and clinical

observation a patient with infantile G(M1) gagliosidosis. Brain Dev 1999:559–62.
4. Amaducci L, Sorbi S, Piacentini S, Bick KL. The first Alzheimer disease case: a metachromatic leukodystrophy? Dev Neurosci 1991; 13:186–7.
5. Amaral O, Fortuna AM, Lacerda I, et al. Molecular characterization of type 1 Gaucher disease families and patients: intrafamilial heterogeneity at the clinical level. J Med Genet 1994; 31:401–4.
6. Andersson U, Smith D, Jeyakumar M, et al. Improved outcome of *N*-butyldeoxygalactonojirimycin-mediated substrate reduction thereapy in a mouse model of Sandhoff disease. Neurobiol Dis 2004:506–15.
7. Ashton-Prolla P, Tong B, Shabbeer J, et al. 22 novel mutations in the a-galactosidase A gene and genotype/phenotype correlations including mild hemizygotes and severely effected heterozygotes. J Invest Med 2000; 48: 227–35.
8. Assman GSU. Acid lipase deficiency: wolman disease and cholesteryl ester storage disease. In: Beaudet S, Valle, ed. The Metabolic and Molecular Bases for Inherited Disease. New York, NY: McGraw-Hill, 2001.
9. Austin JH, Armstrong D, Shearer L. Metachromatic forms of diffuse cerebral sclerosis. V. The nature and significance of low sulfatase activity: a controlled study of brain, liver and kidney in four patients with metachromatic leukodystrophy (MLD). Arch Neurol 1996; 14:259–69.
10. Bambach BJ, Moser HW, Blakemore KJ, et al. Engraftment following in utero bone marrow transplantation for globoid cell leukodystrophy. Bone Marrow Transpl 1997; 19:399–402.
11. Barone R, Bruhl K, Stoeter P, et al. Clinical and neuroradiological findings in classic infantile and late onset globoid-cell leukodystrophy (Krabbe disease). Am J Med Genet 1996; 63:209–17.
12. Batta AK, Shefer S, Batta M, Salen G. Effect of chenodeoxycholic acid on biliary and urinary bile acids and bile alcohols in CTX: monitoring by high performance liquid chromatography. J Lipid Res 1985; 26:690–8.
13. Batten FE, Mayou MS. Family cerebral degeneration with macular changes. Proc Roy Soc Med 1915; 8:70–90.
14. Bauer P, Knoblich R, Bauer C, et al. NPC1: complete genomic sequence, mutation analysis, and characterization of haplotypes. Hum Mutat 2002; 19:30–8.
15. Becker AE, Schoori R, Balk AG, van der Heide RM. Cardiac manifestations of Fabry's disease. Report of a case with mitral insufficiency and electrocardiographic evidence of myocardial infarction. Am J Cardiol 1975; 36:829–35.
16. Bernardini GL, Herrera DG, Carson D, et al. Adult-onset Krabbe's disease in siblings with novel mutations in the galactocerebrosidase gene. Ann Neurol 1997; 41:111–4.
17. Besley GT, Elleder M. Enzyme activities and phospholipid storage patterns in brain and spleen samples from Niemann–Pick disease variants: A comparison of neurophathic and non-neuropathic forms. J Inherit Metab Dis 1986; 9:59–71.
18. Bethune J, Landrigan P, Chipman C. Angiokeratoma corporis diffusum (Fabry's disease in two brothers). N Engl J Med 1961; 264:1280.
19. Beutler E, Kuhl W, Sorge J. Cross-reacting material in Gaucher disease fibroblasts. Proc Natl Acad Sci USA 1984; 81:6506–10.
20. Biffi A, De Palma M, Quattrini A, et al. Correction of metachromatic leukodystrophy in the mouse model by transplantation of genetically modified hematopoietic stem cells. J Clin Invest 2004; 113:1108–10 [see comment].
21. Bjorkhem I, Skrede S, East C, Grundy S. Accumulation of 7a-hydroxy-4-cholesen-3-one and cholesta-4, 6-dien-3-one in patients with CTX. Effect of treatment with chenodeoxycholic acid. Hepatology 1987; 7:266–71.
22. Blom S, Habgerg B. EEG findings in late infantile metachromatic and globoid cell leukodystrophy. Electroencephalogr Clin Neurophysiol 1967; 22:253–9.
23. Boot RG, Hollak EE, Verhoek M, et al. Glucocerebrosidase genotype of Gaucher patients in The Netherlands: limitations in prognostic value. Hum Mutat 1997; 10: 348–58.
24. Bosio A, Binczek E, Stoffel W. Functional breakdown of the lipid bilayer of the myelin membrane in central and peripheral nervous system by disrupted galactocerebroside synthesis. Proc Natl Acad Sci USA 1996; 93:13280–5.
25. Boustany R-M, Filipek P. Seizures, depression and dementia in teenagers with Batten disease. J Inher Metab Dis 1993; 16:252–5.
26. Boustany R-M. Batten disease or neuronal ceroid lipofuscinosis. Handbook of Clinical Neurology, Neurodystrophies and Neurolipidoses. Vol. 66. New York, NY: Elsevier, 1996: 671–900.
27. Boustany R-MQW-H, Suzuki K. Mutations in acid beta galactosidase cause GM1-Gangliosidosis in American Patients. Am J Hum Gen 1993; 53:881–8.
28. Brady RO, Kanfer JN, Mock MB, Fredrickson DS. The metabolism of sphingomyelin. II. Evidence of an enzymatic deficiency in Niemann–Pick disease. Proc Natl Acad Sci USA 1966; 55:366–9.
29. Brady RO. The abnormal biochemistry of inherited disorders of lipid metabolism. Fed Proc 1973; 32:1660.
30. Brett EM, Ellis RB, Hass L, et al. Late onset GM2 gangliosidosis: clinical, pathological and biochemical studies in eight patients. Arch Dis Child 1973; 48:775–85.
31. Brownstein S, Carpenter S, Polomeno RC, Little JM. Sandoff's disease (GM2 gangliosidosis type 2). Histopathology and ultrastructure of the eye. Arch Ophthalmol 1980; 98:1089–97.
32. Bullard WN, Southard EE. Diffuse gliosis of the cerebral white matter in a child. J Nerv Ment Dis 1906; 33:188.
33. Cali JJ, Hsieh C-L, Francke U, Russell DW. Mutations in the bile acid biosynthetic enzyme sterol 27-hydroxylase underlie cerebrotendinous xanthomatosis. J Biol Chem 1991; 266:7779–83.
34. Callahan JW, Khalil M. Sphingomelinases in human tissues. III. Expression of Niemann–Pick disease in cultured skin fibroblasts. Pediatr Res 1975; 9:914–8
35. Caniglia M, Rana I, Pinto RM, et al. Allogeneic bone marrow transplantation for infantile globoid-cell leukodystrophy (Krabbe's disease). Pediatr Transplant 2002; 6:427–31.
36. Carlin L, Roach ES, Riela A, et al. Juvenile metachromatic leukodystrophy: evoked potentials and computed tomography. Ann Neurol 1983; 13:105–6.
37. Cho S, Dawson PE, Dawson G. Role of palmitoyl-protein thioesterase in cell death: implications for infantile neuronal ceroid lipofuscinosis. Eur J Paediatr Neurol. 2001; 5 Suppl A:53–5.
38. Choy FYM, Woo M, Potier M. In situ radiation-inactivation size of fibroblast membrane-bound acid beta-glucosidase in Gaucher type 1, type 2 and type 3 disease. Biochim Biophys Acta 1986; 870:76–81.
39. Cogan DG, Chu FC, Barranger JA, Gregg RE. Macula halo syndrome. Variant of Niemann–Pick disease. Arch Ophthalmol 1983; 101:1698–700.
40. Cogan DG, Kuwabara T, Kolodny E, Driscoll S. Gangliosidoses and the fetal retina. Ophthalmology 1984 May; 91:508 12.

41. Collier J, Greenfield JG. The encephalitis periaxialis of Schilder: a clinical and pathological study with an account of two cases, one of which was diagnosed during life. Brain 1924; 47:489.
42. Conzelmann E, Sandhoff K. Partial enzyme deficiencies: residual activities and the development of neurologic disorders. Dev Neurosci 1983/84; 6:58–71.
43. Cormand B, Vilageliu L, Burguera JM, et al. Gaucher disease in Spanish patients: analysis of eight mutations. Hum Mutat 1995; 5:303–9.
44. Cox TM, Lachmann R, Hollak CE, et al. Novel oral treatment of Gaucher's disease with *N*-butyldeoxynojirimycin (OGT 918) to decrease substrate biosynthesis. Lancet 2000; 355:1481–5
45. Crutchfield KE, Patronas NJ, Dambrosia JM, et al. Quantitative analysis of cerebral vasculopathy in patients with Fabry disease. Neurology 1998; 50:1746–9.
46. Das AK, Becerra CHR, Yi W, et al. Molecular genetics of palmitoyl-protein thioesterase deficincy in the US J Clin Invest 1998; 102:361–70.
47. Davies JP, Ioannou YA. Topological analysis of Niemann–Pick C1 protein reveals that the membrane orientation of the putative sterol-sensing domain is identical to thos of 3-hydroxy-3-methylglutarly-CoA reductase and sterol regulatory element binding protein cleavage-activating protein. J Biol Chem 2000; 275:24367–74.
48. Desnick RJ, Bishop DF. Fabry disease: a-Galactosidase A deficiency and Schindler disease: a-*N*-acetylgalactosaminidase deficiency. In Stanbury JB, Wyngaarden JB, Frederickson DS, Goldstein JL, Brown MS, eds. The Metabolic Basis of Inherited Diseases. 6th ed. New York, NY: McGraw-Hill, 1989:1751.
49. Desnick RJ, Sweeley CC. Fabry disease: a-Galactosidase A deficiency. In: Stanbury JB, Fredrickson DS, Goldstein JL, Brown MS, eds. The Metabolic Basis of Inherited Disease. New York, NY: McGraw-Hill, 1983:903.
50. Dhar S, Bitting RL, Rylova SN, et al. Flupirtine blocks apoptosis in Batten patient lymphoblasts and in human postmitotic CLN3- and CLN2-deficient neurons. Ann Neurol 2002; 51:448–66.
51. Dom R, Brucher JM, Ceuterick C, et al. Adult ceroidlipofuscinosis (Kufs disease) in two brothers: retinal and visceral storage in one; diagnostic muscle biopsy in the other. Acta Neuropathol 1979; 45:67–72.
52. Duffy PE, Kornfeld M, Suzuki K. Neurovisceral storage disease with curvilinear bodies. J Neuropathol Exp Neurol 1968:351.
53. EM FRAJBIK. Infantile GM1-gangliosidosis: complete morphology and histochemistry of two autopsy cases with special reference to delayed central nervous system myelination. Pediatr Dev Pathol 2000; 3:73–86.
54. Escolar ML, Poe MD, Provenzale JM, et al. Transplantation of umbilical-cord blood in babies with infantile Krabbe's disease. New Engl J Med 2005; 352: 2069–81.
55. Federico A, Palmeri S, Malandrini A, et al. The clinical aspects of adult hexosaminidase deficiencies. Develop Neurosci 1991; 13:280–7.
56. Ferrans VJ, Hibbs RG, Burda CD. The heart in Fabry's disease. A histochemical and electron microscopic study. Am J Cardiol 1969; 24:95–110.
57. Franceschetti AT. Cornea verticillata (Gruber) and its relation to Fabry's diesease (angiokeratoma corporis diffusum). Ophthalmologica 1968; 156:232–8.
58. Fukumizu MYH, Takashima S, Sakuragawa N, Kurokawa T. Tay–Sachs Disease: Progression of Changes in four cases. Neuroradiology 1992; 34:483–6.
59. Futerman AH, Sussman JL, Horowitz M, et al. New directions in the treatment of Gaucher disease. Trends Pharmacol Sci 2004; 25:147–51.
60. G.M, Marcais C, Tomasetto C, et al. Niemann–Pick C1 disease: correlations between NPC1 mutations, levels of NPC1 protein, and phenotypes emphasize the functional significance of the putative sterol-sensing domain and of the cysteine-rich luminal loop. Am J Hum Genet 2001; 68: 1373–85.
61. Gal AE, Brady RO, Hibbert SR, Pentchev PG. A practical chromogenic procedure for the detection of homozygotes and heterozygous carriers of Niemann–Pick disease. N Engl J Med 1975; 293:632.
62. Gao H, Boustany R-M, Espinola JA, et al. Mutations in a novel CLN6 encoded transmembrane protein cause variant neuronal ceroid lipofuscinosis in mouse and man. Am J Hum Gen 2002; 70:324–35.
63. Gieselmann V, Polten A, Kreysing J, von Figura K. Arylsulfatase A pseudodeficiency: Loss of a polyadenylation signal and *N*-glycosylation site. Proc Natl Acad Sci USA 1989; 86:9436–40.
64. Gieselmann V, Zlotogora J, Harris A, et al. Molecular genetics of metachromatic leukodystrophy. Hum Mutat 1994; 17:500–9.
65. Gieselmann V. An assay for the rapid detection of the arylsulfatase A pseudodeficiency allele facilitates diagnosis and genetic counseling for metachromatic leukodystrophy. Am J Hum Gen 1991; 86:251–5.
66. Ginns EI, Brady RO, Piruccello S, et al. Mutations of glucocerebrosidase: Discrimination of neurologic and non-neurologic phenotypes of Gaucher disease. Proc Natl Acad Sci USA 1982; 79:5607–10.
67. Goebel HH, Mole SE, Lake BD, eds. The neuronal ceroid lipofuscinoses (Batten Disease): Amsterdam: IOS Press, 1999.
68. Goebel HH, Wisniewski KE. Current state of clinical and morphological features in human NCL. Brain Pathol. 2004; 14:61–9.
69. Grabowski GA, Barton NW, Pastores G, et al. Enzyme therapy in type 1 Gaucher disease: comparative efficacy of mannoseterminated glucocerebrosidase from natural and recombinant sources. Ann Intern Med 1995:33–9.
70. Grabowski GA. Gaucher Disease: lessons from a decade of therapy. J Pediatr 2004; 144:S15–9.
71. Gravel RAKM, Proia R, Sandhoff K, Suzuki K, Suzuki K. The GM2-Gangliosidoses. In: Arthur L, Beaudet CRS, William S, Sly, David Valle, eds. The Metabolic and Molecular Bases of Inherited Disease. New York, NY: McGraw-Hill, 2001.
72. Greer WL, Dobson MJ, Girouard GS, et al. Mutations in NPC1 highlight a conserved NPC1-specific cysteine-rich domain. Am J Hum Genet 1999; 65:1252–60.
73. Guffon N, Souillet G, Maire I, et al. Juvenile metachromatic leukodystrophy: neurological outcome two years after bone marrow transplantation. J Inherit Metab Dis 1995; 18:159–61.
74. Hagberg B, Sourander P, Svennerholm L. Late Infantile progressive encephalopathy with distrubed polyunsaturated fat metabolism. Acta Paediatr Scand 1968; 57:495–9.
75. Hagberg B. Clinical symptoms, signs and tests in metachromatic leukodystrophy. In Folch-Pi J, Bauer H eds. Brain Lipids and Lipoproteins and the Leukodystrophies. Amsterdam: Elsevier, 1963:134.
76. Haltia M, Rapola J, Santavuori P, Keranen A. Infantile type of so-called neuronal ceroid-lipofuscinosis. Part 2. Morphological and biochemical studies. J. Neurol. Sci. 1973:269.

77. Haltia M, Rapola J, Santavuori P. Infantile type of so-called neuronal ceroid lipofuscinosis. Part II. Histological and electron microscopic studies. Acta. Neuropathol 1973:157–70.
78. Hannun YA, Bell RM. Lysosphingolipids inhibit protein kinase C: implications for the sphingolipidoses. Science 1987; 235:670—4.
79. Harmon DL, Gardner-Medwin D, Stirling JL. Two new mutations in a late infantile Tay-Sachs patient are both in exon 1 of the B-hexosaminidase a subunit gene. J Med Genet. 1993; 30:123–8.
80. Harris RA, Loh HH. Brain sulfatide and non-lipid sulfate metabolism in hypothyroid rate. Res Commun Chem Pathol 1979; 24:169–79.
81. Harzer K, Paton BC, Poulos A, et al. Sphingolipid activator protein deficiency in a 16 week old atypical Gaucher disease patient and his fetal sibling: biochemical signs of combined deficiency. Eur J Pediatr 1989; 149: 31–9.
82. Hedley-Whyte ET, Boustany R-M, Riskind P, et al. Peripheral neuropathy due to galactosylceramide-B-galactosidase defiency (Krabbe's disease) in a 73 year old woman. Neuropathol Appl Neurobiol 1988; 14:515.
83. Hinek A, Zhang S, Smith AC, Callahan JW. Impaired elastic-fiber assembly by fibroblasts from patients with either Morquio B disease or infantile GM1-gangliosidosis is link deficiency in the 67-kD spliced variant of beta-galactosidase. Am J Hum Genet 2000; 67:23–36.
84. Hong YB, Kim EY, Jung SC. Down-regulation of Bcl-2 in the fetal brain of the Gaucher disease mouse model: a possible role in the neuronal loss. J Hum Genet 2004; 49: 349–54.
85. Hoogerbrugge PM, Suzuki K, Suzuki K, et al. Donor derived cells in the central nervous system of twitcher mouse after bone marrow transplantation. Science 1988; 239:1035–8.
86. Horinouchi K, Erlich S, Perl DP, et al. Acid sphingomyelinase deficient mice: a model of types A and B Niemann–Pick disease. Nat Genet 1995; 10:288–93.
87. Horinouchi K, Sakiyama T, Pereira L, et al. Mouse models of Niemann–Pick disease: mutation analysis and chromosomal mapping rule out the type A and B forms. Genomics 1993; 18:450–1.
88. Hozumi I, Nishizawa M, Ariga T, et al. Accumulation of glycosphingolipids in spinal and sympathetic ganglia of a symptomatic heterozygote of Fabry's disease. J Neurol Sci 1989; 90:273–80.
89. Hugo W, Moser TL, Anthony H. Fensom, Thierry Levade, Konrad Sandhoff. Acid ceramidase deficiency: Farber lipogranulomatosis. In: Scriver CR, Beaudet AL, Sly WS, Valle D, eds. The Metabolic and Molecular Bases of Inherited Disease. New York, NY: McGraw-Hill, 2001.
90. Hulkova H, Cervenkova M, Ledvinova J, et al. A novel mutation in the coding region of the prosaposin gene leads to a complete deficiency of prosaposin and saposins, and is associated with a complex sphingolipidosis dominated by lactosylceramide accumulation. Hum Mol Genet 2001; 10:927–40.
91. Hund E, Grau A, Fogel W, et al. Progressive cerebellar ataxia, proximal neurogenic weakness and ocular motor disturbances: Hexosaminidase A deficiency with late clinical onset in four siblings. J Neurol Sci 1997; 145: 25–31.
92. Ieshima A, Eda S, Matsui A, et al. Computed tomography in Krabbe's disease: comparison with neuropathology. Neuroradiology 1983; 25:323–7.
93. Jansky J. Dosud nepopsany pripad familiarni amazuroticke idiotie komplikovanem a hypoplasii mozeckovou. Sborn Lek 1908; 13:165–96.
94. Jeyakumar M, Thomas R, Elliot-Smith E, et al. Central nervous system inflammation is a hallmark of pathogen in mouse models of GM1 and GM2 gagliosidosis. Brain 2003:974–87.
95. Johnson DW, Speier S, Qian WH, et al. Role of subunit-9 of mitochondrial ATP synthase in Batten disease. Am J Med Genet 1995; 57:350–60.
96. Johnson WG. The clinical spectrum of hexosaminidase deficiency disease. Neurology. 1981; 31:1453–6.
97. Kaminski WE, Klunemann HH, Ibach B, et al. Identification of novel mutations in the NPC1 gene in German patients with Niemann–Pick C disease. J Inherit Metab Dis 2002; 25:385–9.
98. Kamoshita S, Aron AM, Suzuki K. Infantile Niemann–Pick disease. A chemical study with isolation and characterization of membranous cytoplasmic bodies and myelin. Am J Dis Child 1969; 117:379–44.
99. Kasperzyk JL, El-Abbadi MM, Hauser EC, et al. *N*-butyldeoxygalactonojirimycin reduces neonatal brain ganglio content in a mouse model of GM1 gangliosidosis. J Neurochem 2004; 89:645–53.
100. Kivlin JD, Sanborn GE, Myers GG. The cherry-red spot in Tay-Sachs and other storage diseases. Ann Neurol 1985; 17:356–60.
101. Kolodny EH. Niemann–Pick Disease. Curr Opin Hematol 2000; 7:48–52.
102. Krabbe K. A new familial, infantile form of diffuse brain sclerosis. Brain 1916; 37:74.
103. Krivit W, Lockman LA, Watkins PA, et al. The future for treatment by bone marrow transplantation for adrenoleukodystrophy, metachromatic leukodystrophy, globoid cell leukodystrophy and Hurler syndrome. J Inherit Metab Dis 1995; 18:398–412.
104. Kudoh T, Velkoff MA, Wenger DA. Uptake and metabolism of radioactively labeled sphingomyelin in cultured skin fibroblasts from controls and patients with Niemann–Pick disease and other lysosomal storage diseases. Biochim Biophys Acta 1983; 754:82–92.
105. Kustermann-Kuhn B, Poulos A, Carey WF, Harzer K. A case of combined Farber's and Sandhoff's Disease. Eur J Pediatr 1989; 148:558–62.
106. Lerner TJ, Boustant RM, Anderson JW, et al. Isolation of a novel gene underlying Batten disease, CLN3. Cell 1995; 82:949—95.
107. Lever AM, Ryder JB. Cor pulmonale in an adult secondary to Niemann–Pick disease. Thorax 1983; 38:873–4.
108. Lin SM, Dhar S, Boustany R-M. Extracting knowledge from gene expression data: A case study of Batten Disease. Proceedings of Data Mining in Bioinformatics. San Francisco, CA. ACM-KDD. 2001.
109. Liscum L, Ruggiero RM, Faust JR. The intracellular transport of low density lipoprotein-derived cholesterol is defective in Niemann–Pick type C fibroblasts. J Cell Biol 1989; 1085:1625–36.
110. Liscum L. Niemann–Pick type C mutations cause lipid traffic jam. Traffic 2000; 1:218–25.
111. Luzi P, Rafi MA, Victoria T, et al. Characterization of the rhesus monkey galactocerebrosidase (GALC) cDNA and gene and identification of the mutation causing globoid cell leukodystrophy (Krabbe disease) in this primate. Genomics 1997; 42:319–24.
112. MacLeod PM, Wood S, Jan JE, et al. Progressive cerebellar ataxia, splasticity, psychomotor retardation, and

hexosaminidase deficiency in a 10-year old child: Juvenile Sandhoff disease. Neurology. 1977; 27:571–3.
113. Maret A, Potier M, Salvayre R, Douste-Blazy L. Modification of subunit interaction in membrane-bound acid beta-glucosidase from Gaucher disease. FEBS Lett 1983; 160:93–7.
114. Marks HG, Scavina MT, Kolodny EH, et al. Krabbe's disease presenting as a peripheral neuropathy. Muscle Nerve 1997; 20:1024–8.
115. Martin JJ, Ceuterick C, Martin L, et al. Globoid cell leukodystrophy (Krabbe's disease): peripheral nerve lesion. Acta Neurol Belg 1974; 74:356–75.
116. Matsuda J, Suzuki O, Oshima A, et al. B-Galactosidase-deficient mouse as an animal model for GM1-gangliosidosis. Glycoconjugate 1997; 17:729–36.
117. Matzner U, Herbst E, Hedayati KK, et al. Enzyme replacement improves nervous system pathology and function in a mouse model for metachromoatic leukodystrophy. Hum Mol Genet 2005; 14:1139–52.
118. Mayou MS. Cerebral degeneration with symmetrical changes in the maculae in three members of a family. Trans Ophthalmol Soc UK 1904; 24:142–5.
119. McGraw P, Liang L, Escolar M, et al. Krabbe disease treated with hematopoietic stem cell transplantation: serial assessment of anisotropy measurements—initial experience. Radiology 2005; 236:221–30.
120. Mehl E, Jatzkewitz H. Cerebroside-sulfatase and aryl sulfatase A deficiency in metachromatic leukodystrophy (ML). Biochem Biophys Res Commun 1965; 19:407–11.
121. Meiner V, Shpitzen S, Mandel H, et al. Clinical-biochemical correlation in molecularly characterized patients with Niemann–Pick type C. Genet Med 2001; 3:343–8.
122. Menkes JH, O'Brien JS, Okada S, et al. Juvenile GM2 gangliosidosis: Biochemical and ultrastructural studies on a new variant of Tay–Sachs disease. Arch Neurol 1971; 25:14–22.
123. Millat G, Marcais C, Rafi MA, et al. Niemann–Pick C1 disease: the I1061T substitution is a frequent mutant allele in patients of Western European descent and correlates with a classic juvenile phenotype. Am J Hum Genet 1999; 65:1321–9.
124. Miocic S, Filocamo M, Dominissini S, et al. Identification and functional characterization of five novel muta alleles in 58 Italian patients with Gaucher disease type 1. Hum Mutat 2005; 25:100.
125. Mistry PK, Sirrs S, Chan A, et al. Pulmonary hypertension in type 1 Gaucher's disease: genetic and epigenetic determinants of phenotype and response to therapy. Mol Genet Metab 2002; 77:91–8.
126. Mitchison HM, Hofmann SL, Becerra CH, et al. Mutations in the palmitoyl-protein thioesterase genet (PPT, CLN1) causing juvenile neuronal ceroid lipofuscinosis with granular osmiophilic deposits. Hum Mol Genet 1998:291–7.
127. Miyatake T. A study on glycolipids in Fabry's disease. Jpn J Exp Med 1969; 39:35.
128. Miyawaki S, Mitsuoka S, Sakiyama T, Kitagawa T. Sphingomyelinosis, a new mutation in the mouse: a model of Niemann–Pick disease in humans. J Hered 1982; 73:257–63.
129. Mole SE, Mitchison HM, Munroe PB. Molecular basis of the neuronal ceroid lipofuscinoses: mutations in CLN1, CLN2, CLN3, and CLN5. Hum Mutat. 1999; 14: 199–215.
130. Mole SE. The genetic spectrum of human neuronal ceroid-lipofuscinoses. Brain Pathol 2004; 14:70–6.
131. Morgan SH, Rudge P, Smith SJ, et al. The neurological complications of Anderson-Fabry disease (alpha-galactosidase A deficiency)-Investigation of symptomatic and presymptomatic patients. Q J Med 1990; 75:491–507.
132. Moser HW, Sugita M, Snag MD, Williams M. Liver glycolipids, steroid sulfates and steroid sulfatase in a form of metachromatic leukodystrophy associated with multiple sulfatase deficiencies. In Volk BW, Aronson SM eds. Sphingolipids, Sphingolipidoses and Allied Disorders (Advances in Experimental Medicine and Biology). New York, NY: Plenum. 1972; 19:429.
133. Muldoon LL, Neuwelt EA, Pagel MA, Weiss DL. Characterization of the molecular defect in a feline model for type II GM2-gangliosidosis (Sandhoff disease). Am J Pathol 1994; 144:1109–18.
134. Naureckiene SSD, Lackland H, Fensom A, et al. Identification of HE1 as the second gene of Niemann–Pick C disease. Science 2000; 5500:2298–301.
135. Navon R. Molecular and clinical heterogeneity of adult GM2 gangliosidosis. Div Neurosci 1991; 13:295–8.
136. Ogawa KY, Tominaga L, Ohno K, et al. Chemical chaperone therapy for brain pathology in GM1 gangliosidosis. PNAS 2003; 100:15912–7.
137. Oguz KK, Anlar B, Senbil N, Cila A. Diffusion-weighted imaging findings in juvenile metachromatic leukodystrophy. Neuropediatrics 2004; 35:279–82.
138. Orvisky E, Park JK, Parker A, et al. The identification of eight novel glucocerebrosidase (GBA) mutations in patients with Gaucher disease. Hum Mutat 2002; 19: 458–9.
139. Osiecki-Newman KM, Fabbro D, Dinur T, et al. Human acid beta-glucosidase: affinity purification of the normal placental and Gaucher Disease splenic enzymes on *N*-alkyl-deoxynojirmycin-sepharose. Enzyme 1986; 35: 147–53.
140. Pampiglione G, Privett G, Harden A. Tay–Sachs disease: Neurophysiological studies in 20 children. Develop Med Child Neurol 1974; 16:201–6.
141. Pastores GM, Lien YS. Biochemical and molecular genetic basis of Fabry disease. J Am Soc Nephrol 2002:130–3.
142. Pastor-Soler NM, Rafi MA, Hoffman JD, et al. Metachromatic leukodystrophy in the Navajo Indian populations: A splice site mutation in intron 4 of the arylsulfatase A gene. Hum Mutat 1994; 4:199–207.
143. Paulson JA, Marti GE, Fink JK, et al. Richter's transformation of lymphoma complicating Gaucher's disease. Hematol Pathol 1989; 3:91–6.
144. Pentchev P, Boothe A, Kruth H, et al. A genetic storage disorder in BALB/C mice with a metabolic block in esterification of exogenous cholesterol. J Biol Chem 1984; 259:5784–91.
145. Pentchev PC, Comly ME, Kruth HS, et al. A defect in cholesterol esterification in Niemann–Pick disease type C patients. Proc Natl Acad Sci USA 1985; 82: 8247–51.
146. Pentchev PG, Vanier MT, Suzuki K, Patterson M. Niemann–Pick disease type C: a cellular cholesterol lipidosis. In: Scriver CR, Beaudet Al, Sly WS, Valle, D, eds. The Metabolic and Molecular Bases of Inherited Disease. New York, NY: McGraw-Hill, 1995:2625–39.
147. Persaud-Sawin DA, McNamara J, Rylova S, et al. A galactosylceramide binding motif is involved in trafficking of CLN3 from Golgi to rafts via recycling Endosomes. Pediatr Res 2004; 56:449–63.
148. Persaud-Sawin DA, VanDongen A, Boustany R-M. Motifs within the CLN3 protein: modulation of cell growth rates and apoptosis. Hum Mol Genet 2002; 11:2129–42.
149. Pleasure D. New treatments for denervating diseases. J Child Neurol 2005; 20:258–62.

150. Poulos A, Shankaran P, Jones CS, Callahan JW. Enzymatic hydrolysis of sphingomyelin liposomes by normal tissues and tissues from patients with Niemann–Pick disease. Biochim Biophys Acta 1983; 751:428–31.
151. Proia RL. Extensive Homology of intron placement in the alpha-and beta-chain genes. PNAS 1988; 85:1883–7.
152. Puranam K, Lane SC, Qian WH, Boustany R-M. Overexpression of Bcl-2 is associated with apoptosis inneuronal death. J Cell Biochem Suppl 1995; 19B:318.
153. Puranam K, Qian WH, Nikbakht K, et al. Upregulation of Bcl-2 and elevation of ceramide in Batten disease. Neuropediatrics 1997; 28:37–41.
154. Puranam KL, Guo WX, Qian WH, et al. CLN3 defines a novel antiapoptotic pathway operative in neurodegeneration and mediated by ceramide. Mol Genet Metab 1999; 66:294–308.
155. Rafi MA, Luzi P, Zlotogora J, Wenger DA. Two different mutations are responsible for Krabbe disease in the Druze and Moslem Arab populations in Isreal. Hum Genet 1996; 97:304–8.
156. Ranta S, Savukoski M, Santavuori P, Haltia M. Studies of homogenous populations: CLN5 and CLN8. Adv Genet 2001; 45:123–40.
157. Ranta S, Topcu M, Tegelberg S, et al. Variant late infantile neuronal ceroid lipofuscinosis in a subset of Turkish patients is allelic to Northern epilepsy. Hum Mutat 2004; 23:300–5.
158. Ranta S, Zhang Y, Ross B, et al. The neuronal ceroid lipofuscinoses in human EPMR and mnd mutant mice are associated with mutations in CLN8. Nat Genet 1999; 23: 233–6.
159. Rapin I, Suzuki K, Suzuki K, Valsamis MP. Adult (chronic) GM2-gangliosidosis. Atypical spinocerebellar degeneration in a Jewish sibship. Arch Neurol 1976; 33: 120–30.
160. Rattazzi MC, Dobrenis K. Treatment of GM2 gangliosidosis: past experiences, implications, and future prospects. Adv Genet 2001; 44:317–39.
161. Regis S, Filocamo M, Stroppiano M, et al. A 9-bp deletion (2320del9) on the background of the arylsulfatase A pseudodeficiency allele in a metachromatic leukodystrophy patient and in a patient with nonprogressive neurological symptoms. Hum Genet 1998; 102:50–3.
162. Reider-Grosswasser I, Bornstein N. CT and MRI in late-onset metachromatic leukodystrophy. Acta Neurol Scand 1987; 75:646–9.
163. Ribeiro MGST, Pinto RA, Fontes A, et al. Clinical, enzymatic and molecular characterization of a Portuguese family with a chronic form of GM2-gangliosidosis. J Med Genet 1996; 33: 341–3.
164. Riberiro I, Marcao A, Amaral O, et al. Niemann–Pick type C disease: NPC1 mutations associated with severe and mild cellular cholesterol trafficking alterations. Hum Genet 2001; 109:24–32.
165. Rodriguez M, O'Brien JS, Garrett RS, Powell HC. Canine GM1-gangliosidosis. An ultrastructural and biochemical study. J Neuropathol Exp Neurol 1982; 41:618–29.
166. Rodriquez-Lafrasse C, Vanier MT. Spingosyl phosphorylcholine in Niemann–Pick disease brain: accumulation in type A but not type B. Neurochem Res 1999; 24:199–205.
167. Rylova SN, Amalfitano A, Persaud-Sawin DA, et al. The CLN3 gene is a novel molecular target for cancer drug discovery. Cancer Res 2002; 62:801–8.
168. Santavuori P, Haltia M, Rapola J, Raitta C. Infantile type of so-called neuronal ceroid-lipofuscinosis: Part 1, a clinical study of 15 patients. J Neurol Sci 1973; 18:257–67.
169. Sarna JMS, Schuchman EH, Hawkes R. Patterned cerebellar Purkinje cell death in a transgenic mouse model of Niemann–Pick type A/B disease. Euro J Neurosci 2001; 13:1873–980.
170. Sato M, Akaboshi S, Katsumoto T, et al. Accumulation of cholesterol and GM2 ganglioside in cells cultured in the presence of progesterone: an implication for the basic defect in Niemann–Pick disease type C. Brain Dev 1998; 20:50–2.
171. Satoh J-I, Tokumoto H, Kurohara K, et al. Adult-onset Krabbe disease with homozygous T1853C mutation in the galactocerebrosidase gene. Unusual MRI findings of corticospinal tract demyelination. Neurology 1997; 49:1392–9.
172. Savukoski M, Klockars T, Holmberg V, et al. CLN5, a novel gene encoding a putative transmembrane protein mutated in Finnish variant late infantile neuronal ceroid lipofuscinosis. Nat Genet 1998; 19:286–8.
173. Schenk VW, Gluszcz A, Zelman IB. Atypical form of Krabbe-type leucodystrophy in two siblings accompanies by poliodystrophic changes. Neuropathol Pol 1973; 11: 117–25.
174. Schibanoff JM, Kamoshita S, O'Brien JS. Tissue distribution of glycosphingolipids in a case of Fabry's disease. Clinical, morphologic and biochemical studies. Circulation 1969; 10:515–20.
175. Schindler D, Bishop DF, Wolfe DE, et al. Neuroazonal dystrophy due to lysosomal a-*N*-acetylgalactosaminidase deficiency. J Clin Invest. 1989; 320:1735–40.
176. Schmidt B, Selmer T, Ingendoh A, von Figura K. A novel amino acid modification in sulfatases that is defective in multiple sulfatase deficiency. Cell 1995; 82:271–8.
177. Schmitt-Graff A. Manifestation of infantile GM1 gangliosidosis in the fetal eye. Graefes Arch Clin Exp Ophthalmol 1988; 226:84–8.
178. Schriner JE, Yi W, Hofmann SL. cDNA and genomic cloning of human palmitoyl-protein thioesterase (PPT), the enzyme defective in infantile neuronal ceroid lipofuscinosis. Genomics. 1996; 34:317–22.
179. Schulz A, Dhar S, Rylova S, et al. Impaired cell adhesion and apoptosis in the novel *CLN9* Batten Disease variant. Annals of Neurology. 2004; 56:342–50.
180. Scriver CR, Beaudet Al, Sly WS, et al. The Metabolic and Molecular Bases of Inherited Disease. 7th ed. New York, NY: McGraw-Hill, 1995:2693.
181. Shamseddine A, Taher A, Fakhani S, et al. Novel mutation, L371V, causing multigenerational Gaucher disease in a Lebanese family. Am J Med Genet A 2004; 125:257–60.
182. Sheth KJ, Werlin SL, Freeman ME, Hodach AE. Gastrointestinal structure and function in Fabry's disease. Am J Gastroenterol 1981; 76:246–51.
183. Simpson MA, Cross H, Proukakis C, Priestman DA. Infantile-onset symptomatic epilepsy syndrome caused by a homozygous loss-of-function mutation of GM3 synthase. Nat Genet 2004; 36:1225–9.
184. Sleat D, Wiseman J, El-Banna M, et al. A mouse model of classical late-infantile neuronal ceroid lipofuscinosis based on targeted disruption of the CLN2 gene results in a loss of tripeptidyl-peptidase I activity and progressive neurodegeneration. J Neurosci 2004; 24:9117–26.
185. Sleat DE, Donnelly RJ, Lackland H, et al. Associations of mutations in a lysosomal protein with classical late-infantile neuronal ceroid lipofuscinosis. Science 1997; 277: 1802–5.
186. Spaeth GL, Frost P. Fabry's disease. Its ocular manifestations. Arch Ophthalmol 1965; 74:760–9.

187. Spielmeyer W. Familiare amaurotische Idiotie. Zbl Ges Ophthal 1923; 10:161–208.
188. Stengel E. Beretning om et maerkeligt Sygdomstilfoelde hos fire Sodskende i Naerheden af Roraas. Eyr Med Tidskr 1826; 1:347–52.
189. Suzuki K, Hoogerbrugge PM, Poorthuis BJHM, et al. The twitcher mouse: CNS pathology following bone marrow transplantation (BMT). Lab Invest 1988; 58:302–9.
190. Suzuki K. Genetic animal models of Krabbe disease. In: Driscoll P, ed. Genetically-Defined Animal Models of Neurobehavioral Dysfunction. Boston, MA: Birkhauser, 1992:24.
191. Suzuki K. Globoid cell leukodystrophy (Krabbe's disease): update. J Child Neurol 2003; 18:595–603.
192. Suzuki K. The twitcher mouse: a model for Krabbe disease and for experimental therapies. Brain Pathol 1995; 5:249–58.
193. Takakura H, Nakamo C, Kasagi S, et al. Multimodality evoked potentials in progression of metachromatic leukodystrophy. Brain Dev 1985; 7:424–30.
194. Takamoto K, Beppu H, Hirose K, Uono M. Juvenile beta galactosidase deficiency with mental deterioration, dystonic movement, pyramidal symptoms, dysostosis and cherry red spot. Clin Neurol 1980; 20:339–45.
195. Tarugi P, Ballarini G, Bembi B, et al. Niemann–Pick type C disease: mutations of NPC1 gene and evidence of abnormal expression of some mutant alleles in fibroblasts. J Lipid Res 2002; 43:1908–19.
196. Tedeschi G, Bonavita S, Banerjee TK, et al. Diffuse central neuronal involvement in Fabry disease: a proton MRS imaging study. Neurology 1999; 52:1663–7.
197. Teixeira CA, Espinola J, Huo L, et al. Novel mutations in the CLN6 gene causing a variant late infantile neuronal ceroid lipofuscinosis. Hum Mutat 2003; 21:502–8.
198. Topcu M, Tan H, Yalnizoglu D, et al. Evaluation of 36 patients from Turkey with neuronal ceroid lipofuscinosis: clinical, neurophysiological, neuroradiological and histopathologic studies. Turk J Pediatr 2004; 46:1–10.
199. Turazzini M, Beltramello A, Bassi R, et al. Adult onset Krabbe's leukodystrophy: A report of 2 cases. Acta Neurol Scand 1997; 96:413–5.
200. Tyynela J, Palmer DN, Baumann M, Haltia M. Storage of saposins A and D in infantile neuronal ceroid-lipofuscinosis. Fed Eur Biochem Soc 1993; 330:8–12.
201. van der Voorn JP, Kamphorst W, van der Knaap MS, Powers JM. The leukoencephalopathy of infantile GM1 gangliosidosis: oligodendrocytic loss and axonal dysfunction. Acta Neuropathol 2004; 107:539–45.
202. Vanier MT, Millat G. Niemann–Pick disease type C. Clin Genet 2003; 64:269–81.
203. Vanier MT, Rousoon R, Garcia I, et al. Biochemical studies in Niemann–Pick disease. III. In vitro and in vivo assays of sphingomyelin degradation in cultured skin fibroblasts and amniotic fluid cells for the diagnosis of the various forms of the disease. Clin Genet 1985; 27:20–32.
204. Verheijen FW, Palmeri S, Hoogeveen AT, et al. Human placental neuraminidase. Activation, stabilization and association with beta-galactosidase and its protective protein. Eur J Biochem 1985; 149:315–21.
205. Vesa J, Chin MH, Oelgeschlager K, et al. Neuronal ceroid lipofuscinoses are connected at molecular level: interaction of CLN5 protein with CLN2 and CLN3. Mol Biol Cell 2002; 13:2410–20.
206. Vogt H. Familiare amaurotische Idiotie, histologische und histopathologische Studien. Arch Kinderheik 1909; 51: 1–35.
207. Wang AM, Iaonnou YA, Zeidener KM, et al. Generation of a mouse model with a-galactosidase. Am J Hum Genet 1996; 59:A208.
208. Watanabe Y, Akaboshi S, Ishida G, et al. Increased levels of GM2 ganglioside in fibroblasts from a patient with juvenile Niemann–Pick disease type C. Brain Dev 1998; 20:95–7.
209. Watts GF, Mitchell WD, Bending JJ, et al. Cerebrotendinous xanthomatosis: A family study of sterol 27-hydroxylase mutations and pharmacotherapy. QJM 1996; 89:55–63.
210. Weinberg KI. Early use of drastic therapy. N Engl J Med 2005; 352:2124–6 [comment].
211. Weinreb NJ, Charrow J, Andersson HC, et al. Effectiveness of enzyme replacement therapy in 1028 patients with type 1 Gaucher disease after 2 to 5 years of treatment: a report from the Gaucher registry. Am J Med 2002; 113:112–9.
212. Wenger DA. Krabbe disease (globoid cell leukodystrophy). In: Rosenberg RN, Prusiner SB, DiMauro S, Barchi RL, eds. The Molecular and Genetic Basis of Neurological Disease. Boston: Butterworth-Heinemann, 1997:485.
213. Wheeler RB, Sharp JD, Schultz RA, et al. The gene mutated in variant late-infantile neuronal ceroid lipofuscinosis (CLN6) and in nclf mutant mice encodes a novel predicted transmembrane protein. Am J Hum Genet 2002; 70:537–42.
214. Wiegand V, Chang TY, Strauss JF, et al. Transport of plasma membrane-derived cholesterol and the function of Niemann–Pick C1 protein. FASEB J 2003; 17:782–4.
215. Williams RS, Ferrante RJ, Caviness VS Jr. The isolated human cortex. A Golgi analysis of Krabbe's disease. Arch Neurol 1979; 36:134–9.
216. Willner JP, Grabowski GA, Gordon RE, et al. Chronic GM2 gangliosidosis masquerading as atypical Friedreich ataxia: clinical, morphologic and biochemical studies of nine cases. Neurology 1981; 31:787–98.
217. Wisniewski K, Golabek A, Kida E. Classic late-infantile NCL with tripeptidyl-peptidase I deficiency (CLN2). In: Golden J, Harding B, eds. Pathology and Genetics. Developmental Neuropathology. Basel: ISN Neuropath Press, 2004:274–6.
218. Wisniewski K, Golabek A, Kida E. Palmitoyl-protein thioesterase 1 deficiency with granular osmiophilic deposits (CLN1). In: Golden J, Harding B, eds. Pathology and Genetics. Developmental Neuropathology. Basel: ISN Neuropath Press, 2004:271–3.
219. Wisniewski K, Golabek A, Kida E. Rare forms of neuronal ceroid lipofuscinoses. In: Golden J, Harding B, eds. Pathology and Genetics. Developmental Neuropathology. Basel: ISN Neuropath Press, 2004:280–2.
220. Wojtanik KM, Liscum L. The transport of LDL-derived cholesterol to the plasma membrane is defective in NPC1 cells. J Biol Chem 2003; 278:14850–6.
221. Wrobe D, Hensler M, Huettler S, et al. A non-glycosylated and functionally deficient mutant (N215H) of the sphingolipid activator protein B (SAP-B) in a novel case of metachromatic leukodystrophy (MLD). J Inherit Metab Dis 2000; 23:63–76.
222. Yamamoto T, Ninomiya H, Matsumoto M, et al. Genotype-phenotype relationship of Niemann–Pick disease type C: a possible correlation between clinical onset and levels of NPC1 protein in isolated skin fibroblasts. J Med Genet 2000; 37:707–12
223. Yano T, Taniguchi M, Akaboshi S, et al. Accumulation of G M2 ganglioside in Niemann–Pick disease type C. Proc Jpn Acad Series 1996;72.

224. Yoshida K, Oshima A, Sakuraba H, et al. GM1-gangliosidosis in adults. Clinical and Molecular analysis of 16 Japanese patients. Ann Neurol. 1992; 31:328–32.
225. Zeman W, Donahue P, Dyken P, Green J. The neuronal ceroid-lipofuscinoses (Batten-Vogt Syndrome). In: Vinken PJ, Bruyn GW, eds. Handbook of Clinical Neurology. Leukodystrophies and Poliodystrophies. Amsterdam: North-Holland Publishing, 1970; 10:588–687.
226. Zhong N, Moroziewicz DN, Ju W, et al. Heterogeneity of late-infantile neuronal ceroid lipofuscinosis. Genet Med 2000; 2:312–8.
227. Zimran A, Horowitz M. RecTL: a complex allele of the glucocerebrosidase gene associated with a mild clinical course of Gaucher disease. Am J Med Genet 1994; 50: 74–8.
228. Zlotogora J, Bach G, Barak V, Elian E. Metachromatic leukodystrophy in the Habbinite Jews: high frequency in a genetic isolate and screening for heterozygotes. Am J Hum Gen. 1980; 32:663–9.
229. Zlotogora J, Levey-Lahad E, Legum C, et al. Krabbe disease in Isreal. Israel J Med Sci 1991; 27:196–8.

42

Mucolipidoses

Dwight D. Koeberl
Division of Medical Genetics, Duke University, Durham, North Carolina, U.S.A.

INTRODUCTION

First delineated by Spranger and Wiedemann (36) in 1970, the seven or eight entities originally described shared clinical and radiographical features of both the mucopolysaccharidoses (MPSs) (see Chapter 40) and the sphingolipidoses (see Chapter 41); hence, the name *mucolipidosis* was proposed. Excessive storage of lipids as well as complex carbohydrates in many of the mucolipidoses finds its expression in profound ultrastructural changes at the cellular level in both neural and visceral tissues. In the eye, both cornea and neural retina are affected to varying degrees in all these disorders.

The inherited diseases originally classified as mucolipidoses (MLs) are now subdivided according to the specific enzymatic defect (Table 1). The identification of α-neuraminidase deficiency in mucolipidosis type I (ML-I) led to ML-I being renamed *sialidosis.* Two major subtypes of sialidosis are now recognized (27) and designated sialidosis types I and II (39). The only other disorder still classified according to the general terminology, ML, is mucolipidosis IV (ML-IV). As shown in Table 1, two other groups of inherited lysosomal disorders have also been reclassified. The first is known as disorders of glycoprotein degradation and include mannosidosis, fucosidosis, and galactosialidosis. The second group consists of disorders of lysosomal enzyme phosphorylation and localization: I-cell disease [mucolipidosis type II (ML-II)] and pseudo-Hurler polydystrophy [mucolipidosis type III (ML-III)].

SIALIDOSIS (MUCOLIPIDOSIS TYPE I AND MUCOLIPIDOSIS TYPE IV)

Sialidosis

Sialidosis (mucolipidosis type I; MIM #256550) was described by Spranger et al. (36). Additional cases reported in the literature during the ensuing years provided sufficient evidence to distinguish two phenotypic variants, types I and II. However, both

Table 1 Mucolipidoses (MLs) and Selected Disorders of Glycoprotein Degradation

Disorder	Enzymatic and other protein deficiency	Ocular signs
MLs with a deficiency of a single lysosomal enzyme		
Sialidosis I (ML-I)[a]	α-Neuraminidase	Cherry-red spots, loss of visual acuity, punctate corneal opacities
Sialidosis II (ML-I)[b]	α-Neuraminidase	Cherry-red spots, fine corneal opacities
ML-IV	Mucolipin 1	Corneal clouding, retinal degeneraton
Disorders of glycoprotein degradation		
Mannosidosis	α-D-Mannosidase	Spoke-shaped lens opacities
Fucosidosis	α-L-Fucosidase	Venous tortousities
Galactosialidosis	Protective protein/cathepsin A[c]	Cherry-red spots, corneal clouding
Disorders of lysosomal enzyme phosphorylation and localization		
I-cell disease (ML-II)	UDP-*N*-acetylglucosamine: lysosomal enzyme *N*-acetylglucosaminyl-1-phosphotransferase[d]	Corneal opacities
Pseudo-Hurler polydystrophy (ML-III)	UDP-*N*-acetylglucosamine: lysosomal enzyme *N*-acetylglucosaminyl-1-phosphotransferase[d]	Corneal opacities

[a] Cherry-red spot-myoclonus phenotype; onset in second decade of life; normal somatic features.
[b] Onset early in life; dysostosis multiplex and visceromegaly; mental retardation; cherry-red spot in older children.
[c] Defect that leads to deficiencies of both (β-galactosidase and neuraminidase; corneal clouding is found only in the late infantile form).
[d] Required for synthesis of mannose-6-phosphate recognition marker that is essential for targeting of lysosomal enzymes.

of these phenotypes are due to mutations in the *NEU1* gene that encodes neuraminidase.

Sialidosis Type I

The age of onset is variable but usually appears during the second decade in sialidosis type I (MIM #256550), known also as the cherry-red spot-myoclonus syndrome (32). Patients typically present with myoclonus or gait abnormalities (39). There are no skeletal changes or Hurler-like facies, and patients are usually of normal intellect.

Apart from myoclonus, which is usually severe, the major presenting complaint is decreased visual acuity, which may be associated with impaired color vision or night blindness (39). Cherry-red macular spots are present in all cases examined (35). In addition, mild corneal clouding and lens opacities have been reported (14,15).

The biochemical defect is a generalized deficiency of α-neuraminidase, an enzyme that cleaves terminal sialyl linkages in several oligosaccharides and glycoproteins (9,37,40). The enzyme does not hydrolyze this linkage in gangliosides; hence, storage substances that have so far been identified consist of sialic acid-containing oligosaccharides and glycoproteins. Other lysosomal acid hydrolases, including β-galactosidase, are within the normal range of activity. The *NEU1* gene for sialidosis has been mapped to chromosome 6 (6p21), and multiple mutations have been detected in affected patients (39).

Sialidosis Type II

The severe sialidosis type II (MIM #256550) has its onset in early infancy, although congenital as well as juvenile forms have also been described. Similar to sialidosis type I, cherry-red macular spots and myoclonus are the presenting symptoms. In addition, however, this form of sialidosis is accompanied by abnormal somatic features, including coarse facies and other features of dysostosis multiplex (14,15,29).

Joint stiffness, visceromegaly, and mental retardation are frequently seen, although the severity in individual cases is highly variable (11). Tortuosity and saccular aneurysms of conjunctival and retinal blood vessels have also been described (15,35). Death usually occurs during the first or second decade; however, living patients 25 years of age have been reported (29). A high proportion of reported cases are of Japanese origin. The juvenile form of sialidosis type II was initially called Goldberg syndrome (MIM +256540) (16), but this disorder is now classified as galactosialidosis (see the section entitled Galactosialidosis).

Despite the coarse facies and other skeletal changes resembling those found in some of the MPSs, there is no mucopolysacchariduria, nor is there any evidence for storage of glycosaminoglycans (GAGs). The biochemical defect, a deficiency of α-neuraminidase, is similar to that found in sialidosis type I.

Mucolipidosis Type IV

Mucolipidosis type IV (sialolipidosis, MIM #252650, ML-IV) is a lysosomal storage disorder with an autosomal recessive inheritance (2). This disorder was first reported in Israel (8), and although the early cases studied suggested a high frequency among Ashkenazi Jews, several non-Jewish patients have also been described (11,13,33). The true extent of this disorder is difficult to estimate because the presenting manifestations are not always recognized as a distinct clinical entity.

Clinical Features

The clinical spectrum and developmental features of children from 20 Israeli families have been reviewed in detail (2); other cases with similar clinical findings have been reported in the United States (19,31,38).

Psychomotor retardation and visual disturbances during the first year of life are the major presenting signs. Language development during the next few years is severely reduced or nonexistent. However, the patients are not completely devoid of cognitive function. Organomegaly, skeletal abnormalities, and other signs of MPS are absent in ML-IV; however, growth decelerates markedly by two to three years even though food intake is adequate. Facial dysplasia, kyphoscoliosis, and other severe physical changes have been observed in older patients, 21 and 23 years old (31,33). The disorder has a protracted course, and life expectancy may be into the third decade or beyond.

Ocular Manifestations

The most striking presenting sign in virtually all cases of ML-IV is moderate to severe bilateral corneal clouding at birth or in early infancy. The onset of opacities may vary from early infancy to five years of age (2). It remains static in some patients, but in others it may continue to deteriorate or even to improve. The corneal opacification involves mainly the corneal epithelium and anterior stroma and consists of punctate dots extending from the center of the cornea to the periphery (28). There is no corneal edema. The intraocular pressure (IOP) is invariably normal. A prospective natural history study enrolling 22 patients found associated ocular findings (in descending frequency) to include strabismus, corneal erosion, cataract, corneal abnormalities, ocular fundus abnormalities, and ptosis (18).

Although the retina appears normal in most infants, electroretinograms (ERGs) may be severely diminished or extinct (1). Retinal changes are often difficult to evaluate because of the corneal clouding; however, a subnormal (28) or extinguished (31) ERG, involving both the photopic and scotopic components, have been observed in two patients aged 2 and 14 years, respectively. Severe optic atrophy has been observed in several patients (31,33,38).

Apart from corneal and retinal changes, esotropia and photophobia are present in nearly all patients (2). They appear early in the course of the disease.

Transmission electron microscopy (TEM) of the cornea (13,19,28,33) reveals epithelial cells engorged with single-membrane-limited cytoplasmic vacuoles, some of which contain fibrillogranular material, whereas others are optically empty (Fig. 1). The corneal fibroblasts are somewhat distended and contain laminated structures in addition to the single-membrane-limited vacuoles. Bowman layer is normal. The massive involvement of the corneal epithelium, with relative sparing of the keratocytes, is an important feature of ML-IV. Keratoplasty would be of little value because the replacement of donor epithelium by the host would be expected to bring about renewed clouding (19). However, epithelial removal combined with transplantation of healthy conjunctiva in a 28-month-old patient resulted in improved corneal clarity that continued during the one year follow-up period (13).

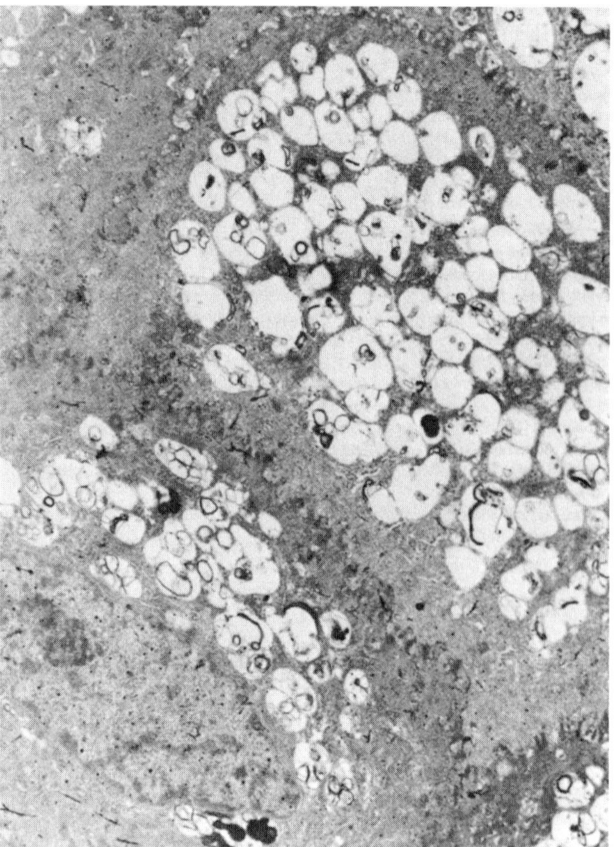

Figure 1 Corneal epithelium in mucolipidosis type IV showing an accumulation of single-membrane-limited vacuoles, most of them optically empty but some of them containing lamellar deposits (×4,600). *Source*: Courtesy of Dr. N. Livni.

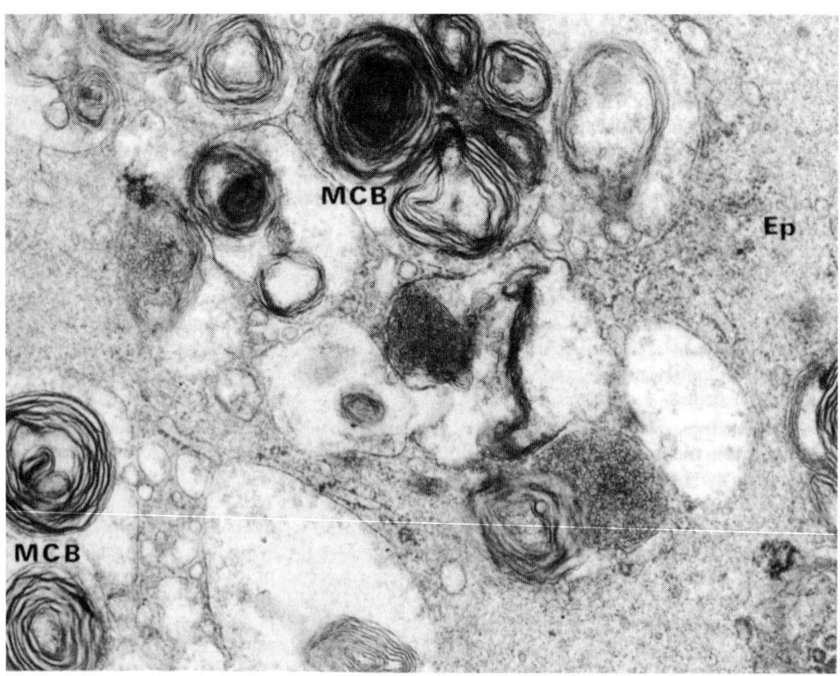

Figure 2 Conjunctival epithelial cell in mucolipidosis type IV filled with single-membrane-limited vacuoles and membranous lamellar bodies (MCBs). Many of the lamellar deposits are contained within the vacuoles (× 26,800). *Abbreviation*: Ep, epithelium. *Source*: From Merin S, Livni N, Berman ER, et al. Mucolipidosis IV: ocular, systemic, and ultrastructural findings. Invest Ophthalmol 1975; 14:437–48.

Striking changes have been noted in the conjunctiva (8,24,33), which provides one of the most reliable tissues for diagnosing this disorder. Epithelial cells as well as fibroblasts are filled with abnormal inclusion bodies similar to those found in the cornea (Fig. 2). The ultrastructural abnormalities are especially prominent in the conjunctival epithelium.

Postmortem examination of an eye from a 23-year-old patient revealed widespread changes, not only in the corneal epithelium and conjunctiva but also in other cells (33). Light microscopy revealed a markedly disorganized and atrophic retina, with loss of photoreceptors together with intraretinal migration of pigment-laden macrophages. TEM revealed two types of storage bodies (membrane-limited vacuoles containing fibrillogranular material and lamellar whorls) in ciliary epithelial cells, Schwann cells, retinal ganglion cells, and vascular endothelial cells. The presence of these characteristic cytoplasmic inclusions is consistent with the storage of GAGs and lipids.

Biochemistry

The basic defect in ML-IV involves the lysosomal storage of a broad spectrum of lipids and GAGs (4). The activities of lysosomal enzymes in leukocytes, plasma, and fibroblasts are within normal limits (8,31,33,38). Those examined include α-fucosidase, β-glucuronidase, β-galactosidase, α-iduronidase, α-mannosidase, hexosaminidases A and B, and sulfatidase. Although the primary storage substances are not known with certainty, excess gangliosides have been detected in brain (38) and in cultured fibroblasts of several patients (5). These have been identified as GM_3 gangliosides and GD_3 gangliosides (Fig. 3). They are classified as hematosides and are normally found mainly in extraneural tissues. In addition, despite a normal excretion of GAGs, there is evidence for an abnormal intracellular metabolism of GAGs in ML-IV.

A specific deficiency of a lysosomal ganglioside sialidase has been demonstrated in cultured fibroblasts of ML-IV patients (6). Measurements of this enzyme activity often yield ambiguous results, however, leaving some doubt about whether this is the primary enzymatic defect (7). Nevertheless, fibroblasts from ML-IV patients consistently accumulate larger amounts of exogenously supplied gangliosides than normal controls (45). This finding provides a basis for diagnosing ML-IV.

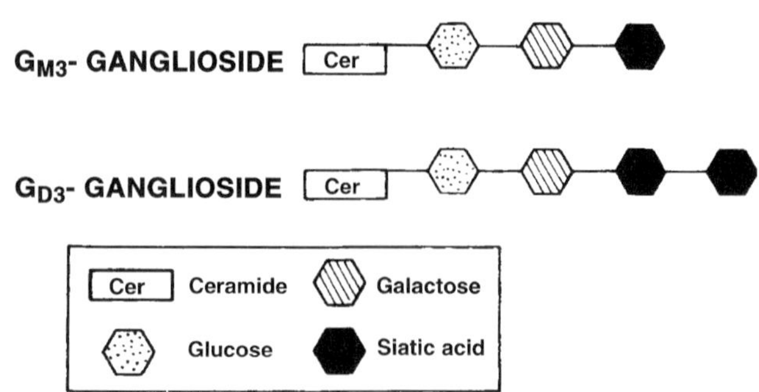

Figure 3 Structural forms of gangliosides accumulating in mucolipidosis type IV.

The basic defect in ML-IV is a mutation in the *MCOLN1* gene on chromosome19 (19p13.2–13.3) that encodes a protein called mucolipin 1 (4). Two mutations account for 95% of Ashkenazi Jewish ML-IV alleles, including an intronic splice-site mutation and an intragenic deletion.

DISORDERS OF GLYCOPROTEIN DEGRADATION

α-Mannosidosis

Clinical Manifestations

At first thought to represent a variant of Hurler syndrome (mucopolysaccharidosis type IH), mannosidosis is recognized clinically by a coarse facies, psychomotor retardation, neural hearing loss, hepatosplenomegaly, gingival hyperplasia, and dysostosis multiplex (39).

Considerable heterogeneity is evident in this autosomal recessive disorder, now classified into two groups: α-mannosidosis type I (MIM #248500) is the severe infantile form with early death, and α-mannosidosis type II is the milder juvenile-adult phenotype with survival into adulthood (39). Vacuolated lymphocytes are present in nearly all cases.

Ocular Manifestations

Ocular findings in α-mannosidosis are distinctive, especially the lenticular lesions, which constitute the major ophthalmological manifestation in both forms of mannosidosis (3,23,30,44). Moreover, the specific appearance of the lens opacity may provide an important tool for distinguishing between the two forms of the disease. A study of 42 cases of mannosidosis (23) showed that the α-mannosidosis type I (severe) form is almost always associated with confluent opacities forming a spokelike pattern in the posterior lens cortex (39,44). This type of opacity is considered pathognomonic for mannosidosis type I by some investigators (Fig. 4). By contrast, only four of 17 patients with mannosidosis type II manifested lenticular changes, and these consisted of punctate opacities scattered randomly throughout the tissue rather than the wheel-like patterns found in α-mannosidosis type I patients.

Other ocular findings are not consistent in all cases of mannosidosis (44). Thus, corneal opacities are occasionally present, whereas fundus changes were noted in only four of 42 patients examined by Letson and Desnick (23). As in all the other MLs and MPSs, the lysosomal nature of the disorder is expressed in the conjunctiva (24,44), where abnormal single-membrane-limited vacuoles containing fibrillogranular material are present in the fibroblasts (Fig. 5). They represent an intralysosomal accumulation of complex carbohydrates. Lipid storage is manifested either in the form of electron-dense globules or as lamellar bodies.

Biochemistry

No mucopolysacchariduria is found in these patients. Instead, there is an increased urinary excretion and tissue accumulation of mannose-rich asparagine-linked oligosaccharides, the principal one having the structure Man(αl→3)-Man(β→4)*N*-acetylglucosamine (1,39). The failure to catabolize oligosaccharides of this type is due to a generalized deficiency of the heat-stable lysosomal acid form of α-mannosidase (20,39).

Another form of this enzyme, a heat-labile cytoplasmic glycosidase with optimum activity at about pH 6, is normal in mannosidosis patients. Most diagnoses have been made using either leukocytes or cultured fibroblasts, with the enzyme assayed at pH 4.0 or lower using substrate concentrations not exceeding 1 mM. Tears are an excellent source of α-mannosidase isoenzymes, in which normal levels are 10-fold higher than in serum or leukocytes. In five proven cases of α-mannosidosis, only about 7% to 20% of normal activity was present in tear fluid (43).

Immunological studies suggest that α-mannosidosis is caused by a defect of a structural gene, leading to the formation of an enzyme with lower, although not totally lacking, affinity for its substrate. Studies with human-mouse and human-Chinese hamster somatic cell hybrids have led to the assignment of the acid α-mannosidase structural gene to chromosome 19 in humans (10), and more recent investigations mapped the gene locus to 19p13.2–q12 (39). The disorder results from a mutation in the *MAN2B1* gene that encodes α-mannosidase class 2B1.

Analysis of the storage products in α-mannosidosis have contributed to our understanding of both the normal pathway(s) of glycoprotein degradation and the aberrant pathways in mannosidosis patients (1). The lysosomal catabolism of glycoproteins containing asparagine-linked oligosaccharides in normal cells proceeds in two steps. First, the polypeptide chain is degraded by the action of endopeptidases (cathepsins), peptidases, and carboxyexopeptidases, resulting in the release of amino acids and asparagine-linked oligosaccharides. The latter are then degraded at the reducing terminus by aspartyl *N*-acetylglucosaminidase and endohexosaminidase and at the nonreducing terminus by exoglycosidases. The lysosomal enzyme α-mannosidase is an exoglycosidase that cleaves α-mannosidic linkages present in complex, hybrid, and high-mannose N-linked oligosaccharides. In the lysosomal storage disease mannosidoses, oligosaccharides with α-linked mannose residues at the non-reducing terminus are not hydrolyzed. As a result, these oligosaccharides accumulate in the tissues and are also excreted in large quantities in the urine.

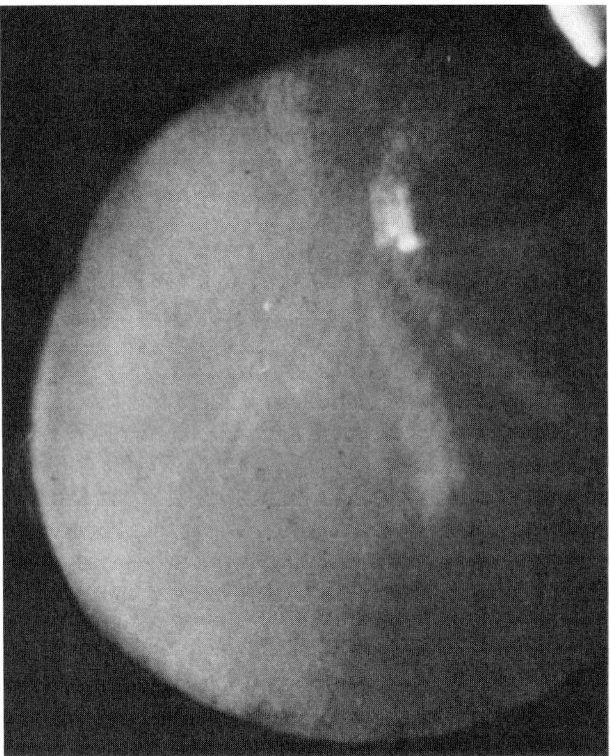

Figure 4 Cataractous lens in mannosidosis as seen by retroillumination with magnification. The opacities, in the form of spokes radiating from a central hub, are composed of small round vacuoles lying at different depths in the lens. *Source*: Courtesy of Dr. A.L. Murphree.

Fucosidosis

Clinical Manifestations

Fucosidosis (MIM +230000) is a rare autosomal recessive disorder characterized by progressive psychomotor retardation, coarse facies, mild dysostosis multiplex, growth retardation, and often but not always mild hepatosplenomegaly and cardiomegaly (39). As in other lysosomal disorders, clinical heterogeneity is also an important feature of fucosidosis. A fatal infantile form, referred to as fucosidosis type I, accounts for about 60% of the patients. The fucosidosis type II phenotype is characterized by psychomotor retardation beginning during the first or second year of life. The other clinical signs are similar to those found in fucosidosis type I, except that angiokeratomatous lesions resembling those in Fabry disease (MIM #301500) are present in fucosidosis type II; moreover, there is longer survival, often to adulthood, and mental retardation appears later than in the fucosidosis type I (25,34).

The major ocular abnormality in fucosidosis is a tortuosity of conjunctival blood vessels, always present in the severe form but not always seen in the adult phenotype (25). The conjunctival blood vessels are dilated and tortuous and have local fusiform and saccular microaneurysms. Similarly, the retinal veins are dilated and tortuous. Corneal opacities are variable and may not be directly related to the disease.

Several specific ultrastructural changes that may be pathognomonic for fucosidosis are found in the conjunctiva by TEM (25). The epithelial cells contain numerous single-membrane-bound inclusion bodies filled with both fibrillogranular and concentric lamellar material (Fig. 6). Conjunctival fibroblasts are distended and contain two types of abnormal storage bodies (Fig. 7). The most abundant appear as clear vacuoles containing delicate reticular material. They are similar in structure to those found in both the epithelium and connective tissue cells of the conjunctiva in the MPSs. The second type of inclusion body is unique to fucosidosis and consists of dark, dense granules with homogeneous matrices. The latter are not generally found in other MLs or in the sphingolipidoses. Two types of membrane-limited vacuoles also accumulate in the endothelial cells of

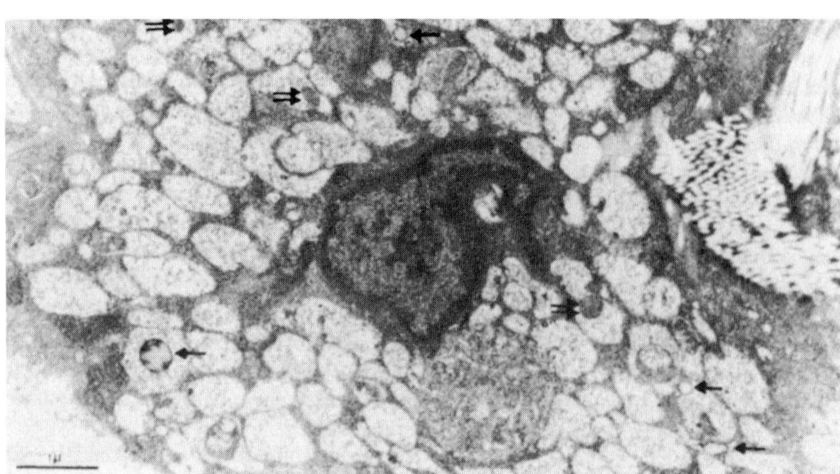

Figure 5 Conjunctival fibroblast in a 25-year-old patient with a mild type of mannosidosis. The cytoplasm is engorged with single-membrane-limited vacuoles containing fibrillogranular material. Opaque lipid deposits (*arrows*) and dense round bodies (*double arrows*) are also found inside the vacuoles (×10,000). *Source*: From Ref. 24.

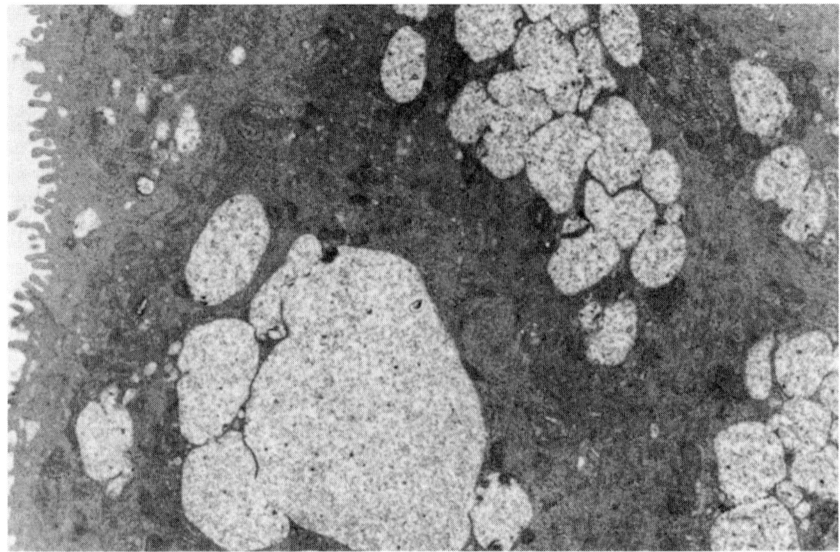

Figure 6 Superficial layer of the conjunctival epithelium in a child with the severe form of fucosidosis. The cytoplasm contains numerous single-membrane-limited vacuoles filled with fibrillogranular material. (× 8,300) *Source*: From Libert I, van Hoof F, Tondeur M. Fucosidosis: ultrastructural study of conjunctiva and skin and enzyme analysis of tears. Invest Ophthalmol 1976; 15:626–39.

the conjunctival capillaries. The most common of these consist of electron-lucent inclusion bodies often containing fine reticular material. The other less frequent type appears as round or oval electron-dense vacuoles. Lamellar material is occasionally present in both types. These changes are probably responsible for the vascular tortuosities in the mild phenotype of fucosidosis. The important and specific changes present in the conjunctiva provide an easily accessible tissue for biopsy and a tissue diagnosis of fucosidosis (25). Cytoplasmic inclusion bodies are also found in conjunctival and corneal epithelium, conjunctival, corneal, and scleral fibroblasts, corneal endothelium, and other ocular tissues, but the lysosomal swelling is not as severe and hence causes no functional impairment.

Biochemistry and Molecular Genetics

In both types of fucosidosis, there is a generalized deficiency of the lysosomal enzyme α-L-fucosidase, with a concomitant accumulation of fucose-containing sphingolipids and oligosaccharides in body tissues. Ultrastructural studies of biopsy specimens from liver reveal foamy cytoplasm in hepatocytes and in Kupffer cells; these cells contain vacuoles that are heterogeneous in appearance, as in conjunctiva described earlier.

The major glycolipid accumulating is the H antigen glycolipid: Fuc(α1→2)Gal(β1→4)*N*-acetyl-glucosamine-α-Gal-ceramide (39). At least 22 other oligosaccharides and asparagine-linked oligosaccharides have also been isolated and identified in urine and tissues of fucosidosis patients. Blood group substances

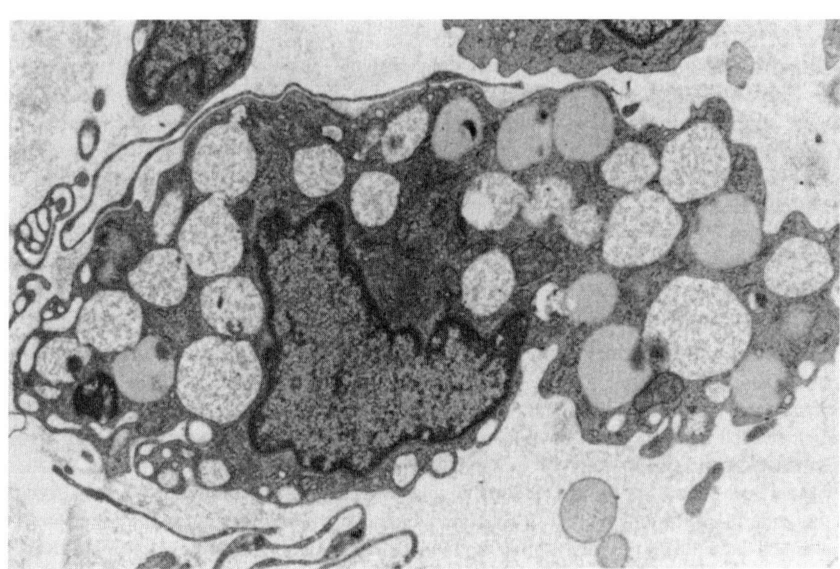

Figure 7 Conjunctival fibroblasts in a child with the severe form of fucosidosis. Two abnormal types of inclusion bodies are present: single-membrane-limited vacuoles filled with fibrillogranular material, and dense inclusion bodies with homogeneous matrix often containing small dense aggregates within (× 9,200). *Source*: From Libert J, van Hoof F, Tondeur M. Fucosidosis: ultrastructural study of conjunctiva and skin and enzyme analysis of tears. Invest Ophthalmol 1976; 15:626–39.

are determined by oligosaccharide chains linked to proteins or lipids. The H, Le^a, and Le^b antigens are determined by the presence of fucosyltransferases. The genotype at these loci may determine the exact nature of the stored material in fucosidosis patients and could in part explain the heterogeneous types of material stored in these patients.

Studies with cDNA clones have established that the lysosomal enzyme α-L-fucosidase is a tetramer composed of four identical 50 kDa subunits (39). A detailed kinetic analysis has revealed four active sites per tetrameric complex. The gene for the enzyme (*FUCA1*) is located on chromosome 1 (1p24).

Galactosialidosis

Clinical Features

Galactosialidosis (MIM +256540) has often been misdiagnosed as either GM_1 gangliosidosis or juvenile-onset sialidosis type II (11,15). It has also been termed the cherry-red spot with dementia syndrome. The finding that this specific phenotype is associated with a combined deficiency of β-galactosidase and α-neuraminidase, as discussed later, has greatly enhanced our understanding of this disorder, now known to be transmitted as an autosomal recessive trait.

Galactosialidosis, like virtually all other inherited lysosomal disorders, is heterogeneous in clinical signs, age of onset, and severity (11). Myoclonus is found in all cases, but other clinical features are variable. The presenting signs in the early infantile form include edema, ascites, skeletal dysplasia, and macular cherry-red spots. A late infantile form that develops after 6 or 12 months of age is characterized by dysostosis multiplex, mild mental retardation, visceromegaly, and macular cherry-red spots. The largest number of patients observed to date have a late juvenile form with onset at any time between infancy and adulthood. These patients, mainly of Japanese origin, have somewhat different presenting signs from those found in the first two phenotypes. The major features of the late juvenile form are skeletal dysplasia, Hurler-like facies, dysmorphism, progressive neurological deterioration, angiokeratomatous rash, corneal clouding, and macular cherry-red spots. Survival is usually into adulthood.

Ocular Manifestations

Macular cherry-red spots are typical of all forms of galactosialidosis. Corneal clouding is observed only in the late infantile type. Detailed histochemical and TEM studies in a 13-year-old patient with this form of galactosialidosis disclosed an extensive loss of ganglion cells and optic atrophy (42). The ganglion cells that remained were swollen and had numerous cytoplasmic inclusion bodies and abnormal accumulations of lipids and proteins that were tentatively characterized as phospholipids and lipofuscinlike substances. Amacrine cells had similar storage substances. Rather unexpectedly, macular cherry-red spots were not observed in this patient before death. Usui et al. (42) reasoned that the cherry-red spots were probably present at an early age, while abnormal storage substances were accumulating. Afterwards they may have faded owing to the extensive loss of ganglion cells. The optic atrophy was considered secondary to ganglion cell death.

Biochemistry and Molecular Genetics

All forms of galactosialidosis are characterized by deficiencies in two lysosomal enzymes, β-galactosidase and α-neuraminidase, which results from a deficiency of protective protein/cathepsin A (11,15). In normal cells this protective protein, which is coded by a locus on chromosome 22, is thought to form a multimolecular aggregate with β-galactosidase and α-neuraminidase that stabilizes the enzymes and prevents their proteolysis. In its absence, the two enzymes may be partially degraded and hence lose their catalytic activity. The disorder was distinguished from GM_1 gangliosidosis on the basis of complementation analyses using somatic cell hybridization, which showed that the two diseases resulted from different gene mutations (11). Other studies using human-mouse somatic cell hybrids have in addition differentiated sialidosis from galactosialidosis; the former results from a mutation on chromosome 10 that encodes the neuraminidase structural gene and the latter from a mutation in a gene on chromosome 20 (20q13.1) that is required for neuraminidase expression (11,29).

DISORDERS OF LYSOSOMAL ENZYME PHOSPHORYLATION AND LOCALIZATION

Two disorders, I-cell disease (ML-II) and pseudo-Hurler polydystrophy (ML-III) are now recognized as belonging to a distinct subgroup of ML (Table 1). They are inherited as autosomal recessive traits, and although closely linked biochemically, with both phenotypes manifesting multiple lysosomal enzyme deficiencies, the clinical features of the two disorders are strikingly different.

Mucolipidosis Type II

Clinical Features

Mucolipidosis II (I-cell disease, MIM #252500, ML-II) is a very severe neurodegenerative disorder having many features in common with mucopolysaccharidosis type IH (Hurler syndrome, MIM #607014). A unique characteristic of ML-II, noted in its first description as a clinical entity, is the presence of inclusion bodies throughout the cytoplasm of fibroblasts from affected individuals (21). The cells were termed inclusion cells (I-cells), and the disorder was subsequently named I-cell disease. Evidence, albeit indirect, for storage of both lipids and complex carbohydrates led to its classification as a mucolipidosis (36). This disorder is characterized by an early onset of psychomotor retardation, craniofacial abnormalities, course facial features, severe skeletal abnormalities, restricted joint movement, visceromegaly, and gingival hyperplasia. There is no mucopolysacchariduria. In the next few years, developmental delay and failure to thrive are prominent features; facial and skeletal changes become more pronounced. Cardiorespiratory complications usually lead to death during the fifth to seventh years, although cases of longer survival have been reported (21).

Ocular Manifestations

Corneal clouding is not always obvious in ML-II; for example, mild opacities consisting of diffuse stromal granularities were seen on slit-lamp examination in only 14 of 35 ML-II patients (26). They generally appear as a late clinical development. This correlates well with ultrastructural changes, since the keratocytes are not extensively swollen and Bowman layer is normal in infants under 8 months of age; moreover, extracellular deposits in the stroma are not observed and the collagen fibrils are regularly arranged. However, the keratocytes are grossly distended by the accumulation of membrane-limited inclusion bodies in older patients (Fig. 8) with ophthalmoscopically visible corneal clouding (26).

As in other MLs and in the MPSs, the genetic defeat is expressed in characteristic ultrastructural changes in the conjunctiva (Fig. 9). Connective tissue cells are ballooned and packed with two types of storage vacuole, single-membrane-limited inclusions with fibrillogranular material similar to those found in the MPSs and membranous lamellar bodies (MCBs) resembling the inclusion bodies in the sphingolipidoses. The severity of the conjunctival abnormalities is not related to the corneal changes, since corneal clouding, even when present, is relatively mild in ML-II.

Mucolipidosis Type III

Clinical Features

Mucolipidosis type III (pseudo-Hurler polydystrophy, MIM #252600, ML-III) is a relatively mild condition, without obvious neurological signs, and compatible with a reasonably long lifespan (21). Onset is usually between two and four years of age. Stiffness of hands and restriction of shoulder movements are among the earliest signs. About 50% of ML-III patients have learning disabilities, and mild mental retardation is thought to be present in all patients. The disease is slowly progressive, and by about six years of age, claw-hand deformities, scoliosis, and short stature are obvious. Progressive destruction of the hip joints develops early, and skeletal dysplasia is also apparent in hands, elbows, and shoulders. Severe pelvic and vertebral changes develop during the second decade of life and are considered characteristic of ML-III; they

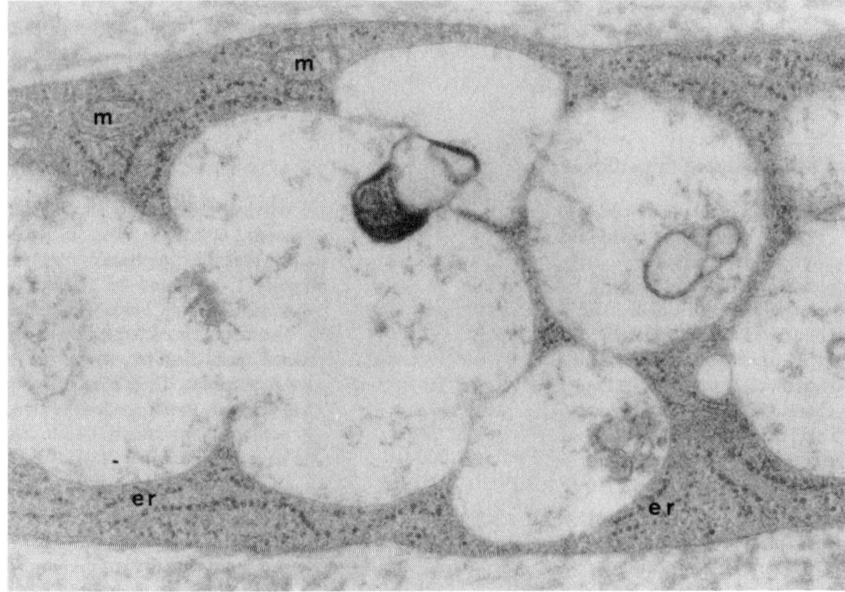

Figure 8 Corneal fibroblasts in mucolipidosis type II are distended by clear single-membrane-limited vacuoles containing fine fibrillogranular material nonhomogeneously dispersed and occasional lamellar whorls. Both the mitochondria (m) and the endoplasmic reticulum (er) are normal in appearance (× 34,000). *Source*: From Ref. 26.

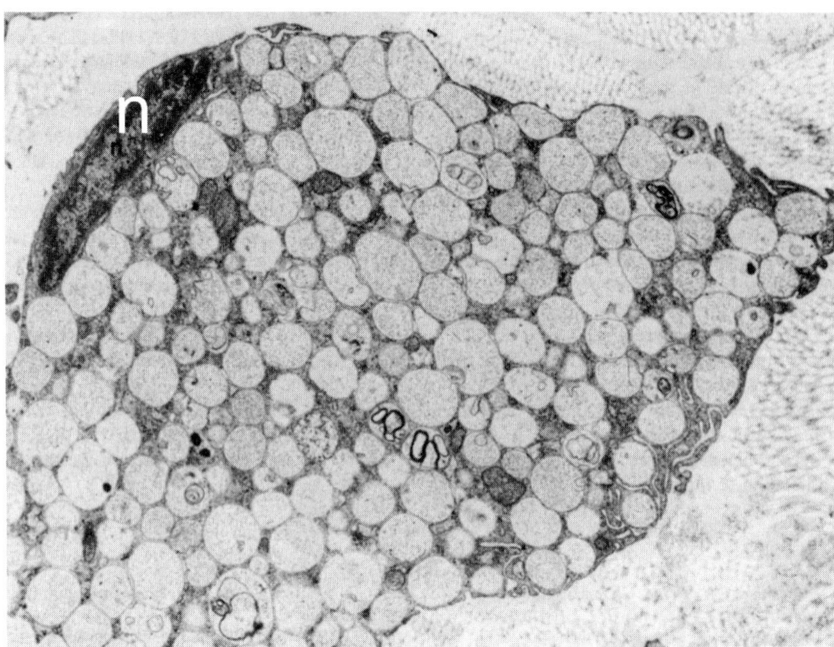

Figure 9 Distended conjunctival fibroblast from a patient with mucolipidosis II. The cell is engorged with single-membrane-limited inclusion bodies containing fine granular material of various density. The nucleus (n) of the fibroblast is displaced to the periphery (× 10,200). *Source*: From Ref. 26.

are more severe in males than in females, for unknown reasons (21). Survival is into the fourth or fifth decade.

Ocular Manifestations

Fine discrete stromal opacities, observable by slit-lamp biomicroscopy and best seen with scleral scatter illumination, are found in virtually all ML-III patients (14,41). The opacities involve both the central and peripheral regions of the cornea but do not interfere with vision. No ultrastructural studies of the cornea are available, but conjunctival biopsies have revealed changes similar, although not completely identical, to those found in ML-II (41). The conjunctival fibroblasts are filled to varying degrees with single-membrane-limited inclusion bodies containing fibrillogranular material. Lamellar inclusions are seen only rarely in the fibroblasts but are abundant in the capillary endothelial cells. The conjunctival epithelium is normal.

There appears to be no obvious relationship between the severity of the ultrastructural changes in the conjunctiva and the degree of corneal clouding in ML-II and ML-III. Conjunctival abnormalities are considered more severe in ML-II than in ML-III, yet corneal clouding, which is a constant feature of ML-III, is either mild or totally absent in ML-II (26). It is curious that despite the similar biochemical defect in these two MLs, the clinical signs in the cornea and the pathological changes in the conjunctiva are distinctly different.

Hyperopic astigmatism, optic disc edema, and surface wrinkling maculopathy have been described in several ML-III patients (41). Visual field defects were found in three of four patients examined; visual acuity is relatively stable despite mild retinopathy.

Biochemistry and Molecular Genetics

Early studies using cultured fibroblasts from ML-II (17) and ML-III (8) patients showed a striking intracellular deficiency of eight or more lysosomal acid hydrolases and a concomitant excess, extracellularly, in the culture medium. Similarly, in patients with these disorders cells of mesenchymal origin show the same pattern of intracellular enzyme deficiency combined with greatly elevated levels of acid hydrolases in serum, body fluids, and urine (22). This is one of the most striking biochemical features of ML-II and ML-III and provides the basis for diagnosis of affected individuals (21). Serum lysosomal enzyme levels in these patients are 10 to 20 times higher than in normal controls; cultured fibroblasts can also be used, and in this case the ratios of extracellular to intracellular enzyme activities are a reliable parameter in the diagnosis.

A key observation by Hickman and Neufeld (17) led to the hypothesis that the major defect in ML-II fibroblasts is the inability to internalize lysosomal enzymes secreted into the medium. These experiments suggested that lysosomal enzymes contain a recognition marker for uptake and transport from the extracellular medium to the lysosomes and that the lysosomal hydrolases from ML-II fibroblasts lacked the required marker. This hypothesis proved to be correct, and a decade or more of investigations in many laboratories has elucidated not only the normal pathway(s) for lysosomal enzyme biogenesis, but also the specific defect in ML-II and ML-III patients.

A detailed summary of the biogenesis of soluble lysosomal acid hydrolases has been presented (21). The major steps in the biosynthesis and transport of lysosomal enzymes are presented here. Lysosomal enzymes, together with many membrane proteins and proteins destined for secretion, are synthesized on endoplasmic reticulum(ER)-bound ribosomes. They contain a specific "signal sequence" that promotes the formation of a complex with a signal recognition particle (SRP). This complex then binds to an SRP and is transported into the lumen of the ER. The signal peptide is then cleaved, and the acid hydrolases are modified in the ER by the addition of high-mannose oligosaccharides. These enzymes are trimmed and modified and are then transferred to the Golgi apparatus for further processing. It is in the cis (or early) Golgi apparatus (12) that many acid hydrolases are specifically modified by the addition of the mannose 6-phosphate (Man-6-P) marker. This addition occurs in two enzymatic steps. The first is the addition of an α-*N*-acetylglucosamine-1-phosphate residue to the 6 position of mannose, resulting in the formation of a phosphodiester intermediate. This step is catalyzed by a lysosomal UDP-*N*-acetylglucosamine; lysosomal enzyme *N*-acetylglucosamine-1-phosphotransferase, the phosphotransferase. The second step involves removal of the *N*-acetylglucosamine residue to expose the Man-6-P marker.

Only acid hydrolases containing the Man-6-P marker can be recognized by specific membrane receptors that direct their transfer to lysosomes. One, which does not require divalent cations for binding activity, is called the cation-independent Man-6-P receptor. The cDNA for this receptor has been cloned, and amino acid sequencing studies indicate a molecular mass of about 270 kDa (12). The second receptor has a smaller mass, 46 kDa, and requires divalent cations; it has also been cloned and sequenced. The cation-independent Man-6-P receptor binds lysomal enzymes, and these complexes are transferred to a prelysosomal compartment thought to be an endosome-like vesicle, in which the Man-6-P-containing lysosomal enzyme is dissociated from the receptors (21). The latter are recycled to the Golgi apparatus, and the acid hydrolases are transported to lysosomes to form primary lysosomes.

In certain cell types, such as fibroblasts, lysosomal enzymes may be internalized from the medium, a process mediated by cation-independent Man-6-P receptors (12). These plasma membrane-associated receptors account for only about 10% to 20% of the total cellular complement of receptors in fibroblasts and are negligible in most other cell types (12). However, it was the discovery of the plasma membrane receptors that led to the identification of a defect in this pathway in ML-II (and, later, in ML-III).

The primary enzymatic defect in all ML-II and ML-III patients is lysosomal UDP-*N*-acetylglucosamine; lysosomal enzyme *N*-acetylglucosamine-1-phosphotransferase, characterized as an enzyme complex of three subunits, $\alpha 2\beta 2\gamma 2$ (21). All other steps in the complex biogenesis of lysosomal enzymes in these patients are normal. The phosphotransferase enzyme can now be assayed in fibroblasts: there is little or no detectable activity in ML-II patients, whereas in ML-III patients, residual activity representing about 2% to 20% of that found in normal fibroblasts has been detected (21). Defects in either of two genes, one encoding the α/β subunits and the other encoding the γ-subunit, underlie the differentiation of patient fibroblasts into either the group A or C complementation groups.

ACKNOWLEDGEMENT

This chapter is a revision of the one originally written by Elaine Berman for the first two editions.

REFERENCES

1. al Daher S, De Gasperi R, Daniel P, et al. The substrate-specificity of human lysosomal alpha-D-mannosidase in relation to genetic alpha-mannosidosis. Biochem J 1991; 277:743–51.
2. Amir N, Zlotogora J, Bach, G. Mucolipidosis type IV: clinical spectrum and natural history. Pediatrics 1987; 79: 953–9.
3. Arbisser AI, Murphree AL, Garcia CA, Howell RR. Ocular findings in mannosidosis. Am J Ophthalmol 1976; 82: 465–71.
4. Bach G. Mucolipidosis type IV. Mol Genet Metab 2001; 73: 197–203.
5. Bach G, Cohen MM, Kohn G. Abnormal ganglioside accumulation in cultured fibroblasts from patients with mucolipidosis IV. Biochem Biophys Res Commun 1975; 66:1483–90.
6. Bach G, Zeigler M, Schaap T, Kohn G. Mucolipidosis type IV: ganglioside sialidase deficiency. Biochem Biophys Res Commun 1979; 90:1341–7.
7. Bargal R, Bach G. Phospholipids accumulation in mucolipidosis IV cultured fibroblasts. J Inherit Metab Dis 1988; 11:144–50.
8. Berman ER, Livni N, Shapira E, et al. Congenital corneal clouding with abnormal systemic storage bodies: a new variant of mucolipidosis. J Pediatr 1974; 84:519–26.
9. Cantz M, Gehler J, Spranger J. Mucolipidosis I: increased sialic acid content and deficiency of an alpha-N-acetylneuraminidase in cultured fibroblasts. Biochem Biophys Res Commun 1977; 74:732–8.
10. Champion MJ, Shows TB. Mannosidosis: assignment of the lysosomal alpha-mannosidase B gene to chromosome 19 in man. Proc Natl Acad Sci U S A 1977; 74:2968–72.
11. D'Azzo A, Andria G, Strisciuglio P, Galjaard H. Galactosialidosis. In: Scriver CR, Beaudet AL, Sly WS, Valle D, eds. The Metabolic and Molecular Bases of Inherited Disease. New York: McGraw-Hill, 2001:3811–26.

12. Dahms NM, Lobel P, Kornfeld S. Mannose 6-phosphate receptors and lysosomal enzyme targeting. J Biol Chem 1989; 264:12115–8.
13. Dangel ME, Bremer DL, Rogers GL. Treatment of corneal opacification in mucolipidosis IV with conjunctival transplantation. Am J Ophthalmol 1985; 99:137–41.
14. Dangel ME, Mauger T. Mucolipidoses. In: Gold DA, Weingeist TA, eds. The Eye in Systemic Disease. Philadelphia: JB Lippincott, 1990:369–72.
15. Deutsch JA, Asbell PA. Sialidosis and galactosialidosis. In: Gold DA, Weingeist TA, eds. The Eye in Systemic Disease. Philadelphia: JB Lippincott, 1990:376–7.
16. Goldberg MF, Cotlier E, Fichenscher LG, et al. Macular cherry-red spot, corneal clouding, and beta-galactosidase deficiency. Clinical, biochemical, and electron microscopic study of a new autosomal recessive storage disease. Arch Intern Med 1971; 128:387–98.
17. Hickman S, Neufeld E. A hypothesis for I-cell disease: Defective hydrolases that do not enter lysosomes. Biochem Biophys Res Commun 1972; 49:992–9.
18. Jeyakumar M, Smith D, Eliott-Smith E, et al. An inducible mouse model of late onset Tay-Sachs disease. Neurobiol Dis 2002; 10:201–10.
19. Kenyon KR, Maumenee IH, Green WR, et al. Mucolipidosis IV. Histopathology of conjunctiva, cornea, and skin. Arch Ophthalmol 1979; 97:1106–11.
20. Kistler JP, Lott IT, Kolodny EH, et al. Mannosidosis. New clinical presentation, enzyme studied, and carbohydrate analysis. Arch Neurol 1977; 34:45–51.
21. Kornfield. S, Sly WS. I-Cell disease and Pseudo-Hurler polydystrophy: disorders of lysosomal enzyme phosphorylation and localization. In: Scriver CR, Beaudet AL, Sly WS, Valle D eds. The Metabolic and Molecular Bases of Inherited Disease. New York: McGraw-Hill, 2001: 3469–82.
22. Kress BC, Miller AL. Urinary lysosomal hydrolases in mucolipidosis II and mucolipidosis III. Biochem J 1979; 177:409–15.
23. Letson RD, Desnick RJ. Punctate lenticular opacities in type II mannosidosis. Am J Ophthalmol 1978; 85:218–24.
24. Libert J. Discussion. Birth Defects 1976; 12:329–30.
25. Libert J. Fucosidosis. In: Gold DA, Weingeist TA, eds. The Eye in Systemic Disease. Philadelphia: JB Lippincott, 1990: 358–60.
26. Libert J, Van Hoof F, Farriaux JP, Toussaint D. Ocular findings in I-cell disease (mucolipidosis type II). Am J Ophthalmol 1977; 83:617–28.
27. Lowden JA, O'Brien JS. Sialidosis: a review of human neuraminidase deficiency. Am J Hum. Genet 1979; 31:1–18.
28. Merin S, Nemet P, Livni N, Lazar M. The cornea in mucolipidosis IV. J Pediatr Ophthalmol 1976; 13:289–95.
29. Mueller OT, Henry WM, Haley LL, et al. Sialidosis and galactosialidosis: chromosomal assignment of two genes associated with neuraminidase-deficiency disorders. Proc Natl Acad Sci U S A 1986; 83:1817–21.
30. Murphree AL, Beaudet AL, Palmer EA, Nichols BL Jr. Cataract in mannosidosis. Birth Defects 1976; 12:319–34.
31. Newell FW, Matalon R, Meyer S. A new mucolipidosis with psychomotor retardation, corneal clouding, and retinal degeneration. Trans Am Ophthalmol Soc 1975; 73: 172–86.
32. O'Brien JS. The cherry red spot-myoclonus syndrome: a newly recognized inherited lysosomal storage disease due to acid neuraminidase deficiency. Clin Genet 1978; 14: 55–60.
33. Riedel KG, Zwaan J, Kenyon KR, et al. Ocular abnormalities in mucolipidosis IV. Am J Ophthalmol 1985; 99:125–36.
34. Snyder RD, Carlow TJ, Ledman J, Wenger DA. Ocular findings in fucosidosis. Birth Defects Orig Artic Ser 1976; 12:241–56.
35. Sogg RL, Steinman L, Rathjen B, et al. Cherry-red spot-myoclonus syndrome. Ophthalmology 1979; 86:1861–74.
36. Spranger JW, Wiedemann HR. The genetic mucolipidoses. Diagnosis and differential diagnosis. Humangenetik 1970; 9:113–39.
37. Swallow DM, Evans L, Stewart G, et al. Sialidosis type 1: cherry red spot-myoclonus syndrome with sialidase deficiency and altered electrophoretic mobility of some enzymes known to be glycoproteins. II. Enzymes studies. Ann Hum Genet 1979; 43:27–35.
38. Tellez-Nagel I, Rapin I, Iwamoto T, et al. Mucolipidosis IV. Clinical, ultrastructural, histochemical, and chemical studies of a case, including a brain biopsy. Arch Neurol 1976; 33:828–35.
39. Thomas GH. Disorders of glycoprotein degradation: α-mannosidosis, β-mannosidosis, fucosidosis, and sialidosis. In: Scriver CR, Beaudet AL, Sly WS, Valle D, eds. The Metabolic and Molecular Bases of Inherited Disease. New York: McGraw-Hill, 2001:3507–33.
40. Thomas GH, Tipton RE, Ch'ien LT, et al. Sialidase (alpha-n-acetyl neuraminidase) deficiency: the enzyme defect in an adult with macular cherry-red spots and myoclonus without dementia. Clin Genet 1978; 13:369–79.
41. Traboulsi EI, Maumenee IH. Ophthalmologic findings in mucolipidosis III (pseudo-Hurler polydystrophy). Am J Ophthalmol 1986; 102:592–7.
42. Usui T, Sawaguchi S, Abe H, et al. Late-infantile type galactosialidosis. Histopathology of the retina and optic nerve. Arch Ophthalmol 1991; 109:542–6.
43. Van Hoof F, Libert J, Aubert-Tulkens G, Serra MV. The assay of lacrimal enzymes and the ultrastructural analysis of conjunctival biopsies: New techniques for the study of inborn lysosomal diseases. Metab Ophthalmol 1977; 1: 165–71.
44. Weiss AH. Mannosidosis. In: Gold DA, Weingeist TA, eds. The Eye in Systemic Disease. Philadelphia: JB Lippincott, 1990:368–9.
45. Zeigler M, Bach G. Internalization of exogenous gangliosides in cultured skin fibroblasts for the diagnosis of mucolipidosis IV. Clin Chim Acta 1986; 157:183–9.

43

Disorders of Amino Acid Metabolism

Dwight D. Koeberl, Sarah Young, and David Millington
Division of Medical Genetics, Duke University, Durham, North Carolina, U.S.A.

Gordon K. Klintworth
Departments of Pathology and Ophthalmology, Duke University, Durham, North Carolina, U.S.A.

DISORDERS OF PHENYLALANINE AND TYROSINE METABOLISM

Of the many genetic disorders that express themselves as specific defects of amino acid metabolism, some, including two of Garrod's four original "inborn errors of metabolism" (albinism, alkaptonuria), produce significant abnormalities in the ocular tissues (92). Several abnormalities in the metabolism of the essential amino acid phenylalanine and its oxidized derivative tyrosine are recognized. From the standpoint of the eye, albinism, alkaptonuria, and tyrosinemia are the most important.

Albinism

The appellation albinism (latin, *albus* = white) embraces a heterogeneous collection of genetically determined conditions typified by decreased melanin pigmentation in the eye and skin (162,166,305,318). Albinism is common and its various forms affect about one in 10,000 births in the United States. An additional 1% to 2% of the population has normal pigmentation, but is heterozygous for a recessive allele for albinism (162). Albinism exemplifies an inherited deficiency of a metabolic product (a partial or total reduction of melanin deposition on melanosomes). Of the various forms of human albinism, some affect all melanins, others only eumelanin. The distribution of the abnormality also varies in different types of albinism, with melanin being deficient in the eye (ocular albinism, OA) or in the most severe forms the skin and hair of the entire body as well as the eyes (oculocutaneous albinism, OCA).

Melanin and Melanogenesis

Albinism has been recognized since antiquity and an understanding of it requires an appreciation of melanogenesis. A review of melanin and its synthesis is beyond the scope of this chapter, so only a few salient points will be stressed. Melanins range in color from brown to black, but not all pigments with these colors are melanin. Eumelanin is a black or brown polymer of high-molecular weight with many quinone groups and a complicated molecular structure. It is insoluble in virtually all solvents, but can be solubilized in 0.1 M sodium dodecyl sulfate and 8 M urea without degrading the proteinaceous components (119). In contrast to the yellow and red phaeomelanins, eumelanin is insoluble in dilute alkali and resistant to degradation by other chemicals. Eumelanin and the phaeomelanins are derived from the same precursors [tyrosine and 3,4-dihydroxyphenylalanine (dopa)] and their synthesis is interrelated, although they are end products of separate metabolic pathways controlled by different genetic loci.

Tyrosinase, a copper-containing oxidase within melanosomes, is encoded by the *TYR* gene on human chromosome 11 (11q14–21). It is believed to mediate two of the metabolic steps between tyrosine and melanin: the oxidation of tyrosine to dopa, and its conversion to dopaquinone (Fig. 1). Much is known about the biosynthetic pathway of melanin in nature and many alleles at different loci on different chromosomes influence it. The regulation of pigmentation is governed at numerous disparate steps. For instance, more than 150 distinct mutations are known to affect pigmentation in the mouse and these involve more than 50 separate genetic loci (120).

Melanosomes form in two ways. Tyrosinase and the structural proteins of melanosomes are synthesized by the ribosomes of the rough endoplasmic reticulum (ER) and then transferred through its cisternae to the Golgi apparatus where the proteins segregate within membrane-limited vesicles. An alternative method of melanosome development takes place in some cells, including the retinal pigment epithelium (RPE), where premelanosomes appear to form in the cisternae of a specialized hydrolase-rich region of the smooth ER (198,211). In such cases the tyrosinase is closely associated with acid phosphatase and other lysosomal enzymes, and although melanin granules in such situations are often designated "melanolysosomes," the melanin is probably not being degraded by the lysosomes.

The stages of melanosome formation have been numbered I–IV. Stage I consists of a spherical membrane-delineated vesicle with tyrosinase activity or filaments with the distinctive melanosomal periodicity. Stage II is an oval organelle with numerous membranous filaments of distinctive periodicity.

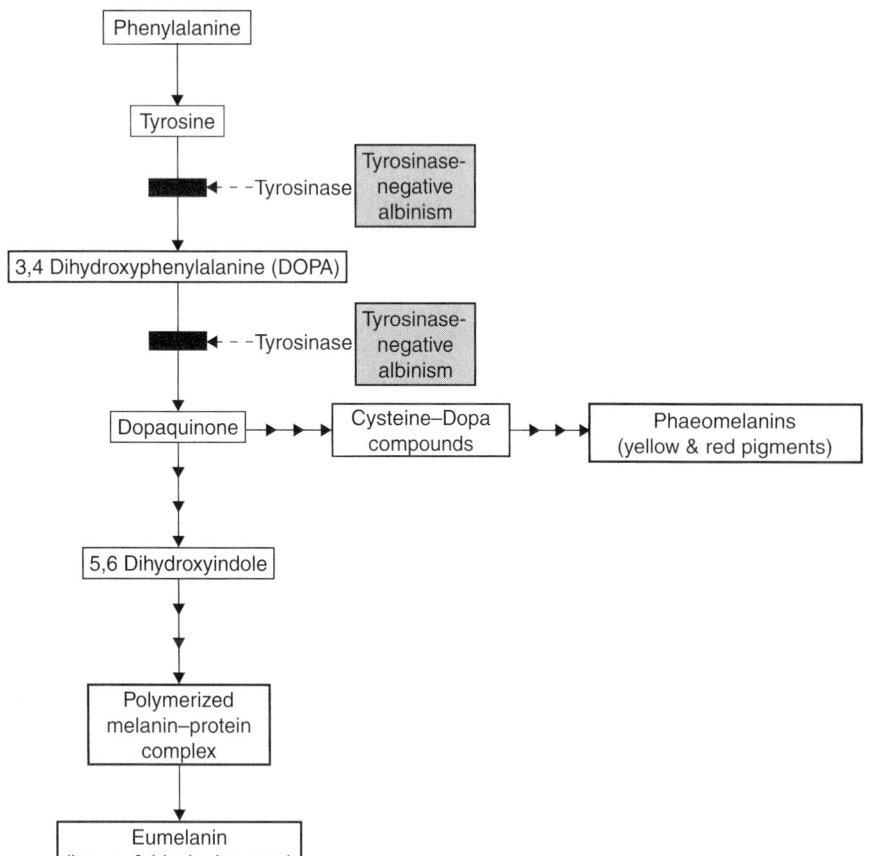

Figure 1 Site of metabolic defect in albinism. *Source*: Modified from Klintworth GK, Landers MB III. The Eye: Structure and Function in Disease. Baltimore: Williams & Wilkins, 1976.

Stage III is a further advancement in which the inner structure is partly obscured by electron-dense material, and stage IV is an electron-opaque oval organelle without discernible internal structure in routine preparations (Fig. 2) (243).

Melanin is synthesized predominantly by melanocytes derived from the neural crest. These cells migrate throughout the embryo and settle in many tissues, including the skin. In the ocular tissues, where melanin is a significant constituent, this pigment is found especially in the eyelids, conjunctiva, and stroma of the iris, ciliary body, and choroid. Melanin is also produced within the eye by another cell population derived embryologically from neuroectoderm (the pigment epithelium of the retina, ciliary body, and iris). The normal melanosomes of the ocular pigmented epithelia range in shape from oval to spherical and tend to be larger than those within the uveal melanocytes.

Classification of Albinism

Albinism is traditionally divided into OCA, in which the melanin deficiency is manifest in both the skin and eyes, and OA in which the skin and hair is clinically of normal color. However, the connotation of OA is a misnomer as melanogenesis is affected in the integument in "ocular" albinism despite the predominant ocular involvement and the apparent lack of participation of the hair and skin (212,213). Hypopigmented skin patches occur in OA and macromelanosomes are present even in clinically unremarkable skin (Figs. 3 and 4) (11–13). Nevertheless, the terms OCA and OA are so entrenched in the literature that authorities on the subject still retain the terms and for that reason they are considered separately in this chapter.

An additional semantic difficulty stems from the traditional, but oversimplified, restriction of the term albinism for congenital heritable hypomelanosis that is apparently limited to the eye, or that involves the eye and integument and in which nystagmus, photophobia, and decreased visual acuity is present. Because of this some disorders with impaired pigmentation, such as the Cross–McKusick–Breen syndrome (MIM %257800) (11,67) and the black locks-albinism-deafness syndrome (MIM 227010) (320), do not fit this strict definition of albinism.

The designation "albinoidism" pertains to hypomelanotic disorders that lack photophobia, nystagmus, and diminished visual acuity (162). Oculocutaneous albinoidism or partial albinism may occur in the Menke disease (X-linked copper malabsorption syndrome; MIM #309400) (see Chapter 48) and the Waardenburg–Klein syndromes (interoculo-iridic-dermato-auditive dysplasia; MIM #148820).

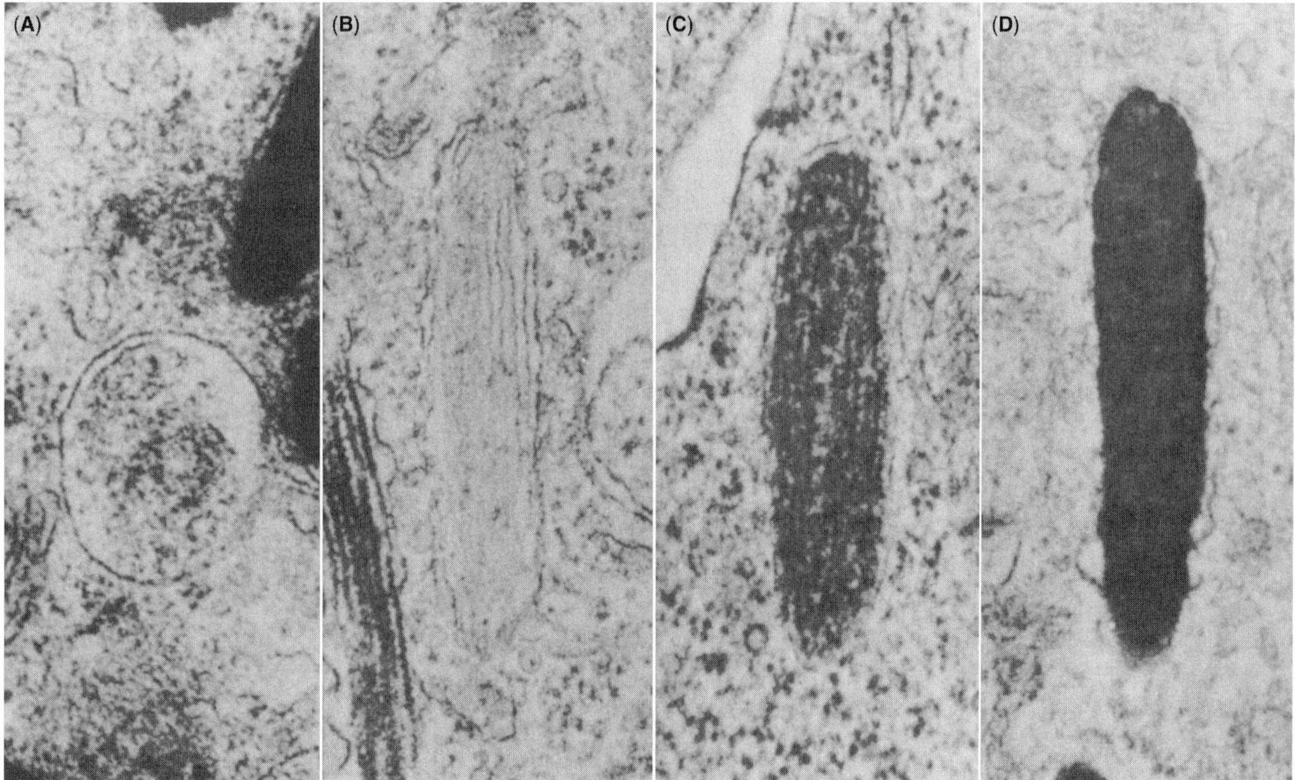

Figure 2 Stages of melanosomes. (**A**) Stage I, (**B**) Stage II, (**C**) Stage III, and (**D**) Stage IV melanosomes. *Source*: From Ref. 243.

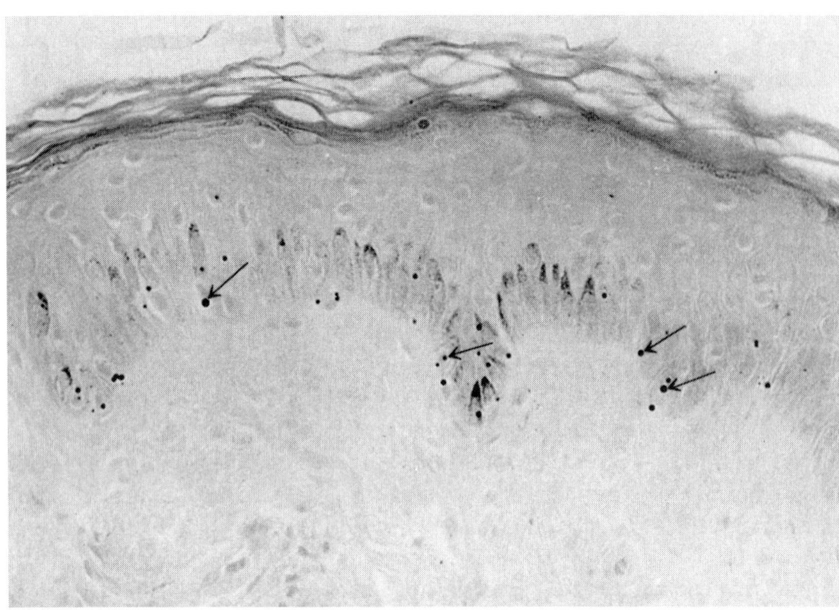

Figure 3 Giant melanin granules (*arrows*) in the basal epidermis of a patient with ocular albinism (Fontana stain, ×430). *Source*: Courtesy of Professor A. Garner.

Albinoidism is also an inconstant finding in acrocephalosyndactyly (Apert syndrome) (exophthalmos, exotropia, optic atrophy, partial ophthalmoplegia and cataracts) (MIM #101200) (188). Other forms of albinoidism include piebaldism (leukism), which may be associated with heterochromia irides (56).

OCA

An absence or diminution of melanin in the skin, hair, and eyes in OCA gives rise to a congenital pink-white skin, snow-white hair, photophobia, nystagmus, and decreased visual acuity.

Ten varieties of OCA can be differentiated on clinical, biochemical, genetic, and morphologic features; however, the identification of the responsible gene defects has provided a genetic classification of OCA, further clarifying the underlying cause of albinism in each entity. An additional four disorders (oculocerebral hypopigmentation/hypopigmentation-microphthalmos/Cross–McKusick–Breen syndrome, albinism with immune deficiency, black locks-albinism-deafness syndrome, and X-linked albinism-deafness syndrome) that have been lumped with OCA in the past are not designated as specific types of

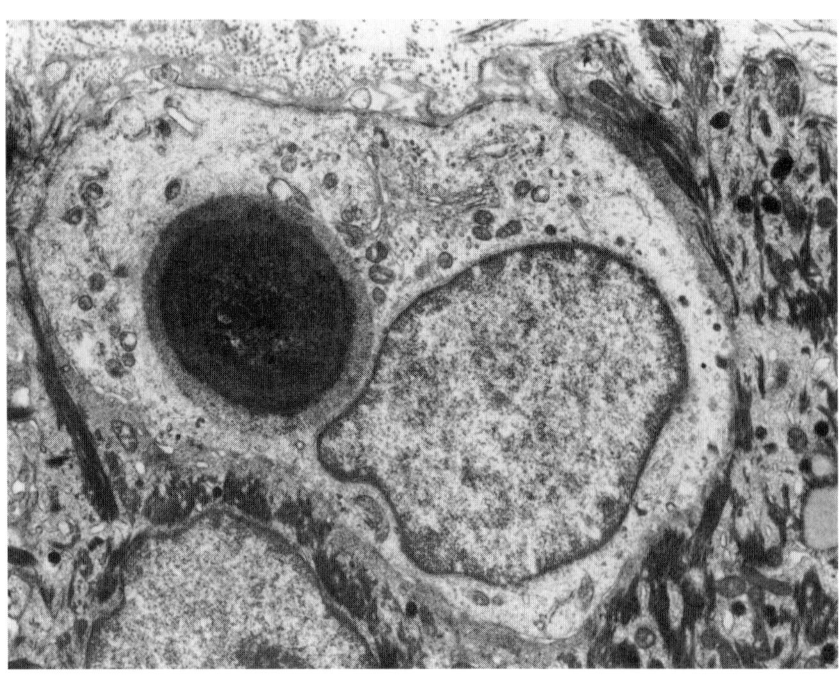

Figure 4 Transmission electron micrograph of giant melanosome in skin of patient with ocular albinism (×86,000). *Source*: Courtesy of Professor A. Garner.

OCA, but are regarded as albinoidism by some investigators.

With the exception of autosomal dominant OCA, other varieties of OCA are inherited as autosomal recessive traits.

Animal models for OCA assisted the finding of human genes for several of these disorders. In several cases mutations involving the human gene were detected after the discovery of the mouse gene. For instance, OCA2 and OCA3 were differentiated following the cloning of the gene for each disorder (52,175,205,246).

The lack of skin pigment predisposes individuals with albinism, especially in the tropics, to sun-induced neoplasms, such as lentigines, solar keratoses, and well-differentiated squamous cell carcinoma (SCC) of the skin, but it is noteworthy that the prevalence of melanomas in albinos is low (162).

OCA Type 1A (OCA1A, Tyrosinase-negative OCA, Imperfect Albinism, MIM #203100). In OCA1A the irides appear gray to blue-gray and the retinal fundus is readily seen through it. The macula is hypoplastic and visual acuity is markedly diminished. Ultraviolet (UV) light causes the hair to become yellow presumably because of its affect on keratin. According to most authorities the melanocytes only contain stage I and II premelanosomes (162), but type IV mature melanosomes have been observed by transmission electron microscopy (TEM) in the iris from a tyrosinase-negative human albino (192).

OCA Type 1B (OCA1B, Yellow Mutant Albinism; MIM #606952). At birth individuals affected with OCA1B, also termed yellow or xanthous albinism, lack pigment at birth, have fair skin, and are indistinguishable from other tyrosinase negative albinos. The condition is common in Amish and some other communities. These albinos eventually develop yellow to yellow-red or yellow-brown hair and yellow-brown irises. Sunlight tans the skin slightly. Stage I, II, and III melanocytes are evident by TEM in affected persons, but the matrices of these organelles, which are unevenly pigmented, resemble phaeomelanosomes (243) and are probably derived from the interaction between dopaquinone and cysteine. Incubation of melanosomes from yellow mutant albinos with L-tyrosine and cysteine intensifies the yellow or red phaeomelanin. Nevocellular nevi in yellow mutant albinos are pigmented.

OCA Type 1B Variants (OCA Type 1C, Platinum Albinism; Minimal Pigment Albinism; Brown Albinism; MIM #606952). At birth, persons suffering from minimal pigment albinism lack pigment in the skin and eye, and their hair is white and their irises are blue. Minimal quantities of pigment accumulate in the iris during the first decade of life. The ultrastructure of cutaneous melanocytes is unremarkable and variations in premelanosomal pigmentation correlate with tyrosinase activity. In contrast to other forms of OCA, the tyrosinase activity may be low in one parent, but normal in the other parent (164).

Albinos in pigmented races with the tyrosinase positive OCA1b have a tan to olive skin, which contains all stages of melanosomes (164). A faint tan develops with sun exposure (163). This has been termed brown albinism, due to the degree of pigment formation, and is undetected in the Caucasian population.

The irises are blue, hazel, or light brown with a punctate and radial translucency (163). The color in their peripheral and central portions may differ. Other ocular abnormalities include an impaired visual acuity, a moderate pendular nystagmus, exotropia, a muted foveal reflex, and reduced retinal pigment. Genetic analysis has demonstrated missense mutations in the *TYR* gene for individuals with brown albinism (162).

In contrast to the white hair of tyrosinase negative albinos, the hair of some albinos have a color reminiscent of platinum. These so-called platinum albinos acquire small quantities of pigment in their eyes and hair during late childhood. The melanosomes in platinum albinism are predominantly of the early stage III variety with faint linear pigmentation of the matrix. Mutation analysis has designated platinum albinism as a form of OCA1B (162).

OCA Type 2 (OCA2, Tyrosinase-Positive Albinism, MIM #203200). OCA2 (formerly called complete perfect albinism) is the most common type of albinism in the United States and in several other countries (162). Because individuals with this variety of albinism form some melanin granules in their hair, skin, and eyes they may appear darker than normal blond Caucasians. In such individuals a red color follows illumination of the fundus (red reflex), but in albinos of heavily pigmented races this may be absent. The presence of some iris pigment imparts a blue, yellow, hazel, or brown color to the eye. Some pigment accumulates with age and cutaneous melanocytes contain abundant stage I to III premelanosomes, but rarely stage IV melanosomes. However, the premelanosomes mature to stage IV on incubation with L-tyrosine. Mutations in the *P* gene cause OCA2 (175,246).

OCA Type 1C (OCA3, Red or Rufous Albinism, MIM #203290). A mahogany-red-brown skin is associated with deep mahogany to sandy red hair in some African-American albinos in the United States and in some albinos in New Guinea. The iris in persons with OCA3 is red-brown in color. OCA3 is caused by mutations in the *TRP1* gene (52,205).

OCA Type 4 (OCA4, Type 4, MIM #606574). OCA4 has recently been defined by mutations in the *MATP* gene (131,209), and it causes approximately 24% of albinism in Japan.

Hermansky–Pudlak Syndrome (OCA Type 6A, Albinism-Hemorrhagic Diathesis, MIM #203300). The Hermansky–Pudlak syndrome consists of the triad of tyrosinase positive OCA, a hemorrhagic diathesis, and a widespread accumulation of a ceroid-like substance. While rare in most parts of the world the gene and heterozygote frequencies for this syndrome are, respectively, 1:12 and 1:6 in a small village in the Valais canton of Switzerland (173).

The epidermal melanocyte population is of normal density and incubation of hairbulbs and epidermis in L-dopa reveals tyrosinase activity (82). Stage I to III melanosomes are found, but stage IV melanosomes are rare. A striking feature of the Hermansky–Pudlak syndrome is the presence of numerous atypical large, irregularly pigmented round melanosomes with spotted pigment that resemble phaeomelanosomes and vacuolated melanocytes (82,173). The giant melanosomes resemble those reported in various hyperpigmented skin lesions (82).

The hemorrhagic diathesis is manifest by a susceptibility to bruises, epistaxis, gingival hemorrhage, hemoptysis, and excessive bleeding after tooth extraction and childbirth. The platelet count is normal, but the function of these cellular elements is defective as a consequence of an impaired storage of normal components of their dense granules (Ca^{++}, nucleotides, amines) (82,173). TEM and fluorescence microscopy have disclosed a lack of dense granules within platelets as well as in the megakaryocytes (173). A ceroid-like substance accumulates in macrophages, lymphocytes, and several other cell types in the oral and intestinal mucosa, lung, liver, kidney, and other organs that become discolored. The ceroid-like substance is also excreted in the urine. Interstitial pulmonary fibrosis is associated with the deposition of this material in alveolar macrophages (289). Pseudomelanosis coli, ulcerative colitis, as well as renal and cardiac failure are frequent manifestations of the condition.

The basic defect in the Hermansky–Pudlak syndrome is poorly understood and, as in many other inherited syndromes, it remains to be determined whether the manifestations reflect different expressions of the same gene or the combined effects of defective closely linked genes. Because the ceroid-like pigment accumulates within lysosomes, the possibility of a deficient lysosomal enzyme has been raised (289). The chromosomal loci for seven human gene defects have been discovered in Hermansky–Pudlasky syndrome, corresponding to specific strains of mutant mice; furthermore, there are 15 strains of Hermansky–Pudlak mice implying that at least eight additional genes could underlie this disorder (Table 1). Mutations in the *HPS1, HPS3, HPS4, HPS5, HPS6, AB3B1, DTNBP1, and BLOC1S3* genes have been identified in patients with Hermansky–Pudlak syndrome.

Chédiak–Higashi Syndrome (MIM #214500). The Chédiak–Higashi syndrome is a rare autosomal recessive disease of childhood characterized by partial OCA; the presence of giant granules in most, but not all, granule-containing cells; a marked susceptibility to recurrent pyogenic infection from an early age; and a hemorrhagic diathesis (17,27,169,282). Subjects with the Chédiak–Higashi syndrome exhibit a peripheral granulocytopenia, defective granulocyte regulation, and intramedullary granulocyte destruction (25). Affected individuals have an accelerated lymphoma-like phase of the disease and death almost invariably occurs during childhood or in early teens from infection, hemorrhage, or malignant lymphomas (291).

This form of partial OCA is of interest to ophthalmologists, as it causes irises that are blue-violet to brown in color, photophobia, nystagmus, decreased retinal pigmentation, and sometimes strabismus. Tissue examinations of the eye have disclosed a diminished amount of pigment within the pigmented epithelia and melanocytes, and an inflammatory cell infiltrate in the choroid, optic nerve, and other ocular structures (31,138,280).

Histologic observations of skin, hair, and eyes have disclosed the basis of the partial albinism to be a clumping of melanosomes and a pigmentary dilution. Some melanosomes are of normal size; others are abnormally large probably as a result of fusion between melanosomes and are apparently not created as giant melanosomes (202). The melanocytes are of normal size and number and contain fully melanized stage IV melanosomes. Such granules are also found in hair follicles (201), RPE, the choroid plexus, as well as in the pia-arachnoid mater covering the CNS (16,312). Despite its rarity the disease has attracted much attention, as reflected by the voluminous bibliography that has accumulated on the subject. Like many other inherited diseases, the Chédiak–Higashi syndrome provides the investigator with an opportunity to study basic mechanisms and functions of tissues, cells, and organelles. This feat is facilitated by the availability of suitable animal models of this disease (227).

Aside from humans, a variety of animal species including mink (174,229) and cattle (229) are known

Table 1 Summary of Types of Albinism

Disorder	Human gene	Chromosomal location	Inheritance	Associated abnormalities	Animal model	Ref.
OCA1A: (tyrosinase-negative albinism; MIM #203100)	*TYR*	11q14–21	AR	Hair color at birth: white	Albino mouse	2,19
OCA1B: (platinum/minimal pigment/brown albinism; MIM #606952)	*TYR*	11q14–21	AR	Hair color at birth: white, blond, light brown	Wistar rat	2,20
OCATS: (temperature-sensitive OCA; MIM #606952)	*TYR*	11q14–21	AR	Hair color at birth: light brown, brown	Siamese cat, Himalayan mouse	2
OOCA2: (tyrosinase-positive albinism; MIM #203200)	*OCA2/P*	15q11.2–q12	AR	Hair color at birth: white, blond, light brown	Pink-eyed dilution mouse	21–24
OCA3: (red/rufous albinism; MIM #203290)	*TRP1*	9q23	AR	Light brown	Brown mouse	25–27
OCA4: (MIM #606574)	*MATP*	5p13.3	AR	White, blond, light brown	Underwhite mouse	28,29
Hermansky–Pudlak syndrome: (MIM #203300)			AR	Variable, including: OCA, bleeding diathesis, pulmonary fibrosis, and colitis	17 mouse models	30,31
Hermansky–Pudlak syndrome type 1: (HPS1; MIM #604982)	*HPS1*	10q23.1	AR	OCA, bleeding diathesis, pulmonary fibrosis, and colitis	Pale ear mouse	32
Hermansky–Pudlak syndrome type 2: (HPS2; MIM #608233)	*HPS2/ ADTB3A/ AP3B1*	5q14.1	AR	OCA, bleeding diathesis	Pearl mouse	33
Hermansky–Pudlak syndrome type 3; (HPS3, MIM *606118)	*HPS3*	3q24	AR	OCA, bleeding diathesis, and colitis	Cocoa mouse	34
Hermansky–Pudlak syndrome type 4 (HPS4; MIM *606682)	*HPS4*	22q11.2–q12.2	AR	OCA, bleeding diathesis, pulmonary fibrosis, and colitis	Light-ear mouse	35
Hermansky–Pudlak syndrome type 5 (HPS5; MIM *607521) Genetics	*HPS5*	11p15–p13	AR	OCA, bleeding diathesis	Ruby eye 2 mouse	36,329
Hermansky–Pudlak syndrome type 6 (HPS6; MIM *607522)	*HPS6*	10q24.32	AR	OCA, bleeding diathesis	Ruby eye mouse	36
Hermansky–Pudlak syndrome type 7 (HPS7; MIM *607145)	*DTNBP1*	6p22.3	AR	OCA, bleeding diathesis		37
Hermansky–Pudlak syndrome type 8 (HPS8)	*BLOC1S3*	19q13	AR	Incomplete OCA, bleeding diathesis		38
Chédiak–Higashi syndrome: (MIM #214500)	*CHS1*	1q34	AR	Severe immune deficiency, OCA (silvery gray hair), bleeding tendency, progressive neurologic defects, and lymphoproliferative syndrome	Beige mouse	39,40

(*Continued*)

Table 1 Summary of Types of Albinism (*Continued*)

Disorder	Human gene	Chromosomal location	Inheritance	Associated abnormalities	Animal model	Ref.
Ocular albinism: (MIM #300500)	*OA1*	Xp22	XR	OCA with pigmented hair	Oa1 knockout mouse	2,41,42
Griscelli syndrome type 1: (GS1; MIM #214450)	*MYO5A*	15q21	AR	Albinism, developmental delay	Ashen mouse	43,44
Griscelli syndrome type 2: (GS2; MIM #607624)	*RAB27A*	15q21	AR	Albinism, hemophagocytic syndrome	Dilute mouse	45
Griscelli syndrome type 3: (GS3; MIM #609227)	*MLPH* or *MYO5A*	2q37 15q21	AR	Albinism		46

Abbreviations: AR, autosomal recessive; XR, X-linked recessive.

to develop the Chédiak–Higashi syndrome. Homology between the syndrome in some of these species has been established (72,228).

Most investigators have failed to demonstrate a reduced amount of lysosomal enzymes in granulocytes from subjects with the Chédiak–Higashi syndrome. Partly because of this the lysosomal defect in this disease has been thought to involve the membrane of the various granules rather than their content (228,311).

The Chédiak–Higashi syndrome has provided insight into such varied phenomena as polymorphonuclear leukocyte (PMN) migration (221,321), bactericidal activity, and the function of platelets (19,33,57). The PMNs of affected individuals manifest impaired chemotaxis and defective lysosomal degranulation following phagocytosis (227). Although most granules in these cells are morphologically normal, some are extremely large (308) and apparently represent secondary lysosomes formed by the fusion of primary granules with ingested or autophagocytosed material rather than enlarged primary granules or multiple fused lysosomes (70). Experimental evidence supports the hypothesis that the abnormalities of PMNs in Chédiak–Higashi syndrome reflect defective microtubules (221).

The giant cytoplasmic inclusions are maintained in culture (26,69) and can be exaggerated by growing fibroblasts from affected subjects for several days after they reach confluence (222).

The discovery of a severe reduction in the levels of elastase in azurophilic granules within PMNs of both humans and mice with the Chédiak–Higashi syndrome suggests that this enzyme may contribute to the killing of certain microorganisms to which patients with the Chédiak–Higashi syndrome are susceptible.

The beige mouse, an animal model of the Chédiak–Higashi syndrome, offers opportunities to investigate the interrelationships between the RPE and the photoreceptors. Using this mutant of the C57 black mouse, Robinson et al. (225) concluded that the primary lysosomes fuse with the enlarged melanin granules. Many cell types, including the RPE, manifest a defective lysosomal degradation of substances ingested by endocytosis (228). By crossbreeding, Robinson and Kuwabara (254) obtained albino-beige mice with giant granules, which should be particularly useful for studying the possible roles of the RPE in the maintenance of photoreceptors and in their recovery from light damage and other injuries. The RPE also contains enlarged granules of variable size and shape (255). Aside from containing structural evidence of melanin, such granules also exhibit acid phosphatase activity, indicating lysosomal activity.

The defect underlying Chédiak–Higashi syndrome affects the *CHS1* gene (165).

Oculocutaneous Albinoidism (Autosomal Dominant Albinism). In the rare autosomal dominant inherited oculocutaneous albinoidism (77), the skin, hair, and eyes contain less melanin than normal. The skin is white to cream and their hair bulbs form melanin from tyrosine. Hair ranges in color from white to yellow or red. The irises are gray to blue, nystagmus is mild or absent, and visual acuity is normal. A defect in melanosomal membranes has been proposed but not confirmed (162).

Oculocerebral Hypopigmentation (Hypopigmentation-Microphthalmos) Syndrome, Cross–McKusick–Breen syndrome, MIM %257800). A unique syndrome was detected in three members of an Amish family with multiple consanguineous marriages from the state of Ohio in the United States (67). This Cross–McKusick–Breen syndrome, named after its discoverers, has been found elsewhere in the United States, as well as in Italy (11) and Uruguay. The syndrome is characterized by retarded growth, tyrosinase negative OCA, impaired cerebral function (athetoid movements and mental retardation), dental defects, and ocular abnormalities (including bilateral microphthalmos with cloudy corneas, iris atrophy, cataracts, and a jerky nystagmus). The fundamental defect in this syndrome remains unknown, but melanosomes are scarce in the skin and small clusters of them in all stages of development have been found in the few melanocytes that are present. Tyrosinemia has been detected in one case, but the significance, if any, of this observation remains to be determined (11).

Griscelli Syndrome Types 1–3 (Albinism with Immune Deficiency; MIM #214450, #607624, #609227). Separate families have been documented with pigment dilution, frequent pyogenic infections, neutropenia, thrombocytopenia, hepatosplenomegaly, and impaired immunity (hypogammaglobulinemia, defective antibody synthesis, impaired delayed hypersensitivity and deficient helper T lymphocytes) (103). Individuals with the Griscelli syndrome have pale skin, sometimes with a tinge of gray, and their hair is silvery-gray. The melanocytes contain unremarkable melanosomes, but lack dendrites that normally transfer melanosomes into the epidermis. This together with a relatively higher number of melanosomes in melanocytes compared to keratinocyte than normal hints at defective melanosome transfer (242). Griscelli syndrome has been classified as types 1–3, with gene defects in the *MYO5A*, *RAB27A*, and *MLPH* or *MYO5A* genes, respectively (Table 1).

Black Locks, Albinism, Deafness Syndrome. At least two kindreds have been documented with a syndrome consisting of congenital sensory deafness, OCA, and some pigmentation. Almost all of the skin and hair lacks melanin pigment, but affected individuals have locks of black hair and brown cutaneous macules. Ocular involvement includes marked nystagmus, poor visual acuity, gray irides, and hyperpigmented and hypopigmented zones on fundoscopy (317).

X-Linked Albinism-Deafness Syndrome. The X-linked albinism-deafness syndrome, which may affect the migration of neural crest-derived precursors of the melanocytes, is characterized by congenital nerve deafness and piebaldness. A linkage analysis together with hybridization studies suggest that the locus for the accountable gene is on the long arm of the X chromosome (Xq26) (259).

Other Possible Types of Albinism. The aforementioned clearly does not reflect the entire story of OCA, as other incompletely characterized varieties of albinism have been documented. Other cases of OCA have been observed in association with microcephaly, hypoplasia of the distal phalanx of several fingers of both hands and agenesis of the distal end of the big toe (41), and infantile neuroaxonal dystrophy (316), but time will tell if these connections are more than fortuitous.

OA

Six types of OA have been documented (192,212, 213,214).

1. Nettleship–Falls or Vogt type of OA (OA type 1)
2. Forsius–Eriksson type of OA (Åland Island Eye Disease, OA type 2)
3. OA cum pigmento (OA type 3)
4. Punctate OA
5. Autosomal dominant OA
6. OA with sensorineural deafness

Four of these varieties of OA (Nettleship–Falls or Vogt Type, Forsius–Eriksson type, OA cum pigmento, and OA with sensorineural deafness) are inherited as X-linked disorders. The other types of OA have autosomal dominant modes of transmission.

Ocular Abinism Type 1 (OA1, Nettleship–Falls or Vogt Type, MIM +300500). OA type 1, the most common variety of OA, is typified by normal or minimally diminished ocular pigmentation, variable degrees of photophobia, horizontal nystagmus, strabismus, impaired visual acuity, and foveal hypoplasia (212,213), but these clinical manifestations vary considerably even within the same sibship (288). A moderately pigmented fundus and lack of iris translucency have been noted in affected Japanese with OA type 1 (114). Female carriers manifest a normal visual acuity, but have an abnormal mosaic pattern of the retinal pigment (288).

Fewer melanosomes than normal and giant melanosomes (up to 12 μm in diameter) are present in the neuroepithelium-derived pigmented epithelia of the eye, as well as within melanocytes and keratinocytes of the skin (114,213,275). Melanocytes of the uvea are lightly pigmented, but macromelanosomes are present in them. Dopa oxidase-positive giant pigment granules are found within melanocytes in the epidermis and dermis, with slate-colored parts of skin having numerous macromelanosomes and hypopigmented areas containing very few granules (213). In black individuals with OA type I, hypomelanotic macules and vitiligo have been observed, although macromelanosomes have not been noted in the hypomelanotic macules, which contain only a few melanosomes (243).

The mutant gene for OA type 1, *OA1* is located at the Xp22.3 locus on the short arm of the X chromosome close to the Xg blood group (112,236).

Ocular Abinism Type 2 (OA2, Forsius–Eriksson Type, Åland Island Eye Disease; MIM %300600). The so-called X-linked OA type 2 was originally reported in 1964 in a family on the Åland Islands (78). This condition is typified by hypopigmentation of the fundus (less severe than in OA type 1), diminished visual acuity, progressive axial myopia (see Chapter 26), astigmatism, nystagmus, foveal hypoplasia, defective dark adaptation, and protanomalous red-green color blindness.

At one time this disorder was regarded as a type of OA, but the skin melanocytes are normal. Also, in contrast to OA type I, female heterozygotes do not manifest mosaic retinal patterns but have a latent nystagmus and mild defects in color discrimination (303). Furthermore, in contradistinction to other forms of OA and OCA, there is no misrouting of the optic pathway (see ophthalmic manifestations of albinism below), and the opticokinetic nystagmus does not resemble that of most albinos. The ocular abnormalities in this X-linked disorder are probably due to a high-grade axial myopia with stretching of the RPE.

Åland Island eye disease differs from congenital stationary night blindness with myopia (also an X-linked recessive disorder) in that the scotopic functions are only moderately affected and the peripheral photopic visual fields are not restricted (303). However, congenital stationary night blindness and Åland Island eye disease may be caused by mutations in the same gene (2).

Linkage studies indicate that the location of the responsible gene is probably in the pericentromeric region of the long arm of the X chromosome (Xq13–q21) (2). An individual with Åland Island eye disease has also expressed a contiguous gene syndrome with features of congenital adrenal hypoplasia, glycerol kinase deficiency, and Duchenne muscular dystrophy (240). Using molecular genetic techniques this deletion has been mapped to the Xp21.3–21.2 portion of the X chromosome (2).

Ocular Abinism Type 3 OA (OA3, OA Cum Pigmento, MIM #203310). Macromelanosomes occur in the skin in darkly pigmented individuals with an X-linked recessive type of OA in which the fundus is often moderately pigmented (212).

Ocular Abinism Type 4 OA (OA4, Punctate Ocular Albinism). A diffuse, fine punctate depigmentation of the iris and RPE have been documented in a woman and two of her children with light-colored skin and hair (22). Other associated abnormalities in this autosomal dominant condition are reduced visual acuity and elevated central cone thresholds. The hairbulb test was positive for tyrosinase.

Autosomal Dominant Ocular Abinism. A predisposition to multiple sun-induced brownish cutaneous spots (lentigines) may be inherited in an autosomal dominant fashion with congenital sensory deafness and vestibular abnormalities (108). In this entity macromelanosomes are detected in the lentigines, but not in the normal skin.

Ocular Albinism with Neural Deafness. Winship and colleagues detected a large Afrikaner kindred in South Africa with an X-linked recessive type of OA and late-onset neural deafness (313).

Nature of Melanosomes in Albinism

In most forms of albinism melanocytes in the skin are present in normal numbers, contain morphologically normal premelanosomes, but lack mature melanosomes. There are usually fewer melanin granules than normal, but Masson–Fontana and Dopa positive giant melanin granules (macromelanosomes, melanin macroglobules) are present in keratinocytes and melanocytes of the skin of most albinos (Hermansky–Pudlak syndrome, Chédiak–Higashi syndrome, OA types 1 and 3, and X-linked OA with deafness) (114,212,213,289) and even in heterozygotes with some types of albinism (OA type 1, and X-linked OA with deafness) (288). Ultrastructurally, macromelanosomes are composed of a dense core and a less profuse surrounding mantle (328). Although absent in the normal skin, such macromelanosomes are present in the lentigines of autosomal dominant albinism as well as in numerous other disorders including neurofibromatosis and xeroderma pigmentosum (202).

The number of giant melanocytic cells is increased in intradermal, compound, and junctional nevi of patients with both tyrosinase negative and tyrosinase positive OCA, and presumably as a reflection of skin sensitivity to UV light, marked solar elastosis surrounds the nevi, even when the lesions are covered by clothing (237).

Pathobiology of Albinism

The basic pathobiology of almost all varieties of albinism is poorly understood. The defect in OCA1A, which is also termed imperfect albinism, is an inability to synthesize tyrosinase. Some forms of tyrosinase-positive albinism are conceivably due to one or more inhibitors of this enzyme. Tyrosinase uses tyrosine as a substrate, and almost any peptide or protein with an exposed tyrosine or phenylalanine residue can function as a competitive inhibitor (120). Indeed, several endogenous melanogenic inhibitors of this enzyme have been purified and partially characterized (120), but such substances have not yet been detected in albinos. Tyrosinase is synthesized in OCA2, but evidence for an inhibitor of this enzyme in OCA2 is lacking (243). Some types of tyrosinase positive albinism may result from an impaired transfer of melanin to cells that normally acquire it like keratinocytes in the skin. The latter mechanism may be involved in Griscelli syndrome (243). Defects in melanosome synthesis can also lead to albinism. Arrested melanosomal development with a partial block in the distal eumelanin pathway has been proposed to occur on the basis of ultrastructural findings in the skin in OCA4 (163). Defective melanosomal membranes may lead to diminished pigmentation, as has been suggested, but not shown, in autosomal dominant OCA7 (162). Pigment dilution due to the presence of fewer melanosomes than normal can account at least in part for the hypopigmentation of the Chédiak–Higashi syndrome. Other potential reasons for albinism include failure of melanocytes to migrate to target tissues or their failure to survive in hypopigmented regions.

Ophthalmic Features of Albinism

The eye is hypopigmented in both OCA and OA. The melanocytes in the conjunctiva, eyelid, iris, ciliary body, choroid, and orbit, and the melanin containing pigment epithelia (of retina, ciliary body, and iris) are hypopigmented. The iris is usually abnormally translucent, light gray to blue in color (but sometimes dark), and is often hypoplastic. Iris pigmentation increases with age in OA. Albinism is manifest clinically in the most severe cases by nystagmus, photophobia, and decreased visual acuity. The severity of these manifestations varies in the different types of albinism and they are most marked in those forms having a marked deficiency of ocular pigment (OCA1A and OCA2, the black locks-albinism-deafness syndrome, and OA1). In the other varieties of albinism individual variations in the ocular abnormalities are conspicuous and in some albinos these are often relatively mild (OCA3, Griscelli syndrome), or absent (autosomal dominant OCA7). In several forms of OCA (OCA1B and OCA2) clinical examination of the translucent iris discloses radial opacities, but such "cartwheeling" is absent in some types of albinism, such as OCA1A.

In OA the melanin in the pigment epithelium of the retina, ciliary body, and iris is absent or severely reduced. In OCA, melanin is usually present in the pigment epithelia of the retina, ciliary body, and iris, although it is diminished in quantity. The paucity of pigment in the RPE and choroid enables the choroidal blood vessels to be visualized with the ophthalmoscope, and illumination of the fundus commonly imparts a red color (red reflex).

Heterozygous females with some types of X-linked OA (OA type 1, X-linked OA with deafness), have a characteristic mosaic pattern of pigmentation in their fundi due to the random inactivation of one X chromosome in each cell during development (Lyon hypothesis) (see Chapter 31) (259). This aids in the recognition of the carrier state and in the clinical diagnosis of X-linked albinism.

The presence of melanin within the eye influences several biological phenomena that separate albinos from individuals with normal melanin pigmentation. These events include a failure of the fovea centralis to develop, the projection of retinal axons from the temporal retina to the contralateral side of the brain, the retinal-light mediated suppression of the synthesis of the pineal gland hormone melatonin, and perhaps anterior chamber angle development.

The albinotic macula is abnormal, owing possibly to the failure of the fovea centralis to develop because of the inability of the RPE to absorb light.

The optic fibers decussate in the optic chiasm in all vertebrates with laterally placed eyes (241). With the appearance of both eyes in a frontal position and the evolution of stereoptic vision, some fibers from the temporal retina project to the brain on the same side as the eye from which they arose. The extent of the uncrossed-over fibers varies in different species. In humans almost half of the axons fail to decussate and those arising in the ganglion cells of the temporal retina normally project to neurons in the CNS on the same side as the eye of origin. However, in virtually all types of human (8,9,28,29,39,54,57,59-63,65,107,161) and animal albinism (64,74,94,95,105,106,108,179, 184,264,265) evaluated an abnormal decussation of the optic tracts has been detected, and nerve fibers from the temporal retina cross to the opposite side of the brain (lateral geniculate body in humans and that site or the optic tectum in animals). The apparent exception to this rule, based on neurophysiologic observations, is OA type 2 but as pointed out above this entity is not really a type of albinism (303). The anomalous decussation of axons in the optic tract of albinos results in an inability to perceive binocular vision. This abnormal decussation has been shown with neurophysiological, morphological, and/or horseradish peroxidase tracer studies (74,162).

At one time the abnormal axonal projections were thought perhaps to be secondary to the loss of a nonmelanin neuronal function of tyrosinase or to a separate mutation in the region of the tyrosinase gene. However, anatomical studies of brains from both tyrosinase negative and tyrosinase positive human albinos have disclosed that the anomalous decussations are independent of the type of albinism (104,107). Several investigators have postulated that the anomalous chiasmatic decussation is a sequel to any defect that results in an absence of pigment in the developing optic cup during the critical stage of ontogeny when optic cup neurons normally become programmed to approach targets within the growing brain (162). But the development of abnormal retino-geniculo-cortical pathways is apparently not specific for the albino state, as it has been observed in both homozygous albino cats and in normally pigmented cats carrying a recessive allele for albinism (179).

Stimulation of the retina by light normally suppresses melatonin synthesis by the pineal gland in rats. Eye pigmentation enhances this reaction, but does not seem to be the critical factor in determining the sensitivity of the rat's pineal gland to retinal photic stimulation (186). Light also suppresses melatonin production by the pineal gland in albino rats, but at higher levels of irradiance than needed for pigmented rats.

Anterior chamber angle imperfections of the Axenfeld type have been documented in too many cases of albinism to be considered a coincidence (21,30,111,114,183,249,302). This developmental anomaly is not related to the type of albinism or to the chromosomal location of the mutant gene. It has been associated with OA (114,249,302), as well as OCA1 (183) and OCA2 (162). Presumably a deficiency of melanin in the developing eye influences significantly the formation of the anterior chamber.

Impaired Hearing in Albinism

Although hearing is usually only mildly affected in albinism, sensory deafness is a prominent feature of some types of albinism (X-linked albinism-deafness syndrome, black locks-albinism-deafness syndrome, OA with late-onset sensorineural deafness) (313) and certain forms of albinoidism (162). The impairment of hearing in albinism is probably not a chance association, but the reason some forms of albinism are more prone to sensory deafness remains to be determined. Melanin is a normal constituent of the inner ear and is believed to protect it from the traumatic effect of noise. Also, as in the visual system, melanin normally influences the neuronal decussation of auditory neurons. In OCA the decussation of nerve fibers from the cochlea is reduced or absent at the level of the superior olive (162). The otic abnormalities in albinism are reviewed by Witkop and colleagues (319).

Alkaptonuria (Ochronosis)

Alkaptonuria (MIM #203500), inherited as an autosomal recessive trait, results from a mutation in the *HGD* gene, which encodes homogentisate 1,2-dioxygenase, an enzyme that exists primarily in the kidney and liver and which oxidizes homogentisic acid (172). Homogentisic acid is an intermediate compound in the metabolic conversion of tyrosine to maleylacetoacetic acid, the latter in turn, being oxidized through the citric acid cycle to yield energy (Fig. 5). A deficiency of homogentisic acid oxidase results in an abnormal accumulation of homogentisic acid, which becomes oxidized to by-products that polymerize to a melanin-like pigment. Because it is rapidly excreted in the urine, the serum levels of homogentisic acid are usually not elevated. The urine is dark or turns dark on standing in affected individuals and the presence of homogentisic aciduria is diagnostic, even in infancy. The condition is often detected later in life, when the progressive deposition of blackish pigment in connective tissue occurs, especially in the cartilage of the nose, ears, and joints.

The most striking ocular abnormalities involve the sclera and peripheral cornea (4,10,13,34,68,81,91, 113,149,225,256,257,260,272,276,277,314), and several reports document microscopic examinations of the ocular tissue in this disease (3,10,68,256,257,272). Triangular-shaped patches of brownish-black scleral pigmentation develop in both eyes midway between the margin of the cornea and the insertions of the horizontal rectus muscles. These lesions usually become evident during the third decade of life. The sclera is pigmented and frequently needs to be bleached to evaluate the underlying tissue. Documented abnormalities include abnormal elastic fibers, loss of cellularity, and the presence of pigment-containing cells in the region of the lateral and medial rectus muscle insertions. Subepithelial pigmented globules that resemble oil drops have been noted near the corneoscleral limbus, and the episclera may contain lesions that resemble pigmented pingueculae. The scleral pigmentation is of practical importance to the ophthalmologist, as it needs to be differentiated from a transscleral extension of a melanoma. Indeed, an only eye has been enucleated from a patient due to such a misdiagnosis (276). A similar scleral pigmentation can occur as an occupational hazard after prolonged ocular exposure to hydroquinones or quinines (5,197). Such exogenous ochronosis can also blacken the skin after the oral or intramuscular administration of quinine and other antimalarial drugs (32) or after the topical treatment of leg ulcers with phenol or the topical use of hydroquinone-containing bleaching creams by black people (128,238). It is noteworthy that these exogenously-induced forms of ochronotic skin pigmentation manifest morphologic similarities to those that accompany alkaptonuria (32,128,238).

A biochemical diagnosis of alkaptonuria relies upon the detection of elevated levels of homogentisic acid in urine using gas chromatography/mass spectrometry or high-performance liquid chromatography (172). Other methods, such as the Benedict sugar reagent or Brigg test lack specificity for homogentisic acid. Darkening of patient urine incubated at room temperature in a specimen cup or wet diaper will occur if the urine is alkaline, which provides a simple office-based screening test.

Treatment of alkaptonuria has been advanced through the development of nitisinone (Orfadin), an inhibitor of 4-dydroxyphenylpyruvic acid

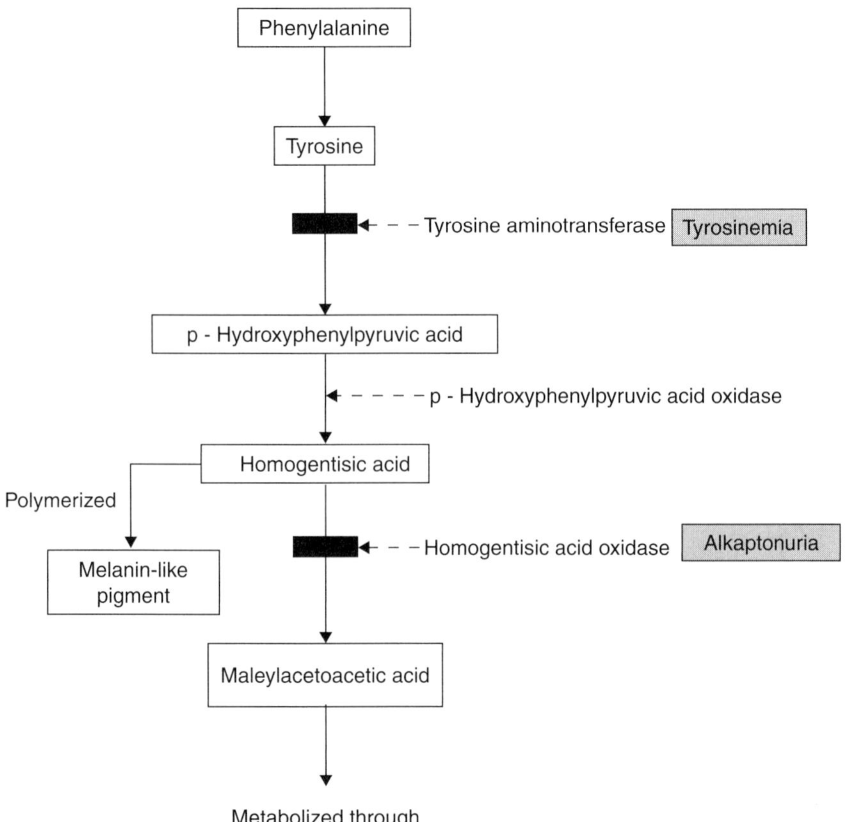

Figure 5 Site of metabolic defect in alkaptonuria and tyrosinemia. *Source*: Reproduced from Klintworth GK, Landers MB III. The Eye: Structure and Function in Disease. Baltimore: Williams & Wilkins, 1976.

dioxygenase (the pentultimate step in homogentisic acid synthesis). Nitisinone effectively reduced homogentisic acid excretion and reduced joint pain in a series of alkaptonuric subjects (239,286). Potential side effects include secondary tyrosinemia; however, no corneal toxicity was detected during a pilot study of three months duration (286).

Tyrosinemia

Tyrosinemia and tyrosinuria are manifestations of several metabolic disorders and the two main types of tyrosinemia have an autosomal recessive mode of inheritance (98,199).

Tyrosinemia Type I (Tyrosinosis, Congenital Tyrosinosis, Hepatorenal Tyrosinemia, Fumarylacetoacetate Hydrolase Deficiency, MIM #276700). Tyrosinemia type I occurs as a consequence of a defect in tyrosine catabolism caused by a mutation in the *FAH* gene on human chromosome 15 (15q23–q25) resulting in a deficiency of fumarylacetoacetate hydrolase. This leads to elevated levels of fumarylacetoacetate and maleylacetoacetate and the formation of succinylacetoacetate and succinylacetone. Succinylacetone has toxic effects on the kidney and liver, and the acute and chronic manifestations of tyrosinemia type I include liver failure and renal Fanconi syndrome. Plasma tyrosine elevations are insufficient to cause tyrosine deposition in the cornea; hence, eye involvement is absent in tyrosinemia type I.

Tyrosinemia Type II [Richner–Hanhart Syndrome, Tyrosinosis (Oregon), MIM +276600]. In tyrosinemia type II tyrosine accumulates in the blood due to the deficiency of the liver enzyme tyrosine aminotransferase (Fig. 5) (159). The *TAT* gene encoding for this enzyme, which converts tyrosine to p-hydroxyphenylpyruvic acid, is located on human chromosome 16 (16q22.1–q22.3) (15). The deficiency of this catabolic enzyme of tyrosine results in markedly elevated plasma tyrosine and this is followed by a rise in tyrosine metabolites in the urine.

The high-plasma tyrosine results in a distinct syndrome with prominent ocular and cutaneous manifestations (23,36,38,42,53,79,99,100,124,136,285). Tyrosine crystallizes in the cornea, producing photophobia with shallow dendritic corneal erosions that resemble herpetic keratitis, and sometimes a corneal epithelial proliferation. In the epidermis of the palms and soles, tyrosine leads to erosions, crusting, and then punctate hyperkeratotic lesions. Mental retardation occurs in approximately 50% of the patients with this disorder. It is important for clinicians to make an early diagnosis as the severity of tyrosinemia can be diminished by a dietary restriction of phenylalanine and tyrosine and of proteins containing them (199,210).

Corneal crystals are not specific for tyrosinemia type II, as they have been observed as a temporary phenomenon in a neonate with tyrosinemia due to other causes. For example, transient neonatal tyrosinemia is relatively common in infants that are premature or ingest a high-protein diet or both (72).

Tyrosinemia type II occurs in mink (44,45,53,101) and dogs (170) and a disorder with almost identical features can be produced in rats by feeding them a high-tyrosine, low-protein diet (37,38,96,250,253). When tyrosinemia is reproduced in young rats by a high-tyrosine diet, pinpoint corneal epithelial opacities evolve into larger ones resembling snowflakes. The earliest morphologic abnormality occurs in the epithelium, where birefringent crystals are evident in alcohol-fixed and fresh tissue (38). Tyrosine crystals dissolve during tissue processing and in TEM micrographs needle-shaped lucent areas traverse the corneal epithelial cells at sites where crystals were presumably originally located. Epithelial lesions in the cornea are followed by a prominent infiltration of PMNs and blood vessels. In the animal model, the cornea, which initially becomes opaque in the axial region, regains its transparency spontaneously with time. The tyrosine-induced keratopathy in rats can almost be prevented by the induction of tyrosine-aminotransferase with adrenal corticosteroids (55) or by decreasing the PMN infiltrate with cyclophosphamide (253).

Biochemical detection of tyrosinemia type II relies upon the demonstration of elevated tyrosine in plasma amino acids, and elevated tyrosine metabolites in urine organic acids (199). Succinylacetone is absent in the urine of patients with tyrosinemia type II, differentiating it from tyrosinemia type I. While enzyme analysis of homogenized liver confirms tyrosine aminotransferase deficiency, a liver biopsy is infrequently performed to confirm the diagnosis. Mutation detection presents an alternative approach to confirming the diagnosis, especially in the Italian population where a common mutation is found (130,207). Tyrosinemia type II has been detected by tandem mass spectrometry newborn screening, while tyrosinemia type I is missed by screening for elevated blood tyrosine levels (309).

DISORDERS OF SULFUR-CONTAINING AMINO ACIDS

Homocystinuria

The activity of the enzyme cystathionine β-synthase is markedly reduced in homocystinuria (MIM +236200), an autosomal recessive disorder with numerous phenotypical similarities to the Marfan syndrome (76). This enzyme catalyzes an important step in the metabolism of methionine to cysteine (Fig. 6). Pyridoxine-responsive and nonresponsive varieties of homocystinuria are recognized (160) and the mutant alleles accountable for both types are localized to the *CBS* gene on the long arm of chromosome 21 (21q22.3) (Table 2) (204).

Cystathionine β-synthetase requires pyridoxal-5′-phosphate as a cofactor and in pyridoxine responsive homocystinuric individuals the mutant synthase has a markedly reduced affinity for both its coenzyme and cosubstrates (L-homocysteine and L-serine) and is much more thermolabile than the normal enzyme. The molecular abnormality in the pyridoxine-responsive mutant enzyme seems to be in the apoenzyme (catalytically inactive enzyme lacking its cofactor), which impairs coenzyme binding. This results in a reduced total enzyme activity by reducing its holoenzyme (catalytically active enzyme-coenzyme complex) formation and by accelerating apoenzyme degradation. Pharmacologic amounts of pyridoxine presumably increase holoenzyme formation modestly, thereby enhancing catalytic activity and slowing apoenzyme turnover (160).

Detection of homocystinuria hinges upon the demonstration of elevated total homocysteine in plasma, which is not detected by routine methods for physiologic amino acid analysis. In both forms of homocystinuria,

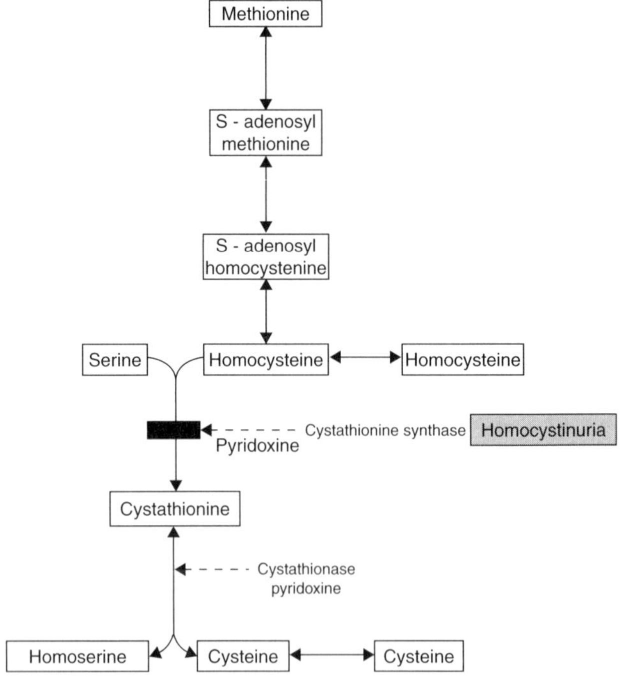

Figure 6 Site of metabolic defect in homocystinuria. *Source*: Reproduced from Klintworth GK, Landers MB III. The Eye: Structure and Function in Disease. Baltimore: Williams & Wilkins, 1976.

Table 2 Amino Acidopathies Featuring Ocular Involvement

Disease	Gene	Biochemical detection	Common mutation (frequency)	Refs.
Alkaptonuria	*HGD*	Urine homogentisic acid	No common mutation	
Tyrosinemia type II	*TAT*	Plasma tyrosine, absence of urine succinylacetone	*R57X* (common in Italian population)	189
Homocystinuria	*CBS*	Plasma homocysteine and methionine	Pyridoxine responsive: 833T>C (29% United Kingdom); pyridoxine resistant: 919G>A (21% United Kingdom/ 71% Ireland)	195,196
Homocystinemia/ methylmalonic aciduria (cblC)	*MMACHC*	Plasma homocysteine, urine methylmalonic acid	271dupA(40%)	197
Cystinosis	*CTNS*	Leukocyte cystine	57 kbp deletion (70% Northern European alleles)	198
Sulfite oxidase deficiency	*SUOX*	Urine S-sulfocysteine	No common mutation	
Molybdenum cofactor deficiency	*MOCS1* and *MOCS2*	Urine S-sulfocysteine	No common mutation	199
Chorioretinal gyrate atrophy	*OAT*	Plasma ornithine	No common mutation	
Familial hyperlysinemia	*AASS*	Plasma lysine/ saccharopine	No common mutation	200
Lowe syndrome	*OCRL*	Urine amino aciduria	No common mutation	
Canavan disease	*ASPA*	Urine/plasma N-aspartic acid	854A>C (85% Ashkenazic); 914C>A (60% European non-Jewish)	

methionine, homocystine, and homocysteine levels are elevated in the serum, excess sulfur-containing amino acids are excreted in the urine, and a cyanide-nitroprusside test of the urine is positive (115). However, confirmation of homocystinuria requires specific analysis of total plasma homocysteine; furthermore, urine organic acid analysis should be done to pursue defects of cobalamin (vitamin B12) metabolism that cause combined homocystinuria and methylmalonic acidemia [methylmalonic acidemia types C (cblC), D (cblD), and F (cblF)]. Newborn screening for homocystinuria has detected affected infants with elevated methionine, although milder forms including pyridoxine-responsive homocystinuria have been missed (204,208,309). Cystathionine synthetase activity in cultured skin fibroblasts is negligible and this activity may increase only slightly with pyridoxine therapy (115).

Ocular manifestations of homocystinuria include subluxated lenses, spherophakia, and high myopia (35,66,178). Ectopia lentis is common and is frequently the presenting clinical manifestation of homocystinuria, with the lens being dislocated usually downward, often into the anterior chamber, and its forward displacement may occlude the pupil and produce pupillary block glaucoma (66,115,148). Occasionally the spherophakic lens becomes cataractous. A single case report documents bilateral band keratopathy decades after bilateral intracapsular cataract extractions (284). Retinal detachment is common even in the absence of cataract surgery, and the globe is often elongated and myopic. Peripheral cystoid degeneration of the retina is marked and evident at an earlier age than usual.

Another important expression in homocystinuria of practical significance to ophthalmologists is the frequent tendency to thrombosis (about 50% of cases) (178). Thromboembolism is a potential postoperative complication of procedures to extract a displaced lens or to treat retinal detachment. Thrombi may develop at a young age in veins (such as the common iliac and deep leg veins) as well as in intermediate-sized arteries throughout the body, including those of the eye, such as the central retinal artery. The thrombotic tendency may lead to embolic complications. Thromboembolic occlusions of retinal vessels may even be the presenting manifestation of the disorder (300).

The thrombotic tendency in individuals with homocystinuria probably results from both platelet activation and abnormalities in blood coagulation. The plasma level of several proteins involved in blood coagulation (antithrombin III, factor VII, protein C antigen) may be lower than normal in homocystinuria (20,231). Evidence of platelet activation (such as an elevated serum β-thromboglobulin) is evident in some cases. These abnormalities may return to normal during pyridoxine therapy and, while the essence of these changes remains unsure, their amelioration during treatment implies that the disordered transsulfuration of homocystinuria affects the production or activity of some liver-dependent coagulation factors (231,204,223,263,274,327). In the pyridoxine-responsive patient, general anesthesia is not hazardous if platelet function can be controlled by the vitamin (115).

How homocystinuria with its autosomal recessive mode of inheritance causes its diverse manifestations remains unknown, but a morphologic explanation for the tendency of the lens to dislocate exists in the region of the zonules and ciliary body. The ciliary body is often small and has been variably interpreted as underdeveloped or atrophic. Deficient zonules recoil onto a markedly thickened basal lamina of the nonpigmented ciliary epithelium (122,247) (Fig. 7). A thickening of this basal lamina is not specific for homocystinuria and also occurs in the Marfan syndrome and Weill–Marchesani syndromes. As cysteine is a normal constituent of zonules (322), a defect in the metabolism of this amino acid may be significant in the genesis of the abnormal zonules. Decreased collagen cross-links have been detected in skin biopsies from 3 patients (150). Intriguingly, fibrillin-1 was aberrantly folded and susceptible to proteolysis when incubated with high-concentration homocysteine, revealing a link to the defective protein implicated in Marfan syndrome (129).

Defects of cobalamin metabolism are detected by combined homocystinuria/methylmalonic aciduria, and eye involvement has been associated with the cblC type including retinal hemorrhages, optic atrophy, and nystagmus with darkly pigmented fundi and sclerotic retinal vessels (75,80,235). The gene defect underlying cblC involves *MMACHC* on chromosome 1p, and a common mutation (271dupA) accounted for 40% of alleles (Table 2) (177). Treatment with hydroxycobalamin and carnitine supplementation, sometimes accompanied by betaine and/or folic acid, has only partially corrected the associated biochemical abnormalities (75,258).

Cystinosis

Another rare autosomal recessive metabolic disorder of amino acid metabolism that affects most parts of the eye is cystinosis (cystine storage disease). Childhood (nephropathic) (MIM #219800), juvenile (MIM #219900), and adult (ocular) (MIM #219750) forms of this condition are recognized (83,86). Cystinosis, leads to the widespread accumulation of cystine crystals in ocular tissues as well as in bone marrow, liver, spleen, lymph nodes, and kidneys. Despite differences in clinical expression, all varieties of cystinosis are characterized by intralysosomal storage of cystine, while plasma cystine and cysteine levels are not consistently elevated. Cystine is stored in leukocytes and other cell types within membrane-bound cytoplasmic vacuoles as fine granular non-crystalline material. The lysosomal identity of the intracytoplasmic inclusions is supported by the associated acid phosphatase activity (324). Available morphologic observations suggest that the storage of cystine precedes its crystallization. The excessive accumulation of cystine within cells is a consequence of impaired transport of cystine from lysosomes (86,88) (see also Chapter 38).

The diagnosis of cystinosis is confirmed by an elevated leukocyte cystine content (86). Cultured fibroblasts from patients with cystinosis accumulate cystine within secondary lysosomes and cystine is depleted with cysteamine (mercaptoamine) (102). This cystine-depleting agent also appears to be beneficial after renal transplantation (87) and, when applied

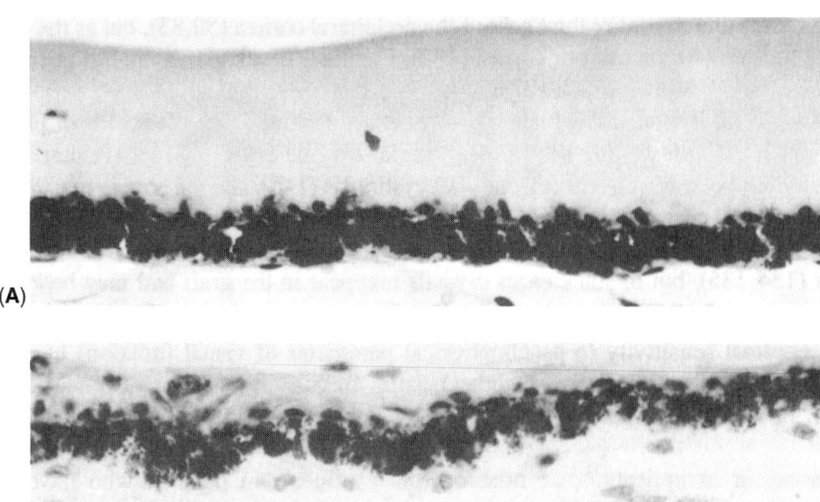

Figure 7 (**A**) Thickened basement membrane of nonpigmented epithelium of ciliary body in Weill–Marchesani syndrome. (**B**) Appearance of normal ciliary body at same magnification (hematoxylin and eosin, ×350).

topically to the eye, such medication may clear the corneal crystals in some (141,146) but not in all patients (187). In a long-term study cysteamine eye-drop therapy relieved symptoms within weeks and cleared the cornea within months (84).

The basic defect in cystinosis involves the *CTNS* gene, which codes for cystinosin and maps to chromosome 17 (17p13) (83,86). The most common mutation consists of a 57-kbp deletion, and 50% of Northern European patients are homozygous for it (Table 2) (294). Patients with milder forms of cystinosis have one severe mutation, such as the 57-kbp deletion, and one missense mutation that confers partial cystinosin function (7,83,86,292).

Childhood cystinosis, the most severe form, is associated with defective renal tubular reabsorption and the Fanconi syndrome (polyuria, generalized aminoaciduria, proteinuria, glycosuria, phosphaturia, and rickets). Renal failure is common, but dialysis and renal transplantation have prolonged the lives of individuals with nephropathic cystinosis, while the availability of cysteamine therapy has preserved renal function into the fourth decade of life and promoted normal growth in many individuals with juvenile cystinosis (86).

The ocular manifestations of cystinosis are well-established (81,242,266). The presence of multiple delicate scintillating crystals in the cornea (chiefly in the region of the corneoscleral limbus and in the anterior corneal stroma) and conjunctiva is characteristic of all forms of cystinosis (49,50,81,86,93, 158,168,331). Crystals may also be present in the iris and other parts of the uvea, retina, and sclera (83,86,306). Although the corneal crystals were once regarded as pathognomonic of cystinosis, other conditions, including hypergammaglobulinemia (discussed in Chapter 36) also produce corneal crystals and need to be differentiated clinically from cystinosis. The corneal crystals are absent at birth and during early infancy, but are usually evident by 1 year of age (86). Early in life the corneal crystals involve the anterior central corneal stroma and the entire thickness of the peripheral cornea (48,86), but as the patient ages the crystals become located in the posterior cornea (193). Pupillary-block glaucoma has been attributed to a cystine accumulation in the iris stroma (306).

From an ocular standpoint, individuals with cystinosis generally complain only of photophobia and glare, which presumably results from the ocular cystine crystals (153). A markedly decreased corneal sensitivity has been detected in persons with cystinosis (152), and the cornea may thicken perhaps as a sequel to subclinical corneal edema (76). The ocular symptoms may necessitate corneal transplantation (143,144,154, 155,156,252). Following keratoplasty the graft may remain free of cystinosis for as long as 2 years (143,144), but in some cases crystals reappear in the graft and may be evident within 6 weeks (154,155). A markedly decreased corneal sensitivity compared to age matched controls has been detected in cystinosis, possibly resulting from an altered function of the basal epithelial neural plexus (152). Loss of contrast sensitivity (a psychophysical parameter of visual function) has been found in individuals with cystinosis, especially at higher spatial frequencies (151), and could result from the corneal, retinal, or CNS abnormalities, although most of the contrast sensitivity probably reflects the corneal lesions.

Long-term ocular complications of nephropathic cystinosis in patients that have survived into adulthood as a result of dialysis and renal transplantation include blepharospasm, photophobia, corneal erosions, posterior synechiae, the deposition of crystals on the anterior lens surface, and reduced visual acuity (86,87,142).

A mottled pigmentary retinopathy is common in cystinosis (251,266,325). The RPE degenerates and this layer of cells may be lost, particularly in the peripheral retina. A patchy depigmentation of the RPE with pigment clumping intensifies from the macula toward the pre-equator area and gives the fundus a 'salt and pepper' appearance (251). Focal depigmentation, atrophy, and hypertrophy of the RPE, without intraretinal pigment migration, has been noted, and the abnormalities of the RPE may precede the corneal crystals. When the RPE is extensively affected, the macula acquires a unique yellow mottling (266). Abnormalities in the RPE begin early in life and vacuoles have been detected in these cells in an 18-week-old fetus with cystinosis (270). The pigmentary retinopathy is absent at birth, but has been noted in a 5-week-old infant girl (39). Crystals have been documented in the retina of at least one case by photography (40).

Cystine crystals are insoluble in absolute ethanol and can be easily seen with polarized light in tissue sections prepared without aqueous solutions that dissolve them. In cystinosis, needle-, rectangular-, or hexagonal-shaped crystals have been found in ocular tissues, with the fusiform crystals being identified only in the cornea and sclera (Fig. 8) (48,266). By TEM intracytoplasmic electron lucencies indicate the sites of crystalline inclusions. They have been identified within membrane-bound vesicles in different cell types in the cornea (158,266), conjunctiva (158,266,281,306,324), iris (306), and in the RPE (266). It is extremely doubtful that cystine crystallizes outside of cells despite reports of extracellular conjunctival crystals by light microscopy (323). In adult cystinosis, profiles of cystine crystals have been identified extracellularly adjacent to degenerated cells (281), but they have apparently not yet been reported

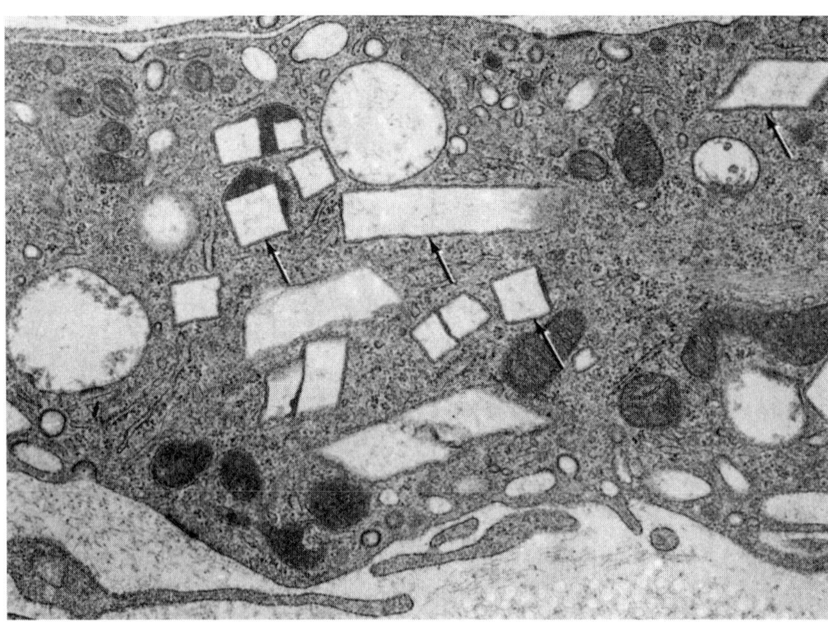

Figure 8 Profiles of crystalline inclusions within the cytoplasm of a histiocyte in cystinosis. *Source*: From Ref. 324.

in this site in childhood cystinosis. Whether this difference is real still needs to be determined. TEM has almost always disclosed profiles of crystalline outlines only within cells.

The eye is not affected in cystinuria (MIM #220100), in contrast to cystinosis, with which it is sometimes confused. The dibasic amino acids, cystine, lysine, arginine, and ornithine, are excreted in excess in cystinuria, a disorder with a transport defect involving renal tubules and the intestinal tract (230).

Sulfite Oxidase Deficiency

Sulfite oxidase, a molybdenum-containing enzyme involved in the oxidation of sulfites to sulfates (51), is deficient in an extremely rare inherited disorder with severe neurological defects, which include severe developmental delay and seizures (135,278). Bilateral dislocated lenses are a prominent clinical feature of sulfite oxidase deficiency (sulfocysteinuria; MIM # 272300), which is caused by mutations in the *SUOX* gene that encodes for sulfite oxidase. Other ocular abnormalities (hypoplasia of ciliary body, diminished ganglion cells and thinning of the nerve fiber layer in the retina, and absence of myelin in the optic nerve) have also been noted. There is an increased urinary excretion of sulfite ions (SO_3=), thiosulfate ions (S_2O_3=), and the amino acid *S*-sulfo-L-cysteine, but sulfate ions in the urine are markedly diminished or absent (203). *S*-sulfo-L-cysteine elevations have been detected by tandem mass spectrometric analysis of urine from patients with isolated sulfite oxidase and molybdenum cofactor deficiency (Table 2) (140). Some patients with mild sulfite oxidase deficiency responded well to a diet low in sulfur-containing amino acids (140).

DISORDERS OF MISCELLANEOUS AMINO ACIDS

Hyperornithinemia

Hyperornithinemia (chorioretinal gyrate atrophy, MIM +258870) is particularly prevalent in Finland and in individuals of Finnish ancestry. This autosomal recessive disorder is characterized by a progressive degenerative disease of the retina and choroid. It is associated with an elevated ornithine (an amino acid not found in protein) in the blood and urine and a reduction or absence of the mitochondrial matrix enzyme ornithine aminotransferase (L-ornithine: 2-oxoacid aminotransferase) (OAT). This enzyme catalyzes the first step of the conversion of ornithine to proline, forming the intermediate glutamic-γ-semialdehyde that spontaneously converts to Δ′-pyrroline 5 carboxylate (Fig. 9) (215,290). Vitamin B6 is required as a coenzyme for ornithine aminotransferase. The clinical picture of gyrate atrophy of the choroid and retina can occur in the absence of hyperornithinemia (137).

The cDNA for human OAT mRNA has been cloned and characterized (125,133,245) and genes encoding for this enzyme have been localized by somatic cell hybrids and in situ hybridization to human chromosome 10 (10q26) as well as to the X chromosome (Xp11.2) (14). The mature protein consists of 407 residues and the amino acid sequence of the enzyme is known (133). Lys292 is the residue that binds the

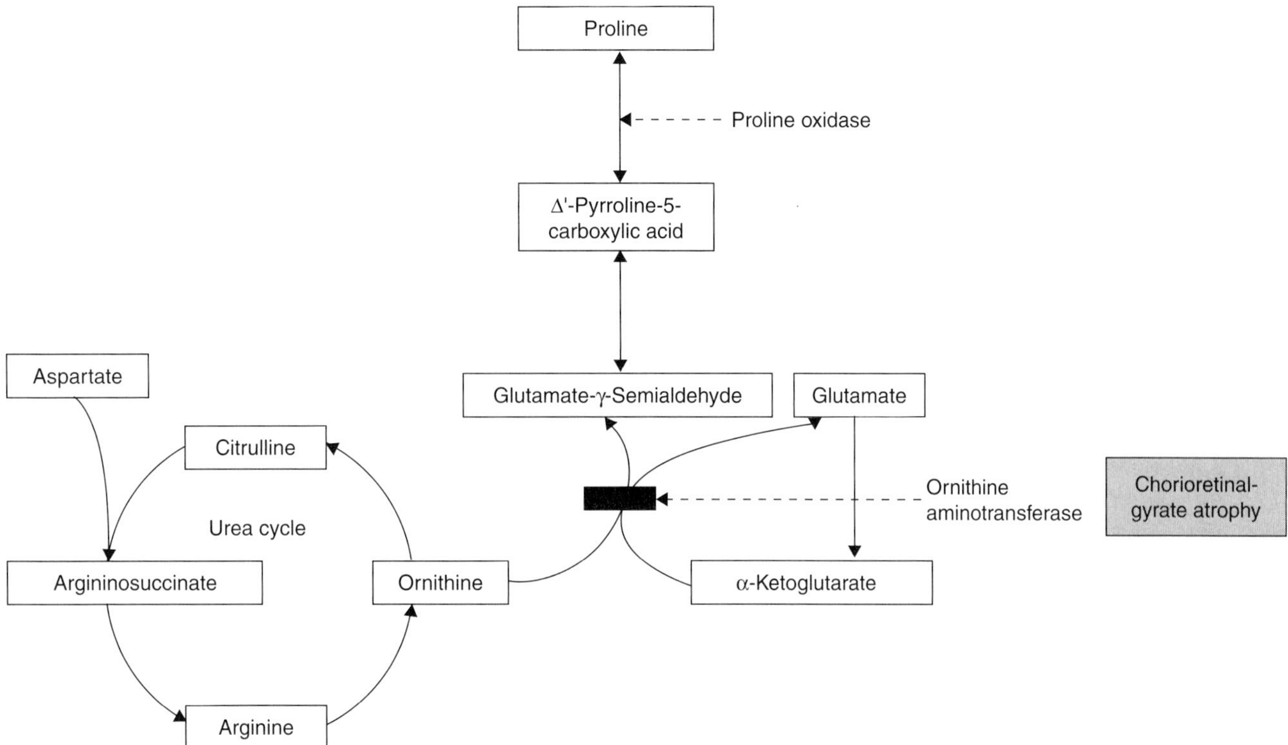

Figure 9 Site of metabolic defect in hyperornithinemia. *Source*: Reproduced from Klintworth GK, Landers MB III. The Eye: Structure and Function in Disease. Baltimore: Williams & Wilkins, 1976.

coenzyme pyridoxal phosphate. The site of posttranslational proteolysis occurs at Ala 25-Thr 26 (273).

Developmental differences of specific ornithine ketoacid aminotransferase activities have been detected between ocular tissues and liver (116). The retina and choroid have a relatively low activity after birth and an increased activity at 2.5 weeks, which remained high thereafter. The ciliary body and iris also manifest relatively low activity at birth and a rapid increase at 1 week, which remains so for about 14 weeks before a gradual decrease occurs (116). Retinoblastoma cells express OAT at a high level (133).

In the early stages of gyrate atrophy, the margins of the atrophic retina appear by fundoscopy as curved circular segments and the term "gyrate atrophy" stems from this clinical appearance (latin, *gyratus* = turned around). The chorioretinal lesions are confined to the peripheral retina in older cases and are minimal in younger patients. However, a macular dystrophy may be a manifestation of gyrate atrophy (123). Electroretino-graphic evidence points to marked involvement of the cone and rod systems (147).

Despite a generalized deficiency of OAT, clinical manifestations are limited to the eye (300). Individuals with gyrate atrophy of the choroid and retina are not weak, but type 2 muscles are atrophic and have tubular aggregates (275) (see Chapter 72). Bizarre-shaped mitochondria have been noted in the liver and in cultured skin fibroblasts of patients with gyrate atrophy (217). Because similar abnormalities can be induced in normal fibroblasts grown in culture media containing a high-ornithine concentration, these are probably a sequel to hyperornithinemia.

TEM studies of the iris in patients with gyrate atrophy have disclosed atrophy, abnormal mitochondria, and tubular aggregates (structures similar to those found in skeletal muscle) in the dilator pupillae. Degenerative changes, such as extracted cellular matrix, dropout of cellular organelles, and dilated intercellular spaces occur in the pigmented posterior epithelium and the anterior iris epithelium (304).

The biochemical detection of OAT deficiency depends upon enzyme analysis of patient fibroblasts and detection of elevated ornithine in body fluids (300). Plasma amino acid quantitation reveals highly elevated ornithine, and urine amino acids reveal markedly elevated ornithine accompanied by moderate elevations of the dibasic amino acids arginine and lysine. Plasma creatine and its precursor guanidinoacetate are reduced; moreover, reduced phosphocreatine detected by ^{31}P-magnetic resonance spectroscopy analysis is associated with abnormal muscle histology in gyrate atrophy patients (121,206,300).

The level of OAT activity in transformed lymphocytes in obligate heterozygous carriers is approximately 50% of the normal value (299).

A deficiency of the enzyme's product proline is unlikely to be important in the pathogenesis of the retinal degeneration, as this amino acid can be derived from other sources (215). Also, proline is an important constituent of collagen, but there is no clinical evidence of a systemic disorder of this ubiquitous protein. A candidate for possible toxicity to the retina in OAT deficiency is glyoxalate (248). Arginine glycine transamidinase activity was not detectable in human retina; thus, a previously postulated creatine phosphate deprivation in OAT deficiency may not be applicable to the pathogenesis of the disease.

Clinical and biochemical heterogeneity has been detected in hyperornithinemia and the response to vitamin B6 also varies (307).

The molecular genetic flaw in gyrate atrophy has been demonstrated by finding a defect in the *OAT* gene, mRNA, and protein (Table 2) (132). Very low levels of the enzyme have been identified in some affected individuals by immunoradioassay (220). Some OAT activity has been detected in homogenates of liver biopsies of some cases of chorioretinal gyrate atrophy (216). However, in these individuals the kinetics of the residual OAT differed from normal OAT, suggesting that an abnormal enzyme rather than an absent one may occur in hyperornithinemia.

The OAT activity in cultured skin fibroblasts from patients with gyrate atrophy is markedly decreased or not detected (215,220,295,297) due not to production of a structurally altered enzyme lacking catalytic activity, but rather to decreased production of enzyme protein (220).

The view that hyperornithinemia is toxic to the retina and choroid and causally related to chorioretinal gyrate atrophy finds support in several observations: The retina and choroid atrophy markedly in both monkeys and rats following an intravitreal injection of ornithine (171). The plasma ornithine level diminished fivefold in an affected individual who was maintained on an arginine-deficient diet for 20 months (145), and this was associated with a subjective improvement in visual function 15 months after institution of the diet.

Some individuals with gyrate atrophy respond to high doses of vitamin B6, by lowering their serum ornithine level and improving their electroretinogram (307). Vitamin B6 responsiveness has been associated with four specific missense mutations in the *OAT* gene (189,196,219,244). Also, with a partial deficiency of OAT activity the residual activity may be stimulated in vitro by high concentrations of pyridoxal phosphate (18). A clinical study of a low-arginine diet to reduce ornithine accumulation effectively reduced plasma ornithine levels and delayed the progression of chorioretinal changes over the course of 26-year follow-up in a patient with no detectable OAT activity (267).

Familial Hyperlysinemia

The protein α-aminoadipic semialdehyde synthase has two enzyme activities: lysine-ketoglutarate reductase and saccharopine dehydrogenase that catabolize L-lysine. Lysine-ketoglutarate reductase is needed for the conversion of lysine to saccharopine, which saccharopine dehydrogenase converts to α-aminoadipic acid semialdehyde (58). In familial hyperlysinemia (MIM #238700) the activity of both of these enzymes is diminished due to mutations in the *AASS* gene on human chromosome 7 (7q31.3), leading to hyperlysinemia and an excess excretion of lysine in the urine (Table 2). An occasional individual with this rare autosomal recessive disorder has bilateral spherophakia or dislocated lenses (279). The question of whether the ocular changes are related to the metabolic defect remains unresolved.

Lowe Syndrome

In 1952, Lowe and colleagues drew attention to the oculocerebrorenal syndrome (MIM #309000), an X-linked recessive disorder with ocular and cerebral abnormalities and an amino aciduria (1,182).

Congenital cataracts in both eyes are characteristic. The lens is small and spherical (spherophakia), and often has a conical-shaped posterior surface (posterior lenticonus). Total, nuclear, or posterior polar cataracts are evident at birth or during early infancy in most cases. Peculiar excrescences on the anterior and equatorial lens capsule (296) resemble those found in trisomy 21 (Down syndrome) and in Miller syndrome.

About 50% of cases have congenital glaucoma and many affected individuals have congenital anomalies of the retina and other ocular structures. Bilateral corneal keloids have been reported in a boy with Lowe syndrome without signs of perforating corneal trauma or iridocorneal incarceration in either eye (46). The cause of the keloids remains obscure and the combination of corneal keloids with Lowe syndrome is probably coincidental in view of the rarity of the association.

The genetic defect in Lowe syndrome is manifest early in embryogenesis as evidenced by the finding of both congenital cataract and irido-corneal angle dysgenesis in the eyes of a fetus obtained from a woman with a previous child having Lowe syndrome (73). All lens cells are presumably affected in males expressing the Lowe syndrome gene, and defective formation and subsequent degeneration of the primary posterior lens fibers account for the characteristic flattened, discoid, or ring-shaped lens opacities. Some lens abnormalities, such as anterior polar cataract, subcapsular fibrous plaque, capsular excrescences, bladder cells, and posterior lenticonus are not specific for Lowe syndrome (301).

Cerebral atrophy that may be detectable clinically by computed tomography (CT) (315) causes mental retardation, hypotonia, and other neurologic manifestations.

Involvement of the kidney accounts for many attributes of Lowe syndrome and many of the systemic effects including proteinuria, excretion of undersulfated chondroitin sulfate A, sialic aciduria, generalized aminoaciduria, renal tubular acidosis, renal rickets, and a reduced ammonia production reflect renal tubular dysfunction.

Other nonocular manifestations include physical retardation and frontal bossing. Studies of skin biopsy specimens in individuals with Lowe syndrome have disclosed cytoplasmic, membrane-bound, electron-lucent vacuoles and some electron-dense membranous inclusion bodies in fibroblasts and Schwann cells, as well as axonal degeneration and vascular changes (315).

As in other X-linked inherited disorders, one of the two X chromosomes is presumably randomly deactivated early in ontogeny in heterozygous female carriers (Lyon hypothesis) (see Chapter 31), who develop punctate opacities in the lens with a relatively high frequency. These opacities in the female lens probably reflect abnormal lens cells that express the mutant gene on the X chromosome. Carriers of Lowe syndrome develop variable-shaped cortical dots that become more numerous with age (47,126,167). Rarely, Lowe syndrome occurs in girls without a positive family history (127,232,262). It may be accompanied by a balanced X autosome translocation, with a breakpoint at Xq25 (127), presumably as resulting from a disruption of the X chromosome within the Lowe syndrome gene locus. In this case nonrandom inactivation of the normal X chromosome would occur that avoids inactivation of autosomal genes associated with the translocation chromosome.

The cDNA for the Lowe syndrome gene encodes a protein, ocrl1, that has phosphatidylinositol 4,5-biphosphate-5-phosphatase activity (12,330). The diagnosis of Lowe syndrome is established by the detection of an inactivating mutation in the *OCRL1* gene (Table 2). An earlier theory postulates that the basic defect in Lowe syndrome involves electron transport in mitochondria prior to the cytochromes (97). This view finds support in the observation of a marked diminution in the respiratory controls of mitochondria from muscle with substrates reducing nicotinamide adenine dinucleotide (glutamate plus malate) and with a flavoprotein-linked substrate (succinate). More recently, the deficiency of ocrl1 was associated with defective actin polymerization in patient fibroblasts, consistent with abnormal formation of tight junctions and adherent junctions—both of which are critical to renal tubule and lens development (283). Most recently, ocrl1 has been localized to clathrin-coated endosomes and implicated in trafficking of proteins from the endosomes to the trans Golgi network (43,298).

Canavan Disease

Canavan disease (spongy degeneration of the brain, MIM #271900) is a rare autosomal recessive lethal disorder of infancy characterized by a spongy state of the white matter in the brain and defective myelination. The salient clinical manifestations include an onset in early infancy of blindness, megalocephaly, severe mental retardation, atonia of the neck muscles, hyperextension of the legs, and flexion of the arms. Death ensues before the end of the second year of life. Congenital, infantile, and late-onset forms of the disorder are recognized (191). Many cases have featured Jewish ancestry and can be traced to eastern Europe (173). Many cases have been identified in Saudi Arabia (226). N-acetylaspartic acid is elevated in the plasma and urine, also in the CSF (190,191), and can be detected in a urine organic acid screen. A deficiency of aspartoacylase has been detected in some affected individuals (Table 2) (190,226). As in many other autosomal recessive disorders, obligate carriers of the mutant gene express enzyme levels of less than 50% of the control values (191). Canavan disease is caused by mutations in the *ASPA* gene on human chromosome 17 (17pter–p13).

Taurine Deficiency

Cholesterol is normally converted into trihydroxycoprostanoate and then into cholyl coenzyme A, an activated intermediate in the synthesis of bile salts. The amino group of the sulfur-containing amino acid taurine, which is not a constituent of any protein, reacts with cholyl coenzyme A to form the bile salt taurocholate. Although it remains uncertain whether taurine has other roles in man, taurine is the most bountiful amino acid in the vertebrate retina (223,305), where it is synthesized. Taurine is particularly abundant in the RPE and the photoreceptors (157,224,305) and it is suspected of having antioxidant, osmoregulatory, and membrane-stabilizing functions in the retina (326). Taurine appears to be important in retinal function at least in the cat, where a deficiency of this amino acid leads to retinal degeneration and blindness (117,269). Cats fed a taurine-free casein diet manifest a central photoreceptor (both rods and cones) degeneration after a plasma and retinal taurine deficiency (117,118,269).

REFERENCES

1. Abbassi V, Lowe CU, Calcagno PL. Oculo–cerebro–renal syndrome. A review. Am J Dis Child 1968; 115:145–68.

2. Alitalo T, Kruse TA, Forsius H, et al. Localization of the Aland Island eye disease locus to the pericentromeric region of the X chromosome by linkage analysis. Am J Hum Genet 1991; 48:31–8.
3. Allen RA, O'Malley C, Straatsma BR. Ocular findings in hereditary ochronosis. Arch Ophthalmol 1961; 65: 657–68.
4. Allen RA, Straatsma BR. Ocular involvement in leukemia and allied disorders. Arch Ophthalmol 1961; 66:490–508.
5. Anderson B. Corneal and conjunctival pigmentation among workers engaged in manufacture of hydroquinone. Arch Ophthalmol 1947; 38:812–26.
6. Anikster Y, Huizing M, White J, et al. Mutation of a new gene causes a unique form of Hermansky–Pudlak syndrome in a genetic isolate of central Puerto Rico. Nat Genet 2001; 28:376–80.
7. Anikster Y, Lucero C, Guo J, et al. Ocular nonnephropathic cystinosis: clinical, biochemical, and molecular correlations. Pediatr Res 2000; 47:17–23.
8. Apkarian P, Reits D, Spekreijse H. Component specificity in albino VEP asymmetry: maturation of the visual pathway anomaly. Exp Brain Res 1984; 53:285–94.
9. Apkarian P, Reits D, Spekreijse H, van Dorp, D. A decisive electrophysiological test for human albinism. Electroencephalogr Clin Neurophysiol 1983; 55:513–31.
10. Ashton N, Kirker JG, Lavery FS. Ocular findings in a case of hereditary ochronosis. Br J Ophthalmol 1964; 48:405–15.
11. Assensio AM, Cascone C, Fracassi A, et al. Albinismo oculocutaneo e tirosinuria. Desrizione di un caso clinico. Minerva Pediatr 1983; 35:99–103.
12. Attree O, Olivos IM, Okabe I, et al. The Lowe's oculocerebrorenal syndrome gene encodes a protein highly homologous to inositol polyphosphate-5-phosphatase. Nature 1992; 358:239–42.
13. Babel J. Rheumatisme. Arch Ophtalmol Rev Gen Ophtalmol 1973; 33:341–54.
14. Barrett DJ, Bateman JB, Sparkes RS, et al. Chromosomal localization of human ornithine aminotransferase gene sequences to 10q26 and Xp11.2. Invest Ophthalmol Vis Sci 1987; 28:1037–42.
15. Barton DE, Yang-Feng TL, Francke U. The human tyrosine aminotransferase gene mapped to the long arm of chromosome 16 (region 16q22-q24) by somatic cell hybrid analysis and in situ hybridization. Hum Genet 1986; 72:221–4.
16. Bedoya V. Pigmentary changes in Chediak–Higashi syndrome. Br J Dermatol 1971; 85:347.
17. Beguez-Cesar A. Neutropenia cronica maligna familiar con granulaciones atipicas de los leucocitos. Bol Soc Cubana Pediatr 1943; 15:900–22.
18. Behrens-Baumann W, Konig U, Schroder K, et al. Biochemical and therapeutical studies in a case of atrophia gyrata. Graefes Arch Clin Exp Ophthalmol 1982; 218:21–4.
19. Bell TG, Meyers KM, Prieur DJ, et al. Decreased nucleotide and serotonin storage associated with defective function in Chediak–Higashi syndrome cattle and human platelets. Blood 1976; 48:175–84.
20. Ben Dridi MF, Karoui S, Kastally R, et al. Homocystinuria. A type with vascular thrombosis and factor VII deficiency. Arch Fr Pediatr 1986; 43:41–4.
21. Benson W. Oculocutaneous albinism with Axenfeld's anomaly. Am J Ophthalmol 1981; 92:133–4.
22. Bergsma DR, Kaiser-Kupfer M. A new form of albinism. Am J Ophthalmol 1974; 77:837–44.
23. Bienfang DC, Kuwabara T, Pueschel SM. The Richner–Hanhart syndrome: report of a case with associated tyrosinemia. Arch Ophthalmol 1976; 94:1133–7.
24. Blaszczyk WM, Arning L, Hoffmann KP, Epplen JT. A tyrosinase missense mutation causes albinism in the Wistar rat. Pigment Cell Res 2005; 18:144–5.
25. Blume RS, Bennett JM, Yankee RA, Wolff SM. Defective granulocyte regulation in the Chediak–Higashi syndrome. N Engl J Med 1968; 279:1009–15.
26. Blume RS, Glade PR, Gralnick HR, et al. The Chediak–Higashi syndrome: continuous suspension cultures derived from peripheral blood. Blood 1969; 33: 821–32.
27. Blume RS, Wolff SM. The Chediak–Higashi syndrome: studies in four patients and a review of the literature. Medicine (Baltimore) 1972; 51:247–80.
28. Boylan C, Clement RA, Harding GF. Lateralization of the flash visual-evoked cortical potential in human albinos. Invest Ophthalmol Vis Sci 1984; 25:1448–50.
29. Boylan C, Harding GF. Investigation of visual pathway abnormalities in human albinos. Ophthalmic Physiol Opt 1983; 3:273–85.
30. Bradley WG, Richardson J, Frew IJ. The familial association of neurofibromatosis, peroneal muscular atrophy, congenital deafness, partial albinism, and Axenfeld's defect. Brain 1974; 97:521–32.
31. Bregeat P, Dhermy P, Hamard H. Manifestations oculaires du syndrome de Chédiak Higashi. Arch Ophtalmol Rev Gen Ophtalmol 1966; 26:661–76.
32. Bruce S, Tschen JA, Chow D. Exogenous ochronosis resulting from quinine injections. J Am Acad Dermatol 1986; 15:357–61.
33. Buchanan GR, Handin RI. Platelet function in the Chediak–Higashi syndrome. Blood 1976; 47:941–8.
34. Bunim JJ, McGuire JS Jr, Hilbish TF, et al. Alcaptonuria; clinical staff conference at the National Institutes of Health. Ann Intern Med 1957; 47:1210–24.
35. Burke JP, O'Keefe M, Bowell R, Naughten ER. Ocular complications in homocystinuria—early and late treated. Br J Ophthalmol 1989; 73:427–31.
36. Burns RP. Soluble tyrosine aminotransferase deficiency: an unusual cause of corneal ulcers. Am J Ophthalmol 1972; 73: 400–2.
37. Burns RP, Beard ME, Weimar VL, Squires EL. Modification of 1-tyrosine-induced keratopathy by adrenal corticosteroids. Invest Ophthalmol 1974; 13:39–45.
38. Burns RP, Gipson IK, Murray MJ. Keratopathy in tyrosinemia. Birth Defects Orig Artic Ser 1976; 12:169–80.
39. Carroll WM, Jay BS, McDonald WI, Halliday AM. Two distinct patterns of visual evoked response asymmetry in human albinism. Nature 1980; 286:604–6.
40. Caruso RC, Kaiser-Kupfer MI, Muenzer J, et al. Electroretinographic findings in the mucopolysaccharidoses. Ophthalmology 1986; 93:1612–6.
41. Castro-Gago M, Pombo M, Novo I, et al. Sindrome familiar de microcefalia con albinismo oculoctáneo y anomalies digitales. An Esp Pediatr 1983; 19:128–31.
42. Charlton KH, Binder PS, Wozniak L, Digby DJ. Pseudodendritic keratitis and systemic tyrosinemia. Ophthalmology 1981; 88:355–60.
43. Choudhury R, Diao A, Zhang F, et al. Lowe syndrome protein OCRL1 interacts with clathrin and regulates protein trafficking between endosomes and the trans-Golgi network. Mol Biol Cell 2005; 16:3467–79.
44. Christensen K, Fischer P, Knudsen KE, et al. A syndrome of hereditary tyrosinemia in mink (Mustela vison Schreb.). Can J Comp Med 1979; 43:333–40.
45. Christensen K, Henriksen P, Sorensen H. New forms of hereditary tyrosinemia type II in mink: hepatic tyrosine aminotransferase defect. Hereditas 1986; 104:215–22.

46. Cibis GW, Tripathi RC, Tripathi BJ, Harris DJ. Corneal keloid in Lowe's syndrome. Arch Ophthalmol 1982; 100:1795–9.
47. Cibis GW, Waeltermann JM, Whitcraft CT, et al. Lenticular opacities in carriers of Lowe's syndrome. Ophthalmology 1986; 93:1041–5.
48. Cogan DG, Kuwabara T. Ocular pathology of cystinosis. Arch Ophthalmol 1960; 63:51–7.
49. Cogan DG, Kuwabara T, Kinoshita J, et al. Cystinosis in an adult. J Am Med Assoc 1957; 164:394–6.
50. Cogan DG, Kuwabara T, Kinoshita J, et al. Ocular manifestations of systemic cystinosis. AMA. Arch Ophthalmol 1956; 55:36–41.
51. Cohen HJ, Betcher-Lange S, Kessler DL, Rajagopalan KV. Hepatic sulfite oxidase. Congruency in mitochondria of prosthetic groups and activity. J Biol Chem 1972; 247:7759–66.
52. Cohen T, Muller RM, Tomita Y, Shibahara S. Nucleotide sequence of the cDNA encoding human tyrosinase-related protein. Nucleic Acids Res 1990; 18:2807–8.
53. Colditz PB, Yu JS, Billson FA, et al. Tyrosinaemia II. Med J Aust 1984; 141:244–5.
54. Coleman J, Sydnor CF, Wolbarsht ML, Bessler M. Abnormal visual pathways in human albinos studied with visually evoked potentials. Exp Neurol 1979; 65:667–79.
55. Comings DE, Amromin GD. Autosomal dominant insensitivity to pain with hyperplastic myelinopathy and autosomal dominant indifference to pain. Neurology 1974; 24:838–48.
56. Comings DE, Odland GF. Partial albinism. JAMA 1966; 195:519–23.
57. Costa JL, Fauci AS, Wolff SM. A platelet abnormality in the Chediak–Higashi syndrome of man. Blood 1976; 48: 517–20.
58. Cox RP. Errors of Lysine Metabolism. In: Scriver CR, Beaudet Al, Valle D, Sly WS, eds. Metabolic and Molecular Bases of Inheritied Disease. New York: McGraw-Hill, 2001:1965–70.
59. Creel D. Problems of ocular miswiring in albinism, Duane's syndrome, and Marcus Gunn phenomenon. Int Ophthalmol Clin 1984; 24:165–76.
60. Creel D, Boxer LA, Fauci AS. Visual and auditory anomalies in Chediak–Higashi syndrome. Electroencephalogr. Clin Neurophysiol 1983; 55:252–7.
61. Creel D, King RA, Witkop CJ, Okoro AN. Visual system anomalies in human albinos. In: Klauss SN, ed. Pigment Cell, Pathophysiology of Melanocytes. New Haven: Karger, 1979:21–7.
62. Creel D, O'Donnell FE Jr, Witkop CJ Jr. Visual system anomalies in human ocular albinos. Science 1978; 201: 931–3.
63. Creel D, Witkop CJ Jr, King RA. Asymmetric visually evoked potentials in human albinos: evidence for visual system anomalies. Invest Ophthalmol 1974; 13:430–40.
64. Creel DJ. Visual system anomaly associated with albinism in the cat. Nature 1971; 231:465–6.
65. Creel DJ, Bendel CM, Wiesner GL, et al. Abnormalities of the central visual pathways in Prader–Willi syndrome associated with hypopigmentation. N Engl J Med 1986; 314:1606–9.
66. Cross HE, Jensen AD. Ocular manifestations in the Marfan syndrome and homocystinuria. Am J Ophthalmol 1973; 75:405–20.
67. Cross HE, McKusick VA, Breen W. A new oculocerebral syndrome with hypopigmentation. J Pediatr 1967; 70: 398–406.
68. Daicker B, Riede UN. Histological and ultrastructural findings in alkaptonuric ocular ochronosis. Ophthalmologica 1974; 169:377–88.
69. Danes BS, Bearn AG. Cell culture and the Chediak–Higashi syndrome. Lancet 1967; 2:65–7.
70. Davis WC, Spicer SS, Greene WB, Padgett GA. Ultrastructure of bone marrow granulocytes in normal mink and mink with the homolog of the Chediak–Higashi trait of humans. I. Origin of the abnormal granules present in the neutrophils of mink with the C-HS trait. Lab Invest 1971; 24:303–17.
71. Dell'Angelica EC, Shotelersuk V, Aguilar RC, et al. Altered trafficking of lysosomal proteins in Hermansky–Pudlak syndrome due to mutations in the beta 3A subunit of the AP-3 adaptor. Mol Cell 1999; 3:11–21.
72. Driscoll DJ, Jabs EW, Alcorn D, et al. Corneal tyrosine crystals in transient neonatal tyrosinemia. J Pediatr 1988; 113:91–3.
73. Dufier JL, Dhermy P, Farriaux JP, et al. Antenatal diagnosis of Lowe's syndrome based on histologic tests of the fetal eyes. J Fr Ophtalmol 1986; 9:361–6.
74. Dunn-Meynell AA, Prasada Rao PD, Sharma SC. The ipsilateral retinotectal projection in normal and albino channel catfish. Neurosci Lett 1983; 36:25–31.
75. Enns GM, Barkovich AJ, Rosenblatt DS, et al. Progressive neurological deterioration and MRI changes in cblC methylmalonic acidaemia treated with hydroxocobalamin. J Inherit Metab Dis 1999; 22:599–607.
76. Finkelstein JD, Mudd SH, Irreverre F, Laster L. Homocystinuria due to cystathione synthetase deficiency: the mode of inheritance. Science 1964; 146: 785–7.
77. Fitzpatrick TB, Jimbow K, Donaldson DD. Dominant oculocutaneous albinism (summary). Br J Dermatol Suppl 1974; 10:23.
78. Forsius H, Eriksson AW. Ein neues Augensyndrom mit X-chromosomaler Transmission. Eine Sippe mit Fundusalbinismus, Foveahypoplasie, Nystagmus, Myopie, Astigmatismus und Dyschromatopsi. Klin Monatsbl Augenheilkd 1964; 144:447–57.
79. Franceschetti AT, Schnyder UW, Felgenhauer WR. Die Cornea beim Richter–Hanhart Syndrom. 9. 1979. Berict uber die 71, Zusammenkuft der Deutchen Ophthalm. Gesellschaft in Heidelburg.
80. Francis PJ, Calver DM, Barnfield P, et al. An infant with methylmalonic aciduria and homocystinuria (cblC) presenting with retinal haemorrhages and subdural haematoma mimicking non-accidental injury. Eur J Pediatr 2004; 163:420–1.
81. Francois J. Ocular manifestations in aminoacidopathies. Adv Ophthalmol 1972; 25:28–103.
82. Frenk E, Lattion F. The melanin pigmentary disorder in a family with Hermansky–Pudlak syndrome. J Invest Dermatol 1982; 78:141–3.
83. Gahl W, Thoene JG, Schneider JA. Cystinosis: A Disorder of Lysosomal Membrane Transport. In: Scriver CR, Beaudet Al, Valle D, Sly WS, eds. Metabolic and Molecular Bases of Inheritied Disease. New York: McGraw-Hill, 2001:5085–108.
84. Gahl WA, Kuehl EM, Iwata F, et al. Corneal crystals in nephropathic cystinosis: natural history and treatment with cysteamine eyedrops. Mol Genet Metab 2000; 71:100–20.
85. Gahl WA, Potterf B, Durham-Pierre D, et al. Melanosomal tyrosine transport in normal and pink-eyed dilution murine melanocytes. Pigment Cell Res 1995; 8:229–33.
86. Gahl WA, Thoene JG, Schneider JA. Cystinosis. N Engl J Med 2002; 347:111–21.
87. Gahl WA, Thoene JG, Schneider JA, et al. NIH conference. Cystinosis: progress in a prototypic disease. Ann Intern Med 1988; 109:557–69.

88. Gahl WA, Tietze F, Bashan N, et al. Defective cystine exodus from isolated lysosome-rich fractions of cystinotic leucocytes. J Biol Chem 1982; 257:9570–75.
89. Gallagher PM, Naughten E, Hanson NQ, et al. Characterization of mutations in the cystathionine beta-synthase gene in Irish patients with homocystinuria. Mol Genet Metab 1998; 65:298–302.
90. Gardner JM, Wildenberg SC, Keiper NM, et al. The mouse pale ear (EP) mutation is the homologue of human Hermansky–Pudlak syndrome. Proc Natl Acad Sci USA 1997; 94:9238–43.
91. Garrett EE. Ocular ochronosis with alkaptonuria. Am J Ophthalmol 1963; 55:617–20.
92. Garrod A. Inborn Errors of Metabolism. London: Frowde, 1909.
93. Garron LK. Cystinosis. Trans Am Acad Ophthalmol Otolaryngol 1959; 63:99–108.
94. Giolli RA, Creel DJ. The primary optic projections in pigmented and albino guinea pigs: an experimental degeneration study. Brain Res 1973; 55:25–39.
95. Giolli RA, Guthrie MD. The primary optic projections in the rabbit. An experimental degeneration study. J Comp Neurol 1969; 136:99–126.
96. Gipson IK, Burns RP, Wolfe-Lande JD. Crystals in corneal epithelial lesions of tyrosine-fed rats. Invest Ophthalmol 1975 14:937–41.
97. Gobernado JM, Lousa M, Gimeno A, Gonsalvez M. Mitochondrial defects in Lowe's oculocerebrorenal syndrome. Arch Neurol 1984; 41:208–9.
98. Goldsmith LA. Tyrosinemia II: lessons in molecular pathophysiology. Pediatr Dermatol 1983; 1:25–34.
99. Goldsmith LA. Tyrosinemia II. Int J Dermatol 1985; 24: 293–4.
100. Goldsmith LA, Kang E, Bienfang DC, et al. Tyrosinemia with plantar and palmar keratosis and keratitis. J Pediatr 1973; 83:798–805.
101. Goldsmith LA, Thorpe JM, Marsh RF. Tyrosine aminotransferase deficiency in mink (Mustela vision): a model for human tyrosinemia II. Biochem Genet 1981; 19:687–93.
102. Greene AA, Jonas AJ, Harms E, et al. A. Lysosomal cystine storage in cystinosis and mucolipidosis type II. Pediatr Res 1985; 19:1170–4.
103. Griscelli C, Durandy A, Guy-Grand D, et al. A syndrome associating partial albinism and immunodeficiency. Am J Med 1978; 65:691–702.
104. Guillery RW. Neuronal abnormalities in albinos. Trend Neurosci 1986; 9:364–7.
105. Guillery RW, Amorn CS, Eighmy BB. Mutants with abnormal visual pathways: an explanation of anomalous geniculate laminae. Science 1971; 174:831–2.
106. Guillery RW, Kaas JH. Genetic abnormality of the visual pathways in a white tiger. Science 1973; 180:1287–9.
107. Guillery RW, Okoro AN, Witkop CJ Jr. Abnormal visual pathways in the brain of a human albino. Brain Res 1975; 96:373–7.
108. Guillery RW, Scott GL, Cattanach BM, Deol MS. Genetic mechanisms determining the central visual pathways of mice. Science 1973; 179:1014–6.
109. Gwynn B, Martina JA, Bonifacino JS, et al. Reduced pigmentation (RP), a mouse model of Hermansky–Pudlak syndrome, encodes a novel component of the BLOC-1 complex. Blood 2004; 104:3181–9.
110. Halaban R, Moellmann G, Tamura A, et al. Tyrosinases of murine melanocytes with mutations at the albino locus. Proc Natl Acad Sci U.S.A. 1988; 85:7241–5.
111. Hales RH. Albinism with Axenfeld's syndrome. Rocky. Mt Med J 1968; 65:51–2.
112. Hamosh A, Scott AF, Amberger J, Valle D, McKusick VA. Online Mendelian Inheritance in Man (OMIM). Hum Mutat 2000; 15:57–61.
113. Hatch JL. Hereditary alkaptonuria with ochronosis. Arch Ophthalmol 1959; 62:575–8.
114. Hayakawa M, Kato K, Nakajima A, et al. Nettleship-Falls X-Linked Ocular Albinism with Axenfelds Anomaly—A Case-Report. Ophthal Paediat Genet 1986; 7:109–14.
115. Hayasaka S. Lens Subluxation in Homocystinuria—A case-report. Acta Ophthalmologica 1984; 62:425–31.
116. Hayasaka S, Shiono T, Mizuno K, et al. Hyperornithinemia, gyrate atrophy, and ornithine ketoacid transaminase. Adv Exp Med Biol 1982; 153:353–8.
117. Hayes KC, Carey RE, Schmidt SY. Retinal degeneration associated with taurine deficiency in the cat. Science 1975; 188:949–51.
118. Hayes KC, Rabin AR, Berson EL. An ultrastructural study of nutritionally induced and reversed retinal degeneration in cats. Am J Pathol 1975; 78:505–24.
119. Hearing VJ, Lutzner MA. Mammalian melanosomal proteins: characterization by polyacrylamide gel electrophoresis. Yale J Biol Med 1973; 46:553–9.
120. Hearing VJ, Tsukamoto K. Enzymatic control of pigmentation in mammals. FASEB J 1991; 5:2902–9.
121. Heinanen K, Nanto-Salonen K, Komu M, et al. Creatine corrects muscle 31P spectrum in gyrate atrophy with hyperornithinaemia. Eur J Clin Invest 1999; 29:1060–5.
122. Henkind P, Ashton N. Ocular pathology in homocystinuria. Trans Ophthalmol Soc UK 1965; 85:21–38.
123. Hennekes R, Gerding H. Atrophia gyrata mit Makuladystrophie. Klin Monatsbl Augenheilkd 1985; 187:216–8.
124. Hill A, Zaleski WA. Tyrosinosis: biochemical studies of an unusual case. Clin Biochem 1971; 4:263–71.
125. Himeno M, Mueckler MM, Gonzalez FJ, Pitot HC. Cloning of DNA Complementary to Ornithine Aminotransferase Messenger-RNA. J Biol Chem 1982; 257:4669–72.
126. Hittner HM, Carroll AJ, Prchal JT. Linkage studies in carriers of Lowe Oculo-Cerebro-Renal syndrome. Am J Hum Genet 1982; 34:966–71.
127. Hodgson SV, Heckmatt JZ, Hughes E, et al. A balanced de novo X/autosome translocation in a girl with manifestations of lowe syndrome. Am J Med Genet 1986; 23:837–47.
128. Hoshaw RA, Zimmerman KG, Menter A. Ochronosislike pigmentation from hydroquinone bleaching creams in American blacks. Archives of Dermatology 1985; 121: 105–8.
129. Hubmacher D, Tiedemann K, Bartels R, et al. Modification of the structure and function of fibrillin-1 by homocysteine suggests a potential pathogenetic mechanism in homocystinuria. J Biol Chem 2005; 280: 34946–55.
130. Huhn R, Stoermer H, Klingele B, et al. Novel and recurrent tyrosine aminotransferase gene mutations in tyrosinemia type II. Hum Genet 1998; 102:305–13.
131. Inagaki K, Suzuki T, Shimizu H, et al. Oculocutaneous albinism type 4 is one of the most common types of albinism in Japan. Am J Hum Genet 2004 74:466–71.
132. Inana G, Hotta Y, Zintz C, et al. Expression defect of ornithine aminotransferase gene in gyrate atrophy. Invest Ophthalmol Vis Sci 1988; 29:1001–5.
133. Inana G, Totsuka S, Redmond M, et al. Molecular cloning of human ornithine aminotransferase mRNA. Proc Natl Acad Sci USA 1986; 83:1203–7.

134. Incerti B, Cortese K, Pizzigoni A, et al. Oa1 knock-out: new insights on the pathogenesis of ocular albinism type 1. Hum Mol Genet 2000; 9:2781–8.
135. Irreverre F, Mudd SH, Heizer WD, Laster L. Sulfite oxidase deficiency: studies of a patient with mental retardation, dislocated ocular lenses, and abnormal urinary excretion of Ssulfo-L-cysteine, sulfite, and thiosulfate. Biochem Med 1967; 1:187–217.
136. Jaeger W, Gallasch G, Schnyder UW, Lutz P, Schmidt H. Tyrosinämie ais Urasche einer doppelseitigen herpetiformen Hornhaut-Spithel-Dystrophie (Richner–Hanhart-Syndrom). Klin Monatsbl Augenheilkd 1978; 173:506–15.
137. Jaeger W, Kettler JV, Hilsdorf C, Lutz P. Gibt es verschiedene Typen der Atrophia gyrata choroideae et retinae? (Atrophie gyrata chorioideae et retinae mit und onhe Ornithinamia). In: W Jaeger. ed. Kunststoffimplantate in der Ophthalmologie. Munich: JF Bermann, 1977:655–63.
138. Johnson DL, Jacobson LW, Toyama R, Monahan RH. Histopathology of eyes in Chediak–Higashi syndrome. Arch Ophthalmol 1966; 75:84–8.
139. Johnson GJ, Gillan JG, Pearce WG. Ocular albinism in Newfoundland. Can J Ophthalmol 1971; 6:237–48.
140. Johnson JL, Duran M. Molybdenum cofactor deficiency and isolated sulfite oxidase deficiency. In: Scriver CR, Beaudet Al, Valle D, Sly WS, eds. Metabolic and Molecular Bases of Inherited Disease. New York: McGraw-Hill, 2001:3163–77.
141. Jones NP, Postlethwaite RJ, Noble JL. Clearance of corneal crystals in nephropathic cystinosis by topical cysteamine 0.5%. Br J Ophthalmol 1991; 75:311–2.
142. Kaiser-Kupfer MI, Caruso RC, Minkler DS, Gahl WA. Long-term ocular manifestations in nephropathic cystinosis. Arch Ophthalmol 1986; 104:706–11.
143. Kaiser-Kupfer MI, Datiles MB, Gahl WA. Corneal transplant in boy with nephropathic cystinosis. Lancet 1987; 1:331.
144. Kaiser-Kupfer MI, Datiles MB, Gahl WA. Clear graft two years after keratoplasty in nephropathic cystinosis. Am J Ophthalmol 1988; 105:318–9.
145. Kaiser-Kupfer MI, de Monasterio FM, Valle D, et al. Gyrate atrophy of the choroid and retina: improved visual function following reduction of plasma ornithine by diet. Science 1980; 210:1128–31.
146. Kaiser-Kupfer MI, Gazzo MA, Datiles MB, et al. A randomized placebo-controlled trial of cysteamine eye drops in nephropathic cystinosis. Arch Ophthalmol 1990; 108:689–93.
147. Kaiser-Kupfer MI, Podgor MJ, McCain L, et al. Correlation of ocular rigidity and blue sclerae in osteogenesis imperfecta. Trans Ophthalmol Soc UK 1985; 104(Pt 2):191–5.
148. Kalra BR, Ghose S, Sood NN. Homocystinuria with bilateral absolute glaucoma. Indian J Ophthalmol 1985; 33:195–7.
149. Kampik A, Sani JN, Green WR. Ocular ochronosis. Clinicopathological, histochemical, and ultrastructural studies. Arch Ophthalmol 1980; 98:1441–7.
150. Kang AH, Trelstad RL. A collagen defect in homocystinuria. J Clin Invest 1973; 52:2571–8.
151. Katz B, Melles RB, Schneider JA. Contrast sensitivity function in nephropathic cystinosis. Arch Ophthalmol 1987; 105:1667–9.
152. Katz B, Melles RB, Schneider JA. Corneal sensitivity in nephropathic cystinosis. Am J Ophthalmol 1987; 104: 413–6.
153. Katz B, Melles RB, Schneider JA. Glare disability in nephropathic cystinosis. Arch Ophthalmol 1987; 105: 1670–1.
154. Katz B, Melles RB, Schneider JA. Recurrent crystal deposition after keratoplasty in nephropathic cystinosis. Am J Ophthalmol 1987; 104:190–1.
155. Katz B, Melles RB, Schneider JA. Crystal deposition following keratoplasty in nephropathic cystinosis. Arch Ophthalmol 1989; 107:1727–8.
156. Katz B, Melles RB, Schneider JA, Rao NA. Corneal thickness in nephropathic cystinosis. Br J Ophthalmol 1989; 73:665–8.
157. Kennedy AJ, Voaden MJ. Free amino acids in the photoreceptor cells of the frog retina. J Neurochem 1974; 23:1093–5.
158. Kenyon KR, Sensenbrenner JA. Electron microscopy of cornea and conjunctiva in childhood cystinosis. Am J Ophthalmol 1974; 78:68–76.
159. Kida K, Takahashi M, Fujisawa Y, et al. Hepatic Tyrosine Aminotransferase in Tyrosinemia Type-Ii. J Inher Metabol Dis 1982; 5:229–30.
160. Kim YJ, Rosenberg LE. On the mechanism of pyridoxine responsive homocystinuria. II. Properties of normal and mutant cystathionine beta-synthase from cultured fibroblasts. Proc Natl Acad Sci USA 1974; 71:4821–5.
161. King RA, Creel D, Cervenka J, et al. Albinism in Nigeria with delineation of new recessive oculocutaneous type. Clin Genet 1980; 17:259–70.
162. King RA, Hearing VJ, Creel DJ, Oetting WS. Albinism. In: Scriver CR, Beaudet Al, Sly WS, Valle D, eds. The Metabolic and Molecular Bases of Inherited Disease. New York: McGraw-Hill, 2001:5587–627.
163. King RA, Lewis RA, Townsend D, et al. Brown oculocutaneous albinism: clinical, ophthalmological, and biochemical characterization. Ophthalmology 1985; 92: 1496–505.
164. King RA, Wirtschafter JD, Olds DP, Brumbaugh J. Minimal pigment: a new type of oculocutaneous albinism. Clin Genet 1986; 29:42–50.
165. Kingsmore SF, Barbosa MD, Tchernev VT, et al. Positional cloning of the Chediak–Higashi syndrome gene: genetic mapping of the beige locus on mouse chromosome 13. J Investig Med 1996; 44:454–61.
166. Kinnear PE, Jay B, Witkop CJ. Albinism. Surv Ophthalmol 1985; 30:75–101.
167. Koniszewski G, Rott HD. The Lyon-Effect in the Lens—Ocular findings in carrier women for X-Linked congenital cataract and Lowes Syndrome. Klinische Monatsblatter fur Augenheilkunde 1985; 187:525–8.
168. Kraus E, Lutz P. Ocular cystine deposits in an adult. Arch Ophthalmol 1971; 85:690–4.
169. Kritzler RA, Terner JY, Lindenbaum J, et al. Chediak–Higashi syndrome. Cytologic and serum lipid observations in a case and family. Am J Med 1964; 36: 583–94.
170. Kunkle GA, Jezyk PF, West CS, et al. Tyrosinemia in a dog. J Am Anim Hosp Assoc 1984; 20:615–20.
171. Kuwabara T, Ishikawa Y, Kaiser-Kupfer MI. Experimental model of gyrate atrophy in animals. Ophthalmology 1981; 88:331–5.
172. La Du BN. Alkaptonuria. In: Scriver CR, Beaudet Al, Valle D, Sly WS, eds. Metabolic and Molecular Bases of Inheritied Disease. New York: McGraw-Hill, 2001: 2109–24.
173. Lattion F, Schneider P, Da Prada M, et al. Syndrome d'Hermansky-Pudlak dans un village valaisan. Helv Paediatr Acta 1983; 38:495–512.
174. Leader RW, Padgett GA, Gorham JR. Studies of abnormal leukocyte bodies in the mink. Blood 1963; 22:477–84.

175. Lee ST, Nicholls RD, Jong MT, et al. Organization and sequence of the human P gene and identification of a new family of transport proteins. Genomics 1995; 26: 354–63.
176. Leimkuhler S, Charcosset M, Latour P, et al. Ten novel mutations in the molybdenum cofactor genes MOCS1 and MOCS2 and in vitro characterization of a MOCS2 mutation that abolishes the binding ability of molybdopterin synthase. Hum Genet 2005; 117:565–70.
177. Lerner-Ellis JP, Tirone JC1, Pawelek PD, et al. Identification of the gene responsible for methylmalonic aciduria and homocystinuria, cblC type. Nat Genet 2006; 38:93–100.
178. Leuenberger S, Faulborn J, Sturrock G, et al. Vasculäre und okuläre Komplikationen bei einem Kind mit Homocystinurie. Schweiz. Med Wochenschr 1984; 114: 793–8.
179. Leventhal AG, Creel DJ. Retinal projections and functional architecture of cortical areas 17 and 18 in the tyrosinase-negative albino cat. J Neurosci 1985; 5:795–807.
180. Lewis RA. Twenty-ninth Annual Meeting of Hum Genet. Vancouver:1978.
181. Li W, Zhang Q, Oiso N, et al. Hermansky–Pudlak syndrome type 7 (HPS-7) results from mutant dysbindin, a member of the biogenesis of lysosome-related organelles complex 1 (BLOC-1). Nat Genet 2003; 35:84–9.
182. Lowe CU, Terrey M, MacLachlan EA. Organic-aciduria, decreased renal ammonia production, hydrophthalmos, and mental retardation; a clinical entity. AMA. Am J Dis Child 1952; 83:164–84.
183. Lubin JR. Oculocutaneous albinism associated with corneal mesodermal dysgenesis. Am J Ophthalmol 1981; 91:347–50.
184. Lund RD. Uncrossed visual pathways of hooded and albino rats. Science 1965; 54:91.
185. Lutzner MA, Lowrie CT, Jordan HW. Giant granules in leukocytes of the beige mouse. J Hered 1967; 58:299–300.
186. Lynch HJ, Deng MH, Wurtman RJ. Light intensities required to suppress nocturnal melatonin secretion in albino and pigmented rats. Life Sci 1984; 35:841–7.
187. MacDonald IM, Noel LP, Mintsioulis G, Clarke WN. The effect of topical cysteamine drops on reducing crystal formation within the cornea of patients affected by nephropathic cystinosis. J Pediatr Ophthalmol Strabismus 1990; 27:272–4.
188. Margolis S, Siegel IM, Choy A, Breinin GM. Oculocutaneous albinism associated with Apert's syndrome. Am J Ophthalmol 1977; 84:830–9.
189. Mashima YG, Weleber RG, Kennaway NG, Inana G. Genotype-phenotype correlation of a pyridoxine-responsive form of gyrate atrophy. Ophthalmic Genet 1999; 20: 219–24.
190. Matalon R, Kaul R, Casanova J, et al. SSIEM Award. Aspartoacylase deficiency: the enzyme defect in Canavan disease. J Inherit Metab Dis 1989; 12(Suppl. 2):329–31.
191. Matalon R, Michals K, Sebesta D, et al. Aspartoacylase deficiency and N-acetylaspartic aciduria in patients with Canavan disease. Am J Med Genet 1988; 29:463–71.
192. McCartney AC, Spalton DJ, Bull TB. Type IV melanosomes of the human albino iris. Br J Ophthalmol 1985; 69: 537–41.
193. Melles RB, Schneider JA, Rao NA, Katz B. Spatial and temporal sequence of corneal crystal deposition in nephropathic cystinosis. Am J Ophthalmol 1987; 104: 598–604.
194. Menasche G, Feldmann J, Houdusse A, et al. Biochemical and functional characterization of Rab27a mutations occurring in Griscelli syndrome patients. Blood 2003; 101:2736–42.
195. Menasche G, Pastural E, Feldmann J, et al. Mutations in RAB27A cause Griscelli syndrome associated with haemophagocytic syndrome. Nat Genet 2000; 25:173–6.
196. Michaud J, Thompson GN, Brody LC, et al. Pyridoxine-responsive gyrate atrophy of the choroid and retina: clinical and biochemical correlates of the mutation A226V. Am J Hum Genet 1995; 56:616–22.
197. Miller SJH. Ocular ochronosis. Trans Ophthalmol Soc UK 2006; 74:349–66.
198. Mishima H, Hasebe H, Fujita H. Melanogenesis in the retinal pigment epithelial cell of the chick embryo. Dopa-reaction and electron microscopic autoradiography of ^{3}H-dopa. Invest Ophthalmol Vis Sci 1978; 17:403–11.
199. Mitchell GA, Grompe M, Lambert M, Tanguay RM. Hypertyrosinemia. In: Scriver CR, Beaudet Al, Valle D, Sly WS, eds. Metabolic and Molecular Bases of Inheritied Disease. New York: McGraw-Hill, 2001:1777–805.
200. Moat SJ, Bao L, Fowler B, et al. The molecular basis of cystathionine beta-synthase (CBS) deficiency in UK and US patients with homocystinuria. Hum Mutat 2004; 23: 206.
201. Morgan NV, Pasha S, Johnson CA, et al. A germline mutation in BLOC1S3/reduced pigmentation causes a novel variant of Hermansky–Pudlak syndrome (HPS8). Am J Hum Genet 2006; 78:160–6.
202. Mosher DB, Fitzpatrick TB, Ortonne JP, Hori Y. Disorders of pigmentation. In: Eisen AZ, Wolff K, Freedberg IM, Austen KF, eds. Dermatology in General Medicine: Textbook and Atlas. New York: McGraw-Hill, 1987: 794–876.
203. Mudd SH, Irreverre F, Laster L. Sulfite oxidase deficiency in man: demonstration of the enzymatic defect. Science 1967; 156:1599–602.
204. Mudd SH, Levy HL, Kraus JP. Disorders of transsulfuration. In: Scriver CR, Beaudet Al, Valle D, Sly WS, eds. Metabolic and Molecular Bases of Inherited Disease. New York: McGraw-Hill, 2001:2007–56.
205. Murty VV, Bouchard B, Mathew S, et al. Assignment of the human TYRP (brown) locus to chromosome region 9p23 by nonradioactive in situ hybridization. Genomics 1992; 13:227–9.
206. Nanto-Salonen K, Komu M, Lundbom N, et al. Reduced brain creatine in gyrate atrophy of the choroid and retina with hyperornithinemia. Neurology 1999; 53:303–7.
207. Natt E, Kida K, Odievre M, et al. Point mutations in the tyrosine aminotransferase gene in tyrosinemia type II. Proc Natl Acad Sci USA 1992; 89:9297–301.
208. Naughten ER, Yap S, Mayne PD. Newborn screening for homocystinuria: Irish and world experience. Eur J Pediatr 1998; 157(Suppl. 2):S84–7.
209. Newton JM, Cohen-Barak O, Hagiwara N, et al. Mutations in the human orthologue of the mouse underwhite gene (UW) underlie a new form of oculocutaneous albinism, OCA4. Am J Hum Genet 2001; 69:981–8.
210. Ney D, Bay C, Schneider JA, Kelts D, Nyhan WL. Dietary management of oculocutaneous tyrosinemia in an 11-year-old child. Am J Dis Child 1983; 137:995–1000.
211. Novikoff AB, Leuenberger PM, Novikoff PM, Quintana N. Retinal pigment epithelium: interrelations of endoplasmic reticulum and melanolysosomes in the black mouse and its beige mutant. Lab Invest 1979; 40: 155–65.
212. O'Donnell FE Jr, Green WR, Fleischman JA, Hambrick GW. X-linked ocular albinism in Blacks. Ocular albinism cum pigmento. Arch Ophthalmol 1978; 96:1189–92.

213. O'Donnell FE Jr, Hambrick GW Jr, Green WR, Iliff WJ, Stone DL. X-linked ocular albinism. An oculocutaneous macromelanosomal disorder. Arch Ophthalmol 1976; 94: 1883–92.
214. O'Donnell FE Jr, King RA, Green WR, Witkop CJ Jr. Autosomal recessively inherited ocular albinism. A new form of ocular albinism affecting females as severely as males. Arch Ophthalmol 1978; 96:1621–5.
215. O'Donnell JJ, Sandman RP, Martin SR. Gyrate atrophy of the retina: inborn error of L-ornithin:2-oxoacid aminotransferase. Science 1978; 200:200–1.
216. O'Donnell JJ, Sipila I, Vannas A, et al. Gyrate atrophy of the retina and choroid. Two methods for prenatal diagnosis. Int Ophthalmol 1981; 4:33–6.
217. O'Donnell JJ, Wood I, Hopkins SR. Mitochondrial abnormalities in cultured fibroblasts from a gyrate atrophy patient. Invest Ophthalmol Vis Sci 1981; 20(Suppl.):79.
218. Oh J, Bailin T, Fukai K, et al. Positional cloning of a gene for Hermansky–Pudlak syndrome, a disorder of cytoplasmic organelles. Nat Genet 1996; 14:300–6.
219. Ohkubo Y, Ueta A, Ito T, et al. Vitamin B6-responsive ornithine aminotransferase deficiency with a novel mutation G237D. Tohoku J Exp Med 2005; 205:335–42.
220. Ohura T, Kominami E, Tada K, Katunuma N. Gyrate atrophy of the choroid and retina: decreased ornithine aminotransferase concentration in cultured skin fibroblasts from patients. Clin Chim Acta 1984; 136:29–37.
221. Oliver JM. Impaired microtubule function correctable by cyclic GMP and cholinergic agonists in the Chediak–Hagashi syndrome. Am J Pathol 1976; 85:395–418.
222. Oliver JM. Cell biology of leukocyte abnormalities—membrane and cytoskeletal function in normal and defective cells: leukocyte abnormalities. Am J Pathol 1978; 93:221–70.
223. Orendac M, Zeman J, Stabler SP, et al. Homocystinuria due to cystathionine beta-synthase deficiency: novel biochemical findings and treatment efficacy. J Inherit Metab Dis 2003; 26:761–73.
224. Orr HT, Cohen AI, Lowry OM. The distribution of taurine in the vertebrate retina. J Neurochem 1976; 26:609–11.
225. Osler W. Ochronosis: the pigmentation of cartilages, sclerotics, and skin in alkaptonuria. Lancet 1904; 1:10–1.
226. Ozand PT, Gascon GG, Dhalla M. Aspartoacylase deficiency and Canavan disease in Saudi Arabia. Am J Med Genet 1990; 35:266–8.
227. Padgett GA. Neutrophilic function in animals with the Chediak–Higashi syndrome. Blood 1967; 29:906–15.
228. Padgett GA, Holland JM, Prieur DJ, et al. The Chediak–Higashi syndrome: a review of the disease in man, mink, cattle, and mice. Anim Models Biomed Res 1970; 3:1–12.
229. Padgett GA, Leader RW, Gorham JR, O'Mary CC. The familial occurrence of the Chediak–Higashi syndrome in mink and cattle. Genetics 1964; 49:505–12.
230. Palacin M, Goodyer P, Nunes V, Gasparini P. Cystinuria. In: Scriver CR, Beaudet Al, Valle D, Sly WS, eds. Metabolic and Molecular Bases of Inheritied Disease. New York: McGraw-Hill, 2001:4909–32.
231. Palareti G, Salardi S, Piazzi S, et al. Blood coagulation changes in homocystinuria: effects of pyridoxine and other specific therapy. J Pediatr 1986; 109:1001–6.
232. Pallisgaard G, Goldschmidt E. Oculo–cerebro–renal syndrome of Lowe in four generations of one family. Acta Paediatr Scand 1971; 60:146–8.
233. Pasantes-Morales H, Kleithi J, Ledig M, Mandel P. Free amino acids of chicken and rat retina. Brain Res 1972; 41: 494–7.
234. Pastural E, Barrat FJ, Dufourcq-Lagelouse, R, et al. Griscelli disease maps to chromosome 15q21 and is associated with mutations in the myosin-Va gene. Nat Genet 1997; 16:289–92.
235. Patton N, Beatty S, Lloyd IC, Wraith JE. Optic atrophy in association with cobalamin C (cblC) disease. Ophthalmic Genet 2000; 21:151–4.
236. Pearce WG, Johnson GJ, Sanger R. Ocular albinism and Xg. Lancet 1971; 1:1072.
237. Perez MI, Sanchez JL. Histopathologic evaluation of melanocytic nervi in oculocutaneous albinism. Am J Dermatopathol 1985; 7(Suppl.):23–8.
238. Phillips JI, Isaacson C, Carman H. Ochronosis in black South Africans who used skin lighteners. Am J Dermatopathol 1986; 8:14–21.
239. Phornphutkul C, Introne WJ, Perry MB, et al. Natural history of alkaptonuria. N Engl J Med 2002; 347:2111–21.
240. Pillers DA, Towbin JA, Chamberlain JS, et al. Deletion mapping of Aland Island eye disease to Xp21 between DXS67 (B24) and Duchenne muscular dystrophy. Am J Hum Genet 1990; 47:795–801.
241. Polyak S. The Vertebrate Visual System. Chicago: University of Chicago Press, 1957.
242. Potterf SB, Furumura M, Sviderskaya EV, et al. Normal tyrosine transport and abnormal tyrosinase routing in pink-eyed dilution melanocytes. Exp Cell Res 1998; 244:319–26.
243. Quevedo WC Jr, Fitzpatrick TB, Szabo B, Jimbow K. Biology of the melanin pigmentary system. In: Fitzpatrick TB, Eisen AZ, Wolff K, Freedberg IM, Austen KF, eds. New York: McGraw-Hill, 1987:224–51.
244. Ramesh V, McClatchey AI, Ramesh N, et al. Molecular basis of ornithine aminotransferase deficiency in B-6-responsive and nonresponsive forms of gyrate atrophy. Proc Natl Acad Sci USA 1988; 85:3777–80.
245. Ramesh V, Shaffer MM, Allaire JM, et al. Investigation of gyrate atrophy using a cDNA clone for human ornithine aminotransferase. DNA 1986; 5:493–501.
246. Ramsay M, Colman MA, Stevens G, et al. The tyrosinase-positive oculocutaneous albinism locus maps to chromosome 15q11.2-q12. Am J Hum Genet 1992; 51:879–84.
247. Ramsey MS, Yanoff M, Fine BS. The ocular histopathology of homocystinuria. A light and electron microscopic study. Am J Ophthalmol 1972; 74:377–85.
248. Rao GN, Cotlier E. Ornithine delta-aminotransferase activity in retina and other tissues. Neurochem Res 1984; 9:555–62.
249. Ricci B, Lacerra F, Lubins JR. Oculocutaneous albinism and corneal mesodermal dysgenesis. Am J Ophthalmol 1987; 92:587.
250. Rich LF, Beard ME, Burns RP. Excess dietary tyrosine and corneal lesions. Exp Eye Res 1973; 17:87–97.
251. Richard G, Kroll P. Netzhautveränderungen bei Zystinose. Ophthalmologica 1983; 186:211–8.
252. Richler M, Milot J, Quigley M, O'Regan S. Ocular manifestations of nephropathic cystinosis. The French-Canadian experience in a genetically homogeneous population. Arch Ophthalmol 1991; 109:359–62.
253. Ripple RE, Lohr KM, Twining SS, et al. Role of leukocytes in ocular inflammation of tyrosinemia II. Invest Ophthalmol Vis Sci 1986; 27:926–31.
254. Robison WG Jr, Kuwabara T, Cogan DG. Lysosomes and melanin granules of the retinal pigment epithelium in a mouse model of the Chediak–Higashi syndrome. Invest Ophthalmol 1975; 14:312–7.
255. Robison WG Jr, Kuwabara T. A new, albino-beige mouse: giant granules in retinal pigment epithelium. Invest Ophthalmol Vis Sci 1978; 17:365–70.

256. Rodenhauser JH. Über die Augenpigmentierung bei Alkaptonurie (Ochronosis oculi). Klin Monatsbl Augenheilkd 1957; 131:202–15.
257. Rones B. Ochronosis oculi in alkaptonuria. Am J Ophthalmol 1960; 49:440–6.
258. Rosenblatt DS, Aspler AL, Shevell MI, et al. Clinical heterogeneity and prognosis in combined methylmalonic aciduria and homocystinuria (cblC). J Inherit Metab Dis 1997; 20:528–38.
259. Rott HD, Rix R. Konduktorinnenstatus bei X-gebundenem, okurärem Albinismus: ein Belegfür die Gültigkeit der Lyon-Hypothese beim Menchen. Klin. Monatsbl. Augenheilkd 1984; 184:128–9.
260. Royer J, Rollin L. Manifestations oculaires de l'ochronose. Bull Soc Ophtalmol Fr 1965; 65:500–2.
261. Sacksteder KA, Biery BJ, Morrell JC, et al. Identification of the alpha-aminoadipic semialdehyde synthase gene, which is defective in familial hyperlysinemia. Am J Hum Genet 2000; 66:1736–43.
262. Sagel I, Ores RO, Yuceoglu AM. Renal function and morphology in a girl with oculocerebrorenal syndrome. J Pediatr 1970; 77:124–7.
263. Sakamoto A, Sakura N. Limited effectiveness of betaine therapy for cystathionine beta synthase deficiency. Pediatr Int 2003; 45:333–8.
264. Salceda R, Carabex A, Pacheco P, Pasantes-Morales H. Taurine levels, uptake, and synthesizing enzyme activities in degenerated rat retinas. Exp Eye Res 1979; 28: 137–146.
265. Sanderson KJ. Normal and abnormal retinogeniculate pathways in rabbits and mink. Anat Rec 1972; 172:389.
266. Sanderson PO, Kuwabara T, Stark WJ, et al. Cystinosis. A clinical, histopathologic, and ultrastructural study. Arch Ophthalmol 1974; 91:270–4.
267. Santinelli R, Costagliola C, Tolone C, et al. Low-protein diet and progression of retinal degeneration in gyrate atrophy of the choroid and retina: a twenty-six-year follow-up. J Inherit Metab Dis 2004; 27:187–96.
268. Sarangarajan R, Zhao Y, Babcock G, et al. Mutant alleles at the brown locus encoding tyrosinase-related protein-1 (TRP-1) affect proliferation of mouse melanocytes in culture. Pigment Cell Res 2000; 13:337–44.
269. Schmidt SY, Berson EL, Hayes KC. Retinal degeneration in cats fed casein. I. taurine deficiency. Invest Ophthalmol 1976; 15:47–52.
270. Schneider JA, Verroust FM, Kroll WA, et al. Prenatal diagnosis of cystinosis. N Engl J Med 1974; 290:878–82.
271. Schnur RE, Nussbaum RL, Anson-Cartwright L, et al. Linkage analysis in X-linked ocular albinism. Genomics 1991; 9:605–13.
272. Seitz R. Über die ochronotischen Pigmentierungen am Auge. Klin Monatsbl Augenheilkd 1954; 125:432–40.
273. Simmaco M, John RA, Barra D, Bossa F. The primary structure of ornithine aminotransferase: identification of active-site sequence and site of post-translational proteolysis. FEBS Lett 1986; 199:39–42.
274. Singh RH, Kruger WD, Wang L, et al. Cystathionine beta-synthase deficiency: effects of betaine supplementation after methionine restriction in B6-nonresponsive homocystinuria. Genet Med 2004; 6:90–5.
275. Sipila I, Simell O, Rapola J, et al. Gyrate atrophy of the choroid and retina with hyperornithinemia: tubular aggregates and type 2 fiber atrophy in muscle. Neurology 1979; 29:996–1005.
276. Skinsnes OK. Generalized ochronosis: report of an instance where it was misdiagnosed as melanosarcoma, with resultant enucleation of eye. Arch Pathol 1948; 45: 552–8.
277. Smith JW. Ochronosis of the cornea and sclera complicating alkaptonuria: review of the literature and report of four cases. JAMA 1946; 120:1282–8.
278. Smith RS. Ocular pathology in sulfite oxidase deficiency. Invest Ophthalmol Vis Sci 1978; 17(Suppl.):247.
279. Smith TH, Holland MG, Woody NC. Ocular manifestations of familial hyperlysinemia. Trans Am Acad Ophthalmol Otolaryngol 1971; 75:355–60.
280. Spencer WH, Hogan MJ. Ocular manifestations of Chediak–Higashi syndrome. Am J Ophthalmol 1960; 50: 1197–203.
281. Stefani FH, Vogel S. Adult cystinosis: electron microscopy of the conjunctiva. Graefes Arch Clin Exp Ophthalmol 1982; 219:143–5.
282. Stigmaier OC, Schneider LA. Chediak–Higashi syndrome. Arch Dermatol 1965; 91:1–9.
283. Suchy SF, Nussbaum RL. The deficiency of PIP2 5-phosphatase in Lowe syndrome affects actin polymerization. Am J Hum Genet 2002; 71:1420–7.
284. Sudarshan A, Kopietz L. Corneal changes in homocystinuria. Ann Ophthalmol 1986; 18:60.
285. Suveges I. Kongenitale Hornhautdysplasie vergesellschaftet mit Richner–Hanhart-Syndrom. Klin Monatsbl Augenheilkd 1970; 157:493–9.
286. Suwannarat P, O'Brien K, Perry MB, et al. Use of nitisinone in patients with alkaptonuria. Metabolism 2005; 54:719–28.
287. Suzuki T, Li W, Zhang Q, et al. Hermansky–Pudlak syndrome is caused by mutations in HPS4, the human homolog of the mouse light-ear gene. Nat Genet 2002; 30: 321–4.
288. Szymanski KA, Boughman JA, Nance WE, et al. Genetic studies of ocular albinism in a large Virginia kindred. Ann Ophthalmol 1984; 16:183–91, 194.
289. Takahashi A, Yokoyama T. Hermansky–Pudlak syndrome with special reference to lysosomal dysfunction. A case report and review of the literature. Virchows Arch. A Pathol Anat Histopathol 1984; 402:247–58.
290. Takki K. Gyrate atrophy of the choroid and retina associated with hyperornithinaemia. Br J Ophthalmol 1974; 58:3–23.
291. Tan C, Etcubanas E, Lieberman P, et al. Chediak–Higashi syndrome in a child with Hodgkin's disease. Am J Dis Child 1971; 121:135–9.
292. Thoene J, Lemons R, Anikster Y, et al. Mutations of CTNS causing intermediate cystinosis. Mol Genet Metab 1999; 67:283–93.
293. Tomita Y, Suzuki T. Genetics of pigmentary disorders. Am J Med Genet Part C-Seminars in Med Genet 2004; 131C:75–81.
294. Touchman JW, Anikster Y, Dietrich NL, et al. The genomic region encompassing the nephropathic cystinosis gene (CTNS): complete sequencing of a 200-kb segment and discovery of a novel gene within the common cystinosis-causing deletion. Genome Res 2000; 10:165–73.
295. Trijbels JM, Sengers RC, Bakkeren JA, et al. L-Ornithine-ketoacid-transaminase deficiency in cultured fibroblasts of a patient with hyperornithinaemia and gyrate atrophy of the choroid and retina. Clin Chim Acta 1977; 79:371–7.
296. Tripathi RC, Cibis GW, Tripathi BJ. Lowe's syndrome. Trans Ophthalmol Soc UK 1980; 100:132–9.
297. Tripathi RC, Cibis GW, Tripathi BJ. Pathogenesis of cataracts in patients with Lowe's syndrome. Ophthalmology 1986; 93:1046–51.

298. Ungewickell A, Ward ME, Ungewickell E, Majerus PW. The inositol polyphosphate 5-phosphatase Ocrl associates with endosomes that are partially coated with clathrin. Proc Natl Acad Sci USA 2004; 101:13501–6.
299. Valle D, Kaiser-Kupfer MI, Del Valle LA. Gyrate atrophy of the choroid and retina: deficiency of ornithine aminotransferase in transformed lymphocytes. Proc Natl Acad Sci USA 1977; 74:5159–61.
300. Valle D, Simell O. The Hyperornithinemias. In: Scriver CR, Beaudet Al, Valle D, Sly WS, eds. Metabolic and Molecular Bases of Inherited Disease. New York: McGraw-Hill, 2001:1857–95.
301. van der Berg W, Verbraak FD, Bos PJ. Homocystinuria presenting as central retinal artery occlusion and long-standing thromboembolic disease. Br J Ophthalmol 1990; 74:696–7.
302. van Dorp DB, Delleman JW, Loewer-Sieger DH. Oculocutaneous albinism and anterior chambre cleavage malformations. Not a coincidence. Clin Genet 1984; 26:440–4.
303. van Dorp DB, Eriksson AW, Delleman JW, et al. Aland eye disease: no albino misrouting. Clin Genet 1985; 28: 526–31.
304. Vannas-Sulonen K, Vannas A, O'Donnell JJ, et al. Pathology of iridectomy specimens in gyrate atrophy of the retina and choroid. Acta Ophthalmol (Copenh) 1983; 61:9–19.
305. Voaden MJ, Lake N, Marshall J, Morjaria B. Studies on the distribution of taurine and other neuroactive amino acids in the retina. Exp Eye Res 1977; 25:249–57.
306. Wan WL, Minckler DS, Rao NA. Pupillary-block glaucoma associated with childhood cystinosis. Am J Ophthalmol 1986; 101:700–5.
307. Weleber RG, Wirtz MK, Kennaway NG. Gyrate atrophy of the choroid and retina: clinical and biochemical heterogeneity and response to vitamin B6. Birth Defects Orig Artic Ser 1982; 18:219–30.
308. White JG. The Chediak–Higashi syndrome: a possible lysosomal disease. Blood 1966; 28:143–56.
309. Wilcken B, Wiley V, Hammond J, Carpenter K. Screening newborns for inborn errors of metabolism by tandem mass spectrometry. N Engl J Med 2003; 348: 2304–12.
310. Wilson SM, Yip R, Swing DA, et al. A mutation in Rab27a causes the vesicle transport defects observed in ashen mice. Proc Natl Acad Sci USA 2000; 97:7933–8.
311. Windhorst DB, Zelickson AS, Good RA. Chediak–Higashi syndrome: hereditary giantism of cytoplasmic organelles. Science 1966; 151:81–3.
312. Windhorst DB, Zelickson AS, Good RA. A human pigmentary dilution based on a heritable subcellular structural defect—the Chediak–Higashi syndrome. J Invest Dermatol 1968; 50:9–18.
313. Winship I, Gericke G, Beighton P. X-linked inheritance of ocular albinism with late-onset sensorineural deafness. Am J Med Genet 1984; 19:797–803.
314. Wirtschafter JD. The eye in alkaptonuria. Birth Defects Orig Artic Ser 1976; 12:279–93.
315. Wisniewski KE, Kieras FJ, French JH, et al. Ultrastructural, neurological, and glycosaminoglycan abnormalities in Lowes syndrome. Annals of Neurology 1984; 16:40–9.
316. Wisniewski KE, Laure-Kamionowska M, Sher J, Pitter J. Infantile neuroaxonal dystrophy in an albino girl. A cliniconeuropathologic study. Acta Neuropathol (Berl) 1985; 66:68–71.
317. Witkop CJ. Depigmentations of the general and oral tissues and their genetic foundations. Ala J Med Sci 1979; 16:330–43.
318. Witkop CJ Jr, Hill CW, Desnick S, et al. Ophthalmologic, biochemical, platelet, and ultrastructural defects in the various types of oculocutaneous albinism. J Invest Dermatol 1973; 60:443–56.
319. Witkop CJ Jr, Jay B, Creel D, Guillery RW. Optic and otic neurologic abnormalities in oculocutaneous and ocular albinism. Birth Defects Orig Artic Ser 1982; 18:299–318.
320. Witkop CJ Jr, White JG, Nance WE, et al. Classification of albinism in man. Birth Defects Orig Artic Ser 1971; 7: 13–25.
321. Wolff SM, Dale DC, Clark RA, et al. The Chediak–Higashi syndrome: studies of host defenses. Ann Intern Med 1972; 76:293–306.
322. Wollensak J. Zonula Zinnii histologische und chemische Untersuchungen, insbesondere uber Zonolysisis enzymatica und Syndroma Marfan. Fortschr Augenheildk 1965; 16:240–335.
323. Wong VG. Ocular manifestations in cystinosis. Birth Defects Orig Artic Ser 1976; 12:181–6.
324. Wong VG, Kuwabara T, Brubaker R, et al. Intralysosomal cystine crystals in cystinosis. Invest Ophthalmol 1970; 9: 83–8.
325. Wong VG, Lietman PS, Seegmiller JE. Alterations of pigment epithelium in cystinosis. Arch Ophthalmol 1967; 77:361–9.
326. Wright CE, Tallan HH, Lin YY. Taurine: biological update. Annu Rev Biochem 1986; 55:427–53.
327. Yap S. Classical homocystinuria: vascular risk and its prevention. J Inherit Metab Dis 2003; 26:259–65.
328. Yoshiike T, Manabe M, Hayakawa M, Ogawa H. Macromelanosomes in X-linked ocular albinism (XLOA). Acta Derm Venereol 1985; 65:66–9.
329. Zhang Q, Zhao B, Li W, et al. Ru2 and Ru encode mouse orthologs of the genes mutated in human Hermansky–Pudlak syndrome types 5 and 6. Nat Genet 2003; 33: 145–53.
330. Zhang X, Jefferson AB, Auethavekiat V, Majerus PW. The protein deficient in Lowe syndrome is a phosphatidylinositol-4,5-bisphosphate 5-phosphatase. Proc Natl Acad Sci USA 1995; 92:4853–6.
331. Zimmerman TJ, Hood CI, Gasset AR. Adolescent cystinosis. A case presentation and review of the recent literature. Arch Ophthalmol 1974; 92:265–8.

44

Disorders of Collagen

Ray P. Boot-Handford and Cay M. Kielty
Faculty of Life Sciences, Wellcome Trust Centre for Cell Matrix Research, University of Manchester, Manchester, U.K.

INTRODUCTION

Collagens are major, predominantly structural, components of the extracellular matrices (ECMs) in multicellular animals. These matrices are either organized into thin sheet-like layers, basement membranes (151) that underlie all epithelia and endothelia including those of the eye, or in interstitial matrices in forms such as cartilage, tendon, ligament, and including the sclera, cornea, and vitreous. It is noteworthy that the principal collagenous components of both basement membrane-like matrices (called collagen type IV in vertebrates) and interstitial matrices (fibril-forming or fibrillar collagens) are a characteristic of multicellular animals and are found in both the simplest sponges and the most complex vertebrates (19). For detailed reviews of collagen structures and disease associations, see Refs. (65,94).

At the time of the first edition of Pathobiology of Ocular Disease in 1982, five different collagen types had been described and this number had risen to 13 by the last edition in 1994 (48). Since 1994, advances in molecular genetic techniques have focused research more on the structure and function of collagens and less on their sequence and biochemistry. To date, in the "post-genome" era, there are 28 distinct types of vertebrate collagen (Table 1) (140). Each new vertebrate collagen has been named using the next available Roman numeral and so the number of the collagen type reflects the order in which the collagens (or, more latterly, the genes encoding novel collagen α-chains) were discovered. Several more "collagen-like" molecules are encoded in the genome and these may be shown eventually to satisfy the criteria (listed below) that are required for a molecule to be considered a fully fledged collagen.

MOLECULAR FEATURES OF A COLLAGEN MOLECULE

Collagen molecules contain three polypeptide chains, each a left-handed helix, which fold together to form the characteristic right-handed triple-helical or collagenous domain. Collagen trimers are composed either of three identical chains (homotrimers) or of two or three distinct but closely related chains (heterotrimers) (19,114). All collagen genes encode one of more peptide domains containing -Gly-X-Y- amino acid repeat sequences that are referred to as collagenous domains. The -X- and -Y- positions in the repeat are frequently proline and hydroxyproline. The hydroxyproline helps to stabilize the triple helix by hydrogen bonding along its axis. Glycine is required at every third position in the repeat, as this is the only amino acid with a small enough side chain (an "H" atom) to allow the residue to be packed into the central core of the collagen triple helix. Classical fibrillar collagens do not tolerate any interruptions in their major collagenous domains composed of 1014–1020 residues (338–340-Gly-X-Y- repeats) (65,71). Other collagen types contain collagenous domains of various lengths (from 1530 residues in collagen VII to ~100 residues for some of the domains in FACIT collagens), many of which have small interruptions in the -Gly-X-Y- repeats. The final distinguishing feature of a "true" collagen molecule is that, upon secretion from the cell, the molecule becomes incorporated into, and forms part of, the insoluble ECM. "Collagen-like" molecules have collagenous triple-helical domains but remain soluble, normally in the plasma. They do not form part of the ECM, but rather function as hormones (e.g., adiponectin), or structural components of enzymes or receptors (C1q and macrophage scavenger receptor, respectively) (65).

COLLAGEN BIOSYNTHESIS

Collagen polypeptides are synthesized in the rough endoplasmic reticulum (ER) and translocated into the lumen of the ER where the unfolded collagenous domains are subject to a series of specific and characteristic post-translational modifications. These modifications include: (*i*) hydroxylation of some proline residues in the Y position of the -Gly-X-Y- repeat; (*ii*) hydroxylation of some lysine residues (hydroxylated forms of proline and lysine are always produced as post-translational modifications as neither modified residue has a codon or tRNA); and (*iii*) glycosylation of some hydroxylysine residues with a disaccharide containing a glucose and galactose moiety (19,65,71). Assembly of the trimeric molecule is driven by chain recognition and association, in most cases occurring at the C-terminal end of the molecule, with the collagenous domain(s) folding linearly in the C- to N-terminal direction (22,73). The folding of the triple-helical domain terminates the post-translational modification of the collagenous triplets. Missense mutations in the collagenous domain that cause a delay or temporary stalling in the folding of the helix result in an increased level of post-translational modification of the residues N-terminal to the mutation (22). Once correctly folded, the collagen molecules are further modified as required in the Golgi apparatus and post-Golgi apparatus compartments, e.g., N-linked glycosylation or the addition of glycosaminoglycan (GAG) side chains and secreted from the cell.

MACROMOLECULAR ASSEMBLY OF COLLAGENS

It is becoming increasingly clear that the assembly of the ECM is a process that is tightly controlled and intricately regulated by the cell (29,151). Some collagen types form macromolecular assemblies in processes that appear to start in the late secretory pathway and which are completed in the extracellular compartment. Whether this is a general feature for macromolecular assembly of all or most collagens is yet to be determined. Once assembled, many of the collagenous macromolecular structures are covalently stabilized by lysine and hydroxylysine-derived cross-links or disulfide bond exchange. The type of macromolecular assembly formed is dependent upon the type of collagen.

COLLAGEN TYPES

Fibril-Forming Collagens

The most abundant and first collagens characterized (collagen types I, II, and III) are fibrillar collagens and there are now four more members of this subfamily (Table 1). The classical fibrillar collagens (collagen types I–III, V, and XI) form the cross-striated fibrils with a 67 nm periodicity apparent in phosphotungstic-stained interstitial matrices. Fibril assembly is catalyzed by the enzymatic cleavage of N- and C-terminal non-collagenous globular domains (N- and C-propeptides) flanking the uninterrupted collagenous domain (28,106). The rod-like collagenous domains then self-assemble in an entropy-driven process by lateral

Table 1 The Collagen Family: Chain Composition, Structure, and Distribution

Collagen type	Molecular composition	Genes	Genomic localization	Structure in ECM	Tissue expression	Function	Related disorders[a]
Fibrillar collagens							
I	$\alpha1(I)_2$, $\alpha2(I)$	*COL1A1* *COL1A2*	17q21.31–q22 7q22.1	67nm banded fibrils often associated with collagen type III	Bone, cornea, ligaments, skin, tendon, vessel walls	Tensile strength	Ehlers–Danlos syndrome type VII, involutional osteoporosis, and osteogenesis imperfecta
II	$\alpha1(II)_3$	*COL2A1*	12q13.11–q13.2	67nm banded fibrils	Cartilage, intervertebral disc, vitreous humor, other tissues in development; splice variant A—embryonic, variant B is marker of mature cartilage	Tensile strength	Kniest dysplasia, spondyloepiphyseal dysplasia, and Stickler syndrome and osteoarthritis
III	$\alpha1(III)_3$	*COL3A1*	2q31	67nm banded fibrils—small diameter	In all tissues with collagen type I except bone	Provides tissue with extensibility	Aortic aneurysms and Ehlers–Danlos syndrome type IV
V	$\alpha1(V)$, $\alpha2(V)$, $\alpha3(V)$, $\alpha1(V)_2$, $\alpha1(V)_1$	*COL5A1* *COL5A2* *COL5A3*	9q34.2–q34.3 2q31 19p13.2	9mm non-banded fibrils; amino terminal domains partially processed; core structure of collagen type I/III/V heterofibrils	Bone, cornea, liver, lung, placenta, skin, tendon, vessel walls	Controls assembly, size, and growth of collagen type I/III/V heterofibrils	Ehlers–Danlos syndrome types I and II
XI	$\alpha1(XI)$, $\alpha2(XI)$, $\alpha3(XI)$	*COL11A1* *COL11A2* *COL11A3* (*COL2A1* product with differing glycosylation and hydroxylation levels)	1p21 6p21.3	Fine non-banded fibrils; amino terminal domains partially processed; core structure of collagen type II/XI heterofibrils	Cartilage, vitreous body	Controls assembly, size, and growth of collagen type II/XI heterofibrils	Mutations in *COL11A1* and *COL11A2* associated with mild chondrodysplasias (e.g., Stickler syndrome), osteoarthritis, and nonsyndromic hearing loss
XXIV	$\alpha1(XXIV)_3$	*COL24A1*	1p22.3		Developing bone and cornea	Predicted function in cell adhesion	
XXVII	$\alpha1(XXVII)_3$	*COL27A1*	9q32		Cartilage, eye ear, gonad, lung, skin, stomach, and tooth	Structural component	
Basement membrane collagen							
IV	$\alpha1(IV)$, $\alpha2(IV)$, $\alpha3(IV)$, $\alpha4(IV)$, $\alpha5(IV)$, $\alpha5(IV)_2$, $\alpha6(IV)$	*COL4A1* *COL4A2* *COL4A3* *COL4A4* *COL4A5* *COL4A6*	13q34 13q34 2q36–q37 2q36–q37 Xq22.3 Xp22.3	Non-fibrillar meshwork stabilized by covalent crosslinks	Basement membrane	Meshwork provides strength and size-selective filtration to basement membrane; non-collagenous domains associated with inhibition of angiogenesis	Mutations in *COL4A3*, *COLA4*, *COLA5*, and *COLA6* are associated with Alport syndrome; *COL4A4* is also associated with familial haematuria; autoimmune response to *COL4A3* NC1 domain associated with glomerular Goodpasture syndrome
Microfibillar collagens							
VI	$\alpha1(VI)$, $\alpha2(VI)$, $\alpha3(VI)$	*COL6A1* *COL6A2* *COL6A3*	21q22.3 21q22.3 2q37	10nm beaded microfibrils	Widespread in all connective tissues	Structural component	Mutations in all chains associated with Bethlem myopathy and Ulrich muscular dystrophy
XXVIII	$\alpha1(XXVIII)_3$	*COL28A1*	7p21.3	Structure of protein similar to that of collagen type VI	Dorsal root ganglia, peripheral nerve, skin, calvaria	Basement membranes surrounding some peripheral nerves, skin, calvaria	

(*Continued*)

Table 1 The Collagen Family: Chain Composition, Structure, and Distribution (*Continued*)

Collagen type	Molecular composition	Genes	Genomic localization	Structure in ECM	Tissue expression	Function	Related disorders[a]
Anchoring fibril collagen							
VII	$\alpha1(VII)_3$	*COL7A1*	3p21.3	Loosely bound fibrous structures associated with collagen type IV network	Dermal-epidermal junctions, cervix, oral mucosa, skin	Structural component of anchoring fibrils that anchor the basement membrane to stromal tissue	Dystrophic forms of epidermolysis bullosa
Short chain collagens							
VIII	$\alpha1(VIII)_3$, $\alpha2(VIII)_3$, $\alpha1(VIII)_2$, $\alpha2(VIII)$	*COL8A1* *COL8A2*	3q12–q13 1p34.3–p32.3	Non-fibrillar hexagonal lattice meshwork	Corneal descemet membrane, endothelia, skin keratinocytes, lens epithelia, mesenchyme surrounding cartilage and calvarial bone, meninges surrounding brain	Membrane stabilization, angiogenesis, interactions with matrix molecules, cell migration, and membrane structural component	Mutations in *COL8A2* gene associated with Fuchs corneal dystrophy and posterior polymorphous corneal dystrophy
X	$\alpha1(X)^3$	*COL10A1*	6q21–q22.3	Non-fibrillar hexagonal lattice meshwork	Hypertrophic cartilage of growth plate	Structural support to calcified matrix	Mutations, mainly in NC1 domain, cause Schmid metaphyseal chondrodysplasia
FACIT collagens (fibril associated collagens with interrupted triple helices)							
IX	$\alpha1(IX)$, $\alpha2(IX)$, $\alpha3(IX)$	*COL9A1* *COL9A2*	6q13 1p33–p32.2	Molecules localize on the surface of collagen fibrils, through lysine covalent crosslinking with the N terminal of collagen type II; hinge in NC3 region causes molecule to reach out and interact with proteoglycans	Cartilage, cornea, invertebral disc, vitreous humor	Links collagen type II molecules, connects collagens to other matrix molecules, and determines size and growth of collagen type II fibrils	Early onset osteoarthritis and various chondrodysplasias (mutations in *COL9A2* associated with multiple epiphyseal dysplasia)
XII	$\alpha1(XII)_3$	*COL12A1*	6q12–q13	Non-fibrillar; interactions similar to collagen type IX	Ligaments, perichondrium, tendon	Connects collagens to other matrix molecules and determines size and growth of collagen type I fibrils	
XIV	$\alpha1(XIV)_3$	*COL14A1*	8q23		Liver, lung, placenta, skin, tendon, vessel wall	Provides strength in tissues under high mechanical stress and determines size and growth of fibrils	
XVI	$\alpha1(XVI)_3$	*COL16A1*	1p34		Widespread in basement membranes		
XIX	$\alpha1(XIX)_3$	*COL19A1*	6q12–q14		Human rhabdomyosarcoma	Determines size and growth of fibrils	
XX	$\alpha1(XX)_3$	*COL20A1*	20q13.33		Corneal epithelium, embryonic skin, sternal cartilage, tendon	Determines size and growth of fibrils	
XXI	$\alpha1(XXI)_3$	*COL21A1*	6p12.3–11.2		Vessel walls		
XXII	$\alpha1(XXII)_3$	*COL22A1*	8q24.3		Tissue junctions		
XXVI	$\alpha1(XXVI)_3$	*COL26A1*	7q22.1	Predicted to be a FACIT collagen as contains two collagenous domains; contains Emi domain	Ovary pre-theca, testis, myoid cells		

Transmembrane collagens							
XIII	$\alpha 1(XIII)_3$	*COL13A1*	10q22	Non-fibrillar	Chondrocytes, epidermis, hair follicle, intestine, liver, lungs, muscle, skin	Transmembrane component of focal adhesion sites	
XVII	$\alpha 1(XVII)_3$	*COL17A1*	10q24.3		Dermal-epidermal junctions		Bullous epithelial disorders
XXIII	$\alpha 1(XXIII)_3$	*COL23A1*	5q35		Metastatic tumor cells		
XXV	$\alpha 1(XXV)_3$	*COL25A1*	4q25		Neurons		
MULTIPLEXINS (multiple triple-helix domains and interruptions)							
XV	$\alpha 1(XV)_3$	*COL15A1*	9q21–q22	Non-fibrillar; distributed throughout basement membrane	Widespread in basement membranes	Stabilizing muscle and microvessel structure; non-collagenous domain associated with inhibition of angiogenesis	
XVIII	$\alpha 1(XVIII)_3$	*COL18A1*	21q22.3		Three variant forms expressed in basement membranes of vessel walls: long unspliced—brain, heart, kidney, liver, lung, skeletal muscle; long spliced—liver; short—kidney	C terminal NC1 domain (endostatin) inhibits angiogenesis; development of vasculature and retina	Knoblach and pigment dispersion syndromes

[a] For Mendelian Inheritance in Man numbers and descriptions, see Online Mendelian Inheritance in Man Web site: http://www.ncbi.nlm.nih.gov/entrez/query.fcgi?db=OMIM
Abbreviation: ECM, extracellular matrix.

aggregation with a 1/4:3/4 stagger. The fibrils formed in vivo are heterotypic with collagen types I, III, and V co-polymerizing together, as do collagen type II and XI. It has become apparent that the inclusion of the quantitatively minor collagen type V (and by implication, its paralogue collagen type XI) is essential for efficient fibrillogenesis in vivo. This is severely curtailed by the ablation of the *Col5a1* gene in the mouse, which prevents the assembly and secretion of a trimeric procollagen type V (145). The newest members of the fibrillar collagen family, collagen types XXIV and XXVII are closely related to each other and may not co-polymerize into fibrils with their classical homologues for a number of reasons. Collagens type XXIV and type XXVII have shorter (by ~21 amino acid residues) collagenous helices than the classical fibrillar collagens and both two conserved interruptions in their -Gly-X-Y- repeat (20,68,101). These cannot be accommodated within the classical fibrillar collagen structures without significant disruption to the structure as seen in diseases such as osteogenesis imperfecta (OI) or Stickler syndrome (71) (see also the section entitled Transmembrane collagens). Preliminary data for collagen type XXVII suggest that it forms thin fibrils that are distinct from the classical cross-striated fibrils of interstitial matrices (105).

Basement Membrane Collagens Forming Meshworks

The main structural component of basement membranes is collagen type IV (Table 1). This collagen assembles into a chicken wire-like network by a combination of dimeric interactions between C-terminal non-collagenous domains, tetrameric parallel/anti-parallel interactions of the N-terminal collagenous domains of interacting molecules (forming the "7S" domain), and lateral aggregation of the triple helices (133,135). The meshwork formed by collagen type IV provides both tensile strength and molecular size-selective filtration properties that play a crucial role in the compartmentalization function of basement membranes (133,151).

Collagen-Associated Microfibrils

Collagen type VI is a heterotrimer composed of three genetically distinct chains. The collagenous domain is relatively short (~330 residues) and is flanked in the trimeric molecule by N- and C-terminal non-collagenous extensions. N-terminal extensions consist of up to 12 von Willebrand factor A (VWF-A) domains, and C-terminal extensions consist of up to 6 VWF-A domains, each depending upon the precise chain composition of the trimer (134). Collagen type VI monomers assemble into dimers by an anti-parallel lateral association between the C-terminal VWF-A domains and the collagenous helices of the binding partners with a 75 nm overlap. Two dimers then laterally aggregate by a similar C-terminal VWF-A domain interaction with anti-parallel collagenous domains to form tetramers prior to secretion from the cell. Upon secretion, tetramers aggregate end-to-end by way of their N-terminal VWF-A domain complexes to form the beaded microfibrils with ~100 nm periodicity (7). These beaded microfibrils are distributed throughout the interstitial matrix (Table 1).

Anchoring Fibrils

Collagen type VII is the major component of fibrils that anchor the basement membrane of specialized epithelia, such as the corneal epithelium, to the underlying stroma (77). The assembly of collagen VII into anchoring fibrils is controlled by proteolytic processing of the C-terminal non-collagenous domain (111), which triggers an anti-parallel lateral dimerization with a 60 nm overlap, followed by lateral aggregation of the dimers.

Short-Chain Collagens Forming Meshworks

The term "short-chain collagens" was coined to describe collagen types VIII and X, related collagen types with distinct expression patterns, but a conserved structure that includes a collagenous domain just less than half the length of the fibrillar collagens (~460 residues). They also have globular C-terminal non-collagenous domains (gC1q domain) that are conserved across a supergene encompassing a large number of "collagen-like" molecules including the C1q component of complement and adiponectin (87). Collagen types VIII and X are thought to assemble into a meshwork with four molecules interacting at their C-terminal gC1q domains to form a tetrahedral complex. The network is completed by anti-parallel dimerization of the collagenous domains of molecules involved in adjacent tetrahedrons (126). Included in this "C1q-like" supergene family is the *CTRP5* gene, which encodes for protein having a collagenous domain of only 69 residues joined to a gC1q-like C-terminus. The mode of assembly of this molecule remains to be established and, at present, CTRP5 is classified as a "collagen-like" molecule, although preliminary evidence suggests it may form part of the ECM (46). A mutation in its gC1q domain has been linked to late-onset retinal degeneration (LORD) (see Chapter 35; see also the section on Multiplexins).

Fibril-Associated Collagens with Interrupted Triple Helices (FACIT Collagens)

FACIT collagens are a group of related collagens that assemble on the surface of collagen fibrils and appear to serve the functions of limiting fibril diameter and linking fibrils to the surrounding matrix (122). The archetypal FACIT, collagen type IX, is a heterotrimer with three distinct chains, whereas the remaining eight members of the subfamily are thought to be homotrimers. In addition, collagen type IX can have a GAG side chain added to its α2(IX) chain. FACIT collagens bind to the surface of collagen fibrils by way of two C-terminal collagenous domains and subsequently become covalently cross-linked (37). The N-terminal domains, which are poorly conserved between FACIT collagens but in general consist of a mixture of collagenous, thrombospondin N-terminal and/or VWF-A domains, appear to protrude from the fibril surface and interact with molecules in the surrounding matrix.

Transmembrane Collagens

The four distinct but related transmembrane collagens are homotrimers with an N-terminal transmembrane domain and a variable number of C-terminal collagenous domains that extend from the plasma membrane and engage with the pericellular matrix (40). Collagen types XIII and XVII have roles in promoting cell adhesion. The extracellular portions of the more recent additions to this subfamily (collagen types XXIII and XXV) can be shed from the plasma membrane by furin (a paired basic amino acid cleaving enzyme) and may therefore play a role in the matrix independent of their membrane function (8,124).

Multiplexins

Collagen types XV and XVIII constitute the multiplexin subfamily of collagens and are named due to their multiple triple-helix domains and interruptions (93,97,113). These homotrimeric collagens are localized to basement membranes, have wide tissue distributions, and are also proteoglycans (4,86). C-terminal proteolytic cleavage of collagen type XVIII yields a non-collagenous fragment, endostatin, which is reported to have anti-angiogenic properties (100). Collagen type XV has a homologous endostatin-like C-terminal domain.

COLLAGENS IN THE EYE

The distributions and functions of various collagens in the eye were recently reviewed (57), and are summarized below. Several ocular collagens are also found in cartilage.

Cornea

The cornea has evolved to enclose and protect the inner eye, as well as focus light onto the retina (90). Within this tissue, epithelial cells, endothelial cells, and fibroblasts synthesize and interact with a variety of collagens and other matrix macromolecules to produce a strong, transparent tissue. The connective tissue elements are organized into four distinct layers: the corneal epithelial basement membrane, Bowman layer, the stroma, and the corneal endothelial basement membrane (Descemet membrane). Chick cornea has provided a valuable model system in which to study corneal collagens (75). A gene expression study of the human eye has confirmed that a number of collagen genes, including *COL5A2*, *COL6A3*, *COL12A1*, *COL17A1*, are expressed in cornea (35). Collagen type XXIV is expressed in both the developing and adult cornea (68).

Epithelial Basement Membrane

The epithelial basement membrane of the cornea is synthesized by the epithelium and contains collagen type IV, laminin and fibronectin, as well as collagen type XVII (bullous pemphigoid antigen) (44). In the central cornea, the basal surface of the epithelium is flat and the basement membrane is composed of a lamina rara and a continuous lamina densa. At the periphery, where the basal surface undulates, the lamina densa is reduplicated, with apparent focal discontinuities. The unilaminar basement membrane of the central cornea is ~100 nm thick at birth and thickens with age at a rate of approximately 3 nm per annum. After the second decade, foci of reduplication are seen, often within excavations of Bowman layer, and eventually the central basement membrane becomes completely multilaminar and markedly thickened. In early life, anchoring filaments based on collagen type VII penetrate deeply (as much as 2μm) into Bowman layer, contributing to epithelial adhesion. Later their length may be insufficient to traverse the multilaminar basement membrane, and bullous separation becomes more frequent.

Bowman Layer

Bowman layer provides a barrier to corneal invasion by tumors and pathogenic organisms. It is a 9–12 μm thick, relatively acellular condensation of the anterior corneal stroma that occurs beneath the epithelial basement membrane (147). Keratocytes are present in Bowman layer and may, together with the corneal epithelium, contribute to its synthesis. Bowman layer contains an abundant, interwoven meshwork of collagen fibrils that are thinner than the aligned lamellar fibrils of the underlying anterior stroma. Bowman layer contains fibrils of collagen types I, III, and V. Collagen type VI, which forms collagen fibril-associated microfibrils, FACIT collagen types XII and XIV collagens, and collagen type XVIII and its anti-angiogenic fragment endostatin, are also present in Bowman layer (80,99), as well as the transforming growth factor–induced protein (TGFBIp) (see Chapter 36).

Corneal Stroma

The stroma occupies about 90% of the thickness of the cornea, and about 80% of its dry weight is collagen. The collagen fibers are arranged in lamellae that appear to extend across the cornea from opposite sides of the corneoscleral limbus. The posterior stromal lamellae are slightly thicker than those in the anterior one-third (0.2–2.5 versus 0.2–2.1 μm) and have a more definite orientation parallel to the corneal surface. This may explain the greater ease of dissection in the posterior stroma during lamellar keratoplasty. In the center of the cornea, there is little or no interweaving of collagen fibers from adjacent lamellae, but interweaving does occur peripherally and thereby contributes to the greater interlamellar adhesive strength in this region. Between the lamellae there is a planar network of fibroblastic cells (keratocytes). Along the optical axis adjacent lamellae are arranged at an angle of slightly less than 90°; in humans the collagen lamellae of the anterior stroma manifest little preferred orientation, but a more orthogonal pattern is seen in the posterior stroma.

The morphology of the individual collagen fibers has been the subject of many investigations. A recent study showed the stromal fibrils in the corneal stroma to have a high degree of uniformity and precision of diameter and spatial arrangement, but also showed substantial variations in diameter, as measured by interfibrillar distribution of mass per unit length, both between fibrils and along individual fibrils (50). A significant proportion of collagen fibrils running across the cornea change direction near the corneoscleral limbus and fuse with the circumferential limbal collagen (90). Fibrillar collagen in the human cornea is arranged anisotropically, and in a highly specific manner, with left and right corneas structurally distinct (21). Studies of genetically engineered mice that lack lumican (lumican-null mice) indicate a role for lumican in the neonatal development of the corneal stroma (11).

In chick, the corneal epithelium lays down a primary stroma of collagen types I and II (about 40%), which overlap in distribution. Some collagen type II is left in the subepithelial stroma (and Descemet membrane), but this gradually decreases with time. The epithelium also synthesizes and secretes the FACIT collagen type IX, but this disappears relatively early in development, possibly triggering stromal swelling and subsequent infiltration by mesenchymal cells. The fibers of the primary stroma are arranged orthogonally and the mesenchymal cells align themselves with a corresponding orthogonal orientation of the cell processes. The deposition of the collagen fibers of the secondary stroma occurs close to the cell surface, and the disposition of the cell processes ensures an orthogonal pattern of fibers as the lamellae form. The secondary stroma shows a uniform distribution of fibrillar collagen type I, together with collagen types III and V, and microfibrillar collagen type VI.

The morphogenesis of the mammalian corneal stroma is simpler in that there is no primary stroma. The mesenchymal cells destined to be keratocytes migrate from the lip of the optic vesicle between the differentiating epithelia of lens and cornea. The keratocytes deposit an orthogonal matrix of collagen fibrils based on collagen types I, III, and V, which are closely associated within the same fiber. Collagen type I is the most abundant collagen in corneal stroma, which is also the richest source of collagen type V in the body (146). Other collagens of the corneal stroma are collagen type VI and membrane-bound collagen type XIII (117). Targeted disruption of collagen type VIII in a mouse model has revealed altered anterior eye development, including formation of the corneal stroma (51).

Descemet Membrane

Although similar to other basement membranes in that it contains collagen type IV, it is also rich in collagen type VIII, and contains small amounts of fibrillar collagen types I, II, and V. Descemet membrane is appreciably thicker than most basement membranes and, in man, its thickness increases from 3 μm at birth to 12.5 μm or more in old age. The provision of mechanical strength to the anterior segment of the eye appears to be a major function of Descemet membrane. Genetically engineered mice that lack collagen type VIII (collagen type VIII null mice) have markedly thinned Descemet membranes (51).

An ultrastructural analysis of the anterior part of Descemet membrane reveals a regular hexagonal array of electron-dense nodes connected by thick filaments, based on the short-chain collagen type VIII, with an internodal distance of approximately 107 nm. Transverse sections indicate that hexagonal arrays are stacked upon each other with the nodes aligned perpendicularly. In human Descemet membrane, the anterior 3 μm (the anterior banded zone), which is deposited during fetal life, is composed of 30–40 compacted lamellae, each a hexagonal array, held in alignment by fine interlamellar fibrils 170 nm long, 40 nm wide, and 110–120 nm apart. Postnatally, the basement membrane thickens by the apposition of non-banded material, although occasional collagen fibers with characteristic 64 nm periodicity are seen.

Sclera

The sclera is composed of irregularly arranged lamellae of collagen fibrils interspersed with proteoglycans and non-collagenous glycoproteins, and with scleral fibroblasts between the lamellae (109,142). It is important in protecting delicate intraocular structures and in preventing distortion of the light-sensitive elements during movement of the globe.

In the sixth week of human embryonic development, the sclera differentiates from neural crest. Maturation proceeds in an anteroposterior direction and from the inner to the outer surface. By the fourth month, the scleral spur appears as circularly oriented fibers. By the fifth month, scleral fibers around the axons of the optic nerve form the lamina cribrosa. Immature collagen is seen in the sixth week as patches of small fibrils. As fiber diameter gradually increases, the fibers become organized into lamellae. By 13 weeks of gestation, histological differences between the pre- and post-equatorial sclera have disappeared, and the adult organization is evident by 24 weeks. At this time, the fiber diameter is the same in the inner and outer sclera; sometime thereafter, this changes so that in the adult sclera the outer fibers are thicker than the inner. Scleral collagen fibril diameter is less consistent than in cornea. A differential gene expression study on mouse sclera has revealed changes in collagen gene expression during ocular development (152).

Collagen type I is the major component in sclera, accounting for over 90% of the total fibrillar collagen, the remainder being collagen types III and V (146). Collagen type II is found in the hyaline cartilage of the avian posterior sclera (146,150) and embryonic mice (118), but not in human sclera. In addition to collagen type I, the human sclera has been shown to contain collagen types III, IV, V, VI, VIII, XII, and XIII (117,144,150). Proteoglycans, some of which are important modulators of collagen fibril assembly and organization, are also found in abundance throughout the sclera (108). Scleral GAGs (dermatan sulfate, chondroitin sulfate, hyaluronan) are different from those in cornea (keratan sulfate, chondroitin), and may influence scleral collagen fiber diameter.

Trabecular Meshwork

The major resistance to aqueous humor outflow occurs at the trabecular meshwork that comprises connective tissue beams lined by endothelial cells (78,79) and an impaired drainage occurs in some types of glaucoma (see Chapter 20). Trabecular meshwork cells from a variety of species have been cultured and shown to synthesize many collagens, including collagen types I, III, IV, V, and VI, as well as non-collagenous glycoproteins (laminin and fibronectin) and proteoglycans (78).

The major components of the trabecular meshwork matrix, include a focally discontinuous subendothelial basal lamina, containing collagen type IV as well as fibrillar collagen types I and III, loose granular connective tissue containing banded collagen fibrils, and electron-dense cores surrounded by a sheath of "wide-spacing" collagen based on collagen type VI microfibrillar arrays. In the basement membrane zone, collagen types III and V, fibronectin, and basement membrane constituents (collagen type IV, laminin, and heparan sulfate proteoglycan) have been identified. Collagen type III, together with collagen type I and elastin, is present within the central core, although the last two are not found in the juxtracanalicular region. Collagen types VIII, XIII, and XVIII are also present in the trabecular meshwork (41,99,117). The relative contributions of elastin and the collagens to the configurational response of the meshwork to intraocular pressure (IOP) are unclear.

Lamina Cribrosa

The lamina cribrosa may, like the trabecular meshwork, be considered a modification of the scleral coat, also with a considerably lower collagen content. Immunohistochemical studies have indicated similarities in the collagen composition of the lamina cribrosa and trabecular meshwork (collagen types I, III, and IV) (142), which is different from that of sclera (mainly collagen type I). The extracellular matrix of the lamina cribrosa comprises a core of elastin, collagen types I, III, and VI, and a fine filamentous network of collagen type IV. Collagen type VI is found at the edge of the laminar plates, which are covered by a basement membrane of presumed glial origin composed of collagen type IV and laminin. The collagenous components of the laminar plates appear to increase with age, although the basement membrane covering the plates does not thicken.

The retrolaminar pial septa of the optic nerve show considerable similarities in composition to the cribriform plates of the lamina cribrosa. The major macromolecular components appear to be collagen types I and III, with collagen type IV being in the basement membranes of the blood vessels and covering the septa. Collagen type VI has been identified at the edge of the pial septa. The elastin and collagen types I and III contents of the septa increase with age.

Uvea

Collagen types I and III appear to be the major components of the iris and choroidal stroma. Collagen type I occurs with collagen type IV in the endothelial and pericyte basement membranes of the blood vessel walls with collagen type III in the tunica adventitia. In the aged human eye, the basement membranes of the non-pigmented and pigmented ciliary epithelia and the ciliary muscle contain not only collagen types I and IV, but also collagen type III, possibly reflecting the exposure of these structures to biomechanical forces. The ciliary zonules are based on the glycoprotein fibrillin, but collagen type IV has also been identified within these filaments (76).

Lens Capsule

The capsule of the crystalline lens is the thickest basement membrane of the body, some 20–25 μm thick in the central anterior region, and turns over slowly. Its collagenous nature was originally established by chemical analysis and X-ray diffraction. Lens capsule filaments are based on collagen type IV, which is synthesized by anterior subcapsular epithelial cells that also incorporate heparan sulfate proteoglycan into the basement membrane. The thinner posterior capsule has a chemical composition identical to that of the anterior capsule, but appears to be secreted by nucleated cortical fiber cells at a much slower rate. Lens capsule collagen type IV α-chain composition changes during development. In the embryo, α1(IV), α2(IV), α5(IV), and α6(IV) chains are present in the basement membrane surrounding the lens vesicle, and persist in the capsule until adulthood, but α3(IV) and α4(IV) chains only appear postnatally (62,98). Thus, in early development, collagen type IV networks may be more flexible [$(\alpha1(IV))_2\alpha2(IV)$ or $\alpha5(IV)_2\alpha6(IV)$], but may later contain a more cross-linked [(α1(IV)α2(IV)α3(IV)] heterotrimer (62). Collagen type XVIII is also present in the lens capsule and its anti-angiogenic fragment endostatin is present in the lens epithelium and extracellularly (80,99). The presence of both collagen types I and III has recently been demonstrated in the lens capsule (120).

Vitreous

The structure, function, and diseases of the vitreous are reviewed elsewhere (14,16,57) (see Chapter 29).

A characteristic property of vitreous is its gel-like consistency, resulting from the trapping of water within a fibrillar network formed by the interaction of collagen fibers with the high-molecular-weight polyanion hyaluronic acid. The collagenous fibers in normal vitreous are based on fibrillar collagen types II and V/XI (23) and are of narrow diameter (7–23 nm), with a major axial period of 62 nm. The thermal stability of vitreous collagen is less than that of articular cartilage collagen, probably because of the greater abundance of proteoglycans in the cartilage matrix. The major reducible cross-links of vitreous collagen, dihydroxylysinonorleucine and hydroxylysinonorleucine, are only half as numerous as in cartilage. Their numbers diminish with age as they mature into pyridinoline. The thin collagen fibrils have a coating of non-covalently attached macromolecules that also contributes to maintaining gel stability. They include the small leucine-rich repeat molecules opticin and decorin (74). Together, they may maintain the short-range spacing of the fibrils and link them to form a continuous network. The FACIT collagen type IX, with its chondroitin sulfate chains, is another important collagen of the vitreous. In addition, the FACIT collagen type XII is found in vitreous (23). Vitreous proteins are derived from several different cell types, especially the posterior non-pigmented ciliary epithelium (15). The vitreous base normally contains the highest density of collagen fibers in the vitreous, with progressive diminution in the posterior vitreous cortex, anterior vitreous cortex, and central vitreous.

Bruch Membrane and Retinal Pigment Epithelium

Bruch membrane is the connective tissue boundary between retinal pigment epithelium (RPE) and the choriocapillaris (107). It is approximately 3 μm thick (2.3–4.2 μm) and is composed of five layers: (*i*) the basal lamina of the RPE cells, 40–100 nm thick; (*ii*) an inner collagenous zone composed of tightly woven fibers of uniform diameter (70 nm); (*iii*) a fenestrated layer of mature elastic fibers through which collagen fibers from the inner collagenous zone pass; (*iv*) an outer collagenous zone of looser texture than the inner collagenous zone; and (*v*) the basal lamina of the endothelium of the choriocapillaris. This appearance, characteristic of eyes in persons <20 years old changes with age, particularly in the macular region with the accumulation of membranous debris in the inner and outer collagenous zones (see the section entitled Multiplexins). Bruch membrane contains elastic fibers, but also fibrillar collagen types I, III, V, basement membrane collagen type IV and microfibrillar collagen type VI, as well as laminin and fibronectin. In culture adult human RPE deposit a matrix containing collagen types I–IV, together with laminin, fibronectin, and fibrillin (116,141).

Retina

The major collagenous structures in the retina are blood vessels and the inner limiting membrane, which is composed of the basement membranes of Müller cell processes.

Segments of retinal capillaries can be isolated by forcing lightly homogenized retina through a nylon sieve with pores 86 μm in diameter. The segments that are retained by the sieve are essentially devoid of non-vascular elements and are metabolically active. Morphological examination indicates that many are not true capillaries but rather arterioles and venules. Retinal capillaries are composed of endothelium with one or more layers of pericytes, as well as the investing basement membrane matrix (55,136). Isolation of the matrix from these segments by treatment with detergents reveals layers of collagen-rich basement membrane. The presence of collagen types I and IV, together with collagen type V, in the basement membranes of retinal capillaries, arteries, and venules has been demonstrated by immunohistochemistry and immunoelectron microscopy. In addition, collagen types III and VI are present in larger blood vessels, hyalinization of which is accompanied by increased deposition of collagen types I, VI, and IV, the last reflecting duplication of basal lamina.

Ultrastructural analyses of isolated retinal capillaries have confirmed the contribution of three cell types to the matrix. The vascular endothelium is separated by a discontinuous, subendothelial basal lamina (70 nm thick) from one or more layers of pericytes that are surrounded by their own basal laminae (each 80–110 nm thick). The presence of fenestrae in the subendothelial basal laminae reflects contact between endothelial and pericyte cell processes. An irregular layer of collagen fibers and pericyte matrix is surrounded by a continuous basal lamina (80–110 nm thick) laid down by perivascular Müller cells. For both pericytes and endothelial cells, collagen types I and IV are the major biosynthetic products, with collagen type III being a minor product. The presence of collagen types IV and V has also been demonstrated in the inner limiting membrane. Although under certain conditions, regeneration of the inner limiting membrane may occur, breaks in the basement membrane are usually complicated by epiretinal membrane formation. Collagen fibers within epiretinal membranes generally have diameters in the range of 10–15 and 20–25 nm, although occasionally thicker fibers may be present (49). The finest fibers may represent incorporated vitreous collagen or collagen type II synthesized by RPE. There does not appear to be a significant diminution in the collagen type II content when vitrectomy has been previously performed. Several collagen types occur within epiretinal membranes: collagen types I and III appear to predominate, with lesser amounts of collagen types II and IV. The presence of collagen type IV reflects the presence of segments of inner limiting membrane and blood vessels within the epiretinal membranes.

Recently, several additional collagens have been shown to contribute to the retinal blood vessels. The anti-angiogenic peptide endostatin, which is a fragment of collagen type XVIII, may modulate some of the effects of vascular endothelial growth factor (VEGF) in the retina (24). Collagen type XVIII is important in the early phase of retinal vascular development and for the regression of the primary vasculature in the vitreous and its homologue, collagen type XV, is a regulator of perivascular glial cell recruitment (56). In addition, collagen type XVII and bullous pemphigoid antigen 1 (BPAG1) colocalize with laminins at photoreceptor synapses and around photoreceptor outer segments; both molecules are expressed by rods, whereas cones express collagen type XVII but not BPAG1 (32).

COLLAGEN DISEASES OF THE EYE

Cornea

Epithelial Basement Membrane

Corneal epithelial basement membrane thickening occurs in diabetes mellitus and as a secondary effect in certain corneal epithelial disorders, such as Meesmann dystrophy and Fuchs corneal dystrophy (FCD), and map-dot-fingerprint dystrophy (see Chapter 30). Basement membrane discontinuities in buphthalmos may account for diminished epithelial integrity. Recent studies, in mice, of the effects of mutations in the gene for the α1 chain of collagen type IV (*COL4A1*) have been shown to cause anterior segment dysgenesis (139).

Bowman Layer

Bowman layer formation can be affected by developmental abnormalities. In addition to its congenital absence, Bowman layer dysgenesis is a cause of congenital corneal opacification characterized by uniform thickening with or without the presence of keratocytes and without apparent disturbance of the collagenous organization. The thickening is not always associated with corneal opacification, as in Smith–Lemni–Opitz syndrome (MIM #270400) (70). Absence of the central part of Bowman layer occurs in various forms of anterior segment dysgenesis, including Peters anomaly (MIM #604229) and sclerocornea. Other acquired abnormalities of Bowman layer include Salzmann nodular degeneration.

Although Thiel-Behnke corneal dystrophy, (MIM #602082) which is caused by mutations in the *TGFBI* gene (see Chapter 32), is associated with an abnormal subepithelial accumulation of "curly" collagen fibrils, there is no evidence that a mutation in the *COL17A1* gene causes generalized atrophic benign epidermolysis bullosa (MIM #226650), which has some similar features to this inherited corneal disorder.

A recent study identified a defect in anchoring fibrils as the cause of corneal epithelial loss in cases of traumatic recurrent corneal erosions and hemidesmosomes were not apparently impaired (30).

Corneal Stroma

Profound ocular morbidity is associated with the degeneration of the corneal stroma that accompanies corneal infection and ulceration, usually due to altered collagenase activity causing stromal degradation. Some organisms, such as *Acanthamoeba castellani* and *Lasiodiplodia theobromae*, which cause severe corneal injury, are able to produce collagenase (47,112), but other organisms, such as *Pseudomonas aeruginosa*, do not. However, the injured keratocytes themselves and the infiltrating neutrophils (PMNs) may be major sources of collagenase (33). Collagenase activity is generally present in the stroma of ulcerated tissues. Tissue inhibitor of metallo proteinase 1 (TIMP1), a natural inhibitor of collagenase, affords some protection against *Pseudomonas aeruginosa* induced corneal destruction (64). Tetracyclines inhibit collagenolytic degradation of the cornea after moderate to severe ocular chemical injuries (110).

Descemet Membrane

Focal interruptions of the Descemet membrane–endothelial cell complex, as in anterior segment dysgenesis, may result in localized corneal scarring and the production of abnormally thick stromal fibrils. Although Descemet membrane is unusual among basement membranes in that it does not thicken in diabetes mellitus, it frequently thickens in response to a corneal endothelial disturbance. Associated with the complicated developmental changes within the normal Descemet membrane, with formation of two zones of different structure and peripheral guttae (Hassal–Henle warts), a variety of different patterns of Descemet membrane thickening can take place. Collagenous tissue posterior to the normal Descemet membrane is termed a posterior collagenous layer and is classified into three ultrastructural categories: (*i*) banded, containing long-spacing material with a macroperiod of 55 or 110 nm; (*ii*) fibrillar, containing non-banded collagenous fibrils of diameter 20 nm; and (*iii*) fibrocellular, containing fibroblastic cells in a compact mesh of banded collagen fibers 30–64 nm in diameter. Fuchs corneal dystrophy provides a good example of a banded posterior collagenous layer that may occur as simple guttate excrescences (see Chapter 32). In this disease, the posterior non-banded zone is generally thin, suggesting that endothelial dysfunction has already commenced by the age of about 20 years. In posterior polymorphous dystrophy, both the anterior banded zone and the posterior non-banded zone may be abnormally thin, suggesting that an endothelial disturbance during intrauterine life resumes in early childhood. The normal overall thickness of Descemet membrane may be attributed to a posterior collagenous layer, generally of the fibrillar category. At least some individuals with the clinical phenotypes of both of these disorders of the corneal endothelium have been found to have mutations in the *COL8A2* gene (17,45). Indeed, Descemet membrane in FCD often has accumulations of abnormal collagen type VIII assemblies. This collagen is an important cell adhesion molecule (137) and in FCD it apparently influences the terminal differentiation of neural crest derived corneal endothelial cells, possibly by integrin-mediated interactions with endothelial cells (137).

In most patients with posterior polymorphous corneal dystrophy (PPCD), pathogenetic mutations have not been identified in the *COL8A2* gene, indicating that additional genetic factors are involved in the development of this autosomal dominant corneal disorder (see Chapter 32) (148). It is noteworthy that one type of PPCD (PPCD type III) (MIM #609141) is caused by mutations in the *TCF8* gene (69), because the encoded transcription factor binds to the promoter of the *COL4A3* gene, which encodes the α3(IV) chain of collagen type IV. Mutations in the *COL4A3* gene cause autosomal recessive Alport syndrome (MIM #203780).

Sclera

Myopia is frequently caused by lengthening of the posterior segment of the eye, so that the retina comes to lie behind the focal plane, where images are focused by the cornea and crystalline lens (see Chapter 26). Changes observed in the sclera include posterior thinning, which is associated with loss of collagen fibril bundles, reduction in size of individual collagen fibrils, predominant loss of collagen I rather than collagen types III and V, abnormal fibrils associated with amorphous cementing substance, and the presence of fissured or star-shaped fibrils (42,109). The scleral thickness is reduced by 35% to 45%, and this is greater than can be accounted for by stretching alone, so there may be an alteration in fibrillogenesis (142), although it is unclear whether these collagen fibril changes are a consequence or a cause of myopia (89). Myopia associated with scleral fragility and rupture occurs in Ehlers–Danlos syndrome type VI (MIM #225400) (see the section on Collagen Types).

A major anatomical disorder of the sclera is the staphyloma, defined as local scleral ectasia lined by uveal tissue. It occurs frequently between the corneoscleral limbus and the ocular equator as a result of prolonged raised IOP. Spontaneous scleral thinning may also occur in the paralimbal region (scleromalacia perforans). No peculiarities of the collagen fibers in this region have been described, although the difference in average fiber diameter between the inner and outer wall is less marked in this area. A localized accumulation of alcianophilic material within the inner sclera can be accompanied by scleral collagen fibers with diameters up to twice normal size. Deposition of GAGs within the sclera may result in disturbed collagen fibrillogenesis.

The sclera is markedly thickened in nanophthalmos. In this syndrome the eye is also small, with a shallow anterior chamber and a tendency to uveal effusion, perhaps through compression of the vortex veins by the thick sclera. Partial-thickness sclerectomy has indicated a disturbance of the lamellar arrangement of the collagen bundles, the severity of which correlates with the reduction in ocular diameter.

Trabecular Meshwork

Primary open angle glaucoma is a leading cause of late onset, progressive, and irreversible blindness (12,38). A major contributory factor is elevated IOP caused by abnormally increased resistance to drainage of aqueous humor through the outflow system, which comprises the trabecular meshwork and Schlemm canal.

Lamina Cribrosa

In glaucoma, the distribution of collagen fiber diameters in the lamina cribrosa (normal mean 50 nm) is shifted toward that of sclera (normal mean 75 nm). These architectural features of the lamina cribrosa may contribute to the pattern of neural degeneration in glaucoma (see Chapter 21). In primary open-angle glaucoma, major changes are often detected in respect to collagen types IV and VI, the amounts of which increase in the cores of the cribriform plates. Collagen type IV is also increased in the prelaminar region of the optic nerve head, where it is produced by glial cells. The extent of this change is proportional to the severity of the glaucoma. The ECM of the lamina cribrosa in both normal and glaucomatous eyes comprises a core of elastin, as well as collagen types I, III, IV, and VI.

Uvea

All parts of the uvea undergo some degree of sclerosis with age, particularly the blood vessels. Atrophy of ciliary muscle in glaucoma is accompanied by atrophy of the connective tissue stroma of the ciliary body and processes. Proliferation of non-pigmented ciliary epithelial cells in a coronal adenoma, benign epithelial tumors of the ciliary processes (9), is accompanied by deposition of a periodic acid Schiff-positive matrix containing predominantly collagen type IV with some collagen type I.

Lens Capsule

Alport Syndrome

Alport syndrome (MIM #301050) is caused by *COL4A5* mutations in its X-linked form, and by *COL4A3* and *COL4A4* mutations in its autosomal forms, which impair formation of the α3(IV)α4(IV)α5 (IV) heterotrimer (53,54). Mutations in *COL4A5* are common and lead to X-linked Alport syndrome. Its major clinical features are familial progressive nephritis and neural deafness, although there is considerable phenotypic and genetic heterogeneity. The principal ocular manifestation is anterior lenticonus, which may occur in as many as 50% of patients. A spontaneous rupture of the anterior lens capsule at the site of the cone may lead to an anterior subcapsular cataract. Marked thinning of the central anterior lens capsule (4 μm versus 16 μm in control lens) associated with lack of immunostaining of α3–α5 collagen type IV chains, is accompanied by the appearance of channels contain 3–64 nm filaments (slightly larger than normal lens capsule filaments) and membranous debris.

Exfoliation of Lens Capsule

Tangential splitting of the capsule may occur in "true exfoliation," or lamellar delamination of the lens capsule. This is a rare disorder in which the lens capsule is thickened and the superficial portion of the lens capsule splits from the deeper layer and extends into the anterior chamber (61). The pathogenesis of this disorder is not clear, but infrared radiation may be a contributory factor to a condition that, once mainly found in workers exposed to hot open furnaces, may also be seen in advanced age irrespective of occupation.

Age-Related Cataract

Although age-related cataract is not accompanied by any specific capsular abnormalities, the thickness of the capsule at the anterior pole increases with advancing age, and lamination of the capsule becomes less prominent (see Chapter 19).

Anterior Subcapsular Cataract

In anterior subcapsular cataracts (see Chapter 23), the subcapsular epithelial cells assume a spindle shape and become embedded in a fibrous matrix. The cells assume characteristics of myofibroblasts, with basal lamina and subplasmalemmal bundles of fine (7 nm diameter) filaments containing electron-dense bodies: intercellular junctions can be seen, except where the cells are widely separated within the plaque. The presence of a collagenous plaque containing contractile cells corrugates the overlying anterior capsule. The collagenous fibers are generally thin (average diameter 15–21 nm) and arranged in strata with alternating layers of basement membrane material. Broad fibrillar aggregates (>1000 nm in diameter) are also seen, which resemble amianthoid collagen, with irregular and angular fibers with a granular appearance in cross-section, and a disintegrated character with some loss of periodicity in longitudinal section, from degenerate cartilage. A recent study has shown that anterior subcapsular cataracts contain collagen types I, IV, V, and VI, as well as fibronectin, fibrillin-1, and LTBP-1 (58).

A Rho GTPase functional knockout transgenic mouse model has recently revealed that disruption of Rho GTPase function in the developing mouse lens causes abnormal cytoskeletal organization, fiber cell interactions, impaired lens fiber cell morphology, and altered gene expression of cellular proteins (83).

Vitreous

During aging, the vitreous liquefies and, in up to 30% of the population, the residual gel structure collapses away from the posterior retina in a process called posterior vitreous detachment (14) (see Chapter 29). This process plays a major role in conditions such as rhegmatogenous retinal detachment (RRD) and macular hole formation (see Chapter 28). The gradual but progressive liquefaction of the human vitreous (synchysis) begins in the central vitreous where the collagen fibers aggregate into thick bundles of parallel fibers.

Penetrating ocular injuries may be complicated by fibrous tissue deposition within the vitreous. The collagen may be in the form of dense fibrous sheets continuous with the scleral perforation and is believed to be deposited by proliferating scleral fibroblasts. The contribution of vitreous hemorrhage to the fibrotic process is unclear. The resorption of vitreous blood clots is slow and is accompanied by the formation of vitreous membranes composed of condensed vitreous collagen.

Bruch Membrane and Retinal Pigment Epithelium

The most significant lesions that form in Bruch membrane are drusen on the inner aspect of Bruch membrane, as a component of age-related macular degeneration (AMD) (see Chapter 18) (31,132). Drusen are formed from extension of the RPE cytoplasm into Bruch membrane with subsequent degeneration, and include remnants of phagocytosed photoreceptor outer segments. The presence of such lipid-rich material in Bruch membrane may produce a hydrophobic barrier limiting water transport and predisposing to RPE detachment. In advanced stages, the basal lamina separating the RPE and the extracellular deposit may disappear completely. Various types of drusen have been identified, and their molecular composition is being defined (59,138). The contribution of connective tissue macromolecules to drusen remains unclear, although several collagens and fibulin-3 (a non-collagenous glycoprotein) are present (18).

RPE, together with fibroblasts, contribute to the subretinal neovascular membrane in AMD that has been shown, by immunoelectron microscopy, to contain collagen types I, III, IV, V, and VI, as well as laminin and fibronectin. In the choroid of aged control eyes, collagen type XVIII (and endostatin, a C-terminal fragment of this collagen) localize to blood vessels, Bruch membrane, and the RPE basal lamina (13). In the retina and choroid of eyes with AMD the pattern of immunostaining of collagen type XVIII is similar, but reduced levels of endostatin in Bruch membrane, RPE basal lamina, intercapillary septa, and choriocapillaris may be permissive for choroidal neovascularization (CNV) (13). It is noteworthy that genetically engineered mice that do not express collagen type XVIII (collagen type XVIII null mice) have iris changes similar to those patients with LORD (MIM #605670) caused by mutations in the *CTRP5* gene, discussed below and in Chapter 35, whilst mice lacking collagen type XVIII/endostatin have a prominent accumulation of subretinal deposits and an age-related loss of vision (84,85). Collagen type VI microfibrillar aggregates have also been identified in Bruch membrane aggregates in AMD (67).

Retina

Thickening of the capillary basement membrane in diabetes mellitus has been linked to the formation and accumulation of advanced glycation end-products (AGEs), especially on collagen fibrils (129,130).

LORD, an autosomal dominant retinal disorder with similar clinical and histopathologic features as AMD (6,46), manifests as delayed dark adaptation and impaired night vision in middle life and later progresses to severe visual impairment (131). It is caused by mutations in the *CTRP5* gene, which encodes a novel short-chain collagen involved in basement membrane function. Mutations occur in the C-terminal globular "C1q" domain of CTRP5 and result in abnormal high-molecular-weight aggregate formation, as well as abnormal extracellular deposits of protein and lipid between the RPE and the Bruch membrane. This is followed by loss of photoreceptors, thinning of RPE, and CNV.

OCULAR MANIFESTATIONS OF GENERALIZED DISORDERS OF COLLAGEN

Keratoconus

Keratoconus (KC) a non-inflammatory corneal disease, causes corneal thinning, cone formation, and scarring (123). It is a bilateral disorder of corneal shape associated with reduced corneal tensile strength, and multiple ruptures and scarring of Bowman layer. The cause and pathogenesis remains unknown (see Chapter 32) (143). Keratoconus may involve matrix metalloproteinases, particularly gelatinase A (MMP-2), the major protease constitutively synthesized and secreted by keratocytes (81). MMP-2 can degrade collagen type IV, newly secreted collagen type I molecules, and partially degraded collagen fibrils. Promatrix metalloproteinase-2 (ProMMP-2) is over-expressed in keratoconic cornea stromal cells without a concomitant increase in TIMP1 or TIMP2 production (123), and the resultant imbalance in proMMP-2/TIMP may facilitate MMP-2 activation.

X-ray diffraction studies reveal that the organization of the stromal laminae is dramatically altered in KC, with uneven distribution of the collagen fibrils, especially around the cone apex (91). These changes may reflect significant interlamellar displacement and slippage, leading to thinning of the central cornea.

Relapsing Polychondritis

Relapsing polychondritis is a rare, generally lethal systemic autoimmune disease affecting primarily cartilage and proteoglycan-rich tissues (see Chapter 6) (1,103) . Episcleritis and intractable scleritis are the most frequent ocular manifestations. Approximately one-third of patients have circulating antibodies to collagen type II, the titer correlating with the severity of inflammation. Since there is no cartilage or collagen type II in human sclera, an indirect mechanism has been invoked for the scleritis, namely, an immune complex vasculitis (see Chapter 5).

Epidermolysis Bullosa

Epidermolysis bullosa comprises a large group of clinically distinct entities characterized by a tendency to blister formation after minor trauma (25). Three major subgroups are recognized, depending on the location of the bullae: (*i*) autosomal dominant "epidermolytic epidermolysis bullosa," in which the bullae form within the epidermis; (*ii*) autosomal recessive "junctional epidermolysis bullosa," in which separation occurs within the lamina rara of the subepidermal basal lamina; and (*iii*) dominant and recessive "dystrophic epidermolysis bullosa," which is caused by mutations in the *COL17A1* gene that encodes for α1(VII) collagen type VII (63) in which the blister forms below the lamina densa. Ocular complications of inherited epidermolysis bullosa occur principally in the recessive dystrophic form and generally take the form of recurrent corneal erosions and blisters (39,119). Blistering of the cornea is accompanied by loss of Bowman layer and anterior stromal scarring.

Ocular manifestations of autoimmune bullous diseases are common and potentially sight-threatening (72), with significant conjunctival involvement in mucous membrane pemphigoid (cicatricial pemphigoid), epidermolysis bullosa acquisita—a chronic subepidermal blistering disease associated with autoimmunity to collagen type VII within anchoring fibrils (34), linear IgA bullous disease, pemphigus vulgaris and paraneoplastic pemphigus.

Osteogenesis Imperfecta

Mutations in the two genes for collagen type I (*COL1A1*, *COL1A2*) cause OI (27,104). Common mutations are substitution of a single glycine residue at one of several positions along the pro-α1(I) chains. OI type I (MIM #166200), a relatively mild condition, is caused by mutations that lead to a reduced production of otherwise normal collagen type I. These patients often have blue sclerae, probably due to a reduction in collagen fiber diameter that increases the visibility of uveal pigment and blood through the sclera. Changes in fiber structure and size may also account for a diminution in ocular rigidity. Patients with OI type II (MIM #166210) have moderately severely affected bone, but generally have white sclerae. Nwosu et al. (96) documented the first description of ocular anterior chamber abnormalities with OI in a patient with features of Ehlers–Danlos syndrome (EDS) and Rieger anomaly carrying an unusual *COL1A1* mutation.

Syndromes resembling OI have ocular complications. They include Cole-Carpenter syndrome (MIM #112240) osteoporosis pseudoglioma syndrome (MIM #259770) and two other syndromes: one with optic atrophy, retinopathy (2), and another with cataracts (26). Patients with Cole-Carpenter syndrome develop multiple metaphyseal fractures, ocular proptosis, and facial dysmorphism (104). Patients with osteoporosis pseudoglioma syndrome have a mild to moderate OI with blindness due to persistent primary hyperplastic vitreous, corneal opacification, and secondary glaucoma. The ocular abnormalities may be a consequence of failed regression of the primary fetal vitreal vasculature.

Ehlers–Danlos Syndrome

The Ehlers–Danlos syndrome is characterized by hyperextensibility and/or fragility of the skin with hypermobility of joints and a tendency to bruising. At least 10 types are recognized, and there is genetic and biochemical heterogeneity within some of the clinical types (128). Although a reduction in fiber diameter and imperfect alignment of fibers within bundles have been described in several types, for most the underlying abnormality is not known. The best characterized type is EDS type IV, (MIM #130050) which results from a deficiency of collagen type III. In EDS type VI the cutaneous and joint lesions are accompanied by prominent ocular abnormalities, including scleral fragility and retinal detachment. The cornea may also be abnormally small and thin. The biochemical defect in some cases of EDS type VI is a deficiency of lysyl hydroxylase that results in fewer hydroxylysine residues in collagen, increases solubility of dermal collagen, and changes in reducible cross-links. Not all cases of apparent

EDS type VI, however, have diminished lysyl hydroxylase.

Collagen type V, which forms heterotypic fibrils with collagen type I, accounts for 10–20% of corneal collagen, and mutations in *COL5A1* and *COL5A2* cause classical EDS due to haploinsufficiency. Using both patient material and a Col5A1-haploinsufficient mouse model of classic EDS, *COL5A1* and *COL5A2* mutations have been shown to manifest as abnormally thin and steep corneas with floppy eyelids (121). These phenotypic changes may reflect altered collagen fibrillogenesis.

Brittle Cornea Syndrome

Blue sclerae, red hair, corneal rupture following minor trauma, KC or keratoglobus, hyperelasticity of the skin without excessive fragility, and hypermobility of the joints have been linked in the autosomal recessive brittle cornea syndrome (BCS) (MIM %229200) (3). The underlying genetic defect remains undetermined. The only tissue abnormalities recognized so far have been a slight reduction in collagen fiber diameter in the dermis and the presence of areas within the dermis that are completely devoid of collagen fibers.

Although there are similarities between BCS and the kyphoscoliotic type of EDS (EDS type VI), they are distinct diseases. BCS patients have biochemical findings reflective of normal activity of lysyl hydroxylase, characteristically deficient in EDS type VI, such as normal urinary total pyridinoline ratios and/or normal electrophoretic migration of collagen chains produced by dermal fibroblasts (3).

Stickler Syndrome and Related Disorders

Stickler Syndrome

Stickler syndrome (MIM #108300) is an autosomal dominant hereditary progressive arthro-ophthalmopathy (52,115). Affected individuals suffer from myopia and congenital vitreous detachment (82). Other features include certain presenile cataracts and ectopia lentis, anterior chamber angle anomalies, open angle glaucoma, and congenital glaucoma.

The Stickler syndrome of premature osteoarthritis and vitreoretinal degeneration (see Chapter 35) is caused in some, but not all, families by mutations in the *COL2A1* gene encoding collagen type II (52,95). Mutations involving exon 2 of this gene are characterized by a predominantly ocular variant of this disorder, consistent with the major form of procollagen type II in non-ocular tissues having exon 2 spliced out. Such patients are all at high risk of retinal detachment (115). A patient with Stickler syndrome type I, with a mutation in the *COL2A1* gene, has been described who had significant retinal abnormalities, including vitreous collagen encased within glial strands on the inner surface of an atrophic and gliotic detached retina (82). Mutations in collagen type XI, a minor component of cartilage collagen, can cause Stickler syndrome type II (MIM #604841) (88,125). A heterozygous mouse model of Stickler syndrome has shown how type II (pro)collagen of collagen type XI influences eye structures (60), including decreased folding of ciliary processes, increased vacuolization of the ciliary process stromal ECM, and lens subcapsular ECM changes.

Rhegmatogenous Retinal Detachment

Rhegmatogenous retinal detachment (see Chapter 28) can occur as a spontaneous event resulting from posterior vitreous detachment (115) and is also a feature of Stickler syndrome. In two large families with autosomal dominant RRD, linkage has been found at the COL2A1 locus. In one of these families, an Arg453Ter mutation was identified that, together with other protein-truncating mutations in the helical domain of COL2A1, have been associated with classic Stickler syndrome (143).

Kniest Dysplasia and Epiphyseal Dysplasias

Kniest dysplasia (MIM #156550) and epiphyseal dysplasias (MIM #132400), also caused by mutations in the *COL2A1* gene for collagen II (95,115), may have ocular features that include severe myopia associated with astigmatism, vitreoretinal degeneration, areas of perivascular lattice degeneration, trophic holes and vitreous traction in the peripheral retina, and cataract.

Wagner Syndrome

Wagner syndrome (MIM #143200) is a rare vitreoretinal degeneration inherited as an autosomal dominant trait without clinically apparent systemic involvement (115), and it is distinct from Stickler syndrome in terms of its characteristic changes in vitreous and RPE, and difficulties in night vision. Wagner syndrome has been mapped to the long arm of chromosome 5 (5q14.3), and is caused by mutations in the versican gene (*CSP62*) (66). Complications include mild myopia, absence of vitreous gel in the retrolental space and avascular membranes, vitreoretinal degeneration and retinal detachment, narrowing of retinal blood vessels, patchy areas of thinned RPE, and presenile cataracts.

Marshall Syndrome

Marshall syndrome (MIM #154780), which is characterized by cataracts, a stable or progressive myopia, sparse, irregularly thickened bundles of collagen fibers throughout the vitreous space, and some similarities with Stickler syndrome, has an autosomal dominant mode of inheritance. Mutations in the *COL11A1* gene for collagen type XI have been identified in this syndrome (5,115).

Knobloch Syndrome

Knobloch syndrome (MIM #267750) is a rare recessive disorder with some similarities to Stickler syndrome (115,127). It is associated with high myopia and retinal detachment. Mutations in the *COL8A1* gene for collagen type XVIII accounts for some cases but, since linkage to the COL18A1 locus has been excluded in one family, provides evidence for the existence of a second KNO locus (92,102).

Thyroid-Associated Ophthalmopathy

Thyroid-associated ophthalmopathy is an autoimmune disorder caused by immune reactivity between orbital and thyroid antigens (see Chapter 47), often in the context of Graves disease (36). Antibodies against collagen type XIII, and other collagen types, may be associated with the congestive subtype of this disorder (10,36).

REFERENCES

1. Afshari NA, Afshari MA, Foster CS. Inflammatory conditions of the eye associated with rheumatic diseases. Curr Rheumatol Rep 2001; 3:453–8.
2. al Gazali LI, Sabrinathan K, Nair KG. A syndrome of osteogenesis imperfecta, optic atrophy, retinopathy and severe developmental delay in two sibs of consanguineous parents. Clin Dysmorphol 1994; 3:55–62.
3. Al-Hussain H, Zeisberger SM, Huber PR, et al. Brittle cornea syndrome and its delineation from the kyphoscoliotic type of Ehlers-Danlos syndrome (EDS VI): report on 23 patients and review of the literature. Am J Med Genet A 2004; 124:28–34.
4. Amenta PS, Scivoletti NA, Newman ND, et al. Proteoglycan-collagen XV in human tissues is seen linking banded collagen fibers subjacent to the basement membrane. J Histochem Cytochem 2005; 53(2):165–76.
5. Annunen S, Korkko J, Czarny M, et al. Splicing mutations of 54-bp exons in the COL11A1 gene cause Marshall syndrome, but other mutations cause overlapping Marshall/Stickler phenotypes. Am J Hum Genet 1999; 65:974–83.
6. Ayyagari R, Mandal MN, Karoukis AJ, et al. Late-onset macular degeneration and long anterior lens zonules result from a CTRP5 gene mutation. Invest Ophthalmol Vis Sci 2005; 46:3363–71.
7. Baldock C, Sherratt MJ, Shuttleworth CA, et al. The supramolecular organization of collagen VI microfibrils. J Mol Biol 2003; 330:297–307.
8. Banyard J, Bao L, Zetter BR. Type XXIII collagen, a new transmembrane collagen identified in metastatic tumor cells. J Biol Chem 2003; 278:20989–94.
9. Bateman JB, Foos RY. Coronal adenomas. Arch Ophthalmol 1979; 97:2379–84.
10. Bednarczuk T, Stolarski C, Pawlik E, et al. Autoantibodies reactive with extracellular matrix proteins in patients with thyroid-associated ophthalmopathy. Thyroid 1999; 9:289–95.
11. Beecher N, Chakravarti S, Joyce S, et al. Neonatal development of the corneal stroma in wild-type and lumican-null mice. Invest Ophthalmol Vis Sci 2006; 47: 146–50.
12. Bhattacharya SK, Peachey NS, Crabb JW. Cochlin and glaucoma: a mini-review. Vis Neurosci 2005; 22: 605–13.
13. Bhutto IA, Kim SY, McLeod DS, et al. Localization of collagen XVIII and the endostatin portion of collagen XVIII in aged human control eyes and eyes with age-related macular degeneration. Invest Ophthalmol Vis Sci 2004; 45:1544–52.
14. Bishop PN. Structural macromolecules and supramolecular organisation of the vitreous gel. Prog Retin Eye Res 2000; 19:323–44.
15. Bishop PN, Takanosu M, Le Goff M, Mayne R. The role of the posterior ciliary body in the biosynthesis of vitreous humour. Eye 2002; 16:454–60.
16. Bishop PN, Holmes DF, Kadler KE, et al. Age-related changes on the surface of vitreous collagen fibrils. Invest Ophthalmol Vis Sci 2004; 45:1041–6.
17. Biswas S, Munier FL, Yardley J, et al. Missense mutations in COL8A2, the gene encoding the alpha2 chain of type VIII collagen, cause two forms of corneal endothelial dystrophy. Hum Mol Genet 2001; 10:2415–23.
18. Blackburn J, Tarttelin EE, Gregory-Evans CY, et al. Transcriptional regulation and expression of the dominant drusen gene FBLN3 (EFEMP1) in mammalian retina. Invest Ophthalmol Vis Sci 2003; 44:4613–21.
19. Boot-Handford RP, Tuckwell DS. Fibrillar collagen: the key to vertebrate evolution? A tale of molecular incest. BioEssays 2003; 25:142–51.
20. Boot-Handford RP, Tuckwell D, Plumb DA, Farrington Rock C, Poulsom R. A novel and highly conserved collagen [pro α1(XXVII)] with a unique expression pattern and unusual molecular characteristics establishes a new clade within the vertebrate fibrillar collagen family. J Biol Chem 2003; 278:31067–77.
21. Boote C, Hayes S, Abahussin M, Meek KM. Mapping collagen organization in the human cornea: left and right eyes are structurally distinct. Invest Ophthalmol Vis Sci 2006; 47:901–8.
22. Bonadio J, Byers PH. Subtle structural alterations in the chains of type I procollagen produce osteogenesis imperfecta type II. Nature 1985; 316:363–6.
23. Bos KJ, Holmes DF, Meadows RS, et al. Collagen fibril organisation in mammalian vitreous by freeze etch/ rotary shadowing electron microscopy. Micron 2001; 32: 301–6.
24. Brankin B, Campbell M, Canning P, et al. Endostatin modulates VEGF-mediated barrier dysfunction in the retinal microvascular endothelium. Exp Eye Res 2005; 81: 22–31.
25. Bruckner-Tuderman L. Epidermolysis bullosa. In: Royce PM, Steinmann B, eds. Connective Tissue and its Heritable Disorders. New York: Wiley-Liss, 2002:687–726.
26. Buyse M, Bull MJ. A syndrome of osteogenesis imperfecta, microcephaly, and cataracts. Birth Defects Orig Artic Ser 1978; 14:95–8.
27. Byers PH, Cole WG. Osteogenesis imperfecta. In Royce PM, Steinmann B eds., Connective Tissue and its Heritable Disorders, Wiley-Liss, New York, 2002:385–430.
28. Canty EG, Kadler KE. Procollagen trafficking, processing and fibrillogenesis. J Cell Sci 2005; 118:1341–53.
29. Canty EG, Lu Y, Meadows RS, et al. Coalignment of plasma membrane channels and protrusions (fibripositors) specifies the parallelism of tendon. J Cell Biol 2004; 165:553–63.
30. Chen YT, Huang CW, Huang FC, et al. The cleavage plane of corneal epithelial adhesion complex in traumatic recurrent corneal erosion. Mol Vis 2006; 12:196–204.

31. Chong NH, Keonin J, Luthert PJ, et al. Decreased thickness and integrity of the macular elastic layer of Bruch's membrane correspond to the distribution of lesions associated with age-related macular degeneration. Am J Pathol 2005; 166:241–51.
32. Claudepierre T, Manglapus MK, Marengi N, et al. Collagen XVII and BPAG1 expression in the retina: evidence for an anchoring complex in the central nervous system. J Comp Neurol 2005; 487:190–203.
33. Collier SA. Is the corneal degradation in keratoconus caused by natrix-metalloproteinases? Clin Exp Ophthalmol 2001; 29:340–4
34. Das JK, Sengupta S, Gangopadhyay AK. Epidermolysis bullosa acquisita. Indian J Dermatol Venereol Leprol 2006; 72:86.
35. Diehn JJ, Diehn M, Marmor MF, Brown PO. Differential gene expression in anatomical compartments of the human eye. Genome Biol. 2005; 6:R74.
36. El-Kaissi S, Frauman AG, Wall JR. Thyroid-associated ophthalmopathy: a practical guide to classification, natural history and management. Intern Med J 2004; 34: 482–91.
37. Eyre DR, Wu J-J, Fernandes RJ, et al. Recent developments in cartilage research: matrix biology of the collagen II/IX/XI heterofibril network. Biochem Soc Trans 2002; 30:894–9.
38. Ferrer E. Trabecular meshwork as a new target for the treatment of glaucoma. Drug News Perspect 2006; 19: 151–8.
39. Fine JD, Johnson LB, Weiner M, et al. Eye involvement in inherited epidermolysis bullosa: experience of the National Epidermolysis Bullosa Registry. Am J Ophthalmol 2004; 138:254–62.
40. Franzke CW, Bruckner P, Bruckner-Tuderman L. Collagenous transmembrane proteins: recent insights into biology and pathology. J Biol Chem 2005; 280:4005–8.
41. Fuchshofer R, Welge-Lussen U, Lutjen-Drecoll E, Birke M. Biochemical and morphological analysis of basement membrane component expression in corneoscleral and cribriform human trabecular meshwork cells. Invest Ophthalmol Vis Sci 2006; 47:794–801.
42. Gentle A, Liu Y, Martin JE, et al. Collagen gene expression and the altered accumulation of scleral collagen during the development of high myopia. J Biol Chem 2003; 278: 16587–94.
43. Go SL, Maugeri A, Mulder JJ, et al. Autosomal dominant rhegmatogenous retinal detachment associated with an Arg453Ter mutation in the COL2A1 gene. Invest Ophthalmol Vis Sci 2003; 44:4035–43.
44. Gordon MK, Fitch JM, Foley JW, et al. Type XVII collagen (BP 180) in the developing avian cornea. Invest Ophthalmol Vis Sci 1997; 38:153–66.
45. Gottsch JD, Zhang C, Sundin OH, et al. Fuchs corneal dystrophy: aberrant collagen distribution in an L450W mutant of the COL8A2 gene. Invest Ophthalmol Vis Sci 2005; 46:4504–11.
46. Hayward C, Shu X, Cideciyan AV, et al. Mutation in a short-chain collagen gene, CTRP5, results in extracellular deposit formation in late-onset retinal degeneration: a genetic model for age-related macular degeneration. Hum Mol Genet 2003; 12(20):2657–67.
47. He YG, Niederkom JY, McCulley JP, et al. In vivo and in vitro collagenolytic activity of *Acanthamoeba castellanii*. Invest Ophthalmol Vis Sci 1990; 31:2235–40.
48. Heathcote JG. Collagen and its disorders. In Garner A, Klintworth GK, eds. Pathobiology of Ocular Disease: A Dynamic Approach. 2nd ed. Chapter 33. New York: Marcel Dekker, 1994:1033–84.
49. Hiscott P, Hagan S, Heathcote L, et al. Pathobiology of epiretinal and subretinal membranes: possible roles for the matricellular proteins thrombospondin 1 and osteonectin (SPARC). Eye 2002; 16:393–403.
50. Holmes DF, Kadler KE. The precision of lateral size control in the assembly of corneal collagen fibrils. J Mol Biol 2005; 345:773–84.
51. Hopfer U, Fukai N, Hopfer H, et al. Targeted disruption of Col8a1 and Col8a2 genes in mice leads to anterior segment abnormalities in the eye. FASEB J 2005; 19: 1232–44.
52. Horton WA, Hecht JT. Chondrodysplasias: disorders of cartilage matrix proteins. In: Royce PM, Steinmann B, eds. Connective Tissue and its Heritable Diseases; Molecular, Genetic and Medical Aspects. New York: Wiley-Liss, 2002:909–38.
53. Hudson BG, Tryggvason K, Sundaramoorthy M, Neilson EG. Alport's syndrome, Goodpasture's syndrome, and type IV collagen. N Engl J Med 2003; 348:2543–56.
54. Hudson BG. The molecular basis of Goodpasture and Alport syndromes: beacons for the discovery of the collagen IV family. J Am Soc Nephrol 2004; 15:2514–27.
55. Hughes S, Chan-Ling TR. Characterization of smooth muscle cell and pericyte differentiation in the rat retina in vivo. Invest Ophthalmol Vis Sci 2004; 45:2795–806.
56. Hurskainen M, Eklund L, Hagg PO, et al. Abnormal maturation of the retinal vasculature in type XVIII collagen/endostatin deficient mice and changes in retinal glial cells due to lack of collagen types XV and XVIII. FASEB J 2005; 19:1564–6.
57. Ihanamäki T, Pelliniemi LJ, Vuorio E. Collagens and collagen-related matrix components in the human and mouse eye. Prog Retin Eye Res 2004; 23:403–34.
58. Ishida I, Saika S, Okada Y, Ohnishi Y. Growth factor deposition in anterior subcapsular cataract. J Cataract Refract Surg 2005; 31:1219–25.
59. Johnson PT, Lewis GP, Talaga KC, et al. Drusen-associated degeneration in the retina. Invest Ophthalmol Vis Sci 2003; 44:4481–8.
60. Kaarniranta K, Ihanamaki T, Sahlman J, et al. A mouse model for Stickler's syndrome: Ocular phenotype of mice carrying a targeted heterozygous inactivation of type II (pro)collagen gene (Col2a1). Exp Eye Res (in press) 2006.
61. Karp CL, Fazio JR, Culbertson WW, Green WR. True exfoliation of the lens capsule. Arch Ophthalmol 1999; 117:1078–80.
62. Kelley PB, Sado Y, Duncan MK. Collagen IV in the developing lens capsule. Matrix Biol 2002; 21:415–23.
63. Kern JS, Kohlhase J, Bruckner-Tuderman L, Has C. Expanding the COL7A1 Mutation Database: novel and recurrent mutations and unusual genotype—phenotype constellations in 41 patients with dystrophic epidermolysis bullosa. J Invest Dermatol 2006; 126:1006–12.
64. Kernacki KA, Chunta JL, Barrett RP, Hazlett LD. TIMP-1 role in protection against *Pseudomonas aeruginosa*-induced corneal destruction. Exp Eye Res 2004; 78:1155–62.
65. Kielty CM, Grant ME. The collagen family: structure, assembly and organization in the extracellular matrix. In: Royce PM, Steinmann B, eds. Connective Tissue and its Heritable Diseases; Molecular, Genetic and Medical Aspects, Wiley-Liss, New York, 2002:159–221.
66. Kloeckener-Gruissem B, Bartholdi D, Abdou MT, et al. Identification of the genetic defect in the original Wagner syndrome family. Mol Vis 2006; 12:350–5.

67. Knupp C, Amin SZ, Munro PM, et al. Collagen VI assemblies in age-related macular degeneration. J Struct Biol 2002; 139:181–9.
68. Koch M, Laub F, Zhou P, et al. Collagen XXIV, a vertebrate fibrillar collagen with structural features of invertebrate collagens: selective expression in developing cornea and bone. J Biol Chem 2003; 278:43236–44.
69. Krafchak CM, Pawar H, Moroi SE, et al. Mutations in TCF8 cause posterior polymorphous corneal dystrophy and ectopic expression of COL4A3 by corneal endothelial cells. Am J Hum Genet 2005; 77:694–708.
70. Kretzer FL, Hittner HM, Mehta RS. Ocular manifestations of the Smith-Lemli-Opitz syndrome. Arch Ophthalmol 1981; 99:2000–6.
71. Kuivaniemi H, Tromp G, Prockop DJ. Mutations in fibrillar collagens (types I, II, III, and XI), fibril-associated collagen (type IX), and network-forming collagen (type X) cause a spectrum of diseases of bone, cartilage, and blood vessels. Hum Mutat 1997; 9:300–15.
72. Laforest C, Huilgol SC, Casson R, et al. Autoimmune bullous diseases: ocular manifestations and management. Drugs 2005; 65(13):1767–79.
73. Lees JF, Tasab M, Bulleid NJ. Identification of the molecular recognition sequence which determines the type-specific assembly of procollagen. EMBO J 1997; 16: 908–16.
74. Le Goff MM, Hindson VJ, Jowitt TA, et al. Characterization of opticin and evidence of stable dimerization in solution. J Biol Chem 2003; 278:45280–7.
75. Linsenmayer TF, Fitch JM, Gordon MK, et al. Development and roles of collagenous matrices in the embryonic avian cornea. Prog Retin Eye Res 1998; 17: 231–65.
76. Los LI, van der Worp RJ, van Luyn MJ, Hooymans JM. Presence of collagen IV in the ciliary zonules of the human eye: an immunohistochemical study by LM and TEM. J Histochem Cytochem 2004; 52:789–95.
77. Lunstrum GP, Sakai LY, Keene DR, et al. Large complex globular domains of type VII procollagen contribute to the structure of anchoring fibrils. J Biol Chem 1986; 261: 9042–8.
78. Lutjen-Drecoll E. Functional morphology of the trabecular meshwork in primate eyes. Prog Retin Eye Res 1999; 18:91–119.
79. Lutjen-Drecoll E. Importance of trabecular meshwork changes in the pathogenesis of primary open-angle glaucoma. J Glaucoma 2000; 9:417–8.
80. Maatta M, Heljasvaara R, Sormunen R, et al. Differential expression of collagen types XVIII/endostatin and XV in normal, keratoconus, and scarred human corneas. Cornea 2006; 25:341–9.
81. Mackiewicz Z, Maatta M, Stenman M, et al. Collagenolytic proteinases in keratoconus. Cornea 2006; 25:603–10.
82. Macrae ME, Patel DV, Richards AJ, et al. Type 1 Stickler syndrome: a histological and ultrastructural study of an untreated globe. Eye (in press) 2006.
83. Maddala R, Deng PF, Costello JM, et al. Impaired cytoskeletal organization and membrane integrity in lens fibers of a Rho GTPase functional knockout transgenic mouse. Lab Invest 2004; 84:679–92.
84. Marks DS, Gregory CA, Wallis GA, et al. (1999) Metaphyseal chondrodysplasia type Schmid mutations are predicted to occur in two distinct three-dimensional clusters within type X collagen NC1 domains which retain the ability to trimerise. J Biol Chem 274, 3632–41.
85. Marneros AG, Keene DR, Hansen U, et al. Collagen XVIII/endostatin is essential for vision and retinal pigment epithelial function. EMBO J 2004; 23:89–99.
86. Marneros AG, Olsen BR. Age-dependent iris abnormalities in collagen XVIII/endostatin deficient mice with similarities to human pigment dispersion syndrome. Invest Ophthalmol Vis Sci 2003; 44:2367–72.
87. Marneros AG, Olsen BR. Physiological role of collagen XVIII and endostatin. FASEB J 2005; 19:716–28.
88. Martin S, Richards AJ, Yates JR, et al. Stickler syndrome: further mutations in COL11A1 and evidence for additional locus heterogeneity. Eur J Hum Genet 1999; 7: 807–14.
89. McBrien NA, Cornell LM, Gentle A. Structural and ultrastructural changes to the sclera in a mammalian model of high myopia. Invest Ophthalmol Vis Sci 2001; 42:2179–87.
90. Meek KM, Boote C. The organization of collagen in the corneal stroma. Exp Eye Res 2004; 78:503–12.
91. Meek KM, Tuft SJ, Huang Y, et al. Changes in collagen orientation and distribution in keratoconus corneas. Invest Ophthalmol Vis Sci 2005; 46:1948–56.
92. Menzel O, Bekkeheien RC, Reymond A, et al. Knobloch syndrome: novel mutations in COL18A1, evidence for genetic heterogeneity, and a functionally impaired polymorphism in endostatin. Hum Mutat 2004; 23:77–84.
93. Myers JC, Kivirikko S, Gordon MK, et al. Identification of a previously unknown human collagen chain, α1(XV), characterized by extensive interruptions in the triple-helical region. Proc Natl Acad Sci U S A 1992; 89:10144–8.
94. Myllyharju J, Kivirikko KI. Collagens and collagen-related diseases. Ann Med 2001; 33:7–21.
95. Nishimura G, Haga N, Kitoh H, et al. The phenotypic spectrum of COL2A1 mutations. Hum Mutat 2005; 26: 36–43.
96. Nwosu BU, Raygada M, Tsilou ET, et al. Rieger's anomaly and other ocular abnormalities in association with osteogenesis imperfecta and a COL1A1 mutation. Ophthalmic Genet 2005; 26:135–8.
97. Oh SP, Warman ML, Seldin MF, et al. Cloning of cDNA and genomic DNA encoding human type XVIII collagen and localization of the α1(XVIII) collagen gene to mouse chromosome 10 and human chromosome 21. Genomics 1994; 19:494–9.
98. Ohkubo S, Takeda H, Higashide T, et al. Immunohistochemical and molecular genetic evidence for type IV collagen alpha5 chain abnormality in the anterior lenticonus associated with Alport syndrome. Arch Ophthalmol 2003; 121:846–50.
99. Ohlmann AV, Ohlmann A, Welge-Lussen U, May CA. Localization of collagen XVIII and endostatin in the human eye. Curr Eye Res 2005; 30:27–34.
100. O'Reilly MS, Boehm T, Shing Y, et al. Endostatin: an endogenous inhibitor of angiogenesis and tumor growth. Cell 1997; 88:277–85.
101. Pace JM, Corrado M, Missero C, Byers PH. Identification, characterization and expression analysis of a new fibrillar collagen gene, COL27A1. Matrix Biol 2003; 22:3–14.
102. Passos-Bueno MR, Suzuki OT, Armelin-Correa LM, et al. Mutations in collagen 18A1 and their relevance to the human phenotype. An Acad Bras Cienc 2006; 78:123–31.
103. Peebo BB, Peebo M, Frennesson C. Relapsing polychondritis: a rare disease with varying symptoms. Acta Ophthalmol Scand 2004; 82:472–5.
104. Plotkin H. Syndromes with congenital brittle bones. BMC Pediatr 2004; 4:16.

105. Plumb D, Boot-Handford RP. Collagen type XVII forms distinct thin fibrils (unpublished observations).
106. Prockop DJ, Sieron AL, Li SW. Procollagen N-proteinase and procollagen C-proteinase. Two unusual metalloproteinases that are essential for procollagen processing probably have important roles in development and cell signaling. Matrix Biol 1998; 16:399–408.
107. Provis JM, Penfold PL, Cornish EE, et al. Anatomy and development of the macula: specialisation and the vulnerability to macular degeneration. Clin Exp Optom 2005; 88:269–81.
108. Rada JA, Achen VR, Perry CA, Fox PW. Proteoglycans in the human sclera. Evidence for the presence of aggrecan. Invest Ophthalmol Vis Sci 1997; 38:1740–51.
109. Rada JA, Shelton S, Norton TT. The sclera and myopia. Exp Eye Res 2006; 82:185–200.
110. Ralph RA. Tetracyclines and the treatment of corneal stromal ulceration: a review. Cornea 2000; 19(3):274–7.
111. Rattenholl A, Pappano WN, Koch M, et al. Proteinases of the bone morphogenetic protein-1 family convert procollagen VII to mature anchoring fibril collagen. J Biol Chem 2002; 277:26372–8.
112. Rebell G, Forster RK. *Lasiodiplodia theobromae* as a cause of keratomycoses. Sabouraudia 1976; 14:155–70.
113. Rehn M, Pihlajaniemi T. α1(XVIII), a collagen chain with frequent interruptions in the collagenous sequence, a distinct tissue distribution, and homology with type XV collagen. Proc. Natl. Acad. Sci U S A 1994; 91:4234–8.
114. Ricard-Blum S, Ruggiero F The collagen superfamily: from the extracellular matrix to the cell membrane. Pathol Biol 2005; 53:430–42.
115. Richards AJ, Scott JD, Snead MP. Molecular genetics of rhegmatogenous retinal detachment. Eye 2002; 16:388–92.
116. Robb BW, Wachi H, Schaub T, et al. Characterization of an in vitro model of elastic fiber assembly. Mol Biol Cell 1999; 10:3595–605.
117. Sandberg-Lall M, Hagg PO, Wahlstrom I, Pihlajaniemi T. Type XIII collagen is widely expressed in the adult and developing human eye and accentuated in the ciliary muscle, the optic nerve and the neural retina. Exp Eye Res. 2000; 70:401–10.
118. Savontaus M, Ihanamäki T, Metsaranta M, et al. Localization of type II collagen mRNA isoforms in the developing eyes of normal and transgenic mice with a mutation in type II collagen gene. Invest Ophthalmol Vis Sci 1997; 38:930–42.
119. Sawamura D, Sato-Matsumura K, Shibata S, et al. COL7A1 mutation G2037E causes epidermal retention of type VII collagen. J Hum Genet (in press) 2006.
120. Sawhney RS. Immunological identification of types I and III collagen in bovine lens epithelium and its anterior lens capsule. Cell Biol Int 2005; 29:133–7.
121. Segev F, Heon E, Cole WG, et al. Structural abnormalities of the cornea and lid resulting from collagen V mutations. Invest Ophthalmol Vis Sci 2006; 47:565–73.
122. Shaw LM, Olsen BR. FACIT collagens: diverse molecular bridges in extracellular matrices. Trens Biochem Sci 1991; 16:191–4.
123. Smith VA, Matthews FJ, Majid MA, Cook SD. Keratoconus: matrix metalloproteinase-2 activation and TIMP modulation. Biochim Biophys Acta 2006; 1762:431–9.
124. Soderberg L, Kakuyama H, Moller A, et al. Characterization of the Alzheimer's disease-associated CLAC protein and identification of an amyloid beta-peptide-binding site. J Biol Chem 2005; 280:1007–15.
125. Spranger J. The type XI collagenopathies. Pediatr Radiol 1998; 28:745–50.
126. Stephan S, Sherratt MJ, Hodson N, et al. Expression and supramolecular assembly of recombinant alpha1(viii) and alpha2(viii) collagen homotrimers. J Biol Chem 2004; 279: 21469–77.
127. Steinmann B, Royce PM. Knobloch syndrome. In: Royce PM, Steinmann B, eds. Connective Tissue and its Heritable Disorders, Wiley-Liss, New York, 2002:1129–30.
128. Steinmann B, Royce PM, Superti-Furga A. The Ehlers-Danlos syndrome. In: Royce PM, Steinmann B, eds. Connective Tissue and Its Heritable Disorders. New York: Wiley-Liss, 2002:431–524.
129. Stitt AW, Frizzell N, Thorpe SR. Advanced glycation and advanced lipoxidation: possible role in initiation and progression of diabetic retinopathy. Curr Pharm Des 2004; 10:3349–60.
130. Stitt AW, Curtis TM. Advanced glycation and retinal pathology during diabetes. Pharmacol Rep 2005; 57 (Suppl.):156–68.
131. Subrayan V, Morris B, Armbrecht AM, et al. Long anterior lens zonules in late-onset retinal degeneration (L-ORD). Am J Ophthalmol 2005; 140:1127–9.
132. Sugino IK, Wang H, Zarbin MA. Age-related macular degeneration and retinal pigment epithelium wound healing. Mol Neurobiol 2003; 28:177–94.
133. Timpl R, Brown JC. Supramolecular assembly of basement membranes. BioEssays 1996; 18:123–32.
134. Timpl R, Chu M-L. Type VI collagen. In Yurchenko PD, Birk D, Mecham RP, eds. Extracellular Matrix Assembly and Structure, Academic Press, New York, 1994:207–42.
135. Timpl R, Wiedemann H, van Delden V, et al. A network model for the organization of type IV collagen molecules in basement membranes. Eur J Biochem 1981; 120:203–11.
136. Tomasek JJ, Haaksma CJ, Schwartz RJ, et al. Deletion of smooth muscle alpha-actin alters blood-retina barrier permeability and retinal function. Invest Ophthalmol Vis Sci 2006; 47:2693–700.
137. Turner NJ, Murphy MO, Kielty CM, et al. α2(VIII) collagen substrata support endothelial cell attachment and enhance cell retention under acute shear stress flow in vitro and in vivo via an α2β1 integrin dependent mechanism. Circulation (in press) 2006.
138. Umeda S, Suzuki MT, Okamoto H, et al. Molecular composition of drusen and possible involvement of anti-retinal autoimmunity in two different forms of macular degeneration in cynomolgus monkey (*Macaca fascicularis*). FASEB J 2005; 19:1683–5.
139. Van Agtmael T, Schlotzer-Schrehardt U, McKie L, et al. Dominant mutations of Col4a1 result in basement membrane defects which lead to anterior segment dysgenesis and glomerulopathy. Hum Mol Genet 2005; 14:3161–8.
140. Veit G, Kobbe B, Keene DR, et al. Collagen XXVIII, a novel von Willebrand factor. A domain-containing protein with many imperfections in the collagenous domain. J Biol Chem 2006; 281:3494–504.
141. Wachi H, Sato F, Murata H, et al. Development of a new in vitro model of elastic fiber assembly in human pigmented epithelial cells. Clin Biochem 2005; 38:643–53.
142. Watson PG, Young RD. Scleral structure, organisation and disease. A review. Exp Eye Res 2004; 78:609–23.
143. Weed KH, Macewen CJ, Cox A, McGhee CN. Quantitative analysis of corneal microstructure in keratoconus utilising in vivo confocal microscopy. Eye (in press) 2006.

144. Wenstrup RJ, Florer JB, Brunskill EW, et al. Type V collagen controls the initiation of collagen fibril assembly. J Biol Chem 2004; 279:53331–7.
145. Wessel H, Anderson S, Fite D, et al. Type XII collagen contributes to diversities in human corneal and limbal extracellular matrices. Invest Ophthalmol Vis Sci 1997; 38: 2408–22.
146. White J, Werkmeister JA, Ramshaw JA, Birk DE. Organization of fibrillar collagen in the human and bovine cornea: collagen types V and III. Connect Tissue Res 1997; 36:165–74.
147. Wilson SE, Hong JW. Bowman's layer structure and function: critical or dispensable to corneal function? A hypothesis. Cornea 2000; 19:417–20.
148. Yellore VS, Rayner SA, Emmert-Buck L, et al. No pathogenic mutations identified in the COL8A2 gene or four positional candidate genes in patients with posterior polymorphous corneal dystrophy. Invest Ophthalmol Vis Sci 2005; 46:1599–603.
149. Young BB, Zhang G, Koch M, Birk DE. The roles of types XII and XIV collagen in fibrillogenesis and matrix assembly in the developing cornea. J Cell Biochem 2000; 87:208–20.
150. Young TL, Guo XD, King RA, et al. Identification of genes expressed in a human scleral cDNA library. Mol Vis 2003; 9:508–14.
151. Yurchenco PD, Amenta PS, Patton BL. Basement membrane assembly, stability and activities observed through a developmental lens. Matrix Biol 2004; 22:521–38.
152. Zhou J, Rappaport EF, Tobias JW, Young TL. Differential Gene Expression in Mouse Sclera during Ocular Development. Invest Ophthalmol Vis Sci 2006; 47: 1794–802.

45

Disorders of Monosaccharide Metabolism

Jennifer B. Green
Division of Endocrinology, Department of Medicine, Duke University, Durham, North Carolina, U.S.A.

INTRODUCTION

Humans are largely dependent upon glucose—and to a lesser extent, the monosaccharides galactose and fructose—to provide fuel for cellular metabolism. Levels of blood glucose are maintained fairly precisely through a balance of dietary intake, breakdown of established glycogen stores, and gluconeogenesis. Given the importance of normal metabolism of these carbohydrates, it is readily understandable that abnormalities in monosaccharide metabolism are associated with significant disease processes. This section will review the inborn errors associated with altered metabolism of galactose and fructose, as well as the more common disorders associated with defects in glucose metabolism.

Dietary sources of glucose are many, including galactose and fructose; the disaccharides sucrose, maltose, and lactose; and polysaccharides (starches). In the normal state, both galactose and fructose are converted through a variety of enzymatic processes to the metabolically important substrate glucose-1-phosphate. Galactose is primarily derived from the intestinal hydrolysis of lactose present in milk and dairy products, but is also present in lesser amounts in a variety of other foods, including fruits, vegetables, and nuts. Fructose is present in fruits, vegetables, and honey, but is also derived from the widely used sweetener sucrose (11).

GALACTOSE METABOLISM

Galactose is converted to glucose-1-phosphate via the enzymes of the Leloir pathway, as outlined in Figure 1. The first of these enzymes, galactose mutarotase, epimerizes beta-D-galactose to alpha-D-galactose. As no human diseases have been associated with mutations in this enzyme, the remainder of this discussion will concentrate on the subsequent three enzymes in the pathway. Deficiencies in these enzymes result in accumulation of galactose and its metabolites, and in the associated rare diseases referred to as the galactosemias (11). The second enzyme, galactokinase

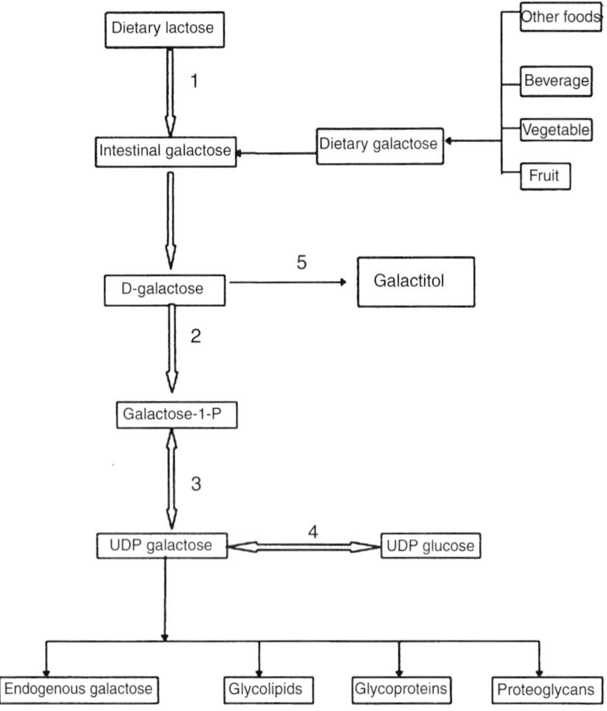

Figure 1 Galactose metabolism (2–4, major pathway; 5, minor pathway). 1 = lactase; 2 = galactokinase; 3 = galactose-1-phosphate uridyltransferase; 4 = UDP-4-epimerase; 5 = aldose reductase. *Source*: From Ref. 22.

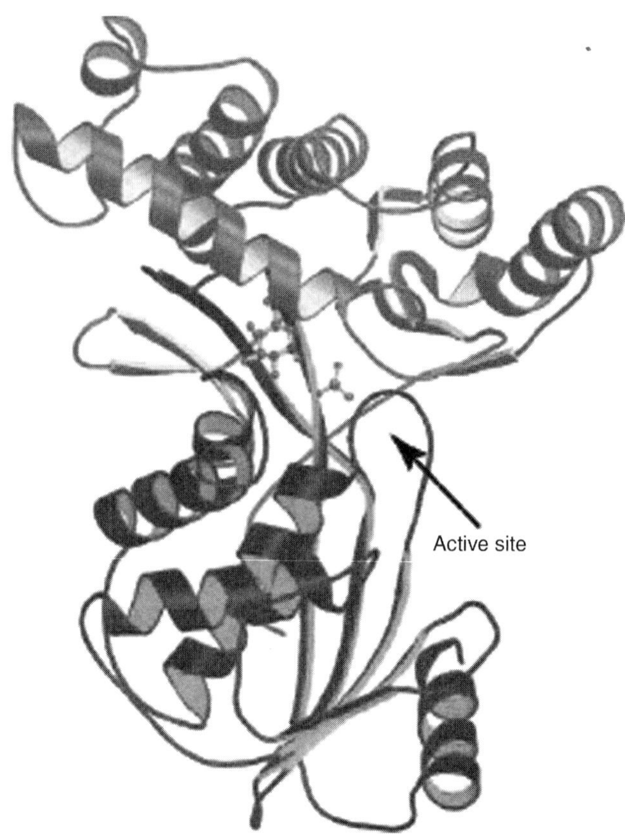

Figure 2 Ribbon representation of galactokinase from *L. lactis*. *Source*: From Ref. 16.

converts galactose to galactose-1-phosphate via ATP-dependent phosphorylation. This enzyme belongs to the GHMP (*G*alactokinase, *H*omoserine kinase, *M*evalonate kinase, *P*hosphomevalonate kinase) enzyme superfamily. Deficiency of this enzyme is associated with the disease known as galactosemia II. The structure of galactokinase has been determined in *Lactococcus lactis*, and is shown in the ribbon representation in Figure 2 as complexed with galactose and inorganic phosphate. This structure is considered to have reasonable similarity to the human form of the enzyme.

The next enzyme, galactose-1-phosphate-uridyltransferase, is involved in the conversion of galactose-1-phosphate to glucose-1-phosphate and UDP-galactose. This enzyme is a member of the histidine triad superfamily of enzymes. Deficiency of this enzyme results in the severe disease known as "classic" galactosemia, or galactosemia I. A ribbon representation of the enzyme from *Escherichia coli* is shown in Figure 3. The final step in the metabolism of galactose involves the conversion of UDP galactose to UDP glucose via the enzyme UDP-galactose-4-epimerase. This enzyme belongs to the short chain dehydrogenase/reductase superfamily. Defects in this enzyme result in the condition referred to as galactosemia III. A ribbon representation of the human enzyme is shown in Figure 4.

Organ system dysfunction in galactosemia is due to the accumulation of galactose and its metabolites, including galactitol. As indicated in Figure 1, galactose is converted to galactitol via the enzyme aldose reductase. This pathway generally does not result in the production of large amounts of galactitol unless high levels of intracellular levels of galactose are present, as in the galactosemias. As previously noted, multiple genetic mutations resulting in deficiencies of galactokinase, galactose-1-phosphate-uridyltransferase, and UDP-galactose-4-epimerase from mutations in the GALK, gut-associated lymphoid tissue (GALT), and *GALE* genes, respectively, have been described. For the most part, deficiencies in these three enzymes are associated with distinct phenotypes. However, considerable genetic and phenotypic variability exists, particularly within the group of individuals with GALT deficiency and classic galactosemia.

Galactose-1-Phosphate Uridyl Transferase Deficiency (Galactosemia Type I, Classic Galactosemia, MIM #230400)

A complete deficiency of galactose-1-phosphate-uridyltransferase due to mutations in the GALT gene

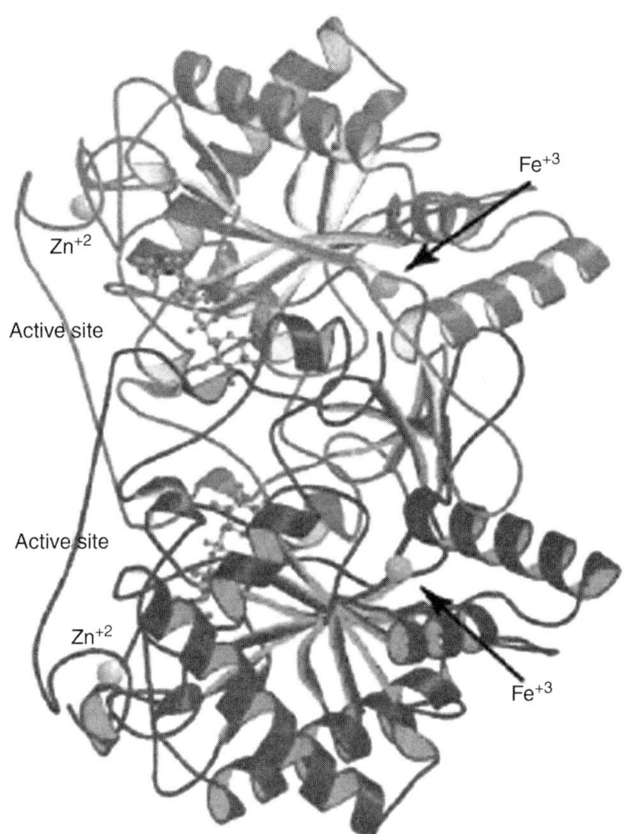

Figure 3 Ribbon representation of galactose-1-phosphate uridylyltransferase from *E. coli. Source*: From Ref. 16.

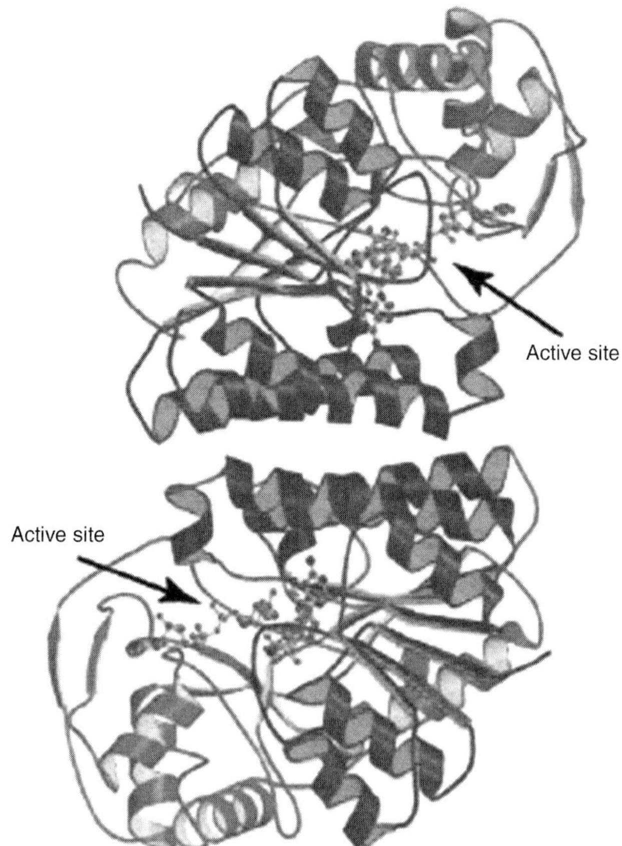

Figure 4 Ribbon representation of human UDP-galactose 4-epimerase. *Source*: From Ref. 16.

results in the most common form of galactosemia, often referred to as "classic" galactosemia or galactosemia type I. This is a severe condition, with affected infants generally presenting within the first few days of life. A newborn infant generally consumes 20% of its calories as lactose (glucose plus galactose). In galactosemia type I, the infant is unable to metabolize galactose-1-phosphate, which accumulates in and causes damage to multiple organs including the liver, brain, and kidneys. Neurologic, hepatic, and renal compromise are common at presentation, with manifestations including lethargy, poor feeding, jaundice, hepatosplenomegaly, and ascites. Infants may bruise/bleed easily, and have ocular involvement manifesting as vitreous hemorrhage, hemolytic anemia, aminoaciduria, or albuminuria. Affected infants are predisposed to *E. coli* sepsis, which may precede the diagnosis of galactosemia. Cataracts generally appear at two weeks of age due to the accumulation of galactitol in the lens, but may occasionally be present at birth (11). The hyperosmotic effect of galactitol results in lens opacification with vacuole formation and swelling of lens fibers (18).

Screening for galactosemia is now a routine part of newborn testing in many countries. Erythrocyte galactose-1-phosphate levels are always elevated in galactosemia, and definitive testing can be performed by demonstrating decreased activity of GALT in erythrocytes (12). Most often a fluorimetric assay is used to perform this testing. Unfortunately, false positive results are common and may be due to the exposure of blood samples to heat or humidity, or in the case of certain benign phenotypes (14). False negative results may occur following transfusion or in glucose-6-phosphate dehydrogenase deficiency (33). In the event of a positive test, or a negative test with a suspicious clinical presentation, additional DNA analysis should be performed on the original sample.

Management of galactosemia is through supportive care and the lifelong dietary restriction of galactose. The elimination of galactose from the diet will reverse the organ system dysfunction, cataract formation, and allow normal growth. Although galactose-1-phosphate levels should be monitored to ensure that the level improves from the very high level seen at presentation, the level generally does not completely normalize with dietary modification. This likely reflects some degree of ongoing endogenous production of galactose (33). Unfortunately, despite appropriate dietary intervention, most galactosemic individuals will have progressive long-term neurologic complications. These generally include developmental delay, learning and speech disorders, and poor motor function with possible tremor and/or ataxia. In one study, levels of galactose-1-phosphate, UDP-galactose, and plasma/urine galactitol were not found to be associated with the Intelligence Quotient (IQ) of affected individuals (27). As galactose is important in many aspects of growth, including that of the nervous system, it is theorized that these longer-term complications might be due to in utero effects of altered galactose metabolism (25,30). Cataract formation, while estimated to occur in 30% of affected individuals, responds to dietary modification. In one survey of 350 galactosemic patients with cataracts, half had resolution of the cataracts with dietary modification, while two required surgery (32). Other treatment modalities are under investigation—several animal studies suggest that galactitol-mediated cataract formation may be slowed by the administration of antioxidants or a free radical scavenger (22). Additionally, aldose reductase inhibitors may have some promise in ameliorating galactitol-mediated changes in the lens.

Ovarian dysfunction is also a well-described complication of galactosemia, and is estimated to affect 75% to 96% of galactosemic females. Amenorrhea may occur at any time during the reproductive phase. This is probably due to the toxic accumulation of galactose metabolites within the ovary. Laboratory evaluation reveals hypergonadotropic hypogonadism, with elevated levels of luteinizing hormone and follicle-stimulating hormone and low levels of estradiol (22). Should primary amenorrhea occur, hormone replacement therapy is recommended starting at 12 years of age (33). Puberty and fertility appear to be unaffected in galactosemic males.

Galactosemia due to galactose-1-phosphate-uridyltransferase deficiency is inherited as an autosomal recessive trait, with the *GALT* gene located on chromosome 9p13. The incidence of this condition varies greatly among populations, with a U.S. incidence estimated at 1/60,000 but an incidence of only 1/1,000,000 in Japan. There is considerable allelic heterogeneity among galactosemics, with several variants of the condition known to exist. The most common disease-associated mutations include Q188R, K285N, S135L, and N314D (30). The Q188R mutation is the most frequently identified mutation in Caucasian populations, accounting for 54% to 70% of all abnormalities. This mutation has also been identified in African-American populations, but at a lesser frequency (23). Those individuals who are homo-allelic for Q188R have essentially no galactose-1-phosphate-uridyltransferase activity, and an associated severe phenotype. The K285N mutation is less common, but may account for 25% to 40% of mutations among certain eastern and central European populations—some individuals heterozygous for this mutation have developed presenile cataracts (19). S135L is confined almost exclusively to African Americans, with this mutation being responsible for approximately 50% of mutant alleles in this group. Interestingly, galactosemic individuals with this mutation may have less severe disease, as galactose-1-phosphate-uridyltransferase activity may be preserved in certain tissues and/or leukocytes. The Duarte (D1) and Los Angeles (LA or D2) variants are characterized by the same N314D mutation (23). However, the D1 variant is associated with increased erythrocyte galactose-1-phosphate-uridyltransferase activity, while the D2 variant demonstrates decreased activity of the enzyme. D2 individuals are thought to have a thermally unstable form of galactose-1-phosphate-uridyltransferase with a reduced half-life. Due to increased newborn screening practices, it has been discovered that approximately 5% to 6% of the non-galactosemic population in North America carries the Duarte allele (30). Distinction between the classic and Duarte alleles may be made through GALT electrophoresis/isoelectric focusing.

Galactokinase Deficiency (GALK Deficiency, Galactosemia Type II, GALK Deficiency, MIM #230200)

Galactosemia due to deficiency of galactokinase is a less common and less severe manifestation of the disease. In this disorder, blood galactose levels are elevated due to an absence of erythrocyte galactokinase activity (11). Subsequent galactitol accumulation and osmotic swelling in the lens results in bilateral cataract formation. Cataracts develop in all individuals not detected by newborn screening; however, the cataracts will regress or be prevented entirely through the elimination of dietary galactose. Rare cases of pseudotumor cerebri have been reported, presumably due to an increase in cerebrospinal fluid (CSF) oncotic pressure. An association between GALK deficiency and mental retardation has been suggested, but is less clear (6).

Galactokinase deficiency is inherited in an autosomal recessive fashion, and is associated with at least 20 mutations of the *GALK1* gene located on chromosome 17q24 (17). The frequency of galactokinase mutation is estimated to vary from 1/52,000 to 1/1,000,000 within various populations in Europe; however, the incidence of actual disease is less than would be expected from these numbers. The highest incidence of disease is amongst the Roma (gypsy) population of eastern Europe, in which the prevalence of the P28T mutation is estimated to be 5% (23). For unexplained reasons, the heterozygous state as well as the A198V mutation (Osaka variant) have been associated with the development of cataracts later in life (12,17).

Galactose Epimerase Deficiency (GALE Deficiency, MIM #606953)

A deficiency of uridine diphosphate galactose-4-epimerase results in the accumulation of galactose metabolites similar to those found in galactosemia type I, with an additional increase in cellular UDP galactose. Elevated galactose levels will be detected by newborn screening, but assessment of galactose-1-phosphate-uridyltransferase activity will be normal. A variety of phenotypes have been described, but are most commonly divided into benign (peripheral) disease or a more severe phenotype associated with a generalized galactose epimerase deficiency. In peripheral disease, the enzyme deficiency is generally confined to leukocytes and erythrocytes. Most affected individuals have no adverse metabolic sequelae; therefore, galactose restriction is not routinely recommended (11). However, reports of individuals with cataracts and/or mental retardation do exist (28).

Generalized deficiency of uridine diphosphate galactose-4-epimerase is extremely rare and results in a clinical picture similar to that seen in classic galactosemia, with the added manifestations of hypotonia and nerve deafness. Cataracts due to an accumulation of galactose metabolites are common in this condition, and one small study of galactosemic individuals demonstrated decreased uridine diphosphate galactose-4-epimerase activity within the lens itself (28). This condition differs significantly from classic galactosemia in that persons with epimerase deficiency cannot synthesize galactose. Thus, galactose levels will decrease much more quickly with dietary restriction than is seen in classic galactosemia. As galactose is an essential component of multiple nervous system proteins, children with galactose epimerase deficiency are placed on a diet that is galactose-restricted rather than galactose-free (12). This condition should be suspected in a newborn with a clinical picture suggestive of galactosemia, but without evidence of galactose-1-phosphate-uridyltransferase deficiency.

Galactose epimerase deficiency is an autosomal recessive disorder caused by mutations in the *GALE* gene on chromosome 1p36. Both the benign and severe forms of the disease have been associated with several missense mutations. The V94M mutation is seen in generalized severe disease, while the K257R mutation is associated with a peripheral enzyme deficiency in African Americans (23). Assessment of epimerase activity in erythrocytes may identify carriers of this variety of galactosemia, and the severe form of the disease may be identified prenatally via assay of amniotic fluid cell enzyme activity (12).

FRUCTOSE METABOLISM

Deficiencies in the enzymes fructokinase, fructose 1,6-bisphospate aldolase, or fructose 1,6-diphosphatase (FBP1) are responsible for the three known inborn abnormalities of fructose metabolism. Although fructokinase deficiency is a benign condition, deficiencies in the other enzymes are associated with severe disease.

Fructokinase Deficiency (Fructosuria, Ketohexokinase Deficiency, MIM #229800)

Fructokinase catalyses the conversion of dietary fructose to fructose-1-phosphate. Absence of this enzymatic activity results in benign fructosuria, which is characterized by elevated levels of fructose in the blood and urine. As no clinical disease is associated with this condition, no intervention or dietary modification is warranted (11). Affected individuals may be identified through the presence of a reducing substance in the urine that is not glucose—the substance can be identified as fructose via chromatography. Fructosuria has an autosomal recessive mode of inheritance and an incidence of 1/120,000. It is caused by mutations in the *KHK* gene located on chromosome 2p23.3, which codes for fructokinase (12).

Hereditary Fructose Intolerance (Fructose 1,6-Bisphosphate Aldolase B Deficiency, Fructosemia, MIM #229600)

Hereditary fructose intolerance is a severe condition manifested upon ingestion of dietary sources of fructose. Three forms of aldolase are present: aldolase A (present in muscle and erythrocytes); aldolase B (present in liver, kidney, and intestine); and aldolase C (present in brain). Aldolase B is the isoenzyme primarily responsible for the glycolytic conversion of fructose-1-phosphate and fructose-1,6-bisphosphate into 3 carbon intermediates, as well as the reverse reaction in gluconeogenesis. Deficiency of aldolase B results in a toxic accumulation of fructose-1-phosphate in addition to reductions in the available pools of phosphate and ATP (Fig. 5). The condition becomes apparent early in life, upon ingestion of dietary fructose or sucrose (commonly found in fruit, fruit juice, table sugar, or sweetened cereals). This generally occurs at the age of weaning, but may occur earlier due to the use of fructose- or sucrose-containing formulas. Infants commonly present with lethargy, growth failure, hypoglycemia, hepatic dysfunction, and metabolic acidosis caused by renal tubular acidosis and lactate accumulation. Aldolase

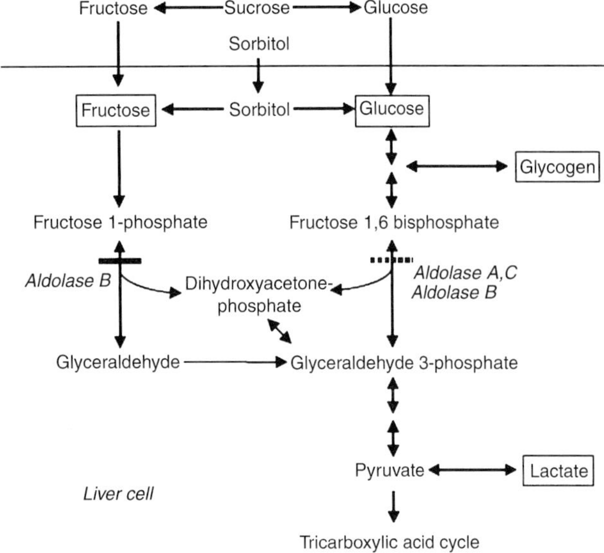

Figure 5 Hepatic fructose metabolism in hereditary fructose intolerance (aldolase B deficiency). *Source*: From Ref. 34.

B deficiency itself (as well as the resultant toxic levels of fructose-1-phosphate) causes hypoglycemia through inhibition of both glycogenolysis and gluconeogenesis (11,34). Affected persons will have a reducing substance present in their urine after an attack—the diagnosis may be confirmed via intravenous fructose tolerance testing. This testing will result in a reduction in plasma phosphate levels, followed by hypoglycemia and then elevations in magnesium and uric acid. Oral fructose loading should be avoided as it may precipitate severe symptoms. The gold standard for diagnosis is the demonstration of decreased enzyme activity in a liver biopsy specimen. Treatment involves the elimination of all dietary sources of fructose, sucrose, and sorbitol—such intervention ameliorating organ dysfunction and permitting normal growth (11). Theoretically, modest degrees of aldolase B and C activity in the liver may permit normal glycogenolysis/gluconeogenesis once dietary fructose is eliminated (34).

The incidence of hereditary fructose intolerance is estimated to be 1/23,000 based upon studies performed in the United Kingdom. Three mutations for the aldolase B gene (*ALDO2*) on chromosome 9q22.3 have been identified (A149P, A174D, N334K), and are responsible for 80% to 85% of cases in the United States and Europe (34). Carriers can be identified by DNA analysis, and prenatal diagnosis is made via cells obtained through amniocentesis/chorionic villus sampling (12). As the use of sorbitol-containing artificial sweeteners becomes more widespread amongst populations, the clinical disease associated with aldolase B deficiency may become more common.

Deficiency of Fructose 1,6-Diphosphatase (MIM #229700)

Deficiency of fructose 1,6-diphosphatase is a rare disorder of gluconeogenesis, which essentially results in the absence of glycogen stores. In contrast to hereditary fructose intolerance, glycogenolysis is unaffected so that hypoglycemia occurs only in the fasting state. Affected individuals are asymptomatic as long as a regular supply of dietary carbohydrate is ingested. However, in the absence of food intake, characteristic episodes of hypoglycemia, lactic and ketoacidosis, hyperventilation, and seizures may occur. Inappropriately managed episodes may result in coma and/or death. As would be expected, glucagon administration is ineffective in this circumstance. Episodes must be treated with an administration of intravenous glucose and management of the metabolic acidosis. Long-term management should include the frequent intake of high carbohydrate meals and snacks, and avoidance of fasting. Provision of a constant source of dietary carbohydrate will permit normal growth and development. Surprisingly, symptoms often become much less severe or may resolve completely in adulthood. A demonstration of the enzyme deficiency in a liver or intestinal biopsy specimen provides definitive diagnosis of this condition. The responsible gene (*FBP1*) is located on chromosome 9q22: identification of carriers and prenatal diagnosis of disease may be performed via DNA analysis (11).

GLUCOSE METABOLISM

In the normal state, blood glucose levels are generally tightly regulated through a balance of glucose utilization in peripheral tissues (such as muscle and adipose stores), hepatic glucose output, and the effects of insulin and other counter-regulatory hormones such as glucagon. Preproinsulin, the precursor to insulin, is produced in the beta cells of the pancreatic islets and is cleaved in several steps to form insulin. The hormone is stored in secretory granules, and is secreted in response to an increase in glucose levels. Glucose influx will result in increased glucose transport into beta cells, mediated by the glucose transport protein GLUT2. Subsequent glycolysis, generation of ATP, and inhibition of the ATP-sensitive potassium channels of the beta cell membrane results in an influx of cellular calcium and increased insulin secretion from the storage granules (Fig. 6). In addition to this immediate response, prolonged glucose-dependent stimulation will also promote active synthesis of insulin within the cell. Insulin is an anabolic hormone which acts primarily to increase glucose uptake into peripheral tissues, although it is also involved in aspects of cellular growth, differentiation, and synthetic function. The effects of insulin action depend upon the site of action. For example, insulin mediates glucose uptake, increases protein synthesis, and promotes the formation of glycogen stores within muscle. Alternatively, it will facilitate lipid synthesis and inhibit lipolysis in adipose tissue (Fig. 7). Insulin is a hormone essential to life: conditions which result in insulin deficiency or impaired insulin action generally result in a significant metabolic disturbance (1).

Diabetes Mellitus

The term diabetes mellitus refers to the variety of conditions associated with disordered glucose metabolism and hyperglycemia. This group of conditions includes disease states caused by insulin deficiency, an alteration in insulin activity, or both. Traditionally, diabetes has been broadly classified as either type 1 or type 2 primarily based upon the presence or absence of endogenous insulin production. However, it is increasingly obvious that diabetes is a significantly heterogenous condition, and that many individuals are not easily classified into one of these two groups. Because there are apparent genetic and environmental factors predisposing to the development of both types of disease, the ability to predict the likelihood of disease based upon genetic testing remains limited at present. Aside from the genetic and environmental effects, a large number of pancreatic conditions, drugs, infectious agents, and endocrine/metabolic conditions have been associated with the development of diabetes (1). These are outlined extensively in Table 1. For the purposes of this text, discussion will primarily focus upon the commonly recognized features of diabetes types 1 and 2. Although these conditions may vary considerably with respect to their pathophysiology, presentation, and management options, it is important to recognize that the complications of both types are the same and may be severe.

At present, diabetes is estimated to affect 170 million individuals worldwide, with the number of affected individuals estimated to rise to 300 million by the year 2025. Major increases in cases of diabetes are expected to occur in developing areas of Asia, South America, and Africa—the majority of these cases will be diabetes type 2 (10,29). Among developed countries, the prevalence of diabetes is estimated to currently be 6% to 7%; however, certain ethnic groups such as African Americans, Native Americans, and Hispanics are disproportionately affected (1). As the prevalence of diabetes has arguably increased by 600% between the years 1958–1993, it is reasoned that environmental factors—rather than genetic changes—have prompted this increase (26). Excess caloric consumption and decreased physical activity have contributed significantly to the increase in numbers of overweight and diabetic individuals.

Diabetes Mellitus Type 1

Diabetes type 1 is characterized by severe insulin deficiency secondary to an autoimmune destruction of the pancreatic beta cells. Although this condition is usually diagnosed in childhood, it is known to occur at any age. Diabetes type 1 comprises only 10% of the population in the United States with diabetes; however, the incidence of this disease has increased since

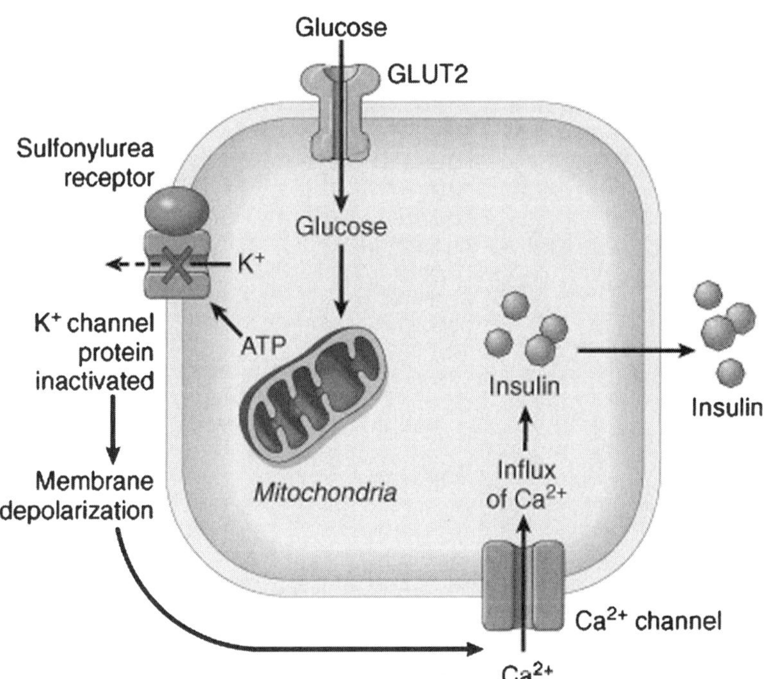

Figure 6 Insulin synthesis and secretion. Intracellular transport of glucose is mediated by GLUT2, an insulin-independent glucose transporter in beta cells. Glucose undergoes oxidated metabolism in the beta cell to yield ATP. ATP inhibits an inward rectifying potassium channel receptor on the beta cell surface; the receptor itself is a dimeric complex of the sulfonylurea receptor and a K+ channel protein. Inhibition of this receptor leads to membrane depolarization, influx of Ca^{2+} ions, and release of stored insulin from beta cells. *Source*: From Ref. 1.

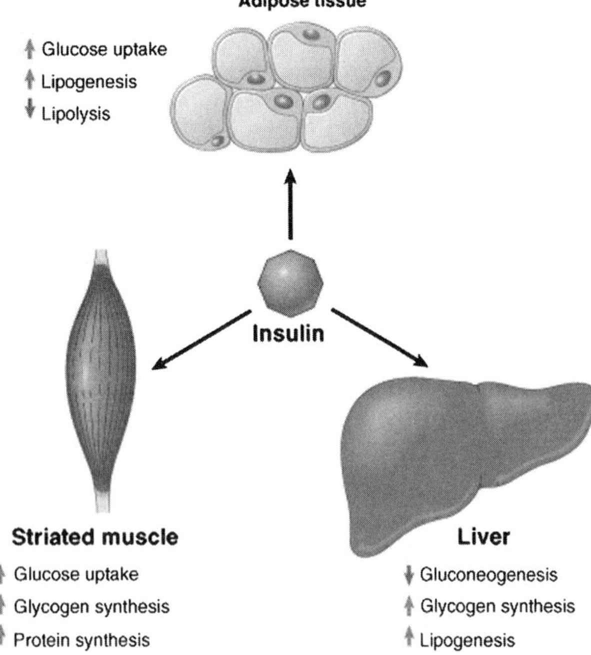

Figure 7 Metabolic actions of insulin in striated muscle, adipose tissue, and liver. *Source*: From Ref. 1.

the 1960s. In this condition, an immune-mediated destruction of the islet cells, with an associated lymphocytic tissue infiltration and cellular necrosis, is mediated by T lymphocytes reacting to beta cell autoantigens. Antibodies to islet cell autoantigens are present in 70% to 80% of individuals with this condition. Clinical disease does not occur until at least 90% of the beta cells have been destroyed, at which point most individuals will develop the abrupt onset of symptoms. These most commonly include polydipsia, polyuria, polyphagia, weight loss, and perhaps diabetic ketoacidosis. Insulin deficiency will alter the metabolism of glucose, fat, and protein: these effects include hyperglycemia through decreased uptake of glucose into peripheral tissues, increased gluconeogenesis, decreased synthesis of glycogen, and increases in proteolysis/lipolysis. Hyperglycemia and glycosuria promote a severe osmotic diuresis, with significant renal losses of water and electrolytes. Diabetic ketoacidosis is a severe complication in which increased breakdown of adipose stores results in elevated levels of free fatty acids, which are metabolized in the liver to the ketone bodies acetoacetate and beta hydroxybutarate. Accumulation of these substances results in ketonemia, ketonuria, and a potentially life-threatening metabolic acidosis (Fig. 8).

A genetic predisposition to diabetes type 1 is clear, with a sibling's risk of developing disease being 100 times that of the general population (24). The

Table 1 Etiologic Classification of Diabetes Mellitus

I. Diabetes type 1 (β-cell destruction, usually leading to absolute insulin deficiency)
  A. Immune mediated
  B. Idiopathic
II. Diabetes type 2 (may range from predominantly insulin resistance with relative insulin deficiency to a predominantly secretory defect with insulin resistance)
III. Other specific types
  A. Genetic defects of β-cell function
    1. Chromosome 2, neuroD1 (MODY6)
    2. Chromosome 7, glucokinase (MODY2)
    3. Chromosome 12, HNF-1 (MODY3)
    4. Chromosome 13, insulin promoter factor-1 (IPF1; MODY4)
    5. Chromosome 17, HNF-1β (MODY5)
    6. Chromosome 20, HNF4 (MODY1)
    7. Mitochondrial DNA
    8. Others
  B. Genetic defects in insulin action
    1. Type A insulin resistance
    2. Leprechaunism
    3. Lipoatrophic diabetes
    4. Rabson–Mendenhall syndrome
    5. Others
  C. Diseases of the exocrine pancreas
    1. Cystic fibrosis
    2. Fibrocalculous pancreatopathy
    3. Hemochromatosis
    4. Neoplasia
    5. Pancreatitis
    6. Trauma/pancreatectomy
    7. Others
  D. Endocrinopathies
    1. Acromegaly
    2. Aldosteronoma
    3. Cushing syndrome
    4. Glucagonoma
    5. Hyperthyroidism
    6. Pheochromocytoma
    7. Somatostatinoma
    8. Others
  E. Drug- or chemical-induced
    1. β-adrenergic agonists
    2. Diazoxide
    3. Dilantin
    4. Glucocorticoids
    5. Alpha-interferon
    6. Nicotinic acid
    7. Pentamidine
    8. Thiazides
    9. Thyroid hormone
    10. Vacor
    11. Others
  F. Infections
    1. Congenital rubella
    2. Cytomegalovirus
    3. Others
  G. Uncommon forms of immune-mediated diabetes
    1. Anti-insulin receptor antibodies
    2. "Stiff-man" syndrome
    3. Others

(*Continued*)

Table 1 Etiologic Classification of Diabetes Mellitus (*Continued*)

III. Other specific types
  H. Other genetic syndromes sometimes associated with diabetes mellitus
    1. Down syndrome
    2. Friedreich ataxia
    3. Huntington disease
    4. Klinefelter syndrome
    5. Laurence–Moon–Biedl syndrome
    6. Myotonic dystrophy
    7. Porphyria
    8. Prader–Willi syndrome
    9. Turner syndrome
    10. Wolfram syndrome
    11. Others
IV. Gestational diabetes mellitus (GDM)

Source: Modified from Ref. 2.

human leukocyte antigen (HLA) locus contributes the most significant genetic risk for diabetes type 1, with the majority of affected individuals having HLA-DR3, HLA-DR4, or both. Susceptibility to or protection from disease is attributed to linked DQ alleles. However, the predictive ability of this testing is poor, as most persons with "susceptible" alleles will not develop clinical disease (1). Genome-wide scans have identified two additional susceptibility loci outside of the HLA locus; however, these appear to contribute insignificantly to risk (3). Environmental factors—in particular viruses, such as the group B coxsackie viruses; cytomegalovirus, rubella, mononucleosis, measles, and mumps viruses—may trigger the autoimmune response which causes diabetes type 1. This type of diabetes is associated with an increased risk of other autoimmune diseases, particularly auto-immune thyroid disease and celiac disease (15). A variant of diabetes type 1 which is not immune-mediated has been described among African Americans and Asians; interestingly, these individuals may not consistently require insulin therapy (2).

As would be expected, individuals with diabetes type 1 are dependent upon exogenous insulin therapy. Although this condition is largely auto-immune in origin, trials of immunosuppressive drugs including cyclosporine, prednisone, azathioprine, and methotrexate have been ineffective in the treatment of diabetes (15). As is also seen in diabetes type 2, tight glycemic control in diabetes type 1 has been associated with a reduction in the microvascular complications of retinopathy, nephropathy, and neuropathy (13). However, strict glycemic management is generally associated with an increased incidence of hypoglycemic events. Intensive insulin management via insulin pump therapy or the administration of multiple daily injections has rapidly become the standard of care in management. Fortunately, the human insulin analogues used in today's therapy have a more physiologic action profile than do older insulins. This often permits acceptable glycemic control without excessive hypoglycemia. Pramlintide acetate, a synthetic analog of human amylin, has recently been approved as an adjunct to insulin therapy in diabetes types 1 and 2. Administration of this substance results in improved postprandial glycemia, and may permit reduction in mealtime insulin doses. Physiologic cure of diabetes, or a significant reduction in insulin requirements, may be achieved via transplantation of pancreatic islet cells or following transplantation of the organ itself. However, the disease may recur due to either rejection of the transplanted tissue, or less likely due to recurrence of the primary autoimmune process (15).

Type 2 Diabetes Mellitus

Diabetes type 2 is a complex metabolic condition presently estimated to affect 5% to 7% of the U.S. population. The pathophysiology is less clear than in diabetes type 1; however, the disease is generally characterized by a resistance to insulin action as well as a relative insulin deficiency. Conditions including overweight/obesity, inactivity, and aging all contribute significantly to the risk of diabetes type 2, but genetic factors are also important. For example, concordance among identical twins is 50% to 90%, and 20% to 40% among first degree relatives (1). This condition is most prevalent in overweight or obese individuals over 40 yrs of age; however, an increasing number of children and adolescents are also affected by diabetes type 2. In fact, diabetes type 2 may now be more common in this age group than is diabetes type 1.

An increase in insulin resistance is thought to occur most likely with aging, weight gain, and decreased physical activity. Insulin resistance is manifest by a decrease in peripheral glucose uptake and utilization, as well as an ineffective suppression of hepatic glucose production. The pancreas is able to compensate for the insulin resistance for some time by producing a compensatory hyperinsulinism. Eventually, however, such compensation proves inadequate, resulting in hyperglycemia. Some studies suggest that defects in insulin secretion may also play a significant role, particularly among certain ethnic groups (29). Affected individuals often have central—or visceral—obesity, a condition associated with abnormal insulin signaling, insulin resistance, and alterations in levels of adipokines such as resistin, adiponectin, and leptin. This metabolic disarray is likely exacerbated by concomitant elevations in circulating free fatty acids, glycerol, and intracellular triglycerides (Fig. 9). Diabetes type 2 in particular is associated with an unfavorable metabolic profile including hypertension; a prothrombotic tendency with elevation in plasminogen activator inhibitor 1

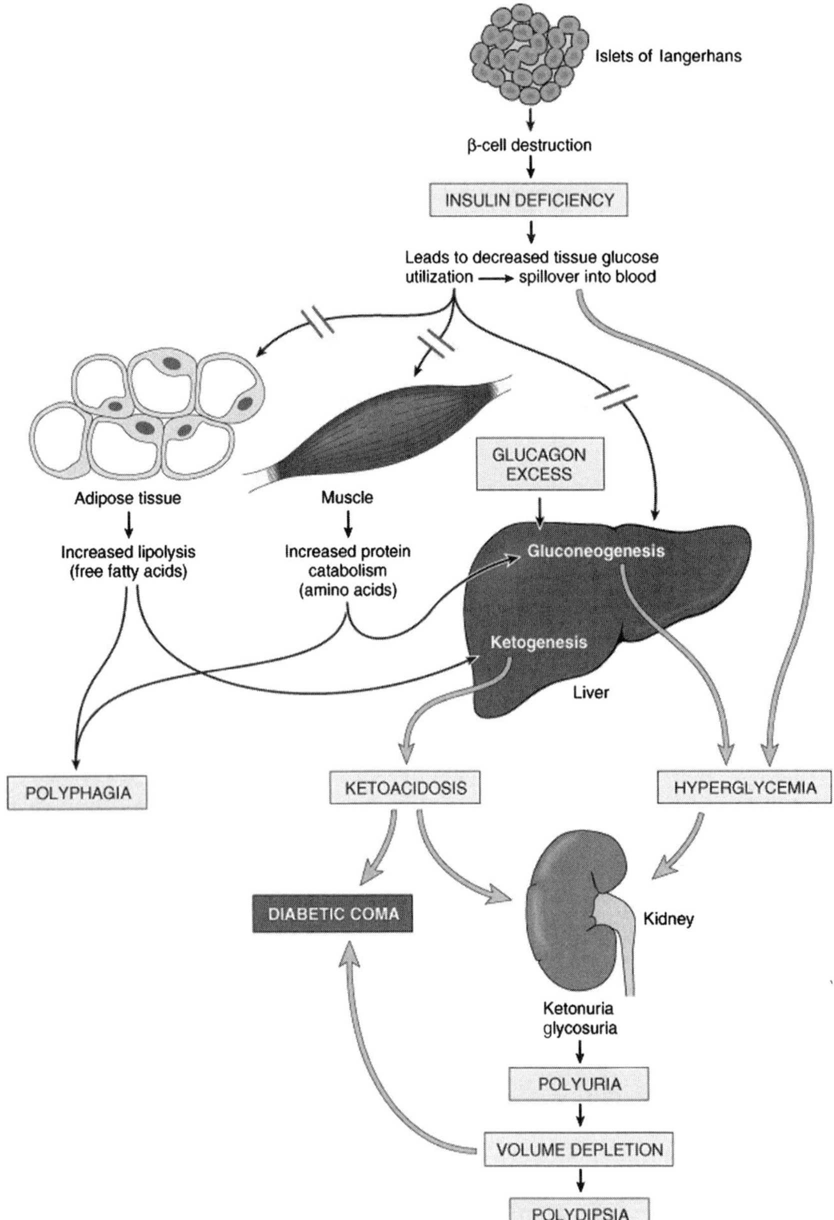

Figure 8 Sequence of metabolic derangements leading to diabetic coma in diabetes type 1 mellitus. An absolute insulin deficiency leads to a catabolic state, eventuating in ketoacidosis and severe volume depletion. These cause sufficient central nervous system compromise to lead to coma and eventual death if left untreated. *Source*: From Ref. 1.

and platelet dysfunction; and a dyslipidemia characterized by low levels of high density lipoprotein cholesterol, elevated triglycerides, and an increase in small, dense, atherogenic low density lipoprotein cholesterol particles (1).

In general, post-prandial blood sugars tend to become abnormal some time before an individual experiences fasting hyperglycemia. This makes screening via fasting blood glucose testing somewhat problematic, and may result in significant delays in diagnosis—in fact, many individuals may have established complications of diabetes at the time of diagnosis. The American Diabetes Association suggests that screening for diabetes type 2 (via fasting blood sugar or oral glucose tolerance testing) be performed every three years starting at age 45 years. However, glucose tolerance testing should be performed earlier for those at increased risk, including those persons with risk factors such as overweight/obesity, dyslipidemia, hypertension, a family history of diabetes, history of gestational diabetes, known previous hyperglycemia, polycystic ovary syndrome, or belonging to high risk ethnic groups (2). The most current criteria for the diagnosis of diabetes include at least two fasting blood sugars of 126 mg/dL or above, a random blood sugar of 200 mg/dL or higher with symptoms of diabetes, or a blood sugar of 200 mg/dL or higher at the two-hour point of oral glucose tolerance testing. A lesser but still significant condition termed impaired glucose tolerance is defined as

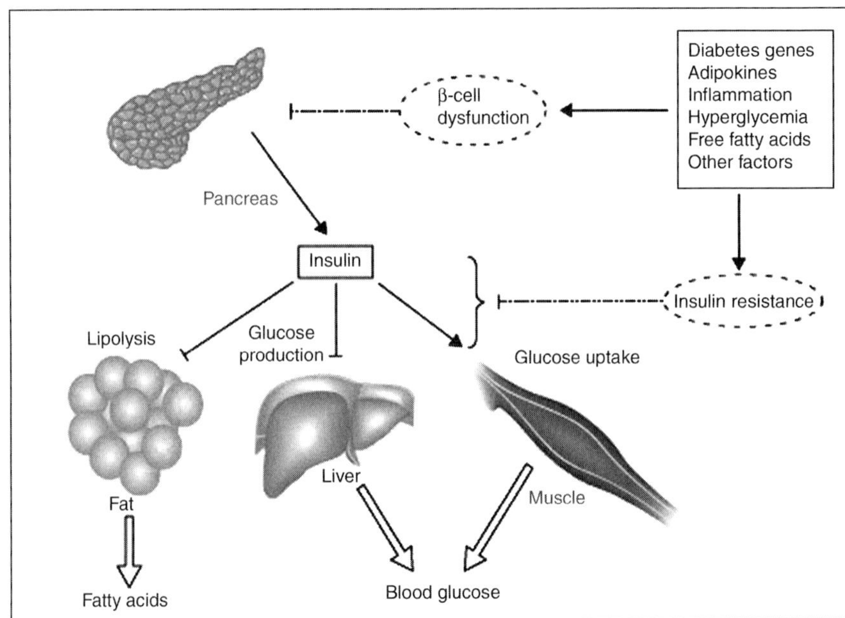

Figure 9 Pathophysiology of hyperglycemia and increased circulating fatty acids in diabetes type 2. Decreased insulin secretion and insulin resistance in target tissues leads to increases in circulating fatty acids and hyperglycemia, which may in turn further impair insulin production and sensitivity. *Source*: From Ref. 29.

fasting blood sugar between 100 and 125 mg/dL and/or a two-hour post-load blood glucose level of 140 to 199 mg/dL (2).

As previously noted, both genetic and environmental factors contribute to the development of diabetes type 2. Aggregation of disease among certain families, and ethnic groups such as the Pima Indians of Arizona, suggests a genetic predisposition. It is noteworthy that diabetes type 2 of relatively young onset seems more strongly heritable than that of later onset (4). Interactions between multiple genes, and between genes and the environment, likely contribute to the complex pattern of heritability (26). A variety of possible genetic defects have been postulated, including possible defects in genes involved in adipocyte differentiation, the insulin and sulfonylurea receptors, and in insulin-like growth factor (29). Several monogenic causes of diabetes have been well characterized, the mutations for which result in defects in beta cell function or the insulin receptor. These conditions, however, account for only a small percentage of individuals with diabetes. For example, the well-described maturity onset diabetes of the young (MODY) comprises only 5% of the diabetic population (1). The monogenic forms of diabetes are generally not characterized as either type 1 or type 2.

The effect of environmental factors, however, is undeniable. It is widely believed that we have inherited a genome most appropriate to a high-fiber diet and sustained levels of physical activity (26). Our increasingly inactive lifestyles, and high-calorie, highly processed foods may mesh poorly with our genetic makeup. As an example, Pima peoples living in Mexico and adhering to traditional lifestyles have much lower rates of disease than do their U.S. counterparts. An increase in diabetes risk is also seen among immigrants to the United States from Asian countries, in whom the risk gradually increases to that of their adopted country (26). Around the globe, industrialization and adaptation of Western lifestyles has generally been followed by increased levels of diabetes type 2.

The United Kingdom Prospective Diabetes Study (UKPDS) trial has clearly demonstrated a reduction in micro-vascular complications associated with tight glycemic control of diabetes type 2 (31). A reduction in cardiovascular events was also seen, but did not reach statistical significance: further studies to determine the relationship between glycemic lowering and cardio-vascular disease are ongoing. As individuals with diabetes type 2 are generally insulin deficient in a relative rather than absolute sense, insulin therapy is not always necessary. However, most persons with diabetes type 2 will eventually require insulin therapy to manage glycemia adequately. Given some degree of intrinsic insulin production, diabetic ketoacidosis is not commonly seen in diabetes type 2. It may occur, however, in conditions that cause a significant increase in insulin requirements—for example, during serious infections, or following surgery or myocardial infarction (1). A variety of classes of oral diabetes medications are currently available, which work through mechanisms including an increase in insulin production, improved insulin sensitivity, or slowed absorption of dietary carbohydrates. Newer injectable agents are available which mimic the effects of naturally occurring pancreatic or small intestinal hormones. In addition, all currently available insulins may be used in the management of diabetes type 2. A complete review of these drugs and their uses is beyond the scope of this text.

Given the complexity of the condition that is diabetes type 2, potentially curative interventions are presently limited. Meaningful weight loss achieved through lifestyle, medical, or surgical intervention has been associated with significant improvements in glycemia. Perhaps most importantly, the Diabetes Prevention Program trial found that lifestyle modification significantly reduced the development of diabetes in an at-risk group of individuals. A reduction in risk was also found with the use of the insulin-sensitizing agent metformin, but to a lesser degree than was seen with dietary and exercise intervention (20). Additionally, troglitazone therapy significantly reduced the likelihood of diabetes in at-risk women who had been previously diagnosed with gestational diabetes (9). Ongoing studies will assess the ability of other agents, such as angiotensin converting enzyme inhibitors and angiotensin receptor blocking agents, to reduce diabetes risk. It is clear, however, that regular physical activity and maintenance of a normal body weight are probably the most effective prevention strategies.

Complications of Diabetes Mellitus

Although the manifestations of diabetes may vary considerably among affected individuals, the potential complications of longstanding diabetes are similar in both diabetes types 1 and 2. Years of hyperglycemia result in dysfunction of and damage to large and small arteries. Endothelial cells are likely highly vulnerable to glucose-mediated cell damage, as these cells are unable to limit glucose uptake in the setting of hyperglycemia (8). Damage to the vasculature is broadly classified as either macrovascular disease (characterized by accelerated atherosclerosis and an increased risk of myocardial infarction, stroke, and peripheral vascular disease), or microvascular disease (with associated damage to the retina, kidneys, and nerves). The development of these complications is complex, but appears to involve multiple mechanisms including the formation of advanced glycation end products, pro-coagulant effects mediated by increased protein kinase C activity, and alterations in the polyol pathway that ultimately increase cellular susceptibility to oxidative stress (1). Cardiovascular risk reduction via smoking cessation, anti-platelet therapy, blood pressure control, and management of dyslipidemia is essential. The role of glycemic control in reducing cardiovascular risk is unclear, but is under further investigation.

The effects of diabetes on the eye may be extensive, as most ocular structures may be affected. Although the visual loss associated with diabetes is largely preventable, it is still the leading cause of blindness among working-age adults in the United States (8). Diabetic retinopathy is a progressive condition characterized by proliferation of the retinal vessels (perhaps secondary to capillary occlusion and ischemia), and increased vasopermeability (5). Visual loss occurs subsequent to macular involvement, vitreal hemorrhage, and/or retinal detachment. Cataract formation is a significant late complication of diabetes. Increased utilization of the polyol metabolic pathway results in osmotic lens changes due to sorbitol accumulation. The osmotic effect in the lens is not as great as that seen in galactosemia: sorbitol is further metabolized to fructose, which leaks passively from the lens (21). Increased oxidative stress, as well as glycation of proteins within the crystalline lens, are also contributing mechanisms. Other ocular manifestations of diabetes include mononeuropathies involving extraocular muscle function, a predisposition to the development of open-angle glaucoma, an increased risk of corneal ulceration, and the potentially life-threatening orbital fungal infection mucomycosis (phycomycosis) (see Chapter 11) (8). Good glycemic and blood pressure control, as well as regular ophthalmologic evaluation, are essential to the preservation of vision. Other management strategies, including the use of glycation inhibitors, aldose reductase inhibitors, non-steroidal anti-inflammatory drugs (NSAIDS), or anti-oxidants hold some promise but are not routinely recommended at present (21). Ophthalmologic screening should begin at the time of diagnosis of diabetes type 2, or five years after the onset of diabetes type 1. Very close follow up during pregnancy is recommended, as retinopathy may progress more rapidly during gestation (2).

Diabetic nephropathy is the primary cause of kidney failure among many developed countries in North America, Europe, and Asia (8). Extensive vascular and other changes occur within the kidney, including damage to the glomeruli, basement membrane, collecting tubules, and interstitium. Early and frequent screening for the presence of albuminuria is essential in monitoring the progression of disease. As in diabetic retinopathy, control of glycemia and hypertension are of proven benefit in both prevention and management of this complication. Individuals who have evidence of nephropathy or are hypertensive should be started preferentially on either an inhibitor of angiotensin converting enzyme or an angiotensin receptor blocking agent (2).

Documentation of nephropathy should prompt an evaluation for cardiovascular disease and retinopathy, as these complications are closely linked. Certain ethnic groups, such as African Americans and Latinos, have disproportionately high rates of nephropathy—it is unclear, however, whether this represents a genetic susceptibility or is a consequence of inadequate access to health care (8).

Most cases of neuropathy in the developed world are secondary to diabetes. In fact, this complication is responsible for the majority of diabetes-related hospitalizations, as well as the majority of non-traumatic amputations. A distal symmetric sensorimotor polyneuropathy is the most common presentation (7). Small fiber neuropathy may cause a painful syndrome of hypersensitivity and hyperalgesia, which may progress to complete sensory loss. Peripheral neuropathy—particularly in association with peripheral vascular disease—predisposes to foot injury, foot deformity, ulceration, and limb loss. Nerve conduction studies are the most sensitive diagnostic test (5); however, a thorough physical examination will also often reveal abnormalities in deep tendon reflexes, proprioception, nociception, temperature sensation, or vibratory sensation. The development of autonomic nerve dysfunction, present in an estimated 50% of individuals with diabetes, may result in a significant deterioration in the quality of life. This complication is commonly manifested as nausea or emesis due to gastroparesis, constipation due to altered colonic motility, erectile dysfunction, or orthostatic hypotension with resting tachycardia. Altered cardiac sympathetic innervation is associated with a significantly increased risk of sudden death. This condition should be suspected in persons with unexplained dyspnea, cough, fatigue, syncope, tachycardia, or bradycardia. A prolonged QT interval—a risk factor for arrhythmia—is characteristic of this condition. Heart rate variability measurement may be used as a means of formal diagnosis (8).

REFERENCES

1. Abbas AK, Frausto N, Kumar V. The endocrine pancreas. In: Robbins and Cotran Pathologic Basis of Disease. 7th ed. Philadelphia: Suangers, 2005:1189–205.
2. American Diabetes Association. Clinical practice recommendations 2005. Diabetes Care 2005; 28(Suppl. 1):S1–79.
3. Anjos S, Polychronakos C. Mechanisms of genetic susceptibility to type I diabetes: beyond HLA. Mol Genet Metab 2004; 81:187–95.
4. Barroso I. Genetics of type 2 diabetes. Diabet Med 2005; 22: 517–35.
5. Bloomgarden ZT. Diabetic retinopathy and neuropathy. Diabetes Care 2005; 28(4):963–70.
6. Bosch AM, Bakker HD, Van Gennip AH, et al. Clinical features of galactokinase deficiency: a review of the literature. J Inherit Metab Dis 2002; 25:629–34.
7. Boulton AJ, Vinik AI, Arezzo JC, et al. Diabetic neuropathies. Diabetes Care 2005; 28(4):956–62.
8. Brownlee M, Aiello LP, Friedman E, et al. Complications of diabetes mellitus. In: Larsen PR, ed. Williams Textbook of Endocrinology. 10th ed. Philadelphia: Saunders, 2003: 1509–65.
9. Buchanan TA, Xiang AH, Peters RK, et al. Preservation of pancreatic beta-cell function and prevention of type 2 diabetes by pharmacological treatment of insulin resistance in high-risk hispanic women. Diabetes 2002; 51: 2796–803.
10. Buse JB, Polonsky KS, Burant CF. Type 2 diabetes mellitus. In: Larsen PR, ed. Williams Textbook of Endocrinology. 10th ed. Philadelphia: Saunders, 2003:1427–68.
11. Chen Y. Glycogen storage diseases and other inherited disorders of carbohydrate metabolism. In: Braunwald E, Hauser SL, Fauci AS, Longo DL, Kasper DL, Jameson JL, eds. Harrison's Principles of Internal Medicine. 15th ed. New York: McGraw-Hill, 2001:2281–9.
12. Chen Y. Defects in fructose metabolism. In: Behrman RE, Kliegman RM, Jenson HB, eds. Nelson Textbook of Pediatrics. 17th ed. Philadelphia: Saunders, 2004:476–7.
13. The Diabetes Control and Complications Trial Research Group. The effect of intensive treatment of diabetes on the development and progression of long-term complications in insulin-dependent diabetes mellitus. N Engl J Med 1993; 329:977–86.
14. Dobrowolski SF, Banas RA, Suzow JG, et al. Analysis of common mutations in the galactose-1-phosphate uridyl transferase gene. J Mol Diagn 2003; 5(1):42–7.
15. Eisenbarth GS, Polonsky KS, Buse JB. Type 1 diabetes mellitus. In: Larsen PR, ed. Williams Textbook of Endocrinology. 10th ed. Philadelphia: Saunders, 2003: 1485–504.
16. Holden HM, Rayment I, Thoden JB. Structure and function of enzymes of the leloir pathway for galactose metabolism. J Biol Chem 2003; 278(45):43885–8.
17. Holden HM, Thoden JB, Timson DJ, et al. Galactokinase: structure, function and role in type II galactosemia. Cell Mol Life Sci 2004; 61:2471–84.
18. Kador PF, Kinoshita JH. Diabetic and galactosemic cataracts. Ciba Found Symp 1984; 106:110–31.
19. Karas N, Gobec L, Pfeifer B, et al. Mutations in galactose-1-phosphate uridyltransferase gene in patients with idiopathic presenile cataract. J Inherit Metab Dis 2003; 26:699–704.
20. Knowler WC, Barrett-Connor E, Fowler SE, et al. Reduction in the incidence of type 2 diabetes with lifestyle intervention or metformin. N Engl J Med 2002; 346:393–403.
21. Kyselova Z, Stefek M, Bauer V. Pharmacological prevention of diabetic cataract. J Diabetes Complications 2004; 18: 129–40.
22. Liu G, Hale GE, Hughes CL. Galactose metabolism and ovarian toxicity. Reprod Toxicol 2000; 14:377–284.
23. Novelli G, Reichardt JKV. Molecular basis of disorders of human galactose metabolism: past, present, and future. Mol Genet Metab 2000; 71:62–5.
24. Permutt MA, Wasson J, Cox N. Genetic epidemiology of diabetes. J Clin Invest 2005; 115(6):1431–9.
25. Petry KG, Reichardt JKV. The fundamental importance of human galactose metabolism: lessons from genetics and biochemistry. TIG 1998; 14(3):98–102.
26. Roberts CK, Barnard RJ. Effects of exercise and diet on chronic disease. J Appl Phys 2005; 98:3–30.
27. Schweitzer S, Shin Y, Jakobs C, et al. Long-term outcome in 134 patients with galactosemia. Eur J Pediatr 1993; 152(1): 36–43.
28. Shin YS, Korenke GC, Huppke P, et al. UDPgalactose epimerase in lens and fibroblasts: activity expression in patients with cataracts and mental retardation. J Inherit Metab Dis 2000; 23:383–6.
29. Stumvoll M, Goldstein BJ, Van Haeften TW. Type 2 diabetes: principles of pathogenesis and therapy. Lancet 2005; 365:1333–46.

30. Tyfield L, Reichardt J, Fridovich-Keil J, et al. Classical galactosemia and mutations at the galactose-1-phosphate uridyl transferase (GALT) gene. Hum Mutat 1999; 13:417–30.
31. UK Prospective Diabetes Study (UKPDS) Group. Intensive blood-glucose control with sulphonylureas or insulin compared with conventional treatment and risk of complications in patients with type 2 diabetes (UKPDS 33). Lancet 1998; 352:837–53.
32. Waggoner DD, Buist NR, Donnell GN. Long-term prognosis in galactosemia: results of a survey of 350 cases. J Inherit Metab Dis 1990; 13:802–18.
33. Walter JG, Collins JE, Leonard JV. Recommendations for the management of galactosaemia. Arch Dis Child 1999; 80:93–6.
34. Wong D. Hereditary fructose intolerance. Mol Genet Metab 2005; 85:165–7.

46

Disorders of Lipid and Lipoprotein Metabolism

John R. Guyton
Department of Medicine, Duke University, Durham, North Carolina, U.S.A.

INTRODUCTION

This chapter briefly describes systemic lipoprotein metabolism and specific disorders of lipid metabolism. Lipid-related abnormalities of the ocular tissues are covered in some depth. Atherosclerosis, the prototypical lipid-related disease, is a disorder of large arteries and therefore affects the eye only indirectly. The ocular sequelae of atherosclerosis, embolism and ischemia, are covered elsewhere in this volume (see Chapter 67).

LIPID AND LIPOPROTEIN METABOLISM

Lipids

Most of the body's fuel needs are supplied by fatty acids, which are efficiently stored and transported as triacylglycerol, or simply, triglyceride. Lipoproteins function primarily to transport triglyceride and cholesterol in plasma. Cholesterol is a component of cell membranes and a precursor for steroid and sex hormones. The heterocyclic structure of cholesterol can be modified but not be degraded in mammalian metabolism. Because cholesterol cannot be degraded, its transport requires both "forward" movement from central organs to peripheral tissues and also "reverse" movement from sites of excess in the periphery back to the liver. Recently it has become clear that most cholesterol synthesis occurs in peripheral tissues (71). Therefore, "reverse cholesterol transport" is the dominant process.

Lipoproteins

Most lipoproteins share a common spherical structure comprising a hydrophobic, oily core of triglyceride and cholesteryl ester, and a surface monolayer of amphiphilic molecules—phospholipid, unesterified cholesterol, and one or more proteins termed apolipoproteins. Apolipoproteins characteristically have alpha helical domains in which one side of the helix exposes hydrophobic amino acids and the other side hydrophilic amino acids. These domains thus bind preferentially to a lipid-aqueous interface. Other domains in apolipoproteins contain binding sites for cellular lipoprotein receptors or lipolytic enzymes. In these binding sites apolipoproteins contain the information necessary to direct and regulate fatty acid and cholesterol delivery to appropriate locations.

Five classes of lipoproteins [high density lipoproteins (HDL), low density lipoproteins (LDL), intermediate density lipoproteins (IDL), very low density lipoproteins (VLDL), and chylomicrons] are separable by ultracentrifugation according to their buoyant density. Density is dictated by the ratio of surface components (more dense) to core components (more buoyant), and thus density is inversely related to particle radius. The smallest lipoproteins are HDL and almost all contain apolipoprotein A1 (apoA1). All lipoproteins larger than HDL contain apolipoprotein B (apoB), which is a huge monomeric protein of 4,536 amino acids, more than 20 times the size of apoA1. LDL have cholesteryl ester as their dominant core lipid. Larger lipoproteins—chylomicrons and VLDL—contain predominantly triglycerides.

The plasma lipoproteins exhibit a variety of genetic and acquired abnormalities, such that the total lipid content of plasma can vary 100-fold in humans. The effects of these abnormalities on the eye and visual function likewise vary.

ApoB is bound noncovalently to lipid in the rough endoplasmic reticulum of hepatocytes and intestinal mucosal cells. The process requires mediation by microsomal triglyceride transfer protein. Intestinal mucosal cells secrete very large, apoB-containing lipoproteins called chylomicrons, formed predominantly of fat absorbed from the diet (triglyceride). Chylomicrons circulate via lymphatics and the bloodstream to peripheral tissues, where their triglyceride is hydrolyzed by an endothelial surface enzyme, lipoprotein lipase. The free fatty acids released by hydrolysis traverse endothelial cell membranes and enter peripheral tissue cells. The remaining material in the lipoproteins forms chylomicron remnant particles, which are rapidly cleared from blood by hepatocytes (50).

VLDL are similar to chylomicrons in carrying predominantly triglyceride in association with apoB, but VLDL are smaller and are secreted by hepatocytes. The VLDL deliver fatty acids to peripheral tissues via lipoprotein lipase just as chylomicrons do. VLDL remnants are called IDL and these are rapidly metabolized by the liver (50) (Fig. 1).

Approximately half of IDL are taken up by hepatocytes via the LDL receptor and the other half undergoes further lipolytic processing by hepatic lipase to form LDL. Thus LDL are not secreted directly from the liver, but arise from VLDL in a precursor-product relationship. Plasma LDL have 3 basic fates. Half are taken up by hepatocytes via LDL receptors. Other LDL particles are internalized via LDL receptors and delivered to lysosomes in peripheral tissue cells. Still others become trapped in certain tissues such as the arterial wall. This occurs in various ways, including binding to elastin and proteoglycans (PGs) extracellular aggregation and fusion of particles, and uptake of "damaged" lipoproteins (oxidized, proteolyzed, or aggregated) via scavenger receptors on phagocytes (53,76,94).

Lipoprotein(a) is a distinct apoB-containing lipoprotein. This LDL-like particle is produced by

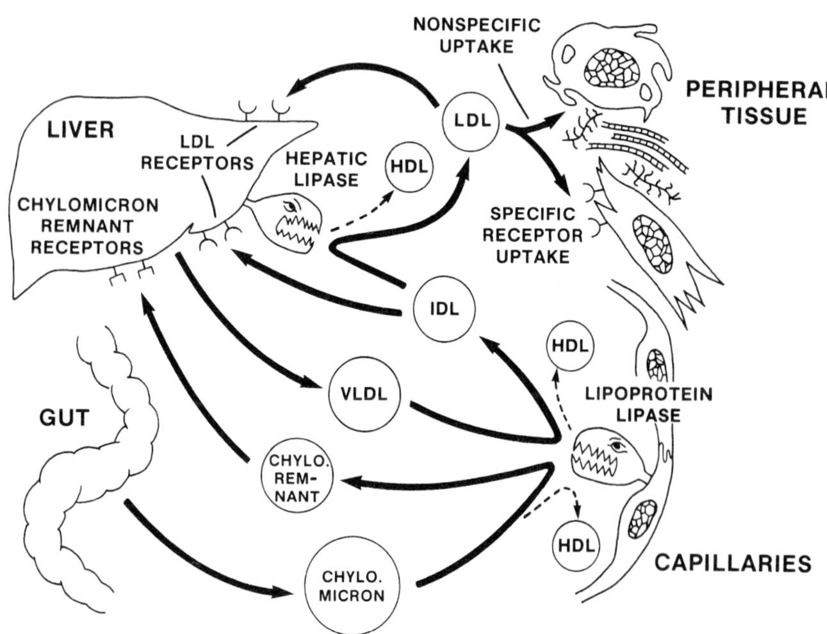

Figure 1 The major pathways of lipoprotein metabolism. *Abbreviations*: HDL, high density lipoproteins; IDL, intermediate density lipoproteins; LDL, low density lipoproteins; VLDL, very low density lipoproteins. *Source*: Guyton JR. Chapter 13. In: Loscalzo J, Creager MA, Dzau VJ, eds. Vascular Medicine: A Textbook of Vascular Biology and Diseases, 2nd ed. Boston: Little, Brown, 1996.

the extracellular formation of a disulfide bridge between apoB on LDL and a very large nonlipid-binding protein, called apolipoprotein(a) [Apo(a)]. The presence of free apo(a) indicates that it can be secreted independently of LDL (64). Apo(a) is genetically hypervariable with regard to the number of repeats of a kringle motif (named for a Danish pastry). The kringle structure is similar to that found in a highly homologous plasma protein – plasminogen. Lipoprotein(a) may contribute to atherosclerotic events not only by forming cholesterol-rich deposits in arteries, but also by competing at various plasminogen binding sites and thus inhibiting physiologic fibrinolysis (122). Lipoprotein(a) has not been implicated in ocular disease.

The Dyslipidemic Triad and the Metabolic Syndrome

A disorder associated with a high risk of atherosclerotic vascular disease is the dyslipidemic triad (the combination of high triglycerides, low HDL-C, and small dense LDL), which occurs in obesity, diabetes, and the metabolic syndrome. This atherogenic lipoprotein patterns begins with high numbers of VLDL particles. Cholesteryl ester transfer protein exchanges triglyceride from VLDL with cholesteryl ester from HDL, leading to HDL particles enriched in triglyceride (i.e., 10–15% of core lipids instead of the usual 7%). The triglyceride-enriched HDL in turn exchange with LDL, leading to similar triglyceride enrichment of LDL. The triglyceride in HDL and LDL is then subject to hydrolysis by lipolytic enzymes, particularly hepatic lipase. In this process, HDL particles become subject to more rapid removal from plasma, and thus HDL cholesterol levels drop. The LDL particles have a net loss of core lipids and therefore shrink in size, becoming smaller and more dense (86).

GENETIC DISORDERS OF LIPOPROTEINS

Disorders with a Deficiency of ApoB-Containing Lipoproteins

A genetic deficiency of apoB-containing lipoproteins may occur from an absence of a microsomal triglyceride transfer protein (abetalipoproteinemia) or from deletions or impaired transcription in the *APOB* gene (hypobetalipoproteinemia). Chylomicron retention disease is another disorder presenting with deficiency of apoB-containing lipoproteins. These disorders involved impaired expression of forms of apoB in plasma, with effects on circulating lipoproteins and their functions notably transport of dietary fat and fat-soluble vitamins, particularly vitamin E (21). Deficiency of these vitamins is likely to be the essential cause of any ophthalmological and particularly retinal features. In these disorders the normal mechanisms of lipid transport from the intestine and liver are impaired, and chylomicrons, VLDL, and LDL are variably absent from plasma or reduced (9,11). Some vitamin E is transported in HDL: in normal plasma much greater amounts are transported in LDL.

Abetaliporoteinemia

Abetalipoproteinemia (Bassen–Kornzweig syndrome, MIM #200100) is a rare autosomal recessive disorder characterized by a near absence of plasma lipoproteins containing apoB and by very low plasma concentrations of triglyceride and cholesterol. It results from mutations in the *MTP* gene encoding the 97 kDa subunit of microsomal triglyceride transfer protein, a dimeric protein that also includes protein disulfide isomerase. Loss of this protein causes a failure of apoB lipidation and an absence of apoB-containing lipoprotein secretion. The disturbance in lipid metabolism extends to HDL as well, since HDL containing apoA1 carry about half the usual amount of cholesterol. Ratios of unesterified to esterified cholesterol and of sphingomyelin to lecithin are increased in the HDL fraction. Downstream effects include malnutrition, lipid-soluble vitamin deficiencies (see Chapter 49), acanthocyte formation and hemolysis of erythryocytes, a pigmentary retinopathy (see Chapter 35) and spinocerebellar degeneration (see Chapter 70). Obligate heterozygotes for abetalipoproteinemia generally have normal lipid levels and are clinically unaffected (8,62).

This disorder usually presents during the months after birth with diarrhea and steatorrhea. A lipid-poor diet is often selected by parents and health-care providers, and the digestive signs can abate with time. A lipid-soluble vitamin deficiency ensues, however, because circulatory transport and distribution of these vitamins depend almost entirely (vitamin E, beta-carotene) or partly (vitamins A, D, and K) on apoB-containing lipoproteins. The clinical features of abetalipoproteinemia—spinocerebellar ataxia and peripheral neuropathy, myopathy with ceroid or lipofuscin deposits in the muscle fibers, retinal degeneration—are thought to result largely from vitamin deficiencies, particularly vitamin E. Lipid peroxidation may proceed unchecked in the absence of vitamin E, giving the characteristic lipofuscin deposits. Hemolytic anemia and acanthocytosis may be driven by shifts in erythrocyte membrane lipid composition (62). Vitamin K deficiency can lead to hemorrhage. Intellectual impairment, skeletal abnormalities, and cardiomyopathy with dysrhythmias may also be present. Without treatment the disorder has a poor prognosis, with increasing visual and neuromuscular defects and death in early adult life (8).

Ophthalmological manifestations begin with alterations in the night and color vision, as well as decrease in peripheral vision. On fundoscopic examination, atypical pigmentation of the retina is found, characterized by brilliant small, white spots, irregularly distributed, and usually sparing the macula. Angioid streaks have been reported in some cases. Electroretinographic evidence of damage may precede the visible changes. Although few histological studies have been performed, widespread destruction of rods and cones has been described, and invasion of the retina by retinal pigment epithelium (RPE) with lipofuscin accumulation. As part of the neuromuscular process, isolated oculomotor paresis, ptosis, and anisocoria may also occur (8).

Combined early treatment with vitamins A and E, in some cases with polyunsaturated lipids, has produced clear evidence of stabilization or improvement in symptoms relating to nerve, muscle, and vision. Prevention of retinopathy and stabilization of, or improvement in, retinal electrophysiological responses and dark adaptation have also been described. Massive oral doses of vitamin E are utilized, while vitamin A needs only to be given orally at 2 to 4 times the usual daily requirement. In some cases neurological and ophthalmological signs may appear despite early and adequate treatment with vitamins. Vitamin D does not require supplementation, because its transport properties and metabolism differ from the other lipid-soluble vitamins (8,62).

Histopathology. Histological studies in a case with ophthalmoplegia suggested that the defects in that case were not myopathic in origin (136), although ceroid inclusions in muscle fibers have been reported (75). Histological data on the retinal changes are available only for the late stages of the disease (124).

Pathogenesis. Cellular aspects of abetalipoproteinemia have been approached by studies of the composition and properties of the spiny erythrocytes (acanthocytes). The lipid composition of erythrocytes and their membranes is abnormal, with a relative increase in sphingomyelin, a reduction in phosphatidylcholine and other phospholipids, and very little linoleate (22,129). The abnormalities of shape and composition are not changed by incubation in normal plasma, and normal erythrocytes are not modified by incubation in affected serum. Acanthocytosis is likely to be a response to abnormal membrane composition; the anemia is probably a less specific consequence of malabsorption and nutritional imbalance. Activities in the plasma of the enzymes LPL, HTGL, and lecithin cholesterol acyltransferase (LCAT) are reduced to about half-normal, but this is probably secondary and unlikely to be of pathological significance because substantial activity remains. Plasma retinol binding protein is also reduced below normal, but this is also likely to be secondary, not significant, because levels tend to increase toward normal on vitamin A supplementation. An increased accumulation of lipofuscin in various tissues, including the heart, suggests that lipid peroxidation is a feature of abetalipoproteinemia. Vitamin E protects the erythrocytes of abetalipoproteinemic patients from hydrogen peroxide-induced hemolysis (31), but the decrease in red cell membrane fluidity is not affected by vitamin E and is therefore unlikely to result from fatty acid peroxidation (21).

Hypobetalipoproteinemia

Hypobetalipoproteinemia is defined as a plasma apoB level <5th percentile of the population. Familial cases of hypobetalipoproteinemia (familial hypobetalipoproteinemia type 1, MIM +107730) are usually heterozygotes with truncations within the coding sequence of the *APOB* gene (18,66), but others (hypobetalipoproteinemia type 2, MIM %605019) have been mapped to chromosome 3 (3p22–p2.11). The condition is relatively benign and the main consequence may be a reduced risk of atherosclerosis (46).

Most heterozygotes have no obvious neuromuscular problems, but posterior column and cerebellar lesions and peripheral neuropathy have been described, with clinical effects in early childhood. Some also contain a few acanthocytes, described as reverting to normal shape on exposure to normal plasma. Fundus changes in the form of a slight irregularity and clumping of the RPE may occur, but significant effects on acuity have not been reported (47,62,137). Homozygosity or compound heterozygosity can lead to a clinical syndrome similar to abetalipoproteinemia, though usually not as severe (62,107). Hypobetalipoproteinemia can also be secondary to a wide spectrum of other disorders (83), including fat malabsorption, hyperthyroidism, and impaired synthetic function of the liver.

Chylomicron Retention Disease

Autosomal recessive inherited disorders with severe fat malabsorption and failure to thrive in infancy are chylomicron retention disease (lipid transport defect of intestine) (MIM #246700), chylomicron retention disease with Marinesco–Sjögren syndrome (MIM #607692) and Anderson disease (MIM #607689). All of these disorders are caused by mutations in the *SARA2* gene (72), a member of the Sar1 GTPase gene family (52) and this leads primarily to fat malabsorption, but hypocholesterolemia and deficiencies of vitamins A and E are also found. Plasma triglyceride levels are normal, and liver-derived apoB-100 is present, but intestinally-derived apoB-48 is absent. The translation product, Sar1b, participates in the transport of chylomicron-containing coat complex II (COPII) vesicles from the endoplasmic reticulum to the Golgi apparatus. Neuromuscular abnormalities have been described in association with chylomicron retention disease (1) and some cases have had defects in color vision or other aspects of retinal function, but not retinitis pigmentosa. Chylomicron retention disease with Marinesco–Sjögren syndrome (1) not only involves the *SARA2* gene, but also the adjacent *SIL1* gene that is responsible for Marinesco–Sjögren syndrome (MIM #248800). The cardinal features of the Marinesco–Sjögren syndrome are congenital cataracts, cerebellar ataxia, and impaired mental and somatic development.

Disorders with Hypercholesterolemia

Low Density Lipoprotein Receptor Deficiency

Heterozygous LDL receptor deficiency (MIM #143890), occurring in approximately 1 in 500 persons worldwide, leads to plasma LDL cholesterol levels approximately twice normal (usually over 200 mg/dL in adult, over 140 mg/dL in children). It also leads to increased IDL levels. Patients often have an early appearance of corneal arcus lipoides and develop xanthomas in the metacarpal, Achilles or other tendons by the fourth or fifth decade of life. Coronary atherosclerosis leads to clinical events in half of untreated males by age 50 years and half of untreated females by age 60 years. The rare homozygote (one in 1,000,000) has extremely high LDL cholesterol (over 700 mg/dL) and dies from the consequences of atherosclerosis by 20 years of age if untreated. For historical reasons, LDL receptor deficiency is called familial hypercholesterolemia (48), although strong familial patterns emerge in polygenic hypercholesterolemia as well (14).

Two other monogenic disorders resemble LDL receptor deficiency clinically, but are less common and less severe. In people with familial defective apoB (MIM #144010), one allele of apoB is defective in binding to the LDL receptor (67). The *ARH* gene for a rare disorder, autosomal recessive hypercholesterolemia (MIM #603813), encodes an adaptor protein that facilitates the localization of the LDL receptor in coated pits (43). This disorder is less severe than homozygous familial hypercholesterolemia (93).

Familial Combined Hyperlipidemia

The most common genetic lipoprotein disorder in patients with early coronary heart disease is familial combined hyperlipidemia (FCH) (MIM #144250). This genetically heterogeneous disorder has been mapped to human chromosome 1 (1q21–q23) and chromosome 8 (8p22) and there is evidence for a locus on chromosome 11. The locus on chromosome 1 is associated with single nucleotide polymorphisms (SNPs) in the *USF1* gene. In most families with FCH, the essential problem is an overproduction of VLDL, which can result in high VLDL (triglyceride), high LDL (cholesterol), or both in a given patient.

Dysbetalipoproteinemia

In dysbetalipoproteinemia (also known as hyperlipoproteinemia type III) (MIM +107741), the metabolic defect is a lack of hepatic uptake of remnant lipoproteins, which accumulate to very high levels. Both plasma cholesterol and triglyceride levels can be very high and nearly equal, mirroring the composition of remnant particles. Allelic variation or mutation of apoE genotype (especially apoE2/apoE2) is an essential feature of this disorder (81).

Extreme Hypertriglyceridemia

Extreme hypertriglyceridemia with defective clearance of chylomicrons from the circulation occurs in recessive disorders related to a deficiency of lipoprotein lipase (*LPL* gene mutation, MIM #238600) or of its essential co-factor, apoC-2. ApoC-2 deficiency (hyperlipoproteinemia type IB) (MIM #207750) is caused by a mutation in the *APOC2* gene. Uncontrolled diabetes mellitus, excessive ethanol ingestion, or polygenic traits can cause a functional lipoprotein lipase deficiency with the same result. Lipemia retinalis may occur in these disorders if plasma triglyceride levels exceed 4,000 mg/dl (16).

Disorders of High Density Lipoprotein

ApoA1 is found in plasma and tissue fluids in three types of particles: spherical HDL (alpha mobility on electrophoresis), discoid particles, and lipid-poor apoA1 (pre-beta mobility). Alpha, or spherical HDL is the predominant species in plasma; the others play important, but short-lived, roles in reverse cholesterol transport. Pre-beta HDL (lipid-poor apoA1) interacts with a specific cell surface protein, the ATP-binding cassette proteinA1 (ABCA1), to remove excess cholesterol from peripheral tissue cells in a regulated manner. Elevated plasma HDL and apoA1 levels are strongly associated with protection from atherosclerosis.

Tangier Disease

A recessive deficiency of ABCA1 is responsible for Tangier disease (familial high-density lipoprotein deficiency) (MIM #205400). In this rare condition involving the *ABC1* gene, most of the patient's apoA1 never forms mature spherical HDL, leading to very low HDL cholesterol levels and high rates of apoA1 catabolism. Despite this abnormality atherogenesis is either not increased or only moderately increased in affected families (3). In plasma, HDL is present in traces only and is of abnormal composition, with levels of apoA1 and apoA2 measuring <1 and <10%, respectively, of reference levels. LDL and total cholesterol are low but with a normal proportion in the ester form, and triglyceride-rich chylomicrons and VLDL may be in moderate excess. All components of HDL are present though very low, and apoA1 and apoA2 are of normal structure. From studies in tissue culture, defects of intracellular lipid and lipoprotein trafficking may be involved (100,105). Any accelerated HDL catabolism does not seem to involve adipose tissue (41). Tissues accumulate phospholipid and cholesterol mainly in ester form consequent to defective mobilization and transport through the virtually absent HDL system. The extent to which ingestion of modified lipoprotein or local synthesis contributes to the accumulation of lipid is not known, but abnormal circulating particles are more obvious after splenectomy and become less numerous after a restriction of dietary fat (63). Uptake of such particles by phagocytosis into macrophages and impaired mobilization of tissue lipid is therefore likely: deposits in most tissues are intracellular as evidenced by a vacuolated cytoplasm ("foam cells"). In homozygotes major sites of lipid accumulation include the spleen, liver, lymphatic and reticuloendothelial systems, tonsils, and cornea. Peripheral neuropathy with various clinical manifestations is an important feature. Lipid deposits in Schwann cells and extracellularly within nerve bundles may explain occasional cardiac abnormalities, including conduction defects.

Corneal involvement with punctate panstromal extracellular deposits without an obvious clear zone at the periphery is a feature, but may not become manifest until adult life. Vision is usually not significantly affected, but impairment can arise through ectropion of the eyelid, incomplete eyelid closure, exposure keratopathy, and corneal infiltration and ulceration (41,98). Refractory strabismus (40) and raised yellow linear conjunctival deposits, presumably lipid, may also occur. Tonsillar enlargement with yellow discoloration is a striking feature, possibly accentuated by the ambient coolness of the oropharynx, which could restrict melting and mobilization of the cholesterol esters present, since the transition temperatures of these liquid crystal deposits are close to body temperature (28,113). Spaeth noted that the deposits in the peripheral cornea were more evident in the 3 o'clock position (114), although this distribution is not necessarily obvious with older patients, particularly when secondary corneal abnormalities have arisen (41). This pattern differs from the 6 and 12 o'clock pattern of early corneal arcus and is consistent with a temperature-dependent accumulation. Thus arcus forms at sites of insudation promoted by temperature (35). Tangier deposits reflect a failure of mobilization accentuated at reduced temperature. The proposed Tangier effect has been directly supported by a chemical and thermographic analysis of the corneas of a patient (41). The presence of myelin figures with accumulated phospholipid, and cholesterol with a normal proportion in ester form, confirmed that lipid was in excess as at other sites and that this excess was the basis of the corneal opacification (134). Tangier material also showed additional transition temperatures in the range 30 to 35°C compared to normal cornea (134), consistent with the idea that the lipid accumulation is influenced by the relationship between lipid transition temperatures and ambient corneal temperature, which like tonsil is below body core temperature in the affected corneal areas.

Tangier disease is relatively benign and despite disability many patients survive beyond 50 years. Accelerated coronary heart disease is a minor feature of homozygotes only, perhaps because levels of LDL are low. Heterozygotes are clinically unaffected, although abnormal storage of lipid may be detected by rectal biopsy and plasma levels of HDL are often reduced, whereas apoA1 levels are lower than normal. In contrast to LCAT deficiency (see later), the proportion of cholesterol present in plasma in ester form is almost normal.

Deficiency of LCAT

Lethicin-cholesterol acyltransferase (LCAT) is a plasma enzyme that resides primarily on HDL, but can act upon both HDL and LDL. It transfers a fatty acyl group from lecithin (phosphatidylcholine) to cholesterol. As a result, cholesterol in the surface lipid monolayer of the lipoprotein becomes cholesteryl ester and enters the hydrophobic core of the lipoprotein. This reaction allows the lipoprotein to carry cholesterol more efficiently. By removing unesterified cholesterol from the lipoprotein surface, the reaction also produces a favorable chemical potential for acquiring additional cholesterol from surrounding cells or lipid deposits. Thus LCAT participates in reverse cholesterol transport.

LCAT deficiency (Norum disease, MIM #245500) and fish eye disease, in which the corneas were likened to boiled fish in the first description (MIM #136120) result from mutations in the same gene (*LCAT*). The biochemical hallmark of genetic LCAT deficiency is a markedly reduced fraction of esterified cholesterol in blood plasma (normally 60-80% of total cholesterol). The routine lipid panel often shows very low HDL cholesterol and sometimes very high total cholesterol. Close examination of the plasma lipoproteins by chromatography and transmission electron microscopy (TEM) reveals nascent particles with disc shapes instead of spheres (due to lack of the fatty core), as well as an accumulation of liposomes and multilamellar vesicles with an overabundance of phospholipid and cholesterol, but little cholesteryl ester (103).

The cornea is susceptible to lipid deposition in LCAT deficiency (103). Corneal opacities appear in early childhood. Numerous tiny gray dots are observed in the entire corneal stroma giving a misty appearance. By TEM membranous material, sometimes multilamellar, is found in an extracellular location (17). Surprisingly, the arterial wall seems to be only mildly susceptible, and early atherosclerosis is uncommon despite the presumed impairment of reverse cholesterol transport and the low levels of HDL (77).

Complete LCAT deficiency, caused either by null mutations in the *LCAT* gene that result in an absence of the protein or by missense mutations that reduce activity, leads to a clinical syndrome of corneal opacities, anemia, proteinuria, and renal failure. A partial LCAT deficiency caused by less critical mutations in the *LCAT* gene can present with corneal opacities alone. Low HDL is a feature of this disorder, and some of the males have had early coronary artery disease (77).

Mutant Apoplipoprotein A1

A mutant apoA called apoA Milano is associated with very low HDL cholesterol levels due to rapid turnover, often with high plasma triglycerides. For reasons that are unclear it seems to protect against atherosclerosis. On the other hand, patients with a genetic absence of apoA1 develop severe and early atherosclerosis accompanied by extremely low HDL cholesterol levels. These individuals may also have corneal clouding (104,118).

Amyloidosis

Some mutations in the genes that encode apoA1 (*APOA1*), apoA2 (*APOA2*), and apoA4 (*APOA4*) cause amyloidosis (see Chapter 37).

DISORDERS WITH DEFECTIVE OXIDATION OF LONG-CHAIN FATTY ACIDS

Overview

Disorders with defective oxidation of long-chain fatty acids includes Refsum syndrome (discussed below), Zellweger syndrome (cerebrohepatorenal syndrome) (MIM #214100) (see Chapter 48), forms of adrenoleukodystrophy (MIM #300100) (see Chapter 70), and hyperpipecolic acidemia (hyperpipecolatemia) (MIM 239400). These conditions are caused mainly by impaired peroxisomal biogenesis (49,127) and are characterized by dysmorphic, neurological, hepatic, and ocular features. The biochemical abnormalities are similar, but the entities differ in the pattern and extent of organ involvement. Peroxisomal defects produce a very wide range of overlapping clinical effects, perhaps substantially because lipids enriched with long-chain acyl species accumulate in brain, nerve and elsewhere (111). Prenatal diagnosis is possible (95,97).

Refsum Disease

Refsum disease (phytanic acid α-hydroxylase deficiency, MIM #266500) is a rare autosomal recessive disorder in which activity of the mitochondrial enzyme catalyzing an early stage in the oxidation and degradation of phytanic acid either is absent or is present at less than 5% of normal activity (127). Classic Refsum disease is a mitochondrial disorder resulting from a mutation in the *PHYH* gene encoding phytanoxyl-coA hydroxylase. Infantile Refsum syndrome is caused by a mutation in the *PEX7* gene that codes peroxin-7. The clinical and biochemical background is consistent with autosomal recessive inheritance. The branched-chain phytanic acid is a normal trace component of plasma, with an apparently entirely exogenous origin related to dietary intake of phytanate and phytol precursor, derived particularly from ruminants and thus dairy products. Further metabolism of phytanate involves peroxisomal processes that are not defective in classical Refsum syndrome. Phytol may also be released from cooked green vegetables, but little absorption occurs in the human. The defect gives a progressive but fluctuating disorder with a variable clinical presentation from childhood to late adulthood (96) and a latency associated with demyelination. Most cases present by age 20 years, with a range from childhood to late adulthood. The essential features are motor and sensory peripheral neuropathy, cerebellar ataxia and an excess of protein in the cerebrospinal fluid (CSF). Characteristically, lipid accumulates in various organs, particularly in the liver, kidney, and parts of the brain (2,15,38,127). An interstitial neuropathy develops, and cardiac deposition may form the basis of myocardial fibrosis and of electrocardiographic (EKG) changes, disorders of rhythm, and occasionally sudden death (2).

Ophthalmological changes include an atypical pigmentary retinopathy with variable early fundoscopic appearances and other ocular defects. Night blindness may precede any pigmentary change, although this may not be obvious if impaired pupillary dilatation in the dark is taken into account and cone function may be unimpaired (58). Cataract, generally posterior subcapsular and bilateral, occurs in about one-third of cases (99). Diminished pupillary reactions, glaucoma and a keratopathy, nystagmus, and optic nerve degeneration may also occur. The sensory retina and RPE are laden with lipid in which phytanate can be identified (25), and lipid deposits are also found in the sclera, trabecular meshwork, and pupillary muscles (129). Xanthomata, when present, have also been shown to contain phytanate. The ocular morphological alterations during the early stages of classic Refsum disease have not been reported.

Structural effects on lipids incorporating phytanate in place of other lipid, such as the linear-chain congener palmitate, may be involved—the antimetabolite hypothesis—although tissue levels of phytanate at post-mortem examination have in some cases been surprisingly low (127). Phytanic acid bears some structural resemblance to the aminophenoxyalkanes, particularly diaminophenoxyalkane, the most potent of this group of agents associated with an experimental degenerative pigmentary retinopathy (12).

Lipid analysis of extracts of blood or tissue samples by thin-layer chromatography readily demonstrates the major excess components, and phytanate can be specifically confirmed by gas-liquid chromatography and mass spectroscopy (127). Antenatal diagnosis can be made on amniotic cells (127). Heterozygote carriers of the responsible mutant gene are asymptomatic.

MISCELLANEOUS DISORDERS

Cerebrotendinous Xanthomatosis

Cerebrotendinous xanthomatosis (MIM #213700) is an autosomal recessive disorder characterized by cataracts, cerebellar ataxia, dementia, spinal cord paresis, tendinous and tuberous xanthomas, and early atherosclerosis. It is the only metabolic disorder of lipid known to cause cataracts and other ophthalmic manifestations have been documented (optic disc pallor, premature retinal senescence (33). Cerebrotendinous xanthomatosis is caused by mutations in the *CYP27A1* gene which encodes sterol 27-hydroxylase. Initially, this enzyme was thought to facilitate reverse cholesterol transport in the central nervous system (CNS), by making the cholesterol molecule relatively more water-soluble. However, sterol 27-hydroxylase is largely absent from the brain, and the 24-hydroxylase has been shown to be the relevant enzyme in the CNS (29).

Serum cholesterol levels are usually normal, but serum levels of cholestanol are markedly increased (10). High levels of sterol 27-hydroxylase have been found in tendons, where a specific role for the enzyme is postulated (123).

Lipoid Proteinosis

Hyaline material which stains with lipophilic dyes, such as Sudan red and oil red O, as well as with histochemical methods for proteins is a feature of lipoid proteinosis (Urbach–Wiethe syndrome) (MIM 247100). Hyaline material accumulates in the skin, mucous membranes, various organs, and at other sites, with hoarseness, stiffening and thickening of the lips and tongue, and blotchy cutaneous lesions, particularly of the elbows, knees, face, and scalp. Neurological involvement, particularly psychomotor epilepsy and rage attacks, may stem from calcified intracerebral lesions (89). Although sometimes present in infancy or early childhood, this chronic disorder has a generally benign course with low direct mortality except when severe laryngeal obstruction is not controlled. The periocular tissues are characteristically involved, with numerous waxy nodules forming in the eyelid margins in more than 60% of cases, together with loss of eyelashes (39). Infiltration less commonly involves the cornea, conjunctiva, and Bruch membrane.

Histologically, the characteristic lesion is an extracellular accumulation of hyaline material, which produces indurated tissue, regarded as the physical basis for the clinical signs (88). The basal lamina of small blood vessels in the dermis are multilaminated from a neighboring deposition of fibrillar material, giving an onionskin appearance (36). The hyaline material is diastase resistant and reacts positively with the periodic acid Schiff sequence and with lipophilic stains, such as Sudan red and oil red O (39,70). This rare multisystem disorder with an autosomal recessive inheritance is caused by a mutation in an extracellular matrix protein gene (*ECM1*). Despite the affinity of the hyaline deposits for lipid stains there is no established local or systemic lipid disorder. There is now extensive evidence of disordered production of collagen subunits and of excess production of normal associated noncollagenous proteins (36,60,61,88,90).

Phytosterolemia

Phytosterolemia (sitosterolemia, MIM #210250) is a rare recessive disorder caused by mutations in the *ABCG8* or *ABCG5* genes. In contrast to normal individuals, who only absorb <1% of noncholesterol dietary sterols derived from plant and shellfish sterols from the intestine, persons with sitosterolemia absorb significant amounts of these sterols and are prone to accelerated atherosclerosis (10).

LIPID DISORDERS OF SPECIFIC OCULAR TISSUES

Corneal arcus lipoides and xanthelasma are cosmetic abnormalities that have significance as physical signs of dyslipidemia and as settings in which to elucidate the interactions of lipids in connective tissue.

Corneal Lipid Deposition

Corneal lipid deposition may be divided into three categories: corneal arcus (arcus lipoides), diffuse corneal lipid deposition (LCAT deficiency and very low HDL syndromes), and an inherited disorder—Schnyder corneal dystrophy (SCD)—that includes both peripheral and central corneal opacity. For an extensive review of the corneal aspects of lipid disorders see Barchiesi et al. (5).

Corneal Arcus Lipoides

Corneal arcus is an extracellular lipid-rich deposit involving predominantly the stroma of the peripheral cornea. Lipid can be demonstrated by light microscopy of suitably stained frozen sections (Fig. 2). Lipid is evident in the periphery of Bowman layer and extracellularly in the adjacent stroma between and occasionally within the corneal fibroblasts, as well as extending into the deeper cornea to the periphery of Descemet membrane. Lipid also accumulates in the adjacent sclera and often also in the ciliary processes and iris.

Corneal arcus characteristically appears first in the upper or lower segment. In time it may extend to a full circle; an outer clear zone is also characteristic. Corneal arcus can occur in young adults, but in Western Europe and North America it is a common aging event. Several studies have shown that its accelerated development is a feature of hyperlipoproteinemia, particularly excess of LDL, although it may arise in the absence of any overt disorder of lipoprotein metabolism (7,42,92,101,108). Premature corneal arcus has also been associated with accelerated coronary heart disease, although this not a simple relationship (20,80). Any contribution of additional variables, such as HDL or Lp(a), is not known. Further marked ethnic and individual variation, even within the severe genetic LDL excess syndromes, such as homozygous familial hypercholesterolemia (130), confirms that factors other than the nature, extent, and duration of any associated dyslipoproteinemia are involved.

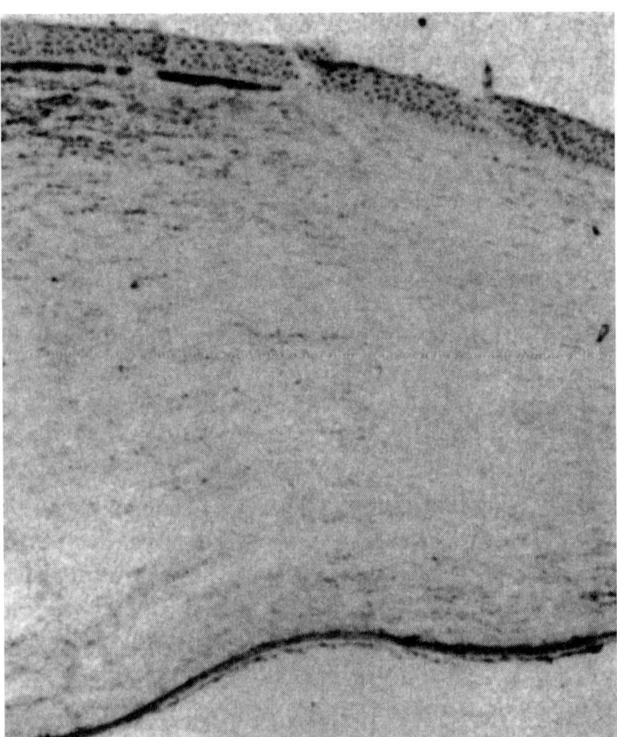

Figure 2 Corneal arcus is characterized histologically by extracellular sudanophilic lipid deposits in the corneal stroma, particularly in Descemet membrane and the periphery of Bowman zone (oil red O, ×105). *Source*: Courtesy of Dr. G.K. Klintworth.

Studies within familial hypercholesterolemia have been informative in the context of the clinical associations of corneal arcus with LDL excess (7,42,108,130,131,132). Homozygotes can develop arcus during early infancy, and arcus is common in heterozygotes by age 30 years, with an incidence in one large family of 100% (108). In another study of over 200 unselected and predominantly unrelated heterozygotes, the mean age for both sexes at which arcus was detected in 50% of cases was 33 years (132). The extent or rate of progression of arcus does not differentiate between those with and without clinical or EKG evidence of coronary heart disease in this high-risk group. The extent and progression of arcus is also strongly correlated with age rather than with the extent of LDL excess, which varied widely between the patients studied. This suggests that in markedly hyperbetalipoproteinemic individuals arcus formation is time dependent rather than dose dependent and that the relevant processes are saturated (131,132). Unilateral arcus can arise in association with contralateral carotid artery stenosis, presumably as the reduced blood flow on the contralateral side restricts the processes leading to the accumulation of lipid within the cornea (36,114). That insudation of lipoproteins at the corneoscleral limbus is a key element in these processes may be inferred from the altered pattern of arcus forming in the presence of anomalous vasculature at the corneoscleral limbus and by direct chemical analysis of the peripheral cornea. When intact human corneas with and without arcus obtained at postmortem are exposed to fluorescein-labeled antibody raised against human LDL (apoB), fluorescence is observed in the areas containing lipid deposits (125). ApoB can be readily identified in peripheral corneas within 6 hours of death, and the extent of reaction is unrelated to the presence or extent of corneal arcus (101). The lipids present in human peripheral cornea with arcus involvement are of a more saturated pattern than those carried in plasma lipoprotein (13,120); neither does the lipid-protein composition of saline extracts of peripheral cornea suggest a recent origin from plasma or a simple relationship with LDL (112). The single major component extracted is of lower molecular weight and lipid-protein ratio than LDL and does not bind to glycosaminoglycans (GAGs), and most preparations fail to react with antibody to apoB/LDL (112).

These clinical and laboratory studies on corneal arcus suggest that insudation of macromolecules at the corneoscleral limbus is a continuous process matched by clearance, some further process being required to build up a lipid-rich but not necessarily apoB- enriched arcus. Secondary processes are involved because the lipid present appears to originate from LDL, which has then been metabolized, with degradation of LDL apoB. Eyelid temperatures favor insudation at the upper and lower segments, and LDL-GAG interaction could trap LDL for modification as is proposed for other tissue deposits (69,115). The peripheral cornea is enriched with dermatan sulfate (44), shown to interact with LDL in vitro, but specific corneal trapping effects are not described. Local lipid metabolism may also be involved, because although the deposits of corneal arcus are predominantly extracellular, their composition differs from that in plasma and LDL. A similar biochemical difference between plasma and cornea has also been detected with LCAT deficiency, compatible with as yet undefined metabolic activity in the cornea (135). Resolution of corneal arcus on control of associated dyslipoproteinemia is described anecdotally in the human. Such regression may be impaired by the temperature gradient across the corneoscleral limbus as demonstrated by infrared thermography (Fig. 3). The accumulation of cholesterol esters becomes modified to include more long-chain saturated acyl residues, which are then trapped in an avascular area below their transition temperatures, as discussed for Tangier disease.

Corneal arcus lipoides is characterized histologically by the formation of extracellular cholesterol ester droplets enmeshed among collagen fibrils in the peripheral cornea (26,44). Foam cells are absent, signifying that cholesterol ester-rich lipid deposits can develop extracellularly without a preliminary step of lipoprotein uptake into cells. The cholesterol ester lipid droplets may arise from the fusion of low density lipoprotein particles in the extracellular space (52,53). As the particles enlarge, the apoB initially present on LDL may be degraded or lost.

Corneal arcus and xanthelasma, which may occur concomitantly in young people, are associated with hypercholesterolemia and specifically with high levels of low density lipoproteins or, less commonly, remnant lipoproteins (hyperlipoproteinemia type III).

Low levels of HDL, but not hypertriglyceridemia, may also be associated with the presence of corneal arcus (85,108). In the Lipid Research Clinics population survey corneal arcus and xanthelasma were both increased in the ischemic heart disease compared to the control group (108). However, corneal arcus can appear in the absence of any systemic lipid disorder, especially in the elderly and in people of color (19,74).

(A)

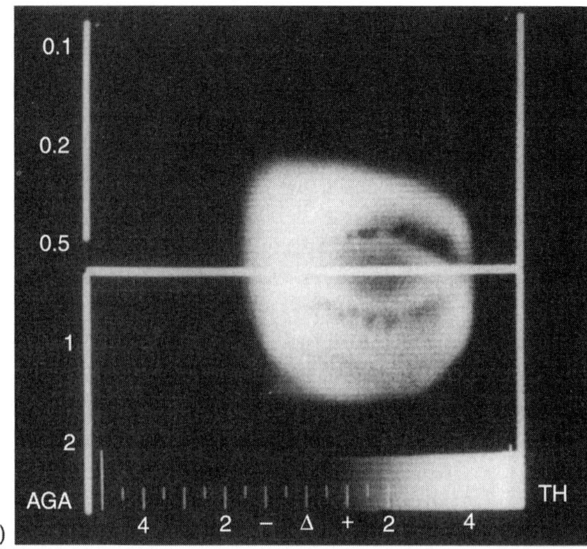

(B)

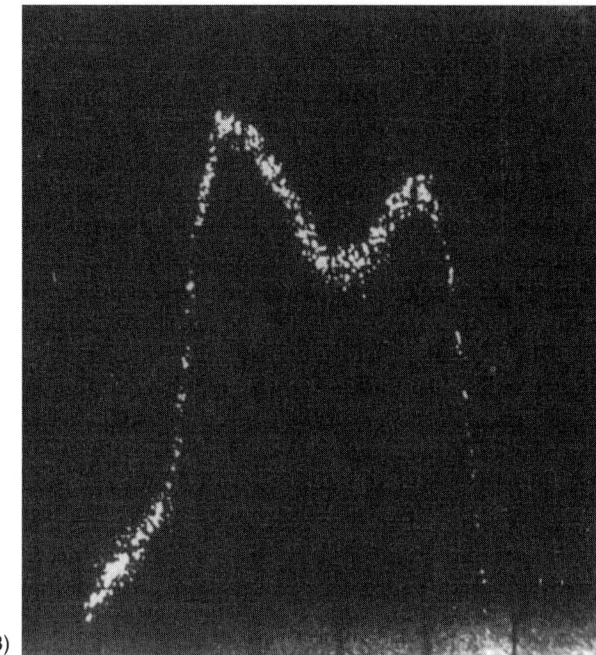

Figure 3 (**A**) Gray tone thermogram of the anterior surface of the eye. (**B**) Single-line temperature profile along the horizontal line shown in the upper part. The central trough corresponds to the relatively cool corneal center. *Source*: Reproduced with permission from Fielder AR, Winder AF, Cooke ED, et al. Arcus senilis and corneal temperature in man. In: The Cornea in Health and Disease. VI Congress European Society for Ophthalmology, Royal Society of Medicine and Academic Press; London, 1981:1015–20.

Diffuse Corneal Lipid Deposition

As discussed above, LCAT deficiency and its variant, fish eye disease, cause diffuse corneal lipid deposition with opacification of the cornea. Milder instances of corneal opacification are found in other patients with very low or absent HDL. Absence of apoA1 due to gene deletions or other mutations gives a mild corneal clouding, early atherosclerosis, and sometimes unusual planar xanthomas of the skin. Tangier disease, due to a recessive deficiency of ABCA1 (see above), gives mild corneal lipid deposits evident on slit lamp biomicroscopy in almost half the cases. ApoA1 Milano is not accompanied with corneal abnormalities (104). Focal areas of diffuse corneal vascularization may be associated with a lipid keratopathy and such lesions can be readily produced experimentally by inducing new blood vessels to invade the cornea in an animal with hypercholesterolemia.

Schnyder Corneal Dystrophy

SCD (MIM %121800), which presents with corneal clouding and often crystalline deposits in the cornea has an autosomal dominant mode of inheritance and results from a mutation in the *UBIAD1* gene (see Chapter 32). The corneal deposits in SCD, as in other lipid disorders with generalized corneal clouding, comprise mainly multilamellar vesicles containing unesterified cholesterol and phospholipids, with a lesser contribution of cholesteryl ester lipid droplets (84). ApoA1, apoA2, and apoE are present, but not apoB (45). Many patients with SCD do not have hyperlipidemia, but because some do, SCD is suspected of being a systemic disorder. Support for this notion comes from the finding that skin fibroblasts from one patient showed abnormal cytoplasmic deposits that were fluorescent after staining with filipin, a reagent apparently specific for unesterified cholesterol (6).

Retina

Age-Related Macular Degeneration

Evidence is mounting that local pathologic lipid metabolism may be involved in the pathogenesis of age-related macular degeneration (AMD) (see Chapter 18). In the aging human eye, lipofuscin deposits in the RPE and extracellular lipid deposits within the retinal aspect of Bruch membrane give evidence of pathologic lipid accumulation. The source of this lipid is probably the phospholipid-containing discs of the retinal photoreceptor outer segment, which are normally phagocytosed by RPE in the course of normal retinal physiology. Lipofuscin is common in aging tissues throughout the body, but especially in lipid-rich tissues, such as the brain, sites of pathologic lipid accumulation (atherosclerosis), and sites of high oxidative metabolism (myocardium). Cross-linking of lipids and other molecules, ascribed to aldehydic products of lipid peroxidation, makes the complex lipofuscin polymers highly insoluble and resistant to removal.

Lipid accumulation in Bruch membrane is likely to be the result of multiple mechanisms. The early characterization of lipids isolated from Bruch membrane described phospholipid, triglyceride, fatty acids, and free cholesterol, but little cholesteryl ester (65). However, the former lipid classes are simply those of normal tissues and it seems possible that pathologic cholesteryl ester deposits in the inner part of Bruch membrane were missed. The presence of droplets of neutral lipid composed substantially of cholesteryl ester has now been confirmed (27,55,78,102). Previous ultrastructural studies had described only membranous material, but the differentiation between membranous lipid vesicles and oily phase lipid droplets requires special cytochemical preparation to preserve the latter (52). An age-related accumulation of cholesteryl ester droplets is found adjacent to elastin in the deep intima of large arteries (51) and elastin is a major component of Bruch membrane. It is enriched in hydrophobic amino acids, and lipoproteins bind to elastin isolated from human aorta with high affinity (94). Along with cross-linked phospholipids (lipofuscin), cholesterol and cholesteryl ester are key elements of pathologic extracellular lipid accumulation, because physiologic mechanisms for their removal are relatively inefficient. There is no clear precedent for pathologic accumulation of triglyceride in extracellular locations. The evidence for cholesteryl ester in Bruch membrane is strong, while the hypothesis that triglyceride also accumulates can be neither accepted nor dismissed at present. In either case, the lipid deposits may eventually impede the transport of critical metabolites between retinal cells and the choriocapillaris (102). This would coincide with the demonstrated decline in hydraulic conductivity of Bruch membrane with aging (116).

The pattern of expression of gene transcripts and peptides in the retina suggests that an active lipid transport system supports the specialized cells and organelles of photoreception. The RPE synthesizes apoE in vivo and in vitro. ApoE secretion from cultured RPE was upregulated by ligands for three transcription factors: liver-X-receptor, retinoid-X-receptor, and thyroid hormone receptor (68). This behavior is similar to that in other peripheral tissues, where apoE is thought to function in local, cell-to-cell transport of cholesterol. Pathologic lipid deposits in Bruch membrane similar to those of AMD have been demonstrated in genetically apoE-deficient mice (30). In addition to apoE, apoA1 has been localized to Bruch membrane by immunohistochemistry. ApoA1 was thought to be synthesized only by the liver and the intestine, but reports of apoA1 transcription in brain capillary endothelium and in retina have appeared (68,87) and apoA1 is a key contributor to reverse cholesterol transport in a number of tissues.

ApoE and apoA1 are the major apolipoproteins found in CSF (54).

A unique role for apoB in the transport of lipids in the retina has been suggested on the basis of immunostaining as well as reverse transcriptase-polymerase chain reaction of mRNA extracted from human retina (82). The hypothesis for local formation of apoB-containing lipoproteins was supported by finding retinal gene expression of microsomal triglyceride transfer protein (79) which operates in concert with apoB to produce triglyceride-rich lipoproteins in liver and intestine. The intriguing possibility that there is apoB-containing lipoprotein formation in the retina awaits further confirmation, conceivably in the form of ultrastructural and biochemical characterization of putative retina-or RPE derived lipoproteins in the endoplasmic reticulum as well as the culture medium.

Drusen are focal collections of lipid-rich material that elevate RPE and separate them from the underlying Bruch membrane, and some forms are an early sign of AMD on ophthalmoscopic examination. The examination of drusen by qualitative histochemical techniques has revealed abundant unesterified and esterified cholesterol (26,55) and apoA1, apoB, and apoE have been identified by immunohistochemical procedures (78,82). Other findings have included evidence of complement activation and lipid peroxidation (23,121). It is not known whether the accumulating material derives from secretion by the overlying RPE, or exudation of plasma constituents from leaky choroidal capillaries, or both. The latter hypothesis would fit with a concept of pathogenesis that postulates deprivation of nutrients to retinal cells as a result of clogging of Bruch membrane (138,139). In response to nutrient deprivation, the RPE may secrete angiogenic factors, such as vascular endothelial growth factor (VEGF), which are known to cause vascular permeability as well as angiogenesis (57) (see Chapter 68). The hypothesis of vascular permeability as a key process in drusen formation would explain apoB immunoreactivity in the material, although the de novo synthesis of apoB by the RPE is an alternative explanation. Activation of plasma-derived complement factors may exacerbate the process, especially since deposits of unesterified cholesterol are known to activate complement (59,109). This theory brings together recent findings on the genetic predispositions to AMD conferred by allelic variations in the *APOE*, complement H (*CFH*), and *VEGF* genes (56,57,73).

Lipemia Retinalis

Lipemia retinalis, despite its striking appearance by fundoscopy, is significant primarily as a physical sign of fasting chylomicronemia, since visual function is little affected.

Eyelid

Xanthelasmata

Xanthelasmata represent intracellular deposits of mixed lipids in which cholesterol esters predominate, forming superficially in the loose skin in and around the eyelids (Fig. 4). They are a common feature of prolonged hyperlipoproteinemia,

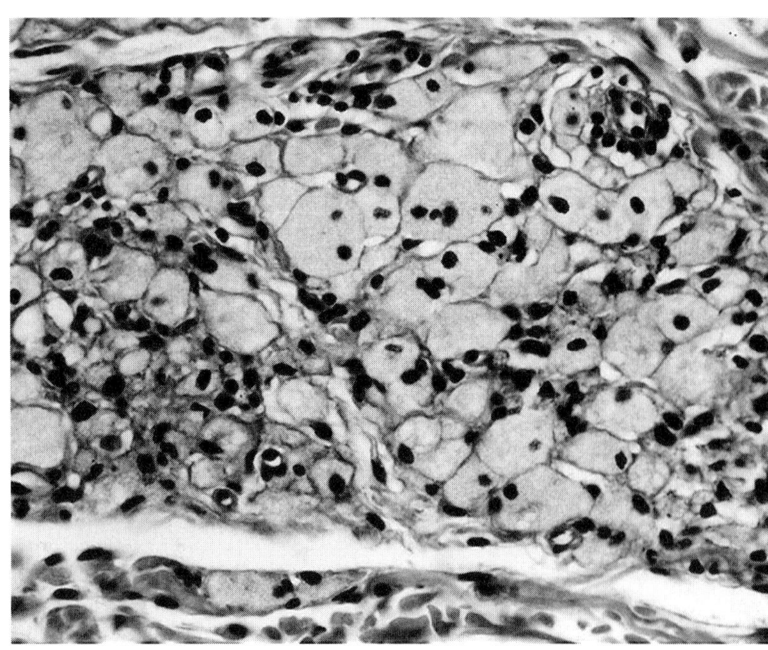

Figure 4 Histologic section of a xanthelasma demonstrating cholesteryl ester-laden foam cells (×400). *Source*: Reproduced from Klintworth GK, Landers MB III. The Eye: Structure and Function in Disease. Baltimore: Williams & Wilkins, 1976.

particularly when an element of hypertriglyceridemia and VLDL excess is also involved. In one series (34), 16 of 35 patients with xanthelasmata were hypercholesterolemic, with levels of cholesterol in plasma in excess of 7.8 mM (300 mg per 100 ml), and in a second series of heterozygotes for familial hypercholesterolemia, those with xanthelasmata had moderate but significant excess of plasma triglycerides and by implication of VLDL (130). About 50% of subjects with xanthelasmata are broadly normolipemic, although detailed investigation may reveal some abnormalities of lipoproteins in the plasma, including reduced levels of HDL and some enrichment of LDL with triglycerides (128). Modified triglyceride-rich lipoproteins may be particularly prone to cellular uptake by scavenger pathways of lipoprotein metabolism. Xanthelasmata can be regarded as one form of xanthomata, and as at other sites development may be accentuated by minor local trauma facilitating extravasation of lipoprotein (126), possibly here involving effects on periorbital skin blood vessels by frequent blinking and eye movements. Complete regression may be achieved by control of obese or lipemic subjects by diet or medication, particularly if the lesions have not been evident for more than a few months, after which partial regression with a darkening of color is more common. The rather variable relationship with patterns of lipoproteins in plasma suggests that local factors are important.

Previous studies on the lipid composition of various forms of xanthomata, including xanthelasmata, showed that in lesions present for a few months or less the lipid content closely resembles that in plasma, particularly that of any component in plasma present in excess (4,37,91). With time, the composition of the accumulations progressively differs from that in plasma. Apoprotein is lost, much triglyceride and other lipid disappears, and the residue is enriched with cholesterol esters, also progressively modified to incorporate acyl residues, which are more saturated and of longer chain length than predominant components in plasma. Similar changes are involved in the natural history of corneal arcus, as discussed, and as with corneal arcus these changes and the relationship with local temperature may also contribute to the chronicity of established xanthelasmata. Studies of a mature xanthelasma by differential scanning calorimetry over the range 30 to 40°C are shown in Figure 5. This material, enriched with saturated cholesterol esters, manifests transition temperatures (lipid-phase transitions analogous to melting points) above local skin temperatures, suggesting that the physical form of this matured lipid is not compatible with remobilization (133).

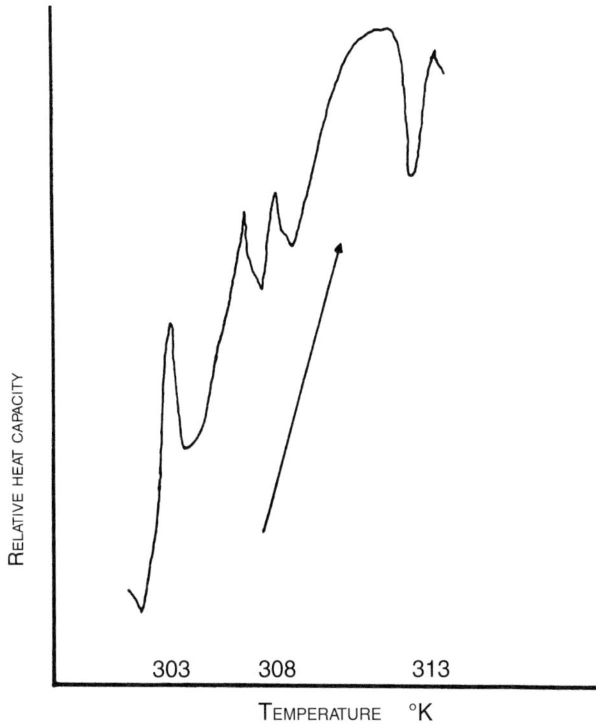

Figure 5 Examination of xanthelasma material by differential scanning calorimetry, expressing change in enthalpy as a function of temperature in relative units. Measurements were in single-channel mode, and the baseline shift is shown. Peaks of deviation from this baseline trend indicate the midpoint temperature of phase changes occurring over the range 308–313°K. *Source*: Reproduced with permission from Winder AF, Bruckdorfer KR, Fielder AR. Thermal transition studies of a mature xanthelasma by differential scanning calorimetry. Clin Chim Acta 1985; 151:253–7.

ACKNOWLEDGMENT

This chapter is a revision of the chapter previously prepared by Dr. Anthony F. Winder for the first two editions.

REFERENCES

1. Aguglia U, Annesi G, Pasquinelli G, et al. Vitamin E deficiency due to chylomicron retention disease in Marinesco-Sjogren syndrome. Ann Neurol 2000; 47: 260–26.
2. Allen IV, Swallow M, Nevin NC, McCormick D. Clinicopathological study of Refsum's disease with particular reference to fatal complications. J Neurol Neurosurg Psychiatr 1978; 41:323–32.
3. Assmann G, Von Eckardstein A, Brewer HB Jr. Familial analphalipoproteinemia: Tangier disease. In: Scriver CR, Beaudet AL, Sly WS, Valle D, Childs B, Kinzler KW, Vogelstein B, eds. The Metabolic and Molecular Bases of Inherited Disease, 8th ed. New York: McGraw-Hill, 2001, Volume II, Chapter 122, part 12, pp. 2937–60.
4. Baes H, Van Gent, CM, Pries C. Lipid composition of various types of xanthomata. J Invest Dermatol 1968; 51: 286–93.

5. Barchiesi BJ, Eckel RH, Ellis PP. The cornea and disorders of lipid metabolism. Surv Ophthalmol 1991; 36: 1–22.
6. Battisti C, Dotti MT, Malandrini A, et al. Schnyder corneal crystalline dystrophy: description of a new family with evidence of abnormal lipid storage in skin fibroblasts. Am J Med Genet 1998; 75:35–9.
7. Beaumont V, Jacotot B, Beaumont J-L. Ischaemic disease in men and women with familial hyper-cholesterolaemia and xanthomatosis. Atherosclerosis 1976; 24:441–50.
8. Berriot-Varoqueaux N, Aggerbeck LP, Samson-Bouma M, Wetterau JR. The role of the microsomal triglygeride transfer protein in abetalipoproteinemia. Annu Rev Nutr 2000; 20:663–97.
9. Bieri JG, Hoeg JM, Schaefer EJ, et al. Vitamin A and vitamin E replacement in abetalipoproteinaemia. Ann Inter Med 1984; 100:238–39.
10. Björkhem I, Boberg KM, Leitersdorf E. Inborn errors in bile acid biosynthesis and storage of sterols other than cholesterol. In: Scriver CR, Beaudet AL, Sly WS, Valle D, Childs B, Kinzler KW, Vogelstein B, eds. The Metabolic and Molecular Bases of Inherited Disease, 8th ed. New York: McGraw-Hill, 2001, Volume II, Chapter 123, part 12, pp. 2961–88.
11. Blum CB, Deckelbaum RJ, Witte LD, et al. Role of apolipoprotein E-containing lipoproteins in abetalipoproteinemia. J Clin Invest 1982; 70:1151–69.
12. Botermans CH. Primary pigmentary retinal degeneration and its association with neurological disease. In Handbook of Clinical Neurology, Vol. 13, Neuroretinal Degenerations, HJ Vincken and GW Bruyn (Eds.), North Holland, Amsterdam 1975; pp. 148–399.
13. Broeckhuyse RM. Lipids in tissues of the eye 14 (corneoscleral lipids during ageing and in arcus senilis). Doc Ophthalmol 1976; 7:313–22.
14. Brown MS, Goldstein JL. A receptor-mediated pathway for cholesterol homeostasis. Science 1986; 232:34–47.
15. Cammermeyer J. Refsum's disease, neuropathological aspects. In Handbook of Clinical Neurology, Vol 21 Part 1, Systemic Disorders and Atrophies, HJ Vincken and GW Bruyn (Eds.), North Holland, Amsterdam 1975; pp. 231–61.
16. Chait A, Brunzell JD. Chylomicronemia syndrome. Adv Intern Med 1992; 37:249–73.
17. Cogan DG, Kruth HS, Datilis MB, Martin N. Corneal opacity in LCAT disease. Cornea 1992; 11:595–9.
18. Collins DR, Knott TJ, Pease RJ, et al. Truncated variants of apolipoprotein B cause hypobetalipoproteinaemia. Nucleic Acids Res 1988; 16:8361–75.
19. Cook GC, Kanyerezi BR. Corneal arcus in the Ugandan African. Am Heart J 1970; 79:718–20.
20. Cooke NT. Significance of arcus senilis in Caucasians. JR Soc Med 1981; 74:1322–4.
21. Cooper RA, Durocher JR, Leslie MH. Decreased fluidity of red cell membrane lipids in abetalipoproteinaemia. J Clin Invest 1977; 60:115–21.
22. Cooper RA, Gulbrandsen CL. The relationship between serum lipoproteins and red cell membranes in abetalipoproteinaemia: Deficiency of lecithinxholesterol acyltransferase. J Lab Clin Med 1971; 78:323–35.
23. Crabb JW, Miyagi M, Gu X, et al. Drusen proteome analysis: an approach to the etiology of age-related macular degeneration. Proc Natl Acad Sci USA 2002; 99: 14682–7.
24. Crispin S. Ocular lipid deposition and hyperlipoproteinaemia. Prog Retin Eye Res 2002; 21:169–224.
25. Cumings JN. Inborn errors of metabolism in neurology (Wilson's disease, Refsum's disease and lipodoses). Proc R Soc Med 1971; 64:313–22.
26. Curcio CA, Presley JB, Malek G, et al. Esterified and unesterified cholesterol in drusen and basal deposits of eyes with age-related maculopathy. Exp Eye Res 2005; 81:731–41.
27. Curcio CA, Presley JB, Millican CL, Medeiros NE. Basal deposits and drusen in eyes with age-related maculopathy: evidence for solid lipid particles. Exp Eye Res 2005; 80:761–75.
28. Davis GJ, Porter RS, Steiner JW, Small DM. Thermal transitions of cholesterol esters of cholesterol esters of C18 aliphatic acids. Mol Crystals Liquid Crystals 1970; 10: 331–6.
29. Dietschy JM, Turley SD. Thematic review series: brain lipids. cholesterol metabolism in the central nervous system during early development and in the mature animal. J Lipid Res 2004; 45:1375–97.
30. Dithmar S, Curcio CA, Le NA, et al. Ultrastructural changes in Bruch's membrane of apolipoprotein E-deficient mice. Invest Ophthalmol Vis Sci 2000; 41: 2035–42.
31. Dodge JT, Cohen G, Kayden HJ, Phillips GP. Peroxidative haemolysis of red blood cells from patients with abetalipoproteinaemia (acanthocytosis). J Clin Invest 1967; 46:357–68.
32. Dodson PM, Galton DJ, Winder AF. Retinal vascular abnormalities in the hyperlipidaemias. Trans Ophthalmol Soc UK 1981; 101:17–21.
33. Dotti MT, Rufa A, Federico A. Cerebrotendinous xanthomatosis: Heterogeneity of clinical phenotype with evidence of previously undescribed ophthalmological findings. Journal of Inherited Metabolic Disease 2001; 24:696–706.
34. Epstein M, Rosenmann RH, Gofman JW. Serum lipids and cholesterol metabolism in xanthelasmata. Arch Dermatol Syphilol 1952; 65:70–81.
35. Fielder AR, Winder AF, Cooke ED, Bowcock SA. Arcus senilis and corneal temperature in man. In The Cornea in Health and Disease VI Congress European Society for Ophthalmology, Royal Society of Medicine and Academic Press, London 1981; pp. 1015–20.
36. Fleischmajer R, Krieg T, Dziadek M, et al. Ultrastructure and composition of connective tissue in hyalinosis cutis et mucosae skin. J Invest Dermatol 1984; 82:252–8.
37. Fletcher RF. Lipid composition of xanthomas of different types. Nutr Metab 1973; 15:97–106.
38. Francois J. Ocular manifestations of inborn errors of carbohydrate and lipid metabolism. V. Primary hyperlipoproteinaemias (hyperlipidaemias). Bibl Ophthalmol 1975; 84:150–9.
39. Francois J, Bacskulin J, Follmann P. Manifestations oculaires du syndrome d'Urbach-Wiethe. Hyalinosis cutis et mucosae. Ophthalmologica 1968; 155:433–48.
40. Fredrickson DS. Hereditary diseases of metabolism that affect the eye. In The Eye and Systemic Disease, F.A. Mausolt (Ed.), C.V. Mosby, St Louis 1975; pp. 8–33.
41. Frohlich J, Fong B, Mien P, et al. Interaction of high-density lipoprotein with adipocytes in a new patient with Tangier disease. Clin Invest Med 1987; 10:377–82.
42. Gagne C, Moorjani S, Brun D, et al. Heterozygous familial hyper- cholesterolemia: Relationship between plasma lipids, lipoproteins, clinical manifestations and ischaemic heart disease in men and women. Atherosclerosis 1979; 34:13–24.

43. Garuti R, Jones C, Li WP, et al. The modular adaptor protein autosomal recessive hypercholesterolemia (ARH) promotes low density lipoprotein receptor clustering into clathrin-coated pits. J Biol Chem 2005; 280:40996–1004.
44. Gaynor PM, Zhang WY, Salehizadeh B, et al. Cholesterol accumulation in human cornea: evidence that extra-cellular cholesteryl ester-rich lipid particles deposit independently of foam cells. J Lipid Res 1996; 37: 1849–61.
45. Gaynor PM, Zhang WY, Weiss JS, et al. Accumulation of HDL apolipoproteins accompanies abnormal cholesterol accumulation in Schnyder's corneal dystrophy. Arterioscler Thromb Vasc Biol 1996; 16:992–9.
46. Glueck CJ, Gartside P, Fallat RW, et al. Longevity syndromes: Familial hypobeta- and familial hyperalpha-lipoproteinemia. J Lab Clin Med 1976; 88:941–57.
47. Glueck CJ, Mellies MJ, Tsang RC, et al. Neonatal hypobetalipoproteinemia. Pediatr Res 1978; 12: 655–68.
48. Goldstein JL, Brown MS. Familial hypercholesterolemia In: Scriver CR, Beaudet AL, Sly WS, Valle D, Childs B, Kinzler KW, Vogelstein B, eds. The Metabolic and Molecular Bases of Inherited Disease, 8th ed. New York: McGraw-Hill, 2001, Volume II, Chapter 120, part 12, pp. 2863–913.
49. Gould SJ, Raymond CV, Valle D. The peroxisosome biogenesis disorders. In: Scriver CR, Beaudet AL, Sly WS, Valle D, Childs B, Kinzler KW, Vogelstein B, eds. The Metabolic and Molecular Bases of Inherited Disease, 8th ed. New York: McGraw-Hill, 2001, Volume II, Chapter 129, part 15, pp. 3181–217.
50. Grundy SM. Hypertriglyceridemia: mechanisms, clinical significance, and treatment. Med Clin North Am 1982; 66: 519–35.
51. Guyton JR, Bocan TM. Quantitative ultrastructural analysis of perifibrous lipid and its association with elastin in nonatherosclerotic human aorta. Arteriosclerosis 1985; 5:644–52.
52. Guyton JR, Klemp KF. Ultrastructural discrimination of lipid droplets and vesicles in atherosclerosis: value of osmium-thiocarbohydrazide-osmium and tannic acid-paraphenylenediamine techniques. J Histochem Cytochem 1988; 36:1319–28.
53. Guyton JR, Klemp KF, Mims MP. Altered ultrastructural morphology of self-aggregated low density lipoproteins: coalescence of lipid domains forming droplets and vesicles. J Lipid Res 1991; 32:953–62.
54. Guyton JR, Miller SE, Martin ME, et al. Novel large apolipoprotein E-containing lipoproteins of density of 1.006–1.060 g/ml in human cerebrospinal fluid. Journal of Neurochemistry 1998; 70:1235–40.
55. Haimovici R, Gantz DL, Rumelt S, et al. The lipid composition of drusen, Bruch's membrane, and sclera by hot stage polarizing light microscopy. Invest Ophthalmol Vis Sci 2001; 42:1592–9.
56. Haines JL, Hauser MA, Schmidt S, et al. Complement factor H variant increases the risk of age-related macular degeneration. Science 2005; 308:419–21.
57. Haines JL, Schnetz-Boutaud N, Schmidt S, et al. Functional candidate genes in age-related macular degeneration: significant association with VEGF, VLDLR, and LRP6. Invest Ophthalmol Vis Sci 2006; 47:329–5.
58. Hansen E, Bachen NI, Flage T. Refsum's disease: Eye manifestations in a patient treated with a low phytol low phytanic acid diet. Acta Ophthalmol (Copenh) 1979; 57: 899–913.
59. Hansson GK, Seifert PS. Complement receptors and regulatory proteins in human atherosclerotic lesions. Arteriosclerosis 1989; 9:802–11.
60. Harper JL, Duance VC, Sims TJ, Light ND Lipoid proteinosis: An inherited disorder of collagen metabolism? Br J Dermatol 1985; 113:145–51.
61. Hausser I, Blitz S, Rauterberg E, et al. Hyalinosis cutis et mucosae (Morbus Urbach-Wiethe). Ultrastrukturelle und immunologische Merkmale. Hautarzt 1991; 42:28–33.
62. Havel RC, Kane JP. Disorders of the biogenesis and secretion of lipoproteins containing the B apolipoproteins. In: Scriver CR, Beaudet AL, Sly WS, Valle D, Childs B, Kinzler KW, Vogelstein B, eds. The Metabolic and Molecular Bases of Inherited Disease, 8th ed. New York: McGraw-Hill, 2001, Volume II, Chapter 114, part 12, pp. 2705–16.
63. Herbert PN, Forte T, Heinen RJ, Fredrickson DS. Tangier disease: One explanation of lipid storage. N Engl J Med 1978; 299:519–21.
64. Holmquist L, Hamsten A, Dahlen GH. Free apolipoprotein (a) in abetalipoproteinaemia. J Intern Med 1989; 225: 285–6.
65. Holz FG, Sheraidah G, Pauleikhoff D, Bird AC. Analysis of lipid deposits extracted from human macular and peripheral Bruch's membrane. Arch Ophthalmol 1994; 112:402–6.
66. Huang L-S, Ripps ME, Korman SH, et al. Hypobetalipoproteinemiadue to an apolipoprotein B gene exon 21 deletion derived by Alu-Alu combination. J Biol Chem 1989; 264:11394–400.
67. Innerarity TL, Mahley RW, Weisgraber KH, et al. Familial defective apolipoprotein B-100: a mutation of apolipoprotein B that causes hypercholesterolemia. J Lipid Res 1990; 31:1337–49.
68. Ishida BY, Bailey KR, Duncan KG, et al. Regulated expression of apolipoprotein E by human retinal pigment epithelial cells. J Lipid Res 2004; 45:263–71.
69. Iverius PH. The interaction between human plasma lipoproteins and connective tissue glycosaminoglycans. J Biol Chem 1972; 247:2607–13.
70. Jensen AD, Khodadoust AA, Emery JM. Lipid proteinosis: Report of a case with electron microscopic findings. Arch Ophthalmol 1972; 88:273–7.
71. Jolley CD, Woollett LA, Turley SD, Dietschy JM. Centripetal cholesterol flux to the liver is dictated by events in the peripheral organs and not by the plasma high density lipoprotein or apolipoprotein A-I concentration. J Lipid Res 1998; 39:2143–9.
72. Jones B, Jones EL, Bonney SA, et al. Mutations in a Sar1 GTPase of COPII vesicles are associated with lipid absorption disorders. Nature Genetics 2003; 34:29–31.
73. Klaver CC, Kliffen M, van Duijn CM, et al. Genetic association of apolipoprotein E with age-related macular degeneration. Am J Hum Genet 1988; 63:200–6.
74. Klein B, Klein R, Haseman J, et al. Corneal arcus and cardiovascular disease in Evans County, Georgia. Arch Intern Med 1975; 135:509–11.
75. Kott E, Delpre G, Kadish U, et al. Abetalipoproteinemia (Batten-Kornzweig syndrome). Acta Neuropathol (Berl) 1977; 37:255–8.
76. Krieger M, Herz J. Structures and functions of multi-ligand lipoprotein receptors: macrophage scavenger receptors and LDL receptor-related protein (LRP). Rev Biochem 1994; 63:601–37.
77. Kuivenhoven JA, Pritchard H, Hill J, et al. The molecular pathology of lecithin:cholesterol acyltransferase (LCAT) deficiency syndromes. J Lipid Res 1997; 38:191–205.

78. Li CM, Chung BH, Presley JB, et al. Lipoprotein-like particles and cholesteryl esters in human Bruch's membrane: initial characterization. Invest Ophthalmol Vis Sci 2005; 46:2576–86.
79. Li CM, Presley JB, Zhang X, et al. Retina expresses microsomal triglyceride transfer protein: implications for age-related maculopathy. J Lipid Res 2005; 46:628–40.
80. Macaraeg PVJ, Lasagna L, Snyder B. Arcus not so senilis. Ann Intern Med 1968; 68:345–54.
81. Mahley RW, Rall SC, Jr. Type III hyperlipoproteinemia (dysbetalipoproteinemia): the role of apolipoprotein E in normal and abnormal lipoprotein metabolism. In: Scriver CR, Beaudet AL, Sly WS, Valle D, Childs B, Kinzler KW, Vogelstein B, eds. The Metabolic and Molecular Bases of Inherited Disease, 8th ed. New York: McGraw-Hill, 2001, Volume II, Chapter 122, part 12, pp. 2835–62.
82. Malek G, Li CM, Guidry C, et al. Apolipoprotein B in cholesterol-containing drusen and basal deposits of human eyes with age-related maculopathy. Am J Pathol 2003; 162:413–25.
83. Malloy MJ, Kane JP. Hypolipidemia. Med Clin North Am 1982; 66:469–84.
84. McCarthy M, Innis S, Dubord P, White V. Panstromal Schnyder corneal dystrophy. A clinical pathologic report with quantitative analysis of corneal lipid composition. Ophthalmology 1994; 101:895–901.
85. Meyer D, Liebenberg PH, Maritz FJ. Serum lipid parameters and the prevalence of corneal arcus in a dyslipidaemic patient population. Cardiovasc J S Afr 2004; 15:166–9.
86. Miranda PJ, DeFronzo RA, Califf RM, Guyton JR. Metabolic syndrome: definition, pathophysiology, and mechanisms. Am Heart J 2005; 149(1):33–45.
87. Mockel B, Zinke H, Flach R, et al. Expression of apolipoprotein A-I in porcine brain endothelium in vitro. J Neurochem 1994; 62:788–98.
88. Moy LS, Moy RL, Matsuoka LY, et al. Lipoid proteinosis: Ultrastructural and biochemical studies. J Am Acad Dermatol 1987; 16:1193–201.
89. Newton FH, Rosenberg RN, Lampert PW, O'Brien JS. Neurological involvement in Urbach-Wiethe's disease (lipoid proteinosis): A clinical, ultrastructural, and chemical study. Neurology 1971; 21:1205–13.
90. Olsen DR, Chu ML, Uitto J. Expression of basement zone genes coding for type IV procollagen and laminin by human skin fibroblasts in vitro: Elevated alpha 1(IV) collagen mRNA levels in lipoid proteinosis. J Invest Dermatol 1988; 900:734–8.
91. Parker F, Short FM. Xanthomatosis associated with hyperlipoproteinaemia. J Invest Dermatol 1970; 55:71–88.
92. Parwaresch MR, Haacke H, Mader CH, Godt CH. Arcus lipoides corneae und Hyperlipoproteinaemia. Klin Wochenschr 1976; 54:495–7.
93. Pisciotta L, Oliva CP, Pes GM, et al. Autosomal recessive hypercholesterolemia (ARH) and homozygous familial hypercholesterolemia (FH): A phenotypic comparison. Atherosclerosis 2006; 188:398–405.
94. Podet EJ, Shaffer DR, Gianturco SH, et al. Interaction of low density lipoproteins with human aortic elastin. Arterioscl Thrombos 1991; 11:116–22.
95. Poll-The BT, Saudubray JM, Rocchiccioli F, et al. Prenatal diagnosis and confirmation of infantile Refsum's disease. J Inherited Metab Dis 1987; 10(Suppl. 2):229–32.
96. Poulos A, Pollard AC, Mitchell JD, et al. Patterns of Refsum's disease: Phytanic acid oxidase deficiency. Arch Dis Child 1984; 59:222–9.
97. Poulos A, Van Crugten C, Sharp P, et al. Prenatal diagnosis of Zellweger syndrome and related disorders: Impaired degradation of phytanic acid. Eur J Paediatr 1986; 145:507–10.
98. Pressly TA, Scott WJ, Ide CH, Winkler A, Reams GR, Ocular complications of Tangier disease. Am J Med 1978; 83:991–4.
99. Refsum S. Heredopathia atactica polyneuritiformis: Phytanic acid storage disease (Refsum's disease). In Handbook of Clinical Neurology, Vol. 21, Part 1, Systemic Disorders and Atrophies, HJ Vincken and GW Bruyn (Eds.), North Holland, Amsterdam, 1975, pp. 181–229.
100. Robenek H, Schmitz G. Abnormal processing of Golgi elements and lysosomes in Tangier disease. Arteriosclerosis Thrombosis 1991; 11:1007–20.
101. Rosenman RH, Brand RJ, Scholtz MS., Jenkins CD. Relation of corneal arcus to cardiovascular risk factors and the incidence of coronary disease. N Engl J Med 1974; 291:1322–4.
102. Ruberti JW, Curcio CA, Millican CL, et al. Quick-freeze/deep-etch visualization of age-related lipid accumulation in Bruch's membrane. Invest Ophthalmol Vis Sci 2003; 44: 1753–9.
103. Santamarina-Fojo S, Hoeg JM, Assman G, Brewer HB, Jr. Lecithin cholesterol acyltransferase deficiency and fish eye disease. In: Scriver CR, Beaudet AL, Sly WS, Valle D, Childs B, Kinzler KW, Vogelstein B, eds. The Metabolic and Molecular Bases of Inherited Disease, 8th ed. New York: McGraw-Hill, 2001, Volume II, Chapter 118, part 12, pp. 2817–33.
104. Schaefer EJ. Clinical, biochemical, and genetic features in familial disorders of high density lipoprotein deficiency. Arteriosclerosis 1984; 4:303–22.
105. Schmitz G, Fischer H, Beuck M, et al. Dysregulation of lipid metabolism in Tangier monocyte-derived macrophages. Arteriosclerosis 1990; 10:1010–9.
106. Schonfeld G, Lin X, Yue P. Familial hypobetalipoproteinemia: genetics and metabolism. Cell Mol Life Sci 2005; 62:1372–8.
107. Schrott AG, Goldstein JL, Hazzard WR, et al. Familial hyper- cholesterolemia in a large kindred: Evidence for a monogenic mechanism. Ann Intern Med 1972; 76:711–20.
108. Segal P, Insull W Jr, Chambless LE, et al. The association of dyslipoproteinemia with corneal arcus and xanthelasma. The Lipid Research Clinics Program Prevalence Study. Circulation 1986; 73:1108–18.
109. Seifert PS, Kazatchkine MD. The complement system in atherosclerosis. Atherosclerosis 1988; 73:91–104.
110. Sharp P, Johnson D, Poulos A. Molecular species of phosphatidylcholine containing very long chain fatty acids in human brain: Enrichment in X-linked adrenoleukodystrophy brain and diseases of peroxisosome biogenesis brain. J Neurochem 1991; 56:30–7.
111. Sheraidah GA, Winder AF, Fielder AR. Lipid-protein constituents of human corneal arcus. Atherosclerosis 1981; 40:91–8.
112. Small DM, Progression and regression of atherosclerotic lesions. Insights from lipid physical biochemistry. Arterioscl-erosis 1988; 8:103–29.
113. Smith JL, Susac JO. Unilateral corneal arcus senilis: Sign of occlusive disease of the carotid artery. JAMA 1973; 226: 676–7.
114. Spaeth GL. Ocular manifestations of the lipodoses. In Retinal Disease in Children, W. Tasman (Ed.), Harper and Row, New York 1971; pp. 127–206.

115. Srinivasan SR, Dolan P, Radhakrishnamurthy B, et al. S. Lipoprotein-acid mucopolysaccharide complexes of human atherosclerotic lesions. Biochim Biophys Ada 1975; 388:58–70.
116. Starita C, Hussain AA, Marshall J. Decreasing hydraulic conductivity of Bruch's membrane: relevance to photoreceptor survival and lipofuscinoses. Am J Med Genet 1995; 57:235–7.
117. Sysi R. Xanthoma corneae as hereditary dystrophy. Br J Ophthalmol 1950; 34:369–74.
118. Tall AR, Breslow JL, Rubin EM. Genetic disorders affecting plasma high-density lipoproteins. In: Scriver CR, Beaudet AL, Sly WS, Valle D, Childs B, Kinzler KW, Vogelstein B, eds. The Metabolic and Molecular Bases of Inherited Disease, 8th ed. New York: McGraw-Hill, 2001, Volume II, Chapter 121, part 12, pp. 2915–36.
119. Toussaint D, Davis P. An ocular pathological study of Refsum's syndrome. Am J Ophthalmol 1971; 72:342–7.
120. Tschetter RT. Lipid analysis of the human cornea with and without arcus senilis. Arch Ophthalmol 1966; 76:403–5.
121. Umeda S, Suzuki MT, Okamoto H, et al. Molecular composition of drusen and possible involvement of anti-retinal autoimmunity in two different forms of macular degeneration in cynomolgus monkey (Macaca fascicularis). FASEB J 2005; 19:1683–5.
122. Utermann G. Lipoprotein(a). In: Scriver CR, Beaudet AL, Sly WS, Valle D, Childs B, Kinzler KW, Vogelstein B, eds. The Metabolic and Molecular Bases of Inherited Disease, 8th ed. New York: McGraw-Hill, 2001, Volume II, Chapter 12, part 12, pp. 2753–88.
123. von Bahr S, Movin T, Papadogiannakis N, et al. Mechanism of accumulation of cholesterol and cholestanol in tendons and the role of sterol 27-hydroxylase (CYP27A1). Arterioscler Thromb Vasc Biol 2002; 22: 1129–35.
124. von Sallman L, Gelderman LH, Laster L. Ocular histopathologic changes in a case of abetalipoproteinemia (Bassen-Kornzweig syndrome). Doc Ophthalmol 1969; 26: 451–60.
125. Walton KW. Studies on the pathogenesis of corneal arcus formation. 1. The human corneal arcus and its relation to atherosclerosis as studied by immunofluorescence. J Pathol 1973; 111:263–73.
126. Walton KW, Thomas C, Dunkerley E. The pathogenesis of xanthomata. J Pathol 1973; 109:271–89.
127. Wanders RJS, Jakobs C, Skjeldal OH, Refsum disease. In: Scriver CR, Beaudet AL, Sly WS, Valle D, Childs B, Kinzler KW, Vogelstein B, eds. The Metabolic and Molecular Bases of Inherited Disease, 8th ed. New York: McGraw-Hill, 2001, Volume II, Chapter 132, part 12, pp. 3303–21.
128. Watanabe A, Yoshimuna A, Wakasugi E, et al. Serum lipids, lipoproteins and coronary heart disease in patients with xanthelasma palpebrarum. Atherosclerosis 1980; 58: 283–90.
129. Ways P, Reed CF, Hanahan DJ. Red cell and plasma lipids in acanthocytosis. J Clin Invest 1963; 42:1248–60.
130. Winder AF. Factors influencing the variable expression of xanthelasmata and corneal arcus in familial hypercholesterolaemia. Birth Defects 1982; 18:449–62.
131. Winder AF. Relationship between arcus and hyperlipidaemia is clarified by studies in familial hyper cholesterolaemia. Br J Ophthalmol 1983; 67:789–94.
132. Winder AF. Corneal arcus and prognosis in familial hypercholesterolaemia. Atherosclerosis 1987; 68:273.
133. Winder AF, Bruckdorfer KR, Fielder AR. Thermal transition studies of a mature xanthelasma by differential scanning calorimetry. Clin Chim Acta 1985; 151: 253–7.
134. Winder A, Frohlich J, Garner A, et al. The cornea in familial high density lipoprotein deficiency, Tangier disease. Atherosclerosis 1991; 90:222.
135. Winder AF, Garner A, Sheraidah GA, Barry P. Familial lecithin: cholesterol acyltransferase deficiency. Biochemistry of the cornea. J Lipid Res 1985; 26:283–7.
136. Yee RD, Cogan DB, Zee DS. Ophthalmoplegia and dissociated nystagmus in abetalipoproteinemia. Arch Ophthalmol 1976; 94:571–5.
137. Yee RD, Herbert PN, Bergsma DR, Breimer JJ. Atypical retinitis pigmentosa in familial hypo- betalipoproteinemia. Am J Ophthalmol 1976; 82:64–71.
138. Zarbin MA. Age-related macular degeneration: review of pathogenesis. Eur J Ophthalmol 1998; 8: 199–206.
139. Zarbin MA. Current concepts in the pathogenesis of age-related macular degeneration. Arch Ophthalmol 2004; 122:598–614.

47

Dysthyroid Eye Disease

Brian S. F. Shine
Department of Clinical Biochemistry, John Radcliffe Hospital, and Oxford Centre for Diabetes, Endocrinology, and Metabolism, Oxford, U.K.

INTRODUCTION

Dysthyroid eye disease (thyroid associated ophthalmopathy) is a chronic condition, characterized by inflammation and an increased volume of the retrobulbar orbital contents, particularly the extraocular muscles, with consequent proptosis, limitation of eye movements, periorbital swelling, and the potential for optic nerve compression. More than 25 names are associated with dysthyroid eye disease, including those relating to early detailed clinical descriptions, such as Caleb Parry (1825), Robert Graves (1835), and Carl von Basedow (1840). Dysthyroid eye disease is an autoimmune disease strongly associated with autoimmune thyrotoxicosis. It is part of the spectrum of autoimmune thyroid disease: nearly all patients with ophthalmopathy have a demonstrable thyroid disorder, and most patients with autoimmune Graves thyroid disease have orbital abnormalities. Although severe disease is uncommon, mild disease is present in most patients with autoimmune thyrotoxicosis. The clinical effects are produced by inflammation and glycosaminoglycan (GAG) accumulation within orbital tissues.

The responsible antigen or antigens have proved elusive, but the most likely candidate is the thyroid-stimulating hormone (TSH) receptor protein.

Although not a common disease, thyroid-associated ophthalmopathy has a high impact on the quality of life (39), in both the short and long term (1). While most people experience improvement in the long term, a significant proportion has residual impairment of visual function (about 70%) or visual appearance (about 90%) (126).

EPIDEMIOLOGY

Most dysthyroid eye disease occurs in association with autoimmune thyroid disease, predominantly thyrotoxicosis, less frequently Hashimoto thyroiditis, but occasionally without overt thyroid disease (51).

Surveys of apparently normal populations in the United States (50), Japan (61), and Scandinavia (20) have shown a prevalence of thyroid peroxidase (TPO) antibodies of more than 5% among males and 10% among all females, and about 10% among pregnant women (69). Thyroid dysfunction, as judged by abnormal TSH levels, has been found in about 13% of females and about 4.5% of males over the age of 60 years recruited from a primary care practice (84), while the incidence of hypothyroidism is approximately 1/1000 per year among females and 0.2/1000 per year among males (19). A large survey of a single village in the United Kingdom revealed a history of thyroid disease in 19/1000 women and 1.6/1000 men (113). When this population was followed-up 20 years later, the incidence of spontaneous hypothyroidism was found to be about 3.5/1000 survivors per year in females and about 0.6/1000 survivors per year in males, with a rate of hyperthyroidism of 0.8/1000 per year in females, the main risk factors being presence of anti-thyroid antibodies and the baseline TSH level (118). Another survey in the United Kingdom found an annual incidence of 35.5 women and 9.2 men per 100,000 inhabitants (9). It is estimated that up to 15% of females and 5% of males develop a dysthyroid condition in their lifetime.

Autoimmune thyroid disease is associated with other autoimmune diseases, such as celiac disease (24,25), vitiligo (49), juvenile rheumatoid arthritis (90), presence of antibodies to the pancreas (76), and to insulin (119) and anti-nuclear antibodies (112), while a large proportion of patients with Sjögren syndrome has positive thyroid antibodies (26,97,102).

Thyroid disease is sometimes familial. For instance, in one study, 440/803 patients with autoimmune thyroid disease had at least one relative with thyroid disease. Thirty-three percent had a family history of either autoimmune hyperthyroidism or Hashimoto thyroiditis (109). Approximately 90% of patients with autoimmune hyperthyroidism have evidence of ophthalmic involvement (13). However, only about 2% to 5% develop clinically significant ophthalmopathy (10,51). The age and sex distributions of patients with ophthalmopathy resemble those of patients with autoimmune hyperthyroidism without significant clinical ophthalmopathy (128).

Environmental agents may trigger the development of thyroid-associated ophthalmopathy, especially smoking (48). Treatment with anti-thyroid drugs and thyroidectomy do not appear to affect the severity of the ophthalmopathy, but radioiodine treatment may precipitate the onset of, or worsen existing, ophthalmopathy especially among those who smoke, those with a pre-existing ophthalmopathy or more severe hyperthyroidism, and those who become hypothyroid after therapy (14,87).

The peak incidence of Graves disease is in the fifth to seventh decades, and the female:male ratio is approximately 4:1 (125). It has been suggested that genetic anticipation occurs, that is, the disease presents at a younger age in successive generations (22). There appears to be no seasonal predisposition (32).

CLINICAL FEATURES

Ophthalmic Features

The reader should refer to Prabhakhar et al. (89) for an extensive review of the clinical features of Graves disease and thyroid-associated ophthalmopathy The commonest ophthalmic features are eyelid retraction (in about 90% of cases), exophthalmos (60%), impairment of eye movements controlled by the extraocular muscles (40%) (sometimes accompanied by diplopia) ocular surface irritation associated with lacrimation (20%) and photophobia (15%), and blurred vision (7%) (16). The ophthalmopathy tends to wax and wane, typically becoming inactive after about 2 years, although active disease may persist for 5 years or longer. Severe complications tend to occur within the first 6 to 9 months, and thus patients who do not have sight-threatening complications within this period are unlikely to experience permanent impairment of visual acuity, although residual strabismus and diplopia are common (15).

The most striking clinical feature is usually proptosis, due to an increase in the volume of orbital contents, particularly the extraocular muscles, and the rigid nature of the orbit (Fig. 1). Measurement of proptosis by exophthalmometry is reliable and reproducible (79), although inter-observer variability may be large and the readings tend to be higher than those obtained by computed tomography (CT) (101). Both magnetic resonance imaging (MRI) (83) and ultrasonography (58) are useful in showing increased volume of the orbital structures. The proptosis is usually axial, with little deviation, and any lateral or medial displacement should lead to an intensive search for other causes. An increase in orbital tension is usually demonstrable either by digital pressure or by mechanical measurement (96), and the intra-ocular pressure increases in about 20% of patients on upgaze (3).

Although most patients have bilateral proptosis, unilateral proptosis occurs in 5% to 15% of patients (128). Dysthyroid eye disease is the most common cause of unilateral proptosis (35,68).

The most commonly and earliest affected extraocular muscles are the inferior (approximately 75%) and medial (approximately 50%) recti (58) although any or all of the extraocular muscles may be affected. The inflammation leads to an increase in bulk followed by fibrosis, with a consequent impairment of muscular control of eye movements. Tightness of the affected muscles leads to increased

(A) 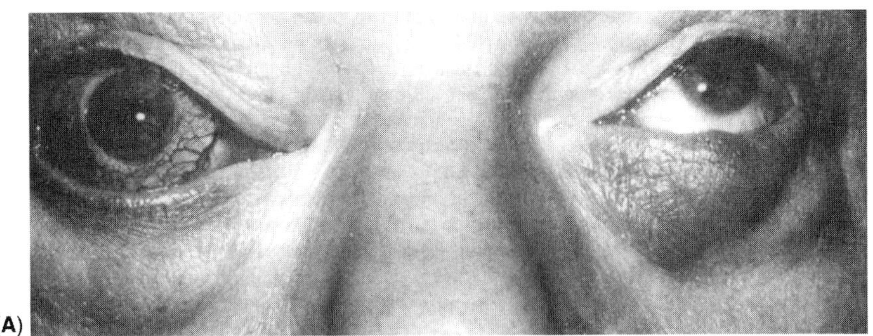

(B) 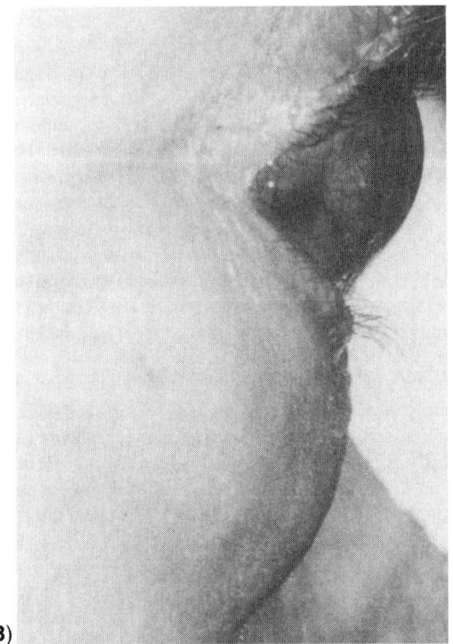

Figure 1 Clinical features of dysthyroid eye disease. (**A**) Conjunctival injection, periorbital edema, superior medial fat herniation, limitation of upgaze in the right eye. (**B**) Proptosis with loss of corneal cover, with injection of conjunctival and prominent veins.

resistance to the action of opposing muscles, resulting in strabismus and diplopia (Fig. 1).

Retraction of the upper and/or lower eyelids is another consistent feature and possible causes for this include sympathetic overactivity due to thyrotoxicosis (although retraction is often present in the absence of toxicosis), hypertrophy of the muscle fibers, inflammatory change with consequent fibrosis, and the mechanical effect of the proptosis. Retraction may lead to reduced corneal and conjunctival cover, particularly when the patient is asleep, and consequent corneal damage. The increased lacrimation may be a reaction to changes in the tear film secondary to a decreased blink rate and widening of the palpebral fissure, and qualitative and quantitative changes in tear proteins have been detected with a change in tear break-up time (60). Superior limbic keratitis, seen as punctate staining with rose Bengal, is also common but by no means universal and its presence does not correlate well with symptoms. Other conjunctival signs include an increased prominence of blood vessels and hyperemia and inflammation of the insertion points of the rectus muscles (Fig. 1).

Periorbital changes include swelling of both upper and lower eyelids, with herniation of fat through the medial part of the aponeurosis of Müller muscle and into the subcutaneous tissue (Fig. 1).

Optic neuropathy is the major vision-threatening complication. It may have a rapid onset and is usually precipitated by increased pressure on the optic nerve from surrounding structures, especially at the orbital apex. Optic neuropathy sometimes occurs without obvious involvement of the extraocular muscles. The earliest sign is often reduction in color saturation, particularly for red targets, often with an increase in the physiological difference between the two eyes in color appreciation. This may be followed by a decrease in visual acuity, with a relative afferent pupillary reaction defect and visual field restriction (45,82). Less severe optic nerve compression may be relatively common, and can be detected by use of visual evoked potentials (4,98). This may mean that active treatment is indicated earlier and in a greater proportion of patients than has previously been appreciated. Occasionally, optic neuropathy appears to be secondary to stretching of the optic nerve as a result of proptosis.

It is important to distinguish between activity and severity (13). A commonly used severity scoring system is that due to Werner (124), the so-called NOSPECS system (N, no signs or symptoms; O, only signs; S, soft tissue swelling; P, proptosis; E, extraocular muscle involvement; C, corneal exposure; S, sight loss). This is convenient and easy to use. However, it does not necessarily give a good guide to whether therapy is required, and so various activity scores have been proposed, such as that described by Mourits et al. (80). This is based upon the presence of pain, redness, swelling and loss of function (namely the cardinal signs of inflammation), and predicts response to therapy (steroids or orbital radiotherapy). Other methods that have been suggested for assessing activity include ultrasound (38), plasma or urine GAGs (54,55,57), octreotide scanning (58), T2-weighted MRI scanning (81,93,114), and single photon emission computer tomography (37).

Thyroid Disease

Many patients with dysthyroid eye disease have a history of autoimmune thyroid disease, and about 50% have clinically apparent thyroid dysfunction at the time of diagnosis of ocular involvement. Thyrotoxicosis is very common, but approximately 5% have primary underactivity, probably due to Hashimoto disease. Most patients with active autoimmune thyrotoxicosis have increased exophthalmometer readings, and ophthalmopathy commonly appears within 18 months of the thyroid condition (51,71,127) but they may be separated by many years. Dysthyroid eye disease may be precipitated by, or worsen after, radioactive iodine treatment of hyperthyroidism (11) but may regress following surgical thyroidectomy (74). Gwinup's group was unable to show any difference between the progress of patients with different levels of thyroid function (44), but DeGroot et al. (29) reported that patients who required multiple doses of radioactive iodine had a greater tendency to develop eye disease.

Treatment for hyperthyroidism differs between Europe and North America. In the former, conventional treatment is with thionamides (such as methimazole, carbimazole, propylthiouracil). In North America, radioiodine treatment is favored. However, this may be associated with the development or worsening of the ophthalmopathy, which may be prevented by steroids (11,12) or by thyroxine (110). In Europe, such treatment tends to be reserved for patients with refractory disease. Smoking (12), high pre-treatment T_3 levels (111), high levels of thyrotropin receptor antibodies (94) or TSH (11,12) are associated with increased risk. Total ablation may result in a lower risk of worsening of ophthalmopathy (28).

The third treatment modality available for thyroid disease is surgery. Since leaving a thyroid remnant may lead to redevelopment of toxicosis, with progression of ophthalmopathy, subtotal thyroidectomy has been replaced by near-total thyroidectomy with which the risk of causing progression appears to be low (13).

Dermopathy

Dysthyroid eye disease is associated with a dermopathy, consisting of non-pitting edema of the skin, most commonly over the pre-tibial area (100). In most cases, this is mild and does not require specific treatment. However, in some instances, usually associated with severe ophthalmopathy, there may also be clubbing, swelling of the fingers and toes, and periosteal reaction affecting bones in the extremities (thyroid acropachy) (34).

LABORATORY INVESTIGATIONS

The aims of laboratory investigations in dysthyroid eye disease are to permit diagnosis, definition of the stage and prognosis of the disease, rational choice of therapy, and assessment of the likelihood of complications requiring intervention. To exclude an orbital tumor, biopsy may be necessary in some patients in whom the diagnosis is not clear and in whom all other investigations are unhelpful. Unless the clinical differential diagnosis includes thyroid disease, the diagnosis may be missed even on biopsy because of the nonspecific nature of the cellular infiltrate.

Thyroid Function Tests

Tests of thyroid function are an essential part of the clinical investigation, since approximately 50% to 60% of patients with dysthyroid eye disease have some functional abnormality of this endocrine gland. TSH is produced in the pituitary gland, and is released in response to the hypothalamic hormone, thyrotropin releasing hormone (TRH) (or thyroliberin). It is inhibited by triiodothyronine (T_3), which is produced by local conversion from tetraiodothyronine (thyroxine, T_4) in the pituitary cells. TSH stimulates T_3 and T_4 production by the thyroid gland and release of these hormones into the peripheral circulation. In the blood, both hormones are extensively bound (T_4 99.97%; T_3 99.7%) to proteins, principally thyroxine binding globulin. Although T_4 concentrations are 30 to 50 times higher than those of T_3, free T_4 levels are only two to three times those of T_3. T_3 is the active metabolic hormone, and approximately 80% of the body's T_3 is produced by peripheral conversion from T_4 rather than in the thyroid gland.

Thyroid activity can be assessed by assaying peripheral levels of T_4 and T_3 and free hormone levels are usually measured, since these are not affected by changes in binding proteins. However, most laboratories use TSH as their front-line test in the assessment of thyroid function. This allows assessment of the control of thyroid function, and is satisfactory for most clinical situations except when the possibility of pituitary disease exists. Free hormones are measured if the TSH is abnormal or where there is reasonable clinical suspicion of an underlying thyroid disorder.

TSH levels are elevated in hypothyroidism of thyroid origin and suppressed in hyperthyroidism due to autonomous secretion (for example by an autonomous thyroid nodule) or autoimmune stimulation (classic Graves disease).

Thyroid Antibody Tests

Stimulating antibodies to the TSH receptor are the cause of Graves hyperthyroidism [see review by McLachlan et al. (77)]. Assays for these antibodies are based either on inhibition of binding by TSH to its receptor or their ability to stimulate functional receptors in isolated thyroid cells or transfected eukaryotic cells. Although these antibodies correlate well with the activity of the thyrotoxicosis and their measurement may be helpful in the differential diagnosis of hyperthyroidism, the assays are not in widespread routine clinical use.

Antibodies to several other thyroid proteins are often present, including thyroglobulin and TPO. Thyroglobulin fills the thyroid colloid vesicles and acts as the reservoir for thyroid hormones previously manufactured inside the thyroid cells. Low levels of anti-thyroglobulin antibodies are present in most patients with thyroid disease.

PATHOGENESIS

The close association between autoimmune thyroid disease and other autoimmune conditions, particularly diabetes mellitus and myasthenia gravis provide strong evidence that dysthyroid eye disease is an autoimmune disorder. About 15% of patients with autoimmune thyroid disease have specific insulin autoantibodies (119). There is a strong association between myasthenia gravis and thyroid-associated ophthalmopathy (123). In one large series, 31 out of 387 patients with dysthyroid eye disease had myasthenia gravis, leading to the hypothesis that there may be a preferential association between the ocular manifestations of dysthyroid eye disease and myasthenia gravis (72). In this section, we will discuss the possible antigens, the mechanisms by which the autoimmune process may occur, and the consequences of these that lead to the clinical features of dysthyroid eye disease.

Antigens

Although it is agreed that the condition is autoimmune in origin, the responsible antigen or antigens have been hard to define. Candidates include the TSH receptor, insulin-like growth factor 1 (IGF1) receptor, muscle proteins, and thyroglobulin.

Most investigators now believe that the TSH receptor is the responsible antigen [see, for example (7)]. TSH receptor expression is greater in orbital adipose tissue in patients with dysthyroid eye disease than in normal subjects (8), and orbital fibroblasts and TSH receptor are recognized by T cells from patients with dysthyroid eye disease. TSH receptor antibodies correlate with clinical activity scores (40).

Another candidate is the IGF1 receptor, which is expressed on orbital fibroblasts (104). IgG in serum from patients with thyroid-associated ophthalmopathy inhibits binding of IGF1 to orbital fibroblasts and binding of IgG to IGF1 receptor on fibroblasts can activate fibroblasts (122,105). It is possible that both the TSH and IGF1 receptors are involved (30).

Several muscle antibodies have been suspected of being involved in the autoimmune reactions associated with dysthyroid eye disease (27,43). A number of antigens have been identified, including a 55 kDa protein called G2s (43) and a 67 kDa flavoprotein (42,65), with antibody levels appearing to predict muscle involvement (42,59), although discrepant results have been obtained in some groups (52).

Kriss hypothesized that thyroglobulin was responsible for dysthyroid eye disease, because of thyroglobulin deposition in the orbit by retrograde lymphatic spread (64). This hypothesis was attractive because dysthyroid eye disease is associated with the presence of thyroglobulin antibodies. However, contrary evidence includes the lack of association between the level of thyroglobulin antibodies and the severity and activity of the ophthalmopathy, and the failure to develop ophthalmopathy in mice immunized with thyroglobulin (73).

Autoimmune Processes

Dysthyroid eye disease affects many orbital components, the most prominent changes occurring in the extraocular muscles and orbital fat. The central actor in this process is a subset of fibroblasts, called preadipocytes. Fibroblasts that can differentiate to form adipocytes can be distinguished by the absence of Thy-1, a glycoprotein found on the cell surface of approximately 50% of orbital fibroblasts. Stimuli for differentiation include activation of peroxisome proliferator-activated receptor γ (PPAR-γ) and cyclic AMP production (116), and thiazolidinediones, which activate PPAR-γ, may induce (70) or worsen (108) dysthyroid eye disease. IL6 appears to stimulate adipogenesis, as judged by TSH receptor expression (53), while transforming growth factor beta (TGFβ), interferon-γ and tumor necrosis factor-alpha (TNFα) inhibit differentiation (117).

Once fibroblasts have differentiated to adipocytes, activation leads to the chain of events resulting in thyroid-associated ophthalmopathy.

1. Differentiation to adipocytes induces expression of functional TSH-receptor (115), although Smith (104) considers that the quantities expressed are not enough to account for the immune response.
2. Interaction between primed T cells and TSH receptors leads to secretion by T cells, antigen presenting cells and T cell-activated macrophages of various cytokines, such as inteferon-γ (IFNγ), IL4, IL1β, and TGFβ, all of which activate fibroblasts. Activation may involve bridging between CD40, a member of the TNFα receptor superfamily present on the surface of orbital fibroblasts, and its ligand, CD154 (104).
3. Orbital fibroblasts respond in an exaggerated manner to proinflammatory cytokines, hormones, prostanoids, gangliosides and protein compared with fibroblasts from other sites (103). Cytokine stimulation of fibroblasts, for instance by IL1β, leads to production of hyaluronan, a GAG, which accumulates in the extracellular space.
4. Activation also leads to increases in prostaglandin endoperoxide H synthase 2 activation, leading to increased PGE2 synthesis (23).
5. Cytokines expressed by orbital fibroblasts, perhaps as a result of B-cell interaction with IGF1 receptors, are important in immune activation and include IL6, IL8, IL16, and regulated upon activation, normal T-cell expressed and secreted (RANTES). These may cause further activation of and infiltration by dendritic antigen-presenting cells, macrophages, and T cells. These are able to produce further cytokines, such as IL1β and TGFβ, which further increase hyaluronan production.
6. Activated T-helper cells are classified as Th1 or Th2 [for review see Ajian and Weetman (2)] depending upon the pattern of cytokines that they secrete. Th1 cells, which produce IFNγ, predominate in the early stages of thyroid associated ophthalmopathy, while Th2 cells, which produce IL4, predominate later (5,46). Th1 cells promote inflammation, cytotoxicity and delayed type hypersensitivity, while Th2 cells promote B-cell differentiation and antibody formation (2).

IgG from patients with dysthyroid eye disease leads to synthesis of hyaluronan in orbital fibroblasts, and this can be reproduced by incubation with IGF1, the effector molecule produced in response to growth hormone (105) [see review by Drexhage (30)]. Moreover, IgG from patients with dysthyroid eye disease also induces production of T cell chemoattractants by fibroblasts from any site (92), probably acting through the IGF1 receptor pathway (91).

Somatostatin receptors may also be involved in the development of dysthyroid eye disease. Somatostatin receptor scanning using labeled octreotide is valuable in defining the activity of dysthyroid eye disease (58): uptake correlates with activity (41,88), and administration of recombinant human TSH may lead to increased uptake in patients with thyroid eye disease, indicating increased numbers of somatostatin receptors and lymphocyte activity (99) [for review of somatostatin receptors and lymphocyte function see (62)].

Somatostatin was named for its inhibitory effect on the pituitary gland, but it also has many other functions, including as a neurohormone and neurotransmitter, regulating endocrine and exocrine secretions and modulating gut motility. The somatostatin receptors (of which five types have been defined) are G-protein coupled receptors [for review see Krassas (63)]. The discovery of somatostatin receptors on fibroblasts (86) and orbital lymphocytes (85) has added evidence that somatostatin may be involved in modulating activity in dysthyroid eye disease [for review see Krantic et al. (62)].

How Do These Processes Lead to Clinical Features?

Differentiation of fibroblasts expressing Thy-1 to adipocytes (66,106) leads to an increase in the volume of cells within the orbit, one of the main causes being the production of hyaluronan by fibroblasts. This GAG is very hydrophilic and its presence leads to a large increase in water and volume (6). Reduced venous and lymphatic drainage may be responsible for the chemosis and periorbital edema. The presence of TSH-receptors in the lacrimal glands of normal subjects suggests a mechanism for the production of reduced or altered tear film in dysthyroid eye disease (31).

Extraocular muscle dysfunction is initially due to swelling and there may be a seven-fold increase in volume. The affected muscles have a firm, rubbery, and variably reddish appearance, and there may be a seven-fold increase in volume. Histologically, the most striking feature in early disease is infiltration of the muscles by lymphocytes (Fig. 2) and an increase in interstitial GAGs. The infiltrate is focal, with groups of cells around the muscle cells, and blood vessels, but little involvement of the orbital fat.

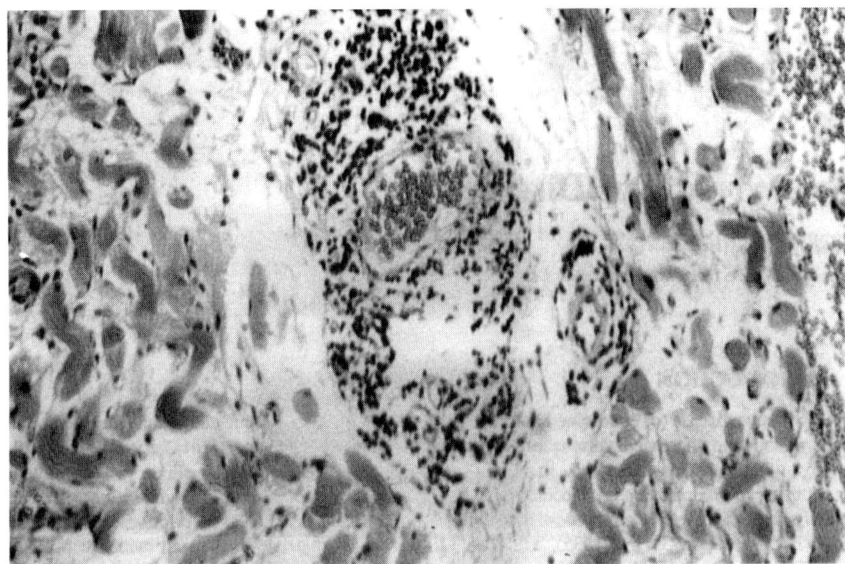

Figure 2 Histological features of active dysthyroid eye disease showing perivascular lymphocytic infiltration with less profuse collections of lymphocytes around muscle cells (hematoxylin and eosin, ×115).

Immunohistochemistry reveals that two-thirds of the infiltrating cells are T cells and one-third B cells, with scattered macrophages (56,121). Some fibroblast proliferation occurs, with increased secretion of GAGs into the intercellular matrix. Inflammation is followed by fibrosis and muscle destruction.

GENETICS

The incidence of dysthyroid eye disease is increased in family members, and the concordance rate in a large Danish study was 0.35 suggesting that inherited factors account for 79% of susceptibility (21). However, identifying genes that may be involved has proved difficult (33,120). Candidates include the major histocompatibilty classes I and II, cytotoxic T lymphocyte antigen 4 (CTLA4), TNFα (18), and thyroglobulin.

ENVIRONMENTAL INFLUENCES

If the evidence for genetic linkage is rather sketchy, a possible alternative is that the environment plays some part in the precipitation of the condition, but research on this topic appears to have been neglected. Studies of antibodies to bacteria have yielded inconclusive results [reviewed in Ref. (95)].

Patients with thyroid associated ophthalmopathy commonly relate the onset or worsening of the condition to some traumatic event and several studies have reported associations between stressful life events and the onset of Graves disease (17,36,47, 67,75,78,107,129).

Several groups have shown a greater frequency of smoking in patients with active thyroid ophthalmopathy than in healthy controls or in patients with Graves disease without ophthalmopathy, although many patients, even those with severe disease, have never smoked [reviewed in Ref. (48)].

REFERENCES

1. Abraham-Nordling M, Torring O, Hamberger B, et al. Graves' disease: a long-term quality-of-life follow up of patients randomized to treatment with antithyroid drugs, radioiodine, or surgery. Thyroid 2005; 15:1279–86.
2. Ajjan RA, Weetman AP. New understanding of the role of cytokines in the pathogenesis of Graves' ophthalmopathy. J Endocrinol Invest 2004; 27:237–45.
3. Allen C, Stetz D, Roman SH, et al. Prevalence and clinical associations of intraocular pressure changes in Graves' disease. J Clin Endocrinol Metab 1985; 61:183–7.
4. Ambrosio G, Ferrara G, Vitale R, et al. Visual evoked potentials in patients with Graves' ophthalmopathy complicated by ocular hypertension and suspect glaucoma or dysthyroid optic neuropathy. Doc Ophthalmol 2003; 106:99–104.
5. Aniszewski JP, Valyasevi RW, Bahn RS. Relationship between disease duration and predominant orbital T cell subset in Graves' ophthalmopathy. J Clin Endocrinol Metab 2000; 85:776–80.
6. Bahn RS. Clinical review 157: pathophysiology of Graves' ophthalmopathy: the cycle of disease. J Clin Endocrinol Metab 2003; 88:1939–46.
7. Bahn RS. TSH receptor expression in orbital tissue and its role in the pathogenesis of Graves' ophthalmopathy. J Endocrinol Invest 2004; 27:216–20.
8. Bahn RS, Dutton CM, Natt N, et al. Thyrotropin receptor expression in Graves' orbital adipose/connective tissues: potential autoantigen in Graves' ophthalmopathy. J Clin Endocrinol Metab 1998; 83:998–1002.
9. Barker DJ, Phillips DI. Current incidence of thyrotoxicosis and past prevalence of goitre in 12 British towns. Lancet 1984; 2:567–70.

10. Bartalena L. Editorial: glucocorticoids for Graves' ophthalmopathy: how and when. J Clin Endocrinol Metab 2005; 90:5497–9.
11. Bartalena L, Marcocci C, Bogazzi F, et al. Use of corticosteroids to prevent progression of Graves' ophthalmopathy after radioiodine therapy for hyperthyroidism. N Engl J Med 1989; 321:1349–52.
12. Bartalena L, Marcocci C, Pinchera A. On the effects of radioiodine therapy on Graves' ophthalmopathy. Thyroid 1998; 8:533–4.
13. Bartalena L, Pinchera A, Marcocci C. Management of Graves' ophthalmopathy: reality and perspectives. Endocr Rev 2000; 21:168–99.
14. Bartalena L, Tanda ML, Piantanida E, et al. Relationship between management of hyperthyroidism and course of the ophthalmopathy. J Endocrinol Invest 2004; 27:288–94.
15. Bartley GB, Fatourechi V, Kadrmas EF, et al. Chronology of Graves' ophthalmopathy in an incidence cohort. Am J Ophthalmol 1996; 121:426–34.
16. Bartley GB, Fatourechi V, Kadrmas EF, et al. Clinical features of Graves' ophthalmopathy in an incidence cohort. Am J Ophthalmol 1996; 121:284–90.
17. Beardsley G, Goldstein MG. Psychological factors affecting physical condition. Endocrine disease literature review. Psychosomatics 1993; 34:12–9.
18. Bednarczuk T, Hiromatsu Y, Seki N, et al. Association of tumor necrosis factor and human leukocyte antigen DRB1 alleles with Graves' ophthalmopathy. Hum Immunol 2004; 65:632–9.
19. Bilous RW, Tunbridge WM. The epidemiology of hypothyroidism–an update. Baillieres Clin Endocrinol Metab 1988; 2:531–40.
20. Bjoro T, Holmen J, Kruger O, et al. Prevalence of thyroid disease, thyroid dysfunction and thyroid peroxidase antibodies in a large, unselected population. The Health Study of Nord-Trondelag (HUNT). Eur J Endocrinol 2000; 143:639–47.
21. Brix TH, Kyvik KO, Christensen K, et al. Evidence for a major role of heredity in Graves' disease: a population-based study of two Danish twin cohorts. J Clin Endocrinol Metab 2001; 86:930–4.
22. Brix TH, Petersen HC, Iachine I, et al. Preliminary evidence of genetic anticipation in Graves' disease. Thyroid 2003; 13:447–51.
23. Cao HJ, Han R, Smith TJ. Robust induction of PGHS-2 by IL-1 in orbital fibroblasts results from low levels of IL-1 receptor antagonist expression. Am J Physiol-Cell Physiol 2003; 284:C1429–37.
24. Ch'ng CL, Biswas M, Benton A, et al. Prospective screening for coeliac disease in patients with Graves' hyperthyroidism using anti-gliadin and tissue transglutaminase antibodies. Clin Endocrinol (Oxf) 2005; 62: 303–6.
25. Cuoco L, Certo M, Jorizzo RA, et al. Prevalence and early diagnosis of coeliac disease in autoimmune thyroid disorders. Ital J Gastroenterol Hepatol 1999; 31:283–7.
26. D'Arbonneau F, Ansart S, Le Berre R, et al. Thyroid dysfunction in primary Sjogren's syndrome: a long-term followup study. Arthritis Rheum 2003; 49:804–9.
27. de Bellis A, Perrino S, Coronella C, et al. Extraocular muscle antibodies and the occurrence of ophthalmopathy in Graves' disease. Clin Endocrinol (Oxf) 2004; 60:694–8.
28. DeGroot LJ. Radioiodine and the immune system. Thyroid 1997; 7:259–64.
29. DeGroot LJ, Mangklabruks A, McCormick M. Comparison of RA 131I treatment protocols for Graves' disease. J Endocrinol Invest 1990; 13:111–8.
30. Drexhage HA. Are there more than antibodies to the thyroid-stimulating hormone receptor that meet the eye in Graves' disease? Endocrinology 2006; 147:9–12.
31. Eckstein AK, Finkenrath A, Heiligenhaus A, et al. Dry eye syndrome in thyroid-associated ophthalmopathy: lacrimal expression of TSH receptor suggests involvement of TSHR-specific autoantibodies. Acta Ophthalmol Scand 2004; 82:291–7.
32. Facciani JM, Kazim M. Absence of seasonal variation in Graves disease. Ophthal Plast Reconstr Surg 2000; 16: 67–71.
33. Farid NR, Marga M. Genetics of thyroid-associated ophthalmopathy: a play in search of a cast of characters. J Endocrinol Invest 2003; 26:570–4.
34. Fatourechi V, Ahmed DD, Schwartz KM. Thyroid acropachy: report of 40 patients treated at a single institution in a 26-year period. J Clin Endocrinol Metab 2002; 87:5435–41.
35. Fells P. Management of dysthyroid eye disease. Br J Ophthalmol 1991; 75:245–6.
36. Fukao A, Takamatsu J, Murakami Y, et al. The relationship of psychological factors to the prognosis of hyperthyroidism in antithyroid drug-treated patients with Graves' disease. Clin Endocrinol (Oxf) 2003; 58: 550–5.
37. Galuska L, Leovey A, Szucs-Farkas Z, et al. Imaging of disease activity in Graves' orbitopathy with different methods: comparison of (99m)Tc-DTPA and (99m)Tc-depreotide single photon emission tomography, magnetic resonance imaging and clinical activity scores. Nucl Med Commun 2005; 26:407–14.
38. Gerding MN, Prummel MF, Wiersinga WM. Assessment of disease activity in Graves' ophthalmopathy by orbital ultrasonography and clinical parameters. Clin Endocrinol (Oxf) 2000; 52:641–6.
39. Gerding MN, Terwee CB, Dekker FW, et al. Quality of life in patients with Graves' ophthalmopathy is markedly decreased: measurement by the medical outcomes study instrument. Thyroid 1997; 7:885–9.
40. Gerding MN, van der Meer JW, Broenink M, et al. Association of thyrotrophin receptor antibodies with the clinical features of Graves' ophthalmopathy. Clin Endocrinol (Oxf) 2000; 52:267–71.
41. Gerding MN, van der Zant FM, van Royen EA, et al. Octreotide-scintigraphy is a disease-activity parameter in Graves' ophthalmopathy. Clin Endocrinol (Oxf) 1999; 50: 373–9.
42. Gunji K, De Bellis A, Kubota S, et al. Serum antibodies against the flavoprotein subunit of succinate dehydrogenase are sensitive markers of eye muscle autoimmunity in patients with Graves' hyperthyroidism. J Clin Endocrinol Metab 1999; 84:1255–62.
43. Gunji K, De Bellis A, Li AW, et al. Cloning and characterization of the novel thyroid and eye muscle shared protein G2s: autoantibodies against G2s are closely associated with ophthalmopathy in patients with Graves' hyperthyroidism. J Clin Endocrinol Metab 2000; 85:1641–7.
44. Gwinup G, Elias AN, Ascher MS. Effect on exophthalmos of various methods of treatment of Graves' disease. JAMA 1982; 247:2135–8.
45. Hallin ES, Feldon SE, Luttrell J. Graves' ophthalmopathy: III. Effect of transantral orbital decompression on optic neuropathy. Br J Ophthalmol 1988; 72:683–7.
46. Han R, Smith TJ. T helper type 1 and type 2 cytokines exert divergent influence on the induction of prostaglandin E-2 and hyaluronan synthesis by interleukin-1 beta in

orbital fibroblasts: Implications for the pathogenesis of thyroid-associated ophthalmopathy. Endocrinology 2006; 147:13–9.
47. Harris T, Creed F, Brugha TS. Stressful life events and Graves' disease. Br J Psychiatry 1992; 161:535–41.
48. Hegedius L, Brix TH, Vestergaard P. Relationship between cigarette smoking and Graves' ophthalmopathy. J Endocrinol Invest 2004; 27:265–71.
49. Hegedus L, Heidenheim M, Gervil M, et al. High frequency of thyroid dysfunction in patients with vitiligo. Acta Derm Venereol 1994; 74:120–3.
50. Hollowell JG, Staehling NW, Flanders WD, et al. Serum TSH, T(4), and thyroid antibodies in the United States population (1988 to 1994): National Health and Nutrition Examination Survey (NHANES III). J Clin Endocrinol Metab 2002; 87:489–99.
51. Jacobson DH, Gorman CA. Endocrine ophthalmopathy: current ideas concerning etiology, pathogenesis, and treatment. Endocr Rev 1984; 5:200–20.
52. Joffe B, Gunji K, Panz V, et al. Thyroid-associated ophthalmopathy in black South African patients with Graves' disease: relationship to antiflavoprotein antibodies. Thyroid 1998; 8:1023–7.
53. Jyonouchi SC, Valyasevi RW, Harteneck DA, et al. Interleukin-6 stimulates thyrotropin receptor expression in human orbital preadipocyte fibroblasts from patients with Graves' ophthalmopathy. Thyroid 2001; 11:929–34.
54. Kahaly G, Forster G, Hansen C. Glycosaminoglycans in thyroid eye disease. Thyroid 1998; 8:429–32.
55. Kahaly G, Hansen C, Beyer J, et al. Plasma glycosaminoglycans in endocrine ophthalmopathy. J Endocrinol Invest 1994; 17:45–50.
56. Kahaly G, Hansen C, Felke B, et al. Immunohistochemical staining of retrobulbar adipose tissue in Graves' ophthalmopathy. Clin Immunol Immunopathol 1994; 73:53–62.
57. Kahaly G, Stover C, Otto E, et al. Glycosaminoglycans in thyroid-associated ophthalmopathy. Autoimmunity 1992; 13:81–88.
58. Kahaly GJ. Recent developments in Graves' ophthalmopathy imaging. J Endocrinol Invest 2004; 27:254–8.
59. Kaspar M, Archibald C, De BA, et al. Eye muscle antibodies and subtype of thyroid-associated ophthalmopathy. Thyroid 2002; 12:187–91.
60. Khurana AK, Sunder S, Ahluwalia BK, et al. Tear film profile in Graves' ophthalmopathy. Acta Ophthalmol (Copenh) 1992; 70:346–9.
61. Konno N, Yuri K, Taguchi H, et al. Screening for thyroid diseases in an iodine sufficient area with sensitive thyrotrophin assays, and serum thyroid autoantibody and urinary iodide determinations. Clin Endocrinol (Oxf) 1993; 38:273–81.
62. Krantic S, Goddard I, Saveanu A, et al. Novel modalities of somatostatin actions. Eur J Endocrinol 2004; 151: 643–55.
63. Krassas GE. Somatostatin analogs: a new tool for the management of Graves' ophthalmopathy. J Endocrinol Invest 2004; 27:281–7.
64. Kriss JP. Radioisotopic thyroidolymphography in patients with Graves' disease. J Clin Endocrinol Metab 1970; 31: 315–23.
65. Kubota S, Gunji K, Ackrell BA, et al. The 64-kilodalton eye muscle protein is the flavoprotein subunit of mitochondrial succinate dehydrogenase: the corresponding serum antibodies are good markers of an immune-mediated damage to the eye muscle in patients with Graves' hyperthyroidism. J Clin Endocrinol Metab 1998; 83:443–7.
66. Kumar S, Coenen MJ, Scherer PE, et al. Evidence for enhanced adipogenesis in the orbits of patients with Graves' ophthalmopathy. J Clin Endocrinol Metab 2004; 89:930–5.
67. Kung AW. Life events, daily stresses and coping in patients with Graves' disease. Clin Endocrinol (Oxf) 1995; 42:303–8.
68. Lawton NF. Exclusion of dysthyroid eye disease as a cause of unilateral proptosis. Trans Ophthalmol Soc UK 1979; 99:226–8.
69. Lazarus JH. Thyroid disorders associated with pregnancy: etiology, diagnosis, and management. Treat Endocrinol 2005; 4:31–41.
70. Levin F, Kazim M, Smith TJ, et al. Rosiglitazone-induced proptosis. Arch Ophthalmol 2005; 123:119–21.
71. Marcocci C, Bartalena L, Bogazzi F, et al. Studies on the occurrence of ophthalmopathy in Graves' disease. Acta Endocrinol (Copenh) 1989; 120:473–8.
72. Marino M, Barbesino G, Pinchera A, et al. Increased frequency of euthyroid ophthalmopathy in patients with Graves' disease associated with myasthenia gravis. Thyroid 2000; 10:799–802.
73. Marino M, Chiovato L, Lisi S, et al. Role of thyroglobulin in the pathogenesis of Graves' ophthalmopathy: the hypothesis of Kriss revisited. J Endocrinol Invest 2004; 27:230–6.
74. Marushak D, Faurschou S, Blichert-Toft M. Regression of ophthalmopathy in Graves' disease following thyroidectomy. A systematic study of changes of ocular signs. Acta Ophthalmol (Copenh) 1984; 62:767–79.
75. Matos-Santos A, Nobre EL, Costa JG, et al. Relationship between the number and impact of stressful life events and the onset of Graves' disease and toxic nodular goitre. Clin Endocrinol (Oxf) 2001; 55:15–9.
76. Maugendre D, Verite F, Guilhem I, et al. Anti-pancreatic autoimmunity and Graves' disease: study of a cohort of 600 Caucasian patients. Eur J Endocrinol 1997; 137: 503–10.
77. McLachlan SM, Nagayama Y, Rapoport B. Insight into Graves' hyperthyroidism from animal models. Endocr Rev 2005; 26:800–32.
78. Mizokami T, Wu Li A, El-Kaissi S, et al. Stress and thyroid autoimmunity. Thyroid 2004; 14:1047–55.
79. Mourits MP, Lombardo SH, van der Sluijs FA, et al. Reliability of exophthalmos measurement and the exophthalmometry value distribution in a healthy Dutch population and in Graves' patients. An exploratory study. Orbit 2004; 23:161–8.
80. Mourits MP, Prummel MF, Wiersinga WM, et al. Clinical activity score as a guide in the management of patients with Graves' ophthalmopathy. Clin Endocrinol (Oxf) 1997; 47:9–14.
81. Nagy EV, Toth J, Kaldi I, et al. Graves' ophthalmopathy: eye muscle involvement in patients with diplopia. Eur J Endocrinol 2000; 142:591–7.
82. Neigel JM, Rootman J, Belkin RI, et al. Dysthyroid optic neuropathy. The crowded orbital apex syndrome. Ophthalmology 1988; 95:1515–21.
83. Nishida Y, Tian S, Isberg B, et al. MRI measurements of orbital tissues in dysthyroid ophthalmopathy. Graefes Arch Clin Exp Ophthalmol 2001; 239:824–31.
84. Parle JV, Franklyn JA, Cross KW, et al. Prevalence and follow-up of abnormal thyrotrophin (TSH) concentrations in the elderly in the United Kingdom. Clin Endocrinol (Oxf) 1991; 34:77–83.
85. Pasquali D, Notaro A, Bonavolonta G, et al. Somatostatin receptor genes are expressed in lymphocytes from

retroorbital tissues in Graves' disease. J Clin Endocrinol Metab 2002; 87:5125–9.
86. Pasquali D, Vassallo P, Esposito D, et al. Somatostatin receptor gene expression and inhibitory effects of octreotide on primary cultures of orbital fibroblasts from Graves' ophthalmopathy. J Mol Endocrinol 2000; 25: 63–71.
87. Perros P, Kendall-Taylor P, Neoh C, et al. A prospective study of the effects of radioiodine therapy for hyperthyroidism in patients with minimally active graves' ophthalmopathy. J Clin Endocrinol Metab 2005; 90:5321–5323.
88. Postema PT, Krenning EP, Wijngaarde R, et al. [111 In-DTPA-D-Phe1] octreotide scintigraphy in thyroidal and orbital Graves' disease: a parameter for disease activity? J Clin Endocrinol Metab 1994; 79:1845–51.
89. Prabhakar BS, Bahn RS, Smith TJ. Current perspective on the pathogenesis of Graves' disease and ophthalmopathy. Endocr Rev 2003; 24:802–35.
90. Prahalad S, Shear ES, Thompson SD, et al. Increased prevalence of familial autoimmunity in simplex and multiplex families with juvenile rheumatoid arthritis. Arthritis Rheum 2002; 46:1851–6.
91. Pritchard J, Han R, Horst N, et al. Immunoglobulin activation of T cell chemoattractant expression in fibroblasts from patients with Graves' disease is mediated through the insulin-like growth factor I receptor pathway. J Immunol 2003; 170:6348–54.
92. Pritchard J, Horst N, Cruikshank W, et al. Igs from patients with Graves' disease induce the expression of T cell chemoattractants in their fibroblasts. J Immunol 2002; 168:942–50.
93. Prummel MF, Gerding MN, Zonneveld FW, et al. The usefulness of quantitative orbital magnetic resonance imaging in Graves' ophthalmopathy. Clin Endocrinol (Oxf) 2001; 54:205–9.
94. Prummel MF, Mourits MP, Berghout A, et al. Prednisone and cyclosporine in the treatment of severe Graves' ophthalmopathy. N Engl J Med 1989; 321:1353–9.
95. Prummel MF, Strieder T, Wiersinga WM. The environment and autoimmune thyroid diseases. Eur J Endocrinol 2004; 150:605–18.
96. Riemann CD, Foster JA, Kosmorsky GS. Direct orbital manometry in patients with thyroid-associated orbitopathy. Ophthalmology 1999; 106:1296–302.
97. Ruggeri RM, Galletti M, Mandolfino MG, et al. Thyroid hormone autoantibodies in primary Sjogren syndrome and rheumatoid arthritis are more prevalent than in autoimmune thyroid disease, becoming progressively more frequent in these diseases. J Endocrinol Invest 2002; 25:447–54.
98. Salvi M, Spaggiari E, Neri F, et al. The study of visual evoked potentials in patients with thyroid-associated ophthalmopathy identifies asymptomatic optic nerve involvement. J Clin Endocrinol Metab 1997; 82: 1027–30.
99. Savastano S, Pivonello R, Acampa W, et al. Recombinant thyrotropin-induced orbital uptake of [111In-diethylene-triamine-pentacetic acid-D-Phe1]octreotide in a patient with inactive Graves' ophthalmopathy. J Clin Endocrinol Metab 2005; 90:2440–4.
100. Schwartz KM, Fatourechi V, Ahmed DD, et al. Dermopathy of Graves' disease (pretibial myxedema): long-term outcome. J Clin Endocrinol Metab 2002; 87: 438–46.
101. Segni M, Bartley GB, Garrity JA, et al. Comparability of proptosis measurements by different techniques. Am J Ophthalmol 2002; 133:813–8.
102. Sharma OP. Sarcoidosis and other autoimmune disorders. Curr Opin Pulm Med 2002; 8:452–6.
103. Smith TJ. Novel aspects of orbital fibroblast pathology. J Endocrinol Invest 2004; 27:246–53.
104. Smith TJ. Insights into the role of fibroblasts in human autoimmune diseases. Clin Exp Immunol 2005; 141: 388–97.
105. Smith TJ, Hoa N. Immunoglobulins from patients with Graves' disease induce hyaluronan synthesis in their orbital fibroblasts through the self-antigen, insulin-like growth factor-I receptor. J Clin Endocrinol Metab 2004; 89:5076–80.
106. Smith TJ, Koumas L, Gagnon A, et al. Orbital fibroblast heterogeneity may determine the clinical presentation of thyroid-associated ophthalmopathy. J Clin Endocrinol Metab 2002; 87:385–92.
107. Sonino N, Girelli ME, Boscaro M, et al. Life events in the pathogenesis of Graves' disease. A controlled study. Acta Endocrinol (Copenh) 1993; 128:293–6.
108. Starkey K, Heufelder A, Baker G, et al. Peroxisome proliferator-activated receptor-gamma in thyroid eye disease: contraindication for thiazolidinedione use? J Clin Endocrinol Metab 2003; 88:55–9.
109. Strieder TG, Prummel MF, Tijssen JG, et al. Risk factors for and prevalence of thyroid disorders in a cross-sectional study among healthy female relatives of patients with autoimmune thyroid disease. Clin Endocrinol (Oxf) 2003; 59:396–401.
110. Tallstedt L, Lundell G, Blomgren H, et al. Does early administration of thyroxine reduce the development of Graves' ophthalmopathy after radioiodine treatment? Eur J Endocrinol 1994; 130:494–7.
111. Tallstedt L, Lundell G, Torring O, et al. Occurrence of ophthalmopathy after treatment for Graves' hyperthyroidism. The Thyroid Study Group. N Engl J Med 1992; 326:1733–8.
112. Tektonidou MG, Anapliotou M, Vlachoyiannopoulos P, et al. Presence of systemic autoimmune disorders in patients with autoimmune thyroid diseases. Ann Rheum Dis 2004; 63:1159–61.
113. Tunbridge WM, Evered DC, Hall R, et al. The spectrum of thyroid disease in a community: the Whickham survey. Clin Endocrinol (Oxf) 1977; 7:481–93.
114. Utech CI, Khatibnia U, Winter PF, et al. MR T2 relaxation time for the assessment of retrobulbar inflammation in Graves' ophthalmopathy. Thyroid 1995; 5:185–93.
115. Valyasevi RW, Erickson DZ, Harteneck DA, et al. Differentiation of human orbital preadipocyte fibroblasts induces expression of functional thyrotropin receptor. J Clin Endocrinol Metab 1999; 84:2557–62.
116. Valyasevi RW, Harteneck DA, Dutton CM, et al. Stimulation of adipogenesis, peroxisome proliferator-activated receptor-gamma (PPARgamma), and thyrotropin receptor by PPARgamma agonist in human orbital preadipocyte fibroblasts. J Clin Endocrinol Metab 2002; 87:2352–8.
117. Valyasevi RW, Jyonouchi SC, Dutton CM, et al. Effect of tumor necrosis factor-alpha, interferon-gamma, and transforming growth factor-beta on adipogenesis and expression of thyrotropin receptor in human orbital preadipocyte fibroblasts. J Clin Endocrinol Metab 2001; 86:903–8.
118. Vanderpump MP, Tunbridge WM, French JM, et al. The incidence of thyroid disorders in the community: a twenty-year follow-up of the Whickham Survey. Clin Endocrinol (Oxf) 1995; 43:55–68.
119. Vardi P, Modan-Mozes D, Ish-Shalom S, et al. Low titer, competitive insulin autoantibodies are spontaneously

produced in autoimmune diseases of the thyroid. Diab Res Clin Pract 1993; 21:161–6.
120. Weetman AP. Determinants of autoimmune thyroid disease. Nat Immunol 2001; 2:769–70.
121. Weetman AP, Cohen S, Gatter KC, et al. Immunohistochemical analysis of the retrobulbar tissues in Graves' ophthalmopathy. Clin Exp Immunol 1989; 75:222–7.
122. Weightman DR, Perros P, Sherif IH, et al. Autoantibodies to IGF-1 binding sites in thyroid associated ophthalmopathy. Autoimmunity 1993; 16:251–7.
123. Weizer JS, Lee AG, Coats DK. Myasthenia gravis with ocular involvement in older patients. Can J Ophthalmol 2001; 36:26–33.
124. Werner SC. Modification of the classification of the eye changes of Graves' disease: recommendations of the Ad Hoc Committee of the American Thyroid Association. J Clin Endocrinol Metab 1977; 44:203–4.
125. Wiersinga WM, Bartalena L. Epidemiology and prevention of Graves' ophthalmopathy. Thyroid 2002; 12:855–60.
126. Wiersinga WM, Prummel MF, Terwee CB. Effects of Graves' ophthalmopathy on quality of life. J Endocrinol Invest 2004; 27:259–64.
127. Wiersinga WM, Smit T, van der Gaag R, et al. Temporal relationship between onset of Graves' ophthalmopathy and onset of thyroidal Graves' disease. J Endocrinol Invest 1988; 11:615–9.
128. Wiersinga WM, Smit T, van der Gaag R, et al. Clinical presentation of Graves' ophthalmopathy. Ophthalmic Res 1989; 21:73–82.
129. Winsa B, Adami HO, Bergstrom R, et al. Stressful life events and Graves' disease. Lancet 1991; 338:1475–9.

48

Metabolic Disorders Involving Metals

Alec Garner
Institute of Ophthalmology, Moorfields Eye Hospital, London, U.K.

George M. Cherian
Departments of Pathology, Pharmacology, and Toxicology, University of Western Ontario, London, Ontario, Canada

J. Godfrey Heathcote
Departments of Pathology and Ophthalmology and Visual Sciences, Dalhousie University, Halifax, Nova Scotia, Canada

INTRODUCTION

Several metals such as zinc, copper, and iron are essential for normal cellular functions and tissue metabolism. However, the accumulation of excessive amounts of these essential metals in cells, as a result of metabolic disorders or abnormal exposure, can cause tissue damage. The eye is a potential target organ for many chemicals including metals. Foreign bodies composed of iron or copper can produce marked degenerative changes in the eye and excessive amounts of cobalt can result in cataractous lens changes in laboratory animals (1). Fumes and salts of metals can act as external irritants giving rise to conjunctivitis and corneal ulceration. In addition, exposure to non-essential metals like gold, silver, and mercury can result in characteristic discoloration of the cornea or lens. Nevertheless, since the eye is protected by two physiological barriers, the blood–retinal and blood–aqueous barriers, the toxicity of metals depends not only on the exposure levels but also on the permeability of these barriers. Certain metabolic disorders either inherited or acquired, can affect the deposition of metals in the eye and cause damage. This chapter will describe ocular disorders caused by either deficiencies or increased amounts of the essential metals.

CALCIUM

Calcium is an essential metal required for several biological functions including signal transduction and apoptosis (see Chapter 2). Ocular lesions can result from either too much or too little calcium in the circulation and tissues.

Hypercalcemia

Hypercalcemia can result from excessive secretion of parathormone (PTH) by a parathyroid tumor or primary hyperplasia or secondarily from hypervitaminosis D, sarcoidosis, multiple myeloma, certain carcinomas, and a number of other disorders. PTH acts primarily on the kidney and on bone where it promotes increased calcium reabsorption by the renal tubules and release of calcium from the skeleton. Vitamin D also acts at a number of sites but dietary excess mainly affects the intestinal absorption of calcium. Sarcoidosis appears to induce an increased sensitivity to vitamin D (111). The hypercalcemia associated with malignant neoplasia is often, but not always, attributable to osteolytic metastases.

Genetic disorders such as the infantile (MIM #241500), childhood (MIM #241510), and adult (MIM #1476300) variants of hypophosphatasia and Alport syndrome (MIM #301050) (82) can result in hypercalcemia with ocular complications. The infantile and childhood types of hypophosphatasia are autosomal recessive disorders with a decreased alkaline phosphatase activity. The associated hypercalcemia reflects reduced incorporation of calcium into bone because of inability to hydrolyze inorganic pyrophosphate, which serves as an inhibitor of hydroxyapatite crystal formation in the absence of adequate levels of alkaline phosphatase (42). Corneal and conjunctival calcification is a recognized complication and other problems include cataract and atypical retinitis pigmentosa (12,70,108). Alport syndrome exhibits a variable pattern of inheritance and is characterized by renal dysfunction, neural deafness, and a range of ocular problems, especially in the lens (49). Calcium deposition in the conjunctiva can occur as renal failure develops and may be associated with a foreign body response (13). Calcium deposition in the conjunctiva and peripheral cornea has been reported in other patients with renal failure and may be associated with both hypercalcemia and hypocalcemia (66).

In general, the ocular complications of hypercalcemia reflect metastatic deposition of hydroxyapatite in the cornea (7), although calcification of the extrinsic muscles of the eye has been described (56). Calcification of the cornea starts at the nasal and temporal peripheries and gradually spreads to form a band-shaped opacity in the line of the interpalpebral fissure (25). Initially, the deposits appear as fine basophilic particles in Bowman layer before extending to the superficial stromal lamellae. This anatomical distribution may reflect loss of carbon dioxide from the interpalpebral region with consequent rise in pH and decreased solubility of calcium salts (23,101).

Sclerochoroidal calcification is an uncommon entity that may be associated with hypercalcemia (Table 1). The condition, which may be bilateral and multifocal, is usually an incidental finding on ophthalmoscopic examination but may be mistaken for a choroidal metastasis, an amelanotic melanocytic lesion, or choroidal lymphoma (60). The lesions are generally circular, yellowish plaques in the post-equatorial and supero-temporal fundus, ranging up to approximately 8 mm in diameter and 3 mm in thickness.

Table 1 Causes of Sclerochoroidal Calcification

Primary, idiopathic
Secondary, dystrophic
Severe ocular trauma
Chronic inflammation
Secondary, metastatic
Hyperparathyroidism
Hypervitaminosis D
Calcium pyrophosphate deposition disease
Inherited renal disorders

They may be associated with RPE changes, particularly atrophy, and occasionally subretinal fluid (60). Some insight into the formation of these calcific plaques has come from the study of metabolic disorders, particularly Bartter syndrome (MIM #601678, #241200, #607364) and Gitelman syndrome (MIM #263800) which have been associated with sclerochoroidal calcification (60,77,119). These renal tubular hypokalemic–metabolic alkalosis syndromes are characterized by hypomagnesemia. Magnesium ions are necessary for the production of calcium pyrophosphate and also increase its solubility; the hypomagnesemia in these syndromes may provoke deposition of calcium pyrophosphate in the eye as well as in the joints (60). The only histopathological description of sclerochoroidal calcification confirmed the presence of calcium pyrophosphate within the deposits (29).

Hypocalcemia

As with hypercalcemia, low levels of serum calcium also result from indirect effects on calcium metabolism produced by hypoparathyroidism, thyroid surgery, or changes in vitamin D concentration, rather than variations in calcium-binding proteins. Chronic renal failure can impair the conversion of 25-hydroxycholecalciferol to its active form 1,25-dihydroxycholecalciferol by the renal tubular epithelium (35) and thereby affect calcium metabolism.

Bilateral cataracts are the most frequent ocular complication of the hypocalcemia associated with hypoparathyroidism (9,94). Typically, the cataracts present as numerous small discrete opacities in the anterior and posterior cortices of the lens. Although the exact mechanisms involved are not understood, osmotic changes resulting from ionic imbalance have been implicated (14) and the ability of parathyroid hormone to regulate lens capsule permeability to calcium has been known for many years (23). Hypocalcemia associated with mild nuclear cataracts and dystrophic calcification of blood vessels has been linked to a missense mutation in the murine *Gprc2a* gene on chromosome 16 (61). The CASR gene encodes an extracellular calcium-sensing receptor (CaSR), which regulates PTH secretion and renal tubular reabsorption of calcium in response to the ambient extracellular concentration of calcium. Other reported ophthalmic effects of hypocalcemia include ptosis and impaired ocular motility, pigmentary retinopathy (36), and optic disc changes suggestive of ischemic optic neuritis (4). Hypocalcemia associated with chronic renal failure can also result in conjunctival calcification that may impinge on the periphery of the cornea (8,54,101). The conjunctival predilection for calcification, the foreign body reaction, and ocular irritation with which it is frequently linked, remain unexplained (8).

COPPER

Copper is an essential metal involved in multiple metabolic processes and is required for growth and development in mammals. At high concentrations, however, it can be toxic. There are two inherited human diseases with defective copper metabolism, one characterized by chronic accumulation of copper in tissues (Wilson disease) and the other by low copper levels because of defects in absorption (Menkes disease). In these diseases, the abnormal copper metabolism is caused by mutations in copper transport proteins, P-type ATPases, which are involved in absorption, distribution, and excretion of copper (97).

Wilson Disease

Wilson disease (hepatolenticular degeneration, MIM #277900) is an autosomal recessive copper toxicosis with an incidence of 1 in 50,000–100,000, depending on the population (31). This disease was first described by Kinnear Wilson in 1912 (53) and is characterized by an accumulation of copper in the liver, followed by deposition in the renal tubules, brain, cornea, and other tissues. Diagnostic copper deposits can be detected in the cornea (described independently in 1903 by Kayser and by Fleischer). In this disease, the biliary excretion of copper is impaired and there is reduced incorporation of copper into ceruloplasmin. Consequently, plasma levels of copper are usually low (<1.0 μmol/L), any circulating copper being only loosely bound to the plasma albumin and readily deposited in the tissues.

The *ATP7B* gene responsible for Wilson disease is located on chromosome 13 (13q14.3) and has been shown to span about 80 kb (99). This gene encodes a copper transport P-type ATPase (127). It has been shown by two different groups that the *ATP7B* gene product is located in the trans-Golgi network of hepatocytes when concentrations of copper are low, distributed to cytoplasmic vesicles when cells are exposed to high concentrations, and then recycled to the trans-Golgi network when copper is removed (63,112). Different types of mutations have been identified in the Wilson disease gene (129). The most frequent missense mutation is His1069Gln and this is present in at least one-third of Wilson disease patients from northern and eastern Europe (75,114). An Asp1270Ser mutation has been found in 61% of patients in Costa Rica and is associated with fulminant hepatic failure (114). Molecular genetic analysis has provided a means to detect carriers and to make an early diagnosis of the disease (76).

The deposition of copper in the cornea to form the characteristic Kayser–Fleischer ring occurs early in the course of the disease and is generally contemporaneous with involvement of the basal ganglia (140). Nevertheless, it may occur in patients who are pre-symptomatic (74,105). The ring begins as an arc at the upper periphery of the cornea, followed by a similar arc in the lower cornea, before a complete circle, variably green to brown, is formed. The copper is incorporated into Descemet membrane, its presence having been confirmed by histochemistry (134) and electron probe analysis (131). The granular metallic deposits tend to be arranged in a linear fashion (Fig. 1), suggesting that copper enters the cornea by diffusion from the anterior chamber (55). The precise nature of the copper in the basement membrane is not known but it appears to be in a chelated form associated with the proteoglycan component. There is also evidence that the formation of discrete granules is preceded by a combination with a sulfur-containing component (65). The initial deposition in superior and inferior arcs has been attributed to slower forward diffusion of fluid in areas of the cornea covered by the eyelids, where surface evaporation is least. This would produce relative stagnation and an increased opportunity for copper deposition (134). Wilson disease can be controlled by treatment with chelating agents such as penicillamine and the corneal changes are reversible. It should be noted that Kayser–Fleischer rings can complicate other acquired disorders where there is high local concentration of copper (144).

A majority of Wilson disease patients develop Kayser–Fleischer rings but a smaller proportion, about 17% in one study, also develop greenish cataracts (140). These are similar to those produced by copper-containing foreign bodies within the eye, in which the distribution of copper in the anterior capsule has been likened to a sunflower (15). However, in a case examined by transmission electron microscopy (TEM) (132), the metallic deposits were most obvious close to the lenticular epithelium, rather than on the free surface of the capsule, suggesting that deposition may be related to cellular activity and not just diffusion. Abnormalities of cellular copper metabolism may also contribute to reversible retinal dysfunction in Wilson disease (109).

Menkes Disease

Menkes disease (X-linked copper malabsorption syndrome, MIM #309400) is an X-linked recessive copper deficiency syndrome first described in 1962 that occurs with a frequency of about 1 in 200,000 (84,130). The genetic defect results in impaired absorption of dietary copper and a severe disturbance in the intracellular transport of copper, resulting in a generalized deficiency (31–33). Enzymes that require copper for their function become inactive or have reduced activity. Characteristically, affected male infants develop whitish, luster-less, short kinky hair within a few weeks of birth, together with skeletal abnormalities and progressive neuromuscular dysfunction. In untreated cases death ensues within 2–3 years. The Menkes disease gene (*ATP7A*) has been mapped to the q13 region of the X-chromosome. Analysis of cDNA reveals that the gene codes for a 1500 amino acid protein, which is a P-type ATPase responsible for the translocation of copper across membranes (19,85,139). Menkes disease mutations occur in the *ATP7A* gene, which is highly expressed in the duodenum and is responsible for transport of copper across intestinal mucosa (26). Central to the metabolic disturbance is abnormal intracellular transport of copper and its excessive retention within fibroblasts and other cells bound to metallothionein, a sulfur-rich 10 kDa protein (69). Thus, there is reduced availability of copper for incorporation into copper-dependent enzyme systems. Both the Menkes and Wilson ATPases have six copper-binding sites (CBS1–CBS6) in their N-terminal region. These sites are not essential for copper transport, although CBS5 and CBS6 are essential for the copper-induced trafficking of the proteins within cells. Paulsen et al. (98) described a patient with an unusually mild form of Menkes disease in which the serum copper and ceruloplasmin were reduced by 50%, rather than the 90% typically seen in the classical form. In this case the mutation in ATP7A resulted in a truncated protein that was partially functional by virtue of reinitiation of translation downstream from the premature termination codon.

In the ophthalmic context, the eyebrows are sparse with twisted and broken hairs, and the eyelashes are variably depigmented, scanty, and stubby. This defect, as with the pathognomonic kinky hair abnormality in general, is attributable to inadequate disulfide bonding because of reduced amine oxidase activity (57). Deficient tyrosinase activity is linked with impaired melanin formation in the skin and RPE (147). Abnormalities of Bruch membrane reflect inadequate cross-linkage of elastin through a deficiency of copper-dependent lysyl oxidase activity. Neuroretinal abnormalities are also common in the form of ganglion cell loss and nerve fiber loss associated with myelin deficiency in the optic nerve (113,147). These changes are reflected in an abnormal electroretinogram (ERG) and diminished visually evoked response (72). The neuronal disturbance is probably multifactorial since copper is needed for cytochrome oxidase-dependent energy metabolism in the mitochondria (72) as well as myelin formation (40). Copper-deficient rats suffer a comparable demyelination affecting the post-laminar part of the optic nerve, together with neuronal swelling and vacuolation in the prelaminar region (30).

Other Abnormalities of Copper Deposition

Ocular copper deposition can result from endogenous or exogenous sources. Pigmented corneal rings with an appearance similar to the Kayser–Fleischer ring have been linked to altered copper metabolism in primary biliary cirrhosis, chronic aggressive hepatitis, and cirrhosis (43). Exogenous copper deposition can result from chalcosis and copper sulfate drops. Chronic chalcosis occurs when ocular foreign bodies have a high (85%) copper content and the affinity of copper for basement membranes results in heterochromia and blue/green-stained corneal endothelium and Descemet membrane. Copper sulfate drops previously used to treat trachoma have been reported to cause greenish deposits in peripheral cornea, as well as lens deposits (10). Golden-brown, metallic dust-like deposits on the central region of Descemet membrane and the anterior and posterior lens capsule, associated with hypergammaglobulinemia and hypercupremia, have been described in patients with multiple myeloma and pulmonary carcinoma (3,39,47,74,79). Goodman et al. (47) reported a case of multiple myeloma with serum copper levels 10–20 times above normal. The central copper deposits in the eye were thought to arise as a result of high levels of a protein–copper complex in the aqueous humor, rather than by diffusion from the corneoscleral limbal circulation as occurs with the peripheral deposits in Descemet membrane in Wilson disease. Lewis et al. (73) described a 41-year-old woman with anemia, asymptomatic multiple myeloma, hypercupremia, and defective color vision. In a 60-year old man with adenocarcinoma of the lung, hypergammaglobulinemia and hypercupremia, pathological examination of a conjunctival biopsy revealed extracellular granules in the substantia propria that stained for copper with rhodamine (79).

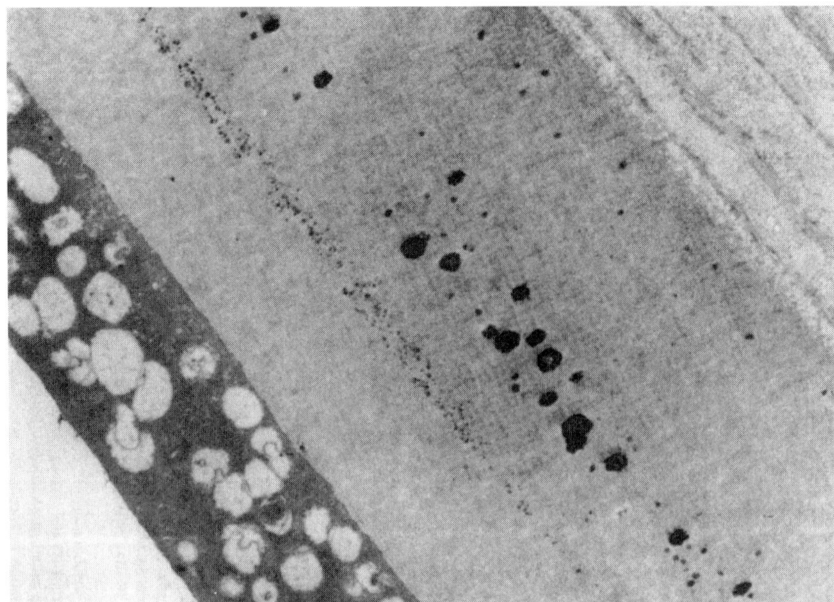

Figure 1 Kayser–Fleischer ring. Electron micrograph of posterior cornea showing granular deposits of copper in Descemet membrane. The linear distribution of the metal with intervening uninvolved areas is suggestive of phasic deposition (Uranyl acetate–lead citrate, ×7,500). *Source*: Courtesy of Harry J, Tripathi RC. Kayser–Fleischer ring: a pathological study. Br J Ophthalmol 1970; 54:794–800.

In addition, TEM demonstrated electron-dense material in the corneal epithelium, the posterior part of Descemet membrane, the fibroblasts and epithelium of the conjunctiva, and the anterior lens capsule. In another case study (102), a patient with blurred vision and a monoclonal gammopathy, but without evidence of underlying malignancy, had bilateral golden-brown, metallic dust-like deposits on the central region of Descemet membrane, and the anterior and posterior lens capsule. Laboratory investigations revealed an elevated serum copper level (10 times greater than normal) and a normal ceruloplasmin level; the major copper-binding fraction was serum IgG. The cause of the hypercupremia in these cases remains uncertain, although three possible mechanisms have been proposed (47): increased intestinal copper absorption alone, increased intestinal copper absorption from abnormal binding of copper to IgG, or the presence of an unusual copper-binding IgG in plasma.

Several childhood copper toxicoses such as Indian childhood cirrhosis have been described and are often associated with excess intake of copper in infancy (123). It has been suggested that this disease is caused by the early introduction of cow or buffalo milk contaminated with copper from brass utensils to children in small rural communities (122). There are no studies on the ocular deposition of copper in these children.

IRON

Local deposition of iron in the corneal epithelium is a relatively common occurrence and in approximately 80% of cases is associated with irregularities of the ocular surface. The tears contain about 80–90 mg/100 mL of iron and they are the likely source of these deposits, since the tears pool within these irregularities (5).

Ocular changes in disorders of iron overload, which may be primary (Table 2) or secondary to conditions such as chronic liver disease, multiple blood transfusions, or long-term hemodialysis, are uncommon but there has been increasing interest in the role of iron in diseases such as age-related macular degeneration (AMD) (see Chapter 18).

Hemochromatosis

Hereditary hemochromatosis (MIM +235200) is a clinical syndrome that affects 1 in 400 and has a carrier frequency of 1 in 10 people of northern European descent. A positive iron balance of 1–2 mg/day leads to iron deposition and eventually multi-organ dysfunction. Hemosiderin deposition in the skin, liver, and pancreas gives rise to the classical triad of skin pigmentation, hepatic cirrhosis, and diabetes mellitus. A distinct male preponderance is likely because of the female capacity to deplete iron stores through menstruation. The condition is treatable if detected early.

Mutations in at least four genes (*HFE, TFR2, SLC40A1, HAMP*) have been shown to give rise to this phenotype but the commonest form of hemochromatosis is an autosomal recessive disorder caused by mutations in the *HFE* gene on human chromosome 6 (6p) and the *HFE* protein is closely related to the major histocompatibility complex class 1 molecules (64,100). Mutations linked to the HFE gene are either homozygous substitutions of a single base resulting in a

Table 2 Causes of Primary Iron Overload

Hemochromatosis
Mutations in the *HFE* gene: encodes HFE protein
Cys282Thr homozygosity
Cys282Thr/His63Asp compound heterozygosity
Hereditary iron overload
Mutation in the *SLC11A3* gene: encodes ferroportin
Mutation in the *TfR2* gene: encodes transferrin receptor 2
Aceruloplasminemia
>30 Mutations in the ceruloplasmin gene
Congenital atransferrinemia
Miscellaneous

change from cysteine to tyrosine at residue 282 (Cys282Tyr) or a compound heterozygous substitution such that Cys282Tyr is accompanied by replacement of a histidine by aspartic acid at a different residue (His63Asp). Cys282Tyr heterozygosity alone is not a significant risk factor for iron overload (87). The mutations prevent the correct folding of the HFE protein, which fails to assemble with β2-macroglobulin and to take up its normal position at the cell surface. The mechanism by which the abnormal protein causes excessive uptake of iron by cells of the intestinal villi is gradually becoming clearer (100). It is important to note that, because of incomplete penetrance, the presence of the mutations does not mean that a person has hemochromatosis but rather is susceptible to developing the phenotype.

It is unclear whether the ocular complications in hemochromatosis are primary or secondary to diabetic retinopathy. In a few cases, iron deposition has been described in the ciliary epithelium and sclera, but with no symptoms or corneal involvement (107). Iron has also been recognized in the RPE in both primary and secondary hemochromatosis (37) and conjunctival microaneurysms have also been reported (59,62). Increased pigmentation of the conjunctiva and eyelid margins caused by melanin in the basal layer of epithelium is a feature in about 30% of cases (34). Iron overload from primary hemochromatosis has been identified as a possible risk factor for rhino-orbito-cerebral zygomycosis (83) (see Chapter 11).

Deferoxamine Therapy and Ocular Toxicity

Deferoxamine is a specific chelating agent of trivalent anions (iron and aluminum), and has been used for more than 30 years for the treatment of hemochromatosis, secondary hemosiderosis, and aluminum intoxication associated with chronic kidney failure. There are a few reports on ocular toxicity during treatment, although the cause is unclear and the toxicity could be due to the underlying disease as well as a direct effect of the drug. Toxic effects have included a gradual loss of visual acuity and pigmentary anomalies near the macula, such as mottling and dispersion, with altered electrophysiological recordings (121). Termination of the treatment did not result in improvement of symptoms but the occurrence of these changes suggests a need for regular ophthalmological monitoring combined with electrophysiological studies before and during treatment with deferoxamine.

Hyperferritinemia–Cataract Syndrome

Hyperferritinemia–cataract syndrome (HCS, MIM #600886) is an autosomal dominant disorder that is characterized by elevated serum ferritin in the absence of iron overload and the early onset of bilateral cataracts (6). Ferritin is a heteropolymer of two subunits: H (heavy)-ferritin and L (light)-ferritin that combine to form a protein shell in which iron atoms are stored. Ferritin synthesis is regulated at translation through the interaction of a cytoplasmic iron regulatory protein (IRP) and an iron-responsive element (IRE) in the mRNA of ferritin, such that when iron is in limited supply, IRP binds to the IRE and ferritin synthesis decreases (116). HCS is caused by a variety of mutations in the IRE of the ferritin light chain gene on chromosome 19 which reduces the binding of IRP and results in increased L-ferritin synthesis (71).

Ophthalmologists should consider this syndrome in patients with congenital or juvenile cataract, since the early onset of bilateral cataracts is the only clinically demonstrable abnormality in HCS (18,89). The cataracts have been described as punctate, white, breadcrumb-like opacities in the lens nucleus and cortex (18) and may be caused by deposition of L-ferritin (89,135). Mumford et al. (89) described amorphous deposits in the lens nucleus that reacted with an antibody to L-ferritin. On TEM these have a square-crystalline appearance. It is still unclear where the L-ferritin deposits originate since L-ferritin does not form aggregates in vitro (71). L-ferritin mRNA is present in normal lens fiber cells and is increased in murine hereditary nuclear cataract (20) so local biosynthesis in conjunction with some conformational change may be needed (89).

Aceruloplasminemia

Aceruloplasminemia (MIM #604290), an autosomal recessive condition, is characterized by virtually complete absence of ceruloplasmin from the serum, neurological degeneration, and the accumulation of iron in the liver, pancreas, and brain (68). It presents by the fourth and fifth decade and is fatal. There have been reports of a pigmentary retinopathy in Japanese families with aceruloplasminemia (86,88) but no histopathological descriptions. A maculopathy, clinically resembling AMD has been observed in a 47-year-old Caucasian male with the condition (38).

Ceruloplasmin is a glycoprotein of MW 132 kDa. The single polypeptide binds six atoms of copper and functions as a copper transport protein in the plasma. In addition, it has a specific role as a ferroxidase and is responsible for converting ferrous (Fe^{2+}) to ferric (Fe^{3+}) iron so that the latter can bind to transferrin (67). It also inhibits Fe^{2+}-stimulated lipid peroxidation and is a scavenger of reactive oxygen species (68). Ceruloplasmin does not cross the blood–brain or blood–retinal barrier but is synthesized locally in retina and brain by perivascular glial cells and it has been identified on the surface of astrocytes in the brain (67,96). It has been suggested that the molecule is responsible for local distribution and oxidation of iron within these tissues; in the absence of ceruloplasmin, ferrous iron accumulates with resultant tissue damage (67). Mice with a mutation in the ceruloplasmin gene (*Cp–/–*) show impaired handling of iron in the liver and brain, but in contrast to the human disease, do not show significant iron overload in the brain or neurological deterioration (52). Hephaestin is another membrane-bound copper ferroxidase with a similar structure to ceruloplasmin and may be able to compensate for the ceruloplasmin deficiency in these mice. A combined deficiency of ceruloplasmin and hephaestin has been shown to result in retinal iron accumulation and after 6–9 months retinal degeneration, with death of RPE cells, loss of the outer nuclear layer, and a subretinal neovascular membrane (52).

Over 30 mutations in the ceruloplasmin gene have now been described in over 40 families with aceruloplasminemia (68). The missense mutation Pro177Arg in a Japanese family results in the biosynthesis of a ceruloplasmin molecule that is retained within the endoplasmic reticulum and does not reach the cell membrane. The missense mutation Gly631Arg described in a Dutch family results in ceruloplasmin that is unable to bind copper.

Cerebrohepatorenal Syndrome

Cerebrohepatorenal syndrome (Zellweger syndrome, MIM #214100) was first described by Zellweger and his colleagues (11), and excessive amounts of iron were found in the tissues. Hence, for a time it was considered that this was fundamental to the pathogenesis of the condition (93,117,137). It has now been established that the condition is a disorder of peroxisomal biogenesis caused by mutations in the *PEX1* gene responsible for the synthesis of peroxisomal proteins (peroxins) (27,141). The condition is incompatible with life beyond a few months and affected infants have a characteristic facial appearance caused by a high forehead with malformed external ears, flat supraorbital ridges, and epicanthal folds (11,46,93,97). A CNS disturbance in the form of hypotonia is a constant feature (93,97), as are hepatomegaly and renal cysts. Among the ocular abnormalities reported are: corneal opacification, glaucoma, cataract, Brushfield spots, and optic nerve atrophy (45,50,118). Cataracts are common, and one report alludes to the presence of curvilinear bodies at the corticonuclear interface in a TEM study of the lens of a heterozygote carrier of the syndrome (58). A rapidly progressive retinal dystrophy associated with extinction of the ERG is a frequent feature and this appears to be due to the loss of photoreceptor outer segments and degeneration of the RPE (24,46).

Unusually large amounts of iron have been reported in a number of tissues, especially the liver and kidneys (93,137), together with raised levels of iron in the serum (117). However, the total body iron in Zellweger syndrome (about 115 mg/kg) represents less than a 50% increase, which is negligible in comparison with the 25- to 50-fold elevation typical of hemochromatosis, and the increased amounts of iron in the tissues may simply reflect deficient utilization secondary to growth retardation (97). In two reported cases in whom appropriate stains were performed, iron was demonstrated in the corneal and non-pigmented ciliary body epithelia in one instance (138) but not in the other (50).

ZINC

High concentrations of zinc are found within the eye, particularly in the retina and choroid. Zinc is required for the maintenance of cellular membrane stability and the biosynthesis of nucleic acids and proteins. It is a structural component of transcription factors with a zinc finger (a DNA-binding protein that resembles a finger with a base binding to a zinc ion). Many of these functions are of ophthalmic importance, such as the maintenance of disc structure in photoreceptor outer segments (48). In addition, several metalloenzymes in the eye are dependent on zinc for their catalytic activity. These include antioxidants such as catalase; retinol dehydrogenase in RPE cells involved in the regeneration of rhodopsin; α-mannosidase, and alkaline phosphatase involved in the metabolism of phagocytosed outer segments; and matrix metalloproteinases involved in the turnover of Bruch membrane (133). Neuronal activity causes release of zinc in synaptic vesicles into the extracellular space in both retina and brain and there is good evidence that the metal modulates neural transmission in the retina (106) and has a neuroprotective function (133).

Despite its essential role in normal neural function, zinc may also cause neurotoxicity in the retina, as well as the brain. The likelihood of toxicity depends not only on the local concentration of the metal but also on its location (intracellular vs. extracellular) and state (free vs. protein-bound). Elevated zinc concentrations appear to expose neurons to increased oxidative stress with resultant accumulation of reactive oxygen species and lipid peroxidation (149). In retinal ischemia there is a loss of zinc homeostasis. Zinc accumulates in the degenerating neurons and its subsequent release into the extracellular space may cause further neuronal death (133).

The adverse effects of high concentrations of zinc must be balanced against its essential metabolic functions. Zinc deficiency has been reported in a wide variety of cultivated plants and animals, with severe effects on all stages of reproduction, growth, and tissue proliferation. In developing countries zinc deficiency is widespread in children. The human health problems associated with zinc deficiency are numerous, and include neurosensory changes, oligospermia, growth retardation, delayed wound healing, immune disorders, and dermatitis. These conditions are generally reversible with zinc supplementation (145).

A low serum concentration of zinc is a common feature of Crohn disease and may be caused by reduced dietary intake and/or impaired absorption. Since almost all zinc is intracellular and serum zinc is bound to albumin, which itself may be reduced in Crohn disease, the low serum concentration may not reflect a true deficiency (80). Nevertheless, retinal dysfunction has been linked to zinc deficiency in Crohn disease. Myung et al. (90) reported the case of a young woman with a severe exacerbation of the inflammatory bowel disease requiring total parenteral nutrition that provided a daily intake of 3 mg of zinc. After 1 week skin lesions characteristic of acrodermatitis enteropathica appeared and these were accompanied by a sudden decline in visual acuity to 20/50 in both eyes. At this time her serum zinc concentration was 58 μg/dL (normal, 70–150 μg/dL). Following intravenous zinc supplementation for 2 weeks, the serum zinc concentration rose to 140 μg/dL and both the skin lesions and the visual dysfunction resolved completely.

Acrodermatitis enteropathica (MIM #201100) is an autosomal recessive condition that presents in early infancy with dermatitis and persistent diarrhea. It is caused by mutations in the *SLC39A4* gene on chromosome 8 (8q24.3) that controls zinc absorption from the intestine (120). The skin lesions develop in a symmetrical pattern around the body orifices and on the fingers and toes and take the form of a bullous pustular dermatitis. Recurrent infections reflect impaired immune efficiency associated with thymic atrophy and T-cell dysfunction (2,120). In the absence of treatment in the form of zinc supplementation, the disease is usually fatal.

Photophobia, impaired dark adaptation, and reduced visual acuity are the principal ocular symptoms (17), and histological examination may reveal RPE degeneration at the posterior pole (16). The eyelids share in the general skin disturbance, presenting with a vesicular eruption that later becomes psoriasiform, and accompanying conjunctivitis is usual (17). Less commonly, the corneal epithelium is affected and erosion of Bowman zone can result with scarring of the immediately subjacent stroma (81,143,146). An unexplained clinical finding in each of these reports has been the presence of linear opacities radiating from the center of the cornea, which disappear following treatment of the underlying condition. Cataract formation has also been reported (17,103).

An understanding of the mutations in the *SLC39A4* gene, which encodes the intestinal zinc-specific transporter, has made the molecular mechanisms involved in the pathogenesis of acrodermatitis enteropathica clearer (142). The gene encodes Zip4 protein, a member of the ZIP family of metal-ion transporters, which accumulates at the apical surfaces of enterocytes. Comparative studies of six different missense mutations in the gene have revealed a number of mechanisms through which zinc uptake by enterocytes is reduced. These include alterations in the amount of Zip4 synthesized; changes in the molecular size of Zip4 caused by different degrees of N-glycosylation; reduction in transport capacity; failure to respond to changes in zinc concentration, and retention of newly synthesized Zip4 in the endoplasmic reticulum of the enterocytes (142).

MECHANISMS OF METAL TOXICITY AND PROTECTIVE MECHANISMS

The excessive deposition of transition metals such as copper and iron in tissues can generate toxic free radicals by the Fenton reaction and these can oxidize most organic compounds near the site of their generation (128). Reactive oxygen free radicals can disturb the normal redox balance of the cell and shift it to a state of oxidative stress, causing various types of cellular damage. Reactive oxygen intermediates have been implicated in degenerative diseases of the eye, including retinopathy, cataractogenesis, and macular degeneration. However, most tissues, including the eye have defensive mechanisms to control the generation of free radicals. The generation of hydrogen peroxide during phagocytosis may act as an intracellular signal in RPE that leads to increased activity of key antioxidant enzymes, such as superoxide dismutases, catalases, glutathione peroxidase, and thioredoxin peroxidase, and other proteins important for protecting the cells from oxidative stress (104). Most cells can also induce anti-oxidant proteins such as metallothionein which can bind with metals like copper or trap free radicals (21).

Metallothioneins

Metallothionein was first isolated by Margoshes and Vallee in 1957 as a thiol-rich cadmium binding protein from equine renal cortex (78). Since then four different isoforms of metallothionein have been identified in mammals. In addition, metallothioneins have been found in many living systems, including fish, birds, plants, fungi, and yeast. These proteins have a high content of cysteine (about 30%) and a high affinity for all group 11 and 12 metals, especially zinc and copper. They can also bind with divalent mercury and monovalent silver atoms. Mammalian metallothioneins can bind with 7 atoms of zinc or cadmium tetrahedrally and these metals are distributed in two clusters in the protein. The functions proposed for this protein include storage of essential metals, protection against toxic metals such as cadmium and mercury, and protection against free radicals (110).

In mammals, metallothionein is mainly found in liver and kidney, but it is also found in brain, intestine, pancreas, reproductive organs, heart, skin, and eye. High levels of the protein bound to zinc and copper are found in fetal and neonatal liver (95). Metallothionein can sequester copper and thus reduce its toxicity: high concentrations of copper-saturated metallothioneins have been isolated from the livers affected by Wilson disease (91). There are several reports demonstrating the expression of metallothionein isoforms in human RPE (125,126) and also in the retina of *Cynomolgus* monkeys during early onset of macular degeneration (92). These studies suggest that induced synthesis of proteins such as metallothionein may play an important role in protecting retinal cells from oxidative stress induced by metals.

Transition Metals and Retinal Degeneration

As discussed above, free iron is highly toxic and stimulates the production of reactive oxygen species. Iron homeostasis is maintained by a variety of regulatory proteins, of which transferrin, transferrin receptor, and ferritin are the three most important with roles in transport, uptake, and storage of iron, respectively. Ceruloplasmin also contributes in that it stimulates the oxidation of ferrous to ferric iron prior to its binding to transferrin. In human and simian glaucoma there is increased expression of ceruloplasmin, transferrin, and ferritin in the retina and the presence of increased mRNA indicates increased local synthesis (41).

Hahn et al. (51) found increased iron in the RPE, sub-RPE deposits, and Bruch membrane in both exudative and non-exudative types of AMD. The increase was seen in early AMD, suggesting possible involvement in pathogenesis. In the Royal College of Surgeons rat model of retinal degeneration, the accumulation of outer segment tips in the sub-retinal space disrupts the normal interaction of the RPE and the photoreceptors, leading to photoreceptor death through apoptosis (148). Although the mutation in the *Mertk* gene, which encodes a receptor tyrosine kinase in the rat, results in a specific failure of phagocytosis of outer segments by the RPE (28), it is the accumulation of iron within the sub-retinal debris that exerts the toxic effect on the retina. The iron is derived from the breakdown of transferrin that is normally synthesized by the RPE and transports iron into the photoreceptors from which it is later recaptured during phagocytosis. There is evidence that mutations in the *MERTK* gene, the human orthologue of the rat gene, are responsible for some cases of retinitis pigmentosa (44).

Studies of human eyes at different ages indicate that the proteins responsible for regulating transition metals within the retina are not uniformly distributed and are affected by age. The level of both zinc and metallothionein is higher in the peripheral retina than in the macula. The concentration of metallothionein decreases with age and this decrease is more pronounced in the macula (124). Although the zinc concentration in the retina does not diminish with age, in the Beaver Dam Study an increased intake of zinc was associated with less pigmentary change, a risk factor for AMD in the long term (136). Using serial analysis of gene expression, Sharon et al. (115) demonstrated that, compared with the macula, a greater proportion of the mRNA in the peripheral retina was devoted to the synthesis of proteins involved in iron metabolism, such as ferritins and transferrin. The synthesis of transferrin in both the retina and RPE is upregulated in both wet and dry AMD (22). It is hard to avoid the conclusion that these proteins form part of the mechanism to protect the retina from oxidative stress, however imperfectly that mechanism may operate.

REFERENCES

1. Alagna G, D'Aquino S. Alterazioni oculari da cloruro di cobalto. Arch Ottalmol 1956; 60:5–29.
2. Allen JI, Kay NE, McClain CJ. Severe zinc deficiency in humans: association with a reversible T-lymphocyte dysfunction. Ann Intern Med 1981; 95:154–7.
3. Alpern M, Bastian B, Pugh EN Jr, et al. Altered ocular pigments, photostable and labile: two causes of deuteranomalous trichromacy. Mod Probl Ophthalmol 1976; 17:273–91.

4. Bajandas FI, Smith JL. Optic neuritis in hypoparathyroidism. Neurology 1976; 26:451–4.
5. Barraquer-Somers E, Chan CC, Green, WR. Corneal epithelial iron deposition. Ophthalmology 1983; 90:729–34.
6. Beaumont C, Leneuve P, Devaux I, et al. Mutation in the iron responsive element of the L-ferritin mRNA in a family with dominant hyperferritinaemia and cataract. Nat Genet 1995; 11:444–6.
7. Berkow JW, Fine BS, Zimmerman LE. Unusual ocular calcification in hyperparathyroidism. Am J Ophthalmol 1968; 66:812–24.
8. Berlyne GM, Shaw AB. Red eyes in renal failure. Lancet 1967; 1:4–7.
9. Blake J. Eye signs in idiopathic hypoparathyroidism. Trans Ophthalmol Soc UK 1976; 96:448–51.
10. Bouchel MJ, Gerhard JP. Impregnation cuprique du segment anterieur après traitement local ausulfate de cuivre. Confirmation par dosage. Bull Soc Ophthalmol Fr 1964; 64:936–9.
11. Bowen P, Lee CSN, Zellweger H, et al. A familial syndrome of multiple congenital defects. Bull Johns Hopkins Hosp 1964; 114:402–14.
12. Brenner RL, Smith JL, Cleveland WW, et al. Eye signs in hypo-phosphatasia. Arch Ophthalmol 1969; 81:614–7.
13. Buchbinder MC, Gindi JJ, Schanzlin, DJ, et al. Conjunctival crystals in Alport's syndrome. Ophthalmology 1983; 91 (Suppl.):123.
14. Bunce GE. Nutrition and cataract. Nutr Rev 1979; 37: 337–43.
15. Cairns JG, Walshe JM. The Kayser–Fleischer ring. Trans Ophthalmol Soc UK 1970; 90:187–90.
16. Cameron JD, McClain CJ. Ocular histopathology of acrodermatitis enteropathica. Br J Ophthalmol 1986; 70:662–7.
17. Cameron JD, McClain CJ, Doughman DJ. Acrodermatitis enteropathica. In: Gold DH, Weingeist TA, eds. The Eye in Systemic Disease. Philadelphia: Lippincott, 1990:631–2.
18. Chang-Godinich A, Ades S, Schenkein D, et al. Lens changes in hereditary hyperferritinemia-cataract syndrome. Am J Ophthalmol 2001; 132:786–8.
19. Chelly J, Tumer Z, Tonnesen T, et al. Isolation of a candidate gene for Menkes disease that encodes a potential heavy metal binding protein. Nat Genet 1993; 3:14–9.
20. Cheng Q, Gonzalez P, Zigler JS Jr. High level of ferritin light chain mRNA in lens. Biochem Biophys Res Commun 2000; 270:349–55.
21. Cherian MG. Metallothionein and intracellular sequestering of metals. In: Sipes IG, McQueen CA, Gandolf AJ, eds. Comprehensive Toxicology. Vol. 3. New York: Pergamon Elsevier Science, 1997:489–503.
22. Chowers I, Wong R, Dentchev T, et al. The iron carrier transferrin is upregulated in retinas from patients with age-related macular degeneration. Invest Ophthalmol Vis Sci 2006; 47:2135–40.
23. Clark JH. The effect of parathyroid hormone on the permeability of the lens capsule to calcium. Am J Physiol 1939; 126:136–41.
24. Cohen SM, Brown ER, Martyn L, et al. Ocular histopathologic and biochemical studies of the cerebrohepato-renal syndrome (Zellweger's syndrome) and its relationship to neonatal adrenoleukodystrophy. Am J Ophthalmol 1983; 96:488–501.
25. Cogan DG, Albright F, Bartter, FC. Hypercalcemia and band keratopathy. Arch Ophthalmol 1948; 40:624–38.
26. Cox DW, Moore SD. Copper transporting P-type ATPase and human disease. J Bioenerg Biomembr 2002; 34: 333–8.
27. Crane DI, Maxwell MA, Paton BC. *PEX1* mutations in the Zellweger spectrum of the peroxisome biogenesis disorders. Hum Mutat 2005; 26:167–75.
28. D'Cruz PM, Yasamura D, Weir J, et al. Mutation of the receptor tyrosine kinase gene Mertk in the retinal dystrophic RCS rat. Hum Mol Genet 2000; 9:645–51.
29. Daicker B. Tophus-like, conglomerated, crystalline calcification of the sclera. Ophthalmologica 1996; 210:223–8.
30. Dake Y, Amemiya T. Electron microscopic study of the optic nerve in copper deficient rats. Exp Eye Res 1991; 52: 277–81.
31. Danks DM. Disorders of copper transport. In: Scriver CR, Beaudet AL, Sly WS, Valle D, eds. The Metabolic Basis of Inherited Disease. 6th ed. Vol. 1. New York: McGraw-Hill, 1989:1411–31.
32. Danks DM, Campbell PE, Stevens BJ, et al. Menkes' kinky hair syndrome: an inherited defect in the intestinal absorption of copper with widespread effects. Pediatrics 1972; 50:188–201.
33. Danks DM, Cartwright E, Stevens BJ, et al. Menkes' kinky hair disease: further definition of the defect in copper transport. Science 1973; 179:1140–2.
34. Davies G, Dymock I, Harry J, et al. Deposition of melanin and iron in ocular structures in haemochromatosis. Br J Ophthalmol 1972; 56:338–42.
35. DeLuca HF. Recent advances in our understanding of the vitamin D endocrine system. J Lab Clin Med 1976; 87:7–26.
36. Dralands L, Evrard P, Ponchon P, et al. Les complications oculaires de l'hypo-parathyroidie familiale chez l'enfant. Bull Soc Belge Ophthalmol 1971; 157:374–92.
37. Duke JR. Ocular effects of systemic siderosis in the human. Am J Ophthalmol 1957; 44:158–72.
38. Dunaief JL, Richa C, Franks EP, et al. Macular degeneration in a patient with aceruloplasminemia: a disease associated with retinal iron overload. Ophthalmology 2005; 112:1062–5.
39. Ellis PP. Ocular deposition of copper in hypercupremia. Am J Ophthalmol 1969; 68:423–7.
40. Eversen CJ, Schrader RE, and Wang T-I. Chemical and morphological changes in brains of copper deficient guinea pigs. J Nutr 1968; 96:115–25.
41. Farkas RH, Chowers I, Hackam AS, et al. Increased expression of iron-regulating genes in monkey and human glaucoma. Invest Ophthalmol Vis Sci 2004; 45:1410–7.
42. Fleisch H, Russell RGG, Straumann F. Effect of pyrophosphate on hydroxyapatite and its implication in calcium homeostasis. Nature 1966; 212:901–3.
43. Fleming CR, Dickson CR, Wahner HW, et al. Pigmented corneal rings in non-Wilsonian liver disease. Ann Intern Med 1977; 86:285–8.
44. Gal A, Yun L, Thompson DA, et al. Mutations in *MERTK*, the human orthologue of the RCS rat retinal dystrophy gene, cause retinitis pigmentosa. Nat Genet 2000; 26:270–1.
45. Garner A, Fielder AR. Zellweger's syndrome: Cerebrohepatorenal syndrome. In: Gold DH, Weingeist TA, eds. The Eye in Systemic Disease. Philadelphia: Lippincott, 1990:411–3.
46. Garner A, Fielder AR, Primavesi R, et al. Tapetoretinal degeneration in the cerebro-hepato-renal (Zellweger's) syndrome. Br J Ophthalmol 1982; 66:422–31.
47. Goodman SI, Rodgerron DO, Katuman J. Hypercupremia in a patient with multiple myeloma. J Lab Clin Med 1967; 70:52–7.
48. Grahn BH, Paterson PG, Gotttschall-Pass KT, et al. Zinc and the eye. J Am Coll Nutr 2001; 20:106–18.

49. Gregg JB, Becker SE. Concomitant progressive deafness, chronic nephritis, and ocular lens disease. Ann Ophthalmol 1963; 69:293–9.
50. Haddad R, Font RL, Friendly DS. Cerebro-hepato-renal syndrome of Zellweger. Ocular histopathologic findings. Arch Ophthalmol 1976; 94:1927–30.
51. Hahn P, Milam AH, Dunaief JL. Maculas affected by age-related macular degeneration contain increased chelatable iron in the retinal pigment epithelium and Bruch's membrane. Arch Ophthalmol 2003; 121:1099–105.
52. Hahn P, Qian Y, Dentchev T, et al. Disruption of ceruloplasmin and hephaestin in mice causes retinal iron overload and retinal degeneration with features of age-related macular degeneration. Proc Natl Acad Sci USA 2004; 101:13850–5.
53. Harada M. Wilson disease. Med Electron Microsc 2002; 35:61–6.
54. Harris LS, Cohn K, Toyofuku H, et al. Conjunctival and corneal calcific deposits in uremic patients. Am J Ophthalmol 1971; 72:130–3.
55. Harry J, Tripathi RC. Kayser-Fleischer ring: a pathological study. Br J Ophthalmol 1970; 54:794–800.
56. Heath P. Calcinosis oculi. Am J Ophthalmol 1962; 54: 771–81.
57. Hiatt RL Menkes' kinky hair syndrome. In: Gold DH, Weingeist TA, eds. The Eye in Systemic Disease. Philadelphia: Lippincott, 1990:388–90.
58. Hittner HM, Kretzer HL, Mehta RS. Zellweger syndrome: Lenticular opacities indicating carrier status and lens abnormalities characteristic of heterozygotes. Arch Ophthalmol 1981; 99:1977–82.
59. Hoisen H, Kopstad G, Elas, T, et al. Idiopathic haemochromatosis and eye symptoms. A case report. Acta Ophthalmol 1985; 63:192–8.
60. Honavar SG, Shields CL, Demirici H, et al. Sclerochoroidal calcification. Clinical manifestations and systemic associations. Arch Ophthalmol 2001; 119: 833–40.
61. Hough TA, Bogani D, Cheeseman MT, et al. Activating calcium-sensing receptor mutation in the mouse is associated with cataracts and ectopic calcification. Proc Natl Acad Sci USA 2004; 101:13566–71.
62. Hudson JR. Ocular findings in haemochromatosis. Br J Ophthalmol 1953; 37:242–6.
63. Hung IH, Suzuki M, Yamaguchi Y, et al. Biochemical characterization of the Wilson disease protein and functional expression in the yeast *Saccharomyces cerevisiae*. J Biol Chem 1997; 272:21461–6.
64. Jazwinska EC, Lee SC, Webb SI, et al. Localization of the hemochromatosis gene close to D6S105. Am J Hum Genet 1993; 53:347–52.
65. Johnson RE, Campbell RJ. Wilson's disease: Electron microscopic, x-ray energy spectroscopic, and atomic absorption spectroscopic studies of corneal copper deposition and distribution. Lab Invest 1982; 46:564–9.
66. Klaassen-Broeckema N, Bijsterveld OP. Red eyes in renal failure. Br J Ophthalmol 1992; 76:268–71.
67. Klomp LWJ, Gitlin JD. Expression of the ceruloplasmin gene in the human retina and brain: implications for a pathogenic model in aceruloplasminemia. Hum Mol Genet 1996; 5:1989–96.
68. Kono S, Miyajima H. Molecular and pathological basis of aceruloplasminemia. Biol Res 2006; 39:15–23.
69. LaBadie GU, Hirschhorn K, Katz S, et al. Increased copper metallothionein in Menkes' cultured skin fibroblasts. Pediatr Res 1981; 15:257–61.
70. Lessel S, Norton EWD. Band keratopathy and conjunctival calcification in hypophosphatasia. Arch Ophthalmol 1964; 71:497–9.
71. Levi S, Girelli D, Perrone F, et al. Analysis of ferritins in lymphoblastoid cell lines and in the lens of subjects with hereditary hyperferritinemia-cataract syndrome. Blood 1998; 4180–7.
72. Levy NS, Dawson WW, Rhodes BJ, et al. Ocular abnormalities in Menkes' kinky-hair syndrome. Am J Ophthalmol 1974; 77:319–25.
73. Lewis AR, Hultquist DE, Baker BL, et al. Hypercupremia associated with a monoclonal immunoglobulin. J Lab Clin Med 1976; 88:376–88.
74. Liu M, Cohen EJ, Brewer GJ, et al. Kayser–Fleischer ring as the presenting sign of Wilson disease. Am J Ophthalmol 2002; 133:832–4.
75. Maier-Dobersberger T, Ferenci P, Polli, C, et al. Detection of the His106G Gln mutation in Wilson disease by rapid polymerase chain reaction. Ann Intern Med 1997; 127:21–6.
76. Maier-Dobersberger T. Wilson's disease: diagnosis with conventional and molecular-biological methods. Deutsche Medizinische Wochenschrift 1999; 124:493–6.
77. Marchini G, Tosi R, Parolini B, et al. Choroidal calcification in Bartter syndrome. Am J Ophthalmol 1998; 126: 727–9.
78. Margoshes M, Vallee BL. A cadmium protein from equine kidney cortex. J Am Chem Soc 1957; 79:4813–4.
79. Martin NF, Kincaid MC, Sark WJ, et al. Ocular copper deposition associated with pulmonary carcinoma, IgG monoclonal gammopathy and hypercupremia: a clinicopathologic correlation. Ophthalmology 1983; 90:111–5.
80. Matsui T. Zinc deficiency in Crohn's disease. J Gastrenterol 1998; 33:924–5.
81. Matta CS, Felker GV, Ide CH. Eye manifestations in acrodermatitis enteropathica. Arch Ophthalmol 1975; 93: 140–2.
82. McDonnell PJ, Green WR, Schanzlin DJ. Alport's syndrome. In: Gold DH, Weingeist TA, eds. The Eye in Systemic Disease. Philadelphia: Lippincott, 1990:499–502.
83. McNab AA, McKelvie P. Iron overload is a risk factor for zygomycosis. Arch Ophthalmol 1997; 115:919–21.
84. Menkes JH, Alter M, Stiegleder GK, et al. A sex-linked recessive disorder with retardation of growth, peculiar hair and focal cerebral and cerebellar degeneration. Pediatrics 1962; 29:764–79.
85. Mercer JF, Livingston J, Hall B, et al. Isolation of a partial candidate gene for Menkes disease by positional cloning. Nat Genet 1993; 3:20–5.
86. Miyajima H, Nishimura Y, Mizoguchi K, et al. Familial apoceruloplasmin deficiency associated with blepharospasm and retinal degeneration. Neurology 1987; 37: 761–7.
87. Moirand R, Guyader D, Mendler MH, et al. *HFE* based re-evaluation of heterozygous hemochromatosis. Am J Med Genet 2002; 111:356–61.
88. Morita H, Ikeda S, Yamamoto K, et al. Hereditary ceruloplasmin deficiency with hemosiderosis: a clinicopathological study of a Japanese family. Ann Neurol 1995; 37:646–56.
89. Mumford AD, Cree IA, Arnold JD, et al. The lens in hereditary hyperferritinaemia cataract syndrome contains crystalline deposits of L-ferritin. Br J Ophthalmol 2000; 84:697–700.
90. Myung SJ, Yang S-K, Jung H-Y, et al. Zinc deficiency manifested by dermatitis and visual dysfunction in a patient with Crohn's disease. J Gastroenterol 1998; 33:876–9.

91. Nartey NO, Frei JV, Cherian MG. Hepatic copper and metallothionein distribution in Wilson's disease (hepatolenticular degeneration). Lab Invest 1987; 57:397–401.
92. Nicolas MG, Fujiki K, Murayama K, et al. Studies on the mechanism of early onset macular degeneration in Cynomolgus monkeys. II. Suppression of metallothionein synthesis in the retina in oxidative stress. Exp Eye Res 1996; 62:399–408.
93. Opitz JM, ZuRhein GM, Vitale L, et al. The Zellweger syndrome (cerebro-hepato-renal syndrome). Birth Defects 1969; 5:144–58.
94. Pahjola S. Ocular manifestations of idiopathic hypoparathyroidism: case report and review of literature. Acta Ophthalmol (Copenh) 1962; 40:255–65.
95. Panemangalore M, Banerjee D, Onosaka S, et al. Changes in intracellular accumulation and distribution of metallothionein in rat liver and kidney during postnatal development. Dev Biol 1983; 97:95–102.
96. Patel BN, David S. A novel glycosylphosphatidylinositol-anchored form of ceruloplasmin is expressed by mammalian astrocytes. J Biol Chem 1997; 272:20185–90.
97. Patton RG, Christie DL, Smith DW, et al. Cerebro-hepato-renal syndrome of Zellweger: two patients with islet cell hyperplasia, hypoglycemia, and thymic anomalies, and comments on iron metabolism. Am J Dis Child 1972; 124: 840–4.
98. Paulsen M, Lund C, Akram Z, et al. Evidence that translation reinitiation leads to a partially functional Menkes protein containing two copper-binding sites. Am J Hum Genet 2006; 79:214–29.
99. Petrukhin K, Fischer SG, Pirastu M, et al. Mapping, cloning and genetic characterization of the region containing the Wilson disease gene. Nat Genet 1993; 5:338–43.
100. Pietrangelo A. Haemochromatosis. Gut 2003; 52(Suppl. II):23–30.
101. Porter R, Crombie ALI. Corneal and conjunctival calcification in chronic renal failure. Br J Ophthalmol 1975; 57: 339–43.
102. Probst LE, Hoffman E, Cherian MG, et al. Ocular copper deposition associated with benign monoclonal gammopathy and hypercupremia. Cornea 1996; 15:94–8.
103. Racz R, Kovacs B, Varga L, et al. Bilateral cataract in acrodermatitis enteropathica. J Pediatr Ophthalmol Strabismus 1979; 16:180–2.
104. Reiter J. Oxidative processes and antioxidative defence mechanisms in the aging brain. FASEB J 1995; 9:526–33.
105. Rodman R, Burnstine M, Esmaili B, et al. Wilson's disease: presymptomatic patients and Kayser–Fleischer rings. Ophthal Genet 1997; 18:79–85.
106. Rosenstein FJ, Chappell RL. Endogenous zinc as a retinal neuromodulator: evidence from the skate (*Raja erinacea*). Neurosci Lett 2003; 345:81–4.
107. Roth AM, Foos RY. Ocular pathologic changes in primary hemochromatosis. Arch Ophthalmol 1972; 87:507–14.
108. Roxburgh ST. Atypical retinitis pigmentosa with hypophosphatasia. Trans Ophthalmol Soc UK 1983; 103:513–6.
109. Satischandra P, Ravishankar NK. Visual pathway abnormalities in Wilson's disease: an electrophysiological study using electroretinography and visual evoked potentials. J Neurol Sci 2000; 176:13–20.
110. Sato M, Bremner I. Oxygen free radicals and metallothionein. Free Rad Biol Med 1993; 14:325–7.
111. Scadding JF. Sarcoidosis. London: Eyre & Spottiswoode, 1967.
112. Schaefer M, Hopkins RG, Failla ML, et al. Hepatocyte-specific localization and copper-dependent trafficking of the Wilson's disease protein in the liver. Am J Physiol 1999; 276:G639–46.
113. Seelenfreund MH, Gartner S, Vinger F. The ocular pathology of Menkes' disease. Arch Ophthalmol 1968; 80:718–20.
114. Shah AB, Chernov I, Zhang HT, et al. Identification and analysis of mutations in the Wilson disease gene (ATP7B) population frequencies, genotype–phenotype correlation, and functional analysis. Am J Hum Genet 1997; 61: 317–28.
115. Sharon D, Blackshaw S, Cepko CL, et al. Profile of the genes expressed in the human peripheral retina, macula, and retinal pigment epithelium determined through serial analysis of gene expression (SAGE). Proc Natl Acad Sci U S A 2002; 99:315–20.
116. Simsek S, Nanayakkara PWB, Keek JMF, et al. Two Dutch families with hereditary hyperferritinaemia-cataract syndrome and heterozygosity for an HFE-related haemochromatosis gene mutation. The Neth J Med 2003; 61: 291–5.
117. Sommer A, Bradel EJ, Hamondi AB. The cerebro-hepato-renal syndrome (Zellweger's) syndrome. Biol Neonate 1974; 25:219–29.
118. Stanescu B, Dralands L. Cerebro-hepato-renal (Zellweger's) syndrome. Arch Ophthalmol 1972; 87:590–2.
119. Sun H, Demirci H, Shields CL, et al. Sclerochoroidal calcification in a patient with classic Bartter's syndrome. Amer J Ophthalmol 2005; 139:365–6.
120. Sunderman FW. Current status of zinc deficiency in the pathogenesis of neurological, dermatological and musculoskeletal disorders. Am Clin Lab Sci 1975; 5:132–45.
121. Szwareberg J, Mack G, Flament J. Ocular toxicity of deferoxamine: description and analysis of three observations. J Fr Ophtalmol 2002; 25:609–14.
122. Tanner MS, Kantarjian AH, Bhave SA, et al. Early introduction of contaminated animal milk feeds as a possible cause of Indian childhood cirrhosis. Lancet 1983; 2:992–5.
123. Tanner MS, Portmann B, Mowat AP, et al. Increased hepatic copper concentration in Indian childhood cirrhosis. Lancet 1979: 1:1203–5.
124. Tate DJ Jr, Miceli MV, Newsome DA. Expression of metallothionein isoforms in human chorioretinal complex. Curr Eye Res 2002; 24:12–25.
125. Tate DJ Jr, Miceli MV, Newsome DA. Phagocytosis and H_2O_2 induce catalase and metallothionein gene expression in human retinal pigment epithelial cells. Invest Ophthalmol Vis Sci 1995; 36:1271–9.
126. Tate DJ Jr, Newsome DA, Oliver PD. Metallothionein shows an age-related decrease in human macular retinal pigment epithelium. Invest Ophthalmol Vis Sci 1993; 34: 2348–51.
127. Terada K, Schilsky ML, Miura N, et al. ATP7B (WND) protein. Int J Biochem Cell Biol 1998; 30:1063–7.
128. Thannickal VJ, Fanburg BL. Reactive oxygen species in cell signaling. Am J Physiol 2000; 279:L1005–28.
129. Thomas GR, Forbes JR, Roberts EA, et al. The Wilson disease gene: spectrum of mutations and their consequences. Nat Genet 1995; 9:210–7.
130. Tonnesen T, Kleijer WJ, Horn N. Incidence of Menkes disease. Hum Genet 1991; 86:408–10.
131. Tripathi RC, Ashton N. Application of electron microscopy to the study of ocular inborn errors of metabolism. In: Bergsma D, Bron AJ, Cotlier E, eds. The Eye and Inborn Errors of Metabolism. New York: Alan R. Liss, 1976:69–104.

132. Tso MOM, Fine BS, Thorpe HE. Kayser–Fleischer ring and associated cataract in a case of Wilson's disease. Am J Ophthalmol 1975; 79:479–88.
133. Ugarte M, Osborne NN. Zinc in the retina. Progr Neurobiol 2001; 64:219–49.
134. Uzman LL, Jakus MA. The Kayser–Fleischer ring: a histochemical and electron microscope study. Neurology 1957; 7:341–55.
135. Van der Klooster JM. Hereditary hyperferritinaemia-cataract syndrome. Ned Tijdschr Geneeskd 2003; 147: 1923–8.
136. VandenLangenberg GM, Mares-Perlman JA, Klein R, et al. Associations between antioxidant and zinc intake and the 5-year incidence of early age-related maculopathy in the Beaver Dam eye study. Am J Epidemiol 1998; 148:204–14.
137. Vitale L, Opitz JM, Shahidi NT. Congenital and familial iron overload. N Engl J Med 1969; 280:642–5.
138. Volpe JJ, Adams D. Cerebro-hepato-renal syndrome of Zellweger: An inherited disorder of neuronal migration. Acta Neuropathol (Berl) 1972; 20:175–98.
139. Vulpe C, Levinson B, Whitney S, et al. Isolation of a candidate gene for Menkes disease and evidence that it encodes a copper-transporting ATPase. Nat Genet 1993; 3: 7–13.
140. Walshe JM. The eye in Wilson's disease. In: Bergsma D, Bron AJ, Cotlier E, eds. The Eye and Errors of Metabolism. New York: Alan R. Liss, 1976:187–9.
141. Wanders RJA. Metabolic and molecular basis of peroxisomal disorders: a review. Am J Med Genet 2004; 126A:355–75.
142. Wang F, Kim B-E, Dufner-Beattie J, et al. Acrodermatitis enteropathica mutations affect transport activity, localization and zinc-responsive trafficking of the mouse ZIP4 zinc transporter. Hum Mol Genet 2004; 13:563–71.
143. Warshawsky RS, Hill CW, Doughman DJ, et al. Acrodermatitis enteropathica: corneal involvement with histochemical and electron microscopic studies. Arch Ophthalmol 1975; 9:194–7.
144. Wiebers DO, Hollenhorst RW, Goldstein P. The ophthalmologic manifestations of Wilson's disease. Mayo Clin Proc 1977; 52:409–16.
145. WHO/IPCS Environmental Health Criteria 221. Zinc. Geneva: World Health Organization, 2001.
146. Wirsching L. Eye symptoms in acrodermatitis enteropathica. Acta Ophthalmol (Copenh) 1962; 40:567–74.
147. Wray SH, Kuwabara T, Sanderson R. Menkes' kinky hair disease: a light- and electron-microscopic study of the eye. Invest Ophthalmol 1976; 15:128–38.
148. Yefimova MG, Jeanny J-C, Keller N, et al. Impaired retinal iron homeostasis associated with defective phagocytosis in Royal College of Surgeons rats. Invest Ophthalmol Vis Sci 2002; 43:537–45.
149. Yoo MH, Lee J-Y, Lee SE, et al. Protection by pyruvate of rat retinal cells against zinc toxicity in vitro, and pressure-induced ischemia in vivo. Invest Ophthalmol Vis Sci 2004; 45:1523–30.

49

Nutritional Deficiencies and Excesses

Chung-Jung Chiu
Department of Ophthalmology and the Jean Mayer USDA Human Nutrition Research Center on Aging, Tufts University, Boston, Massachusetts, U.S.A.

Gordon K. Klintworth
Departments of Pathology and Ophthalmology, Duke University, Durham, North Carolina, U.S.A.

Allen Taylor
Department of Ophthalmology and the Jean Mayer USDA Human Nutrition Research Center for Aging, Tufts University, Boston, Massachusetts, U.S.A.

INTRODUCTION

Malnutrition and its consequences are a major global problem particularly in the developing parts of the world, where the diet is inadequate and insufficient for many reasons including climate, lack of education, primitive agricultural methods, poverty, lack of imported foods, and food taboos (52). Many studies sought to determine the amino acid and vitamin intake requirements for optimal vision and some of these were translated into practice with dramatic results (139). More recently, problems of excessive food intake have been associated with compromises to vision (26–28,89,109,110). Ironically, often problems of over nutrition occur in the same places where malnutrition exists. This review summarizes relations between nutrient insufficiencies, nutrient surfeit, and the function of major eye tissues. For additional information, readers are referred to texts which deal with these topics in greater detail (118,176).

Viewed from a distance, there appear to be two intervals during which nutrients may affect the function of ocular tissues, possible with differing consequences: (*i*) in utero during organogenesis and renewal, or (*ii*) postsynthesis, during homeostasis. Vitamins play a crucial role in many metabolic reactions and a deficiency of a specific vitamin at critical times during intrauterine development results in congenital anomalies in experimental animals. The timing, duration and the severity of the deficiency are related to the anomalies produced. For example, vitamin A is required initially and continues to be required throughout life, as photoreceptors are assembled. Of the vitamins, only vitamin A and nicotinic acid have been found to be teratogenic in excess (34,186).

Vitamin A

Vitamin A encompasses a large group of compounds that includes vitamin A alcohol (retinol), vitamin A aldehyde (retinal), vitamin A acid (retinoic acid), and the active forms of vitamin A. Vitamin A (all-trans-retinol) is a lipid soluble carotenoid derivative which is formed from beta-carotene and which forms the major phototransduction retinoid (Fig. 1) (14,63,163). Dietary sources of vitamin A include preformed vitamin A in animal foods or newly formed vitamin from beta-carotene in green leafy plants.

The small intestine absorbs both retinyl esters from animal tissues and provitamin A carotenoids from vegetables by diffusion at sites where lipid is taken up (63,208). Retinyl esters are enzymatically converted to retinol in the lumen of the intestine and are then absorbed by intestinal cells (enterocytes) (63,208). Within the walls of the small intestine, beta-carotene or other carotenoids are cleaved by an oxygenase to form retinal (132), which becomes converted to the free retinol. Retinal can also be irreversibly oxidized to retinoic acid (Fig. 2) (47).

Within the enterocytes retinyl esters are re-formed by a reaction of retinol with long-chain fatty acids, such as palmitic acid, and then become incorporated into chylomicrons. The esterification of retinol within the intestine involves acyl coenzyme A:retinol acyltransferase (ARAT) (76,77) and lecithin:retinol acyltransferase (LRAT) (111,133). Within the enterocytes retinol becomes bound to the intestinal intracytoplasmic retinol-binding protein [CRB(II)].

Vitamin A_1 (retinol) with its four unsaturated bonds, is transported in the plasma within chylomicrons mainly to the liver where it becomes stored in relatively large quantities, mainly as retinyl palmitate, within lipid droplets of specialized stellate cells

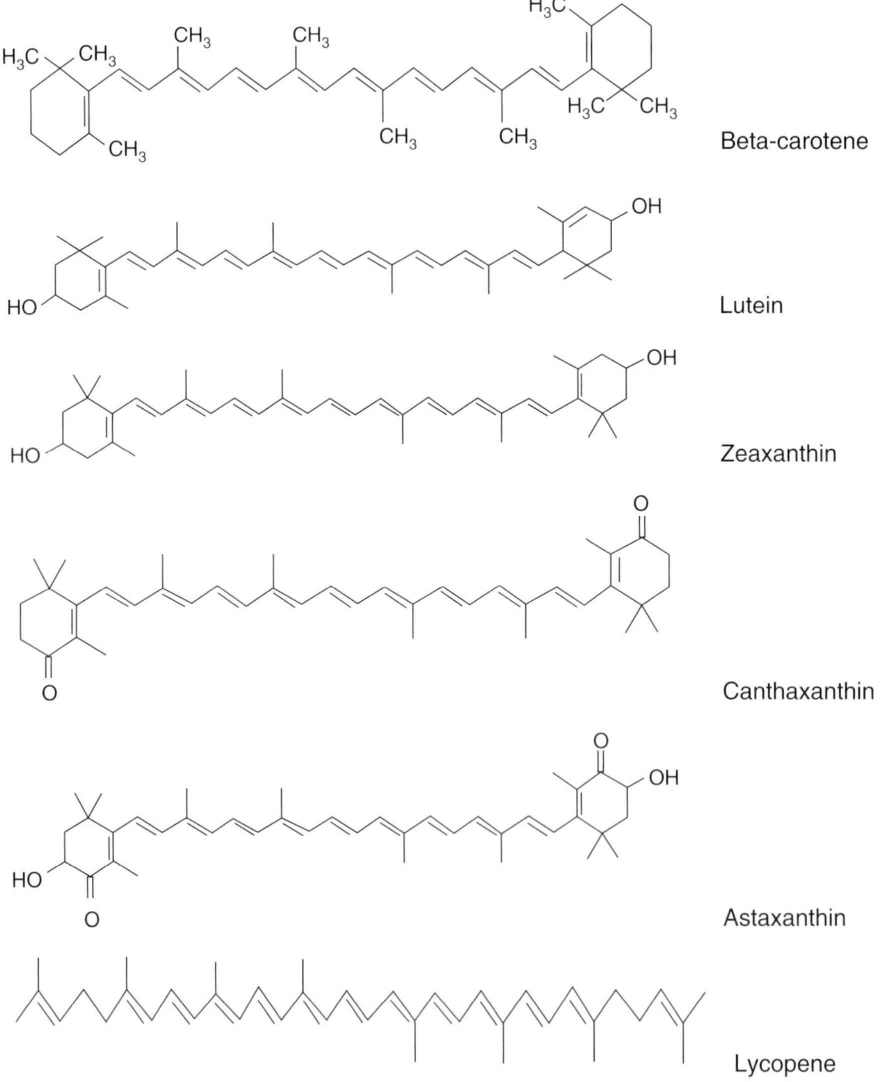

Figure 1 Structures of carotenoids that have been associated with lens or retina health and function.

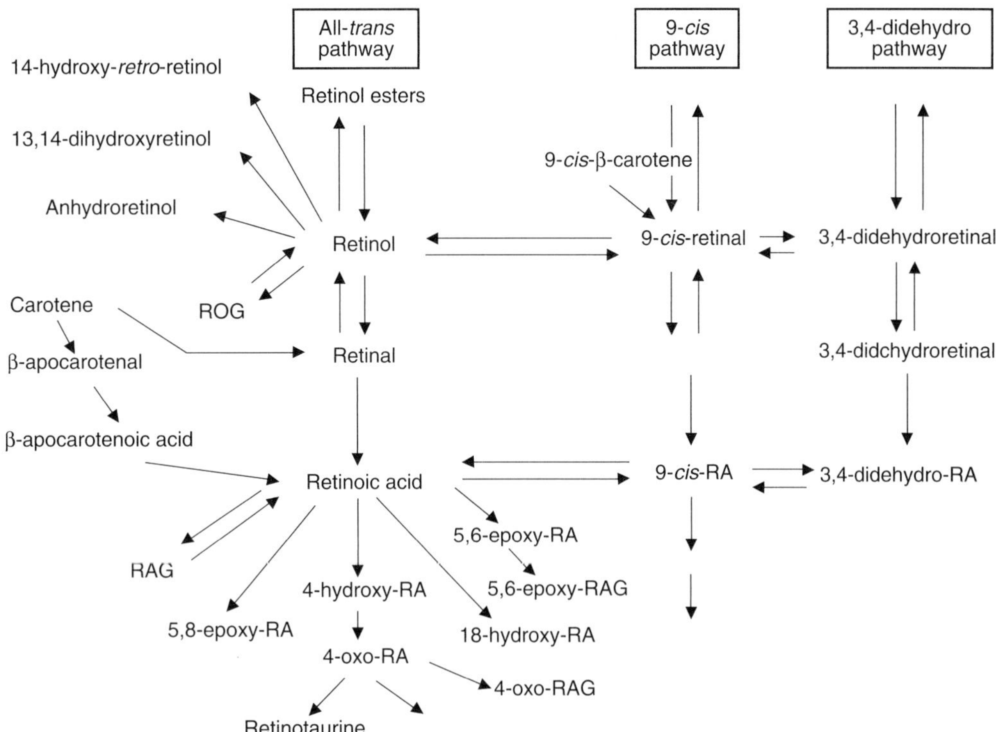

Figure 2 Principle retinoids in the metabolic pathway. The columns represent the various isomerization states, except for the 3,4-didehydro pathway; however, the pathway metabolites are only delineated for the all-*trans* forms. In addition to the 9-*cis* pathway, which is shown, there would also be a 13-*cis* pathway, an 11-*cis* pathway, a 9,13-di-*cis* pathway, etc., which are not shown. In most instances, each of the isomer pathways would have the components shown in the all-*trans* pathway. In general, the *top* has relatively reduced retinoids, whereas the *bottom* has relatively oxidized retinoids. The *arrow* from all-*trans*-4-oxo-RA with no product indicates that there are more oxidized products that are unknown. *Abbreviations*: ROG, all-*trans*-retinyl-β-glucuronide; RAG, all-*trans*-retinoyl-β-glucuronide; RA, retinoic acid. *Source*: Adapted from Ref. 34.

(78,100,193). Of the total vitamin A content of the body, 70–95% is stored in the liver (205) which normally contains sufficient vitamin A to maintain an individual's nutritional needs for nearly a year. The level of retinol in cells may be controlled to some extent through membrane receptors or by excretion from the cell.

Retinol is transported in the plasma by a special retinol-binding protein which is associated with an acidic protein (transthyretin) (135). Mutations in this protein cause a form of amyloidosis (see Chapter 37). Normally the plasma retinol-binding protein is almost saturated with retinol (126,187).

Carotenoids

Human serum contains 30 or more carotenoids but only lutein and zeaxanthin are found in the retina. The only source of lutein and zeaxanthin is diet, especially from leafy green vegetables (113). Several investigations suggest that the level of lutein and zeaxanthin in the macula is related to the intake of foods rich in these carotenoids, such as spinach (70,104). Lens health has also been associated with intake of carotenoids, including the vitamin A precursor (78).

Vitamin A and Vision

Vitamin A plays a crucial role in the vision of all species (160) and all visual pigments are derivatives of it. They include retinaldehyde (also known as retinal and retinene$_1$) and dehydroretinaldehyde (retinene$_2$). All visual pigments are bound as a chromophore to opsin—a protein found in the outer segments of the photoreceptors (Fig. 3). Opsins vary in rods and cones and humans have two main types: rod opsin and cone opsin of which there are three kinds (8,127).

Microsomes isolated from the retinal pigment epithelium (RPE) rapidly convert retinol into retinyl ester (11). If contact between the photoreceptors and RPE is maintained most of retinol leaves the rod outer segments to become esterified and accumulates as all-trans retinyl ester in the oil-droplets of the RPE (21). Retinyl acetate and retinal palmitate (but not retinoic acid) (150) are also taken up into lipid droplets of the RPE where they become esterified and stored and mobilized when needed (20,21,210). Specific receptors for plasma retinol-binding protein seem to be distributed along the basal and lateral surfaces of the RPE (17,199).

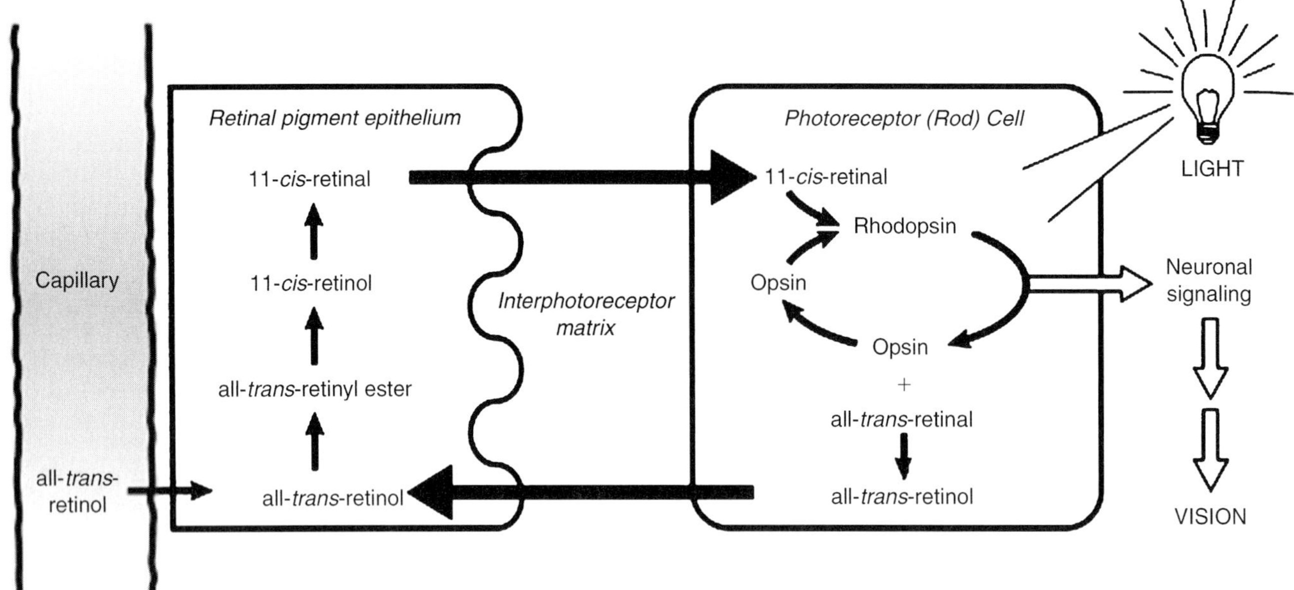

Figure 3 The visual cycle. Retinol is transported to the retina via the circulation, where it moves into retinal pigment epithelial cells. There, retinol is esterified to form a retinyl ester that can be stored. When needed, retinyl esters are broken apart (*hydrolyzed*) and isomerized to form 11-*cis* retinol, which can be oxidized to form 11-*cis* retinal. 11-*cis* retinal can be shuttled to the rod cell, where it binds to a protein called opsin to form the visual pigment, rhodopsin (visual purple). Absorption of a photon of light catalyzes the isomerization of 11-*cis* retinal to all-*trans* retinal and results in its release (194). This isomerization triggers a cascade of events, leading to the generation of an electrical signal to the optic nerve (82,101). The nerve impulse generated by the optic nerve is conveyed to the brain where it can be interpreted as vision. Once released all-*trans* retinal is converted to all-*trans* retinol, which can be transported across the interphotoreceptor matrix to the retinal pigmented epithelial cell to complete the visual cycle. *Source*: Adapted from http://lpi.oregonstate.edu/infocenter/vitamins/vitaminA/visualcycle.html.

Other Functions of Vitamin A

Vitamin A plays a poorly understood role in epithelial cell functions. Vitamin A causes a striking decrease in the production of fucose-containing glycopeptides and it may have a direct action on the mannose-carrying lipid intermediary in glycoprotein synthesis (41). This affect occurs within the corneal epithelium of vitamin A-deficient rats (99). Mucous metaplasia-can be induced with vitamin A (3,86).

Vitamin A lyses lysosomes in vitro (44) and rabbits are depleted of lysosomes by treatment with vitamin A (198). Vitamin A and its analogues (retinoids) have a preventive and therapeutic effect on several experimental tumors in vivo (172). However, under some conditions high doses of vitamin A may enhance tumor production by chemical carcinogens (107,147) and oncogenic viruses (141) .

Vitamin A Deficiency

In most developed countries the vitamin A requirements are satisfactorily met, but cases of deficiency sometimes occur, especially in newborns and pregnant and nursing women, whose nutritional needs are greatest (144,168,182).

Vitamin A deficiency is a public health problem in more than 118 countries and affects more than 140–250 million preschool children worldwide. It is estimated that more than five million children develop xerophthalmia annually and that a quarter million or more become blind from the effects of vitamin A deficiency. It is also a major pathway for measles-associated blindness, particularly in Africa (169). Where this problem exists it is responsible for 25% of child deaths (170). Recent analyses suggest that vitamin A deficiency may also be an important risk factor for maternal mortality (33).

Vitamin A is essential for the immune system function. Giving vitamin A supplements to children who need them increases their resistance to disease, protects against blindness, and improves their chances for survival, growth and development. Because vitamin A can be stored in the liver, high doses can be given through oral supplements once every 4 to 6 months for prevention.

Vitamin A deficiency occurs when body stores are depleted because of an inadequate intake of vitamin A in foods, or where there is too little absorption of this vitamin (as in sprue, celiac disease, cystic fibrosis and other conditions causing steatorrhea) and less often with defective storage (as in liver disease). Vitamin A deficiency can also result from its rapid utilization during illnesses (particularly measles, diarrhea and fevers), pregnancy and lactation, and during phases of rapid growth in young children. Healthy humans on a diet deficient in vitamin A and carotenoids develop evidence of the deficiency after time periods ranging from a few weeks to about a year. Children between the ages of 6 months and 5 years experience more serious effects of vitamin A deficiency than other groups.

The levels of retinol, retinol-binding protein and transthyretin in the blood are directly related. An impaired hepatic release of vitamin A rather than a vitamin A deficiency is important in children. If malnourished children, deficient in vitamin A, are given this vitamin parentally the serum retinol-binding protein does not increase for 24 h (166). On the other hand, when children with kwashiorkor or marasmus receive protein and vitamin A, the serum levels of retinol-binding protein, transthyretin and vitamin A all increase (165).

Retina in Vitamin A Deficiency

Vitamin A deficiency causes a failure of rhodopsin formation from retinal and opsin (194). Initially the time required for dark adaptation increases and eventually night blindness (nyctalopia) ensues due to an impaired function of the retinal rods. Cones are also affected but this is less apparent clinically.

Biochemical, morphological and physiological changes occur in the retina of vitamin A-deficient animals. In rats on a vitamin A deficient diet the first sign of the deficiency is a rise in the threshold and time for eliciting the electroretinogram (ERG) and by 4 to 5 weeks the level of rhodopsin within the retina is decreased (47,131).

Structural degenerative alterations occur in the inner and outer segments of the retina (46,73) as well as in photoreceptor nuclei (46,149). These changes are accompanied by a loss of rhodopsin (24,96). The RPE remains more or less structurally normal, but by transmission electron microscopy (TEM) the lipid droplets appear more homogeneous than in controls (24) and substantially fewer lipofuscin granules accumulate than in non-vitamin A deprived rats (97). This appearance may relate to stored vitamin A or its metabolites, since similar lipid droplets form in mice receiving injections of vitamin A (150). Rods degenerate earlier and with a strikingly greater susceptibility than cones (24). After 7 weeks on a vitamin A-deficient diet, the distal two-thirds of the outer segments stain less intensely with toluidine blue (24), but after 16 weeks some photoreceptor discs become distended with small vesicles (0.19–0.35 μm in diameter) and the normal intimate contact between the RPE and the outer segments is destroyed.

Tadpoles born of vitamin A-deprived mothers and subsequently raised on a vitamin A-free diet sometimes manifest an impaired light-induced electrical response (b-wave of the ERG) and other abnormalities. Morphologic alterations in the rods of these animals are surprisingly subtle and consist of notching of the plasma membrane and, in some instances, invasion of the interdisc space by wedge-shaped clusters of vesicles (206). The biochemical events of insect vision are similar to those in vertebrates and vitamin A deficiency causes decreased visual sensitivity with accompanying ocular morphologic changes (19).

Due to the impression that blindness due to nutritient deficiencies can be delayed or avoided completely, many interventional trials and observational studies have determined optimal intakes of various foods and nutrients, especially for micronutrients (29).

Conjunctiva and Cornea in Vitamin A Deficiency

In vitamin A deficiency the epithelia of the skin and mucous membranes, including the ocular surface, thicken and keratinize. The designation xerophthalmia refers to the external ocular manifestations observed in vitamin A deficiency (xerosis of the conjunctiva and cornea, Bitot spot and keratomalacia). Xerophthalmia is prevalent in many parts of the world and progresses through several recognized stages: conjunctival xerosis (Stage 1A), Bitot spots with conjunctival xerosis (Stage 1B), corneal xerosis (Stage 2), corneal ulceration with xerosis (Stage 3A) and keratomalacia (Stage 3B) (138).

The conjunctiva becomes dry, opaque, thickened, wrinkled and sometimes pigmented. This conjunctival xerosis is often followed by the appearance of small, variable shaped refractile plaques in the superficial bulbar conjunctiva (Bitot spots). These lesions are usually bilateral, in the exposed interpalpebral fissure at the corneoscleral limbus, and especially on the temporal side of the eye. Bitot spots often have a silver gray hue and foamy surface and usually occur in young children with night blindness. The foamy appearance is thought to be due to infection with *Corynebacterium xerosis*.

Xerosis of both corneas follows conjunctival xerosis and is characterized by surfaces which lack their normal luster and have a fine pebbly appearance. The dry corneas become keratinized and are prone to bacterial infection and ulceration. Such cloudy corneas often undergo a characteristic rapidly progressive, usually bilateral, softening (keratomalacia) which results in partial or complete corneal perforation and the transformation of the cornea into a cloudy gelatinous mass. In developing countries this devastating keratomalacia is a major cause of blindness in young children and is usually associated with generalized malnutrition and infections such as measles. Babies born of severely malnourished mothers sometimes have congenital keratomalacia. Since keratomalacia is not a feature of vitamin A deficiency in adults, vitamin A deficiency alone may not be responsible for the condition, but laboratory animals deficient from weaning solely in vitamin A and its precursor beta-carotene develop all the manifestations of xerophthalmia ending with perforation of the cornea and phthisis bulbi (138).

A collagenolytic system exists in xerophthalmic corneas (140). Polymorphonuclear leukocytes (PMNs) infiltrate the ulcerating corneas extensively prior to the capillary invasion and perforation (138) suggesting that enzymes responsible for the melting could be contained in PMNs. This possibility is supported by the fact that PMNs contain several proteolytic enzymes.

In vitamin A-deficient animals the conjunctival goblet cells disappear (18,45,92,207), while the corneal and conjunctival epithelial cells lose their normal surface microprojections and become keratinized (7,207). These changes and the desquamating superficial epithelial cells are dramatically demonstrated by scanning electron microscopy (SEM) (136). Sometimes the corneal stroma becomes invaded by leukocytes (101) and vascularizes (207). In some (7,92), but not other (136), experimental studies corneal ulcers and keratomalacia have developed. Unlike the retinal abnormalities the lesions in the conjunctiva and cornea of vitamin A-deficient animals are prevented by retinoic acid (46).

Vitamin A and Carotenoid Excess

Because the RPE fluorophore, lipofuscin, is associated with the pathobiology of age-related macular degeneration (AMD), considerable attention has been devoted to identifying components of lipofuscin. It is noteworthy that a major lipophilic component of lipofuscin, called A2E, is a metabolite of vitamin A (171).

Excessive ingestion of vegetables containing carotenoids, over prolonged periods may result in the deposition of yellow pigment in the skin (carotenosis) beginning in the nasolabial folds and palms of the hands but in contrast to jaundice, not in the conjunctiva. Excessive vitamin A intake results in benign intracranial hypertension (pseudotumor cerebri) and papilledema (49) (see Chapter 70).

Vitamin A and Developmental Anomalies

Maternal vitamin A deficiency may cause fetal anophthalmia or xerophthalmia. Ocular and various systemic malformations develop in the offspring of vitamin A-deficient pigs (66), rats (85,203), and rabbits (103). The malformations include anophthalmia, microphthalmia, absence of the anterior chamber, iris, and ciliary body, colobomas and disorganization of the retina, failure or impairment of vitreous formation with the development in its place of fibrous retrolental membranes, and failure of the embryonic eyelids to fuse (designated congenital open eye). In calves blindness may follow constriction of the optic nerve caused by anomalous growth of the skeleton (124). In the rat, the offspring born of vitamin A-deficient mothers may manifest abnormalities that resemble in some respects the retinopathy of prematurity (ROP) (see Chapter 67). The abnormality varies considerably in degree in different lines (197), but approximately 75% of the offspring of female rats fed vitamin A-deficient diets prior to or during pregnancy develop ocular anomalies (196).

Hypervitaminosis A during pregnancy is teratogenic with some of its adverse effects reflecting an interference of neural crest cell migration (143). Some of the defects of mandibulofacial dysostosis (Treacher Collins syndrome) develop in all of the offspring of pregnant rats given excess vitamin A at day 8.5 of gestation. Such treatment destroys neural crest cells of the facial and auditory primordia that normally migrate to the first and second branchial arches. The otomandibular defects so produced are identical to those in humans with mandibulofacial dysostosis (142,143).

Embryos exposed to high levels of retinoids, such as vitamin A and retinoic acid, develop characteristic malformations of several structures including the eye (4,61). The pathogenesis of the ocular deformities, which include anophthalmos, microphthalmos, retinal defects, and cataract remains unknown, but their incidence varies with the time of gestation at which the vitamin is administered (9,56,61,160).

An attempt has been made to mimic retinoid-induced teratogenesis in transgenic mice by linking a constitutively active retinoic acid receptor to the αA-crystallin promoter which targets expression of the genes in the crystallin lens. The ocular lens in these genetically engineered mice express the active retinoic acid receptor, but also manifest cataracts in association with microphthalmia (4).

Mechanisms by which retinoic acid manifests its effects are being elucidated (55,173,195). Peroxisomes, the catalase containing cell organelles (see Chapter 1) often occur in close proximity to lipid droplets and may be involved in reactions which remove retinal from the plasma and esterify it (106,150). Giving retinoic acid to rats on a diet deficient in both vitamin A and carotenoids prevents all signs of vitamin A deficiency, including the external ocular changes, except night blindness (146).

VITAMIN B COMPLEX

The vitamin B complex comprises several independent water soluble substances (thiamine, riboflavin, nicotinic acid, pantothenic acid, pyridoxine, choline, biotin, inositol, *p*-aminobenzoic acid, folic acid, and cyanocobalamin). Deficiencies of many of these vitamins produce ocular lesions in experimental animals and deficiencies in some of them are suspected of causing ophthalmic manifestations in humans. It is noteworthy that the normal lens contains unexpectedly large amounts of inositol but the significance of this remains unknown. Recent epidemiologic studies have attempted to identify optimal levels of these nutrients (102,105).

Vitamin B_1 (Thiamine)

A deficiency of thiamine (vitamin B_1), which in its phosphorylated form acts as a coenzyme (cocarboxylase) for the decarboxylation of pyruvate, leads to beriberi and the Wernicke syndrome (ophthalmoplegia, ataxia and mental confusion). Peripheral neuropathy is a frequent complication of beriberi, especially of the chronic form. In beriberi bilateral optic neuritis may occur and diffuse demyelinization of the optic nerve has been observed postmortem (115). Patchy demyelinization of the optic nerves and tracts has also been documented in thiamine deficient rats (152). The prominent nystagmus and ophthalmoplegia of the Wernicke syndrome result from lesions in the brain and disturbances of vision are attributed to involvement of visual pathways. The optic chiasm may be severely gliosed (120) and the optic nerves may also be affected (23).

Vitamin B_2 (Riboflavin)

Riboflavin, a yellow pigment, is a precursor of flavin mononucleotide (FMN) and flavin adenine dinucleotide (FAD), coenzymes in several oxidation-reduction reactions involved in electron transfer (80,119,125). Electrons are transferred from nicotinamide adenine dinucleotide (NADH) to FMN during the chain of reactions in which these negatively charged particles are passed to oxygen.

The flavins are widely distributed throughout the body. Although present in various ocular structures riboflavin, FMN and FAD are particularly abundant in several tissues of the eye and its adnexa (6,137) In cattle they are most copious in the lacrimal and Meibomian glands and the corneal epithelium contains much more riboflavin than the corneal stroma or the aqueous humor (137). In all rabbit ocular tissues the primary flavin is FAD followed by FMN and riboflavin. The ratio of the flavins varies in different tissues. In the rabbit the FAD:FMN: riboflavin ratio has been found to be 6:2:1 in cornea, 42:3:1 in lens cortex, 68:3:1 in lens nucleus and 49:13:1 in retina (6) In the rabbit the cornea has the highest concentration of riboflavin followed by the retina, lens cortex and lens nucleus (6), but FAD and FMN are present in highest concentration in the retina followed by cornea and lens (6).

The flavins are light sensitive and they rapidly degrade following exposure to visible or near ultraviolet light producing inactive and toxic products (68,164). A riboflavin-sensitized production of hydrogen peroxide has been demonstrated in the presence of light and oxygen.

Riboflavin deficiency becomes first manifest clinically in parts of the body exposed to ambient light, namely the skin and eye. Features of riboflavin deficiency include corneal vascularization, photophobia, angular stomatitis, seborrheic dermatitis and growth retardation (63). Studies in riboflavin deficient rats have disclosed corneal vascularization (12), and cataracts have been a feature of some (38,75), but not all such animals (12). Cataracts and keratitis have also been produced in salmon (67) and rabbit (84) fed a riboflavin deficient diet. Cataracts, but not corneal vascularization, have been documented in riboflavin deficient mice (108), pigs (121), cats (57), monkeys (37,193) and chicks (39). The possibility of riboflavin deficiency producing cataracts in man has been raised on nebulous grounds (146). We found elevated dietary riboflavin to be associated with a diminished risk for nuclear opacities, but this was not independent of other nutrients (88). Other lesions noted in experimental animals include: angular blepharoconjunctivitis, "spectacle eye," keratitis, conjunctivitis, and optic atrophy.

The offspring of rodents on a riboflavin deficient diet (65) or treated with the antimetabolite galactoflavin (95,128) develop ocular anomalies, such as microphthalmos, anophthalmos, colobomas of the iris and congenital "open eyes."

Excessively high doses of riboflavin are harmful. An increased fragility of the photoreceptor outer segments has been reported in normal Royal College of Surgeons rats maintained on a high dose (48). Following the ingestion of a lethal dose riboflavin crystallizes in the kidney and death ensues from renal failure (35,116).

Vitamin B_{12} (Cyanocobalamin)

Addisonian pernicious anemia in which the gastric mucosa is atrophic is by far the commonest cause of cyanocobalamin deficiency. Amblyopia may be an early indication of vitamin B_{12} deficiency and Heaton and colleagues (74) found the serum level of this vitamin to be lower than normal in 13 patients suffering from tobacco amblyopia. Freeman and Heaton (53) have suggested that the optic atrophy and "retrobulbar neuritis," which is sometimes found in Addisonian pernicious anemia may be tobacco amblyopia due to cyanide intoxication. This possibility is reinforced by evidence of a link between vitamin B_{12} and the metabolism and detoxification of cyanide (201,202). Some ocular manifestations of vitamin B_{12} deficiency, such as retinal hemorrhages and cotton wool spots, are probably a sequel to severe anemia.

Ocular developmental malformations (microphthalmos, anophthalmos, distortion of lens and retina, colobomas, decreased size of optic cup, extension of everted retinal tissue into the optic nerve) have been reported in the offspring of vitamin B_{12} deficient animals (65).

Folic Acid

Rats maintained on a folic acid deficient diet give birth to pups with deformities of the eye (retinal colobomata, retinal folds and lenticular abnormalities), face and body or do not have viable embryos (60). Deficiencies of folic acid and folate antagonists can also produce anophthalmos, microphthalmos, cataract and coloboma (2).

Pantothenic Acid

Anophthalmia or microphthalmia occur in the offspring of panthothenic acid deficient rats as well as of rats given an antimetabolite to pantothenic acid (16,59,129). A deficiency of this vitamin, which is part of coenzyme A, appears to interfere with the normal inductive process whereby the telencephalon of the brain fails to divide into two hemispheres giving rise to optic cups (47).

VITAMIN C (ASCORBIC ACID)

Only man and the guinea pig are known to require ascorbic acid in the diet; other species can synthesize this compound. Vitamin C is probably the most prevalent and potent dietary antioxidant. The amount of ascorbic acid in different tissues varies considerably amongst species. The lens has a high concentration with its cortex having a higher level than the nucleus (178,179). The corneal epithelium also contains high concentrations of vitamin C (73).

Ascorbic acid, which is reversibly oxidized in the body to ascorbone (dehydroascorbic "acid"), plays an important role in maintaining connective tissues (64,149) being necessary for the hydroxylation of procollagen (5). In addition to its well-established reducing properties, ascorbic acid is aweak acid with metal complexing attributes and in the presence of ferric ions it promotes the generation of free radicals. Hemorrhage caused by the increased capillary fragility is a prominent feature of scurvy, the disorder caused by a deficiency of ascorbic acid, and petechiae or larger hemorrhages can occur in the conjunctiva, eyelids, orbit, anterior chamber, vitreous, or other ocular structures (69). While cataracts are not a feature of natural or experimentally produced scurvy, several animal models of cataract (15,58,179,190,191) suggest that vitamin C can mediate against induced cataracts and many human epidemiologic studies sought to determine optimal levels of this vitamin, with respect to eye health (10,29,90,91,122,177,178).

VITAMIN D (CALCIFEROL)

The principal function of vitamin D is in the control of calcium metabolism and this is accomplished through the mediation of polar hydroxylated metabolites, the most polar being 1,30,31-trihydroxycholecalciferol (40). Both 1,25-dihydroxycholecalciferol and the trihydroxy derivative act on the intestinal mucosa to increase the uptake of calcium ions. A deficiency of vitamin D leads to rickets or osteomalacia and, although significant ocular manifestations are not produced, proptosis may be associated with deformities of the skull.

An excess ingestion of vitamin D causes hypercalcemia and calcium often deposits in the conjunctiva and cornea to produce calcific band keratopathy. Corneal calcification can be induced experimentally in rabbits with vitamin D.

THE VITAMIN E FAMILY (TOCOPHEROLS)

Vitamin E (alpha-tocopherol), which was first recognized as a factor preventing sterility in rats, is a powerful lipophilic antioxidant that protects lipid membranes from attack by free radicals (123). A myriad of studies have demonstrated that vitamin E, glutathione (GSH), and vitamin C act in concert to mitigate against various oxidative stresses (Fig. 4) (176). Since vitamin E is concentrated in the photoreceptor outer segments (44) a specific role in retinal function would be expected and tocopherol may protect the outer segment of photoreceptor cells from excessive lipid peroxidation.

It is not certain that a clinical deficiency of vitamin E exists in man. However, monkeys (71) and rats (151) maintained on a vitamin E-deficient diet develop a retinal degeneration characterized by a focal extensive disruption of photoreceptor outer segments consistent with lipid peroxidation of these lipid rich structures. When rats are maintained on a diet deficient in vitamin E, but adequate in vitamin A, lipofuscin granules become much more numerous in the RPE, the cell that ingests photoreceptor outer segments (151). In the monkey, cones may be even more susceptible to deficiency of vitamin E than of vitamin A and the

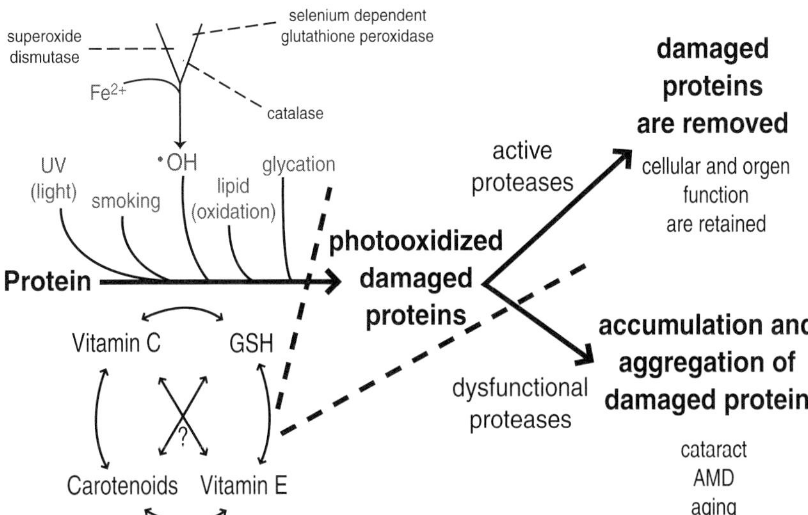

Figure 4 Proposed interaction between proteins, modification of proteins by oxidants, light, smoking, sugars, antioxidants, antioxidant enzymes, and, proteases, as well as resultant effects on tissue function. *Abbreviations*: AMD, age-related macular degeneration; Fe^{2+}, iron; GSH, glutathione; H_2O_2, hydrogen peroxide; •OH, hydroxl iron; O_2^-, oxygen radical; UV, ultraviolet.

macula is more extensively involved than the peripheral retina. Cataract formation has been induced by vitamin E deficiency in the rabbit (43) and turkey embryo (51). Salutary effects with respect to diminishing risk for nuclear cataract have also been reported in persons with higher vitamin E intake (29,88). The ceroid accumulation which occurs in chronic vitamin E deficiency resembles ceroid lipofuscinosis (71).

Ocular developmental anomalies occur in the offspring of rabbits and rats on a vitamin E deficient diet. These malformations include anophthalmos and microphthalmos and retinal abnormalities suggestive of the ROP (22). Indeed, vitamin E is considered to be effective in the prophylaxis of ROP (see Chapter 67) (135). Vitamin E partially retards the cytocidal effect of hyperoxia on rabbit vascular cells in vitro (184). In a double-masked clinical trial of infants with a birth weight less than or equal to 2000 g or a gestational age less than or equal to 36 weeks a decreased incidence of ROP was found in vitamin E-treated infants (94) and vitamin E containing supplements continue to find favor in protecting against many hyperbaric-oxygen-induced conditions. Treatment of moderate and severe ROP with vitamin E above physiologic serum levels appears promising and warrants further investigation. Sepsis and late-onset necrotizing enterocolitis is a potential complication especially in infants weighing 1500 g or less at birth, if the vitamin E treatment continues for at least 8 days.

THE VITAMIN K FAMILY

Since the isolation of vitamin K (1,4-naphthoquinone) several related substances have been recognized to possess the activity of this vitamin: the phylloquinones (vitamin K_1), the menaquinones (vitamin K_2) and the synthetic menadione (vitamin K_3). Vitamin K, which is chemically related to vitamin E, plays an important role in blood coagulation. A deficiency of it results in the synthesis by the liver of an abnormal prothrombin, which lacks the ability to chelate calcium ions essential for the binding of prothrombin to phospholipids and for its activation to thrombin (174). In vitamin K deficiency hemorrhages occur and it has been claimed, on rather nebulous evidence, that retinal hemorrhages in the newborn are less frequent because of the prophylactic administration of vitamin K (145,200).

ESSENTIAL FATTY ACIDS

The essential fatty acids are 18-carbon, polyunsaturated fatty acids that mammals are unable to synthesize. They are derivatives of the dietary precursors alpha-linolenic acid, eicosapentaenoic acid and docosahexaenoic acid (the omega-3 fatty acids) and linoleic acid (the omega-6 fatty acids) (117,209). Because omega-3 and omega-6 fatty acids are apparently important in the development of the brain and retina (18,83,185), their deficiency during infancy may be responsible for visual difficulties in later life (13,79). Essential fatty acids are readily available as over-the-counter nutritional supplements and many individuals use them because of their presumed ability to reduce the immune response in certain human disorders, such as rheumatoid arthritis and some ocular diseases including keratoconjunctivitis sicca and AMD. The ratio of omega-3 to omega-6 fatty acids in the diet is suspected of being important in the anti-inflammatory effort (161,162). While supplemental essential fatty acids may be beneficial and safe, high doses cause adverse effects such as hemorrhage (153). There is also increasing evidence that types of dietary fat affect the risk of both AMD and cataract (110,111,159).

METALS

Several metals, including calcium, iron, manganese, and zinc play essential roles in metabolic pathways and deficiencies of them cause significant disease (see Chapter 48).

NUTRITIONAL AMBLYOPIA

A gradual impairment of central vision commonly develops along with other signs of malnutrition in malnourished individuals of all ages. While the amblyopia is reversible in the early stages it may become permanent in this entity, designated nutritional amblyopia. Impaired vision served by thepapillomacular bundle results in central or paracentral scotomas and fundoscopy discloses pallor of the temporal portions of the optic nerve heads. In a postmortem study of 11 former prisoners-of-war with nutritional amblyopia, Fisher (50) observed degeneration of the papillomacular bundles in four cases.

The cause of nutritional amblyopia, which is generally associated with a deficiency of multiple essential nutrients, remains unknown, but a deficiency of one or more members of the vitamin B complex is believed to be particularly important. While some investigators consider thiamine to be important, others disagree (42). Many individuals with this ocular abnormality have a histamine-fast achlorhydria but the extreme rarity of the condition in persons with true pernicious anemia mitigates against this association.

The so-called tobacco–alcohol amblyopia may be a variant of nutritional amblyopia. Folate deficiency is common in patients with tobacco–alcohol amblyopia, but the role of folic acid in this disorder has been underplayed. The role of cyanide from tobacco smoke, folate and other dietary deficiencies in tobacco–alcohol amblyopia is reviewed by Dang (36). A new hypothesis of the pathogenesis of the amblyopia presumes an alteration of methionine and *S*-adenosyl-L-methionine metabolism.

NUTRITIONAL ASPECTS OF AGE-RELATED MACULOPATHY

AMD is the leading cause of irreversible vision loss in Australian, Western European, and North American elder populations (54,155,183) (see Chapter 18). Dietary intervention with antioxidants, appears to offer a cost-effective means to delay the occurrence and progress of AMD. The hypothesis that micronutrient antioxidants can protect against AMD comes from mounting evidence that oxidative stress plays a causal role in AMD (204) and the observation that diets rich in fruits and vegetables and use of specific antioxidant supplements, are associated with a reduced risk of AMD (29,114,156,159). Specifically, several large observational studies (30–32,51,188,189) and intervention trials (1,130,175,180,181) have focused on the effect of vitamin C, vitamin E, beta-carotene, and zinc in combination or alone on the prevention of AMD.

The macular pigment (MP) is composed of two antioxidant hydroxyl-carotenoids, lutein (L) and zeaxanthin (Z) (98) and is entirely of dietary origin (112). It has been almost three decades since scientists learned that the yellow MP serves as a blue-light filter and it was postulated that L/Z intake may protect against AMD (167). This was corroborated with the finding from Seddon et al. that higher L/Z dietary intake is related to lower risk for AMD (156). Since then, many observational studies have tried to relate dietary or blood L/Z to the risk for AMD (29,114). The results are mixed. Bioavailability is an important issue in this inconsistency. There is considerable interindividual variability with respect to absorption of carotenoids and recently, obesity (157) another risk factor of AMD, has been proposed to interact with L/Z to affect the risk for AMD (93). Currently, no published clinical trial indicates whether or not L/Z supplements prevent or delay the progression of AMD in humans. However, an ongoing multicenter Age-Related Eye Disease clinical trial (AREDS II), which aims to increase our understanding of the role of nutrients as well as potential contributions of L/Z in the development of AMD (25) will provide valuable information.

Overall the available evidence indicates a protective role for antioxidants with respect to a diminished risk for onset or progression of AMD, although the record is neither robust nor consistent (29). Further studies should focus on how these antioxidants are distributed in the body and interact with other risk factors for AMD. Studies on gene–nutrient interaction would be also informative. Such information, together with evidence from large interventional trials of antioxidant supplements using different populations, will provide evidence-based strategies for addressing the emerging significant AMD burden.

There is increasing evidence that types of dietary fat and carbohydrate, which have already been related to the risk of diabetes mellitus and cardiovascular diseases (81,154) affect the risk of AMD (26,158). Since dietary patterns high in antioxidants reduce the risk for major systemic diseases (81,154), persons at high risk of AMD, such as those with early or intermediate signs of AMD (large drusen and pigment abnormalities) or those with a family history of AMD, should be advised to consume more foods containing these antioxidants, such as whole grains (vitamin E, zinc), nuts (vitamin E), dairy products (zinc), kale (beta-carotene, L/Z), spinach (beta-carotene, L/Z), citrus fruits (vitamin C), green peppers (vitamin C), and broccoli (vitamin C, L/Z).

NUTRITIONAL ASPECTS OF CATARACT

Lens health has also been associated with intake of carotenoids, including a vitamin A precursor. Starting in 1991 (87) a variety of studies, suggested that diets rich in fruits and vegetables and/or which provide a high content of vitamin A or beta-carotene, provide protection against cataract (176). What seems clear is that good nutrition, based upon diets which are rich in fruits and vegetables, coupled with healthy lifestyles, which preclude known risk factors for eye diseases such as smoking, overweight, and poverty, must be begun early in life to obtain the benefit of prolonged sight later in life.

For a more thorough review of the recent literature in nutritional and ophthalmic epidemiology, interested readers are refered to the more comprehensive review (29).

REFERENCES

1. Age-Related Eye Disease Study Research Group. A randomized, placebo-controlled, clinical trial of high-dose supplementation with vitamins C and E, beta carotene, and zinc for age-related macular degeneration and vision loss: AREDS report no. 8. Arch Ophthalmol 2001; 119:1417–36.
2. Armstrong RC, Monie IW. Congenital eye defects on rats following maternal folic-acid deficiency during pregnancy. J Embryol Exp Morphol 1966; 16:531–42.
3. Aydelotte MB. The Effects of Vitamin A and citral on epithelial differentiation in Vitro. 2. The chick oesophageal and corneal ppithelia and epidermis. J Embryol Exp Morphol 1963; 11:621–35.
4. Balkan W, Klintworth GK, Bock CB, Linney E. Transgenic mice expressing a constitutively active retinoic acid receptor in the lens exhibit ocular defects. Dev Biol 1992; 151:622–5.
5. Barnes MJ, Kodicek E. Biological hydroxylations and ascorbic acid with special regard to collagen metabolism. Vitam Horm 1972; 30:1–43.
6. Batey DW, Eckhert CD. Analysis of flavins in ocular tissues of the rabbit. Invest Ophthalmol Vis Sci 1987; 32: 1981–5.
7. Beitch I. The induction of keratinization in the corneal epithelium. A comparison of the "dry" and vitamin A-deficient eyes. Invest Ophthalmol 1970; 9:827–43.
8. Bellingham J, Foster RG. Opsins and mammalian photoentrainment. Cell Tissue Res 2002; 309:57–71.
9. Benke PJ. The isotretinoin teratogen syndrome. JAMA 1984; 251:3267–9.
10. Berger J, Shepard D, Morrow F, Taylor A. Relationship between dietary intake and tissue levels of reduced and total vitamin C in the nonscorbutic guinea pig. J Nutr 1989; 119:734–40.
11. Berman ER, Segal N, Horowitz J. Distribution and metabolism of vitamin A in pigment epithelium. Invest Ophthalmol Vis Sci 1979; 18(Suppl.):268.
12. Bessey OAW, SB. Vascularization of the cornea of the rat in riboflavin deficiency, with a note on corneal vascularization in vitamin A deficiency. J Exp Med 1939; 69:1–19.
13. Birch EE, Castaneda YS, Wheaton DH, et al. Visual maturation of term infants fed long-chain polyunsaturated fatty acid-supplemented or control formula for 12 mo. Am J Clin Nutr 2005; 81:871–9.
14. Blomhoff R, Green MH, Berg T, Norum KR. Transport and storage of vitamin A. Science 1990; 250:399–404.
15. Blondin J, Baragi VJ, Schwartz E, et al. Dietary vitamin C delays UV-induced age-related eye lens protein damage. Ann N Y Acad Sci 1987; 498:460–3.
16. Boisselot J. Malformations foetales par insufficiance en acide pantothenique. Arch Franc Pediat 1949; 6: 225–30.
17. Bok D, Heller J. Transport of retinol from the blood to the retina: an autoradiographic study of the pigment epithelial cell surface receptor for plasma retinol-binding protein. Exp Eye Res 1976; 22:395–402.
18. Bourre JM. Roles of unsaturated fatty acids (especially omega-3 fatty acids) in the brain at various ages and during ageing. J Nutr Health Aging 2004; 8:163–74.
19. Brammer JD, White RH. Vitamin A deficiency: effect on mosquito eye ultrastructure. Science 1969; 163:821–3.
20. Bridges CD, Hollyfield JG, Besharse JC, Rayborn ME. Visual pigment loss after light-induced shedding of rod outer segments. Exp Eye Res 1976; 23:637–41.
21. Bridges CD. Vitamin A and the role of the pigment epithelium during bleaching and regeneration of rhodopsin in the frog eye. Exp Eye Res 1976; 22:435–55.
22. Callison EC, Orent-Keiles E. Abnormalities of the eye occurring in young vitamin E-deficient rats. Proc Soc Exp Biol Med 1951; 76:295–7.
23. Campbell ACP, Russell WR. Wernicke's encephalopathy: clinical features and their probable relationship to Vitamin B deficiency. Quart J Med 1941; 34:41–64.
24. Carter-Dawson L, Kuwabara T, O'Brien PJ, Bieri JG. Structural and biochemical changes in vitamin A – deficient rat retinas. Invest Ophthalmol Vis Sci 1979; 18: 437–46.
25. Chew EY, Clemons T. Vitamin E and the age-related eye disease study supplementation for age-related macular degeneration. Arch Ophthalmol 2005; 123:395–6.
26. Chiu CJ, Hubbard LD, Armstrong J, et al. Dietary glycemic index and carbohydrate in relation to early age-related macular degeneration. Am J Clin Nutr 2006; 83:880–6.
27. Chiu CJ, Milton RC, Gensler G, Taylor A. Dietary carbohydrate and glycemic index in relation to cortical and nuclear lens opacities in the Age-Related Eye Disease Study. Am J Clin Nutr 2006; 83:1177–84.
28. Chiu CJ, Morris MS, Rogers G, et al. Carbohydrate intake and glycemic index in relation to the odds of early cortical and nuclear lens opacities. Am J Clin Nutr 2005; 81:1411–6.

29. Chiu CJ, Taylor A. Nutritional antioxidants and age-related cataract and maculopathy. Exp Eye Res 2007; 84:229–45.
30. Cho E, Seddon JM, Rosner B, et al. Prospective study of intake of fruits, vegetables, vitamins, and carotenoids and risk of age-related maculopathy. Arch Ophthalmol 2004; 122:883–92.
31. Cho E, Stampfer MJ, Seddon JM, et al. Prospective study of zinc intake and the risk of age-related macular degeneration. Ann Epidemiol 2001; 11:328–36.
32. Christen WG, Ajani UA, Glynn RJ, et al. Prospective cohort study of antioxidant vitamin supplement use and the risk of age-related maculopathy. Am J Epidemiol 1999; 149:476–84.
33. Christian P. Maternal nutrition, health, and survival. Nutr Rev 2002; 60(5):S59–63.
34. Collins MD, Mao GE. Teratology of retinoids. Annu Rev Pharmacol Toxicol 1999; 39:399–430.
35. Cooperman JM, Lopez R. Riboflavin, In: Machlin LJ, ed. Handbook of Vitamins. Washington DC: National Academy Press, 1991:283–310.
36. Dang CV. Tobacco-alcohol amblyopia: a proposed biochemical basis for pathogenesis. Med Hypotheses 1981; 7: 1317–28.
37. Day PL. Vitamin G deficiency. Am J Publ Health 1934; 24: 603–8.
38. Day PL, Darby WJ, Cosgrove KW. The arrest of nutritional cataract by the use of riboflavin. J Nutr 1938; 15:83–90.
39. Day PL, Langston WC. Further experiments with cataract in albino rats resulting from the withdrawal of Vitamin G (B2) from the diet. J Nutr 1934; 7:97–106.
40. DeLuca HF, Schnoes HK. Metabolism and mechanism of action of vitamin D. Annu Rev Biochem 1976; 45:631–66.
41. DeLuca L, Rosso G, Wolf G. The biosynthesis of a mannolipid that contains a polar metabolite of 15-14c-retinol. Biochem. Biophys. Res. Commun 1970; 41:615–20.
42. Denny-Brown DE. Neurological conditions resulting from prolonged and severe dietary restriction (Case reports in prisoners-of-war and general review.). Medicine 1947; 26:41–113.
43. Devi A, Raina PL, Singh A. Abnormal protein and nucleic acid metabolism as a cause of cataract formation induced by nutritional deficiency in rabbits. Br J Ophthalmol 1965; 49:271–5.
44. Dilley RAM DG. Alpha-tocopherol in the retinal outer segment of bovine eyes. J Mem Biol 1970; 2:317–23.
45. Dohlman CH, Kalevar V. Cornea in hypovitaminosis A and protein deficiency. Isr J Med Sci 1972; 8:1179–83.
46. Dowling JE. The organization of vertebrate visual receptors. In: Allen JM, ed. Molecular Organization and Biological Function. New York: Harper and Row, 1967: 186–210.
47. Dowling JE, Wald G. The biological function of Vitamin A acid. Proc Natl Acad Sci USA 1960; 46:587–608.
48. Eckhert CD, Hsu MH, Batey DW. Effect of dietary riboflavin on retinal density and flavin concentrations in normal and dystrophic RCS rats. Prog Clin Biol Res 1989; 314:331–41.
49. Feldman MH, Schlezinger NS. Benign intracranial hypertension associated with hypervitaminosis A. Arch Neurol 1970; 22:1–7.
50. Fisher M. Residual neuropathological changes in Canadians held prisoners of war by the Japanese; Strachan's disease. Can Serv Med J 1955; 11:157–99.
51. Flood V, Smith W, Wang JJ, Manzi F, et al. Dietary antioxidant intake and incidence of early age-related maculopathy: the Blue Mountains Eye Study. Ophthalmology 2002; 109:2272–8.
52. Follis RH Jr. Deficiency Diseases: Functional and Structural Changes in Mammalia, Which Result from Exogenous or Endogenous Lackof One or More Essential Nutrients. Springfield, IL: Charles C. Thomas, 1958.
53. Freeman AG, Heaton JM. The aetiology of retrobulbar neuritis in Addisonian pernicious anaemia. Lancet 1961; 1:908–11.
54. Friedman DS, O'Colmain BJ, Munoz B, et al. Prevalence of age-related macular degeneration in the United States. Arch Ophthalmol 2004; 122:564–72.
55. Galdones E, Lohnes D, Hales BF. Role of retinoic acid receptors alpha1 and gamma in the response of murine limbs to retinol in vitro. Birth Defects Res A Clin Mol Teratol 2006; 76:39–45.
56. Geelen JA. Hypervitaminosis A induced teratogenesis. CRC Crit Rev Toxicol 1979; 6:351–75.
57. Gershoff SN, Andrus SB, Hegsted DM. The effect of the carbohydrate and fat content of the diet upon the riboflavin requirement of the cat. J Nutr 1959; 68: 75–88.
58. Giblin FJ, Winkler BS, Sasaki H, et al. Reduction of dehydroascorbic acid in lens epithelium by the glutathione redox cycle. Invest Ophthalmol Vis Sci 1993; 34: 1298, ARVO abstract #2929.
59. Giroud A, Delmas A, Prost H, Lefebvres J. Malformations encéphaliques par carenve enacide pantothénique et leur interpretation. Acta Anat (Basel) 1957; 29:209–27.
60. Giroud A, Lefebvres J, Prost H, Dupuis R. Malformations des membres dues a des lesions vasculaires chez le foetus de rat deficient en acide pantothenique. J Embryol Exp Morph 1955; 3:1–12.
61. Giroud A, Martinet M. Tératogenèse par hautes doses de Vitamin A enfonction des stades du développement. Arch Anat Micr 1956; 45:77–98.
62. Goldsmith G. Riboflavin deficiency. In: Rivlin RS, ed., Riboflavin. New York: Plenum Press, 1975:221–38.
63. Goodman DS Vitamin A and retinoids in health and disease. N Engl J Med 1984; 310:1023–31.
64. Gould BS. Ascorbic acid and collagen fiber formation. Vitam Horm 1960; 18:89–120.
65. Grainger RB, O'Dell BL, Hogan AG. Congenital malformations as related to deficiencies of riboflavin and vitamin B12, source of protein, calcium to phosphorus ratio and skeletal phosphorus metabolism. J Nutr 1954; 54:33–48.
66. Hale F. The relation of maternal vitamin A deficiency to microphthalmia in pigs. Tex State Med J 1937; 33: 228–32.
67. Halver JE. Nutrition of salmonoid fishes. III. Water-soluble vitamin requirements of chinook salmon. J Nutr 1974; 62:225–43.
68. Halwer M. The Photochemistry of riboflavin and related compounds. J Am Chem Soc 1951; 73:4870–4.
69. Hamilton JB. Eyes and scurvy. Trans Ophthalmol Soc Aust 1958; 18:83–91.
70. Hammond BR Jr, Johnson EJ, Russell RM, et al. Dietary modification of human macular pigment density. Invest Ophthalmol Vis Sci 1997; 38:1795–801.
71. Hayes KC. Pathophysiology of vitamin E deficiency in monkeys. Am J Clin Nutr 1974; 27:1130–40.
72. Hayes KC. Retinal degeneration in monkeys induced by deficiencies of vitamins E or A. Invest Ophthalmol 1974; 13:499–510.
73. Heath H. The distribution and possible functions of ascorbic acid in the eye. Exp Eye Res 1962; 1:362–7.

74. Heaton JM, Mc CA, Freeman AG. Tobacco amblyopia: a clinical manifestation of vitamin-B12 deficiency. Lancet 1958; 2:286–90.
75. Heffley JD, Williams RJ. The nutritional teamwork approach: prevention and regression of cataracts in rats. Proc Natl Acad Sci U S A 1974; 71:4164–8.
76. Helgerud P, Petersen LB, Norum KR. Retinol esterification by microsomes from the mucosa of human small intestine. Evidence for acyl-Coenzyme A retinol acyltransferase activity. J Clin Invest 1983; 71:747–53.
77. Helgerud P, Petersen LB, Norum KR. Acyl CoA:retinol acyltransferase in rat small intestine: its activity and some properties of the enzymic reaction. J Lipid Res 1982; 23: 609–18.
78. Hirosawa K, Yamada E. The localization of the vitamin A in the mouse liver as revealed by electron microscope radioautography. J Electron Microsc (Tokyo) 1973; 22: 337–46.
79. Hoffman DR, Birch EE, Birch DG, et al. Impact of early dietary intake and blood lipid composition of long-chain polyunsaturated fatty acids on later visual development. J Pediatr Gastroenterol Nutr 2000; 31:540–53.
80. Horwitt MKW LA. Riboflavin biochemical systems—the vitamins. 1967; 5:53–70.
81. Hu FB, Willett WC. Optimal diets for prevention of coronary heart disease. JAMA 2002; 288:2569–78.
82. Hubbard RKA. The action of light on rhodopsin. Proc Natl Acad Sci U S A 1958; 44:130–9.
83. Innis SM. The role of dietary n-6 and n-3 fatty acids in the developing brain. Dev Neurosci 2000; 22:474–80.
84. Irinoda K, Sato S. Contribution to the ocular manifestation of riboflavin deficiency. Tohoku J Exp Med 1954; 61: 93–104.
85. Jackson BK, VE. The relation between maternal vitamin-A intake blood level and ocular abnormalities in the offspring of the rat. Am J Ophthalmol 1946; 29:1234–42.
86. Jackson SFF HB. Epidermal fine structure in embryonic chicken skin during atypical differentiation induced by vitamin A in culture. Dev Biol 1963; 7:394–419.
87. Jacques PF, Chylack LT Jr. Epidemiologic evidence of a role for the antioxidant vitamins and carotenoids in cataract prevention. Am J Clin Nutr 1991; 53:352S–5S.
88. Jacques PF, Chylack LTJ, Hankinson SE, et al. Long-term nutrient intake and early age-related nuclear lens opacities. Arch Ophthalmol 2001; 119:1009–19.
89. Jacques PF, Moeller SM, Hankinson SE, et al. Weight status, abdominal adiposity, diabetes and early age-related lens opacities. Am J Clin Nutr 2003; 78:400–5.
90. Jacques PF, Taylor A, Hankinson SE, et al. Long-term vitamin C supplement use and prevalence of early age-related lens opacities. Am J Clin Nutr 1997; 66:911–6.
91. Jacques PF, Taylor A, Moeller S, et al. Long-term nutrient intake and 5-year change in nuclear lens opacities. Arch Ophthalmol 2005; 123:517–26.
92. Jayaraj AP, Leela R, Rao PB. Studies on cornea and conjunctival mucous metaplasia in vitamin A deficient rats. Exp Eye Res 1971; 12:1–5.
93. Johnson EJ. Obesity, lutein metabolism, and age-related macular degeneration: a web of connections. Nutr Rev 2005; 63:9–15.
94. Johnson L, Quinn GE, Abbasi S, et al. Effect of sustained pharmacologic vitamin E levels on incidence and severity of retinopathy of prematurity: a controlled clinical trial. J Pediatr 1989; 114:827–38.
95. Kalter H, Warkany J. Congenital malformations in inbred strains of mice induced by riboflavin-deficient, galactoflavin-containing diets. J Exp Zool 1957; 136:531–65.
96. Katz ML, Kutryb MJ, Norberg M, et al. Maintenance of opsin density in photoreceptor outer segments of retinoid-deprived rats. Invest Ophthalmol Vis Sci 1991; 32:1968–80.
97. Katz ML, Norberg M, Stientjes HJ. Reduced phagosomal content of the retinal pigment epithelium in response to retinoid deprivation. Invest Ophthalmol Vis Sci 1992; 33: 2612–8.
98. Khachik F, Bernstein PS, Garland DL. Identification of lutein and zeaxanthin oxidation products in human and monkey retinas. Invest Ophthalmol Vis Sci 1997; 38: 1802–11.
99. Kim YCL, Wolf G. Vitamin A deficiency and the glycoproteins of rat corneal epithelium. J. Nutr 1974; 104:710–8.
100. Kobayashi K, Takahashi Y, Shibasaki S. Cytological studies of fat-storing cells in the liver of rats given large doses of vitamin A. Nat New Biol 1973; 243:186–8.
101. Kroft A, Hubbard R. The mechanism of bleaching rhodopsin. Ann N Y Acad Sci 1958; 74:266–80.
102. Kuzniarz M, Mitchell P, Cumming RG, Flood VM. Use of vitamin supplements and cataract: the Blue Mountains Eye Study. Am J Ophthalmol 2001; 132:19–26.
103. Lamming GE, Salisbury GW, Hays RL, Kendall KA. The effect of incipient vitamin A deficiency on reproduction in the rabbit. II. Embryonic and fetal development. J Nutr 1954; 52:227–36.
104. Landrum JT, Bone RA, Joa H, et al. A one year study of the macular pigment: the effect of 140 days of a lutein supplement. Exp Eye Res 1997; 65:57–62.
105. Leske MC, Chylack LTJ, Wu SY. The lens opacities case-control study. Risk factors for cataract. Arch Ophthalmol 1991; 109:244–51.
106. Leuenberger PM, Novikoff AB. Studies on microperoxisomes. VII. Pigment epithelial cells and other cell types in the retina of rodents. J Cell Biol 1975; 65:324–34.
107. Levij IS, Polliack A. Potentiating effect of vitamin A on 9–10 dimethyl 1–2 benzanthracene—carcinogenesis in the hamster cheek pouch. Cancer 1968; 22:300–6.
108. Lippincott SW, Morris HP. Pathologic changes associated with riboflavin deficiency in the mouse. J Nat Cancer Inst 1942; 2:601–10.
109. Lu M, Cho E, Taylor A, Hankinson SE, et al. Prospective study of dietary fat and rsk of cataract extraction among US women. Am J Epidemiol 2005 161:948–59.
110. Lu M, Taylor A, Chylack LTJ, et al. Dietary fat intake and early age-related lens opacities. Am J Clin Nutr 2005; 81: 773–9.
111. MacDonald PN, Ong DE. Evidence for a lecithin-retinol acyltransferase activity in the rat small intestine. J Biol Chem 1988; 263:12478–82.
112. Malinow MR, Feeney-Burns L, Peterson LH, et al. Diet-related macular anomalies in monkeys. Invest Ophthalmol Vis Sci 1980; 19:857–63.
113. Mangels AR, Holden JM, Beecher GR, et al. Carotenoid content of fruits and vegetables: an evaluation of analytic data. J Am Diet Assoc 1993; 93:284–96.
114. Mares-Perlman J, Klein R. Diet and age-related macular degeneration. In: Taylor A, ed. Nutritional and Environmental Influences on the Eye. Boca Raton, FL: CRC Press, 1999: 181–214.
115. Maynard RB. Blindness among prisoners of war. Trans Ophthalmol Soc Aust 1946; 6:92–103.
116. McCormick DB. The fate of riboflavin in the mammal. Nutr Rev 1972; 30:75–9.
117. McCowen KC, Bistrian BR. Essential fatty acids and their derivatives. Curr Opin Gastroenterol 2005; 21:207–15.

118. McLaren DS. Nutritional Ophthalmology. 2nd ed. London: Academic Press, 1980.
119. Merrill AH Jr, Lambeth JD, Edmondson DE, McCormick DB. Formation and mode of action of flavoproteins. Annu Rev Nutr 1981; 1:281–317.
120. Meyer A. The Wernicke syndrome; with special reference to manic syndromes associated with hypothalmic lesions. J Neurol Psychiat 1944; 7:66–75.
121. Miller ER, Johnston RL, Hoefer JA, Luecke RW. The riboflavin requirement of the baby pig. J Nutr 1954; 52: 405–13.
122. Moeller SM, Taylor A, Tucker KL, et al. Overall adherence to the dietary guidelines for americans is associated with reduced prevalence of early age-related nuclear lens opacities in women. J Nutr 2004; 134:1812–9.
123. Molenaar I, Vos J, Hommes FA. Effect of vitamin E deficiency on cellular membranes. Vitam Horm 1972; 30: 45–82.
124. Moore LA. Relationship between carotene, blindness due to constriction of the optic nerve, papillary edema and nyctalopia in calves. J Nutr 1939; 17:443–59.
125. Muller F. Flavin radicals: chemistry and biochemistry. Free Radic Biol Med 1987; 3:215–30.
126. Muto Y, Smith JE, Milch PO, Goodman DS. Regulation of retinol-binding protein metabolism by vitamin A status in the rat. J Biol Chem 1972; 247:2542–50.
127. Nathans J, Thomas D, Hogness DS. Molecular genetics of human color vision: the genes encoding blue, green, and red pigments. Science 1986; 232:193–202.
128. Nelson MM, Baird CD, Wright HV, Evans HM. Multiple congenital abnormalities in the rat resulting from riboflavin deficiency induced by the antimetabolite galactoflavin. J Nutr 1957; 58:125–34.
129. Nelson MM, Wright HV, Baird CD, Evans HM. Teratogenic effects of pantothenic acid deficiency in the rat. J Nutr 1957; 62:395–405.
130. Newsome DA, Swartz M, Leone NC, et al. Oral zinc in macular degeneration. Arch Ophthalmol 1988; 106:192–8.
131. Noell WK, Delmelle MC, Albrecht R. Vitamin A deficiency effect on retina: dependence on light. Science 1971; 172:72–5.
132. Olson JA. Some aspects of vitamin A metabolism. Vitam Horm 1968; 26:1–63.
133. Ong DE, Kakkad B, MacDonald PN. Acyl-CoA-independent esterification of retinol bound to cellular retinol-binding protein (type II) by microsomes from rat small intestine. J Biol Chem 1987; 262:2729–36.
134. Owens WC, Owens EU. Retrolental fibroplasia in premature infants; studies on the prophylaxis of the disease; the use of alpha tocopheryl acetate. Am J Ophthalmol 1949; 32:1631–7.
135. Peterson PA, Berggard I. Isolation and properties of a human retinol-transporting protein. J Biol Chem 1971; 246:25–33.
136. Pfister RR, Renner ME. The corneal and conjunctival surface in vitamin A deficiency: a scanning electron microscopy study. Invest Ophthalmol Vis Sci 1978; 17: 874–83.
137. Philpot FJ, Pirie A. Riboflavin and riboflavin adenine dinucleotide in ox ocular tissues. Biochem J 1943; 37:2504.
138. Pirie A. Xerophthalmia. Invest Ophthalmol 1976; 15: 417–422.
139. Pirie A. Vitamin A deficiency and child blindness in the developing world. Proc Nutr Soc 1983; 42:53–64.
140. Pirie A, Werb Z, Burleigh MC. Collagenase and other proteinases in the cornea of the retinol-deficient rat. Br J Nutr 1975; 34:297–309.
141. Polliak AS, ZB. Enhancing effect of excess topical vitamin A on Rous sarcoma in chicken. J Natl Cancer Inst 1972; 48: 407–16.
142. Poswillo D. The pathogenesis of the Treacher Collins syndrome (mandibulofacial dysostosis). Br J Oral Surg 1975; 13:1–26.
143. Poswillo D. Mechanisms and pathogenesis of malformation. Br Med Bull 1976; 32:59–64.
144. Powell SR, Schwab IR. Nutritional disorders affecting the peripheral cornea. Int Ophthalmol Clin 1986; 26:137–46.
145. Pray LGM, Pokard HS, WE. Hemorrhagic diathesis of the newborn effect of vitamin A prophylaxis and therapy. Am J Obstet Gynec 1941; 42:836–45.
146. Prchal JT, Conrad ME, Skalka HW. Association of presenile cataracts with heterozygosity for galactosaemic states and with riboflavin deficiency. Lancet 1978; 1:12–3.
147. Prutkin L. The effect of vitamin A acid on tumorigenesis and protein production. Cancer Res 1968; 28:1021–30.
148. Ramalingaswami V, Leach EH, Sriramachari S. Ocular structure in vitamin A deficiency in the monkey. Q J Exp Psychol 1955; 40:337–47.
149. Robertson WV. The biochemical role of ascorbic acid in connective tissue. Ann N Y Acad Sci 1961; 92:159–67.
150. Robison WG Jr, Kuwabara T. Vitamin A storage and peroxisomes in retinal pigment epithelium and liver. Invest Ophthalmol Vis Sci 1977; 16:1107–10.
151. Robison WG Jr, Kuwubara T, Bieri JG. Deficiencies of vitamins E and A in the rat: retinal damage and lipofuscin accumulation. Invest Ophthalmol Vis Sci 1980; 19:1030–7.
152. Rodger FC. Experimental thiamin deficiency as a cause of degeneration in the visual pathway of the rat. Br J Ophthalmol 1953; 37:11–29.
153. SanGiovanni JP, Chew EY. The role of omega-3 long-chain polyunsaturated fatty acids in health and disease of the retina. Prog Retin Eye Res 2005; 24:87–138.
154. Schulze MB, Hu FB. Primary prevention of diabetes: what can be done and how much can be prevented? Annu Rev Public Health 2005; 26:445–67.
155. Seddon J, Chen C. Epidemiology of age-related macular degeneration. In: Ryan SJ, ed. Retina. 4th ed. Vol. 2, Chapter 58. St. Louis, MO: Medical Retina. C.V. Mosby, 2005:1017–28.
156. Seddon JM, Ajani UA, Sperduto RD, et al. Dietary carotenoids, vitamins A, C, and E, and advanced age--related macular degeneration. Eye Disease Case-Control Study Group. JAMA 1994; 272:1413–20.
157. Seddon JM, Cote J, Davis N, Rosner B. Progression of age-related macular degeneration: association with body mass index, waist circumference, and waist-hip ratio. Arch Ophthalmol 2003; 121:785–92.
158. Seddon JM, Cote J, Rosner B. Progression of age-related macular degeneration: association with dietary fat, transunsaturated fat, nuts, and fish intake. Arch Ophthalmol 2003; 121:1728–37.
159. Seddon JM, Hennekens CH. Vitamins, minerals, and macular degeneration. Promising but unproven hypotheses. Arch Ophthalmol 1994; 112:176–9.
160. Shenefelt RE. Morphogenesis of malformations in hamsters caused by retinoic acid: relation to dose and stage at treatment. Teratology 1972; 5:103–18.
161. Simopoulos AP. The importance of the ratio of omega-6/omega-3 essential fatty acids. Biomed Pharmacother 2002; 56:365–79.
162. Simopoulos AP. Omega-3 fatty acids in inflammation and autoimmune diseases. J Am Coll Nutr 2002; 21: 495–505.

163. Sklan D. Vitamin A in human nutrition. Prog Food Nutr Sci 1987; 11:39–55.
164. Smith ECM, DE. The photochemical degradation of riboflavin. J Am Chem Soc 1963; 85:3285–8.
165. Smith FR, Goodman DS, Zaklama MS, et al. Serum vitamin A, retinol-binding protein, and prealbumin concentrations in protein-calorie malnutrition. I. A functional defect in hepatic retinol release. Am J Clin Nutr 1973; 26:973–81.
166. Smith FR, Suskind R, Thanangkul O, et al. Plasma vitamin A, retinol-binding protein and prealbumin concentrations in protein-calorie malnutrition. III. Response to varying dietary treatments. Am J Clin Nutr 1975; 28:732–8.
167. Snodderly DM, Auran JD, Delori FC. The macular pigment. II. Spatial distribution in primate retinas. Invest Ophthalmol Vis Sci 1984; 25:674–85.
168. Sommer A. Vitamin A deficiency today: conjunctival xerosis in cystic fibrosis. J R Soc Med 1989; 82:1–2.
169. Sommer A. Xerophthalmia, keratomalacia and nutritional blindness. Int Ophthalmol 1990; 14:195–9.
170. Sommer A. Vitamin A, infectious disease, and childhood mortality: a 2 solution? J Infect Dis 1993; 167:1003–7.
171. Sparrow JR, Fishkin N, Zhou J, et al. A2E, a byproduct of the visual cycle. Vision Res 2003; 43:2983–90.
172. Sporn MB, Dunlop NM, Newton DL, Smith JM. Prevention of chemical carcinogenesis by vitamin A and its synthetic analogs (retinoids). Fed Proc 1976; 35: 1332–8.
173. Sporn MB, Roberts AB. Biological methods for analysis and assay of retinoids: relationships between structure and activity. Retinoids 1984; 1:235–79.
174. Stenflo J. A new vitamin K-dependent protein. Purification from bovine plasma and preliminary characterization. J Biol Chem 1976; 251:355–63.
175. Stur M, Tittl M, Reitner A, Meisinger V. Oral zinc and the second eye in age-related macular degeneration. Invest Ophthalmol Vis Sci 1996; 37:1225–35.
176. Taylor A. Nutritional and environmental influences on the risk for cataract. In: Taylor A, ed. Nutritional and Environmental Influences on the Eye. New York: CRC Press, 1999:53–93.
177. Taylor A, Jacques PF, Nadler D, et al. Relationship in humans between ascorbic acid consumption and levels of total and reduced ascorbic acid in lens, aqueous humor, and plasma. Curr Eye Res 1991; 10:751–9.
178. Taylor A, Jacques PF, Nowell T, et al. Vitamin C in human and guinea pig aqueous, lens and plasma in relation to intake. Curr Eye Res 1997; 16:857–64.
179. Taylor A, Smith DE, Palmer VJ, et al. Relationships between acetone, cataracts, and ascorbate in hairless guinea pigs. Ophthal Res 1993; 25:30–5.
180. Taylor HR, Tikellis G, Robman LD, et al. Vitamin E supplementation and macular degeneration: randomised controlled trial. Br Med J 2002; 325:11–4.
181. Teikari JM, Laatikainen L, Virtamo J, et al. (1998) Six-year supplementation with alpha-tocopherol and beta-carotene and age-related maculopathy. Acta Ophthalmol Scand 2002; 76:224–9.
182. Tielsch JM, Sommer A. The epidemiology of vitamin A deficiency and xerophthalmia. Annu Rev Nutr 1984; 4: 183–205.
183. Tomany SC, Wang JJ, Van Leeuwen R, et al. Risk factors for incident age-related macular degeneration: pooled findings from 3 continents. Ophthalmology 2004; 111:1280–7.
184. Tripathi BJ, Tripathi RC. Cellular and subcellular events in retinopathy of oxygen toxicity with a preliminary report on the preventive role of vitamin E and gamma-aminobutyric acid: a study in vitro. Curr Eye Res 1984; 3: 193–208.
185. Uauy R, Hoffman DR, Peirano P, et al. Essential fatty acids in visual and brain development. Lipids 2001; 36: 885–95.
186. Uyeki EM, Doull J, Cheng CC, Misawa M. Teratogenic and antiteratogenic effects of nicotinamide derivatives in chick embryos. J Toxicol Environ Health 1982; 9:963–73.
187. Vahlquist A, Peterson PA. Comparative studies on the vitamin A transporting protein complex in human and cynomolgus plasma. Biochemistry 1972; 11:4526–32.
188. van Leeuwen R, Boekhoorn S, Vingerling JR, et al. Dietary intake of antioxidants and risk of age-related macular degeneration. JAMA 2005; 294:3101–7.
189. Vanden Langenberg GM, Mares-Perlman JA, Klein R, et al. Associations between antioxidant and zinc intake and the 5-year incidence of early age-related maculopathy in the Beaver Dam Eye Study. Am J Epidemiol 1998; 148:204–14.
190. Varma SD, Richards RD. Ascorbic acid and the eye lens. Ophthalmic Res 1988; 20:164–73.
191. Varma SD, Srivastava VK, Richards RD. Photoperoxidation in lens and cataract formation: preventive role of superoxide dismutase, catalase and vitamin C. Ophthal Res 1982; 14:167–75.
192. Waisman H. Production of riboflavin deficiency in the monkey. Proc Soc Exp Biol Med 1944; 55:69–71.
193. Wake K. Development of vitamin A-rich lipid droplets in multivesicular bodies of rat liver stellate cells. J Cell Biol 1974; 63:683–91.
194. Wald G. Molecular basis of visual excitation. Science 1968; 162:230–9.
195. Ward SJ, Chambon P, Ong DE, Bavik C. A retinol-binding protein receptor-mediated mechanism for uptake of vitamin A to postimplantation rat embryos. Biol Reprod 1997; 57:751–5.
196. Warkany J, Roth CB. Congenital malformations induced in rats by maternal vitamin A deficiency: II. Effects of varying preparatory diet upon yield of abnormal young. J Nutr 1948; 35:1–11.
197. Warkany J, Schraffenberger E. Congenital malformations induced in rats by maternal vitamin A deficiency. I. Defects of the eye. Arch Ophthalmol 1946; 35:150–69.
198. Weissman GT L. Studies on lysosomes. II. The Effect of cortisone on the release of acid hydrolases from a large granule fraction of rabbit liver induced by an excess of vitamin A. J Clin Invest 1963; 42:661–9.
199. Wiggert BO, Bergsma DR, Chader GJ. Retinol receptors of the retina and pigment epithelium: further characterization and species variation. Exp Eye Res 1976; 22:411–8.
200. Wille H. Investigations in the influence of K avitaminosis on the occurrence of retinal hemorrhages in the newborn: a preliminary report. Acta Ophthalmol 1944; 22:261–9.
201. Wilson J, Langman MJ. Relation of sub-acute combined degeneration of the cord to vitamin B 12 deficiency. Nature 1966; 212:787–9.
202. Wilson J, Matthews DM. Metabolic inter-relationships between cyanide, thiocyanate and vitamin B 12 in smokers and non-smokers. Clin Sci 1966; 31:1–7.
203. Wilson JG, Roth CB, Warkany J. An analysis of the syndrome of malformations induced by maternal vitamin A deficiency. Effects of restoration of vitamin A at various times during gestation. Am J Anat 1953; 92: 189–217.

204. Winkler BS, Boulton ME, Gottsch JD, Sternberg P. Oxidative damage and age-related macular degeneration. Mol Vis 1999; 5:32–42.
205. Wiss O, Weber F. The liver and vitamins. In: Rouiller, ed. The Liver, Morphology, Biochemistry, Physiology. Vol. 2. New York: Academic Press, 1964:133–76.
206. Witkovsky P, Gallin E, Hollyfield JG, Ripps H, Bridges CD. Photoreceptor thresholds and visual pigment levels in normal and vitamin A-deprived Xenopus tadpoles. J Neurophysiol 1976; 39:1272–87.
207. Wolbach SBH, PR. Tissue changes following deprivation of fat-soluble A vitamin. J Exp Med 1925; 42:753–78.
208. Wolf G. Multiple functions of vitamin A. Physiol Rev 1984; 64:873–937.
209. Wong KW. Clinical efficacy of *n* 3 fatty acid supplementation in patients with asthma. J Am Diet Assoc 2005; 105: 98–105.
210. Young RW, Bok D. Autoradiographic studies on the metabolism of the retinal pigment epithelium. Invest Ophthalmol 1970; 9:524–36.

50

Toxicology

Devin M. Gattey
Casey Eye Institute, Oregon Health and Science University, Portland, Oregon, U.S.A.

INTRODUCTION

Being an organ that is small, metabolically active, frequently exposed to bright light, and containing many cells that are poor at repairing themselves, the eye is exquisitely sensitive to toxins and especially prone to adverse drug reactions (ADRs). Some structures, including the cornea and lens, are avascular, limiting the ability of these tissues to repair damage.

The purpose of this chapter is not to list every drug and toxin known or suspected to cause ocular damage as this has been expertly accomplished by others (22,28). Rather, the goal is to address substances most clinically relevant with attention to the mechanisms of injury where known. Metal toxicity and defenses against these noxious agents is covered in Chapter 48. As the fields of genetics and molecular biology advance, so is our understanding of ADRs. To date most of our understanding is limited to the level of clinical observations and the light microscope. Surprisingly, very few investigators have studied the pathobiology of substances that are toxic to the ocular tissues. This topic remains a fertile field for investigation particularly with contemporary molecular biologic and genetic techniques.

The eye's response to drug and toxin exposure ranges from blindness to subtle symptoms the patient may not share with the examining ophthalmologist (Table 1). The task of recognizing ocular ADRs and informing the ophthalmic community about them falls to individual practitioners by means of peer-reviewed publications or reporting systems such as the National Registry of Drug-Induced Ocular Side Effects (3). Cases of suspected drug toxicity can be reported on the internet (www.eyedrugregistry.com). Recent advances in magnetic resonance imaging (MRI), ocular coherence tomography (OCT), confocal microscopy, positron emission tomography (PET), and other technologies have aided study of ocular ADRs and toxin damage in the globe and the parts of the central nervous system (CNS) subserving vision (52,58,60).

Table 1 Ocular Adverse Drug Reactions of Common Clinical Concern

Drug	Ocular adverse drug reaction
Amiodarone	Cornea—verticillata (glare, photosensitivity) Lens—subcapsular lens opacities (not visually significant) Optic nerve—NAION-like optic neuropathy (bilateral, may resolve)
Corticosteroids	Anterior segment—impaired aqueous outflow (elevated intraocular pressure, glaucoma) Lens—posterior subcapsular cataract
Ethambutol	Optic Nerve—optic neuropathy (central or peripheral, reversible or permanent)
Hydroxychloroquine and chloroquine	Cornea—verticillata (glare, photosensitivity) Retina—retinopathy (bilateral bull eye maculopathy with central visual field defects and permanent vision loss)
Isotretinoin	Tear film—meibomian gland dysfunction (keratitis sicca, gland atrophy) Conjunctiva—conjunctivitis Optic nerve—papilledema (pseudotumor cerebri) Ocular development—teratogenesis (microphthalmia, visual pathway disturbance)
Pamidronate	Sclera—scleritis, episcleritis (resolves with discontinuation) Uvea—anterior uveitis
Sildenafil	Vision—dyschromatopsia (dose-dependant colored tinge to viewed objects)
Topiramate	Anterior segment—angle closure glaucoma (anterior chamber shallowing, reversible) Vision—myopic shift (may be >6 diopters)

Since the publication of the last edition, many new drugs have been marketed as older pharmaceuticals have become obsolete. Some of the older, now less commonly prescribed drugs, such as phenothiazines, are a shrinking concern for ophthalmologists. Others, such as prostaglandin analogs, are more likely to cause ocular side effects. Another important development has been the huge increase in herbal supplements and homeopathic remedies (25).

FACTORS PREDISPOSING TO DRUG TOXICITY

Individual responses to particular toxic agents may vary due to such factors as the route of administration and metabolism of the toxin, the age of the individual, the presence of underlying disease, and genetic differences between individuals. Factors that influence drug absorption and metabolism predispose infants and the elderly to toxicity. In the pediatric population, adult doses of topically applied ocular medication potentially increase the risk of adverse effects (15,18,48,56). Brimonidine, an alpha agonist eye drop with intraocular pressure (IOP) lowering properties, is well documented to cause CNS depression in certain children and elderly patients (10,19).

Protein Binding

Plasma proteins bind many types of drugs and drug metabolites. The major portion of a drug is usually bound to a protein and only the free portion is pharmacologically active. States of stress such as trauma or infection may increase protein binding and so reduce drug activity at therapeutic dose levels. Hypoalbuminemia or renal or liver disease may increase the fraction of unbound active drug, leading to a higher risk of toxicity. Multiple drugs may compete for a common binding site on a plasma protein, altering levels of free drug, especially for the less tightly bound drugs.

Some drugs have multiple routes of elimination such that the dysfunction of a single route is unlikely to cause a toxic level. Other drugs have only one principal route and if that route is compromised by illness or genetic deficiency, toxic levels are quickly reached. One example of this phenomenon is digoxin which, though initially metabolized by the cytochrome system, relies heavily on *p*-glycoprotein for excretion. Digoxin can reach toxic levels if *p*-glycoprotein becomes unavailable due to competitive binding, illness, or other means.

Ocular Drug Absorption

Numerous variables influence absorption of medications applied topically to the eye and hence possible ADRs, including certain pathological conditions of the ocular structures. For example, conjunctivitis, keratitis, and focal defects in the integrity of the ocular surface epithelium, a dry eye or a decreased tear film may increase drug absorption. Punctal occlusion or simply closing the eye after eye drop installation may also increase ocular drug absorption and therefore possibly toxicity. Some drugs, such as ciprofloxacin eye drops, may partially bind to the corneal epithelium. Others with a favorable chemical makeup may penetrate the cornea readily, leading to a more rapid increase in intraocular concentration.

Preservatives present in contact lens solutions, artificial tears, and topical ocular medications affect the absorption rates of topical medications, as do pH, concentration, lipophilia, and formulation (suspension versus solution) (42,44,47). The most common preservative in these compounds is benzalkonium chloride (BAK). Possessing detergent-like activity, BAK breaks down cell walls and disrupts junctions between superficial epithelial cells of the cornea (38), so inhibiting wound healing and possibly leading to a punctate or toxic epithelial keratopathy (11).

ENZYMATIC DETOXIFICATION

Enzyme systems in the liver and kidney are responsible for the detoxification and excretion of many drugs and toxins, and may be poorly developed in infants. The elderly are prone to toxic reactions because of potential underlying renal, hepatic and/or cardiac diseases as well as drug-drug interactions since they are frequently receiving multiple medications.

Most foreign chemicals (xenobiotics) that gain access to the body are lipophilic, since polar molecules are poorly absorbed through the intestinal wall. Enzyme-mediated reactions detoxify lipophilic xenobiotics utilizing a multiphase system (Fig. 1). The first step involves oxidative, reductive, or hydrolytic processes that add functional side groups such as OH, COOH, and NH_2 to the molecule (Phase I). The next step involves the conjugation of a charged side-group such as glucuronic or sulfuric acid (Phase II). Finally, the original molecule, which has been made more polar and thus more eliminable, is actively transported out of the cell (Phase III). These metabolized molecules, which are often excreted in bile if large or in urine if small, may be more toxic or active than the parent compound.

Phase I reactions which utilize the cytochrome P-450 system are the best characterized (Fig. 2). They mostly take place in the liver, but P-450 enzymes also exist in the corneal epithelium, non-pigmented ciliary epithelium and the retinal pigment epithelium (RPE) (13), so further detoxification often takes place at the site of potential damage. Chronic exposure to certain toxins, such as ethanol, may upregulate or induce the activity of these enzymes.

Intriguingly, drug metabolites may add to the therapeutic effect of the parent drug. For example, once latanoprost, used as a topical agent in the treatment of glaucoma, enters the eye, the free acid form of latanoprost is created by endogenous esterases, giving rise to an active analog of prostaglandin $F_{2\alpha}$.

ACTIVATED OXYGEN SPECIES IN OCULAR TOXICITY

The mechanisms by which many drugs and toxins exert their harmful effects on the eye remain poorly understood. Activated oxygen species play a role in the toxicity of certain compounds. Oxidative phosphorylation, light exposure, and toxin exposure may all lead to the production of reactive oxygen molecules, such as the superoxide anion (O_2^-), hydrogen peroxide (H_2O_2) and the hydroxyl radical (HO^-) (Fig. 3). These compounds may cause cell injury by peroxidation of the phospholipids present in cellular membranes. Fortunately, the body possesses enzymes, such as superoxide dismutase, catalase, and glutathione peroxidase, that limit the damage of these excited oxygen species. For example, superoxide dismutase catalyzes the formation of molecular oxygen and hydrogen peroxide from superoxide radicals (9). Hydrogen peroxide can be reduced to water by both glutathione peroxidase and catalase (Fig. 4). There are also many endogenous scavengers of free radicals, most prominent of which are vitamins C and E (see Chapter 49).

Reactive oxygen species affect proteins, such as the lens crystallins, which will aggregate and precipitate. They are implicated in cataract formation, and certain drugs may act as photosensitizers, which augment the crosslinking of these lens proteins. When in the presence of excessive light, allopurinol may cause cataracts via this method (22). There are high levels of vitamin C and glutathione (GSH) in the human lens (see Chapter 22), which likely resist such damage, and the levels of these compounds decrease with age, perhaps contributing to the increased incidence of cataract in the elderly.

Light exposure seems to induce lipid peroxidation in the retina. Taylor et al. (55) showed that age-related macular degeneration (AMD) was more prevalent in people exposed to higher levels of natural light. Cigarette smoking is also known to increase

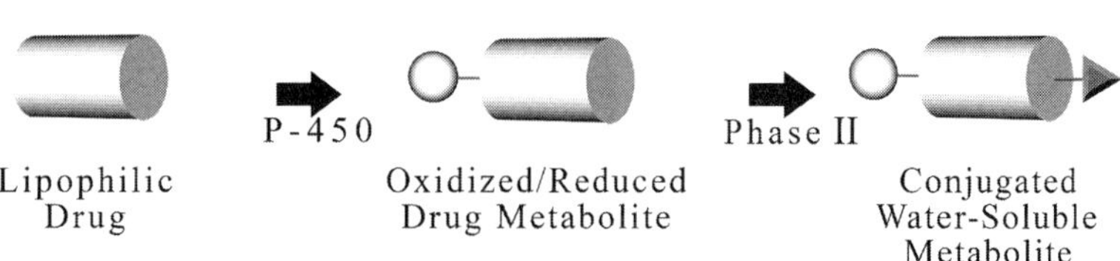

Figure 1 Drug metabolism. Phase I reactions: cytochrome P-450 enzymes add a reactive group, such as a hydroxyl radical, to the lipophilic drug being metabolized. Phase II reactions: various enzymes add a functional side group, such as glucuronic acid, in an effort to make the drug metabolite more hydrophilic and, thus, more eliminable.

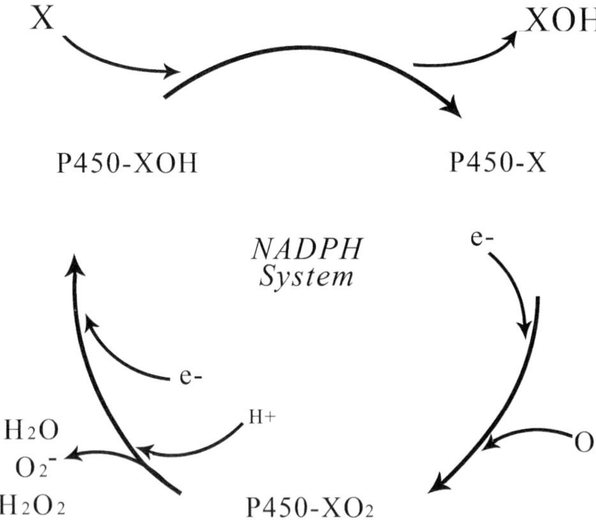

Figure 2 Details of Phase I. Cytochrome P-450 enzymes typically mediate the oxidation or reduction of certain drugs. In a typical reaction, as illustrated here, an atom of oxygen is inserted in the drug being metabolized (X). Electron donation is provided by the reduced nicotinamide adenine dinucleotide phosphate (NADPH) system. The other oxygen atom is reduced to water or reactive oxygen species. The hydroxylated drug (XOH) is now ready for Phase II reactions.

levels of free radical formation, and smokers have higher levels of AMD and cataract. Fortunately, the retina has high levels of glutathione and superoxide dismutase, and much effort has gone into studying the effects on macular health of augmentation of these endogenous antioxidant systems with nutritional supplements.

Hydrogen peroxide is routinely used in certain contact lens disinfectants, but its role in corneal toxicity via the generation of superoxide radicals is unknown. However, exposure of cultured human and rat corneal epithelial cells to hydrogen peroxide or superoxide radicals causes morphologic abnormalities and decreased DNA synthesis. Pre-treatment of corneal epithelial cell cultures with superoxide dismutase and catalase partially counteracts these toxic effects of the superoxide radicals. Exposure of cultured corneal endothelial cells to hydrogen peroxide results in morphologic changes that are blocked by the addition of catalase (32).

OCULAR ADVERSE DRUG REACTIONS

Of the thousands of toxins and medications that cause ADRs, some are of particular clinical significance. The term ADR may be applied to substances and drugs that cause adverse visual, ocular or periocular manifestations in any part of the eye, and CNS structures serving vision. Drugs and toxins causing ADRs may be those applied directly to the eye in the form of drops, gels, or ointments, those injected into or near the globe, and those that are systemic in nature. Many topical, periocularly injected, and systemic therapeutic agents have potential toxic side effects.

Topical Compounds

Chemicals

Caustic chemicals, especially alkaline substances like ammonium, potassium and sodium hydroxides, can severely disrupt the ocular surface and penetrate into the anterior chamber, leading to glaucoma and even phthisis bulbi. Solvents such as toluene and xylene are less damaging, but may lead to corneal edema. Surfactants can be locally irritating and fall into one

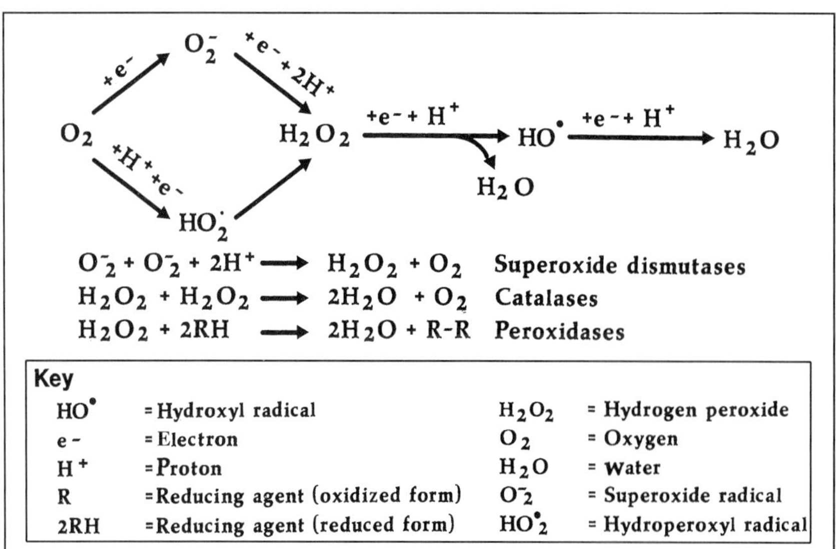

Figure 3 Pathway of oxygen reduction and catalytic scavenging of intermediates.

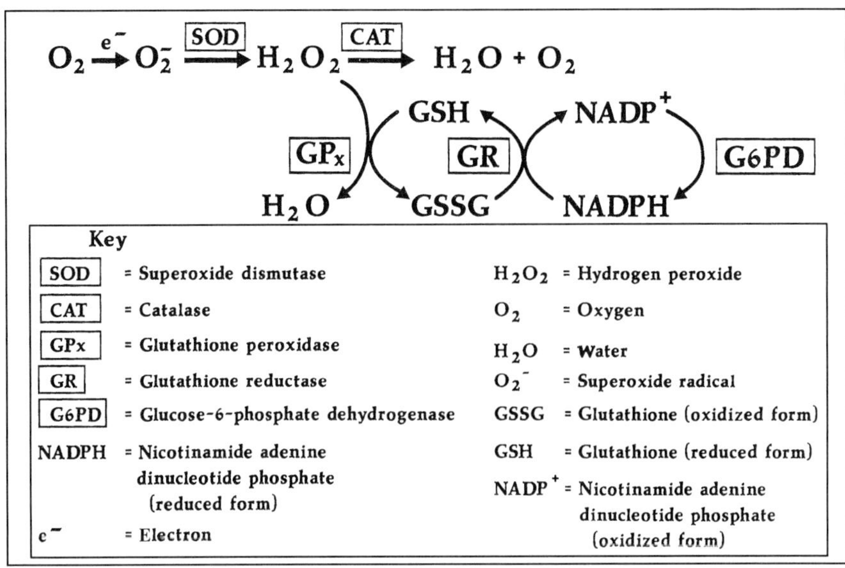

Figure 4 Antioxidant enzyme system.

of three categories—anionic (such as sodium lauryl sulfate and Ivory soap), cationic (like BAK), and nonionic.

Substances that may contact the ocular surface, such as eye drops, cosmetics, shampoos, and soaps, are typically tested for their potential adverse ocular effects. The Draize test has been modified over time, but it remains a common test that drug and cosmetic companies rely when testing the safety of a new topical ocular compound. The test involves the application of the substance in question to the ocular surface of albino rabbits for a specified period of time followed by slit-lamp biomicroscopy at specified intervals (9). International efforts are underway to find acceptable alternatives to animal testing, but after decades, the Draize test remains the gold standard.

Adverse corneal responses to toxins or certain therapeutic agents may occur immediately, but they frequently become manifest only after chronic exposure. To penetrate the normal cornea, topically applied toxic agents must possess particular solubility characteristics. Water soluble compounds enter the corneal stroma, but lipid soluble agents are more likely to enter the lipid rich corneal epithelium.

Drugs

Mostly in the form of prescribed eye drops, contact lens solutions, and artificial tears, millions of people put chemicals onto their eye surfaces every day. Most of these are well tolerated, but allergies and toxic reactions are not rare. Allergies to the preservatives in contact lens solutions are most common, followed by allergies to antibiotics, especially gentamicin. Brimonidine, brinzolamide, and dorzolamide are topical glaucoma medications that can cause a hypersensitivity reaction in the eyelids and conjunctiva which typically clears with cessation of the drugs (31,57) (see Chapter 5). Gentamicin, an aminoglycoside, is frequently used to treat ocular bacterial infections. This agent accumulates in lysosomes where it binds to membrane phospholipids, leading to cell membrane instability and lysosomal rupture (39). Some evidence supports the notion that preservatives account for the toxicity of topical gentamicin. In a study of epithelial healing in rabbits, treatment with either topical gentamicin or its preservative (BAK) significantly retarded epithelial healing rates compared to controls receiving only topical saline (2).

The difference between a therapeutic dose and a toxic one is narrow with certain therapeutic agents, such as trifluridine and related compounds used in the treatment of herpes keratitis. Detecting its toxic effects may be difficult to distinguish from possible progression of the herpetic infection. Eyes with decreased tear production are particularly prone to the trifluridine ocular ADRs of corneal stippling, small epithelial defects, and mild corneal clouding.

Topical non-steroidal anti-inflammatory drugs rarely cause corneal complications, but a few case reports document corneal melting in older patients who used the drops with frequent dosing following ocular surgery (29).

Drops prescribed to lower IOP have a myriad of ADRs, both local and systemic. In addition to its previously mentioned effects, brimonidine may cause a rebound conjunctival hyperemia as with other sympathomimetics. Prostaglandin analogs frequently cause eyelash growth and darken the periocular skin and the terminal differentiation of the fine vellus hair of the eyelid as well as eliciting hypersensitivity

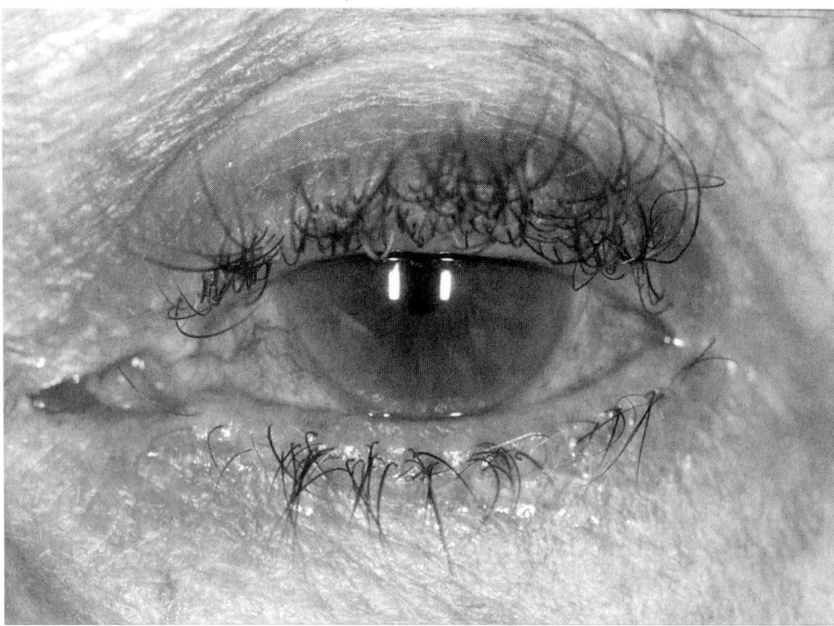

Figure 5 Latanoprost-induced eyelash growth.

reactions (Fig. 5). Hyperpigmentation of the iris is also a frequent ADR of this class of drug (1,53). An increase in tyrosinase activity within the melanocytes is incited after the drugs interact with the cells' prostaglandin $F_{2\alpha}$ ($PGF_{2\alpha}$) receptors. Tissue specimens of iris from patients treated with this class of drug have disclosed an increase in iris freckles rather than nevi and morphologic observations suggest that the absolute number of iris stromal melanocytes is not increased, but that the amount of melanin production is increased. Due to unpleasant side effects and frequent dosing requirements, pilocarpine is now seldom prescribed for glaucoma since the advent of prostaglandin (PG) analogues, but miosis, myopic shift, and brow ache are all common and are due to the status of pilocarpine as a cholinergic agonist. Beta blockers are still commonly used, and though they have few ocular ADRs, systemic effects occur. The topical application of timolol can lead to serum levels similar to that found 6 to 8 hours following a 10 mg oral dose. Accordingly, systemic beta blockade can lead to bronchospasm, bradycardia, depression, and loss of libido. In patients with pre-existing heart disease, these drugs may cause congestive heart failure and exacerbate cardiac conduction defects leading to cardiac arrest (38). Status asthmaticus, which can be fatal, may follow the topical application of timolol to the eye in asthmatic patients.

Like beta blockers, mydriatics and cycloplegics are associated with systemic ADRs. Anticholinergic side effects including delirium, somnolence, flushing, fever, mouth dryness, and tachycardia, are more common when atropine or scopolamine is used in children or the elderly. Fetal tachycardia has been reported when these drugs are used in pregnant women. Contact dermatitis is seen with atropine drops. Assumed to be due to unintentional digital auto-inoculation, monocular dilation has been reported in people using transderm scopolamine patches for sea sickness. Phenylephrine, a sympathomimetic, is typically safe when used in lower concentrations, but there are reports of malignant hypertension and even death when the 10% solution is used (21). Mydriatics and cycloplegics can all precipitate angle closure glaucoma and raise IOP in patients with open angle glaucoma.

Corticosteroid eye drops, similar to systemic corticosteroids, have frequent ADRs. These effects are also noted for the nasal aerosols (24), inhaled forms and injected types of steroids, whether the injection site is intravitreal, periocular or at sites remote from the eye.

Corticosteroids are the drugs most frequently implicated in cataract formation, these being typically subcapsular in type and associated with long-term therapy. Without corticosteroids, posterior subcapsular cataracts form in less than 8% of individuals with rheumatoid arthritis and in 0.2% to 4% of normal individuals. However, in patients with rheumatoid arthritis subjected to 10 mg oral prednisone (or equivalent) for at least two years, the incidence of posterior subcapsular cataracts rises to 30% to 40%. With higher doses (>15 mg of prednisone) and more prolonged therapy (>4 years) the incidence of cataracts approaches 80% to 100% (6). The lens changes develop at all ages. When corticosteroid therapy is withdrawn these cataracts do not regress. Several mechanisms of corticosteroid-induced cataract have been proposed including drug-induced biochemical changes in the lens epithelial cells as well as binding of drug to lens crystallins, but the exact mechanism of steroid-induced posterior subcapsular cataracts is not clear.

The mechanisms leading to glucocorticoid-induced IOP elevation also remain poorly understood. These drugs may decrease outflow facility through a variety of mechanisms (38), which may involve modulation of prostaglandin-adrenergic interactions or the synthesis and cellular distribution of complex carbohydrates, hyaluronic acid, and collagen. Glucocorticoids may reduce phagocytic and extracellular protease activity, alter gene expression, and increase DNA content within trabecular meshwork cells. Cell volume, extracellular matrix volume and cell-to-cell attachment are increased in the trabecular meshwork of eyes exposed to glucocorticoids. Increases in the synthesis of myocilin, a product of the *MYOC* gene believed to be involved in the pathogenesis of certain types of glaucoma (see Chapter 34), follows the time course of steroid-induced IOP rise.

The prolonged administration of systemic corticosteroids has been associated with scleral thinning and darkening. This discoloration probably results from visualization of the underlying uvea through the thinned sclera. Steroids injected into the eyelid may cause skin thinning, depigmentation, and orbital fat atrophy (41).

Injectable and Intraoperative Compounds

Subconjunctival injections of 5-fluorouracil (5-FU) and mitomycin-C have been administered to patients with glaucoma to prevent scar formation following filtering procedures, and the compounds also are used at the time of trabeculectomy. Corneal epithelial defects have been observed following the use of these drugs (51). Late onset tissue thinning has been observed following the use of mitomycin, and this has led to an increased incidence of hypotony, bleb infection, and endophthalmitis.

Retrobulbar injections of mepivacaine, lidocaine or other local anesthetics rarely cause extraocular muscle or visual dysfunction. Retrobulbar anesthesia is more likely to cause complications if the drug is injected directly into one of the rectus muscles or into the optic nerve. In a study of the lateral rectus muscle of rats given a single retrobulbar injection of mepivacaine, ultrastructural analysis disclosed destruction of muscle fibers, activation of myoblasts, phagocytosis and regeneration of muscle fibers (59). Respiratory arrest may complicate retrobulbar injections of the local anesthetics bupivacaine or lidocaine if they are injected into the sheath of the optic nerve. The axons of the nerve itself also may be damaged directly by the needle.

Botulinum toxin, the product of *Clostridium botulinum*, is injected into the facial muscles for blepharospasm and cosmetic indications. It may also be injected into the extraocular muscles themselves to treat certain cases of strabismus. The paralytic action of this neurotoxin involves inhibition of acetylcholine release from the vesicles situated within motor nerve endings. The neurotoxin cleaves SNAP-25, a protein that is integral in the regulation of acetylcholine release. The therapeutic use of botulinum toxin around the eyes has resulted in unintended ptosis and diplopia (16).

During intraocular surgery, various substances are injected or otherwise placed within the anterior chamber or vitreous cavity. These include irrigating solutions possibly containing epinephrine and antibiotics, and they are usually well tolerated. Rarely, an inadvertent inclusion of detergent residues or preservatives occurs when surgical instruments are improperly cleaned or when improper substances are introduced into the eye at the time of surgery. This has led to cases of toxic anterior segment syndrome, which can include corneal endothelial failure (58). Other substances used in surgery include viscosurgical devices, expansible gases, dyes, silicone oil, heavy liquids and corticosteroids. The viscosurgical devices may cause elevated IOP in the postoperative period as they likely interfere with aqueous humor outflow if left behind in the anterior chamber. The gases may lead to cataract and glaucoma while silicone oil has been associated with band keratopathy and retinal toxicity (20) in addition to glaucoma and cataract (Fig. 6). The complications of injectable corticosteroids are dealt with elsewhere in this chapter (see the section entitled Topical Compounds).

Systemic Compounds

Medications administered systemically for non-ocular conditions that lead to significant toxic ocular manifestations usually enter the eye via the circulatory system. The blood–aqueous and the blood–retinal barriers, however, normally prevent many drugs from gaining access to certain parts of the eye by way of the vasculature. The absorption of systemically administered drugs by the eye may increase when these blood-ocular barriers are impaired as during inflammation, and in such settings drugs may reach toxic levels. For example, several reports suggest that a compromised blood–retinal barrier may enhance the entry of chloroquine and vincristine into the eye and exacerbate undesirable side effects.

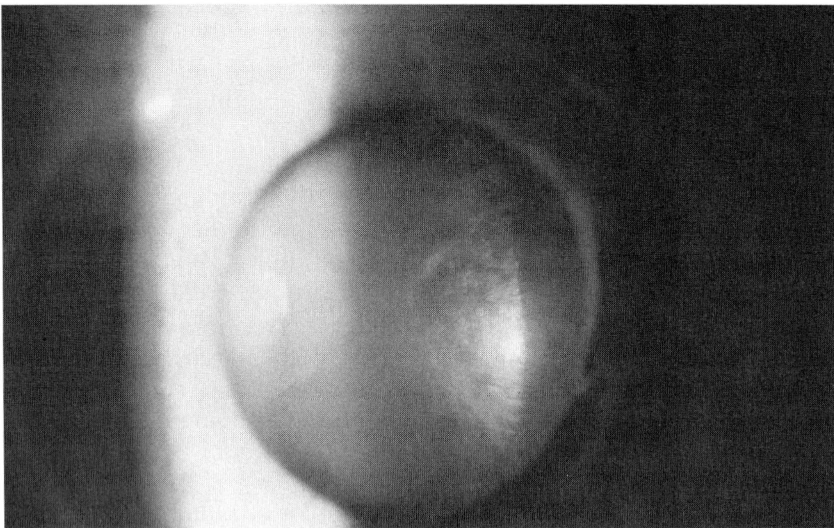

Figure 6 Cataract caused by intravitreal silicone oil.

Ocular Surface

Some systemically administered drugs that are transported to the lacrimal gland and secreted into the tears may be toxic to the ocular surface. An example is isotretinoin, an oral drug used in the treatment of severe cystic acne. This medication commonly causes toxic ocular reactions, such as blepharoconjunctivitis, keratoconjunctivitis sicca, blurred vision and corneal opacities. Users must often forego contact lens wear. Contributing to the surface dysfunction, isotretinoin may cause atrophy of the meibomian gland. The drug also competes with retinoic acid and retinol at binding sites in the retina, causing decreased dark adaptation. Along with many other drugs, including vitamin A, isotretinoin can trigger idiopathic intracranial hypertension (36).

Many other systemic drugs lead to ocular surface disorders. Keratitis sicca is seen with systemic 5-FU administration. Systemic anticholinergics, beta blockers, diuretics, anxiolytics, antineoplastic drugs, and antidepressants can lead to decreased tearing. Tetracycline may lead to yellowing of the conjunctiva or dark brown deposits in the subconjunctival space (11). Minocycline has been associated with scleral pigmentation, and all drugs of the tetracycline class can produce pigmentary changes of the skin, nails and teeth. As with the retinoids, these drugs have also been charged with precipitating idiopathic intracranial hypertension.

Corneal deposits are a frequent ADR of several systemic drugs. Indomethacin has been associated with speckled or whorl-like deposits in up to 16% of patients. Amiodarone and chloroquine also cause whorl-like changes in the cornea (17), resembling the cornea verticillata of Fabry disease (Fig. 7) (see Chapter 41) . These deposits will disappear with the cessation of treatment and may cause transient light sensitivity. The vortex pattern probably follows the differentiation of corneal epithelial cells as they move from peripheral stem cells to the central cornea. Amiodarone has also been associated with visually insignificant, punctate, yellow-white opacities in the crystalline lenses of approximately 50% of chronic users. Additionally, amiodarone is suspected of causing a unique form of bilateral anterior ischemic optic neuropathy that may or may not resolve upon cessation of treatment (40).

Scleral ADRs are rare, perhaps due to the avascular nature of this tissue. Bisphosphonates are commonly used to treat osteolytic malignancies and multiple myeloma. Several cases of scleritis have been reported in conjunction with pamidronate, a drug in this class (27).

Anterior Segment

Acute myopia has been reported in association with sulfa drugs (33). Topiramate, a sulfa-based antiseizure medication, can cause a rapid-onset myopic shift of more than 6 diopters related to shallowing of the anterior chamber and a shifting forward of the lens-iris diaphragm. This is probably due to suprachoroidal effusions causing a forward rotation of the ciliary body. In several cases, this has led to angle closure glaucoma (27). The myopia resolves within a few days after stopping topiramate therapy.

Tamsulosin is an alpha-1A antagonist used to treat prostatic hypertrophy. Patients receiving this drug develop chronic miosis and often a floppy iris syndrome that is particularly evident during cataract extraction (12). This complication persists even after the drug is discontinued for many months prior to surgery.

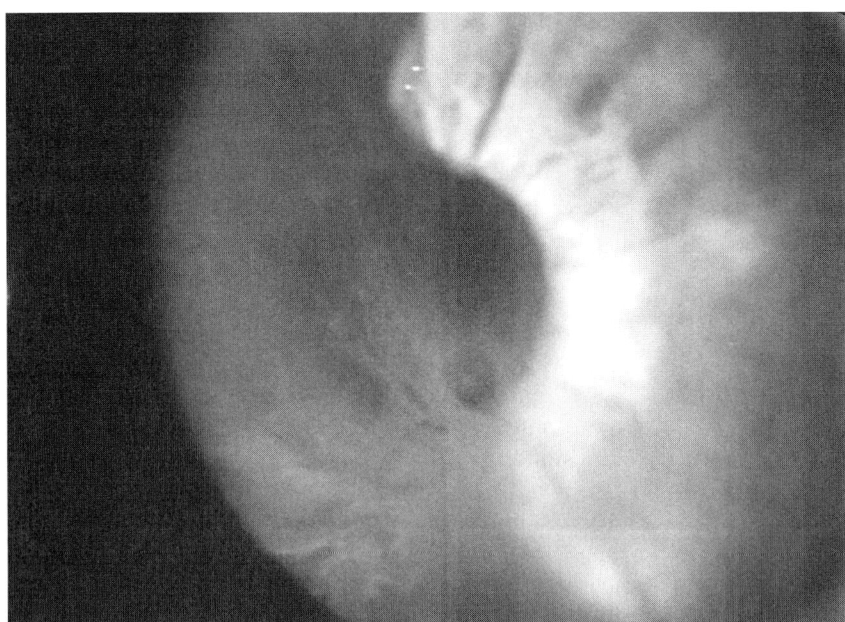

Figure 7 Corneal verticillata from amiodarone use.

Posterior Segment

Retinal hemorrhages have been associated with several compounds, including interferon (IFN), which is used to treat some malignant neoplasms and viral infections (50). Due to its ability to inhibit blood clotting, warfarin also can cause retinal hemorrhage.

Macular edema can be a rare but serious consequence of tamoxifen therapy for metastatic breast carcinoma. A frequent ocular manifestation of this drug is the development of white–yellow refractile opacities in the macula and elsewhere in the retina (35,43). These lesions are found between the nerve fiber layer and the inner plexiform layer and may be associated with reduced vision or subnormal visual fields. In patients on high doses of tamoxifen (>180 mg/day), this ADR can occur within a year and a half, and the vision changes can be permanent. This retinopathy is uncommon and often reversible in patients on chronic low-dose therapy.

Chloroquine and hydroxychloroquine, used in the treatment of malaria and autoimmune disorders, such as rheumatoid arthritis and systemic lupus erythematosus (see Chapter 6), may adversely affect the retina causing decreased visual acuity, blurred vision, diplopia, decreased color and night vision and visual field defects. A devastating retinopathy develops bilaterally and insidiously and is characterized by a fine mottling of the macula, arteriolar narrowing, peripheral retinal pigmentation, and loss of the foveal reflex and, in advanced cases, by a depigmented macula surrounded by a pigmented ring (bull eye maculopathy, Fig. 8). As a consequence of the retinopathy, both the electroretinogram (ERG) and electrooculogram (EOG) are frequently abnormal. Chloroquine/hydroxychloroquine retinopathy is clinically serious and irreversible. This toxic retinopathy is dose related with most cases occurring only after five years or more when used at the recommended doses (36). The maculopathy may persist long after these drugs are stopped as the accumulated drug can take months to clear out of the body.

Chloroquine and hydroxychloroquine retinopathy is characterized morphologically by curvilinear intracytoplasmic bodies within the RPE and clumping of these cells as well as destruction of the adjacent

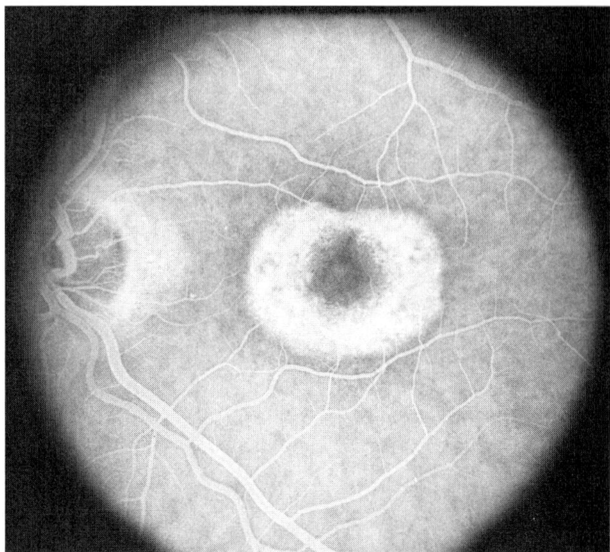

Figure 8 Fluorescein angiogram image of patient with bull eye maculopathy from chloroquine toxicity.

photoreceptors. The mechanisms by which the retina is damaged are poorly understood, but these drugs have an affinity for melanin containing cells, such as the RPE and most investigators contend that RPE damage precedes the degeneration of rods and cones.

Digitalis and its derivatives, such as digoxin, have long been known to be associated with changes in color vision and decreased dark adaptation, and their target is thought to be the cones. Patients may describe snowy vision, yellow tinges to objects, or other dyschromatopsias, and these visual abnormalities usually correlate with toxic serum levels of the drug, but they have been noted at normal serum levels.

Optic Nerve and Central Nervous System

Chemicals with ophthalmic manifestations that affect the optic nerve and/or CNS include methanol, ethanol, and ethambutol. The visual symptoms of methanol intoxication include blurred vision, loss of central vision and complete blindness some 18 to 48 hours after ingestion (5,7). In an investigation of 320 individuals who ingested a mixture containing 35% methanol and 15% ethanol, hyperemia and edema of the optic disc and surrounding retina occurred in some patients who later manifested permanent impairment of vision (7). In persons with marked acidosis, optic atrophy sometimes followed severe retinal edema. A central scotoma was a common visual field defect. Vision recovered partially or completely if improvement began during the first week (7).

Ethanol, the world's most popular recreational drug, is known to cause nystagmus and slowed saccades. Law enforcement officials in the United States use these ocular abnormalities to estimate intoxication levels in suspected drunk drivers. Additionally, ethanol may cause strabismus and a transient lowering of IOP. It is suspected of being responsible for some forms of cataract (74), but as nutritional deficiencies are common in chronic alcoholics, the role of ethanol in cataractogenesis remains uncertain.

Ethambutol suppresses the growth of *Mycobacterium tuberculosis* and *Mycobacterium avium* complex and is used in the treatment of infections caused by those bacteria. This orally administered drug readily accumulates in persons with impaired renal function, and blurred vision, edema of the optic nerve head and macula, visual field defects, and abnormal color vision may occur (6). Optic atrophy and blindness may also develop. If the drug is discontinued at the first sign of visual loss recovery may occur, however, it may take years if it is slowly withdrawn. The visual abnormalities have been attributed to: (*i*) dysfunction of the central fibers of the optic nerve (loss of central vision associated with a central scotoma and a marked decrease in color discrimination, usually with loss of ability to recognize green and sometimes red) and less commonly to (*ii*) impaired function of the peripheral fibers of the optic nerve (defects in the peripheral field isopters). Both the duration and the incidence of visual changes appear to be dose related. Although uncommon, some patients on high doses of ethambutol develop an irreversible optic neuropathy. Ethambutol is the only drug known to create optic chiasmal lesions.

Toxins affecting the CNS may involve visual processing and result in different clinically significant abnormalities. For example, transient cortical blindness occasionally follows the administration of antineoplastic agents, such as intravenous tacrolimus, vincristine and *cis*-platinum (34). Ophthalmoplegia has been associated with some anti-neoplastic drugs (tacrolimus, nitrosureas, vincristine, and methotrexate), anticonvulsants (phenytoin and carbamazepine) and antidepressants (imipramine).

Atypical ocular movements attributed to CNS dysfunction may accompany the use of some therapeutic agents. Ocular dyskinesias, such as ocular skew deviation and nystagmus (down-beating and horizontal) are occasionally associated with the administration of carbamazepine, but do not correlate with serum levels of the drug. Increased catecholaminergic activity in the CNS may account for the carbamazepine-induced ocular dyskinesias. Lithium toxicity may evoke a wide range of ocular motility disturbances, including down-beating or horizontal nystagmus, saccadic pursuit or dysmetria, unilateral gaze palsy, oculogyric crisis and opsoclonus (14). Studies of the brain in rhesus monkeys, as well as in a human case, suggest that lithium causes neuronal degeneration and loss as well as gliosis in neuronal groups beneath the fourth ventricle (medial vestibular and propositus hypoglossi nuclei) that connect to the vestibular nuclei, cerebellum, cerebral cortex and cranial nerve nuclei which innervate the extraocular muscles (14).

Sildenafil is a commonly prescribed drug for erectile dysfunction, and its visual side effects are mostly limited to reversible, dose-related dyschromatopsias (26). Usually, patients report a blue tinge to objects or a sensation of flashing lights with blinking. These effects usually begin 15 to 30 minutes after ingestion and are experienced in up to 50% of patients taking 200 mg (four times the recommended dose). At these higher doses, transient ERG changes have been documented. A few reports of non-arteritic anterior ischemic optic neuropathy (NAION) have surfaced with this drug, but it remains to be determined whether this is an ADR or a coincidental disease in older patients typically at risk for occlusive vascular disease.

Systemic Drugs for the Eye

Nausea is a common ADR of fluorescein angiograms and anaphylactic reactions to this product, including death, have occurred during the procedure (31). Verteporfin is used as part of the photodynamic therapy of choroidal neovascular membranes. This injectable compound can cause headache, visual disturbance, and photosensitization, though it is unclear if permanent ocular damage such as a cataract is due to this.

Anorexia, nausea and abdominal discomfort sometimes follow treatment of glaucoma with carbonic anhydrase inhibitors, such as acetazolamide and methazolamide (24). Aplastic anemia and pancytopenia rarely accompany the administration of these drugs. Carbonic anhydrase inhibitors may also cause metabolic acidosis, which can be worsened by the concurrent use of diuretics. The systemic toxicity of certain medications is exacerbated by drugs that patients receive for other disorders. For example, treatment of glaucoma with carbonic anhydrase inhibitors increases the serum level of non-ionized salicylate and therefore increases the risk of salicylate toxicity in patients concurrently receiving high doses of aspirin. Hence, oral carbonic anhydrase inhibitors should rarely be used for the chronic treatment of glaucoma.

Herbal and Nutritional Supplements

Nutritional supplements have become a multi-billion-dollar industry. In the United States, as elsewhere, these products are mostly unregulated. Several of these substances have ocular side effects. Canthaxanthine used as a tanning pill, is reported to cause a crystalline retinopathy (25). Ironically, chamomile solutions are applied to the eyelids in an effort to ease eyestrain while being notorious for causing allergic conjunctivitis (54). *Datura* is a botanical genus containing atropine and scopolamine. Its extracts are used for bronchial spasms and as analgesics, and as expected, they have anticholinergic side effects including mydriasis.

REFERENCES

1. Albert DM, Gangnon RE, Zimbric ML, et al. A study of iridectomy histopathologic features of latanoprost and non-latanoprost treated patients. Arch Ophthalmol 2004; 122:1680–5.
2. Alfonso EC, Albert DM, Kenyon, KR, et al. In vitro toxicity of gentamicin to corneal epithelial cells. Cornea 1990; 9: 55–61.
3. Altman B. Ocular effects in the newborn from maternal drugs. In: Leopold IH, Burns, RP, eds. Symposium on Ocular Therapy. New York: John Wiley & Sons, 1979:97–9.
4. Barron GJ, Tepper L, Iovine G. Ocular toxicity from ethambutol. Am J Ophthalmol 1974; 77:256–60.
5. Baumbach GL, Cancilla PA, Martin-Amat G, et al. Methyl alcohol poisoning, IV. Alterations of the morphologic findings of the retina and optic nerve. Arch Ophthalmol 1977; 95:1859–65.
6. Becker B. The side effects of corticosteroids. Invest Ophthalmol 1964; 3:492–7.
7. Benton CD, Calhoun FPJ. The ocular effects of methyl alcohol poisoning: report of a catastrophe involving 320 persons. Am J Ophthalmol 1953; 36:1677–89.
8. Bernstein HN. Ocular toxicity of chloroquine. Surv Ophthalmol 1968; 12:415–9.
9. Bhuyan KC, Bhuyan DK. Superoxide dismutase of the eye: relative functions of superoxide dismutase and catalase in protecting the ocular lens from oxidative damage. Biochim Biophys Acta 1978; 542:28–38.
10. Bowman R, Cope J, Nischal K. Ocular and systemic side effects of brimonidine 0.2% eye drops (Alphagan) in children. Eye 2004; 18:24–6.
11. Brothers DM, Hidayat AA. Conjunctival pigmentation associated with tetracyline medication. Ophthalmology 1981; 88:1212–5.
12. Chang DF, Campbell JR, Intraoperative floppy iris syndrome associated with tamsulosin. J Cataract Refract Surg 2005; 31:664–73.
13. Chiou GCY. Ophthalmic toxicology. In: Hayes AW, Thomas JA, Gardner DE, eds. Target Organ Toxicology Series. 2nd ed. Ann Arbor: Taylor & Francis, 1999:366.
14. Corbett JJ, Jacobson DM, Thompson HS, et al. Downbeating nystagmus and other ocular motor defects caused by *lithium toxicity*. Neurology 1989; 39:481–7.
15. Cote TR, Mohan AK, Polder JA, et al. Botulinum toxin type A injections: adverse events reported to the US Food and Drug Administration in therapeutic and cosmetic cases. J Am Acad Ophthalmol 2005; 53:407–15.
16. Coulter R. Pediatric use of topical ophthalmic drugs. Optometry 2004; 75:419–29.
17. D'Amico DJ, Kenyon KR, Rushkin JN. Amiodarone keratopathy: drug induced lipid storage disease. Arch Ophthalmol 1981; 99:257–61.
18. Diamond J. Systemic adverse effects of topical ophthalmic agents. Implications for older patients. Drugs & Aging 1997; 11:352–60.
19. Enyedi L, Freedman S. Safety and efficacy of brimonidine in children with glaucoma. J AAPOS 2001; 5:281–4.
20. Foulks GN, Hatchell DL, Proia AD, Klintworth GK. Histopathology of silicone oil keratopathy in humans. Cornea 1991; 10:29–37.
21. Fraunfelder FT, Scafidi AF. Possible adverse effects from topical ocular 10% phenylephrine. Am J Ophthalmol 1978; 85:447–53.
22. Fraunfelder FT, Fraunfelder FW. Drug-induced Ocular Side Effects. 5th ed. Woburn, MA: Butterworth-Heinemann, 2001:824.
23. Fraunfelder FT, Meyer SM. Posterior subcapsular cataracts associated with nasal or inhalation corticosteroids. Am J Ophthalmol, 1990; 109:489–90.
24. Fraunfelder FT, Meyer SM, Bagby GC Jr, Dreis MW. Hematologic reactions to carbonic anhydrase inhibitors. Am J Ophthalmol 1985; 100:79–81.
25. Fraunfelder FW. Ocular side effects from herbal medicines and nutritional supplements. Am J Ophthalmol 2004; 138: 639–47.

26. Fraunfelder FW. Visual side effects associated with erectile dysfunction agents. Am J Ophthalmol 2005; 140: 723–4.
27. Fraunfelder FW. Fraunfelder FT. Adverse ocular drug reactions recently identified by the National Registry of Drug-Induced Ocular Side Effects. Ophthalmology 2004; 111:1275–9.
28. Grant WM, Schuman JS. Toxicology of the Eye: Effects on the Eyes and Visual System from Chemicals, Drugs, Metals, and Minerals, Plants, Toxins and Venoms; also, Systemic Side Effects from Eye Medications. 4th ed. Springfield: Charles C. Thomas, 1993:1608.
29. Guidera A, Luchs J, Udell I. Keratitis, ulceration, and perforation associated with topical nonsteroidal anti-inflammatory drugs. Ophthalmology 2001; 108:936–44.
30. Hodges GR, Aminoglycoside toxicity. In: Barnes WG, Hodges GR, eds. The Aminoglycoside Antibiotics: A Guide to Therapy. Boca Raton, FL: CRC Press 1984:153–79.
31. Holdiness M. Contact dermatitis to topical drugs for glaucoma. Am J Contact Dermat 2001; 12:217–9.
32. Hull DS, Csukas S, Green K, Livingston V. Hydrogen peroxide and corneal endothelium. Acta Ophthalmologica 1981; 59:409–21.
33. Ikeda N, Ikeda T, Nagata M, Mimura O. Ciliochoroidal effusion syndrome induced by sulfa derivatives. Arch Ophthalmol 2002; 120:1775.
34. Imperia PS, Lazarus HM, Lass JH. Ocular complications of systemic cancer chemotherapy. Surv Ophthalmol 1989; 34: 209–30.
35. Kaiser-Kupfer MI, Kupfer C, Rodrigues MM. Tamoxifen retinopathy: a clinicopathologic report. Ophthalmology 1981; 88:89–93.
36. Kaufman P, Alm A. Adler's Physiology of the Eye. 10th ed. Philadelphia: Mosby, 2003:904.
37. Kwan AS, Barry C, McAllister IL, Constable I. Fluorescein angiography and adverse drug reactions revisited: the Lions Eye experience. Clin Exp Ophthalmol 2006, 34:33–8.
38. Lama P. Systemic reactions associated with ophthalmic medications. Ophthalmol Clin North Am, 2005; 18: 569–84.
39. Lu FC, Kacew S. Lu's basic toxicology: Fundementals, target organs, and risk assessment. In: Lu's Basic Toxicology: Fundamentals, Target Organs, and Risk Assessment. 4th ed. London: Taylor & Francis, 2003:392.
40. Macaluso D, Shults W, Fraunfelder F. Features of amiodarone-induced optic neuropathy. Am J Ophthalmol 1999; 127:610–12.
41. McGhee C, Dean S, Danesh-Meyer H. Locally administered ocular corticosteroids: benefits and risks. Drug Safety 2002; 25:33–55.
42. Mullen W, Shepherd W, Labovitz J. Ophthalmic preservatives and vehicles. Surv Ophthalmol 1973; 17:469–83.
43. Nayfield SG, Gorin MB. Tamoxifen-associated eye disease: a review. J Clin Oncol 1996; 14:1018–26.
44. Noecker R. Effects of common ophthalmic preservatives on ocular health. Adv Ther 2001; 18:205–15.
45. Nuijts RMMA. Ocular Toxicity of Intraoperatively Used Drugs and Solutions. 1st ed. Amsterdam: Kugler Publications, 1995:150.
46. Okland S, Komorowski T, Carlson B. Ultrastructure of mepivacaine-induced damage and regeneration in rat extraocular muscle. Invest Ophthalmol Vis Sci 1989; 30: 1643–51.
47. Pfister RR, Burstein N. The effects of ophthalmic drugs, vehicles, and preservatives on corneal epithelium: a scanning electron microscope study. Invest Ophthalmol Vis Sci 1976; 15:246–59.
48. Routledge PA, O'Mahony MS, Woodhouse KW. Adverse drug reactions in elderly patients. Br J Clin Pharmacol 2003; 57:121–6.
49. Rosenwasser GOD. Complications of topical ocular anesthetics. Int Ophthalmol Clin 1989; 29:153–8.
50. Schulman J, et al. Posterior segment complications in patients with hepatitis C treated with interferon and ribavirin. Ophthalmology 2003; 110:437–42.
51. Shapiro MS, Thoft RA, Friend J, et al. 5-Fluorouracil toxicity to the ocular surface epithelium. Invest Ophthalmol Vis Sci 1985; 26:580–3.
52. Steg RE, Kessinger A, Wszolek ZK. Cortical blindness and seizures in a patient receiving FK506 after bone marrow transplantation. Bone Marrow Transplant, 1999; 23:959–62.
53. Stjernschantz JW, Albert DM, Hu DN, et al. Mechanism and clinical significance of prostaglandin-induced iris pigmentation. Surv Ophthalmol 2002; 47:S162–75.
54. Subiza J, Subiza JL, Alonso M, et al. Allergic conjunctivitis to chamomile tea. Ann Allergy 1990; 65:127–32.
55. Taylor HR, West S, Munoz B, et al. The long-term effects of visible light on the eye. Arch Ophthalmol 1992; 110:99–104.
56. Wallace D, Steinkuller P. Ocular medications in children. Clin Pediatr 1998; 37:645–52.
57. Watts P, Hawksworth N. Delayed hypersensitivity to brimonidine tartrate 0.2% associated with high intraocular pressure. Eye 2002; 16:132–5.
58. Yagmur M, Okay O, Ersoz TR, et al. Confocal microscopic features of amiodarone keratopathy. Toxicol Cutan Ocul Toxicol 2003; 22:243–53.
59. Zeng J, Borchman D, Paterson CA. Acute effect of ethanol on lens cation homeostasis. Alcohol 1998; 16:189–93.
60. Zoumalan CI, Agarwal M, Sadun AA, Optical coherence tomography can measure axonal loss in patients with ethambutol-induced optic neuropathy. Graefe's Arch Clin Exp Ophthalmol 2004; 243:410–6.

51

Embryological Development of the Eye

Duane L. Guernsey
Departments of Pathology, Ophthalmology and Visual Sciences, Surgery, Physiology, and Biophysics, Dalhousie University, Halifax, Nova Scotia, Canada

Johane M. Robitaille
Departments of Ophthalmology and Visual Sciences and Pathology, Dalhousie University, Halifax, Nova Scotia, Canada

J. Douglas Cameron
Department of Ophthalmology, Mayo Clinic, Rochester, Minnesota, U.S.A.

J. Godfrey Heathcote
Departments of Pathology and Ophthalmology and Visual Sciences, Dalhousie University, Halifax, Nova Scotia, Canada

INTRODUCTION

There continues to be much discussion and controversy regarding the evolution of animal eyes: whether eyes evolved once, or at least once in invertebrates and again in vertebrates. Because of the morphological variety in eyes (135) and the different embryological beginnings of the numerous eye structures, the idea that animal eyes arose independently several times during evolution has gained some acceptance. This evolutionary debate is exemplified by the photoreceptor cells. While these cells differ dramatically between invertebrates and vertebrates, both use opsins to catch photons, even though the two opsins are fundamentally different proteins. On the other hand, Arendt et al. reported a surprising similarity between photoreceptors of a marine worm and humans, suggesting that eyes evolved only once (5). Their data show that, in addition to the usual invertebrate opsin, the worm has in the brain another opsin similar to the human protein. This suggests that photosensitive cells in the invertebrate brain could have evolved into vertebrate eyes.

Over the past decade, the monophylogenetic origin of the eye has been supported by the evidence obtained from molecular genetic studies of transcription factors and signaling cascades in eye development (9, 29, 67, 78, 278). Despite their morphological variation, all eyes have in common developmental cascades of transcription factors. An important example is the involvement of the *Pax6* gene in eye morphogenesis in almost all species. Nevertheless, Bailey et al. (9) propose that many of the observations supporting the hypothesis that all eyes developed from a common prototype may have alternative explanations. They emphasize that specific signal cascades thought to be critical for eye development are not found in certain types of eyes. For example, the transcription factor *dachshund* is essential for invertebrate eye formation (152), yet it is apparently unimportant in vertebrate eye development (42). Bailey et al. (9) further suggest that the differential dependence of eye formation on *Rx* genes between insects and vertebrates (43) reflects the different evolutionary origins of these eye types. The debate over the evolution of eyes is scientifically interesting and also serves as a catalyst for research on ocular pathobiology.

MORPHOGENESIS OF THE EYE AND OPTIC STALK

Histological investigations on a series of human embryos by Mann in the mid-20th century established the value of such studies in understanding the disorders of morphogenesis that underlie many congenital malformations (151). The most striking features of embryogenesis are its complexity and reliability and the way in which growth, morphogenesis, and differentiation (histogenesis) underlie the development of the mature organism from the fertilized ovum. Also in the mid-20th century the essential role of genetics in embryogenesis and the tight regulation of development by differential gene expression came to be recognized (89,169).

The normal development of the eye depends on an ordered sequence of morphogenetic events, which themselves rely on processes of growth and selective cell death. In humans much of this development takes place during the embryonic period, the first 8 weeks post-fertilization (183). The sequence of events in this period is governed by the transcription of genetic material and modulated by diffusible growth factors and mechanical mass effects generated by structures developing within and alongside the eye. The ocular anlage is distinguished by the expression of numerous genes including the homeobox transcription factor *Rx* and the paired-box transcription factor *Pax-6*. Important post-embryonic events include the differentiation of the neurosensory retina and the development of the retinal vasculature. Remodeling continues for a while after birth and post-natal growth of the orbit is dependent upon the presence of an intact globe. The young eyeball can also be remodeled by pathological processes, as in buphthalmos.

Specification of the Vertebrate Eye

The specification of the vertebrate eye has been actively investigated (9,29,51,67,78,132,278). The ocular anlage develops at the neural plate stage prior to optic vesicle formation when a group of cells at the anterior end of the plate is specified to form the retina. A group of eye field transcription factors (EFTF) are expressed in the anterior neural plate and the major EFTFs have been identified as *Otx2, Six6, ET, Rx1, Pax6, Six3, Lhx2,* and *tll* (9,278). The homeobox gene *Otx2* is one of the earliest genes expressed in the presumptive eye field and expression is detected only in the periphery, destined to develop into retinal pigment epithelium (RPE), and not the central eye field destined to become the neurosensory retina (9, 156). The importance of the EFTFs in vertebrate eye formation has been clearly demonstrated. Targeted or spontaneous mutations in *Pax6, Six3, Six6, ET, Rx1, Lhx2,* or *tll* result in anophthalmia or abnormal eyes, while overexpression of *Pax6, Six3, Rx1,* and *Six6* can result in the formation of ectopic eye tissue (278). The critical role for *Otx2* is seen in experiments demonstrating that the induction of ectopic eye tissue by overexpression of *Pax6, Six3, Six6,* or *Rx* only occurs in the head region defined by *Otx2* expression (29,30). *ET,* a member of the T-box family of transcription factors, is expressed very early in the eye field (143) and has been shown to be involved in dorso–ventral patterning of the eye (261,278). *Rx1* has been demonstrated to have an early role in eye formation, before the involvement of *Pax6* and *Six3* (273,278). Another layer of complexity is added in that *Wnt4* signaling is required for vertebrate eye development through the expression of *EAF2,* a component of the ELL-mediated RNA polymerase II elongation factor complex (161). *EAF2* is specifically expressed in the eye and expression is dependent on *Wnt4* function. *EAF2* regulates the expression of the eye-specific transcription factor *Rx* and loss of *EAF2* function results in an absence of eyes. All of the aforementioned genes, and more, act in a hierarchical network for specification of the vertebrate eye (192,278).

Role of the Neural Crest in the Formation of Mesenchyme in the Head and Neck

Three distinct elements in the primitive embryo contribute to the development of the human eye: the neural crest, the neuroectoderm, and the surface ectoderm. The mesodermal contribution is largely limited to the formation of the extra-ocular muscles (217) and the endothelium of blood vessels.

The neural crest was recognized as a potential source of mesenchymal tissues in 1888, when Kastschenko (122) claimed that some of the mesenchyme in the head of selachians (sharks) originated from neural crest. Later it became accepted that mesenchyme was a functional entity rather than an anatomical structure derived from one particular embryonic germ layer (the mesoderm). The vertebrate neural crest not only gives rise to melanocytes, Schwann cells, neuroblasts, and ganglion cells of the peripheral nervous system but also contributes extensively to the formation of facial cartilage, bone, and teeth. The only facial structures not of neural crest origin are the skin and other epithelia, vascular endothelia, skeletal muscle, and the retina and the lens (118).

Role of Neuroectoderm in the Formation of the Optic Vesicle

All mammalian eyes arise from an outpouching of the neuroectoderm of the diencephalon that becomes the optic vesicle. The optic primordia initially develop as thickenings of the neural folds at the 18th day of gestation (crown-rump length of 2 mm). Once the sulcus of the neuroectodermal plate deepens and the neural tube forms, the optic evaginations appear as a pair of lateral bulbous projections from the developing forebrain and the neural crest develops from the mesencephalic neuroectoderm (Fig. 1). Subsequently, the neural tube closes and the optic vesicles are pushed out towards the surface ectoderm (170,171). The optic vesicle later invaginates to form the optic cup but remains connected to the cavity of the diencephalon, the third ventricle, by the optic stalk. The optic vesicle becomes ensheathed by neural crest mesenchyme, except for a small central area where the lens and cornea will develop. The processes involved in the induction of the optic cup and the lens placode are thought to be under the influence of such genes as *Otx2*, *Pax6*, *Six3*, *Rx*, and *Lens1* (29).

Induction of the Lens

As the optic vesicle approaches the surface, molecular signals produced by the cells of the vesicle and a specialized region of the surface ectoderm are exchanged. The ectodermal cells in the immediate area of the approaching optic vesicle enlarge and form a plate-like thickening, the lens placode (Fig. 2), separated by its own basal lamina from that of the optic vesicle (207). The placode invaginates to form a lens vesicle that will expand toward the optic vesicle. The lens vesicle in turn makes contact with the cells at the tip of the optic vesicle and, through the influence of fibroblast growth factor (FGF) (193), induces differentiation into neural retina, which is a key factor in the subsequent invagination of the optic vesicle to form the optic cup (Fig. 3) (111). Experiments in chick embryos suggest that the crucial event in this sequence is the contact of the pre-lens ectoderm, i.e.,

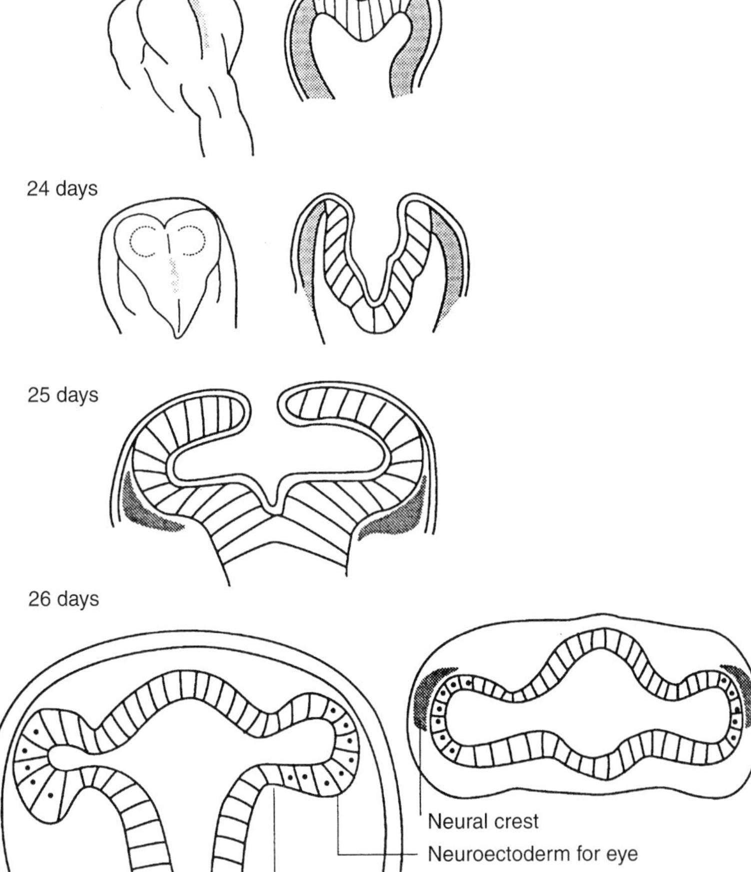

Figure 1 Early development of optic vesicle. At 20 days the neuroectodermal plate has a central depression or sulcus. The lateral ridges grow and converge and by 24 days the sulcus closes and the ridges develop depressions, the optic pits. The convex edge of the neuroectoderm becomes apposed to the surface ectoderm. By 26 days the optic vesicles are well formed, with defined neuroectoderm distinct from the rest of the neural tube. There is rapid apposition of neural crest elements.

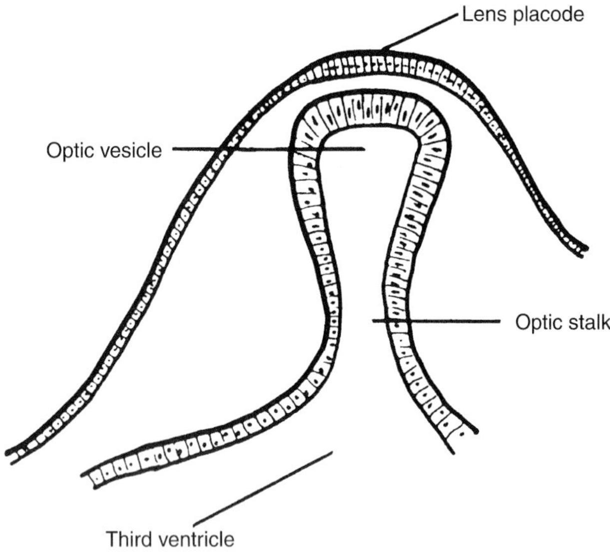

Figure 2 Outpouching of neuroectoderm to form optic vesicle at 25 days gestation in human embryo.

before the formation of the lens placode, with the optic vesicle (111).

The outer layer of the optic cup is destined to become the RPE and the inner layer starts to differentiate towards neurosensory retina. By the end of the embryonic period the retina consists of a pigmented outer layer and a primitive sensory retina with an outer limiting membrane (OLM), a proliferative zone, an external neuroblastic layer, a transient layer, and an internal neuroblastic layer covered by the nerve fiber layer and the inner limiting membrane (ILM).

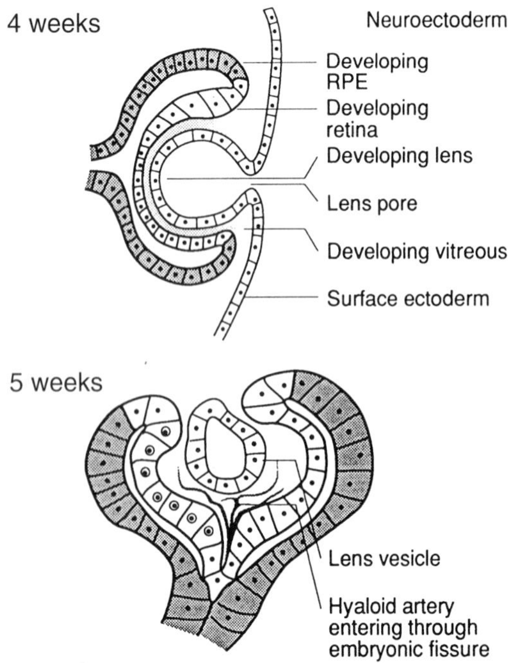

Figure 3 By 4 weeks of gestation, the surface ectoderm has invaginated to form the lens but the lens pore is still open. By 5 weeks the lens vesicle has separated and the hyaloid artery starts to envelop it posteriorly. The embryonic fissure is starting to close. In both diagrams the increasing pigmentation of the retinal pigment epithelium is seen as it differentiates: the inner neural retina remains unpigmented.

Formation of the Optic Stalk and Fissure

During the invagination of the optic vesicle a groove forms in the ventral portion of the tubular optic stalk and this deepens to form the embryonic or optic fissure, through which the hyaloid artery enters the eye. This fissure closes at 5 to 6 weeks of gestation. The proximal section is augmented by the diencephalon to form a cylinder that is subsequently invaded by retinal axons, which obliterate its lumen. The neuroectodermal cells that form the wall of the stalk differentiate into the neuroglia of the optic nerve.

It has been established that the tissue concentrations of the morphogen sonic hedgehog (*Shh*) are crucial for dorsal–ventral patterning of the optic vesicle (27,150,184). During optic vesicle formation a clear dorso–ventral distinction occurs, with the ventral optic stalk separated from the dorsal area destined to become retina. The optic stalk is adjacent to the midline source of the ventralizing morphogen *Shh* and develops into the optic nerve (155). The dorsal area is farther from the source of *Shh* and develops into the neural retina (29). The *Shh* signal that influences the development of the optic nerve acts through induction of the *Pax2* gene proximally and the *Pax6* gene distally (57,150). The effects of *Shh* on ventralization of the visual field are mediated by the two transcription factors encoded by the ventral anterior homeobox (*Vax*) genes *Vax1* and *Vax2* (15,172,173). Vax1 and Vax2 proteins cooperatively ventralize the developing eye field by acting at the midline to repress expression of the *Pax6* gene (173). This allows development of the optic nerve by inhibiting retinal differentiation programs that the *Pax6* gene normally promotes (173). It has recently been demonstrated in neural crest-specific knockout mice that *Pitx2* expression in the neural crest is needed to regulate extrinsic factors required for development of the optic nerve (62); *Pitx2* itself is not expressed in the optic stalk.

HISTOGENESIS OF OCULAR STRUCTURES

Retina

Neurosensory Retina

The primitive optic vesicle consists of ciliated cells arranged as a pseudo-stratified columnar epithelium. The component cells are linked by junctional complexes that form the ILM and OLMs; there are also appositional lateral junctions (194). Before mitosis, the ventricular cells, having replicated their DNA, release their attachments to the ILM and come to lie against the OLM. When division is completed, the daughter cells are found internal to the precursor cells. Initially there is no evidence of differentiation but cells destined to become photoreceptors or radial glia (Müller cells) remain attached to the OLM, whereas other daughter cells migrate to the appropriate level within the retina (107,194). At this point in development the tissue mass of the retina increases by approximately 25% each day (Fig. 4) (92). The Müller cells form a scaffold connecting the ILM and OLMs. Mitosis begins in the central area and ceases first in that area: at about 15 weeks (120 mm) to be followed by differentiation (198,228). Differentiation of the retinal progenitor cells, the retinal neuroblasts, progresses in an orderly manner from outer to inner retina and from posterior to peripheral retina (271). The posterior retina is the first region to differentiate but the last to mature (22). The distinct retinal cell types differentiate in a sequential pattern, with ganglion cells, cone photoreceptors, and horizontal cells appearing first.

Within the retinal neuroblastic layer, some cells begin to undergo differentiation into ganglion cells, with rounded, vesicular nuclei and prominent nucleoli, from which axons begin to sprout (259). The ganglion cells first appear, and are more numerous, superior, and temporal to the optic stalk (151,194). Their axonal outgrowths form a nerve fiber layer that stretches back to the optic stalk (Fig. 5) and they extend to the lateral geniculate body. Those ganglion cells whose axons do not establish contact with the neurons of the lateral geniculate body will undergo apoptosis. The formation of the axons, and the pathways they take to the brain (retinal projections), are heavily influenced by the degree of melanin pigmentation (257). Albino mutations in all species studied, including humans (71), reduce ipsilateral projection by allowing more axons to cross at the optic chiasm. This lack of pigmentation is also associated with a failure of normal foveal development.

Although the ganglion cell and neuroblastic layers are recognizable at this stage, the plexiform layers are not. Retinal cells of dissimilar classes undergoing concurrent neurogenesis are referred to as cohorts, capable of different rates of migration and differentiation. Using thymidine labeling and autoradiography, retinal ganglion cells, type A horizontal cells, and cone photoreceptors have all been shown to form at the same embryological stage. However, although the latter two cell lines are committed, they do not immediately proceed to differentiate (194,271). The definitive layers of the neurosensory retina appear with the migration of ganglion cells and amacrine cell precursors into the neuroblastic layer, leaving cellular processes in the transient layer of Chievitz (Fig. 6). The cell processes may have a role in the final arrangement of the nuclear layers although studies in mice suggest that the trilaminar organization of the neurosensory retina is dependent upon the normal development and orientation of Müller cells (254). The normal development of the Müller cells appears to be directed by the Sonic hedgehog (*Shh*) gene product expressed by the retinal ganglion cells.

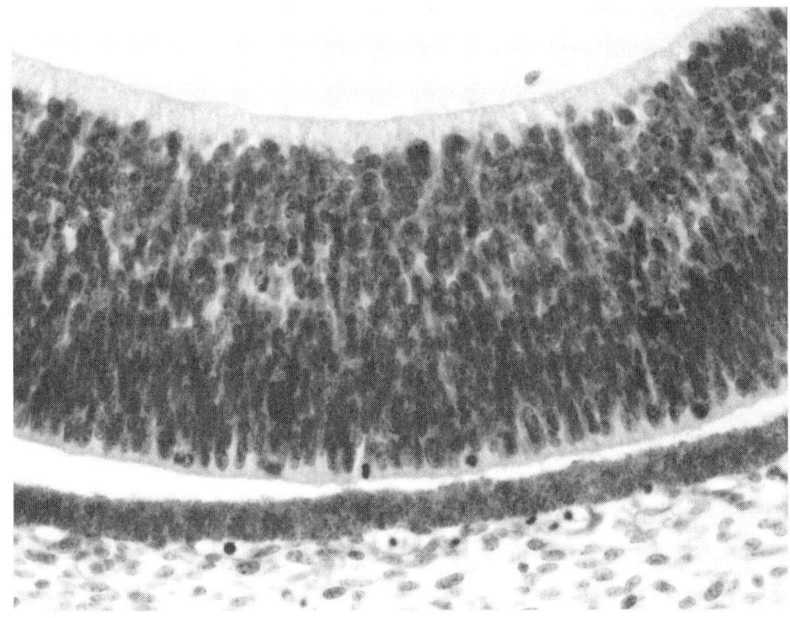

Figure 4 Light photomicrograph of a human eye at 7 weeks of gestation. The retinal pigment epithelium (RPE) has become a single cuboidal layer and has begun to produce melanin. Several vascular channels are present at the basal surface of the RPE cells that will become choriocapillaris, but Bruch membrane is not visible. The cytologic appearance of the neuroblasts is homogeneous and photoreceptor outer segments have not yet formed. The outer and inner limiting membranes are clearly identifiable (hematoxylin and eosin, ×300).

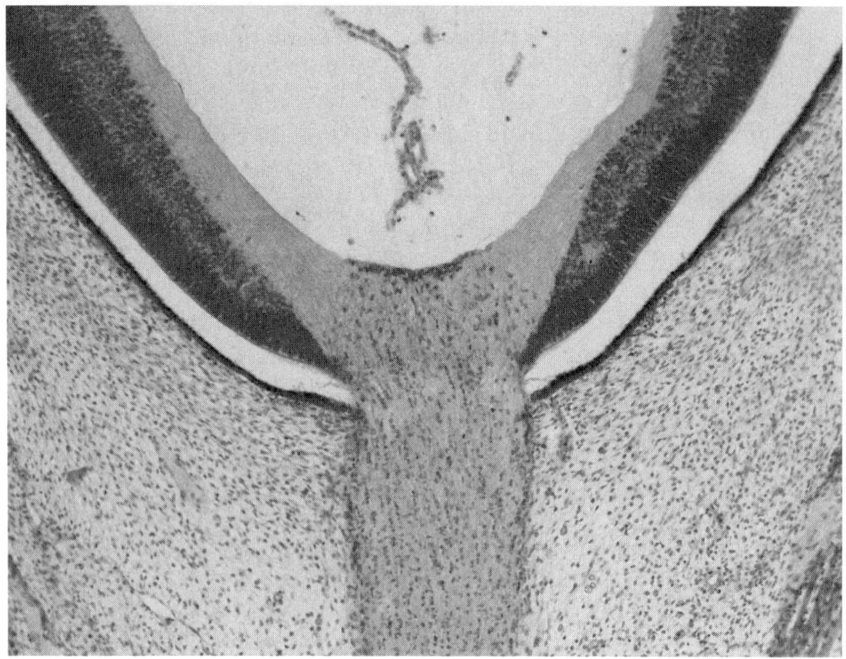

Figure 5 Light photomicrograph of a human eye at 9 weeks of gestation. Bergmeister papilla is in the final stages of involution. Ganglion cells (the lighter stained cells) have migrated toward the inner limiting membrane to become separated from the more darkly staining retinal neuroblasts. The acellular layer between the two cell types is the transient layer of Chievitz, which contains processes from the ganglion cells. Axons from the ganglion cells have begun to extend to the optic disc to form the optic nerve (hematoxylin and eosin, ×100).

Both Müller cells and cone precursors develop after the migration of the ganglion cells and the emergence of the amacrine cells and the radial glia influence the positioning of the rods. Although the nuclei of the Müller cells lie in the inner nuclear layer, the foot processes with associated basal lamina contribute to the structure of the ILM, which provides a smooth inner surface for the neurosensory retina. The demonstration of hyaluronic acid within mature (12 weeks) Müller cell processes has led to the suggestion that these cells may also contribute to the formation of the vitreous (8).

The photoreceptor outer segments are derived from the cilia that project from the outer aspect of the inner layer of the optic vesicle towards the neuroectodermal layer that will form the RPE. In humans, the

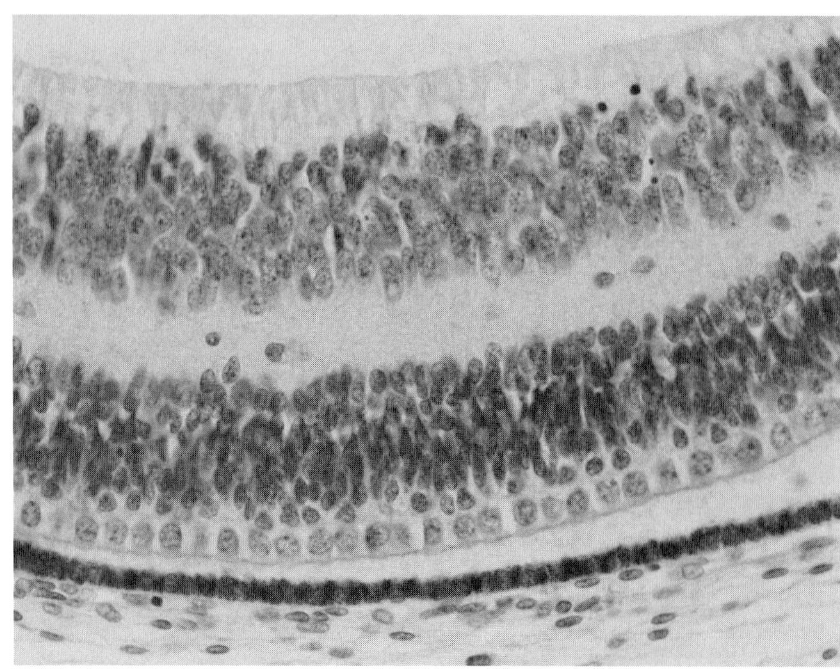

Figure 6 Light photomicrograph of a human eye at 14 weeks of gestation. The lamellar pattern of the retina is becoming established. Cells adjacent to the external limiting membrane are beginning to form differentiated photoreceptor outer segments (hematoxylin and eosin, ×400).

outer segments of the rods develop at about 23 weeks of gestation. Over the subsequent 11 weeks the rods acquire their characteristic stacked lamellar sacs derived from invaginated plasma membranes (220).

Two major families of transcription factors have been implicated in the determination of retinal cell fate: the basic helix-loop-helix (bHLH) and homeodomain (HD) proteins (2,24,56,96,160,189,251). Retinal ontogenesis involves the conversion of neuroepithelial undifferentiated progenitor cells to glia and six classes of retinal neurons. The different retinal cell types are generated in a fixed overlapping temporal sequence (160). The broadly expressed neurogenic bHLH transcription factors are intrinsic regulators of the program that controls proliferation, specification, cell cycle arrest, and differentiation of retinal cells (112,245). The neurogenic bHLH genes expressed in retinal progenitor cells include *Ash1*, *NeuroD*, *Ngn2*, *Hes1*, and *Ath3/5* (2,160) and the earliest cells to differentiate during retinogenesis are the retinal ganglion cells (270). Early in mouse retinal development a subgroup of progenitor cells acquire competence for differentiation into retinal ganglion cells by expressing *Math5* (266). Transcription factors *Ngn2*, *Ash1*, and *Hes*1 have been demonstrated to interact with *Math5* in the selection of retinal ganglion cell precursors and induction of their specific traits (160). The HD protein Pax6 is required for retinal ganglion cell competence (154). A putative downstream target of *Math5* is *Brn3b* (20,110). Brn3b is a transcription factor needed for retinal ganglion cell differentiation, axon outgrowth, and pathfinding (61,75,253). Experimental data suggest that an antagonistic relationship between *Math5* and *Math3/NeuroD* regulates ganglion versus amacrine cell specification (2,20,112,123,252). *Mash1* and *Math3* appear to regulate bipolar versus Müller cell determination, since it has been shown that precursor bipolar cells differentiate towards Müller cells in the absence of *Mash1* and *Math3* expression (97,240). Overexpression of the HD transcription factor *Rx1* promotes differentiation of Müller cells (127,159). Akagi et al. analyzed the mouse retina with three different combinations of triple compound mutations for neurogenic *bHLH* genes (2). They found that rod development is reduced in the *Mash1; Math3; NeuroD* triple mutant retina, whereas horizontal cell development was impaired in the *Mash1; Ngn2; Math3* and *Ngn2; Math3; NeuroD* triple-mutant retinas, suggesting that specification of retinal cell fate depends on the coordinated expression of multiple *bHLH* genes. In other vertebrate experimental systems it has been shown that the HD gene *Otx5b* plays a role in photoreceptor differentiation (246,247), *Chx10* promotes bipolar cell determination (97,241,245) and *Prox1* promotes horizontal cell determination (14,56). It appears that determination of distinct cell types in the vertebrate retina is multifactorial and complicated, with much information yet to be elucidated.

Fovea

The increase in density of ganglion cells at the macula begins at about 18 weeks and continues until the seventh month. At this point there is displacement of ganglion cells and the foveal depression begins to appear. The fovea contains all the adult layers of the neurosensory retina but only cone photoreceptors, the outer segments of which can be distinguished at about 26 weeks of gestation (38,101–103). There is some variation between species. In the monkey at birth a single layer of inner retinal neurons and the cones are stacked three cells deep with elongated inner segments and development continues for the first three months of life. In humans, development is slower by several months and continues until the age of 4 years. This delayed maturation accounts for the dramatic increase in visual function in early childhood, since the fovea mediates color vision and provides high resolution.

The formation of the foveal pit, where the inner retinal layers are absent, is completed after birth and is accompanied by the accumulation of ganglion cells at its periphery, on the foveal slope, where the highest concentration of ganglion cells is to be found (37). The highest concentration of cones occurs within the center of the fovea, in the region called the foveola, where in the human retina there are between 100,000 and 300,000 mm^{-2} (38,39). An area of the human fovea measuring 350 μm in diameter is devoid of rods. Each cone signals to at least two ganglion cells via several bipolar cells and this underlies the high visual acuity and color perception in this region of the retina. The fovea takes longer to mature than any other part of the retina, starting first and finishing last, but the end result is an exquisitely discriminative and sensitive region (102).

Retinal development is therefore determined by three distinct processes: differentiation, lamination, and the emergence of cellular cohorts. The initial mitotic division of the ventricular cell is followed by further proliferation and, after mitosis ceases, the post-mitotic cells undergo neurogenesis, migration, differentiation, and maturation (194,199). The ventricular cells appear to be multipotential: in any given period of neurogenesis, more than one cell type may emerge and these cells form a cohort, with local factors determining post-mitotic commitment. The initial period of neurogenesis is followed by programmed cell death, resulting in the organized adult retina. According to Young (271), the distribution and maturation of any cell within the retina depends on five separate processes:

1. Time and location of the final mitotic division;
2. Morphological differentiation and the extent of surface development of the retina at the time of formation and placement (insertion) of the post-mitotic cell;
3. Subsequent growth and development of the retina after insertion of the post-mitotic cell;
4. Intercellular trophic effects and cell death;
5. Non-uniform expansion of the growing retina.

Within the retina, cell division occurs early and differentiation is initiated at the ILM and OLM into primitive photoreceptors and ganglion cells. Processes emanating from post-mitotic cells grow throughout the retina and guide the placement of other cells. Postnatal metabolic activity includes replacement of the entire outer segment of a rod, about 1000 double membrane discs, every 2 weeks. Since the photoreceptor has lost its ability to disassemble the rods as a result of terminal differentiation, the shed discs are phagocytosed by the RPE (271).

Retinal Pigment Epithelium

RPE cells are derived from the outer layer of the optic cup and normally become pigmented by 5 weeks of gestation (6–7 mm stage), at the same time as the retinal ganglion cells leave the mitotic cycle. Coincidentally with melanogenesis, the cilia present on the inner surface disappear and the RPE becomes a monolayer of cuboidal cells with the apices oriented internally, joined by tight junctions (105). This transformation occurs under the influence of activin, a member of the transforming growth factor beta (TGFβ) superfamily of growth factors (69). Short projections from the apices lie alongside the photoreceptor outer segments that develop from the cilia of the sensory layer. Apposition of the cell layers is essential for normal growth and development. The RPE cells slowly increase in number during fetal development but after birth coverage of the growing eyeball is maintained by cell hypertrophy and mitoses are not seen (188).

The process of neuroectodermal melanogenesis is similar to that seen in neural crest melanocytes, although the melanosomes of all pigment epithelial cells are larger than those of uveal or dermal melanocytes (163). The melanin granules confer calcium buffering properties on the RPE which may influence intercellular communication (52). The lack of melanin within the RPE in albinism results in anomalous organization of the neurosensory retina (71,174).

The basal surface of the developing RPE is covered by a thin but continuous basal lamina and this first element of Bruch membrane is present in the 6-week embryo (188). Initially, the basal lamina abuts the choroidal collagen fibrils but after 13 weeks of gestation the basal lamina of the choriocapillaris and a fenestrated sheet of elastic tissue produced by neural crest-derived fibroblasts are also recognizable (211). The choriocapillaris is itself induced by the RPE in week 4 to 5 of gestation to provide a primitive capillary network surrounding the growing optic cup (210,211).

The molecular mechanisms that specify the RPE have only recently received attention. A comprehensive review has amalgamated the molecular events during development, and provides some hypotheses on the evolutionary origin of RPE cells (157). Signaling molecules from the surface ectoderm and the periocular mesenchyme are important for the early regionalization of the developing optic vesicle into neural retina and RPE (157). Within the developing RPE, the signaling pathways can either induce or suppress networks of transcription factors that will specify RPE differentiation. FGFs, mainly FGF1/FGF2/FGF8/FGF9, from the surface ectoderm normally inhibit RPE formation while activating neural retina specification (180,193,248,277). There is evidence suggesting that the FGF-induced repression of the RPE is mediated by activation of the Ras-Raf-MAPK/ERK kinase (MEK)–mitogen-activated protein kinase (MAPK) pathway (74,275). From the surrounding extraocular mesenchyme members of the TGFβ superfamily provide inductive signals favoring specification of the RPE. TGFβ family members, the activins, are expressed in the extraocular mesenchyme, while their specific receptors are expressed in the developing optic vesicle (63,69). Several studies have indicated the potential role of TGFβ in human RPE in the regulation of various cellular functions such as induction of stearoyl coenzyme A desaturase (209), regulation of nitric oxide production (133), secretion of vascular endothelial growth factor (VEGF) (178) possibly mediated by increased L-type Ca^{2+} channel activity (206), and the production of platelet-derived growth factor (PDGF) (177).

These signaling molecules from surrounding tissues establish RPE by inducing or repressing a transcription factor network composed of microphthalmia-associated transcription factors (*Mitf*), orthodenticle-related transcription factors (*Otx*), and *Pax6* (157). Mitf is a basic helix-loop-helix/leucine zipper (bHLHZip) transcription factor belonging to the Myc superfamily of transcription factors that bind E-box sequences (230,234). *MitfA*, *MitfH*, and *MitfD* are the major isoforms found in the RPE, and are expressed throughout the development of the RPE in vertebrates (83,180,234,236). The genes for the major enzymes responsible for melanin production *Try*,

Tyrp1, and *Dct*, are targets of *Mitf*, suggesting that pigmentation is regulated by *Mitf* activity (230,268). Activation of *Mitf* is necessary for normal development of RPE cells in the optic vesicle (180). *Mitf* deficiency affects cell survival as well as pigmentation, indicating that *Mitf* may target genes other than the enzymes involved in pigmentation (230,249). The regulation of *Mitf* is not well defined, but evidence suggests it may involve the *EMX* homeobox genes (17), and *Wnt* signaling (116,145,267).

Otx1 and *Otx2* are bicoid-type HD genes essential for anterior brain and eye formation in vertebrates (64,222), and for development of photoreceptors and expression of rhodopsin in *Drosophila* (235). During eye development *Otx* genes are expressed in the entire optic vesicle, but subsequently expression becomes restricted to the presumptive RPE where *OTX2* protein interacts with *Mitf* (18,158,222). Furthermore, *Otx2* can directly transactivate the promoter region of the melanogenic genes *Tyr*, *Trp1*, and *Trp2* (17) and there appear to be three different promoters used alternately during development (66). The importance of *OTX2* in human ocular development has recently been clearly demonstrated. Ragge et al. (201) used a candidate-gene approach to identify heterozygous coding-region changes in the *OTX2* gene in eight families with ocular malformations ranging from bilateral anophthalmia to retinal defects resembling congenital amaurosis and pigmentary retinopathy.

The paired HD transcription factors are expressed in the presumptive ocular tissues during development. *Pax2* is expressed mainly in the ventral region of the optic vesicles, while *Pax6* is expressed in the entire optic vesicle and early optic cup (182,250) but is later is lost in the RPE (88). Studies in *Pax2* and *Pax6* null mice have provided evidence that the absence of a functional *Pax6* delays, but does not prevent, the full differentiation of RPE (33,200). Results in double *Pax2/Pax5* null mice demonstrate that the redundant activities of *Pax2* and *Pax6* are required, and sufficient, to effect the determination of RPE (182). This is supported by the observations that the *Pax2* and *Pax6* proteins bind to and activate the promoter of the RPE determinant gene *Mitf* (182).

Retinal Vasculature

The blood supply to the retina is derived from a branch of the internal carotid artery. This primitive ophthalmic artery invades the optic fissure from below at about 28 days (5 mm) and, as the fissure closes, the vessel remains trapped within the optic cup and is referred to thereafter as the hyaloid artery (7). The intraneural portions of the hyaloid vessels later become the definitive central retinal artery and vein. The branches of the hyaloid artery form a network between the marginal zone of the retina and the lens vesicle. This network, together with small vessels from the ophthalmic artery at the optic disc, supply nutrients to the developing retina until primitive retinal vessels begin to form by a combination of vasculogenesis and angiogenesis.[a]

Around the fourth month of gestation spindle-shaped mesenchymal cells from the vascular plexus at the optic disc invade the nerve fiber layer. These cells proliferate, form solid cords that subsequently acquire lumina and contain erythrocytes. This primary network of vessels in the inner retina extends towards the peripheral retina. In the human eye, the angioblasts are confined to the central two-thirds of the retina and are not present in sufficient numbers to create all of the required retinal vessels (25). Consequently, this inner network gives rise through angiogenesis to an outer secondary vascular network and increases the density of the inner network. The vascular networks reach the ora serrata by the eighth month of gestation, a growth rate of approximately 0.1 mm per day (167). VEGF appears to be a major influence on both the angioblasts in the first phase and the endothelial cells in the second phase of vascularization. In the human eye both cell types express its receptor VEGFR2 (*Flk1*) although this may not apply to all mammalian species (25). There is evidence that VEGF is expressed by astrocytes in the ganglion cell layer and by Müller cells in the inner nuclear layer and the influence of astrocytes on retinal vascular development remains controversial (68,208).

While this intra-retinal network is forming, the hyaloid artery enveloped in a sheath of glial cells regresses in an antero-posterior direction. The foveal vasculature has been described in other primates and the avascular zone is apparent at around 125 days of gestation, comparable to 7 months in the human (60). It has been suggested that in humans the avascular zone forms through obliteration of previously formed blood vessels (104). There is substantial post-natal maturation of the retinal vasculature and Ashton postulated that endothelial cell proliferation is promoted by the relative hypoxia of venous blood (7). The retinal vessels have a continuous endothelial lining by birth and pericytes, which begin to appear around the fifth month of gestation, also increase in number at birth.

Physiological retinal angiogenesis is controlled by VEGF which sculpts the developing retinal vasculature

---

[a] Vasculogenesis refers to the formation of blood vessels from precursor cells called angioblasts. These cells coalesce into cords that subsequently canalize to form a vessel lined by endothelial cells. Angiogenesis refers to the sprouting of new blood vessels from pre-existing vessels through the proliferation of endothelial cells.

by numerous means, including spatiotemporal alterations in VEGF and VEGF receptor concentration and differential effects of the several VEGF isoforms (see Chapter 68) (187,197,232). VEGF is a dimeric glycoprotein that is a hypoxia-inducible cytokine. The single gene generates five isoforms in humans (VEGF120, VEGF145, VEGF165, VEGF189, and VEGF206, the numbers referring to the amino acid content) and three in mice (VEGF120, VEGF164, and VEGF188) through alternative splicing (124,179,195,219). Mutant mice have been created to express only one of the isoforms to investigate distinct roles of individual isoforms in retinal vascular growth and development (229). Mice expressing only VEGF164 displayed normal retinal vascularization. In mice expressing only VEGF120, vascular coverage of the retina and development of venules and arterioles were impaired, whereas mice expressing VEGF188 had normal veins but improper arteriolar formation. VEGF regulates endothelial functions involved in proliferation, migration, blood vessel wall assembly, and survival through interaction with endothelial cell-specific receptors (*Flk1*, *Flt1*, and neurophilins 1 and 2). These receptors are expressed in a spatio-temporally distinct manner, adding further ways by which vascular patterning can be achieved (47,76,128,218,238).

Experiments have been reported indicating that normal vascular development proceeds in the absence of blood flow and does not depend on a supply of oxygenated blood to the retina (36). However, hypoxia-inducible factor 1α (HIF1α) and the von Hippel-Lindau disease (VHLD) protein (pVHLD) have been implicated in the mechanisms by which growing vessels sense and respond to varying tissue oxygen levels (50,113,179).

Lens

Development of the lens can be divided into four phases: induction and formation of the lens placode, (135) formation of the lens vesicle, (5) formation of primary fibers, (9) and formation of secondary fibers (29).

Initial dependence on the competence of the cephalic ectoderm to respond to lens inducers during the period of gastrulation of the embryo is followed almost immediately by a phase in which the designated area of surface ectoderm develops a lens-forming bias. It then moves into a period of autonomy, such that the lens ectoderm is able to differentiate on its own. The presence of the optic vesicle ensures that the later phases of differentiation occur at the specified site and the lens-forming bias is suppressed in adjacent sites (81,134). The lens placode arises in a region of the ectoderm that was previously in contact with the neuroectoderm of the optic vesicle (87). Although this contact is a normal requirement, in some species a rudimentary lens may develop in the absence of an optic vesicle. The nature of the interaction between placode and optic vesicle is not clear but it has been suggested that neural crest inhibits lens differentiation and that the optic vesicle may shelter the placode from the influence of the neural crest at this time (87).

The lens placode forms a thickening in the area over the optic vesicle at 27 days of gestation and is induced to move within the lips of the optic vesicle as this structure invaginates (191). The lens placode itself invaginates to form a pit, then a cup, and finally a vesicle (Fig. 7). This is achieved through differential elongation of the ectodermal cells with contraction of their apices producing a series of conical-shaped cells,

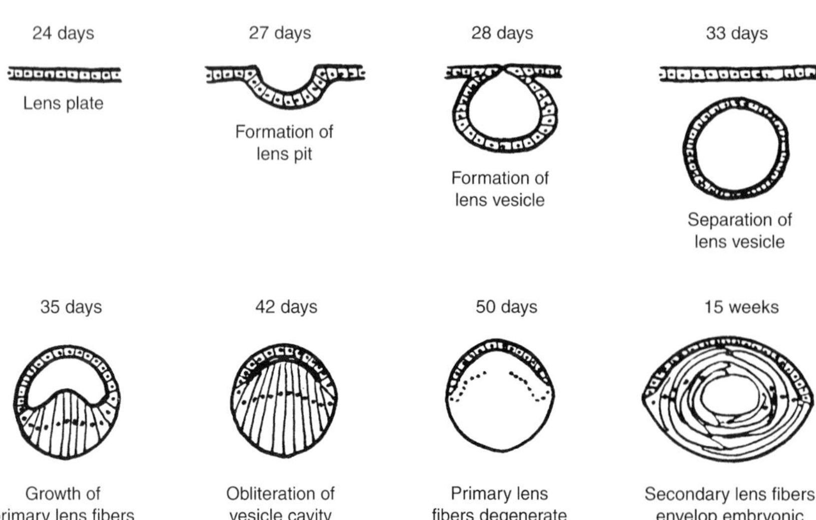

Figure 7 Development of the lens. The lens develops from the surface ectoderm, which invaginates at 27 days to form the lens pit and subsequently the lens vesicle. Separation is achieved by 33 days. The primary lens fibers fill the cavity until they degenerate and are succeeded by the secondary lens fibers, which continue to form throughout life.

each bordered by a basal lamina (221,262). Separation from the surface ectoderm is complete by 33 days (10 mm) and the basal lamina thickens to become the lens capsule, which is recognizable at about 5 weeks of gestation (141). At this stage, and up to 10–12 weeks of gestation, the posterior lens capsule is thicker than the anterior, partly reflecting a contribution from the developing hyaloid vascular network (141).

When the posterior lens cells start to produce the crystallins, they lengthen and the cells become filled with these proteins at the expense of cytoplasmic organelles. These primary lens fibers progressively fill the vesicle and gradually obliterate the lens cavity: their nuclei move forward to create the characteristic lens bow. At this time the anterior lens cells produce secondary fibers that move centrally in successive waves from the lens equator (224). These secondary lens fibers grow forward and backward around the primary lens fibers, meeting at the anterior and posterior sutures. The lens becomes progressively more ellipsoidal as secondary lens fibers are added. The cytoplasmic occupation by the crystallins results in loss of nuclei and by 3 months of gestation no nuclei are visible within the innermost cells of the lens, itself referred to as the nucleus. The number of cell layers within the lens increases from about 400 in the 45 mm fetus to about 1450 in the neonate and 2000 in the adult (54). At birth the lens often has a dimple in its posterior surface but as it grows this is lost and the lens assumes its definitive shape. The subcapsular epithelium is confined to the anterior part of the mature lens and these cells continue to deposit lamellae of collagen type IV within the anterior lens capsule, which thickens gradually throughout life (65).

Lens induction and development is a complex multi-stage process involving multiple molecular pathways (13,26,95,129,136,146,226). Signaling pathways necessary for lens induction and early development include the FGF pathway (146,162), the *Wnt* signaling pathway (26,226,233), and the bone morphogenetic protein (Bmp) signaling pathway (53,255). Critical transcription factors have been identified as part of these pathways or as primary effector targets. The *Pax6* gene is expressed in the lens placode and surrounding surface ectoderm (88). Numerous experiments have indicated that *Pax6* is necessary and sufficient for development of the lens (28,32,70,88,129,136,200). *FoxE3* is a *forkhead* class transcription factor that is regulated by *Pax6* (49). The *FoxE3* mutant mouse (*dysgenic lens, dyl*) demonstrates failure of lens vesicle closure and separation, and suppression of lens epithelial cell proliferation (16,21). *SOX2* transcription factor is a member of the *SOX* family (Sox1, Sox2, Sox3) of proteins that carry a DNA-binding high mobility group domain and additional domains that regulate embryonic development and determination of cell fate (190,258). The importance of *SOX2* in early eye development has been underscored by the report that functional mutations in *SOX2* result in bilateral anophthalmia clinically (90). *Sox1*/*Sox2*/*Sox3* have been implicated in lens development by their regulation of crystallin genes (120,121). *Sox2* cooperatively interacts with *Pax6* to initiate lens differentiation (129). *Mab21l1* (265), *Six3* (85), *Sip1* (269), *Maf* (204), *Pitx3* (125), and *Prox1* (55) transcription factors have also been implicated in the downstream regulation of lens induction and development.

Cornea

The cornea develops from both the surface ectoderm, which gives rise to the epithelial layer and its basal lamina, and the neural crest, from which originates the stroma, Descemet membrane, and the endothelial (posterior epithelial) cells. In contrast to the avian embryo, Bowman layer in primates is thought to develop from the neural crest rather than the anterior stroma secreted by surface epithelium in birds. In a series of transplantation experiments producing chimeric chick-quail embryos, Le Douarin et al. were able to show that most of the connective tissues of the head and neck in birds are of neural crest and not mesodermal origin (138,181). These data have been extrapolated to mammals, including humans, and have led to greater understanding of complex anomalies, although direct evidence is still largely derived from avian studies (93). The diverse morphological expression of tissues derived from neural crest cells depends on the ability of these cells to migrate and disperse, as well as the precision of their localization. Transplantation studies have demonstrated that some cells of the neural crest are pre-committed to differentiate along a certain path but others are capable of differentiating in a different direction in the appropriate environment (81,181,239).

In the 7 mm embryo clusters of neural crest cells destined to form the mesenchyme of the anterior segment are present at the rim of the optic cup. Shortly thereafter (10 mm), these cells give rise to a double layer of cuboidal cells beneath the surface ectoderm that will ultimately form the corneal endothelium (Fig. 8). A further wave of migration at 24 mm gives rise to the corneal stroma and the adjacent sclera and by 8 weeks of gestation there are 8 to 10 layers surrounded by collagen fibers within the developing stroma.

Corneal Epithelium

The area of surface ectoderm destined to give rise to the corneal epithelium is probably determined by some interaction with the neuroectodermal outpouching early in embryogenesis (166). In the 33 mm human embryo, two rows of cells rest on a thin basal lamina

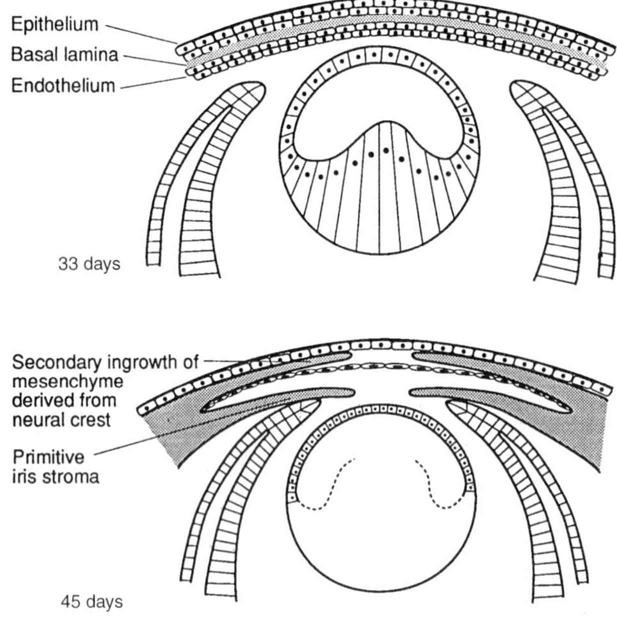

Figure 8 At 33 days (10 mm) the cornea is represented by a double-layered epithelium derived from the surface ectoderm and a posterior epithelial (endothelial) layer of neural crest origin. By 45 days the cornea is further developed and the primitive iris stroma, also derived from neural crest, and pupillary membrane are growing centripetally.

at the 33 mm stage: the outer layer is squamous and the inner columnar. At this stage the eyelids are fused and the developing cornea is protected from amniotic fluid. Wing cells appear in the fourth month of gestation and, when the eyelids separate at about 24 weeks (210 mm), the epithelium is four to five cells thick. In birds, but not in mammals, the corneal epithelial cells secrete the primary corneal stroma (12).

Corneal Stroma

In avian development, the first wave of invading neural crest cells, which forms the endothelium, accumulates posterior to the primary stroma, which contains collagen types I and II and glycosaminoglycans (GAGs) (98). This primary stroma acts as a scaffold for the deposition of the secondary stroma after the arrival of the second wave of neural crest cells. The immigration of the neural crest cells is aided by the hydration of the stroma, largely as a result of abundant hyaluronic acid within it. Subsequent compression of the posterior stromal lamellae in part reflects cessation of hyaluronic acid synthesis (99). In humans where the primary stroma is absent, the second wave of neural crest cells arrives more promptly and posterior compaction of the stromal lamellae occurs relatively earlier in development. At the time when the fused eyelids separate, the central cornea is relatively thin. This has been attributed to its distance from the corneoscleral limbus and the time taken by the incoming neural crest cells to reach there in appropriate numbers. An alternative explanation involves impingement of the lens against the developing corneal stroma, such that the curvature of the cornea matches that of the lens (215).

Given the importance of a precise stromal architecture for the transmission of light through the cornea, the stromal fibroblasts lose their random distribution in the extracellular matrix (ECM) (242). Beginning posteriorly, the cells become spindle-shaped, with their long axes parallel to the corneal surface, and they form a series of lamellar networks around which the stroma is deposited. As the collagen fibers are laid down within each stromal lamella, additional lamellae are also deposited until at birth there are about 30 layers. The collagen fibers are laid down in a spiral orthogonal pattern with the same clockwise rotation in each eye (242).

Descemet Membrane/Corneal Endothelial Complex

The corneal endothelium appears around the seventh week of gestation (17–18 mm) and is originally two cells thick: it represents the first wave of neural crest cell migration into the developing cornea (151). Initially the cells are joined by maculae occludentes but by 12 weeks the cells have formed a monolayer with apical zonulae occludentes and a continuous basement membrane (Descemet membrane) that is recognizable in histological sections. The development of zonulae occludentes also coincides with the onset of secretion of aqueous humor by the developing ciliary apparatus. The number of endothelial cells increases during fetal life and stabilizes at birth at about 5×10^5, with up to 7500 cells mm^{-2}. Mitoses are rarely identifiable in the post-natal endothelium and the total number of cells declines steadily (176).

Descemet membrane first appears as patchy condensations of basal lamina, which gradually become confluent and thicken to form a continuous basement membrane (263,264). At this time, a lucent zone 37 nm thick separates the endothelial cells from a lamina densa of similar thickness. Steady accretion of additional layers throughout gestation results in a basement membrane composed of 30 or more layers at birth, with a thickness of approximately 3 μm (117,215). At birth the predominant type of collagen deposited in the basement membrane matrix changes from collagen type VIII to collagen type IV and the growth rate declines. The consistency of these changes allows dating of pathophysiological insults to the endothelium in a manner akin to the assessment of tree rings (175).

Schwalbe line is a circumferential thickening of the peripheral Descemet membrane that marks the transition to trabecular meshwork. The degree of thickening is variable and, if sufficiently prominent, the ring may be recognizable clinically, e.g., in some forms of anterior segment mesenchymal dysgenesis (ASMD).

Aqueous Humor Outflow Tract

The structures that form the trabecular meshwork originate in the mesenchyme adjacent to the rim of the optic cup in the early embryo. At 12 weeks of gestation the second wave of migrating neural crest cells is seen in a wedge-shaped mass at the junction of the pupillary membrane and the peripheral margin of the cornea. The mesenchymal cells are present in a scanty ECM and a row of small capillaries, thought to be a precursor of the episcleral plexus, is present on its external aspect. Over the following 8–10 weeks the ECM is organized into thin sheets covered by flattened endothelial cells. The small capillaries coalesce into the canal of Schlemm and the giant vacuoles in the canalicular endothelium appear. The scleral spur becomes recognizable during this period and the trabeculum is covered transiently by an extension of the peripheral corneal endothelium (164). In the second half of gestation there is an ongoing remodeling of the trabecular meshwork and anterior chamber angle with integration of uveal and corneoscleral elements.

The forkhead transcription factor genes *Foxc1* and *Foxc2* are expressed in the mesenchyme destined to become the ocular drainage structures (35,48). It has been reported that *Foxc1* heterozygous knockout mutant mice ($Foxc1^{+/-}$) display numerous anterior segment abnormalities that include a small or absent Schlemm canal and aberrantly developed trabecular meshwork (227).

Iris

The formation of a complete iris is dependent on closure of the optic fissure. The iris contains neuroectodermal elements, the pigment epithelium and the dilator and sphincter muscles, and neural crest-derived elements, the stroma and anterior border. At 6 weeks, the anterior chamber is bordered by the corneal endothelium on one side and a lamina composed of connective tissue associated with the tunica vasculosa lentis on the other. Neuroectoderm from the margin of the optic cup extends into this lamina in a centripetal direction around 12 weeks. The sphincter pupillae muscle is derived form the neuroepithelium and starts to form at its farthest limit. By about 30 weeks (250 mm) the sphincter muscle has separated from the neuroepithelium and becomes innervated. The peripheral limit of the sphincter muscle is defined anatomically by a short cuff of pigmented epithelium, the von Michel spur, which also marks the boundary with the dilator muscle. The central portion of the lamina undergoes remodeling to form a pupil and around the sixth month basal extensions of the outer layer of neuroepithelial cells arrange themselves radially around the pupil to form the dilator pupillae muscle. This muscle does not separate completely from the iris pigment epithelium. Early in development the inner layer of the neuroepithelium is continuous with the non-pigmented ciliary epithelium and the neural retina and is amelanotic. Melanin begins to accumulate from about the fourth month and by the eighth month is abundant. During this period the outer neuroepithelial layer loses its intracytoplasmic melanin.

The iris stroma consists of fibroblastic and melanocytic cells of neural crest origin, arranged around blood vessels. As the pupillary membrane is resorbed, its remnants form a ruff around the pupillary margin (the collarette) that persists as the lesser circle of the iris vasculature (186). The anterior border cells migrate in from the neural crest late in human gestation and at birth the stroma is relatively thin and flat. Migration of melanocytes into the stroma continues after birth and pigmentation is dependent on sympathetic innervation (137).

Anterior Segment

The coordination of anterior eye development occurs through interactions between the ocular mesenchyme and cells derived from the surface ectoderm, mediated by transcription factors expressed in both epithelial and mesenchymal cells (40). Fate mapping experiments in chicks have provided evidence that ocular mesenchyme is derived mostly from cranial neural crest, with a minor component from cranial paraxial mesoderm (119,139,140). Gage et al. (72) used binary transgenic systems to demonstrate that the fates of neural crest and mesoderm in mice are similar to those in chick but mesoderm makes a greater contribution to anterior segment structures in the mouse. This finding would indicate that the potential contribution of mesoderm to the anterior segment in humans needs to be re-examined. The primary function of the periocular mesenchyme is to provide cell lineages important for the normal development of the different structures of the anterior segment (40,72,86).

Early studies with chick embryos provided evidence that the differentiation of corneal mesenchymal cells and the development of the anterior chamber are regulated by inductive signals from the developing lens (34,79). *Pitx3* is expressed in presumptive lens ectoderm, the lens placode, and finally the lens itself (225). The human *PITX3* gene encodes a bicoid-like HD transcription factor. Mutations in the gene result in posterior polar cataract and various features of ASMD (see Chapter 52), supporting a key role in lens and anterior segment development (1,212). Double-deletion mutation in the mouse *Pitx3* gene results in arrested development of the lens and anterior chamber at later stages (205,213). *MAF*, a basic region leucine zipper (bZIP) transcription factor, is expressed in lens development and regulates the expression of the crystallins (204). Human patients with a mutation in *MAF* may have pulverulent cataract alone or a cataract associated with microcornea or iris coloboma (114,115). A murine model for this condition has been described (149).

Differentiation of ocular mesenchymal cells and subsequent development of the anterior chamber is also regulated by transcription factors expressed within the mesenchymal cells themselves and some of the important molecules and pathways are known. An almost universal involvement of the *Pax6* gene in eye morphogenesis, as well as the induction of ectopic eyes in flies and frogs with aberrant expression of this gene, strongly suggests a central role in eye development (6,11,29,77,91,131). *Pax6* is expressed in derivatives of neural ectoderm, surface ectoderm, and the ocular tissues derived from it, and mesenchymal tissues (11,88,130). The *Pax6* haploinsufficiency phenotype clearly highlights the crucial role in the differentiation of ocular structures of mesenchymal derivation (11,31,41,82,94,106,202,203). Heterozygosity for *Pax6* deficiency ($PAX6^{+/-}$) in humans results in haploinsufficiency and causes aniridia. Mice with a targeted heterozygous null allele of *Pax6* have small eyes, small anterior chambers, corneal haze, iris hypoplasia, undifferentiated/hypoplastic trabecular meshwork, and absence of Schlemm canal (11). It is noteworthy that *PAX6* gene expression is downregulated in many adult tissues, but remains upregulated in the adult corneal epithelium (33,130), suggesting a role in the maintenance of epithelial and wound healing (203,223). The genetic dissection of *Pax6* dosage requirements in the developing mouse and human eye may help in the design of new treatments for ocular surface disorders (31,40,44,223).

In rodent eyes both *Foxc1* and *Pitx2* are expressed in a similar pattern in periocular mesenchyme and presumptive cornea (72) and mutations in the human *FOXC1* or *PITX2* genes both result in ASMD and a high risk for glaucoma (165,214), suggesting common downstream targets in cells where they are both expressed (72). *FOXC1* is expressed in trabecular meshwork (48), whereas *PITX2* is expressed in eyelids, ocular vasculature, and extraocular muscles (72,144,147,214). $Foxc1^{-/-}$mutant mice display anterior segment abnormalities, such as thickening of the corneal epithelium, stromal disorganization, and absence of endothelium (108,126). *FOXC2* is strongly homologous to *FOXC1* and has a similar expression pattern in the periocular mesenchyme and the tissues derived from it (260). *FOXC1* and *FOXC2* have overlapping functions in ocular development (227), probably through mutual downstream targets (86). *Pitx2* expression in the neural crest is required for specification of corneal endothelium, corneal stroma, sclera, and ocular blood vessels (62) and $Pitx2^{-/-}$ mutant mice have eyes similar to $Foxc1^{-/-}$ mice (73). *LMX1B* encodes a LIM-homeodomain transcription factor expressed in the periocular mesenchyme and presumptive corneal tissues and *LMBX1B* interacts with *FOXC1* in the normal differentiation of keratocytes in the cornea (86,196).

Ciliary Body and Choroid

The ciliary body arises from the tip of the optic cup. Development lags behind that of the retina and it has been proposed that there must be contact between the tip of the cup and the lens for development to proceed (188). At 45 days (20 mm) the tip of the optic cup lies inside a mass of mesenchyme that will give rise to the stromal components of the ciliary body. Although primitive myoblasts form within this mass around the 15th week of gestation, differentiation into tendon and muscle fibers does not occur until the seventh month and is only completed post-partum (151). Blood vessels grow into this region by 4 months and a distinct arterial circle is present by 5 months. At 8 months, anastomoses to the choroidal circulation and branches to the ciliary processes are completely formed (186).

The ciliary processes first begin to appear at about 11 weeks (54 mm), when the outer pigmented cells of the optic cup start to form folds and then meridional ridges, which gain in height and complexity over the next 10 weeks as they develop into the ciliary processes (188). Initially, the ciliary processes lie immediately anterior to the neural retina but over the course of several weeks they become separated as the mass of outer mesenchyme grows forward, dragging the folded epithelium with it, and the pars plana forms.

The stromal elements of the choroid arise after the sclera has enveloped the optic cup and begin as a loose mesenchymal matrix, within which fibroblasts start to secrete collagen fibrils. Muscle elements and elastic tissue, which may later regulate the spatial organization of the choroid during accommodation, are present by 4 months of gestation, by which time the distinct layers of the choroid are recognizable (188). Pigmentation of the choroid occurs late in gestation, around 7 months, when melanocytes arrive from the neural crest, and starts in the outer layer (59). Pigmentation is thought to be induced and maintained by adrenergic nerve fibers present throughout the uvea (137,231).

Blood vessels develop from the mesoderm surrounding the newly formed optic cup and by 35 days (13 mm) capillaries completely encircle the cup. Injection studies indicate that these channels arise as the RPE develops (100), these cells at this age containing mRNA of VEGF (84). RPE expression of angiogenic factors such as VEGF and FGF may be involved in the development and differentiation of the choroidal vasculature (153,208,276) and VEGFR transcripts can also be identified in the choroidal mesenchyme and the endothelial cells of the choriocapillaris (84). The role of RPE in normal choroidal development may involve the production of inductive signals essential for melanocyte differentiation, as well as vascular development (208,276). The vessels of the rudimentary choriocapillaris converge at the lip of the optic cup to form an annular blood vessel that subsequently anastomoses with branches of the posterior ciliary arteries at around 2 months of gestation. The annular blood vessel drains into a choroidal plexus and the vortex veins form from collecting channels draining this plexus at around 4 months. An intermediate layer of arterioles and venules (Sattler layer) develops between the choriocapillaris and the larger arterial branches and veins of the outer (Haller) layer.

Sclera

The sclera is derived from the neural crest and appears as a mesenchymal condensation in the region of the corneoscleral limbus, with growth proceeding in a posterior direction. In contrast to the cornea, the fibroblasts do not become aligned in parallel array and the appositional growth of the collagen fibers is more marked. Elastic tissue also deposits, but the cartilaginous and bony elements seen in birds are not present in humans. The looser episclera and compact sclera can be distinguished in the 7 to 8-week-old (28 mm) human embryo (215). By the fourth month of gestation the connective tissue fibers have penetrated the optic nerve to form the sieve-like lamina cribrosa, which is completed by the eighth month, and a scaffold for the axons. The fibers merge with the tunica adventitia of the hyaloid vessels.

Scleral agenesis was identified in neural crest-specific *Pitx2* knockout mice, suggesting that *Pitx2* expression is necessary for neural crest cells to induce scleral determination (62). Signals from the RPE have been demonstrated to induce scleral fates and it has been suggested that *Pitx2* confers competence on the neural crest cells to respond to inductive signals from the RPE (62).

Vitreous

The primary vascular vitreous, although transitory, is of immense importance in the development of the eye. The arborizing vascular elements of the primary vitreous arise from the hyaloid artery and fill the cavity of the optic vesicle at 7 mm (vasa hyaloidea propria). This network comes to lie behind the developing lens vesicle and interacts with the perilenticular mesenchyme to form the tunica vasculosa lentis. Branches arc around the lens to the annular vessel at the rim of the optic cup and forwards to form the anterior tunica vasculosa lentis and pupillary membrane. Some investigators have suggested that the expression of VEGF in the lens promotes the formation of the tunica vasculosa lentis, since VEGF receptors have been identified within the cells of the developing hyaloid vasculature (84,208). The development of the hyaloid vessels reaches its zenith in the ninth week of gestation (40 mm), at which time the annular vessel appears to function as both artery and vein. A network of small vessels from the lens region and vitreous drains into the choroidal plexus in the region where the ciliary body develops (256).

The connective tissue of the vitreous is first observable at 13 weeks of gestation as a mass of fibrillary material, mesenchymal cells, and primitive blood vessels. Some of the primary vitreous may be of surface ectodermal origin, carried into the cavity with the invaginating lens placode, but neural crest cells at the ventral optic rim, mesenchymal cells accompanying the hyaloid vessels and neuroectodermal cells from the inner layer of the optic cup may all contribute (10,142,188). Initially, there is no discernible orientation of the fibrils but, as part of the development of the secondary (permanent) vitreous, a more ordered, and often parallel, fibrillary structure emerges between the 13 and 70 mm stages.

The fully developed hyaloid vasculature at two months of gestation consists of fenestrated endothelial cells and underlying basement membrane, partially surrounded by connective tissue. Although regression of the hyaloid vascular system appears to be linked to the development of the retinal vasculature and the consequent changes in blood flow within the eye (19), its cause and mechanism remain unclear. Experiments in knockout mice suggest a role for the Norrie disease gene (*NDP*) product (185) (see Chapter 35). Involution begins in the vasa hyaloidea propria when the vessels become occluded by macrophages. The capillaries surrounding the lens atrophy in a centrifugal fashion and finally there is regression of the hyaloid artery itself. Loss of the perilenticular network and atrophy of the mesenchyme, especially in the central portion, creates an opening that becomes part of a funnel-shaped structure within the vitreous. Known as the canal of Cloquet, this structure eventually contains remnants of both the hyaloid artery (in which flow ceases in the seventh month), and the primary vitreous, which retracts as its blood supply fails. At birth Cloquet canal persists, running from a depression in the posterior lens (the patellar fossa) to the optic disc, although resorption of almost all primary vitreous elements and the hyaloid artery has usually occurred. The mechanisms and molecular cues involved in the development of the normal hyaloid vascular system are not well defined but are probably similar to those of the choroidal and retinal vasculatures (208).

The definitive avascular vitreous, the secondary vitreous (Fig. 9), is deposited behind the primary vitreous. In the rabbit, the secondary vitreous is formed by specialized cells (hyalocytes) derived from the immigration of blood-borne macrophages from the ciliary body (10). Such cells may act as facultative phagocytes, ingesting elements of the primary vitreous before passing into a secretory mode, in which they manufacture hyaluronic acid and lay down the collagen fibrils of the secondary vitreous. These fibrils are thicker, with a greater tendency to aggregate at the edge of the optic cup, than those of the primary vitreous (Fig. 10). They merge with the mesenchyme at the lip of the optic cup to form the vitreous base, seen at about 12 weeks (65 mm) as a marginal bundle of Drualt anchoring the vitreous to the internal limiting membrane of the retina.

The tertiary vitreous appears as condensations of the secondary vitreous between the lens and the rim of the optic cup around 12 weeks of gestation. These condensations are firmly attached to the inner surface of the retina where the pars plana will develop and later contribute to the vitreous base. The origin of the zonular fibrils of the tertiary vitreous remains uncertain. They may develop from the neural crest at the rim of the optic cup, with a possible contribution from the tunica vasculosa lentis, with which the immature fibers connect. They may also be derivatives of the tertiary vitreous (Fig. 11) with further contributions from the columnar cells of the nonpigmented ciliary epithelium.

Orbit and Ocular Adnexa

The formation of the ocular adnexal structures involves complex interactions between surface ectodermal derivatives and mesenchyme, much, but not all, of it derived from neural crest.

The eyelids develop as arcuate folds from the ectoderm and mesenchyme above and below the rudimentary eye. At 4 to 5 weeks of gestation (12 mm), there is a proliferation of skin ectoderm at the outer canthus and by 20 mm the eyelids are clearly seen. Mesenchymal proliferation starts at this stage with subsequent invasion of nerve fibers and deposition of collagen. The musculature is derived from second branchial arch mesoderm and differs structurally from the oculomotor muscles. Motor innervations precede sensory innervations at 6 months and specialized nerve endings (Krause corpuscles) are only formed in the seventh month (216).

As the eyelids grow, the margins come into contact at the third month and fusion is complete by 10 weeks (45 mm) (216). Fusion is contingent upon the formation of desmosomes after interdigitation of filopodia on opposing keratinocytes and these remain intact until the fifth month anteriorly and the sixth month posteriorly. Separation is mediated by keratinization of eyelash follicles and the secretion of lipid within them, which serves to disrupt the desmosomes (3,4). Separation takes place over a 2-month period (216) and appears to be hastened by EGF-enhanced keratinization; EGF is present in amniotic fluid from the 20th week of gestation. In mice the transcription factor *c-jun* regulates *EGFR* expression and mice with a *c-jun* deletion have the birth defect of open eyes, resulting from failure of fusion (272). There are fewer and shorter filopodia, the cytoskeletal organization is defective and expression of *EGFR* on keratinocytes is decreased (272). In addition to *Jun*, gene-knockout mutations in several genes have been demonstrated to cause the birth defect of open eyelids: *Tgfa* (148), *Egfr* (168), activin/inhibin βB (*Inhbb*) (244), *Fgfr2b* (23,46), *Fgf10* (237), *MEK kinase 1* (274), and *Foxl2* (243). Mutations in human *FOXL2* are responsible for a rare genetic disease known as the blepharophimosis,

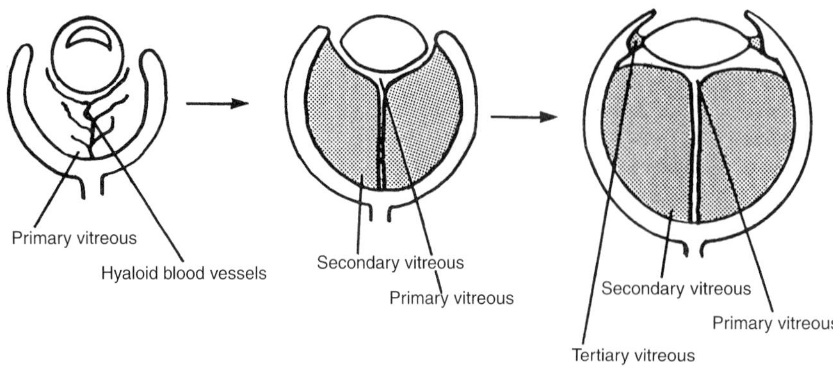

Figure 9 Development of the vitreous. The vascular tissue of the primary vitreous is first apparent at 6 weeks (13 mm) and continues to grow for a further 3 weeks until it involutes and is replaced by the connective tissue elements that form the secondary vitreous. The development of the tertiary vitreous starts at about 12 weeks (65 mm).

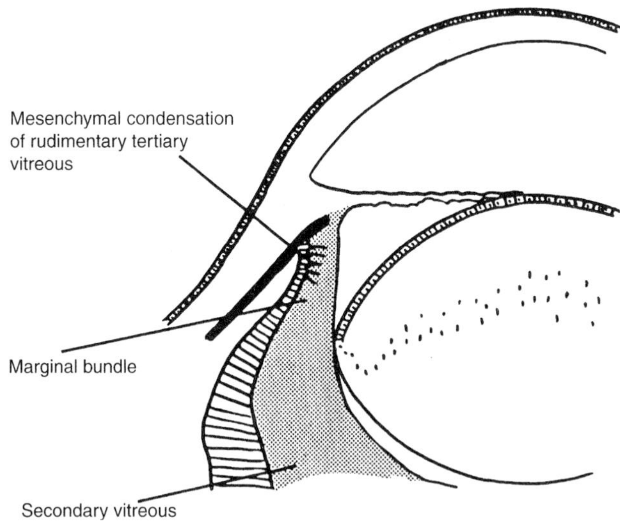

Figure 10 Formation of the tertiary vitreous. At 12 weeks of gestation (65 mm) condensations of mesenchyme at the rim of the optic cup extend towards the lens. Initially these fibrillar deposits run through the margins of the secondary vitreous.

ptosis and epicanthus inversus syndrome (BPES, MIM #110100) (35,45) (see Chapter 52). Heparin-binding EGF-like growth factor (HB-EGF) is a member of the EGF family of growth factors that binds to and activates the EGFR and may also be involved in eyelid closure and separation (58).

The eyelashes are first seen at 9 weeks (40 mm) as epithelial buds extending into the mesenchyme, with the upper eyelid cilia forming in two rows.

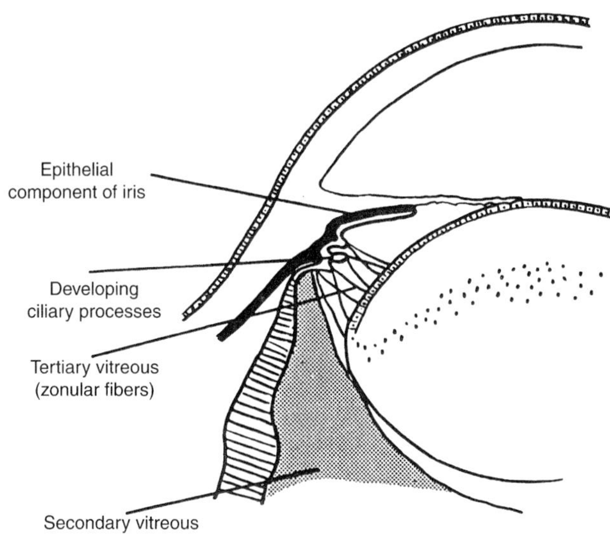

Figure 11 Formation of the lens zonular fibers. During month 4 of gestation, the fibers of the tertiary vitreous become separate from the secondary vitreous, which is subsequently resorbed in their vicinity. Before its involution this annular region of the vitreous is known as the marginal bundle of Drualt.

The Meibomian glands and the apocrine glands of Moll appear at 13 weeks (80 mm) and the glands of Zeis at 14 to 15 weeks (90–100 mm). Lipid production begins shortly thereafter. The tarsus forms from the condensation of basal laminae around the developing glands, with incorporation of adjacent collagen.

The development of the orbit is dependent on the formation of the optic cup. Endochondral ossification of the lesser wing of the sphenoid in the base of the skull is accompanied by membranous ossification of the greater wing and the other orbital bones at 6 months of gestation, with fusion approximately 1 month later. The cartilaginous model of the lesser wing is derived from non-neural crest mesenchyme, whereas the other bones are formed when neural crest mesenchymal cells become osteoblasts and interact with ECM to form osteoid (109). The maxillary process forms the floor and lateral wall of the orbit, as well as the nasal, lacrimal, and ethmoid bones. The ethmoid bone is the first membranous bone formed, at 6 to 8 weeks of gestation. Ossification is not complete at birth and the angle between the orbital axes slowly decreases throughout gestation, from almost 180° to 71° at birth. The adult angle is 68° and this reorientation reflects the accumulation of soft tissue behind and lateral to the globe (188). The continued growth of the orbit after birth is dependent on the presence and normal growth of the globe and the shape of the orbit becomes more conical as the globe matures. Growth of the eye ceases at approximately 3 years of age but the orbit continues to grow with the rest of the facial bones until the final stages of puberty.

The soft tissue of the orbit that protects the globe includes fat and fibrous septa, both of neural crest origin. In the fetus the fat cells are of the primitive brown cell type with a characteristic polygonal shape and prominent nucleus. The extraocular muscles were assumed to be derived from pre-chordal (medial, inferior and superior recti, and inferior oblique muscles) and paraxial (lateral rectus and superior oblique) mesoderm around 5 to 6 weeks of gestation (80), although Sevel (217) has suggested that the development of the extraocular muscle is a result of differentiation within the orbital (neural crest-derived) connective tissues. He contends that there is no ingrowth of mesodermal muscle precursors but that all muscles develop contemporaneously through a sequence of myoblastic induction from mesenchyme into recognizable myotubular elements.

The lacrimal gland appears at 7 weeks (25 mm) as a bud from the conjunctiva in the temporal upper fornix. As this grows, the tendon of the levator palpebrae superioris separates a palpebral lobe from the bulk of the orbital gland. The gland continues to grow for 3 to 4 years after birth and lymphocytic aggregates appear in the interstitium with age.

ACKNOWLEDGMENTS

Portions of this chapter contain material originally presented in the corresponding chapters of the first (Dr. Joan Mullaney) and second (Dr. Alison McCartney) editions.

REFERENCES

1. Addison PK, Berry V, Ionides AC, et al. Posterior polar cataract is the predominant consequence of a recurrent mutation in the *PITX3* gene. Br J Ophthalmol 2005; 89: 138–41.
2. Akagi T, Inoue T, Miyoshi G, et al. Requirement of multiple basic helix-loop-helix genes for retinal neuronal subtype specification. J Biol Chem 2004; 279:28492–8.
3. Andersen H, Ehlers N, Matthiessen ME. Histochemistry and development of the human eyelids. Acta Ophthalmol (Copenh) 1965; 45:642–68.
4. Andersen H, Ehlers N, Matthiessen ME. Histochemistry and development of the human eyelids II. Acta Ophthalmol (Copenh) 1967; 47:288–93.
5. Arendt D, Tessmar-Raible K, Snyman H, et al. Ciliary photoreceptors with a vertebrate-type opsin in an invertebrate brain. Science 2004; 306:869–71.
6. Ashery-Padan R, Gruss P. Pax6 lights-up the way for eye development. Curr Opin Cell Biol 2001; 13:706–14.
7. Ashton N. Retinal angiogenesis in the human embryo. Br Med Bull 1970; 26:103–6.
8. Azuma N, Hida T, Akiya S, et al. Histochemical studies on hyaluronic acid in the developing retina. Graefe's Arch Clin Exp Ophthalmol 1990; 228:158–60.
9. Bailey TJ, El-Hodiri H, Zhang L, et al. Regulation of vertebrate eye development by *Rx* genes. Int J Dev Biol 2004; 48:761–70.
10. Balazs EA, Toth LZ, Ozanics V. Cytological studies on the developing vitreous as related to the hyaloid vessel system. Graefe's Arch Clin Exp Ophthalmol 1980; 213: 71–85.
11. Baulmann DC, Ohlmann A, Flugel-Koch c, et al. Pax6 heterozygous eyes show defects in chamber angle differentiation that are associated with a wide spectrum of other anterior eye segment abnormalities. Mech Dev 2002; 118:3–17.
12. Bee JA. Development and pattern of innervation of the avian cornea. Dev Biol 1982; 92:5–15.
13. Beebe D, Garcia C, Wang X, et al. Contributions by members of the TGFbeta superfamily to lens development. Int J Dev Biol 2004; 48:845–56.
14. Belecky-Adams T, Tomarev S, Li HS, et al. Pax-6, Prox1 and Chx1-homeobox gene expression correlates with phenotypic fate of retinal precursor cells. Invest Ophthalmol Vis Sci 1997; 38:1293–303.
15. Bertuzzi S, Hindges R, Mui SH, et al. The homeodomain protein Vax1 is required for axon guidance and major tract formation in the developing forebrain. Genes Dev 1999; 13:3092–105.
16. Blixt A., Mahlapuu M, Aitola M, et al. A forkhead gene, FoxE3, is essential for lens epithelial proliferation and closure of the lens vesicle. Genes Dev 2000; 14:245–54.
17. Bordogna W, Hudson JD, Buddle J, et al. EMX homeobox genes regulate microphthalmia and alter melanocyte biology. Exp Eye Res 2005; 311:27–38.
18. Bovolenta P, Mallamaci A, Briata P, et al. Implication of OTX2 in pigment epithelium determination and neural retina differentiation. J Neurosci 1997; 17:4243–52.
19. Brown AS, Leamen L, Cucevic V, et al. Quantitation of hemodynamic function during developmental vascular regression in the mouse eye. Invest Ophthalmol Vis Sci 2005; 46:2231–7.
20. Brown NL, Patel S, Brzezinski J, et al. Math5 is required for retinal ganglion cell and optic nerve formation. Development 2001; 128:2497–508.
21. Brownell I, Dirksen M, Jamrich M. Forkhead Foxe3 maps to the dysgenetic lens locus and is critical in lens development and differentiation. Genesis 2000; 27:81–93.
22. Bumsted K, Jasoni C, Szel A, et al. Spatial and temporal expression of cone opsins during monkey retinal development. J Comp Neurol 1997; 378:117–34.
23. Celli G, LaRochelle WJ, Mackem S, et al. Soluble dominant-negative receptor uncovers essential roles for fibroblast growth factors in multi-organ induction and patterning. EMBO J 1998; 17:1642–55.
24. Cepko CL. The roles of intrinsic and extrinsic cues and bHLH genes in the determination of retinal cell fate. Curr Opin Neurobiol 1999; 9:37–46.
25. Chan-Ling T, McLeod DS, Hughes S, et al. Astrocyte-endothelial cell relationships during human retinal vascular development. Invest Ophthalmol Vis Sci 2004; 45:2020–32.
26. Chen Y, Stump RJW, Lovicu FJ, et al. Expression of Frizzleds and secreted frizzled-related proteins (Sfrps) during mammalian lens development. Int J Dev Biol 2004; 48:867–77.
27. Chiang C, Litingtung Y, Lee E, et al. Cyclopia and defective axial patterning in mice lacking Sonic hedgehog gene function. Nature 1996; 383:407–13.
28. Chow R.L., Altmann CR, Lang RA, et al. Pax6 induces ectopic eyes in a vertebrate. Development 1999; 126: 4213–22.
29. Chow RL, Lang RA. Early eye development in vertebrates. Annu Rev Cell Dev Biol 2001; 17:255–96.
30. Chuang JC, Raymond PA. Embryonic origin of the eyes in teleost fish. BioEssays 2002; 24:519–29.
31. Collinson JM, Chanas SA, Hill RE, et al. Corneal development, limbal stem cell function, and corneal epithelial cell migration in the Pax6C/K mouse. Invest Ophthalmol Vis Sci 2004; 45:1101–8.
32. Collinson JM, Hill RE, West JD. Different roles for Pax6 in the optic vesicle and facial epithelium mediate early morphogenesis of the murine eye. Development 1996; 127:945–56.
33. Collinson JM, Quinn JC, Hill RE, et al. The roles of Pax6 in the cornea, retina, and olfactory epithelium of the developing mouse embryo. Dev Biol 2003; 255:303–12.
34. Coulombre AJ, Coulombre JL. Lens development. I. Role of the lens in eye growth. J Exp Zool 1964; 156:39–48.
35. Crisponi L, Deiana M, Loi A, et al. The putative forkhead transcription factor FOXL2 is mutated in blepharophimosis/ptosis/epicanthus inversus syndrome. Nat Genet 2001; 27:159–66.
36. Curatola AM, Moscatelli D, Norris A, et al. Retinal blood vessels develop in response to local VEGF-A signals in the absence of blood flow. Exp Eye Res 2005; 81:147–58.
37. Curcio CA, Allen KA. Topography of ganglion cells in human retina. J Comp Neurol 1990; 300:5–25.
38. Curcio CA, Hendrickson A. Organisation and development of the primate photoreceptor mosaic. In: Osborne

NN, Chader GJ, eds. Progress in Retinal Research. Vol. 10. Oxford: Pergamon Press, 1990:90–120.
39. Cuthbertson RA, Lang RA. Developmental ocular disease in GM-CSF transgenic mice is mediated by autostimulated macrophages. Dev Biol 1989; 134:119–29.
40. Cvekl A, Tamm ER. Anterior eye development and ocular mesenchyme: new insights from mouse models and human disease. BioEssays 2004; 26:374–86.
41. Davis J, Duncan MK, Robison Jr WG, et al. Requirement for Pax6 in corneal morphogenesis: a role in adhesion. J Cell Sci 2003; 116:2157–67.
42. Davis RJ, Shen W, Sandler YI, et al. Dach1 mutant mice bear no gross abnormalities in eye, limb, and brain development and exhibit postnatal lethality. Mol Cell Biol 2001; 21:1484–90.
43. Davis RJ, Tavsanli BC, Dittrich C, et al. *Drosophila* retinal homeobox (drx) is not required for brain and cypeus development. Dev Biol 2003; 259:272–87.
44. Davis-Silberman N, Kalich T, Oron-Karni V, et al. Genetic dissection of Pax6 dosage requirements in the developing mouse eye. Hum Mol Genet 2005; 14:2265–76.
45. De Baere E, Dixon MJ, Small KW, et al. Spectrum of FOXL2 gene mutations in blepharophimosis-ptosis-epicanthus inversus (BPES) families demonstrates a genotype–phenotype correlation. Hum Mol Genet 2001; 10:1591–600.
46. De Moerlooze L, Spencer-Dene B, Revest J, et al. An important role for the IIIb isoform of fibroblast growth factor receptor 2 (FGFR2) in mesenchymal-epithelial signalling during mouse organogenesis. Development 2000; 127:483–92.
47. De Vries C, Escobedo JA, Ueno H, et al. The fms-like tyrosine kinase, a receptor for vascular endothelial growth factor. Science 1992; 255:989–91.
48. Deng KY, Winfrey V, Gould DB, et al. The forkhead/winged helix gene Mf1 is disrupted in the pleotropic mouse mutation congenital hydrocephalus. Cell 1998; 93: 985–96.
49. Dimanlig PV, Faber SC, Auerbach W, et al. The upstream ectoderm enhancer in Pax6 has an important role in lens induction. Development 2001; 128:4415–24.
50. Ding K, Scortegagna M, Seaman R, et al. Retinal disease in mice lacking hypoxia-inducible transcription factor-2±. Invest Ophthalmol Vis Sci 2005; 46:1010–6.
51. Donner AL, Maas RL. Conservation and non-conservation of genetic pathways in eye specification. Int J Dev Biol 2004; 48:743–53.
52. Drager UC. Calcium binding in pigmented and albino eyes. Proc Natl Acad Sci U S A 1985; 82:6716–20.
53. Dudley AT, Robertson EJ. Overlapping expression domains of bone morphogenetic protein family members potentially account for limited tissue defects in BMP7 deficient embryos. Dev Dyn 1997; 208:349–62.
54. Duke-Elder S. Normal and abnormal development, Part 1. System of Ophthalmology. Vol. 3. London: Kimpton, 1964: 1–312.
55. Duncan MK, Cui W, Oh DJ, et al. Prox1 is differentially localized during lens development. Mech Dev 2002; 112: 195–8.
56. Dyer MA. Regulation of proliferation, cell fate specification and differentiation by the homeodomain proteins Prox1, Six3 and Chx10 in the developing retina. Cell Cycle 2003; 2:350–7.
57. Ekker SC, Ungar AR, Greenstein P, et al. Patterning activities of vertebrate hedgehog proteins in the developing eye and brain. Curr Biol 1995; 5:944–55.
58. Elenius K, Paul S, Allison G, et al. Activation of HER4 by heparin-binding EGF-like growth factor stimulates chemotaxis but not proliferation. EMBO J 1997; 16:1268–78.
59. Endo H, Hu F. Pigment cell development in rhesus monkey eyes: an electron microscopic and histochemical study. Dev Biol 1973; 32:69–81.
60. Engerman RL. Development of macular circulation. Invest Ophthalmol Vis Sci 1976; 15:835–843.
61. Erkman L, Yates PA, McLaughlin T, et al. A POU domain transcription factor-dependent program regulates axon pathfinding in the vertebrate visual system. Neuron 2000; 28:779–92.
62. Evans AL, Gage PJ. Expression of the homeobox gene Pitx2 in neural crest is required for optic stalk and ocular anterior segment development. Hum Mol Genet 2005; 14:3347–59.
63. Feijen A, Goumans MJ, van den Eijnden-van Raaij AJ. Expression of activin subunits, activin receptors and follistatin in postimplantation mouse embryos suggests specific developmental functions for different activins. Development 1994; 120:3621–37.
64. Finkelstein R, Boncinelli E. From fly head to mammalian forebrain: the story of otd and Otx. Trends Genet 1994; 10: 310–5.
65. Fisher RF, Pettet BE. The postnatal growth of the capsule of the human lens. J Anat (Lond) 1972; 112:207–14.
66. Fossat N, Courtois V, Chatelain G, et al. Alternative usage of Otx2 promoters during development. Dev Dyn 2005; 233:154–60.
67. Freund C, Horsford DJ, McInnes RR. Transcription factor genes and the developing eye: a genetic perspective. Hum Mol Genet 1996; 5:1471–88.
68. Fruttiger M. Development of the mouse retinal vasculature: angiogenesis versus vasculogenesis. Invest Ophthalmol Vis Sci 2002; 43:522–7.
69. Fuhrmann S, Levine EM, Reh TA. Extraocular mesenchyme patterns the optic vesicle during early eye development in the embryonic chick. Development 2000; 127: 4599–609.
70. Fujiwara M, Uchida T, Osumi-Yamashita N, et al. Uchida rat (rSey): a new mutant rat with craniofacial abnormalities resembling those of the mouse Sey mutant. Differentiation 1994; 57:31–8.
71. Fulton AB, Albert DM, Craft JL. Human albinism. Light and electron microscopic study. Arch Ophthalmol 1978; 96:305–10.
72. Gage PJ, Rhoades W, Prucka SK et al. Fate maps of neural crest and mesoderm in the mammalian eye. Invest Ophthalmol Vis Sci 2005; 46:4200–8.
73. Gage PJ, Suh H, Camper SA. Dosage requirement of Pitx2 for development of multiple organs. Development 1999; 126:4643–51.
74. Galy A, Neron B, Planque N, et al. Activated MAPK/ERK kinase (MEK-1) induces transdifferentiation of pigmented epithelium into neural retina. Dev Biol 2002; 248:251–64.
75. Gan L, Wang SW, Huang Z, et al. POU domain factor Brn-3b is essential for retinal ganglion cell differentiation and survival but not for initial cell fate specification. Dev Biol 1999; 210:469–80.
76. Gariano RF, Hu D, Helms J. Expression of angiogenesis-related genes during retinal development. Gene Expr Patterns 2006; 6:187–92.
77. Gehring WJ, Ikeo K. Pax6: mastering eye morphogenesis and eye evolution. Trends Genet 1999; 15:371–7.
78. Gehring WJ. The genetic control of eye development and its implications for the evolution of the various eye-types. Int J Dev Biol 2002; 46:65–73.

79. Genis-Galvez JM. Role of the lens in morphogenesis of the iris and cornea. Nature 1966; 210:209–10.
80. Gilbert PW. The origin and development of the human extrinsic ocular muscles. Contrib Embryol 1957; 246: 59–78.
81. Gilbert SF. Developmental Biology. 3rd ed. Sunderland, MA: Sinauer Associates, 1991:176–661.
82. Glaser T, Jepeal L, Edwards JG, et al. PAX6 gene dosage effect in a family with congenital cataracts, aniridia, anophthalmia and central nervous system defects. Nat Genet 1994; 7:463–71.
83. Goding CR. Mitf from neural crest to melanoma: signal transduction and transcription in the melanocyte lineage. Genes Dev 2000; 14:1712–28.
84. Gogat K, Le Gat L, Van Den Berghe L, et al. VEGF and KDR gene expression during human embryonic and fetal eye development. Invest Ophthalmol Vis Sci 2004; 45:7–14.
85. Goudreau G, Petrou P, Reneker LW, et al. Mutually regulated expression of Pax6 and Six3 and its implications for the Pax6 haploinsufficient lens phenotype. Proc Natl Acad Sci U S A 2002; 99:8719–24.
86. Gould DB, Smith RS, John SWM. Anterior segment development relevant to glaucoma. Int J Dev Biol 2004; 48:1015–29.
87. Grainger RM, Henry JJ, Saha MS, et al. Recent progress on the mechanisms of embryonic lens formation. Eye 1992; 6: 117–22.
88. Grindley JC, Davidson DR, Hill RE. The role of Pax-6 in eye and nasal development. Development 1995; 121:1433–42.
89. Hadorn E. Developmental Genetics and Lethal Factors. New York: Wiley, 1961.
90. Hagstrom SA, Pauer GJT, Reid J, et al. SOX2 mutation causes anophthalmia, hearing loss, and brain anomalies. Am J Med Genet 2005; 138A:95–8.
91. Halder G, Callaerts P, Gehring WJ. Induction of ectopic eyes by targeted expression of the eyeless gene in *Drosophila*. Science 1995; 267:1788–92.
92. Halfter W, Dong S, Schurer B, et al. Embryonic synthesis of the inner limiting membrane and vitreous body. Invest Ophthalmol Vis Sci 2005; 46:2202–9.
93. Hall BK. The embryonic development of bone. Am Sci 1988; 76:174–81.
94. Hanson IM, Fletcher JM, Jordan T, et al. Mutations at the PAX6 locus are found in heterogeneous anterior segment malformations including Peters' anomaly. Nat Genet 1994; 6:168–73.
95. Hasan MR, Kunio Y. Lens differentiation and crystallin regulation: a chick model. Int J Dev Biol 2004; 48:805–17.
96. Hatakeyama J, Kageyama R. Retinal cell fate determination and bHLH factors. Semin Cell Dev Biol 2004; 15: 39–83.
97. Hatakeyama J, Tomita K, Inoue T, et al. Roles of homeobox and bHLH genes in specification of a retinal cell type. Development 2001; 128:1313–22.
98. Hay ED, Linsenmayer TF, Trelstad RL, et al. Origins and distribution of collagens in the developing avian cornea. Curr Top Eye Res 1982; 1:1–35.
99. Hay ED. Development of the vertebrate cornea. Int Rev Cytol 1980; 63:263–322.
100. Heimann K, Terheggen G. Uber das Vorkommen von choroidalen Blutbildungsherden bei Embryonne and Feten. Ber Zusammenkunft Dtsch Ophthalmol Ges 1969; 70:467–72.
101. Hendrickson A, Kupfer C. The histogenesis of the fovea in the macaque monkey. Invest Ophthalmol Vis Sci 1976; 15:746–56.
102. Hendrickson A, Yuodelis C. The morphological development of the human fovea. Ophthalmology 1984; 91: 603–12.
103. Hendrickson A. A morphological comparison of foveal development in man and monkey. Eye 1992; 6:136–42.
104. Henkind P, Bellhorn RW, Murphy ME, et al. Development of macular vessels in monkey and cat. Br J Ophthalmol 1975; 59:703–9.
105. Hilfer SR, Yang J-JW. Accumulation of CPC-precipitable material at apical cell surfaces during formation of the optic cup. Anat Rec 1980; 197:423–33.
106. Hill RE, Favor J, Hogan BL, et al. Mouse small eye results from mutations in a paired-like homeobox-containing gene. Nature 1991; 354:522–5.
107. Hinds JW, Hinds PL. Development of retinal amacrine cells in the mouse embryo: evidence for two modes of formation. J Comp Neurol 1983; 213:1–23.
108. Hong HK, Lass JH, Chakravarti A. Pleiotropic skeletal and ocular phenotypes of the mouse mutation congenital hydrocephalus (ch/Mf1) arise from a helix/forkhead transcription factor gene. Hum Mol Genet 1999; 8:625–37.
109. Horton WA. The biology of bone growth. Growth Genet Horm 1990; 6:1–3.
110. Hutcheson DA, Vetter ML. The bHLH factors Xath5 and XNeuroD can upregulate the expression of XBrn3d, a POU-homeodomain transcription factor. Dev Biol 2001; 232:327–38.
111. Hyer J, Kuhlman J, Afif E, et al. Optic cup morphogenesis requires pre-lens ectoderm but not lens differentiation. Dev Biol 2003; 259:351–63.
112. Inoue T, Hojo M, Bessho Y, et al. Math3 and NeuroD regulate amacrine cell fate specification in the retina. Development 2002; 129:831–42.
113. Jaakkola P, Mole DR, Tian Y-M, et al. Targeting of HIF-± to the von Hippel-Lindau ubiquitylation complex by O_2-regulated prolyl hydroxylation. Science 2001; 292: 468–72.
114. Jamieson RV, Perveen R, Kerr B, et al. Domain disruption and mutation of the bZIP transcription factor, MAF, associated with cataract, ocular anterior segment dysgenesis and coloboma. Hum Mol Genet 2002; 11:33–42.
115. Jamieson, RV, Munier F, Balmer A, et al. Pulverulent cataract with variably associated microcornea and iris coloboma in a MAF mutation family. Br J Ophthalmol 2003; 87:411–2.
116. Jin EJ, Burrus LW, Erickson CA. The expression patterns of Wnts and their antagonists during avian eye development. Mech Dev 2002; 116:173–6.
117. Johnson DH, Bourne WM, Campbell RJ. The ultrastructure of Descemet's membrane. I. Changes with age in normal corneas. Arch Ophthalmol 1982; 100:1942–7.
118. Johnston MC, Morriss GM, Kushner DC, et al. Abnormal organogenesis of facial structures. In: Wilson JG, Frazer FC, eds. Handbook of Teratology. Vol. 2. New York: Plenum Press, 1977:421–51.
119. Johnston MC, Noden DM, Hazelton RD, et al. Origins of avian ocular and periocular tissues. Exp Eye Res 1979; 29: 27–43.
120. Kamachi Y, Sockanathan S, Liu Q, et al. Involvement of SOX proteins in lens-specific activation of crystallin genes. EMBO J 1995; 14:3510–9.
121. Kamachi Y, Uchikawa M, Collignon J, et al. Involvement of Sox1, 2 and 3 in the early and subsequent molecular events of lens induction. Development 1998; 125:2521–32.
122. Kastschenko N. Zur Entwicklungsgeschichte der Selachierembryos. Anat Anz 1888; 3:445–67.

123. Kay JN, Finger-Baier KC, Roeser T, et al. Retinal ganglion cell genesis requires lakritz, a zebrafish atonal homolog. Neuron 2001; 30:725–36.
124. Keyt BA, Berleau LT, Nguyen HV, et al. The carboxyl-terminal domain [111–165] of vascular endothelial growth factor is critical for its mitogenic potency. J Biol Chem 1996; 271:7788–95.
125. Khosrowshahian F, Wolanski M, Chang WY, et al. Lens and retina formation require expression of Pitx3 in Xenopus pre-lens ectoderm Dev Dyn 2005; 234:577–89.
126. Kidson SH, Kume T, Deng K, et al. The forkhead/winged-helix gene, Mf1, is necessary for the normal development of the cornea and formation of the anterior chamber in the mouse eye. Dev Biol 1999; 211:306–22.
127. Kimura A, Singh D, Wawrousek EF, et al. Both PCE-1/RX and OTX/CRX interactions are necessary for photoreceptor-specific gene expression. J Biol Chem 2000; 275:1152–60.
128. Klagsbrun M, D'Amore PA. Vascular endothelial growth factor and its receptors. Cytokine Growth Factor Rev 1996; 7:259–70.
129. Kondoh H, Uchikawa M, Kamachi Y. Interplay of Pax6 and SOX2 in lens development as a paradigm of genetic switch mechanisms for cell differentiation. Int J Dev Biol 2004; 48:819–27.
130. Koroma BM, Yang JM, Sundin OH. The Pax-6 homeobox gene is expressed throughout the corneal and conjunctival epithelia. Invest Ophthalmol Vis Sci 1997; 38:108–20.
131. Kozmik Z. Pax genes in eye development and evolution. Curr Opin Genet Dev 2005; 13:430–8.
132. Kumar J, Moses K. Transcription factors in eye development: a gorgeous mosaic? Genes Dev 1997; 11:2023–8.
133. Kutty RK, Kutty G, Hooks JJ, et al. Transforming growth factor-beta inhibits the cytokine-mediated expression of the inducible nitric oxide synthase mRNA in human retinal pigment epithelial cells. Biochem Biophys Res Commun 1995; 215:386–93.
134. Kuwabara T. The maturation of lens cells: a morphological study. Exp Eye Res 1975; 20:427–43.
135. Land MF, Nilsson D-E. *Animal Eyes*. New York: Oxford University Press, 2002.
136. Lang RA. Pathways regulating lens induction in the mouse. Int J Dev Biol 2004; 48:783–91.
137. Laties AM. Ocular melanin and the adrenergic innervation to the eye. Trans Am Ophthalmol Soc 1974; 72: 560–605.
138. Le Douarin NM, Cochard P, Vincent M, et al. Nuclear, cytoplasmic and membrane markers to follow neural crest migration. In: Trelstad RL, ed. The Role of the Extracellular Matrix in Development. New York: Alan R Liss, 1984:373–98.
139. Le Douarin NM. The Neural Crest. Cambridge: University Press 1982.
140. Le Lievre CS, Le Douarin NM. Mesenchymal derivatives of the neural crest: analysis of chimaeric quail and chick embryos. J Embryol Exp Morphol 1975; 34:125–54.
141. Lerche W, Wuelle K-G. Electron microscopic studies on the development of the human lens. Ophthalmologica 1969; 158:296–309.
142. Lerche W, Wuelle K-G. Zur Feinstruktur des embryonalen menschlichen Glaskorpers unter besonder Berucksichtigung seiner Beziehung zu Linse und Retina. Ber Zusammenkunft Dtsch Ophthalmol Ges 1967; 68:82–97.
143. Li H, Tierney C, Wen L, et al. A single morphogenic field gives rise to two retina primordia under the influence of the prechordal plate. Development 1997; 124:603–15.
144. Lin CR, Kioussi C, O'Connell S, et al. Pitx2 regulates lung asymmetry, cardiac positioning and pituitary and tooth morphogenesis. Nature 1999; 401:279–82.
145. Liu H, Mohamed O, Dufort D, et al. Characterization of Wnt signalling components and activation of the Wnt canonical pathway in the murine retina. Dev Dyn 2003; 227:323–34.
146. Lovicu FJ, McAvoy LW. Growth factor regulation of lens development. Dev Biol 2005; 280:1–14.
147. Lu MF, Pressman C, Dyer R, et al. Function of Rieger syndrome gene in left-right asymmetry and craniofacial development. Nature 1999; 401:276–78.
148. Luetteke NC, Qiu TH, Peiffer RL, et al. TGF alpha deficiency results in hair follicle and eye abnormalities in targeted and waved-1 mice. Cell 1993; 73:263–78.
149. Lyon MF, Jamieson RV, Perveen R, et al. A dominant mutation within the DNA-binding domain of the bZIP transcription factor Maf causes murine cataract and results in selective alteration in DNA binding. Hum Mol Genet 2003; 12:585–94.
150. Macdonald R, Barth KA, Xu Q, et al. Midline signalling is required for Pax gene regulation and patterning of the eyes. Development 1995; 121:3267–78.
151. Mann I. The Development of the Human Eye. 2nd ed. London: British Medical Association, 1949:1–312.
152. Mardon G, Solomon NM, Rubin GM. *dachshund* encodes a nuclear protein required for normal eye and leg development in *Drosophila*. Development 1994; 120:3473–86.
153. Marneros AG, Fan J, Yokoyama Y, et al. Vascular endothelial growth factor expression in the retinal pigment epithelium is essential for choriocapillaris development and visual function. Am J Pathol 2005; 167:1451–9.
154. Marquardt T, Ashery-Padan R, Andrejewski N, et al. Pax6 is required for the multipotent state of retinal progenitor cells. Cell 2001; 105:43–55.
155. Marti E, Bovolenta P. Sonic hedgehog in CNS development: one signal, multiple outputs. Trends Neurosci 2002; 25:89–96.
156. Martinez-Morales JR, Dolez V, Rodrigo I, et al. OTX2 activates the molecular network underlying retinal pigment epithelium differentiation. J Biol Chem 2003; 278:21721–31.
157. Martinez-Morales JR, Rodrigo I, Bovolenta P. Eye development: a view from the retina pigmented epithelium. BioEssays 2004; 26:766–77.
158. Martinez-Morales JR, Signore M, Acampora D, et al. Otx genes are required for tissue specification in the developing eye. Development 2001; 128:2019–30.
159. Mathers PH, Grinberg A, Mahon KA, et al. The Rx homeobox gene is essential for vertebrate eye development. Nature 1997; 387:603–7.
160. Matter-Sadzinski L, Puzianowska-Kuznicka M, Hernandez J. A bHLH transcriptional network regulating the specification of retinal ganglion cells. Development 2005; 132:3907–21.
161. Maurus D, Heligon C, Burger-Schwarzler A, et al. Noncanonical Wnt-4 signaling and EAF2 required for eye development in *Xenopus laevis*. EMBO J 2005; 24: 1181–91.
162. McAvoy JW, Chamberlain CG, De Iongh RU, et al. The role of fibroblast growth factor in eye lens development. Ann N Y Acad Sci 1991; 638:256–74.
163. McCartney ACE, Bull TB, Spalton DJ. Fuchs' heterochromic cyclitis: an electron microscopic study. Trans Ophthalmol Soc UK 1985; 116:324–9.

164. McMenamin PG. A morphological study of the inner surface of the anterior chamber angle in pre and postnatal eyes. Curr Eye Res 1989; 8:727–39.
165. Mears AJ, Jordan T, Mirzayans F, et al. Mutations of the forkhead/winged-helix gene, FKHL7, in patients with Axenfeld-Rieger anomaly. Am J Hum Genet 1998; 63: 1316–28.
166. Meier S. Initiation of corneal differentiation prior to cornea-lens association. Cell Tissue Res 1977; 184:255–67.
167. Michaelson I. The mode of development of the vascular system of the retina with some observations on its significance for certain retinal diseases. Trans Ophthalmol Soc UK 1948; 68:137–80.
168. Miettinen PJ, Berger JE, Meneses J, et al. Epithelial immaturity and multiorgan failure in mice lacking epidermal growth factor receptor. Nature 1995; 376: 337–41.
169. Morgan TH. Embryology and Genetics. New York: Columbia University Press, 1934.
170. Morriss-Kay GM. Growth and development of pattern in the cranial neuroepithelium of rat embryos during neurulation. J Embryol Exp Morphol (Suppl) 1981; 65: 225–41.
171. Mueller F, O'Rahilly R. The development of the human brain, the closure of the caudal neuropore, and the beginning of secondary neurulation at stage 12. Anat Embryol 1987; 176:413–30.
172. Mui SH, Hindges R, O'Leary DDM, et al. The homeodomain protein Vax2 patterns the dorsoventral and nasotemporal axes of the eye. Development 2002; 129: 797–804.
173. Mui SH, Kim JW, Lemke G, et al. *Vax* genes ventralize the embryonic eye. Genes Dev 2005; 19:1249–59.
174. Murakami D, Sesma MA, Rowe MH. Characteristics of nasal and temporal retina in Siamese and normally pigmented cats. Brain Behav Evol 1982; 21:67–113.
175. Murphy C, Alvarado A, Juster R. Prenatal and postnatal growth of human Descemet's membrane. Invest Ophthalmol Vis Sci 1984; 25:1402–15.
176. Murphy C, Alvarado J, Juster R, et al. Prenatal and postnatal cellularity of the human corneal endothelium: a quantitative histologic study. Invest Ophthalmol Vis Sci 1984; 25:312–20.
177. Nagineni CN, Kutty V, Detrick B, et al. Expression of PDGF and their receptors in human retinal pigment cells and fibroblasts: regulation by TGFβ. J Cell Physiol 2005; 203:35–43.
178. Nagineni CN, Samuel W, Nagineni S, et al. Transforming growth factor-b induces expression of vascular endothelial growth factor in human retinal pigment epithelial cells: involvement of mitogen-activated protein kinases. J Cell Physiol 2003; 197:453–62.
179. Neufeld G, Cohen T, Gitay-Goren H, et al. Similarities and differences between the vascular endothelial growth factor (VEGF) splice variants. Cancer Metastasis Rev 1996; 15:153–8.
180. Nguyen M, Arnheiter H. Signaling and transcriptional regulation in early mammalian eye development: a link between FGF and MITF. Development 2000; 127:3581–91.
181. Noden DM. Origins and patterning of craniofacial mesenchymal tissues. J Craniofac Genet Dev Biol Suppl 1986; 2:15–32.
182. Nornes HO, Dressler GR, Knapik EW, et al. Spatially and temporally restricted expression of Pax2 during murine neurogenesis. Development 1990; 109:797–809.
183. O'Rahilly R. The prenatal development of the human eye. Exp Eye Res 1975; 21:91–112.
184. Ohkubo Y, Chiang C, Rubenstein JL. Coordinate regulation and synergistic actions of BMP4, SHH and FGF8 in the rostral prosencephalon regulate morphogenesis of the telencephalic and optic vesicles. Neuroscience 2002; 111: 1–17.
185. Ohlmann AV, Adamek E, Ohlmann A, et al. Norrie gene product is necessary for regression of hyaloid vessels. Invest Ophthalmol Vis Sci 2004; 45:2384–90.
186. Olver JM, McCartney ACE. Anterior segment casting. Eye 1989; 3:302–7.
187. Ozaki H, Okamoto N, Ortega S, et al. Basic fibroblast growth factor is neither necessary nor sufficient for the development of retinal neovascularization. Am J Pathol 1998; 153:757–65.
188. Ozanics V, Jakobiec FA. Prenatal development of the eye and its adnexae. In: Jakobiec FA, ed. Ocular Anatomy, Embryology and Teratology. Philadelphia: Harper and Row, 1982:11–96.
189. Perron M, Harris WA. Determination of vertebrate retina progenitor cell fate by the Notch pathway and basic helix-loop-helix transcription factors. Cell Mol Life Sci 2000; 52: 215–23.
190. Pevny LH, Lowell-Badge R. Sox genes find their feet. Curr Opin Genet Dev 1997; 7:338–44.
191. Piatigorsky J. Lens differentiation in vertebrates: a review of cellular and molecular features. Differentiation 1981; 19:134–53.
192. Pignoni F, Hu B, Zavitz KH, et al. The eye-specification proteins So and Eya form a complex and regulate multiples steps in *Drosophila* eye development. Cell 1997; 91:881–91.
193. Pittack C, Grunwald GB, Reh TA. Fibroblast growth factors are necessary for neural retina but not pigmented epithelium differentiation in chick embryos. Development 1997; 124:805–16.
194. Polley EH, Zimmerman RP, Fortney RL. Neurogenesis and maturation of cell morphology in the development of the mammalian retina. In: Finlay BL, Sengelaub DR, eds. *Development of the Vertebrate Retina*. New York: Plenum Press, 1989:3–42.
195. Poltorak Z, Cohen T, Sivan R, et al. VEGF145, a secreted vascular endothelial growth factor isoform that binds to extracellular matrix. J Biol Chem 1997; 272:7151–8.
196. Pressman CL, Chen H, Johnson, RL. LMX1B, a LIM homeodomain class transcription factor, is necessary for normal development of multiple tissues in the anterior segment of the murine eye. Genesis 2000; 26:15–25.
197. Provis JM, Leech J, Diaz CM, et al. Development of the human retinal vasculature: cellular relations and VEGF expression. Exp Eye Res 1997; 65:555–68.
198. Provis JM, van Driel D, Billson FA, et al. Development of the human retina: patterns of cell distribution and redistribution in the ganglion cell layer. J Comp Neurol 1985; 233:429–51.
199. Provis JM. Patterns of cell death in the ganglion cell layer of the human retina. J Comp Neurol 1987; 259: 237–46.
200. Quinn JC, West JD, Hill RE. Multiple functions for Pax6 in mouse eye and nasal development. Genes Dev 1996; 10: 435–46.
201. Ragge NK, Brown AG, Poloschek CM, et al. Heterozygous mutations of *OTX2* cause severe ocular malformations. Am J Hum Genet 2005; 76:1008–22.
202. Ramaesh T, Collinson JM, Ramaesh K, et al. Corneal abnormalities in Pax6C/K small eye mice mimic human aniridia-related keratopathy. Invest Ophthalmol Vis Sci 2003; 44:1871–8.

203. Ramaesh T, Ramaesh K, Collinson JM, et al. Developmental and cellular factors underlying corneal epithelial dysgenesis in the Pax6+/− mouse model of aniridia. Exp Eye Res 2005; 81:224–35.
204. Reza HM, Yasuda K. Roles of Maf family proteins in lens development. Dev Dyn 2004; 229:440–8.
205. Rieger DK, Reichenberger E, McLean W, et al. A double-deletion mutation in the Pitx3 gene causes arrested lens development in aphakia mice. Genomics 2001; 72:61–72.
206. Rosenthal R, Malek G, Salomon N, et al. The fibroblast growth factor receptors, FGFR-1 and FGFR-2, mediate two independent signalling pathways in human retinal pigment epithelial cells. Biochem Biophys Res Commun 2005; 337:241–7.
207. Saha M, Spann CL, Grainger RM. Embryonic lens induction: more than meets the optic vesicle. Cell Differ Dev 1989; 28:153–72.
208. Saint-Geniez M, D'Amore PA. Development and pathology of the hyaloid, choroidal and retinal vasculature. Int J Dev Biol 2004; 48:1045–58.
209. Samuel W, Nagineni CN, Kutty RK, et al. Transforming growth factor-beta regulates stearoyl coenzyme A desaturase expression through a SMAD signaling pathway. J Biol Chem 2002; 277:59–66.
210. Sellhayer K, Spitznas M. Morphology of the developing choroidal vasculature in the human fetus. Graefe's Arch Clin Exp Ophthalmol 1988; 226:461–7.
211. Sellhayer K. Development of the choroid and related structures. Eye 1990; 4:255–61.
212. Semina EV, Ferrell RE, Mintz-Hittner HA, et al. A novel homeobox gene PITX3 is mutated in families with autosomal-dominant cataracts and ASMD. Nat Genet 1998; 19:167–70.
213. Semina EV, Murray JC, Reiter R, et al. Deletion in the promoter region and altered expression of Pitx3 homeobox gene in aphakia mice. Hum Mol Genet 2000; 9: 1575–85.
214. Semina EV, Reiter R, Leysens NJ, et al. Cloning and characterization of a novel bicoid-related homeobox transcription factor gene, RIEG, involved in Rieger syndrome. Nat Genet 1996; 14:392–9.
215. Sevel D, Issacs R. A re-evaluation of corneal development. Trans Am Ophthalmol Soc 1988; 34:178–207.
216. Sevel D. A reappraisal of the development of the eyelids. Eye 1988; 2:123–9.
217. Sevel D. Reappraisal of the origin of human extraocular muscles. Ophthalmology 1988; 88:1330–8.
218. Shih SC, Ju M, Liu N, et al. Selective stimulation of VEGFR-1 prevents oxygen-induced retinal vascular degeneration in retinopathy of prematurity. J Clin Invest 2003; 112:50–7.
219. Shima DT, Kuroki M, Deutsch U, et al. The mouse gene for vascular endothelial growth factor. Genomic structure, definition of the transcriptional unit, and characterization of transcriptional and post-transcriptional regulatory sequences. J Biol Chem 1996; 271:3877–83.
220. Sigelman J, Ozanics V. Retina. In: Jakobiec FA, ed. Ocular Anatomy, Embryology and Teratology. Philadelphia: Harper and Row, 1982:441–506.
221. Silver PHS, Wakely J. The initial stage in the development of the lens capsule in chick and mouse embryo. Exp Eye Res 1974; 19:73–7.
222. Simeone A, Puelles E, Acampora D. The Otx family. Curr Opin Genet Dev 2002; 12:409–15.
223. Sivak JM, Mohan R, Rinehart WB, et al. Pax-6 expression and activity are induced in the reepithelializing cornea and control activity of the transcriptional promoter for matrix metalloproteinase gelatinase B. Dev Biol 2000; 222: 41–54.
224. Smelser GK. Embryology and morphology of the lens. Invest Ophthalmol Vis Sci 1965; 4:398–410.
225. Smidt MP, van Schaick HS, Lanctot C, et al. A homeodomain gene Ptx3 has highly restricted brain expression in mesencephalic dopaminergic neurons. Proc Natl Acad Sci U S A 1997; 94:13305–10.
226. Smith A, Miller L-A, Song N, et al. The duality of β-catenin function: a requirement in lens morphogenesis and signaling suppression of lens fate in periocular ectoderm. Dev Biol 2005; 285:477–89.
227. Smith, RS, Zabaleta A, Kume T, et al. Haploinsufficiency of the transcription factors FOXC1 and FOXC2 results in aberrant ocular development. Hum Mol Genet 2000; 9: 1021–32.
228. Spira AW, Hollenberg MJ. Human retinal development: ultrastructure of the inner retinal layers. Dev Biol 1973; 31:1–21.
229. Stalmans I, Ng YS, Rohan R, et al. Arteriolar and venular patterning in retinas of mice selectively expressing VEGF isoforms. J Clin Invest 2002; 109:327–36.
230. Steingrimsson E, Copeland NG, Jenkins NA. Melanocytes and the microphthalmia transcription factor network, Annu Rev Genet 2004; 38:365–411.
231. Stone RA, Ton LP, Iuvone M, et al. Postnatal control of ocular growth: dopaminergic mechanisms. In: Bock G, Widdows K, eds. Myopia and the Control of Eye Growth. Ciba Foundation Symposium 155. Chichester: John Wiley&Sons, 1990:5–62.
232. Stone, J, Itin A, Alon T, et al. Development of retinal vasculature is mediated by hypoxia-induced vascular endothelial growth factor (VEGF) expression by neuroglia. J Neurosci 1995; 15:4738–47.
233. Stump RJW, Ang S, Chen Y, et al. A role for Wnt/β-catenin signaling in lens epithelial differentiation. Dev Biol 2003; 259:48–61.
234. Tachibana M, Perez-Jurado LA, Nakayama A, et al. Cloning of MITF, the human homolog of the mouse microphthalmia gene and assignment to chromosome 3p14.1-p12.3. Hum Mol Genet 1994; 3:553–7.
235. Tahayato A, Sonneville R, Pichaud F, et al. Otd/Crx, a dual regulator for the specification of ommatidia subtypes in the *Drosophila* retina. Dev Cell 2003; 5:391–402.
236. Takeda K, Yasumoto K, Kawaguchi N, et al. Mitf-D, a newly identified isoform, expressed in the retinal pigment epithelium and monocyte-lineage cells affected by Mitf mutations. Biochim Biophys Acta 2002; 1574: 15–23.
237. Tao H, Shimizu M, Kusumoto O, et al. A dual role of FGF10 in proliferation and coordinated migration of epithelial leading edge cells during mouse eyelid development. Development 2005; 132:3217–39.
238. Terman BI, Dougher-Vermazen M, Carrion ME, et al. Identification of the KDR tyrosine kinase as a receptor for vascular endothelial cell growth factor. Biochem Biophys Res Commun 1992; 187:1579–86.
239. Thorogood P. Developmental and evolutionary aspects of the neural crest. Trends Neurosci 1989; 12:38–9.
240. Tomita K, Moriyoshi K, Nakanishi S, et al. Mammalian achaetescute and atonal homologs regulate neuronal versus glial fate determination in the central nervous system. EMBO J 2000; 19:5460–72.
241. Toy J, Norton JS, Jibodh SR, et al. Effects of homeobox genes on the differentiation of photoreceptor and non-photoreceptor neurons. Invest Ophthalmol Vis Sci 2002; 43:3522–9.

242. Trelstad RL. The bilaterally asymmetrical architecture of the submammalian corneal stroma resembles a cholesteric liquid crystal. Dev Biol 1982; 92:133–4.
243. Uda M, Ottolenghi C, Crisponi L, et al. Foxl2 disruption causes mouse ovarian failure by pervasive blockage of follicle development. Hum Mol Genet 2004; 13:1171–81.
244. Vassalli A, Matzuk MM, Gardner HA, et al. Activin/inhibin beta B subunit gene disruption leads to defects in eyelid development and female reproduction. Genes Dev 1994; 8:414–27.
245. Vetter ML, Brown, NL. The role of basic helix-loop-helix genes in vertebrate retinogenesis. Semin Cell Dev Biol 2001; 12:491–8.
246. Viczian AS, Vignali R, Zuber ME, et al. XOtx5b and XOtx2 regulate photoreceptor and bipolar fates in the Xenopus retina. Development 2003; 130:1281–94.
247. Vignali R, Colombetti S, Lupo G, et al. Xotx5b, a new member of the Otx gene family, may be involved in anterior and eye development in *Xenopus laevis*. Mech Dev 2000; 96:3–13.
248. Vogel-Hopker A, Momose T, Rohrer H, et al. Multiple functions of fibroblast growth factor-8 (FGF-8) in chick eye development. Mech Dev 2000; 94:25–36.
249. Wagner SN, Wagner C, Hofler H, et al. Expression cloning of the cDNA encoding a melanoma-associated Ag recognized by mAb HMB-45. Identification as melanocyte specific Pmel 17 cDNA. Lab Invest 1995; 73:229–35.
250. Walther C, Gruss P. Pax-6, a murine paired box gene, is expressed in the developing CNS. Development 1991; 113:1435–49.
251. Wang JC-C, Harris WA. The role of combinational coding by homeodomain and bHLH transcription factors in retinal cell fate specification. Dev Biol 2005; 285:101–15.
252. Wang SW, Kim BS, Ding K, et al. Requirement for math5 in the development of retinal ganglion cells. Genes Dev 2001; 15:24–9.
253. Wang SW, Mu X, Bowers WJ, et al. Brn3b/Brn3c double knockout mice reveal an unsuspected role for Brn3c in retinal ganglion cell axon outgrowth. Development 2002; 129:467–77.
254. Wang YP, Dakubo G, Howley P, et al. Development of normal retinal organization depends on Sonic hedgehog signaling from ganglion cells. Nat Neurosci 2002; 5:831–2.
255. Wawersik S, Purcell P, Rauchman M, et al. BMP7 acts in murine lens placode development. Dev Biol 1999; 207:176–88.
256. Webster EH, Silver AF, Gonsalves NI. The extracellular matrix between the optic vesicle and the presumptive lens during lens morphogenesis in an anophthalmic strain of mice. Dev Biol 1984; 103:142–150.
257. Webster MJ, Drager UC, Silver J. Development of the visual system in hypopigmented mutants. In: Finlay BL, Sengelaub DC, eds. New York: Plenum Press, 1989:69–86.
258. Wegner M. From head to toes: the multiple facets of Sox proteins. Nucleic Acids Res 1999; 27:1409–20.
259. Williams RW, Bastiani MJ, Lia B, et al. Growth cones, dying axons, and developmental fluctuations in the fiber population of the cat's optic nerve. J Comp Neurol 1986; 246:32–69.
260. Winnier GE, Hargett L, Hogan BL. The winged helix transcription factor MFH1 is required for proliferation and patterning of paraxial mesoderm in the mouse embryo. Genes Dev 1997; 11:926–40.
261. Wong K, Peng Y, Kung HF, et al. Retina dorsal/ventral patterning by Xenopus TBX3. Biochem Biophys Res Commun 2002; 290:737–42.
262. Wrenn JT, Wessels NK. An ultrastructural study of lens invagination in the mouse. J Exp Zool 1969; 171:359–67.
263. Wuelle K-G, Lerche W. Electron microscopic observations of the early development of the human corneal endothelium and Descemet's membrane. Ophthalmologica 1969; 157:451–61.
264. Wuelle K-G. Electron microscopy of the fetal development of the corneal endothelium and Descemet's membrane of the human eye. Invest Ophthalmol Vis Sci 1972; 11:897–904.
265. Yamada R, Mizutani-Koseki Y, Hasegawa T, et al. Cell-autonomous involvement of Mab21l1 is essential for lens placode development. Development 2003; 130:1759–70.
266. Yang Z, Ding K, Pan L, et al. Math5 determines the competence state of retinal ganglion cell progenitors. Dev Biol 2003; 264:240–54.
267. Yasumoto K, Takeda K, Saito H, et al. Microphthalmia-associated transcription factor interacts with LEF-1, a mediator of Wnt signaling. EMBO J 2002; 21:2703–14.
268. Yasumoto K, Yokoyama K, Shibata K et al. Microphthalmia-associated transcription factor as a regulator for melanocyte-specific transcription of the human tyrosinase gene. Mol Cell Biol 1994; 14:8058–70.
269. Yoshimoto A, Saigou Y, Higashi Y, et al. Regulation of ocular lens development by Smad-interacting protein 1 involving Foxe3 activation. Development 2005; 132:4437–48.
270. Young RW. Cell differentiation in the retina of the mouse. Anat Rec 1985; 212:199–205.
271. Young RW. The life history of retinal cells. Trans Am Ophthalmol Soc 1983; 81:193–228.
272. Zenz R, Scheuch H, Martin P, et al. c-Jun regulates eyelid closure and skin tumor development through EGFR signaling. Dev Cell 2003; 4:879–89.
273. Zhang L, Mathers PH, Jamrich M. Function of Rx, but not Pax6, is essential for the formation of retinal progenitor cells in mice. Genesis 2000; 28:135–42.
274. Zhang L, Wang W, Hayashi Y, et al. A role for MEK kinase1 in TGF-beta/activin-induced epithelium movement and embryonic eyelid closure. EMBO J 2003; 22:4443–54.
275. Zhao S, Hung FC, Colvin JS, et al. Patterning the optic neuroepithelium by FGF signaling and Ras activation. Development 2001; 128:5051–60.
276. Zhao S, Overbeek PA. Regulation of choroid development by retinal pigment epithelium. Mol Vis 2001; 7:277–82.
277. Zhao S, Overbeek PA. Tyrosinase-related protein 2 promoter targets transgene expression to ocular and neural crest-derived tissues. Dev Biol 1999; 216:154–63.
278. Zuber ME, Gestri G, Viczian AS, et al. Specification of the vertebrate eye by a network of eye field transcription factors. Development 2003; 130:5155–67.

52

Developmental Anomalies of the Eye

Johane M. Robitaille
Departments of Ophthalmology and Visual Sciences and Pathology, Dalhousie University, Halifax, Nova Scotia, Canada

Duane L. Guernsey
Departments of Pathology, Ophthalmology and Visual Sciences, Surgery, Physiology, and Biophysics, Dalhousie University, Halifax, Nova Scotia, Canada

J. Douglas Cameron
Department of Ophthalmology, Mayo Clinic, Rochester, Minnesota, U.S.A.

J. Godfrey Heathcote
Departments of Pathology and Ophthalmology and Visual Sciences, Dalhousie University, Halifax, Nova Scotia, Canada

INTRODUCTION

A wide variety of congenital malformations may arise during development of the eye. Anomalies may involve a single ocular tissue, a region of the eye, or the entire eye. They may be unilateral or bilateral and may occur in association with a constellation of cranial, facial, or systemic abnormalities. When many tissues are affected, the significance of the associations is not always clear, but a chromosomal/genetic abnormality, an intrauterine infection, or maternal toxin is often involved. Overlapping clinical manifestations from different genetic and non-genetic causes occur as a result of spatial and temporal targeting of specific developmental processes and embryonic events. A growing number of developmental genes, mainly transcription factors and genes involved in signaling pathways, are being identified and their regulatory role(s) in vertebrate eye morphogenesis characterized. Depending on the expression pattern of these genes in different tissues, various organs may be affected, resulting in extraocular manifestions.

MECHANISMS OF DISORDERED MORPHOGENESIS

Genetic Factors

Gene Regulation of Morphogenesis

Genes control the development of an individual from conception to maturity. Developmental genes encode proteins that contain DNA binding sites, a feature that allows orchestration of normal development by controlling the production of mRNA by other genes at specific times during the development and differentiation of tissues and organs (496). Such proteins are called transcription factors. Through studies of mutations in developmental genes in *Drosophila*, master control (homeotic) genes were identified and their roles in organ morphogenesis established, with the transformation of middle legs to antennae and vice versa, induced by loss-of-function and gain-of-function mutations respectively, in the *Antennapedia* gene (160,422). Ectopic eye structures were later induced by driving the expression of *Eyeless*, the homologue of the *PAX6* gene in humans, in the wing, antenna and leg of *Drosophila* (186).

A number of DNA binding sites, which code for protein domains capable of influencing the expression of other genes, have been identified over the past two decades. Found in several developmental genes, the homeobox refers to a highly conserved DNA region of 180 base pairs encoding the homeodomain (321). The paired box encodes another domain and is found in all *PAX* genes. In addition to containing a paired box, some *PAX* genes also have a full or partial homeobox (160). Other families of developmental genes include the *POU* genes encoding a POU domain, helix-loop-helix-leucine zipper genes and forkhead box genes (173,496).

In the embryo, cells have the potential to differentiate into many distinct cell types upon further division. Specific cell types distinguish the tissues, organs, and finally the whole organism. With development, pluripotency is lost and a cell of a given type limits its gene activity to produce only those proteins needed for maintenance of its particular functions. Some of the genes involved in development later assume a key role in maintenance once cell differention is completed. The retention of pluripotency is occasionally manifested by the formation of choristomas, although local factors may induce tissues in an abnormal location.

Modification of the genetic information carried by the chromosomes can be caused by a mutation occurring in a single locus or, less commonly, multiple gene loci.

Chromosomal Anomalies

Absence or duplication of a chromosome, deletion of a significant portion of a chromosome and other aberrant forms usually result in mutilating and often lethal defects in the embryo. Spontaneously aborted infants often show major chromosomal abnormalities (217). Monosomy is a universally lethal defect except for the monosomy of females with Turner syndrome where one X chromosome is lost (XO). Trisomies are relatively common and, while many are lethal, individuals with trisomies may lead long lives, though they are frequently developmentally delayed. The most common is trisomy 21 (Down syndrome) (MIM #190685), formerly called mongolism because of the upward slant of the lateral palpebral fissures, and this was the first syndrome in humans to be ascribed to a specific chromosome (243,397,411).

Developmental Events

Some anomalies are clearly related to specific embryonic events, e.g., a typical coloboma results from failure of closure of the embryonic fissure (438). Others, such as retinal dysgenesis, reflect inaccurate timing of the sequential growth and differentiation of embryonic tissue.

Developmental Processes

Embryonic events rely on a complex series of developmental processes such as specification of the prospective eye field, lens induction, patterning or organization of regions that will evolve into specific tissue, such as the sensory retina or retinal pigment epithelium (RPE). These events and processes are critical for proper migration, proliferation, differentiation, apoptosis, remodeling and neuronal connections to yield normal, functional eye structures (144, 183,285,298). The final outcome of these processes depends on a balance between genetic and environmental influences and any disruption can lead to developmental anomalies.

Some of the developmental processes occur almost simultaneously and the genes involved in their regulation may have varying functions and interactions during ocular development (144, 173,298). The spatial and temporal overlap of gene expression and the near synchronous events early in eye morphogenesis explain in part the identical phenotypes caused by mutations in the different regulatory genes (144). For example, determination of the eye field, the region in the anterior neural plate that will give rise to the eyes, is the earliest event in ocular morphogenesis and depends on the expression and interactions of master control genes in this field (173,298). Defects in these regulatory genes can be expected to cause severe ocular malformations, such as panocular malformations seen in aniridia (MIM #106210) from *PAX6* heterozygous mutations (191,489), and anophthalmia (MIM #206900) from compound heterozygous *PAX6* (166) and heterozygous *OTX2* (381) and *SOX2* (136) mutations. The phenotypic variability related to mutations in these genes suggests that the genetic background and/or environmental factors influence the effect of the defective gene (144,191).

Defective Cell Migration

The considerable movement of cells that occurs in embryogenesis is essential to normal development. Early in embryogenesis, neural crest cells migrate to new positions distant from their origin on the crest of the neural folds. The contributions of these cells to the eye and its supporting structures are extensive and interference with the migration of the cells into the new location can be expected to result in abnormalities. Neural crest cells migrate in an extracellular matrix (ECM), which if limited or abnormal may alter migration (239,240). Many craniofacial anomalies are thought to result from faulty migration or abnormal fusion of the cranial neural crest processes. In the arrhinencephalic syndromes, a cleft lip and palate result when the fronto-nasal and maxillary processes fail to meet and fuse inferior and nasal to the globe. Other cellular or tissue movements may be focally impeded as the tips of the optic vesicle grow anteriorly and interact with late waves of neural crest cells to develop the anterior segment of the eye (28).

Impaired Cellular Proliferation

Minor insults to the embryo and fetus that delay proliferation of cells integral to the whole or to a particular structure can be corrected by a subsequent spurt in growth (376). Malformations are prone to arise when the cellular damage occurs at a time, or to such a degree, that compensatory growth is incomplete before the next phase of development. Impaired cellular proliferation can occur, for example, as a result of *CHX10* mutations causing microphthalmia, cataract, and coloboma (MIM #610092) (34,173,285).

Inadequate Differentiation

As pluripotency is lost from the growing embryonic cells, the cells become committed to forming a particular tissue or organ, i.e., they undergo differentiation. Fully differentiate cells are structurally and biochemically mature. Cells which show only partial differentiation or aberrant development are termed dysgenetic or dysplastic. A tissue can be identified histologically when some of the mature features are present. For example, neurosensory retina can be recognized even if one or more nuclear layers are absent, the nuclei form circles or rosettes, or manifest variations in density. These changes constitute retinal dysplasia (dysgenesis) and severely dysgenetic cells and tissues may only function to a limited extent, or not at all (376). Examples of genes responsible for tissue and cell proliferation and differentiation include *WNT* pathway genes and *SHH* in the retina (47,183). In humans, *SHH* mutations cause holoprosencephaly, coloboma and microphthalmia (419). Mutations in *OTX2* cause impaired retinal function in virtually all cases, in addition to anophthalmia, microphthalmia, and optic nerve aplasia, suggesting a role in early retinal differentiation (144,381).

Cell Death

Cells which are part of the ongoing process of development early in embryogenesis may disappear as the organ matures. For example, cells in the stalk connecting the surface ectoderm to the lenticular vesicle disappear as the lenticular vesicle separates (88,89) and suppression of apoptosis (see Chapter 2) leads to faulty separation (367). If residual cells do not die, the migration of neural crest cells to produce the corneal stroma is impaired and the residual primitive cells obstruct later phases of development. On the other hand, when cells are destined to produce all or part of a structure, the loss of a significant number may result in the absence, or limited formation, of that structure (376). In consecutive anophthalmia there is evidence of early development of an eye which subsequently degenerates (144), although anophthalmia can also occur as a result of a failure of retinal progenitor cell proliferation without cell death (285,398,440).

Neuronal Connectivity

As the ocular structures develop, a complex neuronal network must connect the eye to the central nervous system (CNS). Neurodevelopment is an integral part of the evolving visual system and is also guided by genetic factors. In the past decade, the identification of genes causing rare oculomotor diseases, termed congenital cranial dysinnervation disorders, has provided important clues to the mechanisms underlying brainstem oculomotor development and connectivity of cranial motoneurons (129). *ROBO3* was recently identified as causative of horizontal gaze palsy with progressive scoliosis (236). Studies of *Robo3* knockout mice and the homologous *roundabout* genes in *Drosophila* and zebrafish demonstrate anomalous brainstem innervation with aberrant axonal crossing or complete failure of axons to cross the midline brainstem (129,405,424).

Teratogenesis

That so much of what is initially induced as eye-forming tissue completes the entire program resulting in normal, fully functioning eyes attests to the stability of the processes of growth and development from conception to maturity. Nevertheless, internal and external factors may affect the process and result in a defective eye. A teratogen is an agent that produces a defect in the developing embryo or fetus; literally, an inducer of monsters. Although the template for development carried in the genes is relatively constant, the pathways to maldevelopment are many and the same phenotype can result from a variety of teratogens.

In some cases, two factors may be needed for teratogenesis: a predisposing gene defect and an environmental influence. Mice with a genetic predisposition for cleft palate (117) produce some affected offspring. The number of offspring with cleft palate increases if the genetically predisposed female is exposed to diphenylhydantoin which independently produces cleft palate in the offspring (171). However, even in this richly teratogenic milieu, not all offspring are affected. Furthermore, a teratogen may be active only during a limited period in embryogenesis, as demonstrated by Gregg's study of rubella infection (174). Pregnant women infected by the rubella virus in the first trimester produce infants with the rubella syndrome (cataracts, deafness and mental retardation). If the infection occurs later in pregnancy, the infants are less likely to be affected and the severity is reduced (326,503). The extent of the damage may be further influenced by the health of the mother and the nature of the teratogen, whether physical (55,172,434), chemical (324,408,470) or infectious.

Physical Constraint

Amniotic bands have been implicated in the formation of fissures and clefts that do not correspond to the lines of closure in the embryo. Peculiar indentations with adjacent folds, coupled with a malformed eye, ear, nose, or cheek, may result from pressure of an amniotic band on the fetal face. Specific ocular defects reported with the amniotic band syndrome include absent, colobomatous, or foreshortened eyelids, ptosis, ectropion, clefts involving the medial or lateral canthus, extraocular muscle palsies, bony orbital clefts or hypertelorism, lacrimal outflow obstruction, corneal leukomas, and bilateral epibulbar choristomas, as well as anterior segment dysgenesis with absent lens (39,100,197,214,341,342).

Chemicals, Drugs, Toxins

Although many drugs have been linked with developmental defects (36,72,324,408,430,446,465,501,533), convincing evidence through rigorous testing has been presented in only a few: radioactive iodine (430), cyclophosphamide (430,442), coumarin anticoagulants (30,188,192,430,523), diphenylhydantoin (137,218,387,430), 13-cis-retinoic acid (41,105,189,430), lithium (430), alcohol (24,49,456) and thalidomide (533). A human fetus is most susceptible to teratogens during the period of organogenesis (18 to 60 days of gestation).

Infectious Agents

Many infectious agents have been labeled as teratogenic for the human embryo (65,124); yet only a few, cytomegalovirus (152,208,293), herpes virus hominis (3,242), parvovirus B19, rubella virus (174,271,503), *Treponema pallidum* (86,179), *Toxoplasma gondii* (391) and Venezuelan equine encephalitis virus, have been unequivocally implicated as teratogens (430). Varicella has been incriminated as a teratogen (53,74,276,425) and epidemiologic evidence of an association between anophthalmia/microphthalmia has been demonstrated for Coxsackie A9 (261) and influenza (65) viral infections.

Radiation

Maternal exposure to high levels of various forms of radiation during the early stages of embryogenesis can severely damage the fetus (55,131). Timing and dosage are critical (461,502). The earlier in pregnancy that radiation exposure occurs, the more likely is death or malformation to develop. Exposure up to the 11th week is associated with malformations and thereafter the number of anomalies decreases markedly. Radiation damage to the ocular anlage produces anophthalmia, microphthalmia, cataracts, coloboma, eyelid anomalies, and retinal pigmentary changes (55,108). After the 11th week, little damage is produced in the eye except for cataracts or a predisposition to early cataracts. The most serious consequence of maternal radiation when it is not lethal is mental retardation.

Ophthalmic investigations in survivors of the atomic bombing of Hiroshima and Nagasaki, including those exposed in utero, indicate that only axial opacities and polychromatic changes in the posterior subcapsule of the lens were associated with ionizing radiation. Similar findings were detected to a lesser extent in control populations not exposed to ionizing radiation (346). No increase in the number of infants with congenital defects attributable to chromosomal damage has been found in the children of survivors exposed to ionizing radiation in excess of 2 Grey (2 Gy; formerly designated 200 rads) in Hiroshima (345,364). Similarly a study in 16 regions of Europe of the prevalence of congenital anomalies following the Chernobyl accident failed to reveal any teratogenic effects, including cataract and microphthalmia/anophthalmia (119).

Exposure at the current allowable doses of environmental radiation does not increase fetal damage (263,345,363) but diagnostic and therapeutic radiation should be used cautiously in all women of child bearing age as more studies are required to fully assess short-term and long-term safety (131,263).

Maternal Nutrition

According to one estimate, 10% of developmental anomalies are caused by environmental factors, of which 4% can be attributed to deviations in maternal/fetal metabolism or nutrition (56). Recent evidence supports the concept of genome-nutrient interactions producing reversible and irreversible changes in development starting from conception. Metabolic, transcriptional and cell signaling networks can respond and adapt to their environment, with nutrients acting as environmental modifiers. When genomic responses altered during vulnerable periods of development reorganize cellular networks irreversibly (i.e., have a lifelong effect), this is referred to as epigenetic programming or metabolic imprinting. DNA or histone methylation is an epigenetic phenomenon

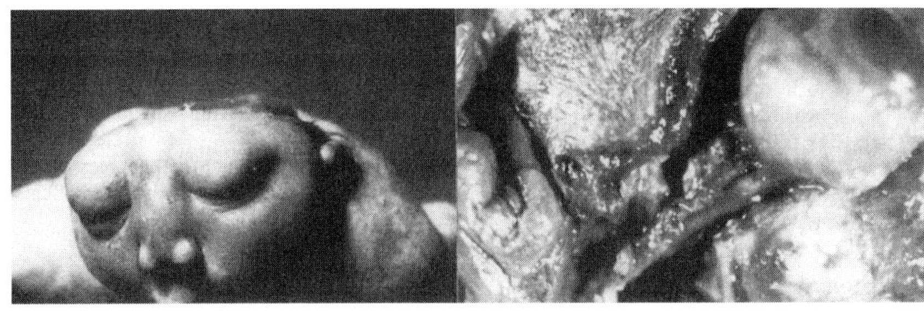

Figure 1 Anencephaly. (*Left*) Eyes and orbits are present despite failed development of the telencephalon. (*Right*) Globe of stillborn with well developed optic nerve that tapers in midline. Interior of globes was normal. *Source*: Courtesy of Dr. S. Young.

that can alter gene expression and is influenced by folate metabolism (460). Deficiencies of folic acid and the use of folate antagonists can produce anophthalmos, microphthalmos, cataract and coloboma (19). Hypervitaminosis A may be teratogenic by interfering with neural crest cell migration (272).

DEVELOPMENTAL ANOMALIES OF THE WHOLE EYE

Abnormalities in Size

Anencephaly

Suppression of development limited to the telencephalon results in anencephaly, with an infant without a forebrain but with eyes (Fig. 1). Anencephaly is uniformally lethal and one pathological study of 11 globes from 7 cases has shown anomalies consisting of atrophy of retinal ganglion cell and nerve fiber layers in all cases, with most demonstrating optic nerve atrophy, and persistent pupillary membrane (44). Other findings included incomplete formation of the anterior chamber, retinal dysgenesis, coloboma, proliferative retinopathy and upper eyelid notch (44,51). Glial nodules (Fig. 2) and intravitreal neovascularization (Fig. 3), which may lead to partial retinal detachment, may be seen in eyes of anencephalics.

Anophthalmia

Anophthalmia is the absence of the eye, but more often the orbit contains a microphthalmic globe, and in those instances the term clinical anophthalmia is appropriate. True anophthalmia occurs when no rudiments of the neuroectoderm of the optic cup are present in the orbit (159). True anophthalmia is a very rare event which results from insults in the third or fourth week of embryogenesis (15). Data from the California Birth Defects Monitoring Program indicates a prevalence of 0.18 per 10,000 live births when cases of holoprosencephaly and chromosomal syndromes are excluded (429). Anophthalmia may exhibit autosomal recessive, autosomal dominant (40) and X-linked (63) patterns of inheritance (212,413).

The diagnosis of true anophthalmia is made histopathologically by serial sectioning of the orbital tissues, a technique almost never undertaken (413). Primary anophthalmia results from the failure of the optic primordium in the earliest stages of embryogenesis. Either no optic anlage develops or a limited ocular primordium is established and fails to grow. Secondary anophthalmia results from widespread failure of development of the anterior neural tube and is lethal since neither brain nor eyes form.

Anophthalmia occurs in a variety of syndromes (310) and has been produced experimentally by a variety of techniques including irradiation of the developing mouse embryo (439). Apparent clustering of cases of anophthalmia is not generally the result of exposure to specific teratogens (294). Anophthalmia

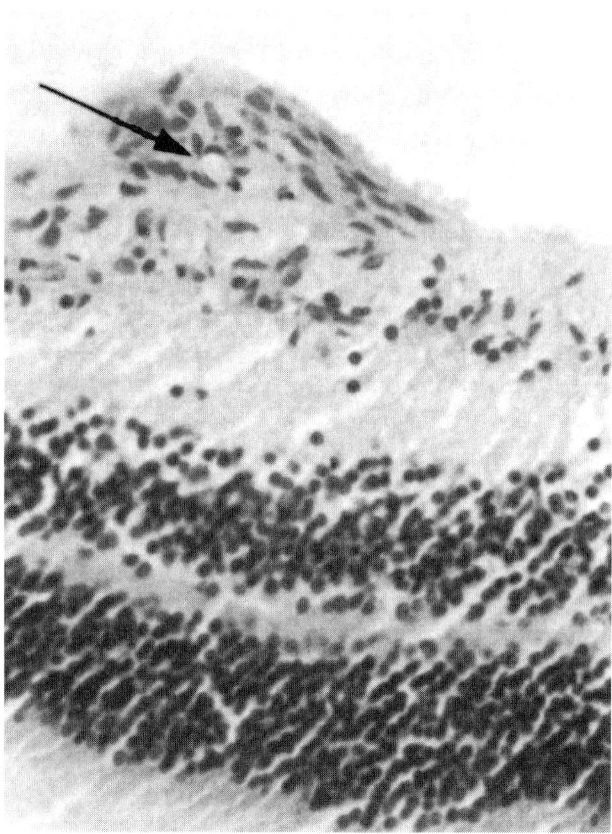

Figure 2 Anencephaly. Nodule of glial tissue, with a blood vessel (*arrow*), on the surface of the retina of an anencephalic fetus (hematoxylin and eosin, ×125). *Source*: Courtesy of Dr. J. Mullaney.

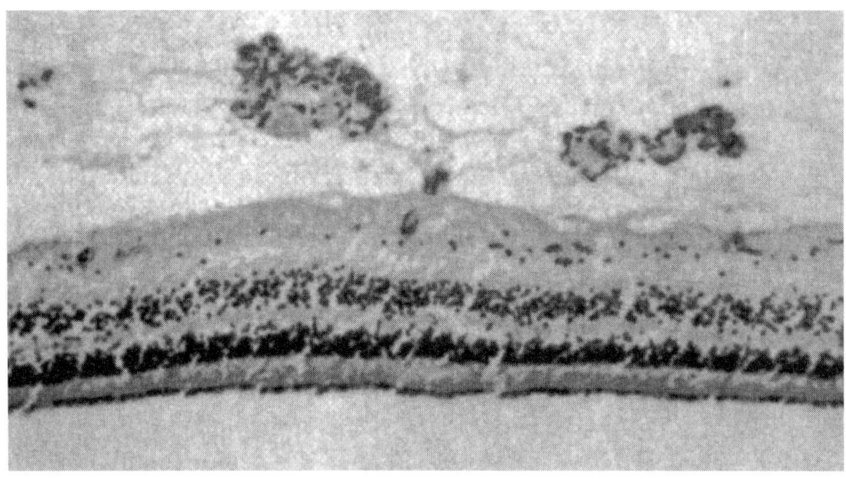

Figure 3 Anencephaly. Intravitreal proliferation of retinal blood vessels (hematoxylin and eosin, ×135). *Source*: Courtesy of Dr. J. Mullaney.

and microphthalmia are often associated with concurrent malformations of the CNS and musculoskeletal system, as well as facial dysmorphism (429). Cases of anophthalmia with other anomalies have been grouped into a *SOX2* anophthalmia syndrome, caused by loss-of-function mutations in the *SOX2* gene, which is important in all stages of development (382). Other genes are involved in syndromic and isolated clinical anophthalmia.

Microphthalmia

Microphthalmia, the small disorganized globe (Fig. 4), is a diverse condition with many causes (142,439). It is defined by an axial length <2 standard deviations below normal for age (527). Microphthalmia may simulate anophthalmia clinically as in microphthalmic syndrome 3 (MIM #206900) (25) and is more common than true anophthalmia.

Weiss and co-workers (526,527) described findings in 62 of 6000 patients seen in a pediatric clinic over six years. Forty patients had small globes with ocular malformations and associated systemic anomalies (complex microphthalmos) (526). Simple microphthalmos occurred in 22 patients (0.36%) (527) who had normal appearing eyes with an axial length less than two standard deviations from the mean (Fig. 5) and vision in the 20/30 to 20/50 range. One patient with simple microphthalmos had vision of 20/100. All eyes were 3 to 4 mm shorter than globes of age matched controls. In the group with complex microphthalmia, severe microcornea correlated with severe microphthalmia, whereas in those with simple microphthalmia, only seven had microcornea (<10.5 mm in diameter). The length of the posterior segment was consistently decreased in the eyes with both complex and simple microphthalmia (Fig. 6). In the simple microphthalmic group the anterior segment lengths were within or just below normal range (Fig. 7), whereas the anterior segment lengths in complex microphthalmia were uniformly at least two standard deviations below the mean.

The mildest changes in the eyes with complex microphthalmia were microcornea and cataracts (526). The more severely involved had colobomas, colobomatous cysts, severe microphthalmia, persistent hyperplastic primary vitreous (PHPV), and facial malformations. The associated systemic disorders included the congenital rubella syndrome, autosomal dominant Weill–Marchesani syndrome (MIM #608328), autosomal recessive Weill–Marchesani syndrome (MIM #277600), deletion of 13q, trisomy 13, the CHARGE (**C**oloboma, **H**eart defects, choanal **A**tresia, mental **R**etardation, **G**enitourinary defects, **E**ar

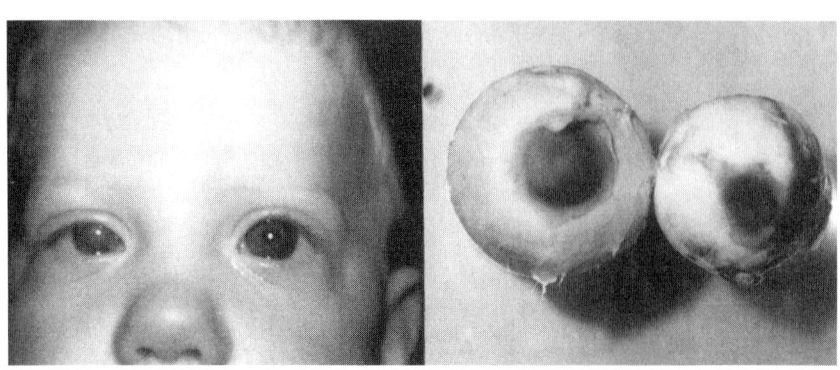

Figure 4 Unilateral microphthalmia. (*Left*) Idiopathic microphthalmia of right eye. (*Right*) Normally sized globe and microphthalmic globe from individual with 13q-syndrome.

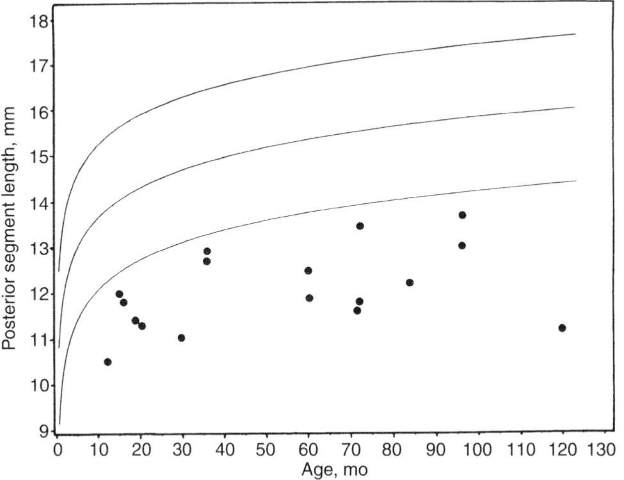

Figure 5 Total axial length in 21 patients with simple microphthalmos. Each dot represents the total axial length of one randomly selected eye of each patient. The mean total axial length values for normal subjects (*middle curve*) and upper and lower 95% confidence bands (*outer curves*) are shown for comparison. *Source*: Reproduced with permission from the American Medical Association and Ref. 527.

anomalies) syndrome (MIM #214800), Lenz syndrome (MIM %309800), incontinentia pigmenti (MIM #308300) and Norrie disease (ND) (MIM #310600). Other associations included achondroplasia, myotonic dystrophy (MIM #160900), diabetic embryopathy, fetal alcohol syndrome, Maroteaux–Lamy syndrome (mucopolysaccharidosis type VI) (MIM #253200) and

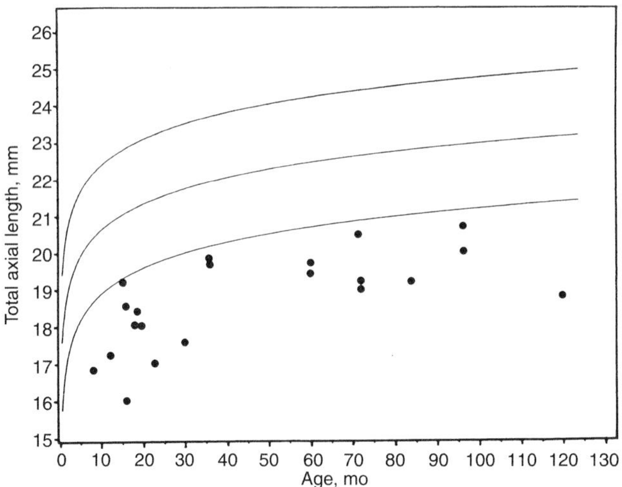

Figure 6 Posterior segment length in 17 patients with simple microphthalmos. Each dot represents the posterior segment length of one randomly selected eye of each patient. The mean posterior segment length values for normal subjects (*middle curve*) and upper and lower 95% confidence bands (*outer curves*) are shown for comparison. *Source*: Reproduced with permission from the American Medical Association and Ref. 527.

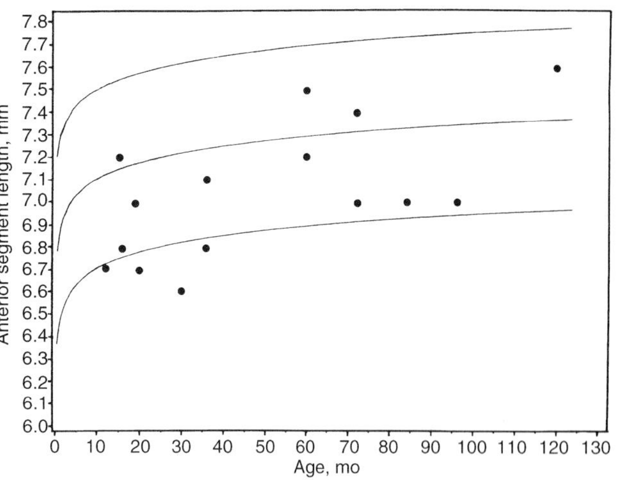

Figure 7 Anterior segment length in 17 patients with simple microphthalmos. Each dot (except one) represents the anterior segment length of one randomly selected eye of each patient. Two pairs of patients with the same anterior segment length are represented by one dot each. The mean anterior segment length of age-similar normal subjects (*middle curve*) with upper and lower 95% confidence bands (*outer curves*) are shown for comparison. *Source*: Reproduced with permission from the American Medical Association and Ref. 527.

isolated growth hormone deficiency (526). Systemic manifestations have been described by other authors (149,164,209), commonly mental retardation (5,91, 209,241,274,340,498) and dwarfism (54,59,485,521).

The microphthalmic globe (266,383) has been associated with numerous ocular anomalies including leukomas (126), anterior segment disorders (122), retinal dysplasia (122), colobomas (209,520), cysts (148,181,286,525,541), and marked internal ocular dysgenesis (149). The associated adnexal abnormalities include a small orbit, shortened palpebral fissure, ptosis, and blepharophimosis. High hyperopia accompanies almost all cases of simple microphthalmos and vitreous development may be faulty in both simple and complex microphthalmos (526,527).

Trisomies or other abnormalities of virtually every chromosome (12,120,159,163,181,339,393,420, 498,525), maternal radiation (55), infections, and toxins are reported in association with microphthalmia (93,134,520). Microphthalmia can be inherited as an autosomal dominant (233), an autosomal recessive (220,233,299,452,498), or as an X-linked (169,498, 517,519) trait and may be an idiopathic phenomenon (54,266). Single defects in the *RX*, *CHX10*, *SOX2*, *SIX6*, *OTX2* and *BCOR* genes have been found in association with the microphthalmia/anophthalmia spectrum (34,136,138,157,184,350,381,382,530).

Nanophthalmos

Nanophthalmos describes a small, functional eye with relatively normal internal structures, although the

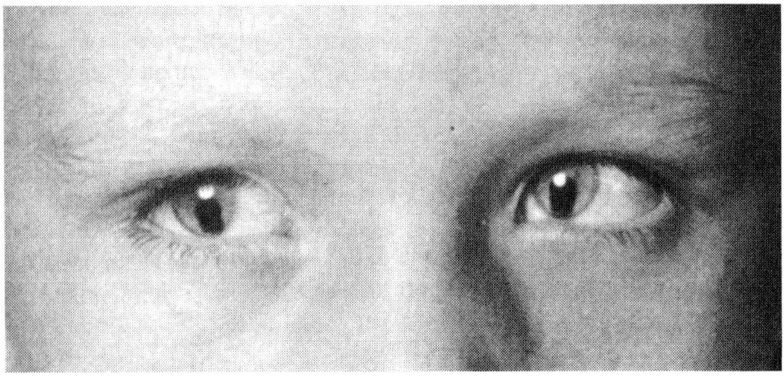

Figure 8 Bilateral iris colobomas in the inferonasal region associated with the embryonic fissure. *Source*: Reproduced from Klintworth GK, Landers MB III. The Eye: Structure and Function in Disease. Baltimore: Williams & Wilkins, 1976.

anterior chamber is crowded and the eye is hyperopic (237,301,527). Familial cases have been reported (118,319) and two types of isolated nanophthalmos are recognized: nanophthalmos type 1 (MIM %600165) and nanophthalmos type 2 (MIM #609549). No gene has been identified for type 1, but type 2 is caused by mutations in the gene that encodes the membrane-type frizzled-related protein (MFRP), a regulator of the WNT signalling pathway. Uveal effusion (102) and exfoliation syndrome (118) may occur. Cataract extraction has been successful despite the small and crowded anterior segment (58). However, post-operative complications such as uveal effusions and choroidal hemorrhages among others are more frequent in small eyes (472). In some cases of nanophthalmos scleral collagen fibers appear abnormal (455), possibly resulting from altered proteoglycan deposition (247,248).

Colobomas

A coloboma is defined as an absence of a part of an ocular structure (301). Colobomas are divided into typical, those associated with aberrant closure of the embryonic fissure of the optic vesicle (Fig. 8), and atypical, those not associated with the fissure closure. They can be complete or incomplete and are frequently associated with microphthalmia and other ocular and non-ocular developmental defects. One of the more common clinically observed congenital ocular anomalies, colobomas are usually bilateral and often asymmetric (126).

Between weeks 5 and 7 of gestation, following invagination of the optic vesicle, fusion of the lips of the embryonic fissure begins centrally and proceeds anteriorly and posteriorly. Failure to complete this process results in defects involving virtually any ocular structure, including the cornea, iris, ciliary body, zonule (giving rise to lenticular notching), choroid, retina, and optic nerve (176,362). Eyelid colobomas can result from failure of fusion of the mesoblastic eyelid folds, usually at the junction of the inner and middle thirds for the upper eyelid and at the junction of the middle and lateral thirds for the lower eyelid (362).

Typical colobomas of the globe occur inferonasally, anywhere along the line of the fissure. In a complete coloboma there is no closure of the fissure and this results in a microphthalmic or cystic eye (Fig. 9). Most typical colobomas are incomplete, being limited to a portion of the fissure. Interrupted closure results in bands of normal appearing tissue, adjacent to the coloboma. The coloboma has well demarcated borders, typically lined by hyperplastic RPE at the edge of the defect where normal tissue begins. The RPE is absent in the coloboma, and the overlying retina is hypoplastic and gliotic, with occasional rosettes detectable histopathologically (Fig. 10). Retinal layers are reversed, with rods and cones facing inward and nerve fiber layer outward toward the sclera. Within the coloboma, the choroid is hypoplastic or absent, and the thinned, ectatic sclera may have cystic spaces filled with glial tissue, occasionally resembling a neoplasm (362). Retinal and choroidal vessels can be seen traversing the coloboma. An iris coloboma is usually full thickness, although a thinned wedge which transilluminates may be present. Typical colobomas of the optic nerve

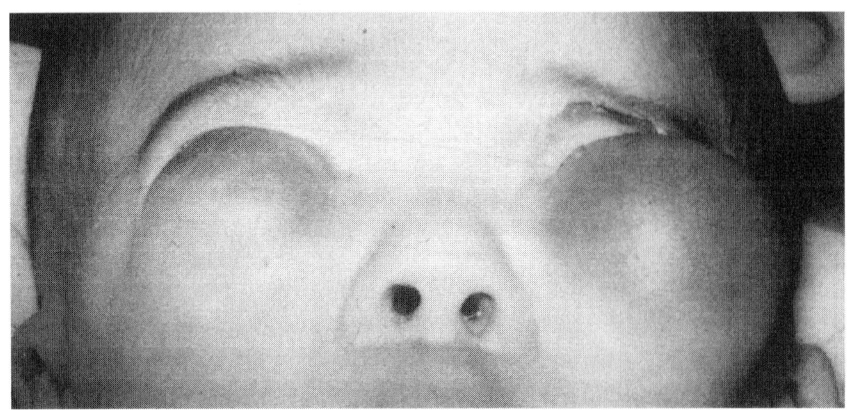

Figure 9 Bilateral cystic eyes. Histopathology showed limited dysgenetic neuroectodermal tissues.

(A) 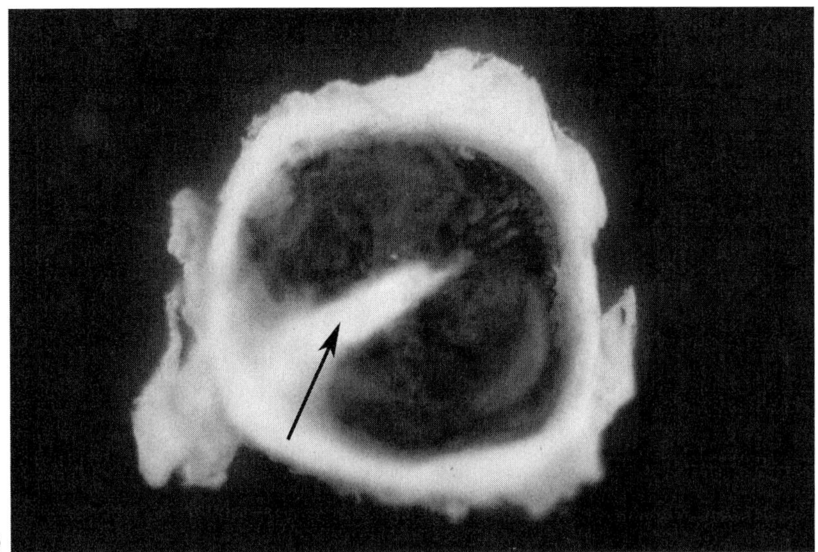

(B) 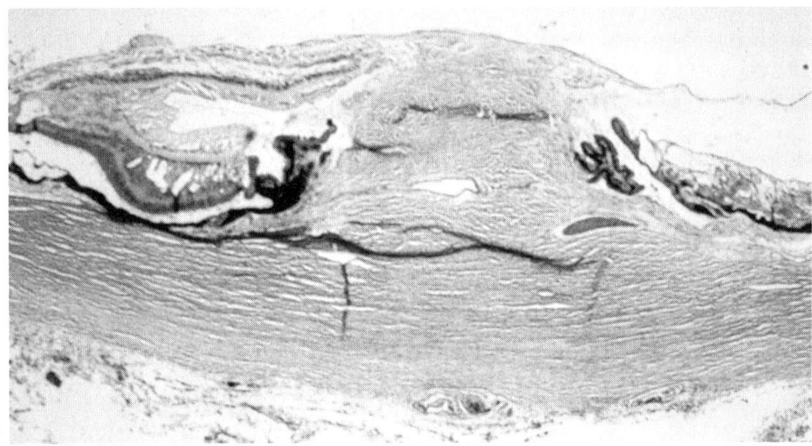

Figure 10 Chorioretinal coloboma. (**A**) A white streak (*arrow*) in the fundus is caused by a defect in the choroid and retinal pigment epithelium (RPE). (**B**) Hyperplastic RPE and dysplastic retina are seen on either side of the defect (hematoxylin and eosin, ×25).

vary from minimal thinning at the posterior termination of a chorioretinal coloboma to involvement of almost the entire nerve so that only a small portion of the superior pole is identifiable as optic disc (Fig. 11). The coloboma of the optic nerve is often continuous with the white defect in the inferior nasal fundus.

Visual acuity depends on the location of the coloboma, such that even large colobomas can be compatible with excellent vision, although an absolute scotoma is expected corresponding to the retinal coloboma. Other factors associated with colobomas that reduce the visual prognosis include the presence of microphthalmia, especially with cysts, and a corneal diameter <6 mm (128,216).

Colobomas are frequently associated with systemic developmental anomalies (78,114,221,228, 362,403), craniofacial syndromes (377,480), focal dermal dysplasia (Goltz syndrome) (MIM #305600) (517), as well as other intraocular malformations (401,449) and occasionally intraocular tumors (glioneuroma, medulloepithelioma, astrocytoma and, in the 13q-syndrome, retinoblastoma) (10). In some systemic conditions, e.g., the CHARGE association (MIM #214800) (1,11,209,403), colobomas of the iris and/or posterior pole are a common feature, occurring in up to 86% of cases.

A large number of genetic causes have been described (176,323), often in association with systemic abnormalities. Autosomal dominant inheritance is most common, followed by autosomal recessive then X-linked recessive (176). Expressivity can be variable: even though one member of a family harbors an isolated coloboma, other members of the pedigree may manifest microphthalmia, cataract, anterior segment dysgenesis (91), aniridia, PHPV and other ocular malformations (66,126). Multiple genes/gene loci, as well as chromosomal abnormalities, have been identified (176). *PAX6* (27), *SHH* (419), and *CHX10* (34,138) mutations have all been identified as causative of non-syndromic ocular colobomas. The cat-eye syndrome (MIM #115470), known to result from incorporation of fragments of chromosomes 13 or 14 into chromosome 22, was originally named because of the constant vertical uveal coloboma (163,297,372).

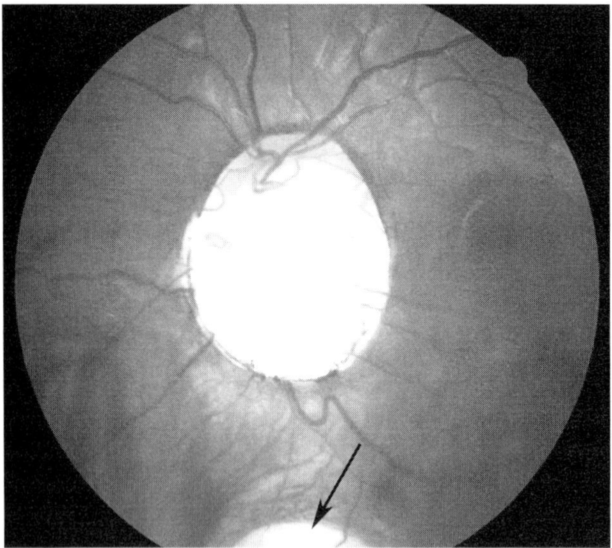

Figure 11 Optic nerve coloboma. Coloboma involves the optic nerve with a separate chorioretinal coloboma inferonasally (*arrow*) along the embryonic fissure. Although reduced vision is common in such patients, this child had a normal foveal reflex and a central visual acuity of 20/20.

Teratogenic influences that have been implicated in the etiology of colobomas include vitamin A deficiency, diphenylhydantoin, carbamazapine, lysergic acid diethylamide (72), thalidomide (284,333,362, 553), cytomegalovirus (152,293), Epstein–Barr virus, varicella-zoster, herpes virus (362), and rubella virus (503). Of these potential teratogens, only thalidomide has been established as a cause of colobomas (362).

Cystic Colobomas and Cystic Eye

Cystic colobomas develop along the line of closure of the embryonic fissure (26) and are serious anomalies that usually result in a blind eye. When the space within the ectopic, folded layers of inner neuroectoderm at the line of expected fusion remains open, either one or both tips of neuroectoderm may expand, one edge into the globe, the other externally (26). The result may be a cystic eye, microphthalmos with cyst (Fig. 12) or coloboma with cyst and the eyes have corneal leukomas, anterior segment dysgenesis, cataracts, PHPV, retinal non-attachment (146), and retinal dysplasia (177,276). The cyst may be larger than the eye, approximately equal in size, or comprise only a small cavity near the optic nerve. Cystic coloboma is associated with a deletion of the long arm of chromosome 13 (13q-) (526), a ring deletion of chromosome 18 (546) and trisomy 18 (Fig. 13) (181).

The congenital cystic eye is diagnosed clinically rather than anatomically. A true cystic eye is rare and represents failure of the optic vesicle to invaginate, the most severe form of congenital non-attachment of the retina. A cystic blue mass, usually distending the eyelids, results from a cystic eye or from a coloboma with cyst (Fig. 9). The opposite eye is typically normal and a number of associated nonocular anomalies have been reported (199). Histopathologic findings include relatively dense connective tissue external to the cyst with a thick layer of neuroglial tissue internally that can obliterate the cyst, cuboidal epithelium, branching cords of epithelium and possibly immature retina in areas. Calcified bodies can be found within the cyst, along with blood vessels, cells containing melanin granules and variable rudimentary ocular structures (199).

Coloboma and Abnormal Intraocular Tissues

In trisomy 13 (212,266,356,383) the microphthalmic eyes often contain a large fibrous coloboma with cartilage, especially if the eyes are <10 mm in

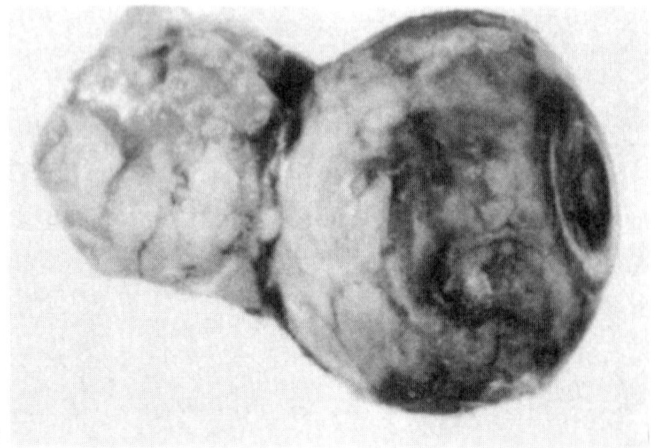

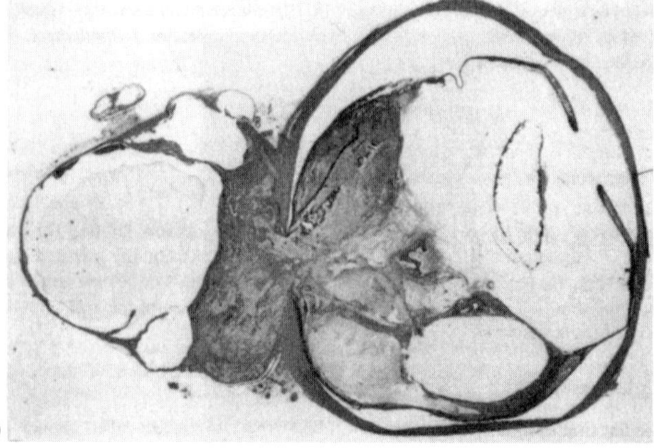

Figure 12 Microphthalmos with a colobomatous cyst. (**A**) A retrobulbar cystic mass is situated adjacent to a small malformed eye (×1.86). (**B**) This horizontal section through specimen in (**A**) demonstrates the cystic nature of the retrobulbar mass and the malformed retina within the microphthalmic eye (hematoxylin and eosin, ×2). *Source*: (**B**) Reproduced from Klintworth GK, Landers MB III. The Eye: Structure and Function in Disease. Baltimore: Williams & Wilkins, 1976.

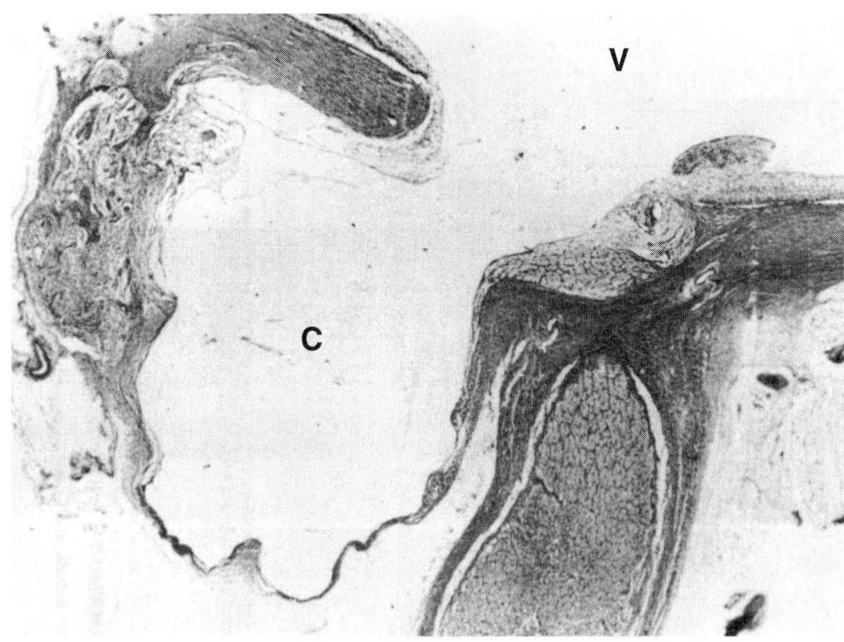

Figure 13 Trisomy 18. Colobomatous cyst (C) is in direct communication with the vitreous cavity (V) (hematoxylin and eosin, ×10). *Source*: Courtesy of Dr. J. Mullaney.

diameter. Intraocular cartilage may be associated with the coloboma in individuals with a ring configuration of chromosome 18 (546), PHPV, and medulloepithelioma. Heterotopic tissues associated with colobomas include smooth muscle (340,546), fibrous tissue, glial tissue, bone, adipose tissue (531), and lacrimal gland (178). Circumferential strands of smooth muscle are occasionally oriented concentrically around the optic disk (145,531). Aberrant locations of pigmented ciliary processes at the margins of a coloboma have been described (304,340). Some of these are explained as heterotopic rests, but the histogenesis of some of these fndings remains unexplained (340).

Atypical Colobomas

Focal defects in ocular tissues in regions distant to the embryonic fissure are called atypical colobomas. Atypical iris colobomas result from strands of the anterior hyaloid system and pupillary membrane which fail to regress spontaneously in late gestation. These exert traction on the edge of the developing iris and produce a notch or indentation. They may occur in any portion of the eye and usually are not as extensive as typical inferonasal colobomas.

Macular colobomas, white, oval patches within the temporal arcade of vessels and sharply demarcated from the surrounding tissues (Fig. 14), are associated with congenital toxoplasmosis, varicella (276), syphilis and may have an autosomal dominant mode of inheritance (414,450,484). Leber congenital amaurosis (313,336), skeletal defects (373), progeria with dwarfism (292) and keratoconus (282) have been associated with macular colobomas. Markedly reduced vision is the rule in such cases.

All manner of deep, wide, elongated, optic discs with vessels displaced to the rim edge and variable pigmentation are called optic disc colobomas, although many are not associated with defective closure of the embryonic fissure. Optic pits, depressions within the optic nerve that usually do not extend to the rim of the optic disc, are generally included in atypical colobomas. Many of these deformities are not strictly colobomatous, which by definition is absence of a part of a structure, but rather a maldevelopment of the whole optic disc and nerve.

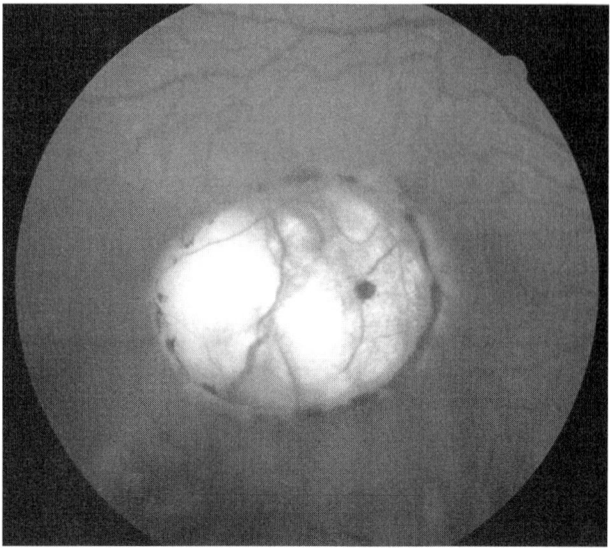

Figure 14 Coloboma of the macula. *Source*: Courtesy of Dr. G.R. LaRoche.

MAJOR CHROMOSOMAL ABNORMALITIES

Trisomy syndromes are caused by an extra functional chromosome. Trisomy of the larger chromosomes is fatal in early embryonic development; however, trisomy of three small chromosomes (chromosomes 13, 18, and 21) may be compatible with postnatal survival. Those afflicted are readily recognizable because of multiple phenotypic and functional abnormalities and a markedly reduced life expectancy. There is a significant association with congenital heart disease (308). The prevalent defect in all forms of trisomy is faulty separation of chromosomal material at meiotic division (meiotic nondisjunction) in the formation of ova or sperm. As a result, three functioning chromosomes or portions of chromosomes are present in the cells of the embryo. The cause of this faulty distribution of genetic material is unknown but it is related to maternal age. Other types of translocation (Robertsonian) and mosaicism may be found in a minority of cases (170).

The presence of the extra chromosome results in a 50% increase in the gene products of that chromosome (309). The genes themselves and the proteins they encode are normal. Chromosome 21, the chromosome most thoroughly studied in this type of abnormality, contains about 350 genes and represents approximately 1.5% of the DNA in a cell. All of the redundant genes appear to be transcribed, although because of dosage compensation the majority of gene products have no apparent effect. A small number of genes located in non-contiguous regions of the long arm of chromosome 21 appear to be responsible for the characteristic phenotype of trisomy 21. It has not yet been established if the phenotype reflects abnormal activity of a few single genes or mild abnormal activity of several interacting genes. No single phenotypic abnormality has been linked to a specific gene product and gene expression differs widely among affected individuals, during different phases of life and in different tissues (17,143,352).

Trisomy 21

Trisomy of chromosome 21 (Down syndrome) is the leading genetic cause of mental retardation. It is associated with the greatest survival, approximately 35 to 50 years, and is thus the most common chromosomal abnormality among live births. The major risk factor is advanced maternal age, with risks of 1 in 1550 live births under the age of 45 years and 1 in 25 over that age. The most common clinical features include hypotonia, hyperextensibility of joints, loose skin on the nape, a flat facial profile, an upward slant of the palpebral fissures, short ears with overhanging helices, dysplastic pelvis, clinodactyly of the fifth fingers and single palmar creases (187). There is a high prevalence of acute childhood leukemia, congenital heart malformations, immunologic abnormalities and early onset Alzheimer disease (70). The most common ocular findings are related to facial soft tissue malformation: upward slanting of the palpebral fissures, which is more prevalent in orientals than occidentals, epicanthus, epiblepharon and nasolacrimal duct obstruction (98). Functional and structural ocular abnormalities include refractive error, strabismus, nystagmus, retinal abnormalities, cataract and, rarely, glaucoma (397). Abnormalities of retinal vasculature may be linked to hemodynamic disturbance (308). The central corneal thickness is reduced by about 13% from normal and this results in a steeper cornea and may be linked to the development of keratoconus (132,198). Among 30 children with Down syndrome institutionalized for mental retardation, keratoconus was found in 9 (30%) (206). Brushfield spots (Fig. 15) on the iris and keratoconus are generally regarded as characteristics of trisomy 21. In a study of 55 children with Down syndrome and

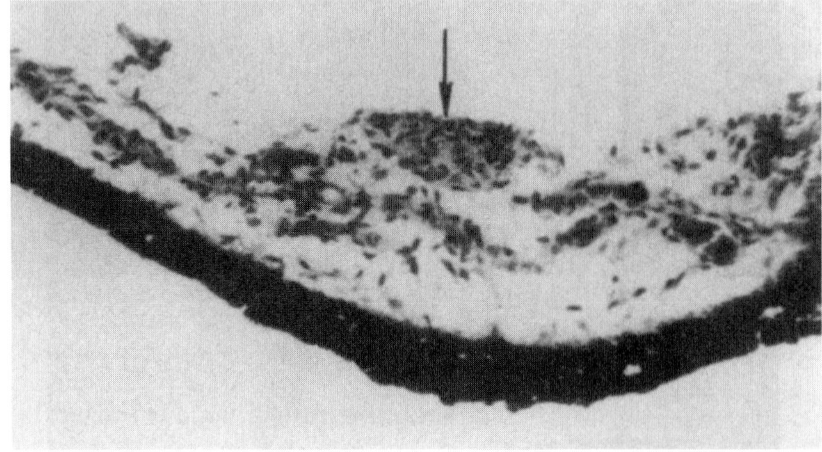

Figure 15 A Brushfield spot (*arrow*) on the anterior surface of the iris represents a focal overgrowth of stromal cells; the adjacent stroma is hypoplastic (hematoxylin and eosin, ×200). *Source*: Courtesy of Dr. J. Mullaney.

lightly pigmented irides, the prevalence of Brushfield spots was found to be 36% (42). However, in two separate evaluations of 140 and 123 Asian children with Down syndrome, none was found to exhibit Brushfield spots or keratoconus (255,536).

Trisomy 13

Trisomy of chromosome 13 (Patau syndrome) occurs in approximately 1 in 14,000 live births and infants rarely survive beyond the neonatal period (386). The syndrome is often associated with severe systemic abnormalities, including cardiac malformations, CNS abnormalities with or without holoprosencephaly, urogenital abnormalities and cleft lip and palate. The few infants who do survive for months or years may be recognized clinically by microphthalmos, an inferonasal iris coloboma and an inferonasal lens opacity (295). More detailed information about the ocular abnormalities has come from histopathological examination of post-mortem eyes and the findings are distinctive and almost always bilateral (Fig. 16) (337). Microphthalmos is universal and the two eyes may be affected to a different degree: it may be mild or sufficiently marked to appear as anophthalmos. As might be expected in a condition associated with impaired cleavage of the prosencephalon, there may be variable fusion of the malformed eyes (synophthalmia) or a single rudimentary eye (cyclopia) (Fig. 17) (264,492). The histopathological features are summarized in Table 1.

Trisomy 18

Trisomy of chromosome 18 (Edwards syndrome) is less common than either trisomy 21 or 13 and the abnormalities may involve all organ systems (386). External ocular abnormalities are not a prominent feature but there is a wide variety of malformations of the globe principally involving the cornea, iris, lens and retina (68).

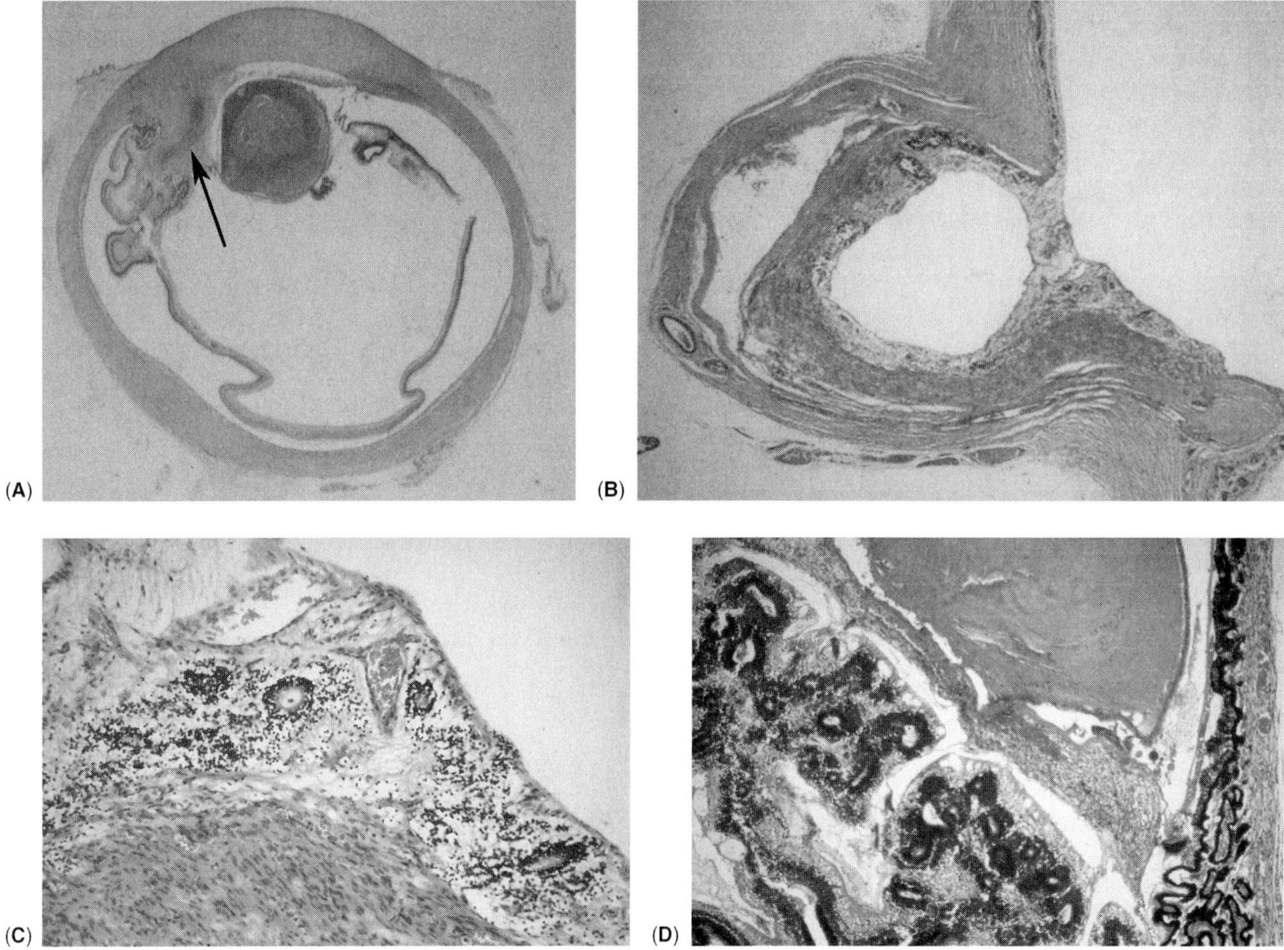

Figure 16 Trisomy 13. Characteristic histopathological features include: (**A**) a small eye with a fibrous coloboma containing cartilage (*arrow*); (**B**) a coloboma of the optic nerve with (**C**) dysplastic rosettes; (**D**) dysplastic retina separated from the cataractous lens by a fibrovascular membrane [hematoxylin and eosin, (**A**) ×4; (**B**) ×10; (**C**) ×60; (**D**) ×60].

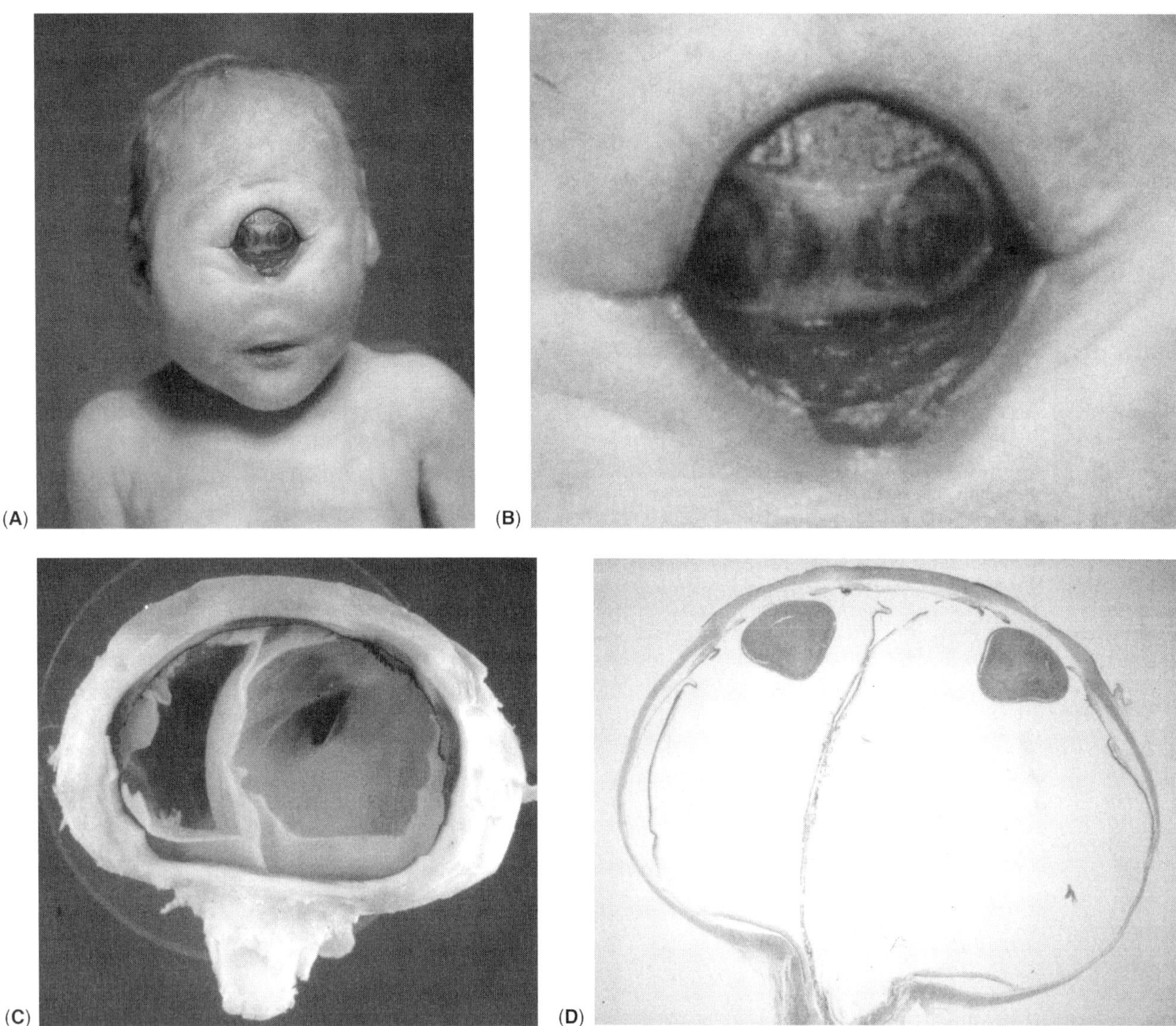

Figure 17 Trisomy 13. (**A,B**) An infant with holoprosencephaly and (**C,D**) fusion of the two eyes.

MENDELIAN DISORDERS

Albinism

Albinism is a group of hereditary disorders associated with reduced vision, foveal hypoplasia, nystagmus, abnormalities of iris transillumination, strabismus, refractive errors and abnormal decussation of the optic nerve fibers at the optic chiasm. All forms of albinism share various degrees of severity of foveal hypoplasia and depigmentation. In albinism the

Table 1 Ocular Histopathological Features of Trisomy 13

Microphthalmos	Usually bilateral; variable
Coloboma	Usually of iris and ciliary body; caused by failure of closure of embryonic fissure at 6 weeks, hence infero-nasal
Intraocular cartilage	Within coloboma at ciliary body region
Persistent hyperplastic primary vitreous	Persistence of the fetal vasculature, especially the posterior tunica vasculosa lentis; elongation of ciliary processes
Retinal dysgenesis (dysplasia)	Disorderly cellular proliferation; loss of cellular stratification; rosette formation
Cataract	Infero-nasal
Anterior chamber anomalies	Iris hypoplasia; rudimentary trabecular meshwork
Synophthalmia	Variable failure to develop two separate eyes; fusion more posteriorly
Cyclopia	Single midline globe; duplication of ocular structures

normal formation of the foveal pit by peripheral migration of the inner retinal layers and central migration of cone photoreceptors fails to occur, leaving foveal cones spaced apart (155). Studies of perifoveal vascularization using intravenous angiography have shown absence of a foveal avascular zone in the majority of cases (451). Occasionally, a retinal vessel may cross the putative fovea. Although not specific for albinism, one of the hallmarks is the abnormal decussation of retinal ganglion cell axons with a higher than normal proportion of fibers from the temporal retina projecting contralaterally. The mechanisms by which the lack or reduction in pigment affects retinal axonal routing remain unknown.

Albinism can be divided into two broad categories: oculocutaneous albinism (OCA) and ocular albinism (OA) (see Chatper 43). OCA variably reduces skin and hair pigmentation in addition to causing ocular manifestations and follows an autosomal recessive mode of inheritance. OA primarily involves the visual system and is inherited in an X-linked recessive fashion. Several syndromes exist in association with albinism, including the Hermansky–Pudlak syndromes type 1 (MIM #203300), Chédiak–Higashi syndrome (MIM #214500) and Cross–McKusick–Breen syndrome (MIM %257800).

Initially, OCA was thought to reflect a single disorder with variable phenotype. The discovery of two biochemical types of albinism led to the "tyrosinase positive" and "tyrosinase negative" classification of OCA (272,357,535), with subtypes later described according to clinical features (323,357). Molecular characterization of albinism since 1989 has broadened our understanding of albinism both in terms of disease classification and pathogenesis (488). OCA types are now defined by their genotype as well as their phenotype. OCA type 1 (OCA1) is caused by mutations in the *TYR* gene that encodes tryrosinase and is further subdivided into three subtypes: OCA type 1A (OCA1A, MIM #203100), OCA type1B (OCA1B, MIM #606952), OCA type 2 (OCA2, #203200), OCA type 3 (OCA3, MIM #203290) and OCA type 4 (OCA4, MIM #606574) are caused by mutations in different genes and comprise the "tyrosinase positive" group.

OCA1A, also known as tyrosinase negative OCA, completely lacks tyrosinase activity with a consequent absence in the formation of melanin. Affected individuals have completely white hair, pink skin and "pink eyes" (from transillumination through a nonpigmented iris). OCA1B refers to the yellow-mutant OCA phenotype and is caused by mutations in the tyrosinase gene (*TYR*) that significantly reduce, but do not completely abolish, its activity. Such patients are born with white hair and pink skin, and may be indistinguishable from the OCA1A patients until later in the first few years of life when they start developing some pigment, manifested clinically by yellowing of hair. Pigment continues to accumulate slowly throughout life in the hair, eyes and skin. Temperature-sensitive OCA patients have the same clinical phenotype as OCA1A and OCA1B initially but, at puberty, develop darker hair in the cooler parts of their body (such as the extremities). Warmer parts of the body, such as the scalp, do not show pigmentation over time. This subtype is caused by a *TYR* gene missense mutation that confers temperature sensitivity on the transcribed enzyme (323,488).

OCA2 is caused by mutations in the *P* gene that result in a variable degree of pigmentation, such that the phenotype can be identical to that seen in OCA1A or OCA1B patients. The exact function of the P protein is not known, but has been hypothesized to direct traffic of melanosomal proteins, including tyrosinase (488).

OCA3 results from mutations in the tyrosinase-related protein 1 (*TRP1*) gene. Described in African, African-American, and Pakistani patients, the skin manifestations are milder, with affected individuals having a lighter skin color than their unaffected relatives (323). TRP1 is an enzyme that catalyzes the polymerization of DHICA (5,6-dihydroxyindole-2-carboxylic acid) to melanin within the melanosomes (488).

OCA4 manifests with a variable phenotype similar to that seen in OCA2 and is caused by mutations in the membrane-associated transporter protein gene (*MATP*). The protein is thought to be a melanosome transporter, similar to the P protein (488).

OCA2 is the most common cause of OCA worldwide with frequencies varying in different populations from 1: 1,100 in Nigeria to 1: 36,000 in North America (280,323,325,360). OCA2 is especially common in African Americans and in certain African and American-Indian populations (259,538). The prevalence of OCA1 is about 1: 39,000 among European Americans but also varies among different populations (259,535).

Ocular albinism type 1 (OA1, also known as Nettleship–Falls type; MIM +300500) is the most common form of OA occurring at an estimated frequency of 1:50,000 (259). Although skin depigmentation is not a feature of OA, giant melanosomes (macromelanosomes) are characteristically found in skin melanocytes and RPE and are suggestive of defective melanosomal synthesis (158,335,418,537). Isolated in 1995, the gene for ocular albinism, *OA1* (35) is expressed temporally and spatially in parallel to *TYR* during development and encodes a G protein-coupled receptor that localizes exclusively to the melanosomal membrane (418). Current evidence suggests that the OA1 protein regulates signals from the melanosomal lumen to the cytosol leading to the proper formation of the melanosome (418). How mutations in *OA1* lead to reduced vision and misrouting of the optic pathways remains to be elucidated.

Clinically, OA1 can appear identical to OCA forms that show only mild reductions in skin pigmentation. Family history may reveal the true type of albinism. However, in the absence of affected relatives, examination of an affected boy's mother can help differentiate OA from OCA. Carriers of OA may show a mud-splattered fundus or tigroid appearance (92%) with anomalous iris transillumination (74% of those with a mud splattered fundus appearance) and macromelanosomes on skin biopsy (84%) (75).

Aniridia

Aniridia (MIM #106200) is a rare panocular disorder with a population frequency ranging from approximately 1 in 60,000 to 100,000 (379). It is characterized by iris and ciliary body hypoplasia (Fig. 18) (312), keratopathy (335,348), cataracts (congenital or progressive) with nuclear and peripheral degeneration (238,302,312,348,417), glaucoma from angle closure secondary to peripheral anterior synechiae (302,312,348), mild optic disc hypoplasia (85,348), and pendular nystagmus with macular hypoplasia (348). Visual acuity is reduced at birth, mainly from macular hypoplasia, but can diminish further over time from glaucoma, keratopathy and cataract formation. The extreme phenotypic variability indicates that aniridia is likely more common than initially thought, with some aniridics demonstrating mild to no iris hypoplasia (Fig. 19) (104,191,335).

Aniridia is caused by mutations in the *PAX6* gene (489). Haploinsufficiency from inactivation of one of the copies of the gene has been shown to cause the disease (379). The condition is familial in about two-thirds of cases and sporadic in the remaining third. The mode of inheritance is autosomal dominant with typically high penetrance and variable expressivity (191,379). Sporadic cases have a 30% chance of developing Wilms tumor in the first 5 years of life (150,210,332) as a result of contiguous deletions encompassing both *PAX6* and *WT1* genes. This mutation is frequently observed with WAGR syndrome (Wilms tumor aniridia-gonadoblastoma-mental retardation, MIM #194072) (15,32,277,312,318,348). Conversely, 1–3% of patients with Wilms tumor have aniridia. This relationship of this neoplasm with aniridia has also been reported in the familial, autosomal dominant mode of inheritance (242,262). A simple test for hemizygosity (only one allele present with deletion of the other) consisting of genotyping using highly polymorphic markers spanning the *PAX6-WT1* region can be performed in cases at risk (180).

The iris may demonstrate a variety of morphological changes that include: stumps of iris occluding the anterior chamber angle (although Schlemm canal can be identified), mesenchymal tissue extending

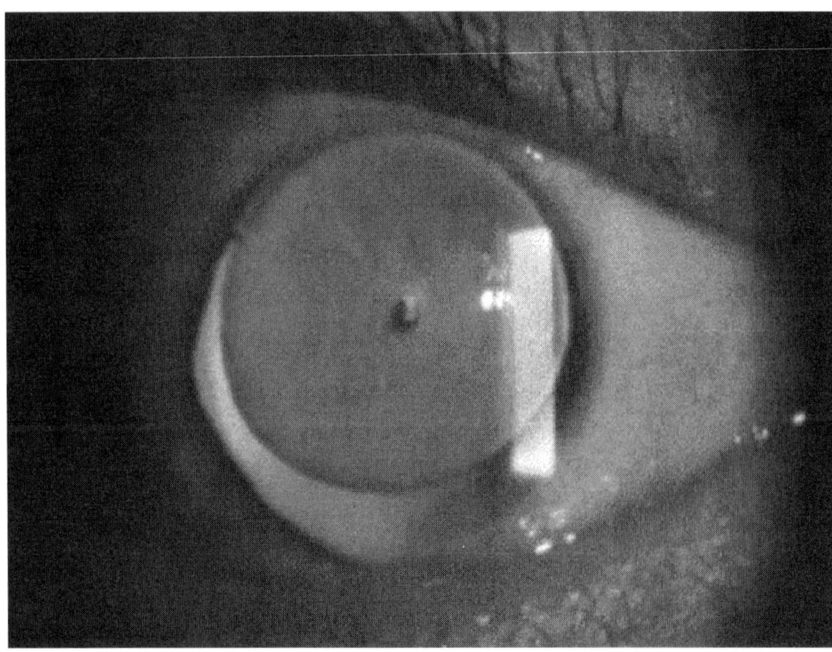

Figure 18 Classic aniridia. No iris is visible on slit-lamp biomicroscopy. A small central lens opacity was present at birth.

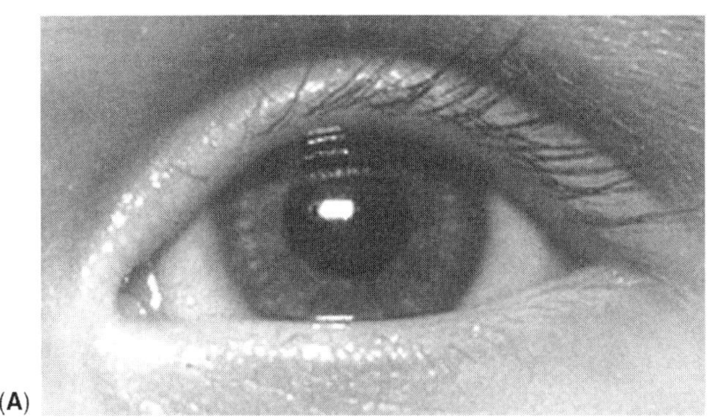

(A)

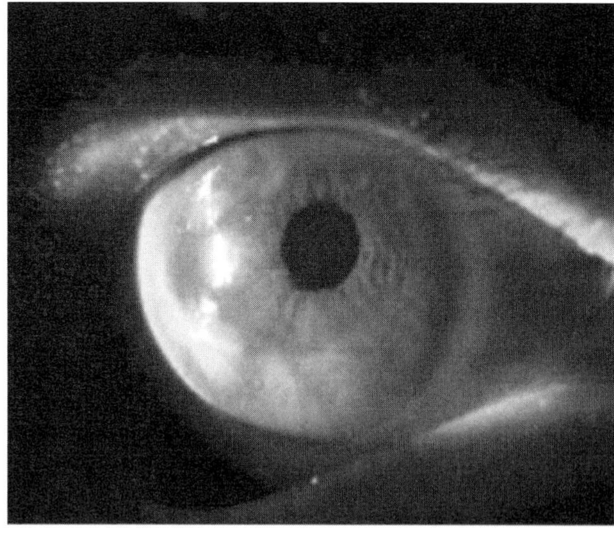

(B)

Figure 19 Aniridia. Phenotypic variability is illustrated by this family with a known *PAX6* mutation. (**A**) The 9-year-old son had congenital nystagmus with macular hypoplasia, a nearly flat electroretinogram, poor vision and a mild corneal pannus but only subtle iris hypoplasia. (**B**) The mother had a history of congenital nystagmus and severe asymmetrical keratopathy but normal irides. *Source*: Courtesy of Drs. I. De Becker and L.-P. Noel.

backward and curving around the pigment layer of the dwarf iris and blood vessels ramifying on the pigmented layer of the iris, blocking further iris growth.

The cornea in aniridia is often clear at birth, with decompensation starting in the teenage years as a result of congenital limbal stem cell deficiency (124,312,353,384). Early changes include ingrowth of blood vessels into the peripheral cornea, with eventual obstruction of the visual axis. Associated changes include the presence of goblet cells in the corneal epithelium (348,353,384), superficial stromal neovascularization, infiltration of the stroma with inflammatory cells and destruction of Bowman layer (312,384). Transplantation of corneal limbal stem cells has been attempted (213), although the long-term results remain poor (384,486).

Glaucoma occurs in 50% to 75% of cases from abnormal differentiation of the trabecular meshwork with or without absence of Schlemm canal (97,348). Electroretinography reveals that most aniridia patients have significantly reduced rod and cone responses, although the range of reduction is wide. The cause of this abnormality remains unknown (499).

Extraocular manifestations have recently come to light, mainly through clues obtained from mouse studies (190). Previously overlooked, impaired olfaction was identified in all but one of 14 aniridia patients tested, with a wide range of defects (443). Also, brain magnetic resonance imaging (MRI) in aniridia has demonstrated a range of anomalies, the significance of which remains unclear (151,443).

Norrie Disease

ND (MIM #310600) is an X-linked recessive disorder characterized by a triad of retinal fibrovascular proliferation (pseudoglioma) and/or retinal dysplasia at birth in all cases, progressive hearing loss by the second decade (40%) and variable mental retardation (50%) (396,515,517). The classic ocular manifestations of ND include a retrolental fibrovascular mass with posterior synechiae, cataract and shallow anterior chamber. Systemic signs of ND usually appear in the first two decades of life.

ND is primarily a disease of abnormal retinal vascular development with ensuing complications. A histopathological study of an 11-week fetus with ND failed to show any abnormality of the ocular structures (369), in keeping with the concept of an abnormality in retinal vascularization, which occurs later than 11 weeks. Reported pathological anomalies include loss of retinal ganglion cells and retinal capillaries, hypoplasia and disorganization of the inner nuclear layers, deposition of hyaline material, vacuolation of the outer nuclear layer and photoreceptors with absence of photoreceptor outer segments (423), severe gliosis and cysts, and compact lamellar bone formation (329). Retinal folding and detachment, a mixture of fibrovascular tissue and retina in the vitreous, microphthalmia and rosettes of immature retinal cells within vascular connective tissue of hyperplastic primary vitreous have also been described (423,516). In a tissue biopsy from a 6-month-old male with bilateral retrolental membranes, retinal neurons were well differentiated with the expression of neuron-specific enolase, and proliferating cells were present in the vitreous while the retina failed to demonstrate proliferative activity (423). Two reports have identified peripheral venous insufficiency associated with ND (329,390).

ND is caused by mutations in the *NDP* gene. X-linked recessive familial exudative vitreoretinopathy (FEVR type 2) (EVR2, MIM #305390) and ND are allelic (323), with significant overlap in the phenotypic appearance. Although ND is commonly described as manifesting a worse phenotype than FEVR, the variability demonstrated through clinical and molecular analyses of large pedigrees with X-linked recessive inheritance of ocular anomalies (9,396,552) and review of pedigrees with autosomal dominant FEVR (9) suggest that diagnostic categorization based on severity of eye findings alone is artificial. Interestingly, mutations in *NDP* have been implicated in Coats disease (48) and retinopathy of prematurity (ROP) (185,207,428,476), two conditions that also show phenotypic overlap with ND and FEVR. Using mouse models, the histopathological anomalies support the hypothesis that Norrin, the protein encoded by *NDP*, and the Norrin-FZD4 pathway play a crucial role in hyaloid regression (296) and angiogenesis during retinal vascular development (296,359,540). Mutations in *FZD4* causing FEVR type 1 (EVR1, MIM #133780) (400) and the gene for its co-receptor, *LRP5* causing FEVR type 4 (EVR4, MIM #601813) (491), have been shown to cause autosomal dominant FEVR and autosomal dominant and recessive FEVR, respectively and both gene products are part of the same developmental pathway, with direct interactions between Norrin, FZD4 and LRP5 (540).

ENVIRONMENTAL EMBRYOPATHIES

Congenital Rubella

Congenital cataracts were the first manifestation of congenital rubella reported by Gregg, following a particularly severe rubella epidemic in Australia in 1941 (174). At the time, the cause of the outbreak of these peculiar cataracts, which involved all but the outermost layers of the lens, was unknown but consultation with colleagues revealed several other cases. Soon it became apparent that the cataracts were associated with heart defects. When Gregg heard two parents discussing the rubella infection they had contracted during the pregnancy, he checked for a history of maternal rubella in the rest of the cases and the association became apparent (524). Vaccination became available only after the mid-1960s epidemic in Europe and the United States that left 30,000 children born with rubella-associated defects. Since the introduction of widespread vaccination in developed countries, the incidence of congenital rubella has fallen dramatically. However, the duration of protection can be variable and a small percentage of those vaccinated show little to no immunity to rubella (20,524). In developing countries, the prevalence of congenital rubella syndrome continues to be significant with 100,000 cases yearly (539).

The risk of fetal infection depends upon the gestational age of the fetus at the time of maternal infection. Fetal infection occurs in 81% of infants exposed in the first trimester. Interestingly, the rate of fetal infection declines during the second trimester to 25% at 23 to 26 weeks gestation but then increases gradually to 100% by 36 weeks to term (524). The development of specific congenital malformations also depends on the timing of maternal rubella infection with respect to the gestational age of the fetus. Infection within the first 16 weeks of gestation commonly causes central or nuclear cataracts (Fig. 20), retinopathy, deafness, cardiovascular malformations (especially patent ductus arteriosus), and neurological damage with microcephaly, mental retardation and spastic diplegia. These manifestations are rare with infection occurring after that period. This reduced susceptibility in the second trimester is possibly related to the development of the fetal immune response and transfer of maternal immunoglobulin G (IgG) through the placenta, although the virus can still be cultured from most organs in neonates (524).

The period of susceptibility to the development of cataract is confined to exposure between days 12 and 43 of gestation (524). Retention of nuclei in lens fibers is characteristic of congenital rubella infection (524). Infected lenses show pyknotic nuclei, cytoplasmic vacuoles and inclusion bodies in the primary lens fibers (90,490) and nuclear necrosis in neonates (52,474). Late changes include signs of active infection in the developing lens fibers (524). Cataracts have been described as nuclear, lamellar, membranous, or mature and are often bilateral (427). The virus can continue to accumulate in the lens and can persist for up to three years (327).

Other ocular manifestations include focal injury to the RPE (Fig. 20), necrosis of the ciliary body and iris, central corneal opacities, microphthalmia, retinopathy (described as "salt and pepper") and glaucoma (52,111,165,510). The susceptibility period for the last two manifestations is longer than for cataract (2 to 117 days gestation) (503). Retinitis and late onset retinal vasculitis have been documented (269,394).

Thalidomide

The thalidomide story illustrates a number of important points in the effort to establish that an agent is teratogenic. In the early 1960s a number of infants, first in Germany and then elsewhere (252), were born with phocomelia, a rare congenital anomaly of absent

(A)
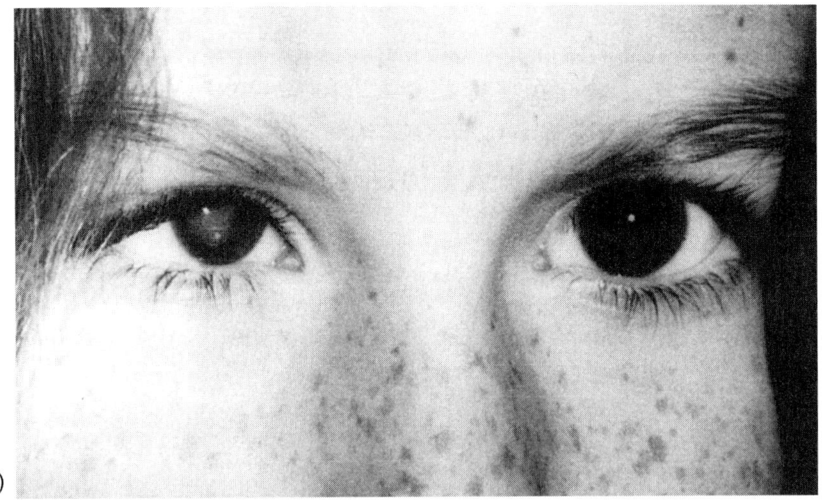

(B)
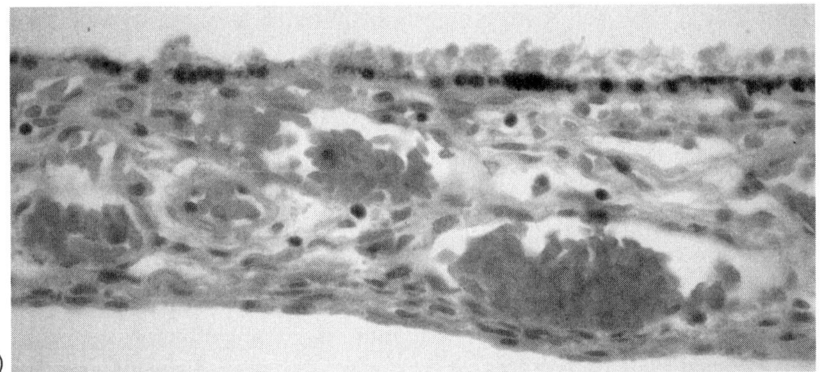

(C)
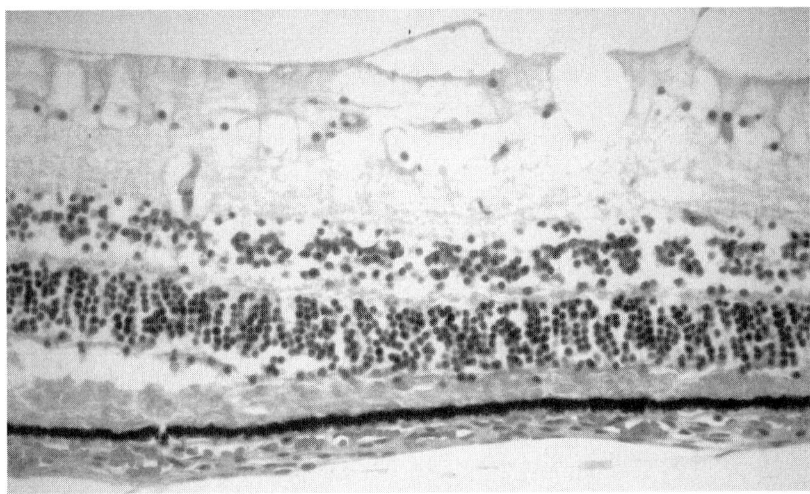

Figure 20 Congenital rubella syndrome. (**A**) Although normal at birth, the eye grew more slowly and the cataract developed by 10 years of age. Histopathological examination of an infant's eye reveals patchy depigmentation of the retinal pigment epithelium at the posterior pole (**B**) compared with the equator (**C**) [hematoxylin and eosin, (**B**) ×350; (**C**) ×200].

or limited limb development (284). Epidemiological studies implicated a recently released sedative, thalidomide. Maternal ingestion of thalidomide between the 27th and 40th day of gestation resulted in complete or partial phocomelia in 20% of the offspring (252). Other defects such as ear anomalies occurred if the drug had been ingested between the 21st and 27th day. Pre-market testing of thalidomide in rats and mice did not reveal the teratogenic potency and it was later learned that rodents are relatively undisturbed by this teratogen. Had rabbits or monkeys been used, the teratogenic potential would have been unmasked. This experience illustrates that the same defect is produced in those exposed to a particular teratogen, that a critical period of susceptibility is present, that there is species variability in response to a teratogen and that the individual ability to withstand the effects of the teratogen is remarkable (430). These principles are paramount to the understanding of teratogenesis and must be considered when any agent is implicated as a possible teratogen. Thalidomide-induced ocular defects were only occasionally found but included microphthalmos, anophthalmos, buphthalmos, lens anomalies, colobomas, disturbances of ocular motility, gaze paresis, facial palsy, and 'crocodile' tears (95,161,284,333,468,553).

Fetal Alcohol Syndrome

In contrast to the detailed and rapidly completed epidemiological studies prompted by the severe and unusual teratogenic effect of thalidomide, many years were required to uncover the teratogenic potential of maternal alcohol ingestion. Although alcohol was suspected as a teratogen almost a century ago (456), it was only in 1968 that Lemoine first described the characteristic findings of the fetal alcohol syndrome (283). The results of his study have been widely confirmed, and it is now recognized that the fetal alcohol syndrome is one of the most widespread teratogenetic disorders. The prevalence of fetal alcohol syndrome and alcohol-related neurodevelopmental disorders is highly variable worldwide. In Japan, the frequency is among the lowest at 1 in 10,000 live births (477), whereas in the Western world, various reports have estimated roughly 9 cases per 1000 live births (300,409). One survey in British Columbia, Canada, disclosed that 190 of 1000 children aged 1 to 18 years were affected in an American Indian community (399) and another in a South African community reported 65 to 74 cases per 1000 primary grade children (511). The mechanisms by which alcohol injures the eyes and visual system remain poorly understood and little is known about the minimum dose required to produce damage. A genetic predisposition to susceptibility to the teratogenic effects has been proposed (469).

A characteristic craniofacial dysmorphism is seen in all patients with the full blown syndrome and partially in those who are less affected (23). The features include short palpebral fissures in 80% of those affected, short up-turned nose, hypoplastic philtrum with thin upper vermillion border of the lip, retrognathia and micrognathia in infancy (283,464). The facial appearance is only mildly modified by a relative prognathism as the infant grows into adulthood. Mental retardation is one of the most prominent and serious manifestations of the syndrome. Affected persons test lower than two standard deviations below the mean on intelligence tests; only occasionally does an affected person have an average or better than average mental ability. Pathological studies demonstrate a variety of alterations in the brain; the most common are cerebellar dysplasias, heterotopic cell clusters on the brain surface, failure or interruption of neuronal and glial migration, microcephaly and hydrocephalus (316). Behavioral features include irritability, hypotonia, hyperactivity, and poor coordination. The infants are small at birth and the low weight and short stature continue throughout life. Affected individuals have a diminished amount of adipose tissue.

All parts of the eyes can be affected. Ocular findings most commonly reported are short palpebral fissures (80%), optic nerve hypoplasia (48%) and tortuosity of retinal vessels (49%) (469). Other features include poor vision, ptosis, telecanthus, epicanthal folds, blepharophimosis, esotropia, microphthalmia, microcornea, Peters anomaly, cataract, PHPV, iris and chorioretinal coloboma, retinal dysplasia, and refractive errors (464,466,467,469).

DEVELOPMENTAL ANOMALIES OF SPECIFIC OCULAR STRUCTURES

Anterior Segment

Corneoscleral Limbus

Choristomas make up 22% of epibulbar tumors in children (96). Limbal dermoids are white-tan, firm, usually solitary nodules in the lower temporal quadrant (Fig. 21). Beneath a keratinized stratified squamous epithelium, there is a mound of dense collagen that contains adipose tissue and sweat glands, as well as hair follicles and sebaceous glands. Occasionally, cartilage or bone (Fig. 21) may be present. Lacrimal gland tissue may be seen with a variety of mesenchymal elements in complex choristomas and these are generally more tan in color and located in the supero-temporal quadrant (13).

Cornea

Abnormalities of Size

With a lower limit of normal of 11.0 mm in men and 10.7 mm in women for "white-to-white" horizontal corneal diameter (402), microcornea (Fig. 22) has usually been defined by a horizontal diameter of <10.5 mm (527). Although it is often associated with microphthalmos (526) or other anterior segment abnormalities (406), this is not always the case and it has also been associated with macrophthalmos in the rare colobomatous macrophthalmia with microcornea syndrome (MIM %602499) (368,487). The failure of corneal growth, reflecting overgrowth of the tips of the optic cup, is generally not accompanied by abnormal histogenesis, although Inoue et al. (224) described an abnormal ultrastructure of Descemet membrane in a 10-year-old boy with microcornea complicated by bullous keratopathy. Microcornea is commonly found with glaucoma, cataract (406) and hyperopia (527) and myopia has also been described (448).

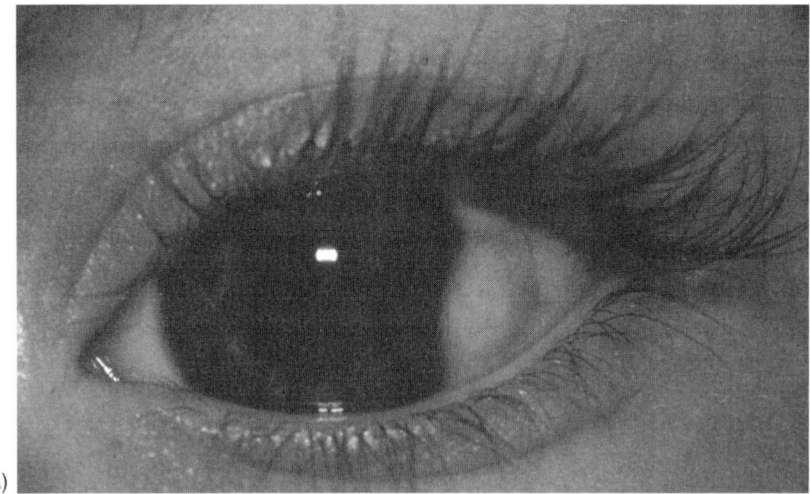

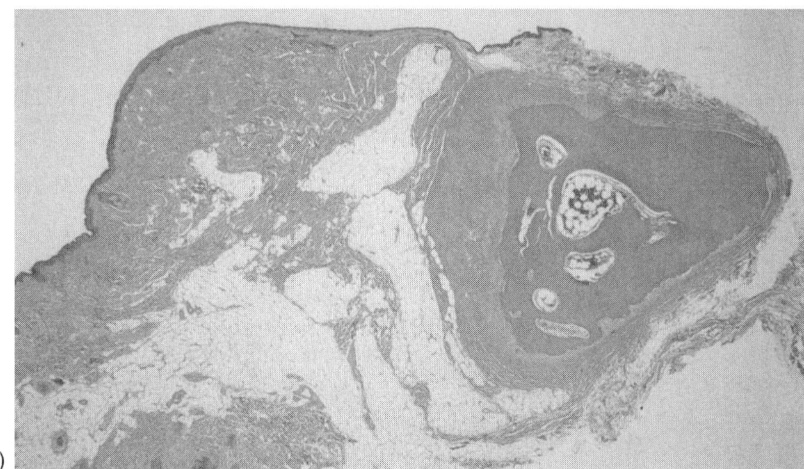

Figure 21 Epibulbar choristoma. (**A**) White nodule at infero-temporal limbus in an infant with Goldenhar syndrome. *Source*: Courtesy of Dr. R.B. Orton. (**B**) Osseous choristoma (hematoxylin and eosin, ×14).

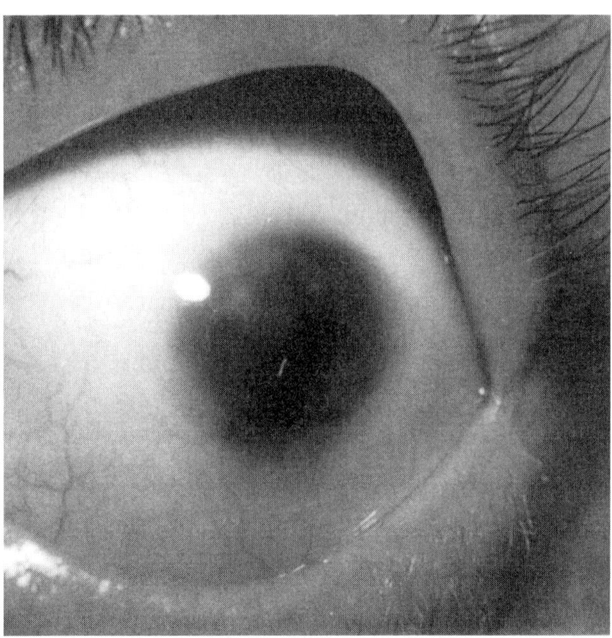

Figure 22 Microcornea illustrating a smaller than normal cornea.

Microcornea may occur sporadically or be inherited in an autosomal dominant or recessive manner. Increasingly, a variety of syndromes of which it is a part are being characterized. Thus, autosomal dominant congenital cataract and microcornea have been associated with missense mutations in the *GJA8* gene, which encodes connexin-50 (115). Jamieson et al. (229) identified a mutation in the DNA-binding domain of the transcription factor MAF in three generations of a family with cataract of early onset and variable microcornea. *MAF* is known to have a role in lens development and may be implicated in anterior segment morphogenesis. Crystallin genes have also been implicated in cataract-microcornea syndromes. Willoughby et al. (532) reported a mutation in the *CRYBB1* gene that is predicted to elongate the COOH-terminal extension of the protein and disrupt β-crystallin interactions. Vanita et al. (507), studying a large Indian family, found a novel fan-shaped cataract associated with microcornea to be caused by a mutation in the αA-crystallin gene *CRYAA*. Autosomal dominant microcornea is also associated with cataract in the microcornea, rod-cone

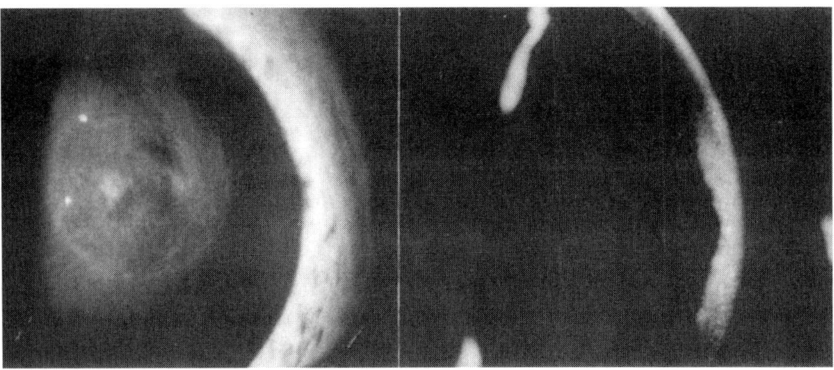

Figure 23 Posterior keratoconus. Amblyopic eye of 45-year-old man. *Left*: Central opacified ring. *Right*: Stromal whitening and posterior excavation of central opacity to right, iris at left. *Source*: Courtesy of Dr. M. Mets.

dystrophy, cataract and posterior staphyloma syndrome (MRCS), which has been linked to a region on chromosome 11 (11q13) close to the nanophthalmos locus (388). Mutations in the *VMD2* gene have been identified in some, but not all, cases of this syndrome (330). Ramprasad et al. (385) have reported a truncating mutation in the *NHS* gene in a four-generation family with Nance-Horan syndrome (MIM #302350), an inherited x-linked developmental lens opacity and microcornea. Little is known about the function of this gene, except that it encodes a protein containing four conserved nuclear localization signals.

In megalocornea, the horizontal corneal diameter is >13 mm but a definitive diagnosis can only be reached after the age of one year when the cornea has reached its adult size. The abnormality results from a failure of the rim of the optic cup to bend towards the axis of the eye and the anterior segment enlarges. Megalocornea is usually bilateral but, when associated with congenital glaucoma, may be unilateral. Congenital glaucoma may be distinguished from primary megalocornea by the elevated intraocular pressure and the presence of breaks in Descemet membrane (211). X-linked megalocornea (MIM %309300) has been mapped to Xq21.3–q22 (77). Megalocornea may be inherited in autosomal recessive manner in association with mental retardation in Neuhauser syndrome (MIM %249310) (109,154,311).

Abnormalities of Shape

Cornea plana refers to flattening of the cornea with a reduction in refractive power. The autosomal dominant form (MIM %121400) is mild but the autosomal recessive form (MIM #217300) is more severe and accompanied by a central corneal opacity and scleralization of the peripheral cornea (147). Both types are linked to overlapping regions of chromosome 12 (12q22) and mutations in the *KERA* gene have been described in the recessive form (127). This gene encodes the protein core of keratocan, a major corneal keratan sulfate proteoglycan that contributes to the regular spacing of collagen fibers within the stroma and appears to have a role in the determination of corneal shape (127).

Posterior keratoconus is characterized by circumscribed thinning of the posterior corneal stroma with a normal anterior surface (Fig. 23). The condition may be unilateral or bilateral and may become manifest before the sixth month of gestation (268). The disorder may coexist with other ocular anomalies (462). Heon et al. (203) found mutations in the *VSX1* gene (visual system homeobox 1) in Canadian patients affected by either anterior keratoconus or posterior polymorphous corneal dystrophy. The involvement of the *VSX1* gene in inherited keratoconus has been confirmed by Bisceglia et al. (46) in a series of unrelated Italian patients.

Anterior Chamber

Since 1920, when Axenfeld described a thickening of the Schwalbe line, many anomalies of the anterior segment have been reported under a variety of different names, such as Axenfeld syndrome, Rieger anomaly, mesodermal dysgenesis, anterior chamber cleavage syndrome and iridogoniodysgenesis (113,175,389,431,432,433). Since these can occur singly or in virtually any combination, the terms Axenfeld-Rieger syndrome (433) or anterior segment dysgenesis (ASD) *(222)* are now commonly used to include the whole spectrum of malformations of the anterior segment (Table 2) (Fig. 24), most of which reflect abnormal growth and distribution of neural crest mesenchyme. Tissues of ectodermal (corneal and lenticular epithelium) and neuroectodermal (iris musculature and pigment epithelium) are also involved.

The phenotypic expression of anterior segment dysgenesis ranges from a simple thickening of the Schwalbe line (Fig. 25), otherwise known as posterior embryotoxon, to extensive disorganization of the anterior segment (Fig. 26) (431,433,534). The eyes of one individual may differ markedly in the degree of disorganization and phenotypic variation in a family

Table 2 Morphological Abnormalities in Anterior Segment Dysgenesis

Anomaly	Specific name	Refs.
Prominent Schwalbe ring	Posterior embryotoxon	
Strands from Schwalbe line to iris	Axenfeld anomaly	
Iris hypoplasia	Rieger anomaly	370
Congenital ectropion iridis		156,534
Polycoria and corectopia	Rieger anomaly	
Abnormal angle structure	Iridogoniodysgenesis	273,432
Posterior keratoconus		268,462
Focal absence of Descemet/endothelial complex with central corneal opacity, adhesion to cataractous lens, and adhesion to iris	Leukoma, Peters anomaly, von Hippel internal ulcer	268,458,494,495

is common (Fig. 27) (64,278,406). Infantile glaucoma is commonly present (110,273,389,432,522) but anomalies of the posterior segment, although occasionally present (459), are not constant features. Systemic features include dental abnormalities, cleft lip/palate and facial dysmorphism, in keeping with a neurocristopathy, as well as cardiac, otological and other abnormalities (67,222,366).

Although the pathogenesis of Axenfeld–Rieger syndrome remains poorly understood, Shields and colleagues postulated developmental arrest as the basic mechanism (431–433). Late in gestation, a layer of endothelial cells of neural crest origin, normally covering or involved in the development of portions of the iris and anterior chamber angle, fails to regress. Some cells lay down abnormal basement membrane material and others crossing the anterior chamber fail to regress completely, leaving residual strands of iridic tissue within the angle. Environmental agents, such as ochratoxin A (435) and alcohol (469), have been shown to produce anterior segment malformations but their mechanism of action is unknown. Isotretinoin has been shown to produce keratolenticular adhesion (Peters anomaly) in rodents (88,89). Histologically, the ectodermal stalk from the corneal surface epithelium to the lens fails to disintegrate and thus prevents complete migration of neural crest cells into the central cornea. These effects are mediated in part by a delayed production of ECM macromolecules, including laminin and fibronectin (88,89). The importance of the interactions of the periocular (neural crest) mesenchymal cells with matrix components and cytokines in anterior segment development has become increasingly apparent (392) and Peters anomaly (Fig. 28) illustrates the importance of the Descemet membrane/endothelial complex in the histogenesis of the corneal stroma. Inactivation of the genes for collagen type VIII in mice (*Col8a1*, *Col8a2*) leads to malformations of the anterior segment including hypoplasia of the corneal stroma, thinning of Descemet membrane and keratoglobus. It has been suggested that collagen type VIII may provide a substrate for migration of the periocular mesenchymal cells (215).

Chromosomal aberrations have been described in cases of ASD. Several have been linked to Peters anomaly (MIM #604229) (260), including ring chromosome 21 (83), partial trisomy 16q (139), the 18q- syndrome, chromosome 13 deletion syndrome (453) and occasionally deletion of 4p16 (Wolf–Hirschhorn syndrome, MIM #194190) (267). However, in a series of 37 patients with this anomaly, many of whom also had systemic anomalies, none of the 34 patients tested had an abnormal karyotype (366). ASD has been described in association with duplication of chromosome 2p21–2p25 (200), a region that includes a locus (GLC3A) for primary congenital glaucoma (457).

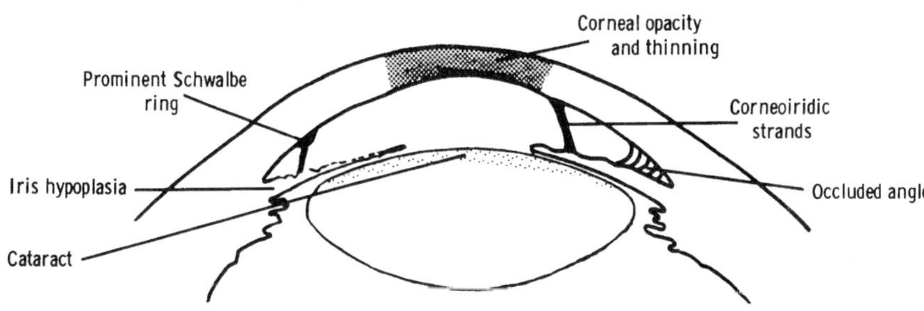

Figure 24 Composite diagram of developmental anomalies encountered in the anterior chamber. *Source*: Courtesy of Dr. J. Mullancy.

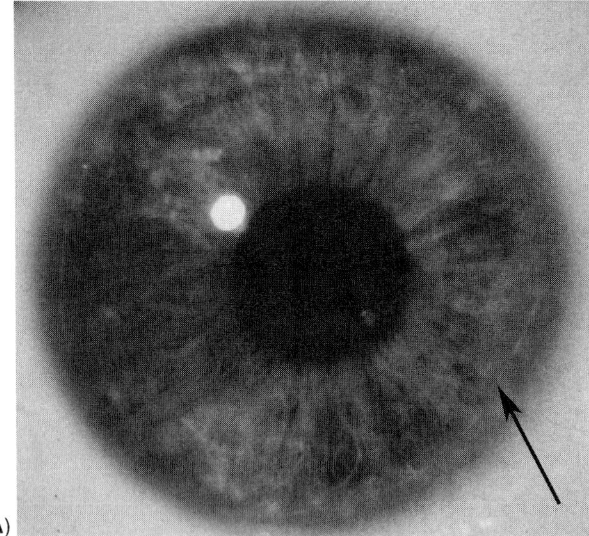

(A)

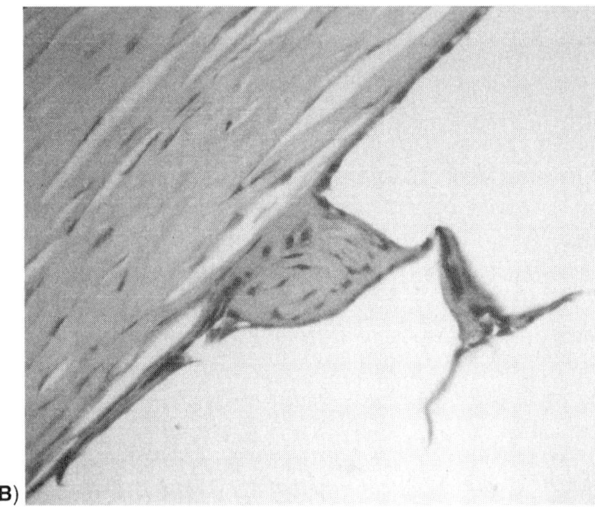

(B)

Figure 25 Schwalbe line. (**A**) A circumferential ring (*arrow*) internal to the corneoscleral limbus is seen through the cornea. (**B**) Prominent mass of connective tissue at terminus of Descemet membrane (hematoxylin and eosin, ×200).

The introduction of fluorescent in situ hydridization and molecular genotyping has allowed the characterization of subtle chromosomal aberrations, as well as mutations, in genes that appear to be important in anterior segment development, many of which encode transcription factors [reviewed in Refs. (97,171)]. Mutations in the *FOXC1* and *PITX2* genes have been identified in 15/19 (79%) patients from 13 families with ASD in a study from Germany (528). The *PITX2* gene is located on chromosome 4 (4q25). The protein belongs to the paired-bicoid family of homeodomain transcription factors and is involved in the differentiation of the ocular mesenchyme, the dental lamina, and the umbilical cord (426). Microdeletions or mutations in *PITX2* have been detected in about 10% of cases of ASD (289). The *FOXC1* gene, located on chromosome 6p25, also encodes a transcription factor. Autosomal dominant iris hypoplasia with early onset glaucoma (familial glaucoma iridogoniodysplasia, MIM #137750) has been associated with duplication of the 6p25 region and other abnormalities of ASD have been linked to a microdeletion in this region (281). Mutations in the transcription factor gene *PITX3* have also been described in cases of ASD in association with posterior polar cataract (2). Additionally, there are reports providing evidence that the *MAF* gene and the *PAX6* gene may be involved in Axenfeld–Rieger syndrome (230,395). Chavarria-Soley et al. (76) have detected causative mutations in the *CYP1B1* gene in individuals suffering from Rieger anomaly. Since mutations in *CYP1B1* are responsible for ~80% of the familial cases of primary congenital glaucoma (412), Chavarria-Soley et al. (76) suggest that anterior segment disorders and primary congenital glaucoma may share a common molecular pathophysiology through this pathway.

Lens

Abnormalities of Formation

Congenital aphakia, the absence of a lens, is rare and may be primary or secondary. Primary congenital aphakia (MIM #610256) occurs when the lens placode fails to form and the lens does not develop; it is accompanied by a complete failure of anterior segment development, such that the iris, outflow tract and ciliary apparatus are also absent. However in a series of human embryos with rubella or parvovirus B19 infection, there was some degree of anterior segment formation (196). Primary congenital aphakia has been linked to a nonsense mutation in the *FOXE3* gene. The expression of this gene is restricted to pre-lenticular and lenticular tissue and in this family the aphakia was, as might be expected, unaccompanied by systemic anomalies (505). In secondary congenital aphakia, the lens is formed to some degree but subsequently resorbed; variable degrees of ASD occur. Reduplication of the lens, biphakia, has also been reported (177). In this case, two well-formed clear lenses lay in the coronal plane behind a large cornea.

Ectopia lentis is often related to defective formation of the zonules (347) and is often bilateral and associated with ectopic pupils (MIM #225200) (167). It occurs in a variety of syndromes, including Marfan syndrome (MIM #154700) (347), autosomal recessive Weill–Marchesani syndrome (MIM #277600), autosomal dominant Weill–Marchesani syndrome (MIM #608328) (551) and Ehlers–Danlos syndrome type I (MIM #130000) (347); it may also occur as an isolated dominant trait (isolated ectopia lentis, MIM

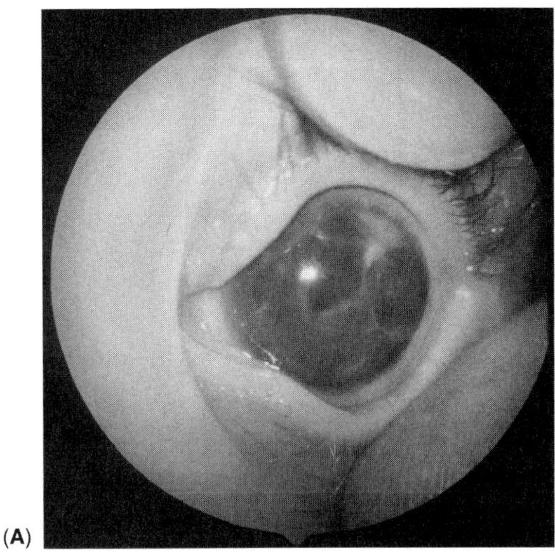
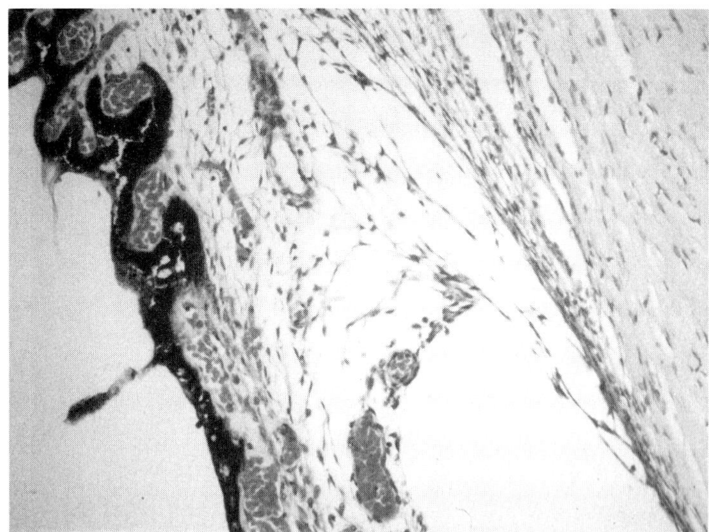

Figure 26 Anterior segment dysgenesis. (**A**) Eye with microcornea, iris stromal hypoplasia, corectopia and central corneal opacification. *Source*: Courtesy of Dr. G.R. LaRoche. (**B**) Mesenchymal strands extend across anterior chamber angle (hematoxylin and eosin, ×150).

#129600) (232). The lens may not become dislocated until the second decade or later (37,347).

Abnormalities of Shape and Size

Microspherophakia refers to a lens that is smaller and more spherical than normal and the condition is usually bilateral. With an increase in antero-posterior dimension, the lens may be closely apposed to the cornea. Microspherophakia may occur as an isolated anomaly and is usually explained by an arrest in lens development at about the fifth month of gestation when the lens is normally spherical. Actinomycin D administered to pregnant rats can produce microphakia in the offspring (501).

In Weill–Marchesani syndrome microspherophakia and ectopia lentis are associated with short stature, joint stiffness and brachydactyly. Although clinically homogeneous, the condition may be inherited in either an autosomal recessive or dominant manner. The dominant form (MIM #608328) has been linked to a deletion in the *FBN1* gene that encodes fibrillin-1 (133) and the recessive form (MIM #277600) has been linked to mutations in the *ADAMTS10* gene, which encodes a metalloprotease involved in connective tissue remodeling (99).

Anterior lenticonus is usually an isolated bilateral anomaly that predominantly affects males and may be inherited as an autosomal recessive trait. The anterior surface of the lens displays a conical projection that causes high myopia and is associated with lens opacities. Anterior lenticonus is pathognomonic of Alport syndrome in which the anterior lens capsule is unusually thin. Based on the mode of inheritance three types of Alport syndrome are recognized: autosomal dominant Alport syndrome (MIM %104200), X-linked recessive Alport syndrome (MIM #301050) and autosomal recessive Alport syndrome (MIM #203780). In one study, absence of collagen type IV α_3–$\alpha_6$chains was accompanied by a mutation in the *COL4A5* gene which encodes part of the α_5(IV) polypeptide (358). Posterior lenticonus is more frequent than anterior lenticonus, is usually a unilateral isolated anomaly and occurs more frequently in females. It may result from central thinning of the posterior lens capsule but this is not proven.

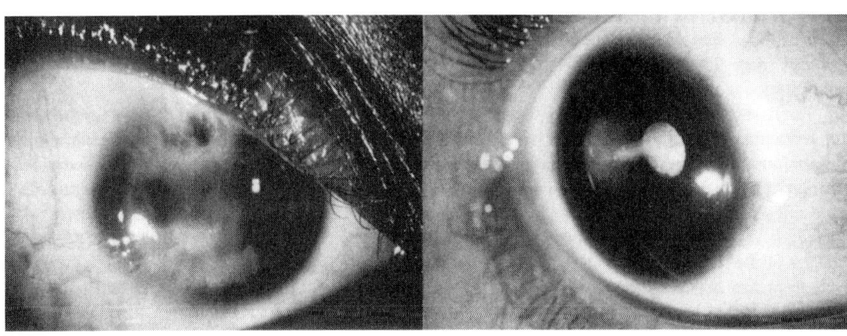

Figure 27 Axenfeld–Rieger syndrome. Familial variation. *Left*: Mother with corneal leukomas and anterior segment dysgenesis. *Right*: Daughter with small corneal leukoma with stalk connected to anterior lens; Peters anomaly.

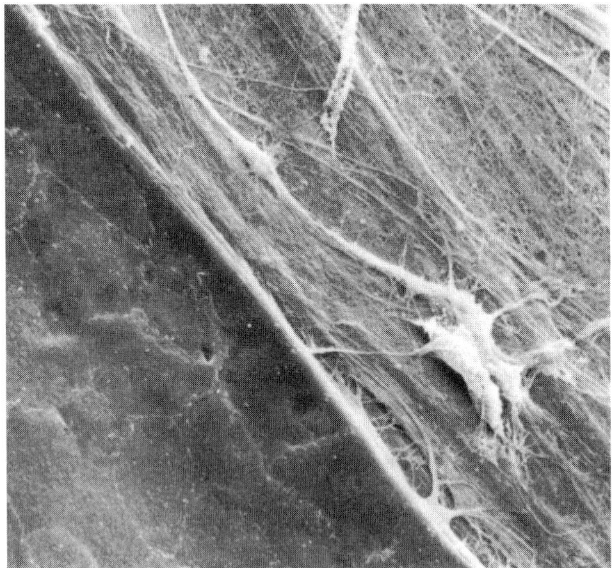

Figure 28 Peters anomaly. Scanning electron micrograph of posterior corneal surface, showing normal endothelial cells on the left. The corneal endothelium and Descemet membrane are missing over a crater in the central cornea (right side) (×900). *Source*: Courtesy of Dr. G.K. Klintworth.

Autosomal dominant inheritance of bilateral posterior lenticonus has been described (421).

Posterior Segment

Vitreous

Persistent Hyperplastic Primary Vitreous

The failure of the primary vitreous to regress is associated with a malformated small eye. The condition known as PHPV is unilateral in 90% of cases with no systemic manifestations. Bilateral cases may be associated with other ocular and systemic anomalies (436). The ocular manifestations may be characterized according to location within the posterior chamber: anterior (25%), posterior (12%) or combined (63%) (436). In the anterior cases, a mass of retrolenticular fibrous tissue is attached to elongated ciliary processes (126) and the iris-lens diaphragm is displaced anteriorly to produce a shallow anterior chamber (Fig. 29). The retrolenticular plaque is associated with a break in the posterior lens capsule and a cataract may form postnatally, suggesting that the tear in the capsule results from organization and contraction of the plaque. In addition to fibrovascular elements, the plaque may contain undifferentiated neural tissue, fat and cartilage (126,303) and the hyaloid artery extends into its posterior aspect. In the purely posterior form of PHPV, the fibrovascular tissue emanates from the optic nerve head, which may be hypoplastic. Foci of glial tissue arising from Müller cells may project into the vitreous (279).

PHPV has been associated with maternal cocaine use (481) and a deficiency of protein C (204). Although not strictly genetic, the condition is a feature of trisomy 13 and has occasionally shown an autosomal dominant pattern of inheritance (288). A study of one consanguineous family with congenital blindness in four generations suggested a linkage of autosomal recessive, non-syndromic PHPV to chromosome 10 (10q11–q21) (250). In certain breeds of dogs it is hereditary (50). Molecular genetic studies in mice have indicated a role for the *Ski* proto-oncogene

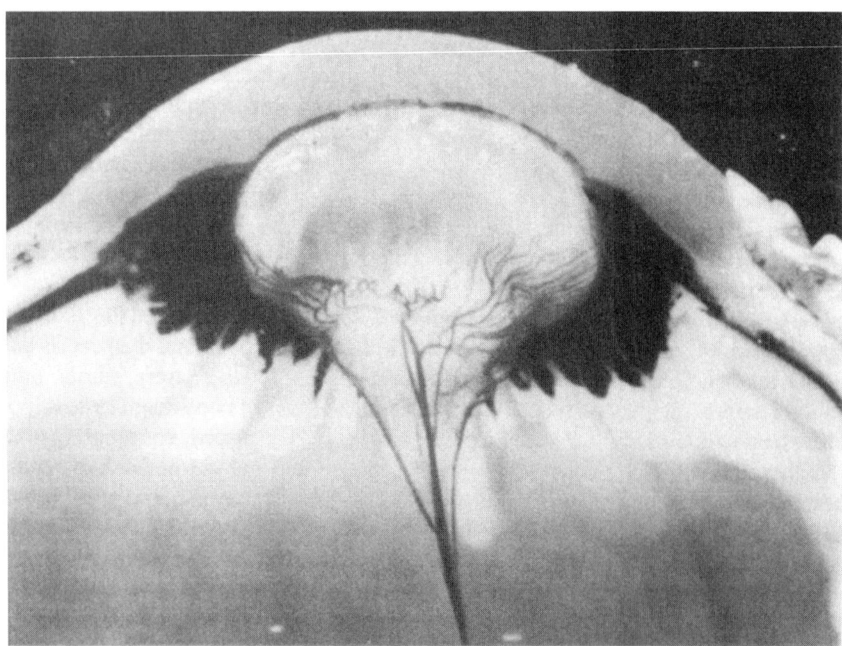

Figure 29 Persistent hyperplastic primary vitreous, showing elongated ciliary processes reaching to the surface of the lens and the persistence of the tunica vasculosa lentis (hematoxylin and eosin, ×10). *Source*: Courtesy of Dr. F. Stefani.

in ocular development. The gene is involved in the regulation of transcription and a null mutation of this gene resulted in PHPV and microphthalmia in 100% of fetuses (320). Mice lacking the *Arf* gene also develop a condition that is identical to PHPV (317). *Arf* encodes a protein that stabilizes p53 and is expressed in the perivascular cells of the developing vitreous. The null mutation appears to interfere with the regression of the normal vitreous vessels, perhaps by inhibiting apoptosis of the endothelial cells, and to predispose to the accumulation of these pericytes on the persistent vascular scaffold.

Miscellaneous Abnormalities

Although the entire hyaloid vascular system is normally resorbed before birth, remnants may be seen. Persistence of the anterior hyaloid system manifests as a small black dot in the red reflex (Mittendorf dot), located slightly infero-nasal to the posterior pole of the lens. A remnant of the posterior hyaloid system on the optic disc is called Bergmeister papilla and includes a segment of the artery surrounded by a glial sheath. Other anomalies include persistent vascular loops (114) and congenital vitreous cysts (290). Cloquet canal normally extends from the patellar fossa, the depression in the anterior vitreous formed by the lens, to the margin of the optic nervehead. An anomalous Cloquet canal, condensed into a vitreous strand and extending to a fine membrane overlying an inferior optic nervehead coloboma, has been described in association with rhegmatogenous retinal detachment in a 10-year-old boy (6). A whiplash motion of the condensed canal on eye movement was thought to have produced a tear in the neurosensory retina adjacent to the optic disc.

Goldberg has attempted to collect many of these anomalies, including classical PHPV, into one entity: persistent fetal vasculature (PFV) (168). These anomalies are commonly associated with a variety of secondary manifestations, such as centrally dragged ciliary processes, cataract and atypical iris colobomas.

Retina

Abnormalities of Formation

Primary retinal aplasia only occurs in true anophthalmos, since the retinal anlage is essential for development of ocular structures, whereas secondary retinal aplasia may result from severe intraocular inflammation in utero. Retinal elements also fail to differentiate when invagination of the optic vesicle fails: in congenital cystic eye the cavity is lined by neuroglial elements (182). Primary generalized hypoplasia of the retina is difficult to identify either clinically or histologically although foveal hypoplasia has been reported (126,361). Secondary hypoplasia may occur in anencephaly, microencephaly and hydranencephaly (305). The axons in the nerve fiber layer form normally but degenerate if they are unable to form synapses in the lateral geniculate body.

Foveal hypoplasia is strongly correlated with optic chiasmal misrouting, i.e., excessive axonal decussation, in albinism (121), although the two anomalies have been identified together in non-albino patients (506). Both appear to result from the effect of abnormal melanin synthesis within the RPE on cell growth in the neural retina (235) and experimental evidence also suggests that local variation in the melanin content of the RPE influences retinal development (162). In aniridia, foveal hypoplasia is not associated with optic chiasmal misrouting (349) and it seems likely, for this reason, and also by virtue of the timing of foveal development, that it is the misrouting that is the primary abnormality in albinism. The projection of retinal ganglion cells appears to be influenced by the winged helix transcription factor Foxd1: in the mouse Foxd1 is only expressed in the ventro-temporal ganglion cells that project ipsilaterally. Foxd1-deficient mice have a higher proportion of fibers that project contralaterally or are arrested in the midline (205).

Retinal Dysgenesis (Dysplasia)

Retinal dysgenesis refers to a heterogeneous group of clinical and histopathological changes caused by abnormal cellular proliferation and stratification within the neurosensory retina (274). It generally occurs in malformed, especially microphthalmic, eyes but may be found as an isolated ocular anomaly, with or without systemic abnormalities (126). Both X-linked recessive and autosomal dominant inheritance have occasionally been described (291). Normal RPE is necessary for the orderly growth and maturation of the retina and experimentally produced separation of the photoreceptor layer and the RPE leads to the formation of rosettes (Fig. 30) (440). Hence, where RPE is lacking or the neural retina is separated from it, dysgenesis can be expected (Fig. 31). In Aicardi syndrome (MIM #304050) dysgenetic retina may overlie foci of attached but unpigmented epithelium (lacunae), as well as areas of apparently normal RPE (4,219). The degree of maturity of the retina seems to be of major importance in its susceptibility to dysgenesis, since these changes do not follow retinal detachment.

Rosettes are the histopathological hallmark of dysgenesis (Fig. 30). They are circular to oval configurations of retinal nuclei and fibrils around a central aperture and the number of layers and degree of differentiation within the rosettes can be variable. Better differentiated rosettes occur in association with systemic abnormalities such as triploidy, trisomy 13, Meckel syndrome (MIM #249000) (299) and Norrie disease (18). Primitive single-layered rosettes are

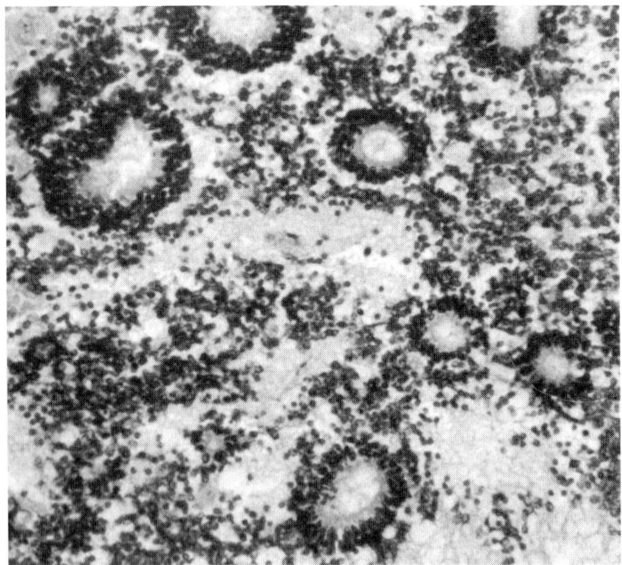

Figure 30 Retinal dysgenesis in trisomy 13. Well formed rosettes are seen in the neurosensory retina (hematoxylin and eosin, ×60).

usually found as isolated abnormalities. Müller cells have been identified in dysgenetic rosettes but not in those of retinoblastoma. The presence of pigment-containing cells in the center of some dysgenetic rosettes has been interpreted as attempted repair involving the phagocytosis of necrotic cell remnants (274). Dysgenetic rosettes are seen in experimental herpetic retinitis, as well as congenital herpetic retinopathy in infants, suggesting that in some circumstances the growth disturbance may reflect the healing of necrotic retina.

A marked reduction in retinal thickness has been noted in cases of retinal dysgenesis produced by certain viruses (7,8) and chemicals (371). In the case of cytosine arabinoside, this is the result of the drug's antimitotic activity (371). Abnormal lamination of the neurosensory retina has been described in *CRB1* mutations (225) that are associated with retinitis pigmentosa and Leber congenital amaurosis. The perifoveal retina was thickened and had a less distinct laminar pattern than normal, possibly as a result of an interruption of the programmed cell death that occurs during normal retinal development.

Sharply demarcated depigmented lesions of different sizes in the peripheral and/or central retina are characteristic features of the microcephaly-lymphedema-chorioretinal dysplasia syndrome (MLCRD, MIM %152950) (69). This condition, which appears to be a composite of a variety of previously recognized microcephaly syndromes (508), is probably inherited in an autosomal dominant manner (287). To date, there have been no reports of the ocular histopathology and the genetic defect is unknown; the karyotype is normal.

Abnormalities of the RPE

The RPE may be absent beneath dysgenetic retina and from large chorioretinal colobomas. Claudin 19 is a tight junction protein involved in electrolyte transport in the renal tubular epithelium and RPE and mutations in the gene (*CLDN19*) are associated with progressive renal dysfunction and macular colobomas (MIM #248190) (265). Bestrophin forms a chloride channel in the basolateral membrane of the RPE cells and is encoded in both developing and adult RPE by the *VMD2* gene. Missense mutations in *VMD2* are responsible for vitelliform macular dystrophy (Best disease, MIM #153700) but other missense mutations that interfere with splicing and result in exon skipping during transcription are linked to an autosomal

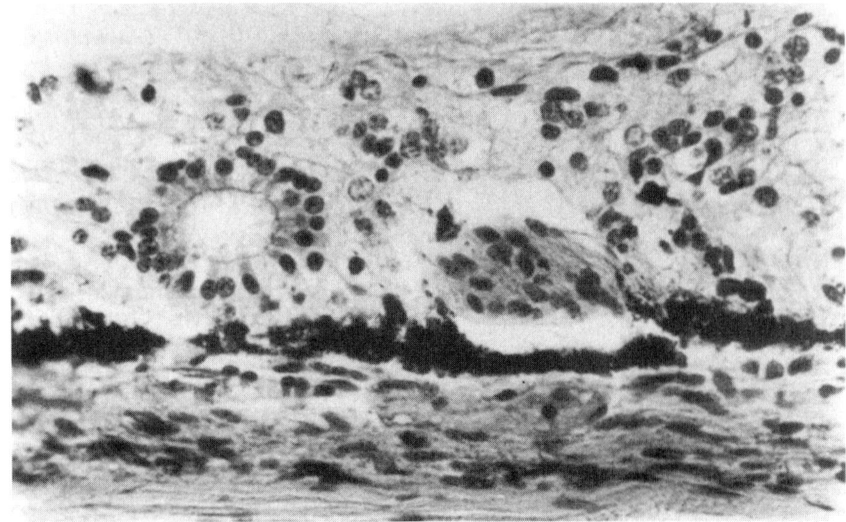

Figure 31 Retinal dysgenesis in Aicardi syndrome. Single-layered rosette in immature retina overlies a partially deficient pigment epithelium (hematoxylin and eosin, ×350). *Source*: Courtesy of Dr. P. Dhermy.

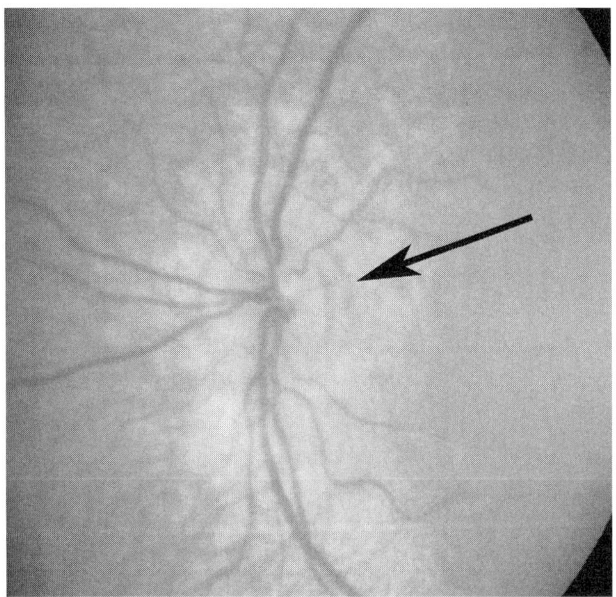

Figure 32 Optic nerve hypoplasia. Double ring sign (*arrow*) is apparent. *Source*: Courtesy of Dr. G.R. LaRoche.

dominant vitreoretinochoroidopathy (MIM #193220) (547). This condition, which is characterized by peripheral circumferential retinal pigmentation anomalies and punctate white retinal opacities, has also been associated with developmental anomalies in some families. With these molecular studies, the boundary between a dystrophy and a dysgenetic process is becoming blurred and the importance of the RPE in neurosensory retinal development is emphasized. The RPE also influences development of the choroidal vasculature and melanocytes through release of VEGF from the basal aspect of the cells and mutant mice that lack expression of VEGF are microphthalmic, have reduced RPE melanin and shorter photoreceptor outer segments (315).

Congenital Retinoschisis

Retinoschisis refers to the formation of a split in the inner layers of the retina. Although there have been occasional reports of autosomal dominant inheritance, most cases are X-linked recessive and X-linked retinoschisis (XLRS, MIM +312700) is the leading cause of macular degeneration in young males (257,436). It is caused by predominantly missense mutations in the *RS1* gene located at Xp22.1, which encodes a protein in photoreceptors and bipolar cells, retinoschisin. Retinoschisin is a secreted protein, which polymerizes to form an active octamer that plays a role in cell adhesion and maintenance of architectural integrity of the retina. Mutations have been described that interfere with both the secretion of retinoschisin, as well as its polymerization and subsequent function (514). However, there is no obvious correlation between the type of mutation and the severity or progression of the condition. Macular schisis is characteristic of the condition but the split can also form in the peripheral inferotemporal retina. Complications include hemorrhage from unsupported blood vessels crossing the schisis cavity and rhegmatogenous retinal detachment. Histopathological studies of XLRS have confirmed the split in the inner retina with gliosis and loss of neurons in the inner wall. Although the outer wall of the retinal cavity may remain attached, there is still degeneration of photoreceptors accompanied by dystrophic calcification (16,306,346). Retinal vessels may become sclerotic with ischemic consequences. On the basis of clinical examination, Conway and Welch (87) suggested that the splitting of the inner retina begins in the vicinity of major vessels. These authors found that, as a vessel is traced centrifugally into an area of schisis, one branch may lie in the deep layer but another branch of the same vessel may run in the inner wall, or travel unsupported in the cavity. In a similar manner, strands of nerve fibers may run obliquely through the schisis cavity. The presence of these intact nerve fibers may explain why the peripheral visual field defects in XLRS are often mild compared with the more severe visual impairment of senile retinoschisis (87).

Optic Nerve

A variety of congenital anomalies of the optic nerves and discs are recognized (125) and different disc anomalies may be found in the eyes of one patient (473).

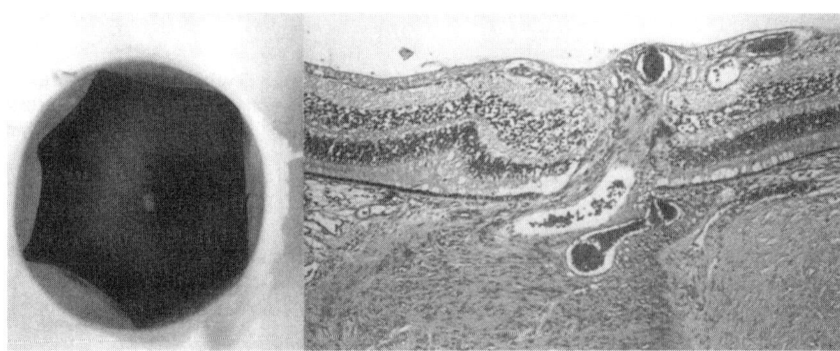

Figure 33 Hypoplasia of optic disc. *Left*: Gross specimen. *Right*: Small opening in pigment epithelium admits only retinal artery. No retinal axons extend into nerve below (hematoxylin and eosin, ×75).

Abnormalities of Size

Optic nerve hypoplasia (MIM #165550) is a congenital, non-progressive reduction in the number of axons in one or both optic nerves (493). It occurs in approximately 7 per 100,000 births and is more common than total aplasia (153,275). Optic nerve hypoplasia is characterized by a small optic disc and a peripapillary halo with a border of dark pigment (Figs. 32 and 33) and may be unilateral or bilateral. Segmental optic nerve hypoplasia has been reported (254). The condition may occur as an isolated finding in up to 40% of patients, or in association with other malformations (338,493). Among the associated malformations are albinism and aniridia, as well as a variety of CNS and endocrine anomalies (444). Septo-optic dysplasia (de Morsier syndrome, MIM #182230) presents with a variable combination of optic nerve hypoplasia, hypoplasia or absence of the septum pellucidum and pituitary-hypothalamic dysfunction (375). Although linked in some cases to inactivating mutations in the *HESX1* gene (101), which is involved in development of the prosencephalon, the condition appears genotypically and phenotypically heterogeneous (375). Risk factors for optic nerve hypoplasia in infants include low maternal age and parity, cigarette smoking in early pregnancy and possibly drug ingestion (493). Anticonvulsants (218) and varicella infections (276) have been implicated and optic nerve hypoplasia is a well-documented feature of the fetal alcohol syndrome (469).

A morphometric comparison of optic nerve hypoplasia with Leber hereditary optic neuropathy (OMIM #535000) supports the view that the condition reflects excessive apoptosis of retinal ganglion cells and their axons and is not the result of axonal degeneration (404), although the hypoplasia associated with periventricular leucomalacia is caused by trans-synaptic degeneration secondary to the lesion in the optic radiation (226). Experimental evidence in rats indicates that high doses of ethanol in the postnatal period may accelerate the normal postnatal loss of axons in the optic nerve and reduce their myelination (195). Other mechanisms almost certainly play a role in some forms of optic nerve hypoplasia. Netrin-1 is an axonal guidance molecule that appears to have a role in the direction of retinal axons into the developing optic nerve and netrin-1 deficient mice show variable degrees of hypoplasia (107). A variety of mutations in the *PAX6* gene have been reported in optic nerve hypoplasia (27).

Complete or partial absence of the chiasm may occur in association with optic nerve aplasia or hypoplasia (410). Achiasmia refers to a condition in which the decussation of retinal ganglion cell axons is reduced during development. It may occur as an isolated anomaly, or in association with septo-optic dysplasia or encephalocele of the skull base (407). Excessive decussation of axons is a recognized feature of albinism.

Abnormalities of Shape

Colobomas of the optic nerve may be found in a wide range of conditions, including the CHARGE association (MIM #214800), Walker–Warburg syndrome (MIM #236670), Aicardi syndrome (MIM %304050), and Goldenhar syndrome (MIM %164210) (125). Bilateral congenital colobomas confined to the optic nerve (MIM #120430) may have an autosomal dominant mode of inheritance and may result in macular or extramacular serous detachment of the retina (416,478,544). The defect in the optic disc may be associated with heterotopic adipose tissue and smooth muscle (531) or medullary epithelium (126). The appearance of a structure resembling a second optic disc in the posterior fundus may be produced by an ectatic peripapillary chorioretinal coloboma (246,509).

An optic disc pit may be seen in the same eye as an optic disc coloboma. A pit is an indentation of the surface usually in the lower temporal quadrant, unlike the typical coloboma. It is usually unilateral but bilateral cases have been reported (61,478) and pits have been reported in association with large discs (241). Macular detachment and subretinal neovascularization may accompany an optic pit (234,447). It is uncertain whether the formation of optic pits is related to an abnormality of embryonic fissure closure (73). A tilted disc is another congenital non-progressive anomaly that is related to abnormal fissure closure. Tilting refers to infero-nasal angulation of the axis of the optic cup with elevation of the superotemporal neuroretinal rim. It is found in 1% to 2% of the population and may be either unilateral or bilateral (512). It may be accompanied by a posterior staphyloma and result in a visual field defect.

The morning glory optic disc anomaly (syndrome) (Fig. 34) refers to a congenital, and funnel-shaped excavation of the posterior fundus that includes the optic disc and is associated with serous retinal detachment (258,447). Abnormalities of the carotid circulation and midline cranial defects may also occur (31,374,380) and lens colobomas and PHPV have been described (71). Imaging studies reveal a cystic abnormality of the nerve optic but there have been few histopathological reports (307). The condition has been described with trisomy 4q (354). Although usually unilateral, bilateral morning glory disc anomaly has been reported in a 5-year-old girl with a mutation in the *PAX6* gene that led to a reduction in its transcription activation potential (27).

In the autosomal dominant papillorenal (renal-coloboma) syndrome (MIM #120330), atypical colobomas of the optic disc are associated with variable, but

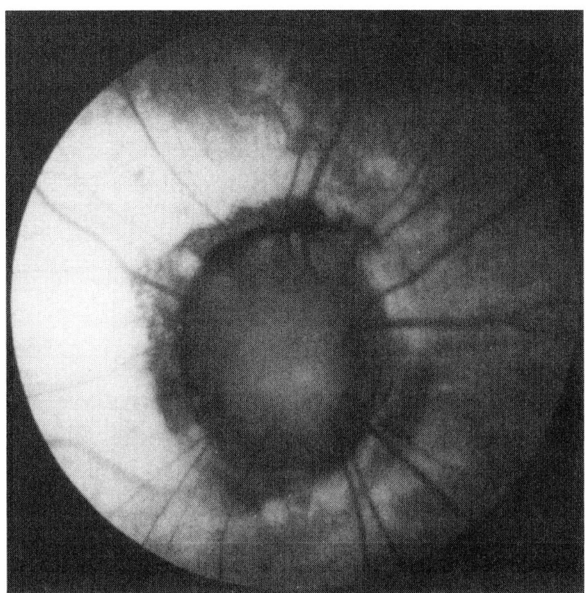

Figure 34 Optic disc in the morning glory syndrome. The optic nerve head is hyperemic, projects anteriorly in a dome-shaped manner, and is surrounded by a raised rim of grayish retina. *Source*: Courtesy of Professor D. Archer.

usually progressive, renal disease. The disc optic characteristically has central excavations and multiple fine cilio-retinal arteries traverse the rim in all quadrants (251). Juxtapapillary depigmentation may be present. Several reports have identified mutations in the *PAX2* gene on chromosome 10 (10q24), which is involved in closure of the embryonic fissure, and the ocular disc phenotype may vary (81,550). Experimental studies indicate that a band of Pax2+ cells of astrocytic lineage normally forms a boundary between the axons that enter the optic nerve head and the surrounding retinal tissue (80).

Ocular Adnexa

Eyelids

Ectodermal Dysplasia

Ectodermal dysplasia refers to a group of over 150 conditions characterized by absence or dysfunction of two or more structures of ectodermal derivation. The abnormalities involve the teeth and skin, including the hair, nails and sweat glands, but ocular surface problems develop in many patients and show a tendency to worsen with age (244). Structural alterations in the Meibomian glands, such as complete or incomplete agenesis and the presence of coarse acini with limited branching, occur in as many as 95% of patients and can be detected by transillumination biomicroscopy (244).

Priolo and Lagani (378) have proposed that the ectodermal dysplasia syndromes be classified in two groups linked to pathogenesis. These authors attribute the first group, which contains the relatively common disorders ectrodactyly–ectodermal dysplasia–cleft lip/palate (EEC, MIM %129900) and ankyloblepharon–ectodermal dysplasia–cleft lip/palate (AEC, MIM #106260) to defects in developmental regulation and epithelial–mesenchymal interaction. The second group, which includes oculo-tricho-dysplasia (MIM 257960) and ectrodactyly–ectodermal dysplasia–macular degeneration (EEM, MIM #225280), appears to be caused by defects in structural proteins involved in the maintenance of the cytoskeleton and intercellular communication. It has become clear that different mutations in the same gene can influence which ectodermal dysplasia becomes manifest and its severity. Missense mutations generating amino acid substitutions in the DNA-binding domain of the *TP73L* gene for p63 have been identified in the EEC syndrome (62,549). Interestingly, missense mutations falling within the p63 exon 13, coding for the sterile alpha motif (SAM) domain (protein-protein interaction module) of the gene, cause the AEC syndrome and these mutations affect only the p63α isoform of the six p63 isoforms (482). A novel 3 bp insertion into the SAM domain resulted in the incorporation of an additional phenylalanine residue into the protein and a form of AEC without ankyloblepharon (500). The variable severity of the keratitis–ichthyosis–deafness syndrome (MIM #148210) appears to reflect the precise mutation in the *GJB2* gene that encodes connexin-26 in gap junctions (231). This condition is characterized by loss of eyebrows and eyelashes, thickened and keratinized eyelids with corneal epithelial defects, stromal scarring and neovascularization and limbal insufficiency (328).

Morphogenetic Anomalies

A variety of abnormalities of the eyelids may occur either sporadically or as part of recognized syndromes. Although given different names, they all represent a failure of normal development of the anterior lamella, the skin and muscle, of the eyelid, possible reflecting congenital hypoplasia of the orbicularis oculi muscle.

Ablepharon is associated with macrostomia, abnormalities of the ears and nose, as well as genital and perhaps CNS abnormalities in the ablepharon-macrostomia syndrome (AMS, MIM 200110) (14). Visual problems largely reflect corneal exposure and resultant opacification (454). Although generally sporadic, the condition has been reported in the father and two daughters in one family (140). Despite its name, small eyelids are recognizable and there is a vertical shortening of the anterior lamella (94). The same reduction in the vertical dimension of all four eyelids is seen in microblepharon, although unilateral microblepharon has been described (43). The condition has also been reported in association with trisomy of chromosome 12p [inv dup(12)(p13.3p12)] (479). Euryblepharon refers to a horizontal widening of the palpebral aperture and again appears to be caused by a short anterior lamella. It may occur as an isolated abnormality but is also a feature of the autosomal dominant blepharocheilodontic syndrome (MIM %119580) (548).

Cryptophthalmos is a relatively frequent anomaly with a prevalence of approximately 11 cases per 100,000 live births (445). It is the single most important diagnostic feature of Fraser syndrome (MIM #219000), which also includes syndactyly, renal and genital abnormalities, as well as ear malformations and laryngeal stenosis. In Fraser syndrome, cryptophthalmos is usually bilateral and complete, with the malformed upper eyelid adherent to the upper cheek with no palpebral fissure and no conjunctival sac (Fig. 35). Incomplete (rudimentary eyelids with a small lateral palpebral fissure and conjunctival sac) and abortive (upper eyelid without a defined margin but adherent to cornea) forms also occur. Other ocular anomalies may accompany cryptophthalmos: eyelid coloboma (17.9%), microphthalmia (21.4%), microcornea or absence of cornea (10.3%) and anterior chamber anomalies (5.1%). In approximately 50% of families with Fraser syndrome there is a mutation in *FRAS1*, a gene on chromosome 4 (4q) that encodes an ECM protein of uncertain function (322). Some other cases have shown mutations in the related gene *FREM2* that would affect the calcium-binding properties of the expressed protein (227).

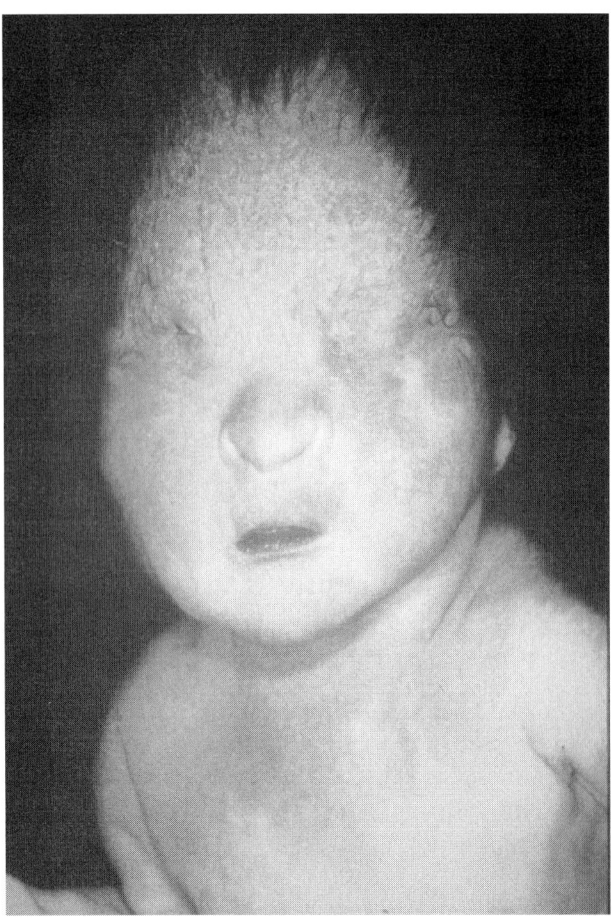

Figure 35 Cryptophthalmos in an infant with Fraser syndrome.

Although there is less information on anomalous development of the posterior lamella, eyelid laxity in classic Ehlers–Danlos syndrome (EDSI, MIM #130000) may reflect thinning of the tarsal plate secondary to abnormal collagen fibrillogenesis. Floppy eyelids were identified in a group of patients with mutations in the *COL5A1* and *COL5A2* genes that encode for the $\alpha1$ and $\alpha2$ chains of collagen type V, respectively (425). Using a murine model of Ehlers–Danlos syndrome, Wenstrup et al. (529) demonstrated that *Col5α1* haploinsufficiency disrupts collagen fibril assembly at multiple stages leading to the connective tissue dysfunction associated with this syndrome.

Epicanthus

Epicanthus is a genetically determined crescentic fold of skin that extends from the upper eyelid to the side of the nose, with its concavity directed to the inner canthus. Anatomically, it results from a Z-shaped kink in the fibers of the orbicularis oculi muscle produced by insertion of the levator tendon nearer the eyelid margin than usual. Epicanthal folds have been reported in a variety of conditions, most notably trisomies 18 (339) and 21 (411) and Smith-Lemli-Opitz syndrome (MIM #270400) (193).

Epicanthus inversus, a small vertical skin fold extending from the lower eyelid to the medial upper eyelid, is a characteristic feature of the blepharophimosis-ptosis-epicanthus inversus syndrome (BPES, MIM #110100). The shortened palpebral fissure is also associated with telecanthus (314), and these children have a high incidence of amblyopia, strabismus, and refractive error (79). Two types of BPES occur, depending on presence (type I) or absence (type II) of premature ovarian failure in addition to the eyelid malformations (103). In both types there are usually mutations in the *FOXL2* gene which encodes one of the forkhead transcription factors (92). Although the condition is inherited in an autosomal dominant manner, approximately 50% of cases represent de novo mutations and some cases result from small deletions on the long arm of chromosome 3 (106), where *FOXL2* is located. Recently, Nallathami et al. (344) have reported the first evidence for a recessive form of blepharophimosis syndrome associated with ovarian dysfunction in an Indian family with a novel polyalanine expansion in *FOXL2*. It has been established that *FOXL2* has a major role in ovarian development (502).

Phakomatous Choristoma of the Eyelid

This congenital tumor, first described by Zimmerman (554), represents a proliferation of ectopic lens tissue in the inferonasal lower eyelid. It is composed of large epithelial cells with the ultrastructural appearance and immunophenotype of lens epithelium arranged in nests, cords and tubules within a fibrous stroma (475,483). There is no mitotic activity and the lesion does not recur after incomplete excision, suggesting it is a choristoma rather than a neoplasm. Three theories have been proposed to account for its formation: (*i*) downgrowth of surface ectoderm into the mesenchyme of the developing eyelid, (*ii*) location of the lens placode in the area destined to become the inferonasal eyelid, (*iii*) migration of primitive lens cells through the embryonic fissure as it closes. The association of a phakomatous choristoma with an eye that contained a colobomatous hypoplastic disc and a staphyloma would support the third pathogenetic mechanism (483).

Congenital Anomalies of the Eyelashes

Absence of the eyelashes is very unusual, although reduced numbers may be seen in a variety of ectodermal dysplasias (244). The association of long eyelashes with pigmentary degeneration of the retina and mental and growth retardation is known as congenital trichomegaly (Oliver–McFarlane syndrome) (MIM %275400), the pathogenesis of which remains unknown (194).

Distichiasis is the name given to the presence of supernumerary eyelashes located along the posterior border of the eyelid margin where the Meibomian glands have their orifices. In familial distichiasis (MIM %126300) the abnormality of the lashes is isolated whereas in lymphedema–distichiasis (LD) syndrome (MIM #153400) the eyelash abnormality is associated with lymphedema, varicose veins, cleft palate and, in 31% of patients, congenital ptosis (57). Both conditions are inherited in an autosomal dominant manner and both are associated with mutations in the forkhead transcription factor gene *FOXC2* (57,60,497). Numerous different mutations have been described and primarily comprise nonsense mutations, insertions or deletions that produce a premature stop codon, and thus a truncated FOXC2 protein (29,38,135,141). It has also been demonstrated that the few *FOXC2* missense mutations are functional nulls and that *FOXC2* haploinsufficiency underlies lymphedema-distichiasis (45). The role of the aberrant transcription factor may be clarified from studies of *Foxc2*$^{+/-}$mice, which also display distichiasis (270). Distichiasis of the upper eyelid with no eyelashes on the lower eyelids is part of Setleis syndrome (MIM %227260), which includes coarse facies, thick lips and chronic conjunctivitis (84).

Lacrimal System

Ectopic lacrimal gland tissue has been reported within the eye (253), the orbit and the epibulbar conjunctiva (13). The epibulbar glandular tissue is frequently part of a complex choristoma but may form a solitary mass; its predominantly temporal location suggests that it is derived in some way from the palpebral lobe of the gland (13).

Congenital alacrima refers to the absence of tears resulting from an anatomical or functional abnormality of the lacrimal gland. The condition may be isolated (MIM %103420) or part of a syndrome and may be inherited in either an autosomal dominant (202) or recessive (201) manner. Lacrimal gland dysfunction may reflect a failure of innervation whereas aplasia of the gland may be partial or complete and is frequently associated with abnormalities of the lacrimal drainage system (256).

Autosomal dominant aplasia of the lacrimal and salivary glands (ALSG, MIM #180920) has been linked to both a deletion of exons 2 and 3 of the *FGF10* gene on chromosome 5 and a stop mutation in exon 3 (130). *Fgf10*$^{+/-}$mice lack lacrimal glands and have hypoplastic salivary glands. When an obstruction exists distally and proximately, the importance of FGF signaling in many aspects of craniofacial development is recognized (351) and mutations in *FGF10* have been identified in the lacrimo-auriculo-dento-digital syndrome (LADD; MIM #149730) (334). In this syndrome a wide variety of phenotypic changes affecting the ears, teeth and digits, as well as genito-urinary abnormalities, are seen in addition to the lacrimal and salivary gland aplasia of ALSG. Both conditions may include abnormalities of the lacrimal drainage system, e.g., punctal agenesis. ALSG and LADD syndrome are allelic disorders demonstrating variable presentations of the same clinical spectrum caused by mutations in *FGF10* (334).

Congenital naso-lacrimal duct obstruction usually represents a failure of the nasal mucous membrane at the lower opening of the duct to rupture, which it normally does between the seventh month of gestation and 2 months after birth. When an obstruction exists distally and proximally, the increased pressure in the nasolacrimal duct gives rise to a dacryocystocele and, sometimes, a bulging cystic mass in the nasal mucosa that may cause respiratory difficulty (112,178). The lumina of the lacrimal canaliculi normally become patent during the fourth month of gestation but the puncta do not open until just before the eyelids separate in the seventh month. Punctal agenesis is usually associated with canalicular agenesis (513) and atresia of the tear ducts is common feature of the EEC syndrome (MIM %129900) (245).

Lacrimal drainage anomalies have been reported in a variety of problems associated with maldevelopment of the face, including the Pierre Robin sequence

(MIM 261800) (21), mandibulofacial dysostosis (MIM 248390) (33), autosomal dominant Robinow syndrome (MIM %180700), autosomal recessive Robinow syndrome (MIM #268310) (3) and oblique facial clefts (463).

Extraocular Muscles

Absence of extraocular muscles may occur in craniofacial syndromes (116) or as an isolated anomaly (223). Agenesis of one extraocular muscle may be accompanied by anomalies of other muscles that arise from the same mesodermal complex in the developing orbit (22,123), e.g., absence of the inferior rectus may be associated with anomalies of the inferior oblique muscle and lateral rectus muscle.

Congenital fibrosis of the extraocular muscles (CFEOM) is now regarded as a cranial dysinnervation disorder. It occurs in at least three forms and the classic autosomal dominant form (CFEOM1, MIM #135700) has been linked to mutations in *KIF21A* on chromosome 12, which encodes a microtubule-associated protein important in neuronal development (129,542). The anomalous innervation may extend beyond the extraocular muscles, since mutations in the same gene appear to contribute to the Marcus Gunn (jaw-winking) phenomenon (MIM 154600) in some cases of CFEOM (543). CFEOM type 2 (CFEOM2, MIM #602078) is inherited in an autosomal recessive fashion and is caused by mutations in the *ARIX* gene. These are thought to lead to defects in the superior and inferior division of the oculomotor nerve (as opposed to the superior division only in CFEOM1) (343).

Similarly, Duane retraction syndrome is also part of the cranial dysinnervation syndromes. Although usually sporadic, up to 10% of cases are familial with autosomal dominant inheritance. Large pedigrees exist and have been utilized to identify two gene loci; Duane retraction syndrome type 1 (MIM %126800) and Duane retraction syndrome type 2 (MIM %604356) (82,323,365). Interestingly, some of the systemic features associated with Duane syndrome suggest the insult occurs mainly in the 4th week gestation and overlap with those caused by thalidomide (333,468).

ACKNOWLEDGMENTS

Portions of the material included in this chapter were originally presented in the corresponding chapter of the first and second editions, written by Joan Mullaney and Elise Torczynski, respectively.

REFERENCES

1. Abruzzo MA, Erickson RP. Re-evaluation of new X-linked syndrome for evidence of CHARGE syndrome or association. Am J Med Genet 1989; 34:397–400.
2. Addison PKF, Berry V, Ionides ACW, et al. Posterior polar cataract is the predominant consequence of a recurrent mutation in the PITX3 gene. Br J Ophthalmol 2005; 89: 138–41.
3. Aguirre-Vila-Coro A, Mazow ML, Drtil SH, et al. Lacrimal anomalies in Robinow's syndome: case report. Arch Ophthalmol 1988; 106:454–6.
4. Aicardi J, Lefebvre J, Lerique-Koechlin A. A new syndrome: spasm in flexion, callosal agenesis and ocular abnormalities. Electronencephalogr Clin Neurophysiol 1965; 19:606–12.
5. Aitchison C, Easty DL, Jancar J. Eye abnormalities in the mentally handicapped. J Ment Defic Res 1990; 34:41–8.
6. Akiba J, Yoshida A, Ohta I, et al. Anomalous Cloquet's canal in a case of optic nervehead coloboma associated with extensive retinal detachment. Br J Ophthalmol 1993; 77:381–2.
7. Albert DM, Lahav M, Carmichael LE, et al. Canine herpes-induced retinal dysplasia and associated ocular anomalies. Invest Ophthalmol 1976; 15:267–78.
8. Albert DM, Lahav M, Colby ED, et al. Retinal neoplasia and dysplasia: induction by feline leukemia virus. Invest Ophthalmol Vis Sci 1977; 16:325–38.
9. Allen RC, Russell SR, Streb LM, et al. Phenotypic heterogeneity associated with a novel mutation (Gly112Glu) in the Norrie disease protein. Eye 2006; 20: 234–41.
10. Allerdyce P, David JG, Miller OJ, et al. The 13q-deletion syndrome. Am J Hum Genet 1969; 12:499–512.
11. Allouche C, Sarda P, Tronc F, et al. The CHARGE association. Pediatrie 1989; 44:391–5.
12. Alvarado M, Bocian M, Walker AP. The interstitial deletion of the long arm of chromosome 3: case report, review, and definition of a phenotype. Am J Med Genet 1987; 27:781–6.
13. Alyahya GA, Bangsgaard R, Prause JU, et al. Occurrence of lacrimal gland tissue outside the lacrimal fossa: comparison of clinical and histopathological findings. Acta Ophthalmol Scand 2005; 83:100–3.
14. Amor DJ, Savarirayan R. Intermediate form of ablepharon-macrostomia syndrome with CNS abnormalities. Amer J Med Genet 2001; 103:252–4.
15. Andersen SR, Geertinger P, Larsen HW, et al. Aniridia, cataract and gonadoblastoma in a mentally retarded girl with deletion of chromosome 11: a clinicopathological case report. Ophthalmologica 1978; 176:171–7.
16. Ando A, Takahashi K, Sho K, et al. Histopathological findings of X-linked retinoschisis with neovascular glaucoma. Graefe's Arch Clin Exp Ophthalmol 2000; 238:1–7.
17. Antonarakis S, Epstein CG. The challenge of Down syndrome. Trends Mol Med 2006; 12:473–9.
18. Apple DJ, Fishman GA, Goldberg MF Ocular histopathology of Norrie's disease. Am J Ophthalmol 1974; 78: 196–203.
19. Armstrong RC, Monie IW. Congenital eye defects on rats following maternal folic-acid deficiency during pregnancy. J Embryol Exp Morphol 1966; 16:531–42.
20. Arnold J. Ocular manifestations of congenital rubella. Curr Opin Ophthalmol 1995; 6:45–50.
21. Arya SK, Chaudhuri Z, Jain R, et al. Congenital alacrima in Pierre Robin sequence. Cornea 2004; 23:632–4.
22. Astle WF, Hill VE, Ells AL, et al. Congenital absence of the inferior rectus muscle — diagnosis and management. J AAPOS 2003; 7:339–4.
23. Astley SJ, Clarren SK. Diagnosing the full spectrum of fetal alcohol-exposed individuals: introducing the 4-digit diagnostic code. Alcohol Alcohol 2000; 35:400–10.

24. Astley SJ, Magnuson SI, Omnell LM, et al. Fetal alcohol syndrome: changes in craniofacial form with age, cognition, and timing of ethanol exposure in the macaque. Teratology 1999; 59:163–72.
25. Aughton DJ. Clinical anophthalmia, dextrocardia, and skeletal anomalies in an infant born to consanguineous parents. Am J Med Genet 1990; 37:178–81.
26. Awan KJ. Intraocular and extraocular colobomatous cysts in adults. Ophthalmologica 1986; 192:76–81.
27. Azuma N, Yamaguchi Y, Handa H, et al. Mutations of the PAX6 gene detected in patients with a variety of optic-nerve malformations. Am J Hum Genet 2003; 72:1565–70.
28. Bahn CF, Falls HF, Varley GA, et al. Classification of corneal endothelial disorders based on neural crest origin. Ophthalmology 1984; 91:558–63.
29. Bahuau M, Houdayer C, Tredano M, et al. FOXC2 truncating mutation in distichiasis, lymphedema, and cleft palate. Clin Genet 2002; 62:470–3.
30. Baillie M, Allen ED, Elkington AR. The congenital warfarin syndrome: a case report. Br J Ophthalmol 1980; 64:533–5.
31. Bakri SJ, Siker D, Masaryk T, et al. Ocular malformations, moyamoya disease, and midline cranial defects: a distinct syndrome. Am J Ophthalmol 1999; 127:356–7.
32. Bartelmez GN, Blount MP. The formation of neural crest from primary optic vesicle in man. Contrib Embryol Carneg Inst 1954; 35:55–71.
33. Bartley GB. Lacrimal drainage anomalies in mandibulofacial dysostosis. Am J Ophthalmol 1990; 109:571–4.
34. Bar-Yosef U, Abuelaish I, Harel T, et al. CHX10 mutations cause non-syndromic microphthalmia/anophthalmia in Arab and Jewish kindreds. Hum Genet 2004; 115:302–9.
35. Bassi MT, Schiaffino MV, Renieri A, et al. Cloning of the gene for ocular albinism type 1 from the distal short arm of the X chromosome. Nat Genet 1995; 10:13–9.
36. Beckman DA, Brent RL. Mechanisms of known environmental teratogens: drugs and chemicals. Clin Perinatol 1986; 13:649–87.
37. Behki R, Noel LP, Clarke WN. Limbal lensectomy in the management of ectopia lentis in children. Arch Ophthalmol 1990; 108:809–11.
38. Bell R, Brice G, Child AH, et al. Analysis of lymphoedema–distichiasis families for FOXC2 mutations reveals small insertions and deletions throughout the gene. Hum Genet 2001; 108:546–51.
39. BenEzra D, Frucht Y, Paez JH, et al. Amniotic band syndrome and strabismus. J Pediatr Ophthalmol Strabismus 1982; 19:33–6.
40. BenEzra D, Sela M, Peter J. Bilateral anophthalmia and unilateral microphthalmia in two siblings. Ophthalmologica 1989; 198:140–4.
41. Benke PJ. The isotretinoin teratogen syndromes. J Am Med Assoc 1984; 251:3267–9.
42. Berk A, Saatci, Ercal M, et al. Ocular findings in 55 patients with Down's syndrome. Ophthalmic Genet 1996; 17:15–19.
43. Bernardini FP, Kersten RC, de Conciliis C, et al. Unilateral microblepharon. Ophthal Plast Reconstr Surg 2004; 20:467–9.
44. Bernardo AI, Kirsch LS, Brownstein S. Ocular anomalies in anencephaly: a clinicopathological study of 11 globes. Can J Ophthalmol 1991; 26:257–63.
45. Berry FB, Tamimi Y, Carle MV, et al. The establishment of a predictive mutational model of the forkhead domain through the analyses of *FOXC2* missense mutations identified in patients with hereditary lymphedema with distichiasis. Hum Mol Genet 2005; 14:2619–27.
46. Bisceglia L, Ciaschetti M, De Bonis P, et al. VSX1 mutational analysis in a series of Italian patients affected by keratoconus: detection of a novel mutation. Invest Ophthalmol Vis Sci 2005; 46:39–45.
47. Black GC, Mazerolle CJ, Wang Y, et al. Abnormalities of the vitreoretinal interface caused by dysregulated Hedgehog signaling during retinal development. Hum Mol Genet 2003; 12:3269–76.
48. Black GCM, Perveen R, Bonshek R, et al. Coats' disease of the retina (unilateral retinal telangiectasis) caused by somatic mutation in the NDP gene: a role for norrin in retinal angiogenesis. Hum Molec Genet 1999; 8:2031–5.
49. Blader P, Strahle U. Ethanol impairs migration of the prechordal plate in the zebrafish embryo. Dev Biol 1998; 201:185–201.
50. Boeve MH, Vrensen GFJM, Willekens BLJC, et al. Early morphogenesis of persistent hyperplastic tunica vasculosa lentis and primary vitreous (PHTVL/PHPV). Graefe's Arch Clin Exp Ophthalmol 1993; 231:29–33.
51. Boniuk V, Ho PK. Ocular findings in anencephaly. Am J Ophthalmol 1979; 88:613–7.
52. Boniuk M, Zimmerman LE. Ocular pathology in the rubella syndrome. Arch Ophthalmol 1967; 77:455–73.
53. Borzyskowski M, Harris RF, Jones RWA. The congenital varicella syndrome. Eur J Pediatr 1981; 137:335–8.
54. Boyntow JR, Phesant TR, Johnson BL, et al. Ocular findings in Kenny's syndrome. Arch Ophthalmol 1979; 97:896–900.
55. Brent RL. Radiations and other physical agents. In: Fraser FC, Wilson JG, eds. Handbook of Teratology. New York: Plenum Press, 1977:153–201.
56. Brent RL, Beckman DA. The contribution of environmental teratogens to embryonic and fetal loss. Clin Obstet Gynecol 1994; 37:646–70.
57. Brice G, Mansour S, Bell R, et al. Analysis of the phenotypic abnormalities in lymphoedema – distichiasis syndrome in 74 patients with FOXC2 mutations or linkage to 16q24. J Med Genet 2002; 39:478–83.
58. Brockhurst RJ. Cataract surgery in nanophthalmic eyes. Arch Ophthalmol 1990; 108:965–7.
59. Brook CG, Sanders MD, Hoare RD. Septo-optic dysplasia. Br Med J 1972; 3:811–3.
60. Brooks BP, Dagenais SL, Nelson CC, et al. Mutation of the *FOXC2* gene in familial distichiasis. J AAPOS 2003; 7: 354–7.
61. Brown GC, Shields, JA, Goldberg RE. Congenital pits of the optic nerve head. II. Clinical studies in humans. Ophthalmology 1980; 87:51–65.
62. Brunner HG, Hamel BC, van Bokhoven HH. p63 gene mutations and human developmental syndromes. Am J Med Genet 2002; 112:284–90.
63. Brunquell PJ, Papale JH, Horton JC, et al. Sex-linked hereditary bilateral anophthalmos. Pathologic and radiologic correlation. Arch Ophthalmol 1984; 102:108–13.
64. Bundy WE, Kaufman PL, Stainer GA, et al. Unilateral Rieger's anomaly. Am J Ophthalmol 1980; 90:725–7.
65. Busby A, Dolk H, Armstrong B. Eye anomalies: seasonal variation and maternal viral infections. Epidemiology 2005; 16:317–22.
66. Butler JM, Raviola G, Miller CD, et al. Fine structural defects in a case of congenital microcoria. Graefe's Arch Clin Exp Ophthalmol 1989; 227:88–94.
67. Calcagni G, Digilio MC, Capolino R, et al. Concordant familial segregation of atrial septal defect and Axenfeld-Rieger anomaly in father and son. Clin Dysmorphol 2006; 15:203–6.

68. Calderone JP, Chess J, Borodic G, et al. Intraocular pathology of trisomy 18 (Edwards's syndrome): report of a case and review of the literature. Br J Ophthalmol 1983; 67:162–9.
69. Casteels I, Devriendt K, Leys A, et al. Autosomal dominant microcephaly-lymphoedema-chorioretinal dysplasia syndrome. Br J Ophthalmol 2001; 85:499–500.
70. Catalano RA. Down syndrome. Surv Ophthalmol 1990; 34:385–8.
71. Cennamo G, Liguori G, Pezone A, et al. Morning glory syndrome associated with marked persistent hyperplastic primary vitreous and lens colobomas Br J Ophthalmol 1989; 73:684–6.
72. Chan CC, Fishman M, Egbert PR. Multiple ocular anomalies associated with maternal LSD ingestion. Arch Ophthalmol 1978; 96:282–5.
73. Chang L, Blain D, Bertuzzi S, et al. Uveal coloboma: clinical and basic science update. Curr Opin Ophthalmol 2006; 17:447–70.
74. Charles NC, Bennett TW, Margolis S. Ocular pathology of the congenital varicella syndrome. Arch Ophthalmol 1977; 95:2034–7.
75. Charles SJ, Moore AT, Grant JW, et al. Genetic counselling in X-linked ocular albinism: clinical features of the carrier state. Eye 1992; 6:75–9.
76. Chavarria-Soley G, Michels-Rautenstrauss K, Caliebe A, et al. Novel CYP1B1 and known PAX6 mutations in anterior segment dysgenesis (ASD). J Glaucoma 2006; 15: 499–504.
77. Chen JD, Mackey D, Fuller H, et al. X-linked megalocornea:close linkage to DXS87 and DXS94. Hum Genet 1989; 83:292–4.
78. Chestler RJ, France TD. Ocular findings in CHARGE syndrome: six case reports and a review. Ophthalmology 1988; 95:1613–9.
79. Choi KH, Kyung S, Oh SY. The factors influencing visual development in blepharophimosis-ptosis-epicanthus inversus syndrome. J Pediatr Ophthalmol Strabismus 2006; 43:285–8.
80. Chu Y, Hughes S, Chan-Ling T. Differentiation and migration of astrocyte precursor cells and astrocytes in human fetal retina: relevance to optic nerve coloboma. FASEB J 2001; 15:2013–5.
81. Chung GW, Edwards AO, Schimmenti LA, et al. Renal-coloboma syndrome: report of a novel *PAX2* gene mutation. Am J Ophthalmol 2001; 132:910–4.
82. Chung M, Stout JT, Borchert MS. Clinical diversity of hereditary Duane's retraction syndrome. Ophthalmology 2000; 107:500–3.
83. Cibis GW, Waeltermann J, Harris DJ. Peters' anomaly in association with ring 21 chromosomal abnormality. Am J Ophthalmol 1985; 100:734–44.
84. Clark RD, Golabi M, Lacassie Y, et al. Expanded phenotype and ethnicity in Setleis syndrome. Am J Med Genet 1989; 34:354–7.
85. Cohen SM, Nelson LB. Aniridia with congenital ptosis and glaucoma: a family study. Ann Ophthalmol 1988; 20: 53–7.
86. Contreras F, Pereda J. Congenital syphilis of the eye with lens involvement. Arch Ophthalmol 1978; 96:1052–3.
87. Conway BP, Welch RB. Juvenile retinoschisis. Am J Ophthalmol 1977; 83:853–6.
88. Cook CS, Sulik KK. Keratolenticular dysgenesis (Peters' anomaly) as a result of acute embryonic insult during gastrulation. J Pediatr Ophthalmol Strab 1988; 25:60–6.
89. Cook CS, Sulik KK. Laminin and fibronectin in retinoid-induced keratolenticular dysgenesis. Invest Ophthalmol Vis Sci 1990; 31:751–7.
90. Cordes FC, Barber A. Changes in the lens of an embryo after rubella. Arch Ophthalmol 1966; 36:135–40.
91. Cotlier E, Reinglass H, Rosenthal I. The eye in partial trisomy 2q syndrome. Am J Ophthalmol 1977; 84:251–9.
92. Crisponi L, Deiana M, Loi A, et al. The putative forkhead transcription factor *FOXL2* is mutated in blepharophimosis/ptosis/epicanthus inversus syndrome. Nat Genet 2001; 27:159–66.
93. Cross HE, Yoder F. Familial nanophthalmos. Am J Ophthalmol 1976; 81:300–7.
94. Cruz AAV, Souza CA, Ferraz VEF, et al. Familial occurrence of ablepharon macrostomia syndrome: eyelid structure and surgical considerations. Arch Ophthalmol 2000; 118:428–30.
95. Cullen BA. Ocular defects in thalidomide babies. Br J Ophthalmol 1964; 48:151–3.
96. Cunha RP, Cunha MC, Shields JA. J Pediatric Ophthalmol Strab 1987; 24:249–54.
97. Cvekl A, Tamm ER. Anterior eye development and ocular mesenchyme: new insights from mouse models and human diseases. Bioessays 2004; 26:374–86.
98. Da Cunha RP, Moreira JB. Ocular findings in Down's syndrome. Am J Ophthalmol 1996; 122:236–44.
99. Dagoneau N, Benoist-Lasselin C, Huber C, et al. *ADAMTS10* mutations in autosomal recessive Weill-Marchesani syndrome. Am J Hum Genet 2004; 75:801–6.
100. Datta H, Datta S. Anterior segment dysgenesis and absent lens caused by amniotic bands. Clin Dysmorphol 2003; 12:69–71.
101. Dattani MT, Robertson IC. HESX1 and septo-optic dysplasia. Rev Endocr Metab Disord 2002; 3:289–300.
102. David T, Chauvaud D, Pouliquen Y. Nanophthalmos with uveal effusion. Bull Soc Ophtalmol Fr 1990; 90:263–5.
103. De Baere E, Dixon MJ, Small KW, et al. Spectrum of *FOXL2* gene mutations in blepharophimosis-ptosis-epicanthus inversus (BPES) families demonstrates a genotype-phenotype correlation. Hum Mol Genet 2001; 10: 1591–600.
104. De Becker I, Walter M, Noel LP. Phenotypic variations in patients with a 1630 A>T point mutation in the PAX6 gene. Can J Ophthalmol 2004; 39:272–8.
105. De La Cruz M, Sun S, Vangvanichyakorn K, et al. Multiple congenital malformations associated with maternal isotretinoin therapy. Pediatrics 1984; 74:428–30.
106. de Ru MH, Gille JJP, Nieuwint AWM, et al. Interstitial deletion in 3q in a patient with blepharophimosis-ptosis-epicanthus inversus syndrome (BPES) and microcephaly, mild mental retardation, and growth delay: clinical report and review of the literature. Amer J Med Genet 2005; 137A:81–7.
107. Deiner MS, Kennedy TE, Fazeli A, et al. Netrin-1 and DCC mediate axon guidance locally at the optic disc: loss of function leads to optic nerve hypoplasia. Neuron 1997; 19:575–89.
108. Dekaban AS. Abnormalities in children exposed to X-radiation during various stages of gestation: tentative timetable of radiation injury to the human fetus, part 1. J Nucl Med 1968; 9:471–7.
109. Del GiudiceE, Sartorio R, Romano A, et al. Megalocornea and mental retardation syndrome: two new cases. Am J Med Gen 1987; 26:417–20.
110. Deluise VP, Anderson DR. Review: primary infantile glaucoma (congenital glaucoma). Surv Ophthalmol 1983; 28:1–19.
111. Deluise VP, Cobo LM, Chandler D. Persistent corneal edema in the congenital rubella syndrome. Ophthalmology 1983; 90:835–9.

112. Denis D. Nasolacrimal duct cysts in congenital dacryocystocele. Graefe's Arch Clin Exp Ophthalmol 1994; 232: 252–5.
113. Denis D, Gabisson P, Saracco JB. Anterior chamber cleavage syndromes. Bull Soc Ophtalmol Fr 1990; 90:557–60.
114. Deutman AF. Vitreoretinal dystrophies. In: Krill AE, ed. Hereditary Retinal and Choroidal Diseases. New York: Harper and Row, 1977,1043–108.
115. Devi RR, Vijayalakshmi P. Novel mutations in GJA8 associated with autosomal dominant congenital cataract and microcornea. Mol Vis 2006; 12:190–5.
116. Diamond GR, Katowitz JA, Whitaker LA, et al. Variations in extraocular muscle number and structure in craniofacial dysostosis. Am J Ophthalmol 1980; 90:416–8.
117. Diehl SR, Erickson RP. Genome scan for teratogen-induced clefting susceptibility loci in the mouse: evidence of both allelic and locus heterogeneity distinguishing cleft lip and cleft palate. Proc Natl Acad Sci USA 1997; 94: 5231–6.
118. Diehl DLC, Feldman F, Tanzer H, et al. Nanophthalmos in sisters, one with exfoliation syndrome. Can J Ophthalmol 1989; 24:327–30.
119. Dolk H, Nichols R. Evaluation of the impact of Chernobyl on the prevalence of congenital anomalies in 16 regions of Europe. EUROCAT Working Group. Int J Epidemiol 1999; 28:941–8.
120. Donnenfeld AE, Graham JMF, Packer RJ, et al. Microphthalmia and chorioretinal lesions in a girl with an Xp22.2-pter deletion and partial 3p trisomy. Am J Med Genet 1990; 37:182–6.
121. Dorey SE, Neveu MM, Burton LC, et al. The clinical features of albinism and their correlation with visual evoked potentials. Br J Ophthalmol 2003; 87: 767–72.
122. Drews RC. Heterochromia iridum with coloboma of the optic disc. Arch Ophthalmol 1973; 90:437.
123. Drummond GT, Keech RV. Absent and anomalous superior oblique and superior rectus muscles. Can J Ophthalmol 1989; 24:275–9.
124. Dudgeon JA. Infective causes of human malformations. Br Med Bull 1976; 32:77–83.
125. Dutton GN. Congenital disorders of the optic nerve: excavations and hypoplasia. Eye 2004; 18:1038–48.
126. Duvall J, Miller SL, Cheatle E, et al. Histopathologic study of ocular changes in a syndrome of multiple congenital anomalies. Am J Ophthalmol 1987; 103:701–5.
127. Ebenezer ND, Patel CB, Hariprasad SM, et al. Clinical and molecular characterization of a family with autosomal recessive cornea plana. Arch Ophthalmol 2005; 123:1248–53.
128. Elder MJ. Aetiology of severe visual impairment and blindness in microphthalmos. Br J Ophthalmol 1994; 78: 332–4.
129. Engle EC. The genetic basis of complex strabismus. Pediatr Res 2006; 59:343–8.
130. Entesarian M, Matsson H, Klar J, et al. Mutations in the gene encoding fibroblast growth factor 10 are associated with aplasia of lacrimal and salivary glands. Nat Genet 2005; 37:125–7.
131. EUROCAT Working Group. Preliminary evaluation of the impact of the Chernobyl radiological contamination on the frequency of central nervous system malformations in 18 regions of Europe. Paediatr Perinat Epidemiol 1988; 2: 253–64.
132. Evereklioglu C, Yilmaz K, Bekir N. Decreased central corneal thickness in children with Down syndrome. J Pediat Ophthalmol Strabismus 2002; 39:274–7.
133. Faivre Gorlin RJ, Wirtz MK, et al. In frame fibrillin-1 gene deletion in autosomal dominant Weill-Marchesani syndrome. J Med Genet 2003; 40:34–6.
134. Falls HF. Chromosomal abnormalities in ophthalmology. In: Beard C, Falls HF, Franceschetti A, Francois J, Goodman G, Krill AE, Scheie H, eds. Symposium on Surgical and Medical Management of Congenital Anomalies of the Eye. Transactions of the New Orleans Academy of Ophthalmology. St. Louis, MO: C. V. Mosby, 1968:14–33.
135. Fang J, Dagenais SL, Erickson RP, et al. Mutations in FOXC2 (MFH-1), a forkhead family transcription factor, are responsible for the hereditary lymphedema–distichiasis syndrome. Am J Hum. Genet 2000; 67:1382–8.
136. Fantes J, Ragge NK, Lynch SA, et al. Mutations in SOX2 cause anophthalmia. Nat Genet 2003: 33:461–3.
137. Feldman GL, Weaver DD, Lovrien EW. The fetal trimethadione syndrome. Am J Dis Child 1977; 131:1389–92.
138. Ferda Percin E, Ploder LA, Yu JJ, et al. Human microphthalmia associated with mutations in the retinal homeobox gene CHX10. Nat Genet 2000; 25:397–401.
139. Ferguson JG, Hicks EL Jr. Rieger's anomaly and glaucoma associated with partial trisomy 16q: case report. Arch. Ophthalmol 1987; 105:323.
140. Ferraz VEF, Melo DG, Hansing SE, et al. Ablepharon-macrostomia syndrome: first report of familial occurrence. Amer J Med Genet 2000; 94:281–3.
141. Finegold DN, Kimak MA, Lawrence EC, et al. Truncating mutations in FOXC2 cause multiple lymphedema syndromes. Hum Mol Genet 2001; 10:1185–9.
142. Fischer G. Abnorme Ciliarkorperanlage in einen Mikrophthalmos. Albrecht von Graefe's Arch Ophthalmol 1934; 132:71–81.
143. FitzPatrick DR. Transcriptional consequences of autosomal trisomy; primary gene dosage with complex downstream effects. Trends Genet 2005; 21:249–53.
144. Fitzpatrick DR, van Heyningen V. Developmental eye disorders. Curr Opin Genet Dev 2005; 15:348–53.
145. Font RL, Zimmerman LE. Optic disc coloboma. Am J Ophthalmol 1971; 72:452–8.
146. Foos FY, Kiechler RJ, Allen RA. Congenital non-attachment of the retina. Am J Ophthalmol 1968; 65: 202–11.
147. Forsius H, Damsten M, Eriksson AW, et al. Autosomal recessive cornea plana. A clinical and genetic study of 78 cases in Finland. Acta Ophthalmol Scand 1998; 76: 196–203.
148. Foxman S, Cameron JD. The clinical implications of bilateral microphthalmos with cyst. Am J Ophthalmol 1984; 97:632–8.
149. Francois J. A new syndrome, dyscephalia with birdface and dental anomalies, nanism, hypotrichosis, cutaneous atrophy, microphthalmia and congenital cataract. Arch Ophthalmol 1958; 60:842–62.
150. Fraumeni JF Jr, Glass AG. Wilms' tumor and congenital aniridia. J Am Med Assoc 1968; 206:825–8.
151. Free SL, Mitchell TN, Williamson KA, et al. Quantitative MR image analysis in subjects with defects in the PAX6 gene. Neuroimage 2003; 20:2281–90.
152. Frenkel LD, Keys MP, Hefferen SJ, et al. Unusual eye abnormalities associated with congenital cytomegalovirus infection. Pediatrics 1980; 66:763–5.
153. Frisen L, Holmegaard L. Spectrum of optic nerve hypoplasia. Br J Ophthalmol 1978; 62:7–15.
154. Frydman M, Berkenstadt M, Raas-Rothschild A, et al. Megalocornea, macrocephaly, mental and motor retardation (MMMR). Clin Genet 1990; 38:149–54.

155. Fulton AB, Albert DM, Craft JL. Human albinism. Light and electron microscopy study. Arch Ophthalmol 1978; 96:305–10.
156. Futterweit W, Ritch R, Teekhasaenee C, et al. Coexistence of Prader-Willi syndrome, congenital ectropion uvea with glaucoma, and factor XI deficiency. J Am Med Assoc 1986; 255:3280–92.
157. Gallardo ME, Rodriguez De Cordoba S, Schneider AS, et al. Analysis of the developmental SIX6 homeobox gene in patients with anophthalmia/microphthalmia. Am J Med Genet 2004; 129A:92–4.
158. Garner A, Jay BS. Macromelanosomes in X-linked ocular albinism. Histopathology 1980; 4:243–54.
159. Gazali LI, Mueller RF, Caine A, et al. Two 46,XX,t(X;Y) females with linear skin defects and congenital microphthalmia: a new syndrome at Xp22.3. J Med Genet 1990; 27:59–63.
160. Gehring WJ. The master control gene for morphogenesis and evolution of the eye. Genes Cells 1996; 1:11–5.
161. Gilkes MJ, Strode M. Ocular anomalies in association with developmental limb abnormalities of drug origin. Lancet 1963; 1:1026–7.
162. Gimenez E, Lavado A, Jeffery G, et al. Regional abnormalities in retinal development are associated with local ocular hypopigmentation. J Comp Neurol 2005; 485: 338–47.
163. Ginsberg J, Dignan P, Soukup S. Ocular abnormality associated with an extra small chromosome. Am J. Ophthalmol 1968; 65:740–6.
164. Girard B, Topouzis F, Saraux H. Microphthalmos in Pierre Robin syndrome: clinical and X-ray computed tomographic study. Bull Soc Ophtalmol Fr 1989; 89:1385–90.
165. Givens KT, Lee DA, Jones T, et al. Congenital rubella syndrome: ophthalmic manifestations and associated systemic disorders. Br J Ophthalmol 1993; 77:358–63.
166. Glaser T, Jepeal L, Edwards JG, et al. PAX6 gene dosage effect in a family with congenital cataracts, aniridia, anophthalmia and central nervous system defects. Nat Genet 1994; 7:463–71.
167. Goldberg MF. Clinical manifestations of ectopia lentis et pupillae in 16 patients. Trans Am Ophthalmol Soc 1988; 86:158–75.
168. Goldberg MF. Persistent fetal vasculature (PFV): an integrated interpretation of signs and symptoms associated with persistent hyperplastic primary vitreous (PHPV). Am J Ophthalmol 1997; 124:587–626.
169. Goldberg MF, McKusick VA. X-linked colobomatous microphthalmos and other congenital anomalies, a disorder resembling Lenz's dysmorphogenetic syndrome. Am J Ophthalmol 1971; 71:1128–33.
170. Gorlin RJ, Cohen MMJ, Hennekam RC. Chromosomal syndromes: common and/or well-known syndromes. In: Gorlin RJ, Cohen MMJ, Hennekam RC, eds. Syndromes of the Head and Neck. 4th ed. New York: Oxford University Press, 2001:35–76.
171. Gould DB, Smith RS, John SWM. Anterior segment development relevant to glaucoma. Int J Dev Biol 2004; 48:1015–29.
172. Graham JM Jr, Marshall J. Edwards: discoverer of maternal hyperthermia as a human teratogen. Birth Defects Res A Clin Mol Teratol 2005; 73:857–64.
173. Graw J. The genetic and molecular basis of congenital eye defects. Nat Rev Genet 2003; 4:876–88.
174. Gregg NM. Congenital cataract following German measles in the mother. Trans Ophthalmol Soc UK 1941; 3:35–46.
175. Gregor Z, Hitchings RA. Rieger's anomaly: 42 year follow up. Br J Ophthalmol 1980; 64:56–8.
176. Gregory-Evans CY, Williams MJ, Halford S, et al. Ocular coloboma: a reassessment in the age of molecular neuroscience. J Med Genet 2004; 41:881–91.
177. Grey RHB, Rice NSC. Congenital duplication of the lens. Br J Ophthalmol 1976; 60:673–6.
178. Grin TR, Mertz JS, Stass-Isern M. Congenital nasolacrimal duct cysts in dacryocystocele. Ophthalmology 1991; 98: 1238–42.
179. Grossman J. Congenital syphilis. Teratology 1977; 16: 217–24.
180. Gupta SK, De Becker I, Guernsey DL, et al. Polymerase chain reaction-based risk assessment for Wilms tumor in sporadic aniridia. Am J Ophthalmol 1998; 125:687–92.
181. Guterman C, Abboud E, Mets MB. Microphthalmos with cyst and Edwards' syndrome. Am J Ophthalmol 1990; 109:228–30.
182. Guthoff R, Klein R, Lieb WE. Congenital cystic eye. Graefe's Arch Clin Exp Ophthalmol 2004; 242:268–71.
183. Hackam AS. The Wnt signaling pathway in retinal degenerations. IUBMB Life 2005; 57:381–8.
184. Hagstrom SA, Pauer GJ, Reid J, et al. SOX2 mutation causes anophthalmia, hearing loss, and brain anomalies. Am J Med Genet 2005; 138 A:95–8.
185. Haider MZ, Devarajan LV, Al-Essa M, et al. A C597→A polymorphism in the Norrie disease gene is associated with advanced retinopathy of prematurity in premature Kuwaiti infants. J Biomed Sci 2002; 9:365–70.
186. Halder G, Callaerts P, Gehring WJ. Induction of ectopic eyes by targeted expression of the eyeless gene in Drosophila. Science 1995; 267:1788–92.
187. Hall B. Mongolism in newborns: clinical and cytogenetic study. Acta Paed Scand 1964; Suppl. 154:1–95.
188. Hall JG, Pauli RM, Wilson KM. Maternal and fetal sequelae of anticoagulation during pregnancy. Am J Med Genet 1980; 68:122–40.
189. Hansen LA, Pearl GS. Isotretinoin teratogenicity. Acta Neuropathol 1985; 65:335–7.
190. Hanson IM. PAX6 and Congenital Eye Malformation. Pediatric Research 2003; 54:791–6.
191. Hanson I, McKie M, Brown A. The Human PAX6 Allelic Variant Database Web Site, 2004. http://pax6.hgu.mrc.ac.uk/ (Accessed November 1, 2007).
192. Hanson JW, Myrianthopoulos NC, Harvey MAS, et al. Risks to the offspring of women treated with hydantoin anticonvulsants with emphasis on the fetal hydantoin syndrome. J Pediatr 1976; 89:662–8.
193. Harbin RL, Katz JI, Frias JL, et al. Sclerocornea and Smith-Lemli-Optiz syndrome. Amer J Ophthalmol 1977; 84:72–5.
194. Haritoglou C, Rudolph G, Kalpadakis P, et al. Congenital trichomegaly (Oliver-McFarlane syndrome): a case report with 9 years' follow up. Br J Ophthalmol 2003; 87:119–20.
195. Harris SJ, Wilce P, Bedi KS. Exposure of rats to a high but not low dose of ethanol during early postnatal life increases the rate of loss of optic nerve axons and decreases the rate of myelination. J Anat 2000; 197:477–5.
196. Hartwig NG, Vermeij-Keers C, Versteeg J. The anterior eye segment in virus induced primary congenital aphakia. Acta Morphol Neerl-Scand 1988/89; 26:283–92.
197. Hashemi K, Traboulsi EI, Chavis R, et al. Chorioretinal lacuna in the amniotic band syndrome. J Pediatr Ophthalmol Strabismus 1991; 28:238–9.
198. Haugen OH, Hivding G, Eide GE. Biometric measurements of the eyes in teenagers and young adults with

Down syndrome. Acta Ophthalmol Scand 2001; 79: 616–25.
199. Hayashi N, Repka MX, Ueno H, et al. Congenital cystic eye: report of two cases and review of the literature. Surv Ophthalmol 1999; 44:173–9.
200. Heathcote JG, Sholdice J, Walton JC, et al. Anterior segment mesenchymal dysgenesis associated with partial duplication of the short arm of chromosome 2. Can J Ophthalmol 1991; 26:35–43.
201. Hegab SM, Al-Mutawa SA. Congenital hereditary autosomal recessive alacrima. Ophthalmic Genet 1996; 17: 35–8.
202. Hegab SM, Sheriff SMM, El-Aasar EM, et al. Congenital alacrima without associated manifestations (AD). Ophthalmic Paediatrics and Genetics 1991; 12:161–3.
203. Heon E, Greenberg A, Kopp KK, et al. *VSX1*: A gene for posterior polymorphous dystrophy and keratoconus. Hum Molec Genet 2002; 11:1029–36.
204. Hermsen VM, Conahan JB, Koops BL, et al. Persistent hyperplastic primary vitreous associated with protein C deficiency. Am J Ophthalmol 1990; 109:608–9.
205. Herrera E, Marcus R, Li S, et al. Foxd1 is required for proper formation of the optic chiasm. Development 2004; 131:5727–39.
206. Hestnes A, Sand T, Fostad K. Ocular findings in Down's syndrome. J Mental Defic Res 1991; 35:194–203.
207. Hiraoka M, Berinstein DM, Trese MT, et al. Insertion and deletion mutations in the dinucleotide repeat region of the Norrie disease gene in patients with advanced retinopathy of prematurity. J Hum Genet 2001; 46:178–81.
208. Hittner H, Desmond MM, Montgomery FR. Optic nerve manifestations of human congenital cytomegalovirus infection. Am J Ophthalmol 1976; 83:661–6.
209. Hittner HM, Hirsch NJ, Kreh GM, et al. Colobomatous microphthalmos, heart disease, hearing loss and mental retardation: a syndrome. J Ped Ophthalmol Strab 1979; 16: 122–8.
210. Hittner HM, Riccardi VM, Francke U. Aniridia caused by a heritable chromosome 11 deletion. Ophthalmology 1979; 86:1173–83.
211. Ho CL, Walton DS. Primary megalocornea: clinical features for differentiation from infantile glaucoma. J Pediatr Ophthalmol Strabismus 2004; 41:11–7.
212. Hoepner J, Yanoff M. Ocular findings in trisomy 13–15. Am J Ophthalmol 1972; 74:729–38.
213. Holland EJ, Djalilian AR, Schwartz GS. Management of aniridic keratopathy with keratolimbal allograft: a limbal stem cell transplantation technique. Ophthalmology 2003; 110:125–30.
214. Hollsten DA, Katowitz JA. The ophthalmic manifestations and treatment of the amniotic band syndrome. Ophthal Plast Reconstr Surg 1990; 6:1–15.
215. Hopfer U, Fukai N, Hopfer H, et al. Targeted disruption of *Col8a1* and *Col8a2* genes in mice leads to anterior segment abnormalities in the eye. FASEB J 19:1232–44.
216. Hornby SJ, Adolph S, Gilbert CE, et al. Visual acuity in children with coloboma: clinical features and a new phenotypic classification system. Ophthalmology 2000; 107:511–20.
217. Howard RO, Boue J, Deluchat C, et al. The eyes of embryos with chromosome abnormalities. Am J Ophthalmol 1974; 78:167–88.
218. Hoyt CS, Billson FS. Maternal anticonvulsants and optic nerve hypoplasia. Br J Ophthalmol 1978; 62:3–6.
219. Hoyt CS, Billson F, Ouvrier R, et al. Ocular features of Aicardi's syndrome. Arch Ophthalmol 1978; 96:291–5.
220. Hsia YE, Bratu M, Herbordt A. Genetics of the Meckel syndrome (dysencephalia splanchnocystica). Pediatrics 1971; 42:237–47.
221. Hunter AGW, Rothman SJ, Hwang WS, et al. Hepatic fibrosis, polycystic kidney, colobomata and encephalopathy in siblings. Clin Genet 1974; 6:82–9.
222. Idrees F, Vaideanu D, Fraser SG, et al. A review of anterior segment dysgeneses. Surv Ophthalmol 2006; 51: 213–31.
223. Ingham PN, McGovern ST, Crompton JL. Congenital absence of the inferior rectus muscle. Aust N Z J Ophthalmol 1986; 14:355–8.
224. Inoue Y, Inoue T, Ishii Y, et al. Histology of microcornea complicated by bullous keratopathy. Acta Ophthalmol Scand 2001; 79:94–6.
225. Jacobsen SG, Cideciyan AV, Aleman TS, et al. *Crumbs homolog 1* (*CRB1*) mutations result in a thick human retina with abnormal lamination. Hum Mol Genet 2003; 12: 1073–8.
226. Jacobson L, Ygge J, Flodmark O. Nystagmus in periventricular leucomalacia. Br J Ophthalmol 1998; 82:1026–32.
227. Jadeja S, Smyth I, Pitera JE, et al. Identification of a new gene mutated in Fraser syndrome and mouse myelencephalic blebs. Nat Genet 2005; 37:520–5.
228. James PM, Karseras AG, Wybar KC. Systemic association of uveal coloboma. Br J Ophthalmol 1974; 58:917–21.
229. Jamieson RV, Munier F, Balmer A, et al. Pulverulent cataract with variably associated microcornea and iris coloboma in a MAF mutation family. Br J Ophthalmol 2003; 87:411–2.
230. Jamieson RV, Perveen R, Kerr B, et al. Domain disruption and mutation of the bZIP transcription factor, MAF, associated with cataract, ocular anterior segment dysgenesis and coloboma. Hum Mol Genet 2000; 11:32–42.
231. Janecke AR, Hennies HC, Guenther B, et al. *GJB2* mutations in keratitis-ichthyosis-deafness syndrome including its fatal form. Amer J Med Genet 2005; 133A: 128–31.
232. Jaureguy BM, Hall JG. Isolated congenital ectopia lentis with autosomal dominant inheritance. Clin Genet 1979; 15:97–109.
233. Jay M. The Eye in Chromosome Duplication and Deficiencies. Ophthalmic Series 2. New York, 1977: 1–249.
234. Jay WM, Pope J, Riffle JE. Juxtapapillary subretinal neovascularization associated with congenital pit of the optic nerve. Am J Ophthalmol 1984; 97:655–7.
235. Jeffery G. The albino retina: an abnormality that provides insight into normal retinal development. Trends Neurosci 1997; 20:165–9.
236. Jen JC, Chan WM, Bosley TM, et al. Mutations in a human ROBO gene disrupt hindbrain axon pathway crossing and morphogenesis. Science 2004; 304:1509–13.
237. Jin JC, Anderson DR. Laser unsutured sclerotomy in nanophthlalmos. Am J Ophthalmol 1990; 109:575–80.
238. Johns KJ, O'Day DM. Posterior chamber intraocular lenses after extracapsular cataract extraction in patients with aniridia. Ophthalmology 1991; 98:1698–702.
239. Johnston MC, Bhakdinaronk A, Reid YC. An expanded role of the neural crest in oral and pharyngeal development. In: Bosma JF, ed. Fourth Symposium on Oral Sensation and Perception. Washington D.C: U.S. Govt. Printing Office, 1973:37–52.
240. Johnston MC, Noden DM, Hazelton RD, et al. Origins of avian ocular and periocular tissues. Exp Eye Res 1979; 29: 27–43.

241. Jonas JB, Naumann GO. Pits of the optic papilla in large optic nerve papillae. Papillometric characteristics in 15 eyes. Klin Monatsbl Augenheilkd 1987; 191:287–91.
242. Jotterand V, Boisjoly HM, Harnois C, et al. 11p13 deletion, Wilms' tumor, and aniridia: unusual genetic, non-ocular and ocular features of three cases. Br J Ophthalmol 1990; 74:568–70.
243. Journel H, Urvoy M, Baudet D, et al. Manifestations oculaires de la trisomie 21. Etude de cinquante-trois cas et revue de la litérature. Ann Pediatr (Paris) 1986; 33:387–92.
244. Kaercher T. Ocular symptoms and signs in patients with ectodermal dysplasia syndromes. Graefe's Arch Clin Exp Ophthalmol 2004; 242:495–500.
245. Kaesmann B, Ruprecht KW. Ocular manifestations in a father and son with EEC syndrome. Graefe's Arch Clin Exp Ophthalmol 1997; 235:512–6.
246. Kamath GG, Prasad S, Patwala YJ, et al. Peripapillary coloboma simulating double optic disc. Br J Ophthalmol 1999; 83:1207.
247. Kawamura M, Tajima S, Azuma N, et al. Biochemical studies of glycosaminoglycans in nanophthalmic sclera. Graefe's Arch Clin Exp Ophthalmol 1995; 233:58–62.
248. Kawamura M, Tajima S, Azuma N, et al. Immunohistochemical studies of glycosaminoglycans in nanophthalmic sclera. Graefe's Arch Clin Exp Ophthalmol 1996; 234:19–24.
249. Keppen LD, Brodsky MC, Michael JM, et al. Hypogonadotropic hypogonadism in mentally retarded adults with microphthalmia and clinical anophthalmia. Am J Med Genet 1990; 36:285–7.
250. Khaliq S, Hameed A, Ismail M, et al. Locus for autosomal recessive nonsyndromic persistent hyperplastic primary vitreous. Invest Ophthalmol Vis Sci 2001; 42:2225–8.
251. Khan AO, Nowilaty SR. Early diagnosis of the papillorenal syndrome by optic disc morphology. J Neuro-Ophthalmol 2005; 25:209–11.
252. Kida M. Thalidomide Embryopathy in Japan. Tokyo: Kodansha Ltd, 1987:143–53.
253. Kim BH, Henderson BA. Intraocular choristoma. Semin. Ophthalmol 2005; 20:223–9.
254. Kim RY, Hoyt WF, Lessell S, et al. Superior segmental optic hypoplasia. Arch Ophthalmol 1989; 107:1312–5.
255. Kim J, Hwang J, Kim H, et al. Characteristic ocular findings in Asian children with Down syndrome. Eye 2002; 16:710–14.
256. Kim SH, Hwang S, Kweon S, et al. Two cases of lacrimal gland agenesis in the same family – clinicoradiologic findings and management. Can J Ophthalmol 2005; 40: 502–5.
257. Kim DY, Neely KA, Sassani JW, et al. X-linked retinoschisis. Novel mutation in the initiation codon of the *XLRS1* gene in a large family. Retina 2006; 26:940–6.
258. Kindler, P. Morning glory syndrome. Am J Ophthalmol 1970; 69:376–84.
259. King RA, Hearing VJ, Creel DJ, et al. Albinism. In: Scriver CR, Beaudet AL, Sly WS, Valle D, eds. The Metabolic and Molecular Bases of Inherited Disease. New York: McGraw, 1995:4353–92.
260. Kivlin J, Fineman RM, Crandall AS, et al. Peters anomaly as a consequence of genetic and nongenetic syndromes. Arch Ophthalmol 1986; 104:1–64.
261. Knox EG, Lancashire RJ. Epidemiology of congenital malformations. London: Her Majesty's Stationary Office, 1991.
262. Knudson AG Jr, Strong LC. Mutation and cancer: a model for Wilm's tumor of the kidney. J Natl Cancer Inst 1972; 48:313–24.
263. Kok RD, de Vries MM, Heerschap A, et al. Absence of harmful effects of magnetic resonance exposure at 1.5 T in utero during the third trimester of pregnancy: a follow-up study. Magn Reson Imaging 2004; 22:851–4.
264. Kokich VG, Ngim C-H, Siebert JR, et al. Cyclopia: an anatomic and histologic study of two specimens. Teratology 1982; 26:105–13.
265. Konrad M, Schaller A, Seelow D, et al. Mutations in the tight-junction gene claudin 19 (*CLDN19*) are associated with renal magnesium wasting, renal failure, and severe ocular involvement. Am J Hum Genet 2006; 79: 949–57.
266. Koole FD, Velzeboer CM, van der Harten JJ. Ocular abnormalities in Patau syndrome (chromosome 13 trisomy syndrome). Ophthalmic Paediatr Genet 1990; 11: 15–21.
267. Kozma C, Hunt M, Meck J, et al. Familial Wolf-Hirschhorn syndrome associated with Rieger anomaly of the eye. Ophthalmic Paediatr Genet 1990; 11:23–30.
268. Krachmer HJ, Rodrigues MM. Posterior keratoconus. Arch Ophthalmol 1978; 95:1867–73.
269. Kresky B, Nauheim JS. Rubella retinitis. Am J Dis Child 1967; 113:305–10.
270. Kriederman BM, Myloyde TL, Witte MH, et al. FOXC2 haploinsufficient mice are a model for human autosomal dominant lymphedema – distichiasis syndrome. Hum Mol Genet 2003; 12:1179–85.
271. Krill AE. The retinal disease of rubella. Arch Ophthalmol 1967; 77:445–9.
272. Kugelman TP, Van Scott EJ. Tyrosinase activity in melanocytes of human albinos. J Invest Dermatol 1961; 37:73–6.
273. Kupfer C, Kaiser-Kupfer MI. Observations on the development of the anterior chamber angle with reference to the pathogenesis of congenital glaucomas. Am J Ophthalmol 1979; 88:424–6.
274. Lahav M, Albert PM, Wyand S. Clinical and histopathologic classification of retinal dysplasia. Am J Ophthalmol 1973; 75:648–67.
275. Lambert SR, Hoyt CS, Narahara MH. Optic nerve hypoplasia. Surv Ophthalmol 1987; 32:1–9.
276. Lambert SR, Taylor D, Kriss A, et al. Ocular manifestations of the congenital varicella syndrome. Arch Ophthalmol 1989; 107:52–6.
277. Lavedan C, Barichard F, Azoulay M, et al. Molecular definition of de novo and genetically transmitted WAGR-associated rearrangements of 11p13. Cytogenet Cell Genet 1989; 50:70–4.
278. Lawin-Brussel, C. and Busse, H. Iridocorneotrabecular dysgenesis in a patient sample of the Munster University Eye Clinic. Clin Fortschr Ophthalmol 1988; 85:101–4.
279. Lee WR, Grierson I. Posterior vitreo-retinal malformation: a clinic-pathological case report. Ophthalmologica 1977; 171:282–90.
280. Lee ST, Nicholls RD, Bundey S, et al. Mutations of the P gene in oculocutaneous albinism, ocular albinism, and Prader-Willi syndrome plus albinism. N Engl J Med 1994; 330:529–34.
281. Lehmann O, Ebenezer ND, Ekong R, et al. Ocular developmental abnormalities and glaucoma associated with interstitial 6p25 duplications and deletions. Invest Ophthalmol Vis Sci 2002; 43:1843–9.
282. Leighton DA, Harris R. Retinal aplasia in association with macular coloboma, keratoconus and cataract. Clin Genet 1973; 4:270–4.
283. Lemoine P, Harousseau H, Borteyru JP, et al. Les enfants de parents alcooliques. Anomalies observees. A propos de 127 cas. Ouest-Medical 1968; 21:476–82.

284. Lenz W. Thalidomide and congenital abnormalities. Lancet 1962; 45:2371–2.
285. Levine EM, Green ES. Cell-intrinsic regulators of proliferation in vertebrate retinal progenitors. Semin Cell Dev Biol 2004; 15:63–74.
286. Lieb W, Rochels R, Gronemeyer U. Microphthalmos with colobomatous orbital cyst: clinical, histological, immunohistological, and electronmicroscopic findings. Br J Ophthalmol 1990; 75:59–62.
287. Limwongse C, Wyszynski R, Dickerman L, et al. Microcephaly-lymphedema-chorioretinal dysplasia: a unique genetic syndrome with variable expression and possible characteristic facial appearance. Am J Med Genet 1999; 86:215–8.
288. Lin AE, Biglan AW, Garver KL. Perisitent hyperplastic primary vitreous with vertical transmission. Ophthalmic Paediatr Genet 1990; 11:121–2.
289. Lines MA, Kozlowski K, Kulak SC, et al. Characterization and prevalence of *PITX2* microdeletions and mutations in Axenfeld-Rieger malformations. Invest Ophthalmol Vis Sci 2004; 45:828–33.
290. Lisch W, Rochels R. Pathogenesis of congenital vitreous cysts. Klin Monatsbl Augenheilkd 1989; 195:375–8.
291. Lloyd IC, Colley A, Tullo AB, et al. Dominantly inherited unilateral retinal dysplasia. Br J Ophthalmol 1993; 77: 378–80.
292. Loh RCK, Tan DSL. Unusual case of progeria-like dwarfism with bilateral macular coloboma. Am J Ophthalmol 1970; 70:968–74.
293. Lonn L. Neonatal cytomegalic inclusion disease chorioretinitis. Arch Ophthalmol 1972; 88:434–8.
294. Lowry RB, Kohut R, Sibbald B, et al. Anophthalmia and microphthalmia in the Alberta Congenital Anomalies Surveillance System. Can J Ophthalmol 2005; 40:38–44.
295. Lueder GT. Clinical ocular abnormalities in infants with trisomy 13. Am J Ophthalmol 2006; 141:1057–60.
296. Luhmann UF, Lin J, Acar N, et al. Role of the Norrie disease pseudoglioma gene in sprouting angiogenesis during development of the retinal vasculature. Invest Ophthalmol Vis Sci 2005; 46:3372–82.
297. Luleci G, Bagci G, Kivran M, et al. A hereditary bisatellite-dicentric supernumerary chromosome in a case of cat-eye syndrome. Hereditas 1989; 111:7–10.
298. Lupo G, Andreazzoli M, Gestri G, et al. Homeobox genes in the genetic control of eye development. Int J Dev Biol 2000; 44:627–36.
299. MacRae DW, Howard RO, Albert DM, et al. Ocular manifestations of the Meckel syndrome. Arch Ophthalmol 1972; 88:106–33.
300. Maillard T, Lamblin D, Lesure JF, et al. Incidence of fetal alcohol syndrome on the southern part of Reunion Island (France). Teratology 1999; 60:51–2.
301. Mann I. Developmental Abnormalities of the Human Eye. London: Cambridge University Press, 1957.
302. Mannens M, Bleeker-Wagemakers EM, Bliek J, et al. Autosomal dominant aniridia linked to the chromosome 11p13 markers catalase and D11S151 in a large Dutch family. Cytogenet Cell Genet 1989; 52:32–6.
303. Manschot WA. Persistent hyperplastic primary vitreous. Arch Ophthalmol 1958; 59:188–203.
304. Manschot WA. Primary congenital aphakia. Arch Ophthalmol 1963; 69:571–7.
305. Manschot WA. Eye findings in hydranencephaly. Ophthalmologica 1971; 162:151–9.
306. Manschot WA. Pathology of hereditary juvenile retinoschisis. Arch Ophthalmol 1972; 88:131–8.
307. Manschot WA. Morning glory syndrome: a histopathological study. Br J Ophthalmol 1990; 74:560–80.
308. Mansour AM, Bitar FF, Traboulsi EI, et al. Ocular pathology in congenital heart disease. Eye 2005; 19:29–34.
309. Mao R, Zielke, CL, Zielke HR, et al. Global up-regulation of chromosome 21 expression in the developing Down syndrome brain. Genomics 2003; 81:457–67.
310. Marcus DM, Shore JW, Albert DM. Anophthalmia in the focal dermal hypoplasia syndrome. Arch Ophthalmol 1990; 108:96–100.
311. Margari L, Presicci A, Ventura P, et al. Megalocornea and mental retardation syndrome: clinical and instrumental follow-up of a case.
312. Margo CE. Congenital Aniridia: a histopathological study of the anterior segment in children. J Ped Ophthal Strab 1983; 20:192–8.
313. Margolis S, Scher BM, Char RE. Macular colobomas in Leber's congenital amaurosis. Am J Ophthalmol 1977; 83: 27–31.
314. Mari F, Giachino D, Russo L, et al. Blepharophimosis, ptosis, epicanthus inversus syndrome: clinical and molecular analysis of a case. J AAPOS 2006; 10:279–80.
315. Marneros AG, Fan J, Yokoyama Y, et al. Vascular endothelial growth factor expression in the retinal pigment epithelium is essential for choriocapillaris development and visual function. Am J Pathol 2005; 167:1451–9.
316. Martin XD, Rabineau PA. Dysgenesis of the neural crest, ectoderm, mesoderm and fetal alcohol syndrome. Klin Monatsbl Augenheilkd 1990; 196:279–84.
317. Martin AC, Thornton JD, Liu J, et al. Pathogenesis of persistent hyperplastic primary vitreous in mice lacking the *Arf* tumor suppressor gene. Invest Ophthalmol Vis Sci 2004; 45:3387–96.
318. Martinez-Mora J, Audi L, Toran N, et al. Ambiguous genitalia, gonadoblastoma, aniridia, and mental retardation with deletion of chromosome 11. J Urol 1989; 142: 1298–300.
319. Martorina M. Familial nanophthalmos. J Fr Ophthalmol 1988; 11:357–61.
320. McGannon P, Miyazaki Y, Gupta P, et al. Ocular abnormalities in mice lacking the *Ski* proto-oncogene. Invest Ophthalmol Vis Sci 2006; 47:4231–7.
321. McGinnis W, Levine MS, Hafen E, et al. A conserved DNA sequence in homoeotic genes of the Drosophila Antennapedia and bithorax complexes. Nature 1984; 308: 428–33.
322. McGregor L, Makela V, Darling SM, et al. Fraser syndrome and mouse blebbed phenotype caused by mutations in *FRAS1*/*Fras1* encoding a putative extracellular matrix protein. Nat Genet 2003; 34:203–8.
323. McKusick VA. On-line Mendelian Inheritance in Man. http://www.ncbi.nlm.nih.gov/entrez/query.fcgi?db=OMIM.
324. McLane NJ, Carroll DM. Ocular manifestations of drug abuse. Surv Ophthalmol 1986; 30:298–313.
325. McLeod R, Lowry RB. Incidence of albinism in British Columbia (B.C.). Separation by hairbulb test. Clin Genet 1976; 9:77–80.
326. Menser MA, Dods L, Harley JD. A twenty-five-year follow-up of congenital rubella. Lancet 1967; 2:1347–50.
327. Menser MA, Harley JD, Hertzberg R, et al. Persistence of virus in lens for three years after prenatal rubella. Lancet 1967; 2:387–8.
328. Messmer EM, Kenyon KR, Rittinger O, et al. Ocular manifestations of keratitis-ichthyosis-deafness (KID) syndrome. Ophthalmology 2005; 112:e1–16.

329. Michaelides M, Luthert PJ, Cooling R, et al. Norrie disease and peripheral venous insufficiency. Br J Ophthalmol 2004; 88:1475.
330. Michaelides M, Urquhart J, Holder GE, et al. Evidence of genetic heterogeneity in MRCS (microcornea, rod-cone dystrophy, cataract, and posterior staphyloma) syndrome. Am J Ophthalmol 2006; 141:418–20.
331. Miller MT, Deutsch TA, Cronin C, et al. Amniotic bands as a cause of ocular anomalies. Am J Ophthalmol 1987; 104:270–9.
332. Miller RW, Fraumeni JF, Manning MD. Association of Wilm's tumor with aniridia, hemihypertrophy and other congenital malformations. N Engl J Med 1964; 270:922–7.
333. Miller MT, Stromland K. Ocular motility in thalidomide embryopathy. J Pediatr Ophthalmol Strab 1991; 28:47–54.
334. Milunsky JM, Zhao G, Maher TA, et al. LADD syndrome is caused by *FGF10* mutations. Clin Genet 2006; 69: 349–54.
335. Mirzayans F, Pearce WG, MacDonald IM, et al. Mutation of the PAX6 gene in patients with autosomal dominant keratitis. Am J Hum Genet 1995; 57:539–48.
336. Mizuno K, Takei Y, Sears ML, et al. Leber's congenital amaurosis. Am J Ophthalmol 1977; 83:32–42.
337. Moerman P, Fryns J-P, van der Steen K, et al. The pathology of trisomy 13 syndrome. A study of 12 cases. Hum Genet 1988; 80:349–56.
338. Mosier MA, Lieberman MF, Green WR, et al. Hypoplasia of the optic nerve. Arch Ophthalmol 1978; 96:1437–43.
339. Mullaney J. Edwards' syndrome. Am J Ophthalmol 1972; 76:246–54.
340. Mullaney J. Complicated sporadic colobomata. Br J Ophthalmol 1978; 62:384–5.
341. Muraskas JK, McDonnell JF, Chudik RJ, et al. Amniotic band syndrome with significant orofacial clefts and disruptions and distortions of craniofacial structures. J Pediatr Surg 2003; 38:635–8.
342. Murata T, Hashimoto S, Ishibashi T, et al. A case of amniotic band syndrome with bilateral epibulbar choristoma. Br J Ophthalmol 1992; 76:685–7.
343. Nakano M, Yamada K, Fain J, et al. Homozygous mutations in ARIX(PHOX2A) result in congenital fibrosis of the extraocular muscles type 2. Nat Genet 2001; 29:315–20.
344. Nallathambi J, Moumne L, De Baere E, et al. A novel polyalanine expansion in FOXL2: first evidence for a recessive form of the blepharophimosis syndrome (BPES) associated with ovarian dysfunction. Hum Genet 2007; 121:107–12.
345. Neel JA. Update on the genetic effects of ionizing radiation. J Am Med Assoc 1991; 266:698–701.
346. Nefzger MD, Miller RJ, Fujino T. Eye findings in atomic bomb survivors of Hiroshima and Nagasaki: 1963–1964. Am J Epidemiol 1968; 89:129–38.
347. Nelson LB. Diagnosis and management of congenital and developmental cataracts. Semin Ophthalmol 1990; 5: 154–65.
348. Nelson LB, Spaeth GL, Nowinski TS, et al. Aniridia: a review. Surv Ophthalmol 1984; 28:621–42.
349. Neveu MM, Holder GE, Sloper JJ, et al. Optic chiasm formation in humans is independent of foveal development. Eur J Neuroscience 2005; 22:1825–9.
350. Ng D, Thakker N, Corcoran CM, et al. Oculofaciocardiodental and Lenz microphthalmia syndromes result from distinct classes of mutations in BCOR. Nat Genet 2004; 36:411–6.
351. Nie X, Luukko K, Kettunen P. FGF signaling in craniofacial development and developmental disorders. Oral Diseases 2006; 12:102–11.
352. Nikolaienko O, Nguyen C, Crinc LS, et al. Human chromosome 21/Down syndrome gene function and pathway database. Gene 2005; 364:90–8.
353. Nishida K, Kinoshita S, Ohashi Y, et al. Ocular surface abnormalities in aniridia. Am J Ophthalmol 1995; 120: 368–75.
354. Nucci P, Mets MB, Gabianelli EB. Trisomy 4q with morning glory disc anomaly. Ophthalmic Paediatr Genet 1990; 11:143–5.
355. O'Donnell FE Jr, Hambrick GW Jr, Green WR, et al. X-linked ocular albinism. An oculocutaneous macromelanosomal disorder. Arch Ophthalmol 1976; 94:1883–92.
356. O'Grady RB, Rothstein TB, Romano PG. D-Group deletion syndromes and retinoblastoma. Am J Ophthalmol 1974; 77:40–5.
357. Oetting WS, Fryer JP, Shriram S, et al. Oculocutaneous albinism type 1: the last 100 years. Pigment Cell Res, 6: 307–11.
358. Ohkubo S, Takeda H, Higashide T, et al. Immunohistochemical and molecular genetic evidence for type IV collagen $\alpha5$ chain abnormality in the anterior lenticonus associated with Alport syndrome. Arch Ophthalmol 2003; 121:846–50.
359. Ohlmann A, Scholz M, Goldwich A, et al. Ectopic norrin induces growth of ocular capillaries and restores normal retinal angiogenesis in Norrie disease mutant mice. J Neurosci 2005; 25:1701–10.
360. Okoro AN. Albinism in Nigeria. A clinical and social study. Br J Dermatol 1975; 92:485–92.
361. Oliver MD, Dotan SA, Chemke J, et al. Isolated foveal hypoplasia. Br J Ophthalmol 1987; 71:926–30.
362. Onwochei BC, Simon JW, Bateman JB, et al. Ocular colobomata. Surv Ophthalmol 2000; 45:175–94.
363. Ornoy A, Patlas N, Schwartz L. The effects of in utero diagnostic X-irradiation on the development of pre-school-age children. Isr J Med Sci 1996; 32:112–5.
364. Otake M, Schull WJ. In utero exposure to A-bomb radiation and mental retardation: a reassessment. Br J Radiol 1984; 57:409–11.
365. Ott S, Borchert M, Chung M, et al. Exclusion of candidate genetic loci for Duane retraction syndrome. Am J Ophthalmol 1999; 127:358–60.
366. Ozeki H, Shirai S, Nozaki M, et al. Ocular and systemic features of Peters'anomaly. Graefe's Arch Clin Exp Ophthalmol 2000; 238:833–9.
367. Ozeki H, Ogura Y, Hirabayashi Y, et al. Suppression of lens stalk cell apoptosis by hyaluronic acid leads to faulty separation of the lens vesicle. Exp Eye Res 2001; 72:63–70.
368. Pallotta R, Fusillis P, Sabatino G, et al. Confirmation of the colobomatous macrophthalmia with microcornea syndrome: report of another family. Am J Med Genet 1998; 76:252–4.
369. Parsons MA, Curtis D, Blank CE, et al. The ocular pathology of Norrie disease in a fetus of 11 weeks' gestational age. Graefe's Arch Clin Exp Ophthalmol 1992; 230:248–51.
370. Pedersen OO, Rushood A, Olsen EG. Anterior mesenchymal dysgenesis of the eye. Acta Ophthalmol 1989; 67: 470–6.
371. Percy DH, Danylchuk KD. Retinal dysplasia and cytosine arabinoside. Invest Ophthalmol Vis Sci 1977; 16:353–64.
372. Petersen RA. Schmid-Fraccaro syndrome ("cat's eye" syndrome). Arch Ophthalmol 1973; 90:287–92.
373. Phillips CI, Griffiths DL. Macular coloboma and skeletal abnormality. Br J Ophthalmol 1969; 53:346–9.
374. Pierre-Filho Pde T, Limeira-Soares PH, Marcondes AM. Morning glory syndrome associated with posterior

pituitary ectopia and hypopituitarism. Acta Ophthalmol Scand 2004; 82:89–92.
375. Polizzi A, Pavone P, Iannetti P, et al. Septo-optic dysplasia complex: a heterogeneous malformation syndrome. Pediat Neurol 2006; 34:66–71.
376. Poswillo D. Mechanisms and pathogenesis of malformations. Br Med Bull 1976; 32:59–64.
377. Poswillo D. Pathogenesis of craniofacial syndromes exhibiting colobomata. Trans Ophthalmol Soc UK 1976; 96:69–72.
378. Priolo M, Lagana C. Ectodermal dysplasia: a new clinical-genetic classification. J Med Genet 2001; 38:579–85.
379. Prosser J, van Heyningen V. PAX6 mutations reviewed. Hum Mutat 1998; 11:93–108.
380. Quah BL, Hamilton J, Blaser S, et al. Morning glory disc anomaly, midline cranial defects and abnormal carotid circulation: an association worth looking for. Pediatr Radiol 2005; 35:525–8.
381. Ragge NK, Brown AG, Poloschek CM, et al. Heterozygous mutations of OTX2 cause severe ocular malformations. Am J Hum Genet 2005; 76:1008–22.
382. Ragge NK, Lorenz B, Schneider A, et al. SOX2 anophthalmia syndrome. Am J Med Genet 2005; 135 A: 1–7.
383. Raizman MB. Ocular abnormalities accompanying chromosome 13 defects. Arch Ophthalmol 1987; 105:744.
384. Ramaesh K, Ramaesh T, Dutton GN, et al. Evolving concepts on the pathogenic mechanisms of aniridia related keratopathy. Int J Biochem Cell Biol 2005; 37: 547–57.
385. Ramprasad VL, Thool A, Murugan S, et al. Truncating mutation in the NHS gene: phenotypic heterogeneity of Nance-Horan Syndrome in an Asian Indian family. Invest Ophthalmol Vis Sci 2005; 46:17–23.
386. Rasmussen SA, Wong LYC, Yang Q, et al. Population-based analyses of mortality in trisomy 13 and trisomy 18. Pediatrics 2003; 111:777–84.
387. Rating D, Nau H, Jäger-Roman E, et al. Teratogenic and pharmacokinetic studies of primidone during pregnancy and in the offspring of epileptic women. Acta Paediatr Scand 1982; 71:301–11.
388. Reddy MA, Francis PJ, Berry V, et al. A clinical and molecular genetic study of a rare dominantly inherited syndrome (MRCS) comprising of microcornea, rod-cone dystrophy, cataract, and posterior staphyloma. Br J Ophthalmol 2003; 87:197–202.
389. Reese AB, Ellsworth RM. The anterior chamber cleavage syndrome. Arch Ophthalmol 1966; 75:307–18.
390. Rehm HL, Gutierrez-Espeleta GA, Garcia R, et al. Norrie disease gene mutation in a large Costa Rican kindred with a novel phenotype including venous insufficiency. Hum Mutat 1997; 9:402–8.
391. Remington JS. Toxoplasmosis and congenital infection. Birth Defects 1968; 4:47–56.
392. Reneker LW, Silversides DW, Xu L, et al. Formation of corneal endothelium is essential for anterior segment development – a transgenic mouse model of anterior segment dysgenesis. Development 2000; 127:533–42.
393. Rethore MO, Dutrillaux B, Giovannelli G. La trisomie 4p. Ann Genet 1974; 17:125–8.
394. Riikonen RS. Retinal vasculitis caused by rubella. Neuropediatrics 1995; 26:174–6.
395. Riise R, Storhaug K, Brondum-Nielsen K. Rieger syndrome is associated with PAX6 deletion. Acta Ophthalmol Scand 2001; 79:201–3.
396. Riveiro-Alvarez R, Trujillo-Tiebas MJ, Gimenez-Pardo A, et al. Genotype-phenotype variations in five Spanish families with Norrie disease or X-linked FEVR. Mol Vis 2005; 11:705–12.
397. Robb RM, Marchevsky A. Pathology of the lens in Down's syndrome. Arch Ophthalmol 1978; 96:1039–43.
398. Robb RM, Silver J, Sullivan RT. Ocular retardation (or) in the mouse. Invest Ophthalmol Vis Sci 1978; 17:468–73.
399. Robinson GC, Conry JL, Conry RF. Clinical profile and prevalence of fetal alcohol syndrome in an isolated community in British Columbia. Can Med Assoc J 1987; 137:203–7.
400. Robitaille J, MacDonald ML, Kaykas A, et al. Mutant frizzled-4 disrupts retinal angiogenesis in familial exudative vitreoretinopathy. Nat Genet 2002; 32:326–30.
401. Rouland JF, Hochart G, Constaninides G. Chorioretinal coloboma and neovascular membrane. Bull Soc Ophtalmol Fr 1990; 90:654–5.
402. Ruefer F, Schroeder A, Erb C. White-to white corneal diameter. Normal values in healthy humans obtained with the Orbscan II topography system.Cornea 2005; 24: 259–61.
403. Russel-Eggit IM, Blake KD, Taylor DS, et al. The eye in the CHARGE association. Br J Ophthalmol 1990; 75:421–26.
404. Saadati HG, Hsu HY, Heller KB, et al. A histopathologic and morphometric differentiation of nerves in optic nerve hypoplasia and Leber hereditary optic neuropathy. Arch Ophthalmol 1998; 116:911–6.
405. Sabatier C, Plump AS, Ma L, et al. The divergent Robo family protein Rig-1/Robo3 is a negative regulator of Slit responsiveness required for midline crossing by commissural axons. Cell 2004; 117:157–69.
406. Salmon JF, Wallis CE, Murray AD. Variable expressivity of autosomal dominant microcornea with cataract. Arch Ophthalmol 1988; 106:505–10.
407. Sami DA, Saunders D, Thompson DA, et al. The achiasmia spectrum: congenitally reduced chiasmal decussation. Br J Ophthalmol 2005; 89:1311–7.
408. Samples JR, Meyer SM. Use of ophthalmic medications in pregnant and nursing women. Am J Ophthalmol 1988; 106:616–23.
409. Sampson PD, Streissguth AP, Bookstein FL, et al. Incidence of fetal alcohol syndrome and prevalence of alcohol-related neurodevelopmental disorder. Teratology 1997; 56:317–26.
410. Sanjari MS, Ghasemi Falavarjani K, Paravaresh MM, et al. Bilateral aplasia of the optic nerve, chiasm and tracts in an otherwise healthy infant. Br J Ophthjalmol 2006; 90: 513–4.
411. Saraux J. Ocular manifestations of disease due to aberrations of non-sexual chromosomes. J Med Genet 1970; 25:227–38.
412. Sarfarazi M. Recent advances in molecular genetics of glaucomas. Hum Molec Genet 1997; 6:1667–77.
413. Sassani JW, Yanoff M. Anophthalmos in an infant with multiple congential anomalies. Am J Ophthalmol 1977; 83:43–51.
414. Satorre J, Lopez JM, Martinez J, et al. Dominant macular colobomata. J Pediatr Ophthalmol Strab 1990; 27:148–52.
415. Savage MO, Moosa A, Gordon RR. Maternal varicella infection as a cause of fetal malformations. Lancet 1973; 1: 352–4.
416. Savell J, Cook R Jr. Optic nerve colobomas of autosomal dominant heredity. Arch Ophthalmol 1975; 94:395–400.
417. Schanzlin DJ, Goldberg DB, Brown SI. Hallerman-Streiff syndrome associated with sclerocornea, aniridia and a chromosomal abnormality. Am J Ophthalmol 1980; 90: 411–5.

418. Schiaffino MV, Tacchetti C. The ocular albinism type 1 (OA1) protein and the evidence for an intracellular signal transduction system involved in melanosome biogenesis. Pigment Cell Res 2005; 18:227–33.
419. Schimmenti LA, de la Cruz J, Lewis RA, et al. Novel mutation in sonic hedgehog in non-syndromic colobomatous microphthalmia. Am J Med Genet 2003; 116 A: 215–21.
420. Schinzel A, Dapuzzo V. Anophthalmia in a retarded infant with partial trisomy 4p and 22 following a maternal translocation, rcp(4;22)(p15.2;q11.2). Ophthalmic Paediatr Genet 1990; 11:139–42.
421. Schipper I, Senn P, Schmid M. Diagnosis and management of bilateral posterior lenticonus in 7 members of the same family. J Cataract Refract Surg 2006; 32:261–3.
422. Schneuwly S, Klemenz R, Gehring WJ. Redesigning the body plan of Drosophila by ectopic expression of the homoeotic gene Antennapedia. Nature 1987; 325: 816–8.
423. Schroeder B, Hesse L, Bruck W, et al. Histopathological and immunohistochemical findings associated with a null mutation in the Norrie disease gene. Ophthalmic Genet 1997; 18:71–7.
424. Seeger M, Tear G, Ferres-Marco D, et al. Mutations affecting growth cone guidance in Drosophila: genes necessary for guidance toward or away from the midline. Neuron 1993; 10:409–26.
425. Segev F, Heon E, Cole WG, et al. Structural abnormalities of the cornea and lid resulting from collagen V mutations. Invest Ophthalmol Vis Sci 2006; 47:565–73.
426. Semina EV, Reiter R, Leysens NJ, et al. Cloning and characterization of a novel bicoid-related transcription factor gene, RGS, involved in Rieger syndrome. Nat Genet 1996; 14:392–9.
427. Sharan S, Sharma S, Billson FA. Congenital rubella cataract: a timely reminder in the new millennium? Clin Exp Ophthalmol 2006; 34:83–4.
428. Shastry BS, Pendergast SD, Hartzer MK, et al. Identification of missense mutations in the Norrie disease gene associated with advanced retinopathy of prematurity. Arch Ophthalmol 1997; 115:651–5.
429. Shaw GM, Carmichael SL, Yang W, et al. Epidemiologic characteristics of anophthalmia and bilateral microphthalmia among 2.5 million births in California, 1989–1997. Am J Med Genet 2005; 137 A:36–40.
430. Shepard TH. Catalog of Teratogenic Agents. 6th ed. Baltimore: Johns Hopkins University Press, 1989.
431. Shields MB. Axenfeld-Rieger syndrome: a theory of mechanism and distinctions from the iridocorneal endothelial syndrome. Trans Am Ophthalmol Soc 1983; 81: 736–84.
432. Shields MB. A common pathway for developmental glaucomas. Trans Am Ophthalmol Soc 1987; 85:222–37.
433. Shields MB, Buckley E, Klintworth GK, et al. Axenfeld-Rieger syndrome: a spectrum of developmental disorders. Surv Ophthalmol 1985; 29:387–409.
434. Shiota K. Neural tube defects and maternal hyperthermia in early pregnancy: epidemiology in a human embryo population. Am J Med Genet 1982; 12:281–8.
435. Shirai S, Ohshika S, Yuguchi S, et al. Ochratoxin A: III. Developmental abnormalities of the anterior segment of the eye induced in mice by ochratoxin A. Acta Soc Ophthalmol Jap 1985; 89:753–60.
436. Sikkink SK, Biswas S, Parry NRA, et al. X-linked retinoschisis: an update. J Med Genet 2007; 44:225–32.
437. Silbert M, Gurwood AS. Persistent hyperplastic primary vitreous. Clin Eye Vision Care 2000; 12:131–7.
438. Silver J, Hughes A. The role of cell death during morphogenesis of the mammalian eye. J Morphol 1973; 140:159–70.
439. Silver J, Hughes AFW. The relationship between morphogenetic cell death and the development of congenital anophthalmia. J Comp Neurol 1974; 157:281–301.
440. Silver J, Robb RM. Studies on the development of the eye cup and optic nerve in normal mice and in mutants with congenital optic nerve aplasia. Dev Biol 1979; 68:175–90.
441. Silverstein AM. Dysplasia and rosettes. Am J Ophthalmol 1974; 77:51–9.
442. Singh S, Sanyal AK. Eye anomalies induced by cyclophosphamide in rat fetuses. Acta Anat 1976; 94:490–500.
443. Sisodiya SM, Free SL, Williamson KA, et al. PAX6 haploinsufficiency causes cerebral malformation and olfactory dysfunction in humans. Nat Genet 2001; 28: 214–6.
444. Skarf B, Hoyt CS. Optic nerve hypoplasia in children: association with anomalies of the endocrine and CNS. Arch Ophthalmol 1984; 102:62–7.
445. Slavotinek AM, Tifft CJ. Fraser syndrome and cryptophthalmos: review of the diagnostic criteria and evidence for phenotypic modules in complex malformation syndromes. J Med Genet 2002; 39:623–33.
446. Smithells RW. Environmental teratogens of man. Br Med Bull 1976; 32:27–33.
447. Sobol WM, Bratton AR, Rivers MB, et al. Morning glory disk syndrome associated with subretinal neovascular membrane formation. Am J Ophthalmol 1990; 110:93–5.
448. Sohajda Z, Hollo D, Berta A, et al. Microcornea associated with myopia. Graefe's Arch Clin Exp Ophthalmol 2006; 244:1211–3.
449. Soong HK, Raizman MB. Corneal changes in familial iris coloboma. Ophthalmology 1986; 93:335–9.
450. Sorsby A. Congenital coloboma of the macula. Br J Ophthalmol 1935; 19:65–74.
451. Spedick MJ, Beauchamp GR. Retinal vascular and optic nerve abnormalities in albinism. J Pediatr Ophthalmol Strabismus 1986; 23:58–63.
452. Stanescu B, Dralands L. Cerebrohepatorenal (Zellweger's) syndrome. Arch Ophthalmol 1972; 87: 590–2.
453. Stathacopoulos RA, Bateman JB, Sparkes RS, et al. The Rieger syndrome and a chromosome 13 deletion. J Pediatr Ophthalmol Strab 1987; 24:198–203.
454. Stevens CA, Sargent LA. Ablepharon-macrostomia syndrome. Amer J Med Genet 2002; 107:30–7.
455. Stewart DH III, Streeten BW, Brockhurst RJ, et al. Abnormal scleral collagen in nanophthalmos. An ultrastructural study. Arch Ophthalmol 1991; 109:1017–25.
456. Stockard CR. The influence of alcohol and other anesthetics on embryonic development. Am J Anatomy 1910; 10:369–92.
457. Stoilov I, Akarsu AN, Sarfarazi M. Identification of three different truncating mutations in cytochrome P4501B1 (CYP1B1) as the principal cause of primary congenital glaucoma (Buphthalmos) in families linked to the GLC3A locus on chromosome 2p21. Hum Mol Genet 1997; 6:641–7.
458. Stone DL, Kenyon KR, Green WR, et al. Congenital central corneal leukoma (Peters' anomaly). Am J Ophthalmol 1976; 81:173–93.
459. Storimans CW, Van Schooneveld MJ. Rieger's eye anomaly and persistent hyperplastic primary vitreous. Ophthalmic Paediatr Genet 1989; 10:257–62.
460. Stover PJ, Garza C. Nutrition and developmental biology—implications for public health. Nutr Rev 2006; 64: S60–71.

461. Strange JR, Murphree RL. Exposure-rate response in the prenatally irradiated rat: effects of 100 R on day of gestation to the developing eye. Radiat Res 1972; 51: 674–84.
462. Streeten BW, Karpik AG, Spitzer KH. Posterior keratoconus associated with systemic abnormalities. Arch Ophthalmol 1983; 101:616–22.
463. Stretch JR, Poole MD. Nasolacrimal abnormalities in oblique facial clefts. Br J Plast Surg 1990; 43:463–7.
464. Stromland K. Ocular involvement in the fetal alcohol syndrome. Surv Ophthalmol 1987; 31:277–83.
465. Stromland K. Ocular malformations in children exposed to drugs during gestation. Clin Pediatr 1988; 27:257–8.
466. Stromland K. Visual impairment and ocular abnormalities in children with fetal alcohol syndrome. Addict Biol 2004; 9:153–7.
467. Stromland K, Miller M, Cook D. Ocular teratology. Surv Ophthalmol 1991; 35:429–46.
468. Stromland K, Miller MT. Thalidomide embryopathy: revisited 27 years later. Acta Ophthalmol (Copenh) 1993; 71:238–45.
469. Stromland K, Pinazo-Duran MD. Ophthalmic involvement in the fetal alcohol syndrome: clinical and animal model studies. Alcohol Alcohol 2002; 37:2–8.
470. Sulik KK. Genesis of alcohol-induced craniofacial dysmorphism. Exp Biol Med (Maywood) 2005; 230: 366–75.
471. Sullivan-Jones P, Hansen DK, Sheehan DM, et al. The effect of teratogens on maternal corticosterone levels and cleft incidence in A/J mice. J Craniofac Genet Dev Biol 1992; 12:183–9.
472. Susanna R Jr. Implantation of an intraocular lens in a case of nanophthalmos. CLAO J 1987; 13:117–8.
473. Suzuki Y, Kawase E, Nishina S, et al. two patients with different features of congenital optic disc anomalies in the two eyes. Graefe's Arch Clin Exp Ophthalmol 2006; 244: 259–61.
474. Swan C. A study of three infants dying from congenital defects following maternal rubella in the early stages of pregnancy. Pathol Bacteriol 1944; 61:289–95.
475. Szyfelbein K, Kozakewicz HPW, Syed NA, et al. Phakomatous choristoma of the eyelid: a report of a case. J Cutan Pathol 2004; 31:506–8.
476. Talks SJ, Ebenezer N, Hykin P, et al. De novo mutations in the 5′ regulatory region of the Norrie disease gene in retinopathy of prematurity. J Med Genet 2001; 38:E46.
477. Tanaka H. Fetal alcohol syndrome: a Japanese perspective. Ann Med 1998; 30:21–6.
478. Taylor DSI. The genetic implications of optic disc anomalies. Trans Ophthalmol Soc UK 1985; 104:853–6.
479. Tekin M, Jackson-Cook C, Pandya A. De novo inverted tandem duplication of the short arm of chromosome 12 in a patient with microblepharon. Amer J Med Genet 2001; 104:42–6.
480. Temple IK, Brunner H, Jones B, et al. Midline facial defects with ocular colobomata. Am J Med Genet 1990; 37:23–7.
481. Teske MP, Trese, MT. Retinopathy of prematurity-like fundus and persistent hyperplastic primary vitreous associated with maternal cocaine use. Am J Ophthalmol 1987; 103:719–20.
482. Testoni B, Mantovani R. Mechanisms of transcriptional repression of cell-cycle G2/M promoters by p63. Nucleic Acids Res 2006; 34:928–38.
483. Thaung C, Bonshek RE, Leatherbarrow B. Phakomatous choristoma of the eyelid: a case with associated eye abnormalities. Br J Ophthalmol 2006; 90:245–6.
484. Thompson EM, Baraitser M. Sorsby syndrome: a report on further generations of the original family. J Med Genet 1988;, 25:313–21.
485. Thompson EM, Winter RM. A child with sclerocornea, short limbs, short stature, and distinct facial appearance. Am J Med Genet 1988; 30:719–24.
486. Tiller AM, Odenthal MT, Verbraak FD, et al. The influence of keratoplasty on visual prognosis in aniridia: a historical review of one large family. Cornea 2003; 22:105–10.
487. Toker E, Elcioglu N, Ozcan E, et al. Colobomatous macrophthalmia with microcornea syndrome: report of a new pedigree. Am J Med Genet 2003; 121A:25–30.
488. Tomita Y, Suzuki T. Genetics of pigmentary disorders. Am J Med Genet Semin Med Genet 2004; 131C:75–81.
489. Ton CC, Hirvonen H, Miwa H, et al. Positional cloning and characterization of a paired box- and homeobox-containing gene from the aniridia region. Cell 1991; 67: 1059–74.
490. Tondury G, Smith DW. Fetal rubella pathology. J Pediatr 1966; 68:867–79.
491. Toomes C, Bottomley HM, Jackson RM, et al. Mutations in LRP5 or FZD4 underlie the common familial exudative vitreoretinopathy locus on chromosome 11q. Am J Hum Genet 2004; 74:721–30.
492. Torczynski E, Jacobiec FA, Johnston MC, et al. Synophthalmia and cyclopia: a histopathologic, radiographic and organogenetic analysis. Doc Ophthalmol 1977; 44:311–78.
493. Tornqvist K, Ericsson A, Kallen B. Optic nerve hypoplasia: risk factors and epidemiology. Acta Ophthalmol Scand 2002; 80:300–4.
494. Townsend WM. Congenital corneal leukomas. 1. Central defect in Descemet's membrane. Am J Ophthalmol 1974; 77:80–7.
495. Townsend WM, Font RL, Zimmerman LE. Congenital corneal leukomas. 2. Histopathologic findings in l9 eyes with central defect in Descemet's membrane. Am J Ophthalmol 1974; 77:192–206.
496. Traboulsi EI. Ocular malformations and developmental genes. J AAPOS 1998; 2:317–23.
497. Traboulsi EI, Al-Khayer K, Matsumoto M, et al. Lymphedema—distichiasis syndrome and *FOXC2* gene mutation. Am J Ophthalmol 2002; 134:592–6.
498. Traboulsi EI, Lenz W, Gonzales-Ramos M, et al. The Lenz microphthalmia syndrome. Am J Ophthalmol 1988; 105: 40–5.
499. Tremblay F, Gupta SK, De Becker I, et al. Effects of PAX6 mutations on retinal function: an electroretinographic study. Am J Ophthalmol 1998; 126:211–8.
500. Tsutsui K, Asai Y, Fujimoto A, et al. A novel *p63* sterile alpha motif (SAM) domain mutation in a Japanese patient with ankyloblepharon, ectodermal defects and cleft lip and palate (AEC) syndrome without ankyloblepharon. Br J Dermatol 2003; 149:395–9.
501. Tuchmann-Duplessis H, Mercier-Parot L. The teratogenic action of the antibiotic actinomycin D. In: Wolstenholme GEW, O'Connor CM, eds. Ciba Foundation Symposium on Congenital Malformations. Boston: Little, Brown, 1960:115–33.
502. Tyndall DA. MRI effects on the teratogenicity of x-irradiation in the C57BL/6J mouse. Magn Reson Imaging 1990; 8:423–33.
503. Ueda K, Nishida Y, Oshima K, et al. Congenital rubella syndrome: correlation of gestational age at time of maternal rubella with type of defect. J Pediatr 1979; 94: 763–5.

504. Uhlenhaut NH, Treier M. Fox12 function in ovarian development. Molec Genet Metab 2006; 88:225–34.
505. Valleix S, Niel F, Nedelc B, et al. Homozygous nonsense mutation in the *FOXE3* gene as a cause of congenital primary aphakia in humans. Am J Hum Genet 2006; 79: 358–64.
506. van Genderen MM, Riemslag FCC, Schull J, et al. Chiasmal misrouting and foveal hypoplasia without albinism. Br J Ophthalmol 2006; 90:1098–102.
507. Vanita V, Singh J, Hejtmancik JF, et al. A novel fan-shaped cataract-microcornea syndrome caused by a mutation of *CRYAA* in an Indian family. Molec Vision 2006; 12:518–22.
508. Vasudevan PC, Garcia-Minaur S, Pilar Botella M, et al. Microcephaly-lymhoedema-chorioretinal dysplasia: three cases to delineate the facial phenotype and review of the literature. Clin Dysmorphol 2005; 14:109–16.
509. Vedantham V. Double optic discs, optic disc coloboma and pit: spectrum of hybrid disc anomalies in a single eye. Arch Ophthalmol 2005; 123:1450–2.
510. Vijayalakshmi P, Srivastava KK, Poornima B, et al. Visual outcome of cataract surgery in children with congenital rubella syndrome. J AAPOS 2003; 7:91–5.
511. Viljoen DL, Gossage JP, Brooke L, et al. Fetal alcohol syndrome epidemiology in a South African community: a second study of a very high prevalence area. J Stud Alcohol 2005; 66:593–604.
512. Vongphanit J, Mitchell P, Wang JJ. Population prevalence of tilted optic disks and the relationship of this sign to refractive error. Am J Ophthalmol 2002; 133:679–85.
513. Wang J-K, Lai P-C, Liao S-L. Punctal and canalicular agenesis presented with congenital nasolacrimal duct obstruction. Graefe's Arch Clin Exp Ophthalmol 2002; 240:960–1.
514. Wang T, Zhou A, Waters CT, et al. Molecular pathology of X linked retinoschisis: mutations interfere with retinoschisin secretion and oligomerisation. Br J Ophthalmol 2006; 90:81–6.
515. Warburg M. Norrie's disease: a new hereditary bilateral pseudotumour of the retina. Acta Ophthalmol 1961; 39: 757–72.
516. Warburg M. Norrie's disease. A congenital progressive oculo-acoustico-cerebral degeneration. Acta Ophthalmol 1966; Suppl 89:1–47.
517. Warburg M. Focal dermal hypoplasia: ocular and general manifestations with a survey of the literature. Acta Ophthalmol 1970; 48:525–36.
518. Warburg M. Norrie's disease: differential diagnosis and treatment. Acta Ophthalmol 1975; 53:217–36.
519. Warburg M. X-linked cataract and x-linked microphthalmos: how many deletion families? Am J Med Genet 1989; 34:451–3.
520. Warburg M, Friedrich U. Coloboma and microphthalmos in chromosomal aberrations: chromosomal aberrations and neural crest cell developmental field. Ophthalmic Paediatr Genet 1987; 81:104–18.
521. Waring GO, Rodrigues MM. Ultrastructure and successful keratoplasty of sclerocornea of Mieten's syndrome. Am J Ophthalmol 1980; 90:469–75.
522. Waring GO, Rodrigues M, Laibson P. Anterior chamber-cleavage syndrome: a stepladder classification. Surv Ophthalmol 1975; 20:3–27.
523. Warkany J. Warfarin embryopathy. Teratology 1976; 14: 205–10.
524. Webster WS. Teratogen update: congenital rubella. Teratology 1998; 58:13–23.
525. Weiss A, Margo CF. Bilateral microphthalmos with cyst and 13q deletion syndrome. Arch Ophthalmol 1987; 105:29.
526. Weiss AH, Kousseff BG, Ross EA, et al. Complex microphthalmos. Arch Ophthalmol 1989; 107:1619–24.
527. Weiss AH, Kousseff BG, Ross EA, et al. Simple microphthalmos. Arch Ophthalmol 1989; 107:1625–30.
528. Weisschuh N, Dressler P, Schuettauf F, et al. Novel mutations of *FOXC1* and *PITX2* in patients with Axenfeld-Rieger malformations. Invest Ophthalmol Vis Sci 2006; 47:3846–52.
529. Wenstrup RJ, Florer JB, Davidson JM, et al. Murine model of the Ehlers-Danlos syndrome. *Col5α1* haploinsufficiency disrupts collagen fibril assembly at multiple stages. J Biol Chem 2006; 281:12888–95.
530. Williamson KA, Hever AM, Rainger J, et al. Mutations in SOX2 cause anophthalmia-esophageal-genital (AEG) syndrome. Hum Mol Genet 2006; 15:1413–22.
531. Willis R, Zimmerman LE, O'Grady R, et al. Heterotopic adipose tissue and smooth muscle in the optic disc. Arch Ophthalmol 1972;, 88:139–46.
532. Willougby CE, Shafiq A, Ferrini W, et al. CRYBB1 mutation associated with congenital cataract and microcornea. Molec Vision 2005; 11:587–93.
533. Wilson JG. Present status of drugs as teratogens in man. Teratology 1973; 73–115.
534. Wilson ME. Congenital iris ectropion and a new classification for anterior segment dysgenesis. J Pediatr Ophthalmol Strab 1990; 27:48–55.
535. Witkop CJ Jr, Nance WE, Rawls RF, et al. Autosomal recessive oculocutaneous albinism in man. Evidence for genetic heterogeneity. Am J Hum Genet 1970; 22:55–74.
536. Wong V, Dickson H. Ocular abnormalities in Down syndrome: an analysis of 140 Chinese children. Pediatr Neurol 1997; 16:311–14.
537. Wong L, O'Donnell FE Jr, Green WR. Giant pigment granules in the retinal pigment epithelium of a fetus with X-linked ocular albinism. Ophthal Paediatr Genet 1983; 2: 47–65.
538. Woolf CM. Albinism (OCA2) in Amerindians. Am J Phys Anthropol 2005; Suppl 41:118–40.
539. World Health Organization. Report of a meeting on preventing congenital rubella syndrome: immunization strategies, surveillance needs. Proceedings of the Department of Vaccines and Biologicals Geneva, Switzerland, 2000:1.
540. Xu Q, Wang Y, Dabdoub A, et al. Vascular development in the retina and inner ear: control by Norrin and Frizzled-4, a high-affinity ligand-receptor pair. Cell 2004; 116:883–95.
541. Yamada E, Ishikawa T. Some observations on the submicroscopic morphogenesis of the human retina. In: Rohen JN, ed. The Structure of the Eye. Stuttgart: Schattauer, 1965; 5–16.
542. Yamada K, Andrews C, Chan WM, et al. Heterozygous mutations of the kinesin KIF21A in congenital fibrosis of the extraocular muscles type 1 (CFEOM1). Nat Genet 2003; 35:318–21.
543. Yamada K, Hunter DG, Andrews C, et al. A novel *KIF21A* mutation in a patient with congenital fibrosis of the extraocular muscles and Marcus Gunn jaw-winking phenomenon. Arch Ophthalmol 2005; 123:1254–9.
544. Yamashita T, Kawano K, Ohba N. Autosomal dominantly inherited optic nerve coloboma. Ophthalmic Paediatr Genet 1988; 9:17–24.
545. Yanoff M, Rahn EK, Zimmerman LE. Histopathology of juvenile retinoschisis. Arch Ophthalmol 1968; 79: 49–53.

546. Yanoff M, Rorke LB, Allman MI. Bilateral optic system aplasia with relatively normal eyes. Arch Ophthalmol 1978; 96:97–101.
547. Yardley J, Leroy BP. Hart-Holden N, et al. Mutations of *VMD2* splicing regulators cause nanophthalmos and autosomal dominant vitreoretinochoroidopathy (ADVIRC). Invest Ophthalmol Vis Sci 2004; 45: 3683–9.
548. Yen MT, Lucca LM, Anderson RL. Management of eyelid anomalies associated with blepharo-cheilodontic syndrome. Am J Ophthalmol 2001; 132:279–80.
549. Ying H, Chang DL, Zheng H, et al. DNA-binding and transactivation activities are essential for TAp63 protein degradation. Mol Cell Biol 2005; 25:6154–64.
550. Yoshimura K, Yoshida S, Yamaji Y, et al. De novo insG619 mutation in PAX2 gene in a Japanese patient with papillorenal syndrome. Am J Ophthalmol 2005; 139:733–5.
551. Young ID, Fielder AR, Casey TA. Weill-Marchesani syndrome in mother and son. Clin Gen 1986; 30:475–80.
552. Zaremba J, Feil S, Juszko J, et al. Intrafamilial variability of the ocular phenotype in a Polish family with a missense mutation (A63D) in the Norrie disease gene. Ophthalmic Genet 1998; 19:157–64.
553. Zetterstrom B. Ocular malformations caused by thalidomide. Acta Ophthalmol 1966; 44:391–5.
554. Zimmerman LE. Phakomatous choristoma of the eyelid: a tumor of lenticular anlage. Am J Ophthalmol 1971; 71: 169–77.

53

Overview of Oncogenesis

D. Cory Adamson
Departments of Neurosurgery and Neurobiology, Duke University, Durham, North Carolina, U.S.A.

Hai Yan
Department of Pathology, Duke University, Durham, North Carolina, U.S.A.

INTRODUCTION

The beginning of this century brought with it an explosion of knowledge in the field of oncogenesis. Perhaps the most prominent aspect of our collective knowledge of carcinogenesis is its heterogeneous nature in every respect, from the gene mutating events that initiate the process to the histological and clinical presentations. Instead of isolated specific carcinogenic culprits, cancer-related research has uncovered a plethora of different contributing factors leading to its pathogenesis. The explosion of studies in this field has taught us that this is a disease with multiple causes, which will likely require a similar multitude of therapeutic approaches.

The heterogeneity of carcinogenesis was first hinted at by the initial scientific inquiries. Almost a hundred years ago, we began to realize that cancer is a multistep process of cellular transformation from a normal cell into a cancerous cell, with successive phases of initiation, promotion, and progression. After the discovery of DNA as the genetic basis for life, we correctly assumed that alterations in DNA provided the genetic basis for cancer. Indeed, the past few decades of research have clearly solidified another key concept in carcinogenesis, namely, that it is a genetic disease that can be described and manipulated genetically. Perhaps the most exciting concept of cancer pathogenesis that has gained tremendous momentum recently is that it may largely be a disease of stem cells. With our current understanding of cancer genetics and tumor stem cell biology, we may have now come full circle and hopefully will begin to elucidate the heterogeneous multistep processes of this deadly disease.

Publication of the Human Genome in 2001 represented one of our greatest achievements in understanding the human genetic design (17,40). Not only did this work greatly increase what we now know about the human genome, but also it facilitated a similar explosion into the genetic study of both normal and abnormal biology. Recent advances in molecular and genetic biology have been similarly revealing. Unsurprisingly, the search for the molecular and genetic mechanisms of malignant transformation of cells has always closely paralleled the search for the molecular mechanisms controlling related, normal cellular processes such as growth, development, differentiation, adaptation, and senescence of cells.

CARCINOGENESIS IS A MULTISTEP DISEASE PROCESS

Studies over half a century ago showed that carcinogenesis is a multistep cellular process. In their classic manuscript in the 1940s, pioneering experiments by Friedewald and Rous introduced the idea that the neoplastic process could be broken down experimentally into two stages, which they termed initiation and promotion (10). Later investigators would add a third stage of progression. These early investigators noted that multiple applications of an extrinsic carcinogenic material (coal tar) to a rabbit's ears induced skin tumors, whereas a single application did not. However, if ears were subjected to chronic wounding after a single application of this material, then tumors would form. Tumors were not induced by wounding alone. The application of the carcinogen was termed initiation, and the regimen of chronic wounding was termed promotion. Later investigations would identify the actual initiating chemical carcinogens in coal tar (15). These early descriptions of the initial steps of carcinogens speculated that initiators were molecules covalently bound to DNA, and they therefore acquired the term mutagens (1,23). These observations strongly supported the hypothesis of initiation as a somatic mutagenic event, such that once a cell was initiated, all of that cell's progeny also became initiated cells. Future discoveries would broaden this definition of carcinogenic initiation to include other ways of altering gene expression. For example, epigenetic mechanisms such as methylation, which may alter gene expression without altering the genetic sequence. In contrast to initiation, the mechanisms by which promotion act were not as clearly defined by these early investigations. Promoting molecules were not always thought to influence DNA directly, but instead, to contribute to the environments supporting or promoting carcinogenesis. For example, molecules that dampen inflammatory reactions (such as certain cytokines), induce angiogenesis (such as growth factors), facilitate cell movement (such as extracellular matrix proteases) or enhance cell proliferation (such as apoptosis inhibitors) could all be considered carcinogenic promoters (6,34). These molecules may not even interact directly with the transformed tumor cell. Alternatively, promoters were also thought to help tumors achieve a malignant phenotype, namely, the ability to invade surrounding tissues locally and metastasize to distant sites. If the promoting influence was removed before full malignant conversion occurred, the growth would remain benign or possibly regress which suggests that the early stages of promotion are reversible and less likely genetic in nature (33). Yet another way of explaining promotion is the selective or stimulated cell growth hypothesis. This theory contends that initiation is a rare event affecting only one or a few cells in the tissue. Initiated cells are selectively stimulated to grow or are inhibited from dying, such that they enjoy a significant growth advantage. Initiated cells first develop into benign tumors which explains the monoclonal nature of many early neoplasms. With this theory, initiation is an event, likely genetic, that directly alters the phenotype of the cell destined to become cancerous. Malignant transformation occurs when additional promoting events occur. Not all tumors undergo malignant transformation; some remain benign in their growth characteristics. In other words malignancy is not a universal, inevitable outcome of carcinogenesis. A benign tumor is one that has undergone events prescribed by initiation and promotion. Regardless, these steps of initiation and promotion introduced decades ago, albeit ill-defined, have clearly provided the basis for regarding carcinogenesis as a multistep process. As modern science has consistently shown, the exact molecular mechanisms underlying initiation and promotion in carcinogenesis vary between different tumor cells and even within the same tumor cells exposed to different environments. Although these processes may not yet be easily described by a simple genetic paradigm with current technology, study of virtually every tissue demonstrating carcinogenesis has shown a multistep process (8).

ENVIRONMENTAL AND CHEMICAL CARCINOGENESIS

The discovery of DNA and subsequent theories of mutation naturally led to the search and characterization of the actual mutagens acting on DNA. The list of mutagens is ever growing and can be divided into two broad categories: exogenous environmental agents, such as chemicals, viruses, irradiation, and endogenous reactive molecules generated by normal cellular processes. Normal cellular processes that can produce mutagens include reactions with reactive oxygen and nitrogen species, alkylation, depurination, and cytidine deamination (19). The early forays into carcinogenic research largely focused on environmental and chemical agents; consequently, there are now extensive epidemiological reviews detailing the hundreds of environmental and chemical factors known to be carcinogens (see Ref. 46 for excellent review). The more recent genetic revolution has enticed many cancer biologists to turn their attention to the endogenous sources of mutagens. However, the list of exogenous environmental and chemical mutagens will continue to grow as technological advances permit the manufacture and discovery of more novel factors capable of altering gene expression. These environmental and chemical agents embrace numerous organic and inorganic agents, most notably viruses. Some of these agents even interact synergistically, markedly increasing the cancer risk. One of the first discovered and most studied examples of such synergy is the interactive relationship between exposure to aflatoxin (a mycotoxin formed by fungi growing on grain products and shown to be an environmental carcinogen in the 1960s) and hepatitis B virus infection in the development of hepatocellular carcinoma (46). Carcinogens from the use of tobacco products (>60 carcinogens), especially nitrosamines, provide another well-founded example of a lifestyle environmental factor that interacts with this virus. Typically, these carcinogens undergo metabolic activation (usually by the cytochrome P_{450} system), leading to the formation of DNA adducts as the metabolites bind covalently to DNA. If adducts escape cellular repair mechanisms, they may lead to miscoding and permanent mutations. For example, carcinogens in tobacco smoke have been linked to mutations in *p53*, a gene product important for the regulation of the cell cycle, in lung cancers. Additionally, environmental and chemical agents can influence the function of enzymes needed to activate or detoxify other agents, thereby indirectly influencing the carcinogenic risk. Because of extensive differences between individuals owing to gene polymorphisms and even between cells of the same tissue type, identical agents may have different effects on different people.

A description of the diverse list of carcinogenic environmental and chemical agents and their interactions is beyond the scope of this chapter; however, one type of environmental factor warrants discussion because of its intimate role in the birth of cancer genetics. The discovery of the role of viruses in carcinogenesis is of particular significance as it paved the way to our current understanding of the process. The existence of oncogenic viruses (viruses that induce cancer formation upon infection; also called tumor viruses) was first documented in the classic paper by Peyton Rous in which he reported the discovery of the Rous sarcoma virus (RSV) and the demonstration that a sarcoma could be transmitted from chicken to chicken through inoculation with a cell-free filtrate, later discovered to contain the RSV (30). In the 1930s he demonstrated the joint action of tars (methylcholanthrene) and human papillomavirus in inducing squamous cell carcinomas in rabbits, providing some of the initial evidence of *co-carcinogenesis*. As illustrated above, co-carcinogenesis is the additive or synergistic effect of two or more agents causing cancer (see Ref. 13 for an excellent review of viruses and co-carcinogenesis). Several other viral co-carcinogenes have been clearly verified since then. They include human papillomavirus and tar exposure in squamous cell cervical cancer, hepatitis B virus and aflatoxins in hepatocellular carcinoma, human herpes virus type 8 and HIV in Kaposi sarcoma, Epstein–Barr virus and malaria in Burkitt lymphoma, and simian virus 40 (SV40) and asbestos in mesothelioma (13). The steps involved in co-carcinogenesis could easily be described within the context of initiation and promotion. The numerous viruses that induce tumors in animals and humans and transform cells in culture fall into two large categories: DNA- and RNA-containing viruses (see Chapter 8). The DNA oncogenic viruses consist primarily of six families: hepatitis viruses, herpes viruses, adenoviruses, SV40 and polyomavirus, papillomaviruses, and pox viruses. There is just one important family of RNA oncogenic viruses, the retroviruses.

The DNA oncogenic viruses are perhaps the most extensively studied. Hepatitis B virus has been clearly linked with human hepatocellular carcinoma. This tumor is rare in the developed countries, but in areas of the world where hepatitis B is endemic, hepatocellular carcinoma is the most common human cancer (4). The mechanism of oncogenic transformation by hepatitis B virus is not completely unraveled, possibly acting through non-specific mechanisms, such as chronic hepatic necrosis, inflammation, and cell replication, and perhaps behaving more as a tumor promoter than initiator. SV40 and polyomavirus transform cells only from species that are not permissive for viral replication. That is, the virus does not transform cells or induce tumors in the animal species which the virus naturally infects, monkeys (SV40) or mice (polyomavirus). In permissive cells, the virus replicates and then kills the infected cells during the lytic cycle of virus release so that no cells are alive to become transformed. In non-permissive cells virus replication is blocked and, in a few cells, the viral DNA becomes permanently integrated into the cellular genome and the viral gene products are expressed. Viral genes expressed early during infection are the genes that are sufficient and necessary for transformation. They are called the large T (SV40) and large and middle T antigens (polyomavirus) (43). The entire function of these gene products is not completely clear, but the protein products may interact with tumor suppressor genes and possibly proto-oncogenes (oncogenes that have a viral origin). The discovery of viruses integrating their own DNA into a host cell's genome was a revolutionary finding that propelled the study of cancer genetics. Papillomaviruses are also known for neoplastic transformation in animals and humans. They are best known for the induction of benign papillomas of the skin, including the eyelid, such as the common wart. They are also implicated in the induction of cervical carcinoma as well as papillomas and some squamous cell carcinomas of the conjunctiva (see Chapter 57). E6 and E7 are the two most elucidated transforming genes of this virus, possibly functioning by increasing the activity of growth factor receptors and interacting with tumor suppressor genes (43). Adenoviruses are also lytic in permissive cells but can transform non-permissive cells. Two genes, E1A and E1B, which encode multiple proteins through alternative splicing, are responsible for transformation. These proteins likely interact with the gene products of tumor suppressor genes (43). Herpes viruses induce a number of malignant tumors in animals and possibly humans. They have larger, more complex genomes than many other viral families, and much less is known about the molecular mechanisms involved in their transformation of cells into tumors. The Epstein–Barr virus is thought to induce African Burkitt lymphoma, nasopharyngeal carcinoma, and several other types of malignant tumors. Pox viruses induce benign neoplasms in rabbits and monkeys, but little is known about the mechanism of action. The RNA viruses, primarily retroviruses, have provided an immense amount of information about normal cell growth, differentiation, and transformation. Most importantly, studies of retroviruses have provided the central unifying concepts in mechanisms of both viral and chemical carcinogenesis. These viruses replicate by making a DNA copy of the viral RNA genome using reverse transcriptase and then actively inserting this *pro*virus into the genome of the cell. There, under the influence of strong promoters, the gene products of the provirus are expressed. The provirus is replicated along with the cellular DNA, and in most cases the release of packaged virus proceeds in a non-lytic manner to transform the cells of the natural host. Some of these viruses are the most potent cell transformation agents known. They induce a wide variety of tumors in numerous mammalian species, including humans. The human T-cell leukemia viruses I and II are thought to induce human adult T-cell leukemia and hairy cell leukemia, respectively. Another retrovirus, HIV, causes the fatal disease known as the acquired immunodeficiency syndrome (AIDS) and may induce tumors as well. Ironically, the early studies of these tumor-causing viruses that provided so much enlightenment into carcinogenesis have led to their exploitation for the development of therapeutic tools. For example, in the 1990s, viral vectors began to be created from herpes simplex virus and used to treat various cancers. These first-generation vectors, which targeted the actively dividing cancer cells, carried recombinant suicide genes that code for such proteins as thymidine kinase (tk) (35). After the administration of this form of gene therapy, patients were given ganciclovic, which is transformed by the viral tk into a monophosphate form that is subsequently converted by endogenous mammalian kinases to a triphosphate that is a potent inhibitor of viral DNA polymerase and a purine analog competing with normal nucleotides for viral DNA replication. Importantly, it also competed with normal nucleotides for DNA replication in mammalian cancer cells and caused cell death. Only cells expressing the viral tk and close neighboring cells (bystander effect) were killed.

CARCINOGENESIS IS A GENETIC DISEASE

Overview

A multitude of ways that gene expression, and thus cellular phenotype, is altered by changes in DNA structure is now known. Mutations in cancer cell DNA cover a wide spectrum, from enormous chromosomal alterations that encompass millions of nucleotides to miniscule point mutations involving only a single or just a few nucleotides (41). Multiple chromosomal alterations have been found in most tumor types and involve aneuploidy (change in the number of whole chromosomes), translocations, deletions, and amplifications of genes. While there are diagnostic chromosomal alterations that occur at high frequencies in certain tumors, such as chromosome 1p and 19q loss in oligodendrogliomas, there is usually enormous heterogeneity of chromosomal alterations in cancer cells, even within the same tumor. Measurements of the number of copies of segments of the genome in tumor cells (DNA copy number) and the loss of pieces of DNA (loss of heterozygosity) have established that most tumors possess as many as 40 chromosomal alterations, potentially involving millions of genes (14).

Regardless of whether or not carcinogenesis starts from an intrinsic molecular or genetic derangement of the precancerous cell (as from a DNA replication error, DNA damage from free radicals, or inherited mutations) or from some extrinsic environmental carcinogenic factor (such as ionizing radiation, ultraviolet radiation, or chemical carcinogens), the true initial inciting event that allows the process of carcinogenesis to unravel is genetic in nature. Malignancies occur when normal cells progressively transform into tumor cells via the acquisition of mutations to their genome. We now realize that the acquisition of these mutations underlies the multistep processes of initiation, promotion, and progression. Cells become tumor cells when they can continue to replicate in the absence of regulatory influences that normally control cell growth, namely, when they acquire the genetic changes for uncontrolled growth (5). There are many opportunities to intervene in the process between intrinsic or extrinsic carcinogenic exposure and the expression of the genetic alteration, but the opportunities to reverse the process after that initial genetic event dramatically lessen during the early growth of the tumor. Despite the recent explosion in our knowledge of normal genetic biology, it has not been paralleled by an ability to devise mechanisms to help cells reverse the molecular processes of carcinogenesis.

Cancer geneticists now divide the critical genes altered in carcinogenesis into three general classes based on their functional phenotype: oncogenes, tumor suppressor genes, and stability genes (41). This classification provides a framework with which to attempt to understand how many of the genes in the human genome (estimated at about 30,000) can contribute to cancer.

Oncogenes and Proto-Oncogenes

In the simplest of terms, oncogenes represent a large class of very diverse genes that when constitutively or inappropriately expressed lead to carcinogenesis. In the astute car analogy described by Vogelstein and Kinzler, oncogenes represent a "stuck accelerator" (41). The products of oncogenes may be any type of cellular protein, but some of the more well known include membrane-bound proteins (such as growth factor receptors), intracellular signaling proteins (such as tyrosine kinases), cell cycle regulators (such as cyclins), and cell survival factors (such as the product of the *BCL2* gene).

Much of our understanding of oncogenes stems from early studies of the oncogenic potential of retroviruses. These viruses integrate their DNA into the genomic DNA, allowing transcription of cellular and viral genes. Originally, the cellular oncogenes that arose from viral integration, often in prior generations, were called proto-oncogenes. One of the earliest studied viral culprits is the RSV, an example of an acute transforming virus (30). Acute transforming viruses transform cells poorly and induce tumors in animals only after extremely long latent periods. The genome of RSV is large and consists of long terminal repeat promoter regions followed by the *gag, pol,* and *env* viral genes; *gag* encodes the major structural proteins, *pol* the reverse transcriptase, and *env* the viral envelope glycoproteins. RSV has an extra gene called *src* (for sarcoma), which was discovered to be solely responsible and sufficient for neoplastic transformation of cells (22).

The discovery of *src* was revolutionary. With the ability to construct molecular probes of the *src* gene came the finding that the *src* gene is contained in all eukaryotic cells probed and is conserved over a large evolutionary range (38). It was recognized that *src* is not a viral gene but a eukaryotic gene picked up by the virus at some point in its evolution. Numerous retroviral oncogenes have now been described (2), many having been found to have normal cellular homologs. The viral proto-oncogenes are not exact duplicates of the cellular gene but frequently are truncated, mutated, or oncogene fusion proteins (such as *gag*-oncogene fusion). The mutation often confers the transforming ability of the expressed product. Nontransforming retroviruses pick up genes from normal cells and change them into some of the most potent oncogenic agents known, some showing almost 100% efficiency of transformation.

The foregoing studies illuminated some of the mechanisms of viral carcinogenesis but shed little light on the mechanisms of chemical, physical, or inherited forms of carcinogenesis. A very simple experiment opened the door to another explosion in two fields of carcinogenesis, control of cell replication and signal transduction. In a pivotal study, the DNA from tumor cells was transfected into NIH-3T3 fibroblasts (32). These cells became immortal and lost their contact inhibition when grown in culture, common characteristics of tumor cells. Normal cells move and proliferate until they come into contact with other cells, and upon cell–cell contact, cell–cell adhesions form and movement stops (contact inhibition). Transformed cells continue proliferating when in contact with others, such as the foci of piled-up transformed cells noted in the exposed plates of the NIH-3T3 fibroblasts. A very low frequency of transformation was noted in plates exposed to DNA from normal cells. This was repeated with bladder tumor cells. DNA from piled-up transformed foci were retransfected into NIH-3T3 cells and a higher frequency of transformation was noted. This procedure was repeated until the frequency of transformation remained constant. Because NIH-3T3 cells were murine and the donor DNA was human, investigators could then search for human-specific sequences and identify the exact stretch of DNA responsible for transformation, which led to the surprising discovery of a sequence almost identical to the *ras* transforming gene of the Harvey sarcoma virus (27). This oncogene resulted from a single point mutation (G to T) in the *ras* gene from the tumor cells at codon 12, which caused valine to be coded instead of glycine (39). Thus, for the first time, a specific alteration in a

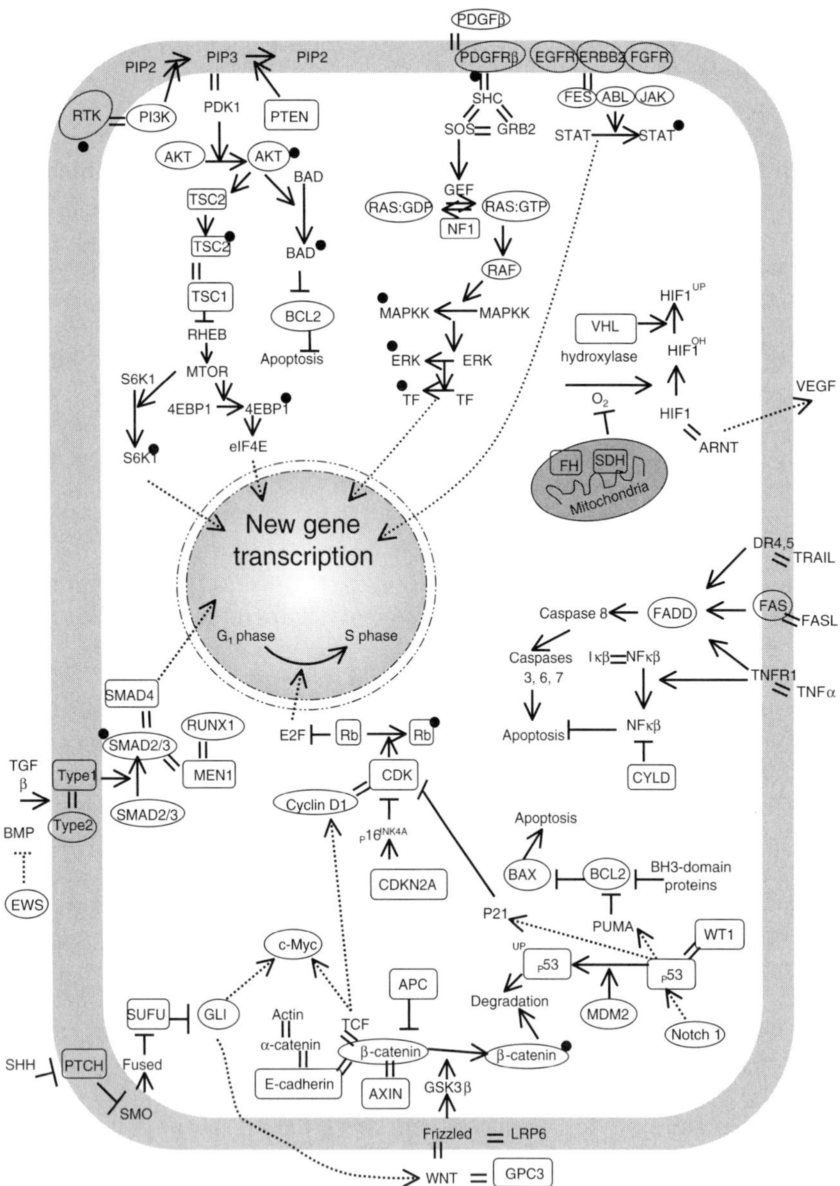

Figure 1 Common signaling pathways implicated in oncogenesis: PTEN and AKT, RTKs, HIF-1, apoptosis, p53, WNT, Rb, SHH, SMAD. The most studied components are included in each pathway—numerous factors are excluded for simplicity. All of these pathways do not occur in all tumor cells simultaneously, but some may interact under unique situations. Generally, only one factor in a pathway is altered in an aberrant fashion (exclusivity principle). Gene products in boxes or circles have been demonstrated to be mutated congenitally or somatically, respectively. Equal signs represent protein-protein interactions. Small solid circles represent covalently attached phosphates, typically indicating activation of protein. Ubiquinated proteins (UP) are destined for degradation. Dotted arrows and "T" bars represent transcription induction or repression, respectively. *Abbreviations*: TF, transcription factor; OH, hydroxylated. See Ref. 41 for details on pathways.

cellular gene was demonstrated to induce transformation. It is now known that *ras* is a family of genes (*H-ras* and *K-ras*) and that mutations at a number of sites can activate these proto-oncogenes.

The next question was whether this was the critical target gene in the cell mediating malignancy. Armed with the knowledge that the cellular homologs of retroviral oncogenes may be directly activated, the search for other oncogenes and the probing of tumors to see if they all had "activated" *ras* began. Activated *ras* is not found in all tumors, but numerous other oncogenes have been found (see Ref. 41 for excellent review and a current listing of oncogenes). The genetic basis for the induction of tumors has turned out to be much more complex and heterogeneous than expected (Fig. 1).

The mechanism of oncogene activation varies considerably. Oncogenes can be activated by gene amplification, gene rearrangements, chromosome translocations, insertion of viral promoters adjacent to proto-oncogenes, or intragenic mutations that alter gene expression. The *myc* oncogene is an excellent example of this heterogeneity. For example, it has been shown to be activated by all of these mechanisms and in many different tumor types. Even within the same tumor type, different mechanisms of activation may exist. In medulloblastomas, it is amplified on double minutes which results in a much higher than normal level of expression. Double minutes are small, paired chromatin bodies consisting of a few mega-base pairs, often, seen in human tumors that are defined as cytogenetic equivalents of amplified DNA sequences (11). These tiny pieces of DNA are passed onto cell progeny in tumors and express functional oncogenes. In plasmacytomas the gene normally found on chromosome 8 is translocated to a specific area of chromosome 14, where it comes under the control of the promoter of immunoglobulin G. This also results in abnormally high expression of the normal gene product. In adult T-cell leukemia-lymphoma, functional long terminal repeats of proviral promoters are inserted upstream of the gene, which causes an abnormally high level of expression. Thus, a number of mechanisms, including abnormal expression of the normal gene product and normal expression of a mutated gene, have been shown to contribute to carcinogenesis.

Functional studies of the proteins encoded by proto-oncogenes have yielded much knowledge on how cells control replication and how they interact with the environment. For example, the *ras* gene protein product was found to be located at the plasma membrane and to be a guanosine triphosphate (GTP) binding protein thought to be involved in signal transduction pathways (31). The specific point mutation described that results in activation of *ras* greatly reduces the ability of the protein to hydrolyze GTP to guanosine diphosphate (21). This results in the protein remaining in the active state for a longer period of time. The *myc* gene product has been found to be located in the nucleus, bind to DNA, and play a role in the regulation of transcription (12). The *erb-B* oncogene product has been shown to be a truncated version of its normal cellular homolog epidermal growth factor receptor, which is a tyrosine kinase (26). The viral oncogene lacks the receptor binding domain contained in the normal cellular gene but retains the tyrosine kinase domain. It is thought to function constitutively without the need for receptor binding. Thus, many oncogenes have been shown to be involved in gene regulation by either directly affecting transcription or altering signal transduction pathways.

Tumor Suppressor Genes

Normal proliferating cells require negative growth signals when growth is no longer appropriate. This is accomplished through the normal expression of genes called tumor suppressors genes (28). These genes are expressed in normal cells under normal conditions and function in various capacities to prevent or suppress the normal cell from becoming a tumor cell. For example, the *TP53* tumor suppressor gene for *p53* is expressed in normal cells to control DNA synthesis, induce cell death, regulate senescence, and control angiogenesis. When *p53* expression is lost, these processes go unchecked and promote tumor development. An alternative mechanism to oncogene activation for the transformation of cells is the loss of gene products that control and limit cell growth, namely, tumor suppressor gene products. Keeping with Vogelstein's car analogy, loss of tumor suppressor gene activity would be like a "dysfunctional brake in an automobile." Support for this concept has come from two lines of evidence. The first was the observation that if malignant cells are fused with normal cells, the resulting hybrid cells usually lose the tumorigenic phenotype, suggesting that normal cells provided some anti-tumor factor (36). These hybrid cells may retain some characteristics of the transformed cell in vitro, but the hybrids cease to form tumors in animals. The observation that with time some of the cells revert to the tumorigenic phenotype and that this correlates with the loss of certain chromosomes from the nontransformed donor strongly suggested that some gene on the lost chromosome was responsible for the loss of tumorigenicity (37). Inactivation of tumor suppressor genes usually arises from a missense mutation at residues critical for activity, from mutations that result in truncated proteins, from deletions or insertions, or from epigenetic silencing such as methylation.

The study of retinoblastoma has provided some of the best evidence for the existence of tumor suppressor genes (see Chapter 60). The disease exists in two forms, inherited and sporadic. Inherited retinoblastomas develop early in life and are frequently bilateral and multicentric. The sporadic form develops later, usually as a unilateral single tumor. Although multiple tumors occur in the hereditary form of retinoblastoma, the vast majority of retinal cells do not develop into tumors. These observations led to the Knudson classic two-hit hypothesis for tumor suppressor genes in the 1970s (16), which is that the first mutation is inherited, but the second occurs as a rare event in some of the cells over a period of time. This hypothesis was based on clinical observations without any knowledge of the genetic defect! On the other hand, oncogenes may need only one copy to be altered for malignant transformation to occur.

The concept of the loss of genes rather than the activation of an oncogene was spawned by research on retinoblastoma, which led to the discovery of tumor suppressor genes (see Chapter 60). More modern studies have now elucidated the role of the product of the retinoblastoma gene. It is located in the nucleus and binds to DNA, acting either as a repressor of transcription of genes that induce proliferation or a transactivator of other genes that repress genes involved in replication. Additionally, several genes of oncogenic viruses that stimulate cell replication also complex with the retinoblastoma gene product and inhibit its binding to cell DNA (44).

Another widely studied tumor suppressor gene is *TP53*, which encodes the nuclear protein *p53* that has been shown to bind to the SV40 transforming gene product (large T antigen) (18). The *TP53* is lost by deletion, gene rearrangement, mutation, or inactivation by proviral insertion in a number of animal and human tumors. Its introduction into transformed cells can reverse the transformed phenotype (3,9). Numerous other notable tumor suppressor genes have clear roles in normal cellular function. BRCA1 is a growth inhibitory factor secreted by breast epithelium that binds to surface receptors of neighboring cells. The *DCC* (deleted in colon cancer) gene encodes a cell surface molecule involved in cell-cell and cell-matrix interactions (5). *NF1* (the gene responsible for neurofibromatosis type 1) (see Chapter 63) is a signal transduction protein that converts active *ras* to inactive *ras*. Candidate tumor suppressor genes have now been found in tumors of most tissues of the human body, and the list will undoubtedly grow (41).

Stability Genes

Oncogenes and tumor suppressor genes produce similar physiological effects. They either promote cell growth or decrease cell death. A third class of genes called stability genes can have the same effect when mutated (see Ref. 41 for excellent review of all three classes). Because of the disparity between the relative infrequency of spontaneous mutations and the large numbers of mutations reported in human tumors, it is postulated that cancers may harbor a cancer predisposition by mutations in these genes that normally function to guarantee genetic stability. The roles of this class include mismatch repair, nucleotide-excision repair, base-excision repair, transcription-coupled repair, chromosomal recombination and segregation of genes, and even direct reversal of DNA damage (41). Because of the enormous number of exogenous and endogenous sources of DNA damage, there is an armamentarium of DNA repair systems that continually monitor the genome stability and repair sites of damage. Over 130 of these DNA repair genes have been identified. Mutations in stability genes presumably arise via random DNA mutations, by environmental or endogenous agents, or from inherited defects. In general, stability genes, like tumor suppressor genes, must be mutated on both alleles to have an effect. Xeroderma pigmentosum is a well-established example, where affected individuals inherit a mutation in genes needed to repair UV-induced DNA damage (7).

DNA repair mechanisms themselves may be prone to error and thus induce mutations or gene rearrangements. In bacteria, for example, when the level of DNA damage is so high that a reasonable amount of repair cannot take place before replication, the cell repairs postreplication DNA by bypassing errors in DNA, by a process called SOS repair (45). This is a complex recombination process involving several gene products in which the cell increases the chance for mutation as the price for enhancing the chance of survival and growth. Clearly, recombination events occur or are increased in mammalian cells following DNA damage. For example, increases in sister chromatid exchanges have been observed in mammalian cells after exposure to DNA-damaging agents in vivo and in vitro (15).

Cancer Epigenetics

Another important contribution to understanding carcinogenesis was the discovery that the expression of non-mutated genes can be altered. The nucleotide sequence of numerous genes implicated in carcinogenesis is normal, but their expression is often influenced by another gene mutation involved in their functional pathway. Alternatively, the expression of carcinogenic genes may be altered not by a mutation in its sequence, but by "epigenetic" changes. Epigenetic phenomena play a critical role in normal cellular biology as well as carcinogenesis (20,24). The modification of gene expression without changing the nucleotide sequence has become appreciated only recently. The most widely recognized epigenetic phenomenon is the methylation of cytosine phosphate guanine dinucleotide (CpG) sites along the DNA sequence, and this change is heritable, because the methylation status of DNA is faithfully transmitted to daughter DNAs by maintenance DNA methyltransferase. While methylated CpG islands in promoter regions of genes are the usual method of silencing gene expression, additional epigenetic functions will likely be uncovered as this new phenomenon is explored further. Genome-wide hypomethylation is widely detected in tumor cells and leads to genomic instability and carcinogenesis.

Aberrant methylation of CpG islands in promoter regions of tumor suppressor genes, such as *RB1*, *p16*, *VHL*, *hMLH1*, *E-cadherin*, and *BRCA1*, is known to be involved in their repression in numerous malignant tumors, including those affecting the stomach, colon, liver, breast, uterus, kidney, renal and hematopoietic systems. Epigenetic mechanisms change the accessibility of chromatin to transcriptional regulation with modifications of the DNA or nucleosomes.

Simple methylating agents, such as dimethylnitrosamine and dimethylsulfate, differ greatly in carcinogenic potency in vivo. The most abundant product induced by both of these chemicals is methylation at the nitrogen atom in position 7 of guanine (^{7}MG). Dimethylnitrosamine induces a higher amount of oxygen methylation, however, especially at position 6 of guanine (O^6MG) and the O^4 position of thymine (O^4MT) (29). These oxygen atoms are involved with base pairing, whereas the nitrogen at position 7 in guanine is not. In vitro studies have shown that if O^6MG or O^4MT is contained in the template, mispairing occurs at high frequency, resulting in the induction of point mutations (29). Early studies of methylation have provided the framework for work currently being done in the role of hypermethylation in carcinogenesis, perhaps one of the most common epigenetic processes of cancer regulation.

TUMOR SIGNALING PATHWAYS

Despite the potential thousands of tumor-related genes and the numerous ways that they can be activated, there may still be a light at the end of the tunnel for curing cancer. Research over the past couple of decades has demonstrated that all of these protean mechanisms may converge in a relatively small number of critical, tumor-related molecular pathways. Regardless of the molecular defect in tumors, it may be more realistic to identify and target the affected pathway instead.

The large variety of mutated cancer genes can have comparable pathophysiological effects by altering similar intracellular signaling pathways. For example, several genes involved in the cell cycle have been found to be mutated in similar tumors. *RB1*, *p16*, *cyclin D1*, *ckd4* are all involved in the transition from G1 to the S phase in the cell cycle, and all have been demonstrated to be mutated in cancers. These mutations often obey an "exclusivity principle," where only one gene in a particular pathway is mutated in any single tumor (41). A major discovery in the 1990s was that most oncogenic DNA viruses inactivate the p53 or Rb pathways (47) and these pathways are affected in a large variety of tumors. Like Rb, p53 is another transcription factor that regulates cell growth by inhibiting growth and stimulating cell death. Mutations in *TP53*, or in other genes, can disrupt the p53 pathway.

Other important genes and proteins implicated in multiple tumors include the adenomatous polyposis coli gene (*APC*), glioma-associated oncogene (*GLI*), hypoxia-inducible transcription factor-1 (*HIF-1*) gene, phosphoinositide 3-kinase, intracytoplasmic proteins critical for transmitting signals from transforming growth factor-β to the nucleus (SMADs), and tyrosine kinase receptors. The discovery that these signaling pathways are involved in multiple tumor types represents one of the greatest achievements in carcinogenic research and bodes well for the development of molecular-based therapies that can target many different tumor types (27).

THE FUTURE

The complexity of oncogenesis is not obvious The conversion of NIH-3T3 cells by a single oncogene superficially suggests a simple one-hit model of carcinogenesis. It is important to note, however, that although NIH-3T3 cells retain contact inhibition and are hence not fully transformed, they are immortal, demonstrating pre-existing genetic change(s). The observation that primary cultures of fibroblasts, without this pre-existing change, could not be transformed by a single oncogene (such as activated *ras* or *myc)* but required the transfection of at least two *(ras* plus *myc)* is supportive of the multistage genetic nature of carcinogenesis observed in vivo and suggests a more complicated model. In this model at least two, and probably more than two, rare genetic events must occur for stable malignant transformation of a cell. The interplay of numerous environmental and host factors, genetic and epigenetic, increases or decreases the probability of these events occurring. The existence of dominant transforming oncogenes, tumor suppressor genes, key stability genes, and the multiple ways of activating or inactivating these genes suggest a number of molecular changes that can result in transformation. This recently realized plethora of genetic events in carcinogenesis will need to be fine-tuned and better characterized for future molecular therapies to succeed. Mapping of the "cancer genome" will be a critical goal for future scientists.

It is important to add that the majority of the studies mentioned here deal with the control or loss of control of cell growth, which is only the initial step in carcinogenesis. The ability to metastasize is perhaps the worst feature of some tumors (see Chapter 54). Locally invasive tumors can frequently be cured surgically, but tumors that spread to distant sites while the primary tumor is still small and difficult to detect are the most lethal. The development of the metastatic phenotype adds another layer of complexity to the phenotypic changes necessary for uncontrolled growth. Thus, understanding the multistep process in which cell changes from normal, to initiated, to benign growth, to invasive growth, to the fully malignant cancer cell, in each of the different cells and tissues of the body, in specific molecular detail, is essential if we are to develop more specific and efficacious methods for diagnosis and treatment.

Surprisingly, cancer cells are more sensitive than normal replicating cells to chemotherapies such as antimetabolites, alkylating agents, DNA intercalators, topoisomerase inhibitors, and apoptosis inducers. This observation has led to a new area of study in carcinogenesis, called cellular addiction, where tumor cells not only result from a specific genetic event, but their survival depends on the continued expression of key tumor-promoting genes. For example, the amplification of an oncogene may initiate tumorigenesis, but the tumor cell may become addicted to downstream factors, such as the expression of antiapoptotic genes. Inhibition of a pathway to which a tumor cell is addicted does not simply revert the cell back to normality; it more likely kills the cell. The genetic basis of this process will need elucidation in the future to better understand how to target it.

The discovery of new cancer-causing genes which contribute to an ever increasing genetically heterogeneous disease, with more powerful techniques, such as DNA arrays (25) and digital karyotyping (42) will be critical. Together with the sequencing of the human genome, new genetic techniques provide the tools to monitor and investigate these complex events underlying carcinogenesis.

REFERENCES

1. Ames BN. Identifying environmental chemicals causing mutations and cancer. Science 1979; 204:587–93.
2. Auersperg N, Roskelley C. Retroviral oncogenes: interrelationships between neoplastic transformation and cell differentiation. Crit Rev Oncog 1991; 2:125–60.
3. Baker SJ, Fearon ER, Nigro JM, et al. Chromosome 17 deletions and *p53* gene mutations in colorectal carcinomas. Science 1989; 244:217–21.
4. Beasley RP, Hwang LY. Hepatocellular carcinoma and hepatitis B virus. Semin Liver Dis 1984; 4:113–21.
5. Bertram JS. The molecular biology of cancer. Mol Aspects Med 2000; 21:167–223.
6. Boutwell RK. Some biological aspects of skin carcinogenisis. Prog Exp Tumor Res 1964; 19:207–50.
7. Cleaver JE, Kraemer KH. Xeroderma pigmentosum. In: Scriver CR, Beaudet AL, Sly WS, Valle D, eds. The Metabolic and Molecular Bases of Inherited Disease. 8th ed. New York: McGraw-Hill, 2001:2949–71.
8. Farber E. Chemical carcinogenesis: a biologic perspective. Am J Pathol 1982; 106:271–96.
9. Finlay CA, Hinds PW, Levine AJ. The *p53* proto-oncogene can act as a suppressor of transformation. Cell 1989; 57: 1083–93.
10. Friedewald WF, Rous P. The initiating and promoting elements in tumor production. J Exp Med 1944; 80: 101–44.
11. Gebhart E. Double minutes, cytogenetic equivalents of gene amplification, in human neoplasia—a review. Clin Transl Oncol 2005; 7:477–85.
12. Hansen MF, Koufos A, Gallie BL, et al. Osteosarcoma and retinoblastoma: a shared chromosomal mechanism revealing recessive predisposition. Proc Natl Acad Sci USA 1985; 82:6216–20.
13. Haverkos HW. Viruses, chemicals and co-carcinogenesis. Oncogene 2004; 23:6492–9.
14. Kallioniemi A, Kallioniemi OP, Piper J, et al. Detection and mapping of amplified DNA sequences in breast cancer by comparative genomic hybridization. Proc Natl Acad Sci USA 1994; 91:2156–60.
15. Kennaway EI. The identification of a carcinogenic compound in coal tar. BMJ 1955; 2:749–52.
16. Knudson AG Jr. Mutation and cancer: statistical study of retinoblastoma. Proc Natl Acad Sci U S A 1971; 68:820–3.
17. Lander ES, Linton LM, Birren B, et al. Initial sequencing and analysis of the human genome. Nature 2001; 409: 860–921.
18. Lane DP, Crawford LV. T antigen is bound to a host protein in SV40-transformed cells. Nature 1979; 278:261–3.
19. Loeb LA. Endogenous carcinogenesis: molecular oncology into the twenty-first century—presidential address. Cancer Res 1989; 49:5489–96.
20. Lund AH, van Lohuizen M. Epigenetics and cancer. Genes Dev 2004; 18:2315–35.
21. Manne V, Bekesi E, Kung HF. Ha-ras proteins exhibit GTPase activity: point mutations that activate Ha-ras gene products result in decreased GTPase activity. Proc Natl Acad Sci U S A 1985; 82:376–80.
22. Martin GS, Duesberg PH. The α subunit in the RNA of transforming avian tumor viruses. I. Occurrence in different virus strains. II. Spontaneous loss resulting in nontransforming variants. Virology 1972; 47:494–7.
23. Miller EC, Miller JA. Mechanisms of chemical carcinogenesis: nature of proximate carcinogens and interactions with macromolecules. Pharmacol Rev 1966; 18:805–38.
24. Miyamoto K, Ushijima T. Diagnostic and therapeutic applications of epigenetics. Jpn J Clin Oncol 2005; 35: 293–301.
25. Mocellin S, Provenzano M, Rossi CR, et al. DNA array-based gene profiling: from surgical specimen to the molecular portrait of cancer. Ann Surg 2005; 241:16–26.
26. Nilsen TW, Maroney PA, Goodwin RG, et al. c-erbB activation in ALV-induced erythroblastosis: novel RNA processing and promoter insertion result in expression of an amino-truncated EGF receptor. Cell 1985; 41: 719–26.
27. Parada LF, Tabin CJ, Shih C, Weinberg RA. Human EJ bladder carcinoma oncogene is homologue of Harvey sarcoma virus *ras* gene. Nature 1982; 297:474–8.
28. Payne SR, Kemp CJ. Tumor suppressor genetics. Carcinogenesis 2005; 26:2031–45.
29. Rideout WM 3rd, Coetzee GA, Olumi AF, Jones PA. 5-Methylcytosine as an endogenous mutagen in the human LDL receptor and *p53* genes. Science 1990; 249:1288–90.
30. Rous P. Transmission of a malignant new growth by means of a cell-free filtrate. JAMA 1911; 56:198–9.
31. Scolnick EM, Papageorge AG, Shih TY. Guanine nucleotide-binding activity as an assay for src protein of rat-derived murine sarcoma viruses. Proc Natl Acad Sci U S A 1979; 76: 5355–9.
32. Shih C, Shilo BZ, Goldfarb MP, et al. Passage of phenotypes of chemically transformed cells via transfection of DNA and chromatin. Proc Natl Acad Sci U S A 1979; 76:5714–8.
33. Slaga TJ. Overview of tumor promotion in animals. Environ Health Perspect 1983; 50:3–14.
34. Slaga TJ, Fischer SM, Weeks CE, et al. Specificity and mechanism(s) of promoter inhibitors in multistage promotion. Carcinog Compr Surv 1982; 7:19–34.
35. St Clair MH, Lambe CU, Furman PA. Inhibition by ganciclovir of cell growth and DNA synthesis of cells biochemically transformed with herpesvirus genetic information. Antimicrob Agents Chemother 1987; 31:844–9.
36. Stanbridge EJ. Suppression of malignancy in human cells. Nature 1976; 260:17–20.
37. Stanbridge EJ, Flandermeyer RR, Daniels DW, Nelson-Rees WA. Specific chromosome loss associated with the expression of tumorigenicity in human cell hybrids. Somatic Cell Genet 1981; 7:699–712.

38. Stehelin D, Varmus HE, Bishop JM, Vogt PK. DNA related to the transforming gene(s) of avian sarcoma viruses is present in normal avian DNA. Nature 1976; 260:170–3.
39. Tabin CJ, Bradley SM, Bargmann CI, et al. Mechanism of activation of a human oncogene. Nature 1982; 300: 143–9.
40. Venter JC, Adams MD, Myers EW, et al. The sequence of the human genome. Science 2001; 291:1304–51.
41. Vogelstein B, Kinzler KW. Cancer genes and the pathways they control. Nat Med 2004; 10:789–99.
42. Wang TL, Maierhofer C, Speicher MR, et al. Digital karyotyping. Proc Natl Acad Sci U S A 2002; 99:16156–61.
43. Weinberg RA. Oncogenes and the Molecular Origins of Cancer. New York: Cold Spring Harbor Press, 1989.
44. Whyte P, Buchkovich KJ, Horowitz JM, et al. Association between an oncogene and an anti-oncogene: the adenovirus E1A proteins bind to the retinoblastoma gene product. Nature 1988; 334:124–9.
45. Witkin EM. Ultraviolet mutagenesis and inducible DNA repair in *Escherichia coli*. Bacteriol Rev 1976; 40:869–907.
46. Wogan GN, Hecht SS, Felton JS, et al. Environmental and chemical carcinogenesis. Semin Cancer Biol 2004; 14:473–86.
47. zur Hausen H. Oncogenic DNA viruses. Oncogene 2001; 20:7820–3.

54

Metastatic Tumors

D. Cory Adamson
Departments of Neurosurgery and Neurobiology, Duke University, Durham, North Carolina, U.S.A.

INTRODUCTION

Carcinogenesis is clearly a heterogeneous and complex biological process that can be described in multiple ways—transcriptional, molecular, histologic, clinical, to name a few. Adding to this complexity, this past decade has revealed the enormous heterogeneity in genetic and epigenetic events that can be used to describe this dysregulated growth of a normal cell into a tumor cell. Throughout this complex process, clearly, the key clinical turning point in carcinoma progression is the establishment by emigrant cells of secondary growth sites, i.e., metastases, which take up residence distant from the primary site of tumor origin. Carcinogenesis undergoes multiple steps to establish the primary tumor; and there are many additional steps needed to establish a metastatic tumor. This "metastatic cascade" that results in tumor spread can be described by a few critical, but discrete steps (Fig. 1) (21,49).

BIOLOGY OF TUMOR METASTASIS

The metastatic cascade begins with the escape of cells from the primary tumor site, often referred to as an "epithelial–mesenchymal transition" (EMT) (87). Once undergoing the EMT, tumor cells then penetrate and migrate through the local extracellular matrix (ECM), intravasate into nearby vascular or lymphatic vessels, aggregate with platelets, survive in turbulent blood or lymph flow, interact with and adhere to distant endothelia, extravasate through the endothelium, migrate through the ECM to a site for recolonization, and then clonally expand into another tumor. During this time, the errant tumor cell must avoid typically effective immune clearance mechanisms, survive the migratory pathway, and successfully trigger events that will support its proliferation into a metastasis, most notably, de novo tumor angiogenesis. The tumor cell cannot act alone. It must have the capacity to interact with numerous stromal molecules and cells, and induce morphogenetic changes in these other elements to be successful (17). Metastases can settle within the same organ or inhabit distant organs,

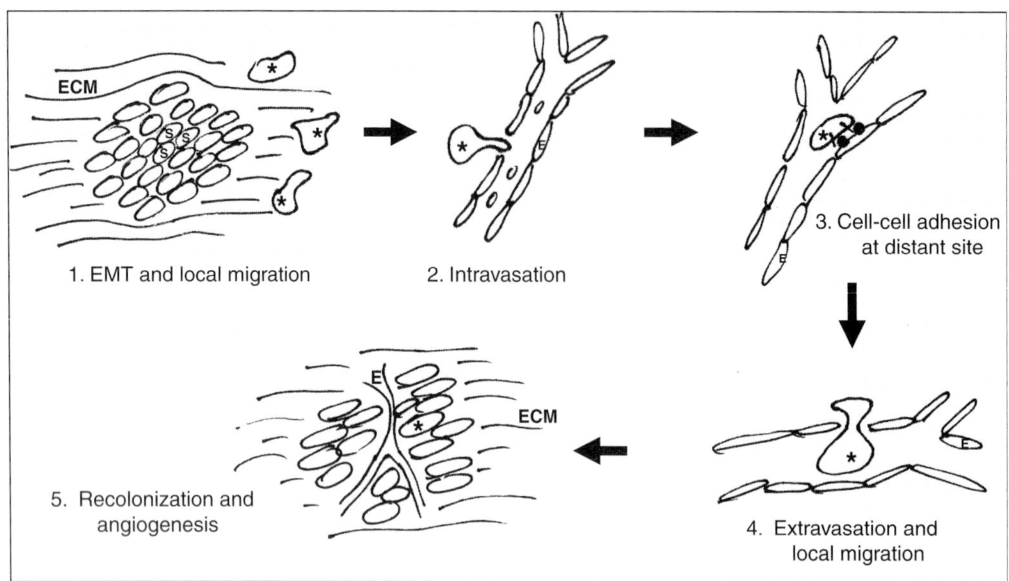

Figure 1 Metastatic cascade (21). (**1**) Cells in periphery of primary tumor undergo epithelial–mesenchymal transition into motile cells. These cells migrate to local blood vessels or lymphatics (49). (**2**) Migrating tumor cells intravasate into vessels and then flow to distant sites (87). (**3**) Tumor cells with appropriate cell surface proteins adhere to complimentary cell surface proteins on endothelium (17). (**4**) Attached tumor cells extravasate through endothelium and migrate to the site of the secondary tumor (74). (**5**) Recolonization occurs when metastatic tumor cells successfully proliferation and trigger pro-angiogenic factors. *Migrating tumor cell. *Abbreviations*: E, endothelial cell; ECM, extracellular matrix; S, primary tumor stem cells that renew primary tumor; EMT epithelial-mesenchymal transition.

as in the case when the primary tumor has been successfully managed.

The EMT is a dramatic switch in cell phenotype that heralds this metastatic cascade. It has been well recognized in developmental biology as instrumental in many of the morphogenetic changes in the embryo (74). For example, the initial development of the primitive neural tube from the overlying neuroectoderm during primary neurulation can be viewed as an example of an EMT. Likewise, the invagination from the surface into the interior of an embryo to form the mesoderm in gastrulation is another illustration (84). Unsurprisingly, metastasis begins with a similar dramatic switch in cell phenotype. The recent explosion in our molecular understanding of carcinogenesis has often highlighted parallels with our molecular understanding of development, so it is no surprise that carcinogenesis utilizes a process like EMT. However, it is important to note that these are different (83). Developmental EMT likely represents a radical change in function, developmental fate and cell identity, whereas carcinoma EMT represents a change in the phenotypic behavior of the same tumor cell. Both involve similar molecular and genetic events. In the simplest of terms, carcinoma cells undergoing an EMT lose their polarity with adjacent tumor cells, cell–cell adhesive architecture, and sedentary existence; and the carcinoma cell transforms into a cell with considerable translocation or migration ability. It is likely that tumor cells in the periphery of the primary tumor undergo this transition, whereas tumor stem cells located in the center of the primary tumor play more of a role in proliferation and self-renewal of the primary tumor. This shift in cell behavior involves many classes of molecules that change in expression, distribution, and function. These have been well characterized in developmental EMT and are now actively investigated in carcinoma EMT. For example, clinical cancer specimens often show a loss or delocalization of junctional E-cadherin (prostate cancers show a switch from N-cadherin to E-cadherin) in carcinoma EMT (59). Notable other examples include growth factors [e.g., transforming growth factor-β, and a family of highly conserved developmental control genes (WNTs involved in a signalling pathway named after wingless (Wg) and, Int)], transcription factors [such as regulators of epithelial–epithelial transition (SNAILs), SMAD, lymphoid enhancer-binding factor, nuclear β-catenin], cell–cell adhesion proteins (cadherins, catenins), cell-ECM adhesion proteins (integrins, focal contact proteins, ECM proteins), cytoskeletal modulators (Rho family), intermediate filaments (cytokeratins, vimentin), and extracellular proteases (matrix metalloproteinases, plasminogen activators) (28,87). Primary tumors are heterogeneous and usually only a small proportion at the periphery, the "invasive front," at any single time will undergo this EMT. Of note numerous examples now exist where epithelial and mesenchymal states of the same cell line show very different cancer activities, with the mesenchymal state typically demonstrating a more motile and invasive phenotype (27). This has been seen in mouse, rat, and human cells from different organ sites, such as the bladder, cervix, mammary, colon, bronchial, prostate, kidney, and skin (27). Despite being a similar process among different species, organs, tissues, and cells; the exact molecular signature of carcinoma EMT will likely vary dramatically among various cancers.

The other steps in the metastatic cascade are critical events and must occur for metastasis to be successful. Cells must be able to express appropriate proteases to degrade the ECM surrounding the primary tumor and the basement membrane lining the endothelium. There must be appropriate cell surface integrins expressed on the tumor cell for it to attach to endothelial cells and pull itself through the endothelial basement membrane and into the vessel. Similarly, specific cell surface proteins must interact between the tumor cell and distant endothelium for the tumor cell to attach and migrate out of the vessel. Once again, there must be appropriate proteases secreted to help degrade the basement membrane and ECM for further migration. Pro-angiogenic factors, such as vascular endothelial growth factor, must be in place for the metastatic tumor to proliferate when it reaches its final destination. These additional molecular events may occur during these respective steps; however, the majority of necessary and sufficient events are likely set in motion during the initial establishment of the EMT. These events likely accumulate over a relatively long time period in the life of the primary tumor until a threshold of necessary and sufficient events have occurred. Once a cell breaks away from the primary site, it quickly intravasates, extravasates, and migrates to a new site for recolonization over a short period of time that precludes a significant number of transcriptional events. If all the morphogenetic events are not in place, it is unlikely that the tumor cell will survive. Clinically, this process seems incredibly efficient since it is the metastatic spread of tumor that leads to most cancer mortality; however, it is more likely that this metastatic cascade is initiated unsuccessfully thousands of times for each primary tumor. In fact, it is clear that most intravascular metastatic emboli do not in fact develop into metastases (30,40). This large number of tumor cells entering the metastatic process, followed by the relatively small numbers of metastases that develop has been previously described as "metastatic inefficiency" (89).

Finally, metastatic tumors recapitulate their birth of origin, demonstrating similar histologic and clinical patterns on which their diagnosis is based. Therefore, the migrating tumor cells from the primary tumor cell must undergo a reversal in their phenotype, from mesenchymal in nature back to a more epithelial-like cell (85), or at least produce progeny that resembles the more nonmotile cells of the primary tumor.

GENETICS OF TUMOR METASTASIS

As might be expected, the genetic revolution at the turn of the century has only added to the complexity of understanding carcinogenesis. However, there are some important islands to be noticed in this new sea of genetic information regarding metastases. Large-scale gene expression studies, such as with cDNA microarrays, have added greatly to this area. This is well illustrated by the study by Montel et al. comparing metastatic and non-metastatic cell lines (55). The most obvious observation seen throughout this literature is that expression profiles of metastatic tumors closely resemble those of the primary tumors. This is not surprising, but it emphasizes that primary tumor cells undergo a fundamental shift in phenotype to migrate and then return to their native phenotype. Therefore, future molecular-based therapies may be equally effective against primary and metastatic tumors. Another important observation, however, is that there is genetic heterogeneity within the primary tumor. "Genetic signatures" can be used to differentiate tumor cells with low metastatic potential from those destined to metastasize. It is obvious that metastasizing cells acquire new expression patterns, but they also decrease important gene expression patterns, namely, those involved in growth and differentiation-controlling genes. These "metastasis suppressor genes" (77) are similar in concept to "tumor suppressor genes" discussed in Chapter 53. Despite the marked similarity between metastatic and primary tumors in gene expression, there are genetic differences that may be exploited in the future for diagnostic and therapeutic purposes. Examples of differentially expressed genes found in multiple microarray studies include those involved in chromosomal stability (kinesins), intracellular signaling (G-protein regulators), vesicular trafficking (the family of small GTP-binding proteins [Rab family]), membrane fusion (syntaxins), and energy production (tricarboxylic acid cycle) (78). Unique transcription factors, such as TWIST, have been shown to turn on genes needed to induce an EMT and regulate metastases in cancer models (90). The genetics of metastasis is in its infancy and will need considerable maturity before the key events can be elucidated.

MECHANISMS OF METASTATIC SPREAD TO THE EYE AND ORBIT

In the past, the eye has not been considered a significant site for metastatic disease, likely because eyes are not examined during routine autopsies nor in patients with metastatic disease. However, recent studies suggest that the eye may be a favored site for metastatic emboli. Weiss has demonstrated that the highly vascularized uvea has one of the highest metastatic efficiency indices (MEI) of any organ (88). The MEI is a ratio of the incidence of metastatic involvement to blood flow. It is now generally accepted that the most frequent intraocular cancers are metastases, and this would likely be more appreciated if physicians looked more often. Even though many emboli likely go to the uvea, only a minority of them will eventually develop into metastases because of the numerous other interactions noted above that must successfully occur. Paget introduced this "seed-and-soil" hypothesis more than a century ago (58).

Metastases to the eye and orbit occur by mechanisms similar to those in other organs, largely hematogenous and contiguous spread. When tumors metastasize to the eye, they are multifocal in 13.2% to 21.4% of cases (19,79). Within the eye, the uveal tract is the most vascular tissue, lying next to the inner surface of the sclera. It is divided into three structures: the choroid, the vascular layer that supplies blood to the outer layers of the retina; the ciliary body, largely muscle tissue, which by its contraction and relaxation alters the focussing of the lens; and the iris, composed mostly of connective tissue and smooth muscle fibers. Because of its vascular nature, the uvea is the site of predilection for most eye metastases (61). Metastatic foci are universally blood-borne and reach the eye via distal branches of the internal carotid artery (ICA). From the ICA, foci travel through the ophthalmic artery to the ciliary blood vessels that penetrate the uvea. In the tiny capillaries, tumor cells become lodged and extravasate into the adjacent uveal structures. Despite the slightly more anatomically direct path from the heart of the left ICA system compared to the right, there appears to be an equal distribution of metastatic foci in the eyes. Ample evidence shows no significant predilection for either eye (1,10,19,20). Unique patterns of focal deposition within the uvea have been observed (20,86). Metastases are more commonly seen in the posterior segment of the uvea because metastatic tumor cells are more likely to travel up the more than 20 short posterior ciliary arteries rather than the two long posterior or the five anterior arteries (19). Ferry and Font found that 11.4% of cases of metastatic carcinoma to the eye involved only the anterior segment, with the ciliary body more affected than the iris (19). Foci are seen more along the meridian of the posterior segment, i.e., more nasal and temporal versus superior and inferior. Near the temporally located macula, the short ciliary arteries are more numerous and larger, and more likely to receive tumor emboli. In the anterior segment, the ciliary zone of the iris is the most affected, compared to the pupillary or mid-zones of the iris. When looking at the entire intraocular space, metastases occur more frequently in lateral (39%) and upper (32%) areas (29). Animal models demonstrate that metastases to the eye are hematogenous, whereas metastases specifically to the orbit migrate along the optic nerve sheath and cranial nerves (35). This is unusual for most orbital metastases from other sites, but is thought to be due to the lack of the blood–brain barrier in cranial nerve ganglia.

Typically, tumor emboli will travel through the lung parenchyma first; however, some may bypass the lung and reach the eye by the Batson vertebral system. The Batson vertebral system is a rich network of venous plexi that surround the spinal cord and base of the brain, where flow is often bidirectional. Emboli have often been postulated to spread from this venous network into structures such as the orbit through the ophthalmic veins. There is an apparent lymphatic drainage from the superficial orbit into cervical lymph nodes; however, this is not demonstrated to play a major role in metastatic spread of tumor to the orbit or other eye structures.

Metastatic tumors to extraocular orbital structures are less common than ocular metastases and are usually from distant sites as well; however, locally aggressive tumors can certainly spread from adjacent structures (66). Only 1% to 3% of orbital neoplasms are metastatic. In adults, almost half of all orbital metastatic tumors come from breast, followed by lung and prostate. Tumors from distant sites typically arrive via hematogenous routes to the bone or fat in the orbit, with very rare deposits to the muscle. Breast carcinoma favors orbital fat, whereas prostate carcinoma favors orbital bones. Orbital invasion from the eyelids is usually related to locally aggressive squamous or basal cell carcinoma (6), while squamous cell carcinoma and malignant melanoma are the usual conjunctival tumors with a propensity to involve the orbit. Tumors of the paranasal sinuses, such as the esthesioneuroblastoma and oncocytic tumors, can invade the adjacent orbit. Intracranial tumors, most notably meningiomas, but also pituitary adenomas, germinomas, medulloblastomas, and glioblastoma multiforme, have been described extending through the orbital apex into the orbit.

METASTATIC TUMORS TO THE EYE AND ORBIT

Ocular involvement is more common than pure orbital involvement by metastatic tumors (66); however, orbital tumors may be diagnosed more often. In older literature looking at pathologic specimens, primary malignant melanoma, usually uveal, has often been reported as the most common ocular malignancy in adults; however, others have argued that metastatic carcinoma may be underdiagnosed and actually be the more common eye tumor (20,36). This is likely due to the fact that surgical removal of the eye was commonly the treatment of choice in the past for malignant melanoma, whereas metastatic carcinoma has been treated systemically or gone undiagnosed until patients succumbed to their systemic disease. Regardless, metastases to the eye or orbit should always be considered in the differential diagnosis for an intraocular or orbital tumor.

The incidence of clinically symptomatic ocular metastatic disease is only about 2% because many metastases are not clinically apparent and individuals with terminal cancer usually do not undergo comprehensive eye examinations (1). Altered vision, usually in the form of decreased acuity, is detected in 80% of patients, with pain the second most common clinical finding in metastases to the eye (20). Typically, ocular metastases appear as a nonpigmented flat thickening of the posterior choroid. The surface of the tumor may appear mottled, its edges are usually ill defined, and there may be an associated overlying shallow serous retinal detachment. The early occurrence of pain, the relatively acute onset of the lesion, its rapid increase in size, and the presence of additional tumors in the same eye aid in the clinical differentiation of metastatic carcinoma from primary malignant melanoma. Primary melanoma and metastatic carcinomas comprise the vast majority of ocular tumors.

As described above, metastatic tumors to the eye favor the vascular uveal tract. Anterior uveal metastatic tumors are more likely to present with visual complaints, mass effect, and redness; whereas, posterior uveal tumors more often present with visual complaints and pain. Metastases to the iris can mimic anterior uveitis, such as inflammation due to tuberculosis, sarcoidosis, and syphilis (70,71,82). Less common signs of metastases to the eye include hyphema and iridocyclitis (especially in anterior uvea involvement), detached retina, or secondary glaucoma (open and closed forms may occur).

As in the orbit, metastatic tumors to the uveal tract are largely from breast, lung, or prostate sites. Metastatic carcinoma in the iris most frequently arises in the lung followed by the breast (32). Although rare, there are numerous other malignant sarcomas that may metastasize to the choroid, including neuroblastoma, Ewing sarcoma, fibrosarcoma, and osteogenic sarcoma (1,42,65,76).

Although a very small fraction of eye metastases in most series, carcinoid tumors arising in the lung or gastrointestinal tract are often cited as having a propensity to go to the eye, mostly to the uvea (4,7–9,31,46,52,62–64,67). In contrast to metastatic carcinoma, metastatic carcinoid tumors have a much more favorable prognosis. These tumors arise from amine precursor uptake decarboxylase cells derived from the primitive foregut, midgut, and hindgut. Although gastrointestinal carcinoid tumors are more common than bronchial carcinoid tumors, most carcinoid tumors in the uvea metastasize from the bronchus. Carcinoid tumors are composed of uniform cells arranged in chords and nests with granular cytoplasm and bland nuclei. Carcinoid tumors of foregut origin (lung, pancreas, stomach, and mediastinum) react with argyrophilic stains (i.e., reduce silver) but usually not with argentaffinophilic stains (i.e., take up reduced silver), whereas those of midgut origin (small intestine and ascending colon) are both argyrophilic and argentaffinophilic; those of hindgut origin (descending colon and rectum) are negative by both reactions. These stains are of practical importance since in some instances the metastasis appears before the primary tumor is recognized. Ultrastructural examination of carcinoid tumors discloses intracytoplasmic dense-core granules. Immunohistochemical stains are positive for neuron-specific enolase, chromogranin and synaptophysin in tumor cells.

Metastatic intraocular melanomas, usually from cutaneous sites, are much less common than primary uveal melanoma. Font et al. found 17 cases in the literature and reported 10 additional examples (25). These tumors are usually diagnosed at a younger age and their prognosis is worse, as compared to metastatic carcinomas in general. The average age of patients when the ocular metastases are detected is 40 years, and the average period of survival following diagnosis is about 5 months. In a histopathological study of the eyes of 15 consecutive patients who died from metastatic malignant melanoma arising in the skin, asymptomatic microscopic intraocular metastases were detected in five patients (22). The microscopic metastases were in multiple sites in both the choroid and retina, were of "epithelioid cell" type, and were minimally pigmented. Large or symptomatic ocular metastases from cutaneous melanoma are rare, but the frequency of microscopic uveal metastases from cutaneous melanomas may be similar to that reported for metastatic breast carcinoma (10). Microscopic metastatic foci tend to be intravascular clusters of epithelioid cells, which together with the lack of adjacent nevi help distinguish metastatic melanoma from primary uveal melanoma. Ciliary body metastasis of cutaneous melanoma has also been observed (60,80).

Lastly, leukemia and lymphoma have also been cited as having a propensity to go to the eye. Leukemic deposits more commonly occur in the acute forms, and they complicate the lymphoblastic disorders more frequently than the myelogenous disorders. It is estimated that 50% to 90% of patients with leukemia have ocular involvement, with leukemic infiltrations occurring in the conjunctiva, corneoscleral limbus, vitreous, retina, uveal tract, optic nerve, and orbit (3,44,48). Clinically, the retina is the most affected ocular structure, but histopathological studies have shown the choroid to be most often involved, with an incidence ranging from 28% to 81.8% of cases (3,45,48,56). Retinal lesions usually include hemorrhages, cotton-wool spots, and white-centered hemorrhages. In a prospective clinical study of the ocular manifestations of 120 patients at the time of diagnosis of leukemia, Schachat et al. observed changes in 66% of the patients, including retinal hemorrhages in 35% (69). Less frequent manifestations included conjunctival hemorrhages, central vein occlusion, vitreous hemorrhages, and choroid hemorrhages. There may be an association between retinal hemorrhages and thrombocytopenia in these patients (33). The presence of anemia may be related to white-centered hemorrhages in patients with acute nonlymphocytic leukemia. Cotton-wool spots are not associated with hematological parameters. Leukemic infiltrates in the choroid are more common in chronic leukemia and can cause drusen, retinal pigment epithelial (RPE) defects and foci of hyperplasia, and serous RPE detachments (44,45). When choroidal leukemic infiltrates precede the diagnosis of chronic leukemia, the features may be mistaken for a choroidal melanoma. Leukemic infiltrates in the iris may be either nodular or diffuse and may or may not be associated with involvement elsewhere in the eye (51,68,81). The nodules have ill-defined borders and extend up to the pupillary margin, but if the infiltration is diffuse, iris discoloration and heterochromia may occur. Secondary glaucoma may result from blockage of aqueous outflow channels by leukemic cells. Other findings include hyphema and the presence of numerous leukemic cells in the anterior chamber (pseudo-hypopyon). In reported cases with involvement of the iris, there was little difficulty in establishing the diagnosis clinically because the presence of systemic disease was already known; however, anterior chamber paracentesis can be utilized to establish a diagnosis (43,68).

It is more common for lymphoma to spread directly from the brain [primary central nervous system (CNS) lymphoma] than to metastasize from the body (see Chapter 66). Intraocular involvement in patients with lymphoma is relatively less common than in those with leukemia (32). Isolated reports document uveal involvement in Burkitt lymphoma, lymphoblastic lymphoma, malignant histiocytosis, Hodgkin disease, mycosis fungoides, and multiple myeloma (12,32,41,72). Uveal involvement is usually widespread, but the iris is rarely affected (3). Perhaps the most common type of lymphoma to involve the uvea is large cell lymphoma (reticulum cell sarcoma), although fewer than 100 cases have been reported (26). In a review of 32 histopathologically proven examples of ocular large cell lymphoma, Freeman et al. found CNS involvement in 56% of patients, isolated ocular involvement in 22%, visceral involvement in 16%, and CNS as well as visceral involvement in 6%. Isolated ocular or combined ocular and CNS involvement is usually associated with subretinal pigment epithelial infiltration, clinically causing a mottled appearance (47). Cytological examination of vitreous aspiration specimens can provide a diagnosis. Large cell lymphoma cells have a large nucleus with one or more nucleoli, nuclear membrane abnormalities, and scant cytoplasm (32). Angiotropic large cell lymphoma is a rare, generally fatal disease characterized by intravascular proliferation of neoplastic B lymphocytes with only minor extravascular lesions (54). Ocular manifestations include choroidal distension, RPE defects and foci of hyperplasia, and serous detachments of the RPE and retina (18).

Most estimates place the incidence of orbital metastases in carcinoma patients between 5% and 10%; however, this will increase as patients live longer with their primary disease (13,20,29,34,57,73, 75). Orbital metastases, tend to present clinically faster than ocular metastases with an average duration of symptoms before presentation of about 3 to 4 months (66). For metastatic tumors from distant sites, proptosis and a motility disturbance causing diplopia predominate as the presenting signs and symptoms due to a mass effect on the globe, extraocular muscles, or nerves innervating the muscles. Tumors invading from contiguous structures tend to present with pain or paresthesia (50). In primary tumors of the orbit, ocular motility limitation and mass effect causing displacement, proptosis, or palpable mass are also common modes of presentation, making it difficult to discern the type of tumor from the clinical presentation alone. Extraocular movement dysfunction was first described by Horner in 1864 (38). Usually, the eye muscles and adjacent orbital structures are both involved, whereas only 5% of orbital metastases involve only the eye muscles (5). Since many orbital metastases have perineural invasion, it is not surprising that pain is a common presentation (15).

With few exceptions, tumors that metastasize to the orbit in adults are carcinomas. Metastatic carcinoma occurs much more frequently than other metastatic tumors and even more frequently than primary intraocular tumors in some autopsy series (1,2,10,56). In adults, numerous primary tumors have been reported to metastasize to the orbit; however, the most frequent are carcinomas of the breast for females and of the lung for men (20). Breast represents the primary tumor in over 70% of females, and lung is the primary tumor in about 50% of men. With the increasing improvement in survival from breast and lung cancer, metastatic disease to the eye will certainly increase for these groups. The next most common sites in men are kidney, testicle, and prostate. Breast metastatic tumors favor fatty periorbital tissue, lung tumors favor muscle, and prostate favors bone; however, these are not exclusive patterns of infiltration. Metastatic tumors, especially from lung, gastrointestinal tract, thyroid gland, and kidney, present with ophthalmic symptoms before the discovery of the primary tumor in about half of the cases (20,24,29). In contrast, though, the vast majority of metastatic breast carcinoma patients have already had treatment for the primary tumor (34). Since clinical presentation of orbital involvement may precede discovery of the primary tumor, diagnosis with fine-needle aspiration is the rule of thumb.

The average age of presentation for orbital metastases of all types is in the sixth decade (20). There is no sex preference, and race distribution parallels that of the primary tumors (20). Unilateral orbital involvement is the rule for the vast majority of cases, with bilateral involvement being slightly more common in cases of breast carcinomas and metastatic tumors to the choroid for unclear reasons (11,29).

Survival after diagnosis of an orbital metastatic lesion is universally dismal, with median survival of a year or less in most series (13,20). The approximate average survival after ocular diagnosis is 13 months for breast carcinoma and 52 months for lung carcinoma (79).

As with most malignant neoplasia, eye and orbital metastases are unusual in childhood and represent only 1% to 2% of all eye and orbital tumors in children. In children, the most common metastatic lesions to the eye are neuroblastoma, arising from adrenal medulla or parasympathetic or sympathetic structures, followed by Ewing tumor (see Chapter 65), extramedullary forms of acute myelogenetic leukemia (chloroma), Langerhans cell histiocytosis, and Wilm tumor (2).

Suspicious signs or symptoms suggestive of any orbital tumor require imaging with magnetic resonance imaging following gadolinium intravenous administration, with 1 mm fine cuts occasionally acquired to better define the lesions (14). Bony involvement can be better assessed by computer tomography. Fine-needle aspiration biopsies are easily performed in outpatient settings and diagnostic in >85% of cases (91).

METASTATIC TUMORS FROM THE EYE, ORBIT, AND ADNEXA

The eye and orbit consists of multiple structures from which various tumors can arise; however, few of them metastasize to distant sites (16,73). Some may aggressively invade nearby structures, causing a significant mass effect. The periosteal lining of the orbit, the periorbita, helps to serve as a barrier to intracranial extension of neoplastic growth and may explain the low incidence of spread. The most common primary eye and orbital tumors that may metastasize are retinoblastoma (Rb) and melanoma followed by much less common malignant tumors of the eyelid and orbit.

More than 80% of retinal tumors are Rbs, and this is the most common intraocular tumor of childhood (23) (see Chapter 60). Rb has seen a remarkable increase in survival with aggressive therapy; however, advanced Rb can invade extraocular structures, infiltrate the optic nerve, and metastasize (37). If untreated, Rb can invade orbital structures. Rb metastasizes in four ways: direct infiltration, dispersion, hematogenous dissemination, and lymphatic spread. The most common form of spread is directly into the optic nerve, and then into the subarachnoid space surrounding the brain, where free tumor cells may circulate throughout the cerebrospinal fluid (CSF). Rb tumor cells, can also invade extraocular structures and tumar cells disseminate hematogenously, or they made invade conjunctival lymphatics. Risk factors for distant metastasis include massive choroidal infiltration, retrolaminar optic nerve invasion, invasion of the optic nerve to transection, scleral infiltration, and extrascleral extension. Metastatic disease at the time of Rb diagnosis is rare; however, when it occurs, the most common sites are regional lymph nodes, CNS, bone, and bone marrow (37).

The most common primary tumor arising from the uvea is malignant melanoma (up to 90% of uveal tumors), which is the most common primary intraocular tumor in Caucasians in some series and is most commonly found in the choroid (53) (see Chapter 59). Uveal melanomas can invade through the sclera, particularly along the course of perforating nerves and blood vessels into the orbit or anteriorly into the conjunctiva. The sclera provides a barrier to extension; however, tumor can egress along the emissaries of the vortex veins and the ciliary arteries and nerves. Hematogenous spread to the liver can then develop from this vascular proximity. Unlike Rb, malignant melanoma tumors are unlikely to spread by lymphatics. Optic nerve invasion and CSF dispersion is also rare. Melanomas that arise in the ciliary body can extend from the eye through aqueous outflow channels from the trabecular meshwork and Schlemm canal. Melanoma is the most common uveal tumor to spread into the rest of the orbit.

About 10% of orbital tumors are meningiomas that arise from arachnoid cap cells of the meninges (34) (see Chapter 63). They usually arise intracranially and expand into the orbit, but can arise within the orbit. These benign tumors cause a significant mass effect and hyperostosis of orbital bones. Although they do not metastasize to distant sites, these slow-growing tumors will invade adjacent tumors and extend intracranially if left untreated. About 10% of meningiomas are atypical or malignant and grow more aggressively.

Some lymphomas derived from the ocular adnexa have a propensity to spread to distant sites (see Chapter 66), but they often arise elsewhere in the body and metastatize to the orbit. Of the other malignant orbital tumors some derived from the lacrimal gland (adenoid cystic carcinoma and other carcinomas) (see Chapter 61), soft tissue (rhabdomyosarcoma and malignant fibrous histiocytoma), hemangiopericytoma (see Chapter 64), nerves [malignant peripheral nerve sheath tumors (MPNST)] (see Chapter 63), bone (osteogenic sarcoma) (see Chapter 65) and cartilage (chondrosarcoma) (see Chapter 65) have a propensity to spread to distant sites (34,39).

Rarely, highly malignant optic nerve gliomas extend intracranially. Conjunctival melanoma, squamous cell carcinoma, and malignant lymphoma are all known to metastasize. Basal cell carcinoma, squamous cell carcinoma, and sebaceous gland carcinoma of the eyelid (see Chapter 56) typically invade local tissues such as the eye and orbit, before spreading by lymphatics or the vasculature to distant sites.

REFERENCES

1. Albert DM, Rubenstein RA, Scheie HG. Tumor metastasis to the eye. I. Incidence in 213 adult patients with generalized malignancy. Am J Ophthalmol 1967; 63:723–6.
2. Albert DM, Rubenstein RA, Scheie HG. Tumor metastasis to the eye. II. Clinical study in infants and children. Am J Ophthalmol 1967; 63:727–32.
3. Allen RA, Straatsma BR. Ocular involvement in leukemia and allied disorders. Arch Ophthalmol 1961; 66:490–508.
4. Archer DB, Gardiner TA. An ultrastructural study of carcinoid tumor of the iris. Am J Ophthalmol 1982; 94: 357–68.
5. Arnold RW, Adams BA, Camoriano JK, Dyer JA. Acquired divergent strabismus: presumed metastatic gastric carcinoma to the medial rectus muscle. J Pediatr Ophthalmol Strabismus 1989; 26:50, 51.
6. Aurora AL, Blodi FC. Reappraisal of basal cell carcinoma of the eyelids. Am J Ophthalmol 1970; 70:329–36.
7. Balestrazzi E, di Tondo U, delle Noci N, Blasi MA. Metastasis of bronchial carcinoid tumour to choroid. Ophthalmologica 1989; 198:104–9.
8. Bardenstein DS, Char DH, Jones C, et al. Metastatic ciliary body carcinoid tumor. Arch Ophthalmol 1990; 8:1590–4.
9. Bell RM, Bullock JD, Albert DM. Solitary choroidal metastasis from bronchial carcinoid. Br J Ophthalmol 1975; 59:155–63.
10. Bloch RS, Gartner S. The incidence of ocular metastatic carcinoma. Arch Ophthalmol 1971; 85:673–5.
11. Carriere VM, Karcioglu ZA, Apple DJ, Insler MS. A case of prostate carcinoma with bilateral orbital metastases and the review of the literature. Ophthalmology 1982; 89:402–6.
12. Chambers JD, Mosher ML Jr. Intraocular involvement in systemic lymphoma. Surv Ophthalmol 1966; 11:562–4.
13. Char DH, Miller T, Kroll S. Orbital metastases: diagnosis and course. Br J Ophthalmol 1997; 81:386–90.
14. Char DH, Sobel D, Kelly WM, et al. Magnetic resonance scanning in orbital tumor diagnosis. Ophthalmology 1985; 92:1305–10.
15. Char DH. Clinical Ocular Oncology. Philadelphia: Raven-Lippincott, 1996.
16. Darsaut TE, Lanzino G, Lopes MB, Newman S. An introductory overview of orbital tumors. Neurosurg Focus 2001; 10:E1.
17. Dawe CJ. Epithelial–mesenchymal interactions in relation to the genesis of polyoma virus-induced tumors of mouse salivary gland. In: Tarin D, ed. Tissue Interactions in Carcinogenesis. London: Academic Press, 1972:305–58.
18. Elner VM, Hidayat AA, Charles NC, et al. Neoplastic angioendotheliomatosis. A variant of malignant lymphoma immunohistochemical and ultrastructural observations of three cases. Ophthalmology 1986; 93:1237–45.
19. Ferry AP, Font RL. Carcinoma metastatic to the eye and orbit. I. A clinicopathologic study of 227 cases. Arch Ophthalmol 1974; 92:276–86.
20. Ferry AP. The biological behavior and pathological features of carcinoma metastatic to the eye and orbit. Trans Am Ophthalmol Soc 1973; 71:373–425.
21. Fidler IJ The pathogenesis of cancer metastasis: the 'seed and soil' hypothesis revisited. Nat Rev Cancer 2003; 3:453–8.
22. Fishman ML, Tomaszewski MM, Kuabara T. Malignant melanoma of the skin metastatic to the eye. Frequency in autopsy series. Arch Ophthalmol 1976; 94:1309–11.
23. Font RL, Croxatto JO, Rao, N. Tumors of the Eye and Ocular Adnexa. Washington, DC: Armed Forces Institute of Pathology, 2006.
24. Font RL, Ferry AP. Carcinoma metastatic to the eye and orbit III. A clinicopathologic study of 28 cases metastatic to the orbit. Cancer 1976; 38:1326–35.
25. Font RL, Naumann G, Zimmerman LE. Primary malignant melanoma of the skin metastatic to the eye and orbit. Report of ten cases and review of the literature. Am J Ophthalmol 1967; 63:738–54.
26. Freeman LN, Schachat AP, Knox DL, et al. Clinical features, laboratory investigations, and survival in ocular reticulum cell sarcoma. Ophthalmology 1987; 94:1631–9.
27. Gilles C, Newgreen D, Sato H, Thompson EW. Matric metalloproteases and epithelial-to mesenchymal transtion: implications for carcinoma metastasis. In: P S, ed. Rise and Fall of Epithelial Phenotype. Georgetown: Landes Bioscience Publishers, 2004:297–315.
28. Gilles C, Polette M, Piette J, et al. Vimentin expression in cervical carcinomas: association with invasive and migratory potential. J Pathol 1996; 180:175–80.
29. Goldberg RA, Rootman J, Cline RA. Tumors metastatic to the orbit: a changing picture. Surv Ophthalmol 1990; 35: 1–24.
30. Goldmann E. Growth of malignant disease in man and the lower animals with special emphasis to the vascular system. Proc R Soc Med 1907; 1:1–13.
31. Gragoudas ES, Carroll JM. Multiple choroidal metastasis from bronchial carcinoid treated with photocoagulation and proton beam irradiation. Am J Ophthalmol 1979; 87:299–304.
32. Green WR. The uveal tract. In: Spencer WH, ed. Ophthalmic Pathology. Philadelphia: W.B. Saunders, 1986:1352–2072.

33. Guyer DR, Schachat AP, Vitale S, et al. Leukemic retinopathy. Relationship between fundus lesions and hematologic parameters at diagnosis. Ophthalmology 1989; 96:860–4.
34. Henderson JW, Campbell RJ, Farrow GM, Garrity JA. Orbital Tumors. New York: Raven Press, 1994.
35. Hochman J, Assaf N, Deckert-Schluter M, et al. Entry routes of malignant lymphoma into the brain and eyes in a mouse model. Cancer Res 2001; 61:5242–7.
36. Hogan MJ, Zimmerman LE. Ophthalmic Pathology. Philadelphia: W.B. Saunders Co., 1962.
37. Honavar SG, Singh AD. Management of advanced retinoblastoma. Ophthalmol Clin North Am 2005; 18: 65–73, viii.
38. Horner F. Case report. Klin Monatsbl Augenheilkd 1864; 2: 186–92.
39. Housepian EM, Trokel SL, Jakobiec FA, et al. Neurological Surgery. Philadelphia: WB Saunders, 1990.
40. Iwasaki T. Histological and experimental observations on the destruction of tumour cells in the blood vessels. J Path Bacteriol 1915; 20:85–105.
41. Jakobiec FA, Jones IS, Tannenbaum M. Leiomyoma. An unusual tumour of the orbit. Br J Ophthalmol 1973; 57: 825–31.
42. Jampol LM, Cottle E, Fischer DS, Albert DM. Metastasis of Ewing's sarcoma to the choroid. Arch Ophthalmol 1973; 89:207–9.
43. Johnston SS, Ware CF. Iris involvement in leukaemia. Br J Ophthalmol 1973; 57:320–4.
44. Kincaid MC, Green WR, Kelley JS. Acute ocular leukemia. Am J Ophthalmol 1979; 87:698–702.
45. Kincaid MC, Green WR. Ocular and orbital involvement in leukemia. Surv Ophthalmol 1983; 27:211–32.
46. Lack EE, Harris GB, Eraklis AJ, Vawter GF. Primary bronchial tumors in childhood. A clinicopathologic study of six cases. Cancer 1983; 51:492–7.
47. Lang GK, Surer JL, Green WR, et al. Ocular reticulum cell sarcoma. Clinicopathologic correlation of a case with multifocal lesions. Retina 1985; 5:79–86.
48. Leonardy NJ, Rupani M, Dent G, Klintworth GK. Analysis of 135 autopsy eyes for ocular involvement in leukemia. Am J Ophthalmol 1990; 109:436–44.
49. Liotta LA, Stetler-Stevenson WG, Steeg PS. Cancer invasion and metastasis: positive and negative regulatory elements. Cancer Invest 1991; 9:543–51.
50. Lowe BA, Mershon C, Mangalik A. Paraneoplastic neurological syndrome in transitional cell carcinoma of the bladder. J Urol 1992; 147:462–4.
51. Martin B. Infiltration of the iris in chronic lymphatic leukaemia. Br J Ophthalmol 1968; 52:781–5.
52. Masek P, Janula J, Rejthar A. Ocular metastasis of bronchial carcinoid (author's transl). Cesk Oftalmol 1981; 37:60–3.
53. McLean IW, Burnier MN, Zimmerman LE, Jakobiec FA. Tumors of the Eye and Ocular Adnexa. Washington, DC: Armed Forces Institute of Pathology, 1994.
54. Molina A, Lombard C, Donlon T, et al. Immuno-histochemical and cytogenetic studies indicate that malignant angioendotheliomatosis is a primary intravascular (angiotropic) lymphoma. Cancer 1990; 66:474–9.
55. Montel V, Huang TY, Mose E, et al. Expression profiling of primary tumors and matched lymphatic and lung metastases in a xenogeneic breast cancer model. Am J Pathol 2005; 166:1565–79.
56. Nelson CC, Hertzberg BS, Klintworth GK. A histopathologic study of 716 unselected eyes in patients with cancer at the time of death. Am J Ophthalmol 1983; 95:788–93.
57. Ohtsuka K, Hashimoto M, Suzuki Y. A review of 244 orbital tumors in Japanese patients during a 21-year period: origins and locations. Jpn J Ophthalmol 2005; 49: 49–55.
58. Paget S. The distribution of secondary growths in cancer of the breast. Lancet 1889; i:571–3.
59. Peinado H, Portillo F, Cano A. Transcriptional regulation of cadherins during development and carcinogenesis. Int J Dev Biol 2004; 48:365–75.
60. Radnot M. Metastatic melanosarcoma of the uvea in both eyes. Klin Monatsblatter Augenheilkd Augenarztl Fortbild 1952; 121:352–4.
61. Reese AB. Tumors of the Eye. New York: Harper and Row, 1963.
62. Ricketts MM, Price T, Thomas M. Choroidal metastasis of bronchial adenoma; adenoid-cystic carcinoma type. Am J Ophthalmol 1955; 39:33–6.
63. Riddle PJ, Font RL, Zimmerman LE. Carcinoid tumors of the eye and orbit: a clinicopathologic study of 15 cases, with histochemical and electron microscopic observations. Hum Pathol 1982; 13:459–69.
64. Rodrigues M, Shields JA. Iris metastasis from a bronchial carcinoid tumor. Arch Ophthalmol 1978; 96:77–83.
65. Rootman J, Carvounis EP, Dolman CL, Dimmick JE. Congenital fibrosarcoma metastatic to the choroid. Am J Ophthalmol 1979; 87:632–8.
66. Rootman J. Diseases of the Orbit. Baltimore: Lippincot Williams & Wilkins, 2003.
67. Rosenbluth J, Laval J, Weil JV. Metastasis of bronchial adenoma to the eye. Arch Ophthalmol 1960; 63: 47–50.
68. Schachat AP, Jabs DA, Graham ML, et al. Leukemic iris infiltration. J Pediatr Ophthalmol Strabismus 1988; 25: 135–8.
69. Schachat AP, Markowitz JA, Guyer DR, et al. Ophthalmic manifestations of leukemia. Arch Ophthalmol 1989; 107: 697–700.
70. Scholz R, Green WR, Baranano EC, et al. Metastatic carcinoma to the iris. Diagnosis by aqueous paracentesis and response to irradiation and chemotherapy. Ophthalmology 1983; 90:1524–7.
71. Scruggs JH. Malignant melanoma of the uvea. Am J Ophthalmol 1960; 49:594–605.
72. Shakin EP, Augsburger JJ, Eagle RC Jr., et al. Multiple myeloma involving the iris. Arch Ophthalmol 1988; 106: 524–6.
73. Shields JA, Shields CL, Scartozzi, R. Survey of 1264 patients with orbital tumors and simulating lesions. The 2002 Montgomery Lecture, part I. Ophthalmology 2004; 111:997–1008.
74. Shook D, Keller R. Mechanisms, mechanics and function of epithelial–mesenchymal transitions in early development. Mech Dev 2003; 120:1351–83.
75. Silva D. Orbital tumors. Am J Ophthalmol 1968; 65:318–39.
76. Spaulding AG, Woodfin MC Jr. Osteogenic sarcoma metastatic to the choroid. Arch Ophthalmol 1968; 80: 84–6.
77. Steeg PS, Ouatas T, Halverson D, et al. Metastasis suppressor genes: basic biology and potential clinical use. Clin Breast Cancer 2003; 4:51–62.
78. Steeg PS. New insights into the tumor metastatic process revealed by gene expression profiling. Am J Pathol 2003; 166:1291–4.
79. Stephens RF, Shields JA. Diagnosis and management of cancer metastatic to the uvea: a study of 70 cases. Ophthalmology 1979; 86:1336–49.

80. Szeps J, Patterson TD. Metastatic malignant melanoma of ciliary body and choroid from a primary melanoma of skin. Can J Ophthalmol 1969; 4:394–9.
81. Tabbara KF, Beckstead JH. Acute promonocytic leukemia with ocular involvement. Arch Ophthalmol 1980; 98: 1055–8.
82. Talegaonkar SK. Anterior uveal tract metastasis as the presenting feature of bronchial carcinoma. Br J Ophthalmol 1969; 53:123–6.
83. Tarin D, Thompson EW, Newgreen DF. The fallacy of epithelial mesenchymal transition in neoplasia. Cancer Res 2005; 65:5996–6000; discussion 5991–6000.
84. Thiery JP, Chopin D. Epithelial cell plasticity in development and tumor progression. Cancer Metastasis Rev 1999; 18:31–42.
85. Thiery JP. Epithelial–mesenchymal transitions in tumour progression. Nat Rev Cancer 2002; 2:442–54.
86. Thomas C, Algan B, Pierson B, Reny A. Metastatic cancer of the anterior uvea. Arch Ophtalmol Rev Gen Ophtalmol 1964; 24:669–84.
87. Thompson EW, Newgreen DF, Tarin D. Carcinoma invasion and metastasis: a role for epithelial–mesenchymal transition? Cancer Res 2005; 65:5991–5; discussion 5995.
88. Weiss L. Analysis of the incidence of intraocular metastasis. Br J Ophthalmol 1993; 77:149–51.
89. Weiss L. Metastatic inefficiency. Adv Cancer Res 1990; 54: 159–211.
90. Yang J, Mani SA, Donaher JL, et al. Twist, a master regulator of morphogenesis, plays an essential role in tumor metastasis. Cell 2004; 117:927–39.
91. Zeppa P, Tranfa F, Errico ME, et al. Fine needle aspiration (FNA) biopsy of orbital masses: a critical review of 51 cases. Cytopathology 1997; 8:366–72.

55

Neoplasia Syndromes

David M. Gamm, Amol D. Kulkarni, and Daniel M. Albert
Department of Ophthalmology and Visual Sciences, University of Wisconsin, Madison, Wisconsin, U.S.A.

INTRODUCTION

Tradition holds that the varied disorders collectively referred to as the phakomatoses be discussed together. However, from a genetic, developmental, and clinical standpoint, the designation has limited usefulness, as can be deduced from efforts to define the term (130,131,145). The phakomatoses comprise a heterogenous group of diseases that feature widespread, tumor like malformations (130,242) consisting of tissue components normally found at the involved site (hamartomas) (5,251). The hamartomas are usually congenital and tend to involve the central nervous system (CNS), retina, and skin, and thus the conditions are also referred to as the "neurocutaneous syndromes" (2,254). The label "phakomatoses," derived from the Greek root for "mother spot" or birthmark, was introduced in 1932 by van der Hoeve (130), who substituted the term "phakoma" in preference to the designation "nevus," which pathologists had previously applied to these conditions (234,235). Originally, three entities were included under the classification of phakomatosis: angiomatosis retinae [von Hippel–Lindau disease (VHLD)]; neurofibromatosis (NF); and tuberous sclerosis (now called tuberous sclerosis complex) (TSC). It is noteworthy that these "original three" phakomatoses have subsequently been shown to develop from mutations in genes involved in the control of cell replication and the suppression of tumor formation (130,145). Thus, scientific discovery established a link between these entities that supports the grouping of at least some of the phakomatoses. However, it is important to realize that the genes involved in VHLD, NF, and TSC differ, and their clinical manifestations are dissimilar (130).

Following van der Hoeve's original description of the phakomatoses, encephalotrigeminal angiomatosis (Sturge–Weber syndrome) (SWS), ataxia telangiectasia, and Wyburn–Mason syndrome were added to the group, although the last does not have cutaneous manifestations. Other disorders, including McCune–Albright syndrome, Carney complex, adenomatous polyposis coli, nevus sebaceus of Jadassohn, nevoid basal cell carcinoma, and the multiple endocrine neoplasia syndromes are also included within the broader designation of the neoplastic syndromes. In this chapter, we provide descriptions of these additional entities.

With our growing understanding of the molecular and developmental causes of the phakomatoses, attempts have been made to re-classify them on pathogenetic grounds. As mentioned previously, a subset of the phakomatoses (NF, TSC, and VHLD) occur from loss-of-function mutations in tumor suppressor genes and, for the most part, adhere to Knudson's "two-hit" hypothesis of tumor formation (128) (see Chapter 60). Others have noted that certain phakomatoses, such as TSC, are known or postulated to disrupt a common intracellular signal transduction pathway linked to the mammalian target of rapamycin (mTOR) kinase (111). Thus, while advances in our understanding of the molecular pathogenesis of the phakomatoses have revealed unsuspected heterogeneity amongst these entities, commonalities have also been found.

From a developmental standpoint, Bolande (20) in 1974 emphasized the wide distribution and multipotential nature of the migratory derivatives of the neural crest and their susceptibility to teratogenic, oncogenic, and mutagenic influences. He coined the term "neurocristopathies" to emphasize his conviction that neuroblastoma, neurofibromatosis, pheochromocytoma, medullary carcinoma of the thyroid, carcinoid tumors, Hirschprung disease and syndromes involving combinations of these abnormalities arise from aberrations in the early migration, growth, and differentiation of neural crest cells. He noted that, because of the extremely variable and complex forms of neurofibromatosis, all of which can be pathogenetically related to primary dysontogenesis of the primitive neuroectoderm and its neural crest derivatives, neurofibromatosis represents "a most pivotal and dramatic representative" of the concept (20). Since his initial description, there has been an increase in the number and variety of neurocristopathies, which continue to show some overlap with the phakomatoses (21).

As the molecular mechanisms and developmental events underlying the phakomatoses are revealed, further revisions in their categorization will surely follow. In addition to their clinical manifestations, future classifications of these disorders will increasingly incorporate genetic knowledge in an effort to predict clinical phenotypes and aid in prognosis and treatment.

PHAKOMATOSES

von Hippel–Lindau Disease

VHLD (MIM #193300) is an autosomal dominant, multisystem, familial cancer syndrome that results from a germline mutation in the *VHL* gene (70,143,190,243). This disease has perpetuated the names of the German ophthalmologist Eugen von Hippel (1867–1939) and the Swedish pathologist Arvid Lindau (1892–1958).

VHLD is an uncommon disease, with an incidence in the general population of about 1 in 36,000 people and its principal clinical findings usually appearing between 18 and 30 years of age (190). The mean age of onset for retinal hemangioblastomas is 25 years, with a reported range of onset from 1 to 67 years of age (143). The frequency of retinal lesions ranges from 25% to 70% (143,215).

Similar to retinoblastoma, the identification of the genetic basis of VHLD has yielded fundamental insights into the mechanisms of tumorigenesis. The *VHL* gene, which contains three exons, was first cloned in 1993 (134,209). The chromosomal location for *VHL* in humans is on chromosome 3 (3p25–26) (85). *VHL* is a tumor suppressor gene, and patients with VHLD harbor a germline mutation or deletion of one copy of the gene. It is generally believed that the familial tumors develop from cells in which the remaining wild-type copy of *VHL* acquires a somatic mutation, resulting in inactivation of both copies of the tumor suppressor gene. This follows Alfred Knudson's two-hit theory (128). The protein encoded by the VHL tumor suppressor gene (*VHL*) plays a key role in the mammalian oxygen-sensing pathway. In the absence of VHL, hypoxia-inducible factor becomes stabilized and induces the expression of its target genes. These, in turn, are important in regulating angiogenesis, cell growth, and cell survival. The exact pathologic mechanisms causing the different phenotypes are not yet fully identified, but it is generally believed that the differential loss of the multiple functions of VHL leads to the different disease presentations. Biallelic inactivation of *VHL* is also believed to be a key factor in the pathogenesis of the sporadic form of these tumors. The cell from which hemangioblastomas derive is still unknown (52,84,124,180).

The major systemic manifestations of VHLD are craniospinal hemangioblastomas (Fig. 1); clear-cell renal cell carcinomas and renal cysts; pheochromocytomas, neuroendocrine pancreatic tumors and pancreatic cysts; and endolymphatic sac tumors. There is a 95% penetrance at age 60 years and a positive family history in up to 75% of cases (189,200). The genotype-phenotype classification in families with VHLD is given in Table 1 (24,38,45,50,103,119,143,255). The hemangioblastomas occurring in VHLD are often multiple and may continue to occur over the course of the patient's life (159). Serial imaging studies indicate that these tumors grow in an unpredictable manner (243).

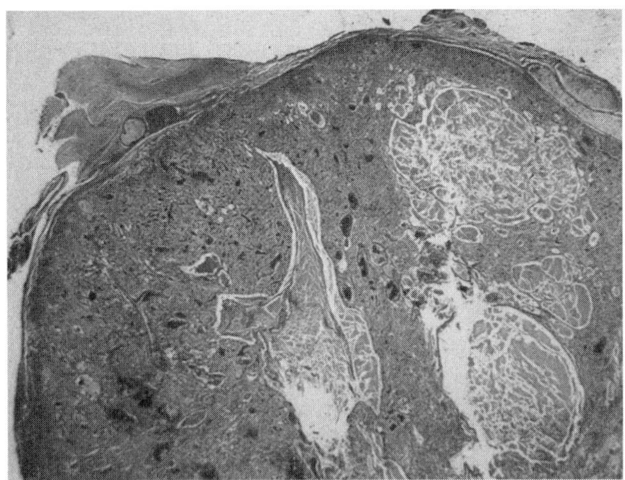

Figure 1 Cerebellar hemangioblastoma composed of capillary vessels intermixed with stromal cells (hematoxylin and eosin, ×45).

With reference to eye findings, retinal hemangioblastomas are the primary ocular lesions of VHLD, typically arising in the retinal periphery (Fig. 2), on or adjacent to the optic disc, or in both locations. The typical appearance of the retinal lesion is a two- to three-optic disc diameter rounded, yellow to red mass usually associated with large dilated and tortuous feeder vessels (Fig. 2). In about 50% of cases, they are multiple and may be bilateral (143). In VHLD, only one third of patients are found to have multiple angiomas at the time of first evaluation, and only half of these have bilateral involvement. In the absence of a family history or medical history of other tumors, molecular genetic testing is the most effective method of diagnosing VHLD (70). Although peripheral retinal tumors are often asymptomatic on initial examination, they usually will cause visual symptoms through growth and an increased vascular permeability, causing the accumulation of subretinal fluid and the development of exudates at the macula. Fluorescein angiography (FA) distinguishes the vein from the arteriole in the feeder vessels and often demonstrates continuous leakage from the angioma. Ultimately, this extravasation leads to the formation of organized fibroglial bands, gliosis, and retinal detachment (79). Iris neovascularization, secondary angle-closure glaucoma, and eventually phthisis bulbi commonly develop.

Regarding the ocular lesions of VHLD, retinal hemanioblastoma is grossly and histologically indistinguishable from the craniospinal hemangioblastomas. By light microscopy, these tumors are composed of plump, lipid-containing cells surrounding capillaries. These cells appear vacuolated in routinely processed specimens and are regarded as endothelial cells, macrophages, neuroglia, pseudoxanthomatous cells, or stromal cells. Solid lesions, composed of masses of angioblastic cells, occur as well and appear to have more growth potential than the lesions composed of capillary spaces. These vacuolated tumor cells resemble the tumor cells seen in clear-cell renal cell carcinomas. In recent studies of hemangioblastomas of the CNS, Hasselblatt and associates found that tumors predominantly composed of densely packed tumor cells, as compared to the large vacuolated stromal cells with a rich capillary network, had more frequent recurrences (102). These investigators suggested that histological subtyping of hemangioblastomas has prognostic implications and may contribute to identifying patients at risk for recurrence.

Neurofibromatosis

Neurofibromatosis was described by the German pathologist von Recklinghausen in 1882 (240). It is now appreciated that neurofibromatosis is a general term that includes several distinct disorders. While these share many features, they have important differences in natural history and management. In the 1980s, Riccardi proposed a classification that included seven types (187,188,197) and Gorlin (90) added two further categories. The most widely accepted classification at the present time is that

Table 1 Genotype–Phenotype Classifications in Families with von Hippel–Lindau Disease

Type	Clinical characteristics	Genotype	Refs.
Type I	Retinal hemangioblastomas, CNS hemangioblastomas, renal cell carcinomas, pancreatic neoplasms, and cysts	Typically deletions or protein-truncating mutations in *VHL*	38,49,146,217
Type 2A	Pheochromocytomas, retinal hemangioblastomas, CNS hemangioblastomas	Typically missense mutations in *VHL* (e.g., Tyr98His mutation)	7,24
Type 2B	Pheochromocytomas, retinal hemangioblastomas, CNS hemangioblastomas, renal cell carcinomas, pancreatic neoplasms, and cysts	Typically missense mutations in *VHL* (e.g., Arg167Gln mutation)	38,49,146
Type 2C	Pheochromocytoma only	Typically missense mutations in *VHL* gene (e.g., Leu188Val and Val84Leu mutations)	1,48,165,191

Note: Endolymphatic sac tumors and cystadenomas of the epididymis and broad ligament have not been assigned to specific von Hippel–Lindau types.

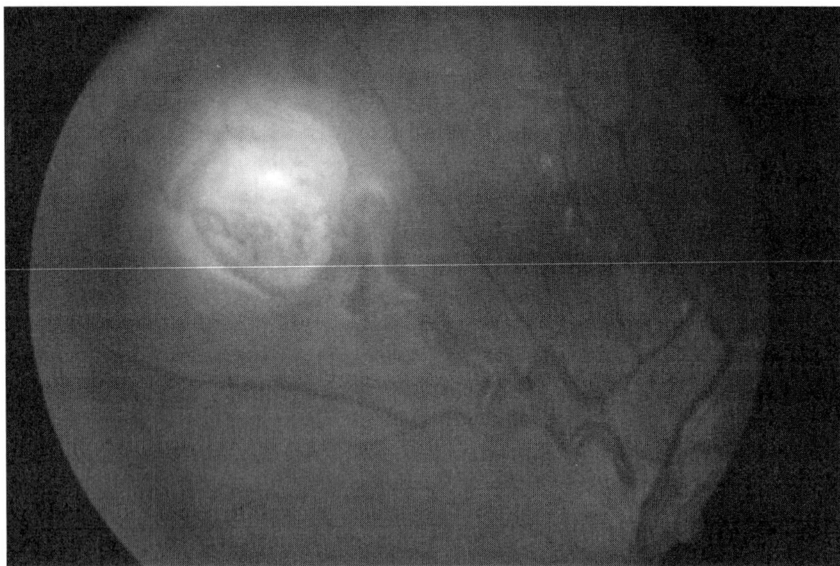

Figure 2 Fundus photograph of retinal hemangioblastoma associated with large, dilated and tortuous feeder vessels.

recommended in 1987 by the National Institutes of Health (NIH) Consensus Conference on Neurofibromatosis (164). According to this classification, neurofibromatosis 1 (NF1) (MIM +162200) replaces the term "von Recklinghausen" or "peripheral neurofibromatosis" or "multiple neurofibromatoses" and neurofibromatosis 2 (NF2) (MIM #101000) replaces "bilateral acoustic neurofibromatosis" or "central neurofibromatosis." The Consensus Conference statement notes that other types exist, which at that time were not adequately defined to be included in the formal classification.

Although both NF1 and NF2 are autosomal dominant disorders of multiple tumor types, they differ significantly in incidence. NF1 is one of the most common inherited diseases in man and the commonest form of neurofibromatosis. Its characteristic features are *café au lait* patches, neurofibromas, CNS tumors, and distinctive bony dysplasia. NF1 has an estimated incidence of 1 per 2,500 births and a prevalence of approximately 1 in 4,500 (109). NF2 is less frequent in the general population, with an incidence of approximately 1 in 33,000 births and a symptomatic prevalence of 1 in 210,000 (197). Approximately half of the cases have no family history of the disease. In common with NF1, there is a high penetrance and variable expressivity. Typically, NF2 patients develop bilateral acoustic neuromas (vestibular schwannomas) and multiple CNS tumors, including schwannomas, gliomas, ependymomas and meningiomas (252). NF2 has a higher morbidity and mortality than other forms of neurofibromatosis.

The genetic bases of both NF1 and NF2 have been established and studied extensively. The *NF1* gene was identified on human chromosome 17 (17q11.2) and encodes neurofibromin (96,97,131), one of the functions of which is to reduce cell proliferation by the cell-signaling molecule Ras (154). If neurofibromin function is lost due to a homozygous mutation, there is an inability to terminate the Ras-mediated signals (43,69).

The *NF2* gene was mapped to human chromosome 22 (22q11.2) and encodes a protein known as merlin or schwannomin (95,195,233). Merlin is a cytoskeletal protein, which links the actin cytoskeleton to cell-surface glycoproteins and is involved in cellular remodeling (95,157). The mechanisms underlying merlin's function as a tumor suppressor in the pathogenesis of schwannomas and other NF2-associated tumors have not been determined (205).

Both NF1 and NF2 exhibit systemic disease. NF1 patients may have involvement of any organ (74,96,110,197). Abnormalities include CNS tumors; including bilateral vestibular schwannomas in 85% to 90% of patients (153), as well as other cranial and spinal tumors.

Ocular and adnexal manifestations are more common in NF1 than in NF2. Lesions may occur in the eyelid, the globe, the optic nerve, or the orbit. Three important diagnostic criteria of NF1 involve these structures: Lisch nodules of the iris, optic glioma, and plexiform neurofibromas of the orbit and eyelid. In addition, *café au lait* spots, choristoma of the conjunctiva, drusen of the optic disc, proliferation of melanocytes and neural cells in the choroid, and retinal astrocytic hamartomas may occur. Congenital and infantile glaucoma are also seen in NF1 patients.

Café au lait spots are pigmented macular lesions of the skin, with ill-defined, serrated edges caused by hyperpigmentation of the basal cell layer, which on histopathologic examination corresponds to an increased number of melanocytes (Figs. 3A and B). Freckle-like spots, or pigmented nevi, are also frequently associated with *café au lait* spots. Although *café au lait* spots develop in 10% of the population, patients with six or more of these lesions, >1.5 cm in diameter, usually have NF1.

Neurofibromas are benign, heterogeneous, peripheral nerve sheath tumors that arise from the endoneurium or connective tissue of peripheral nerve sheaths (see Chapter 63). Fibroma molluscum, a common form of neurofibroma, clinically appears as a pedunculated, pigmented nodule, which histologically is composed of enlarged cutaneous nerves with a proliferation of Schwann cells and other connective tissue elements (Fig. 4). The plexiform neuroma ("bag of worms") consists of enlarged nerves surrounded by thickened perineural sheaths. An additional cutaneous manifestation known as "elephantiasis neuromatosa" is characterized by a diffuse proliferation of the cellular elements of the nerve sheath, resulting in a marked thickening and folding of the skin. Schwannomas are benign encapsulated tumors originating from the Schwann cells of the peripheral nervous system (see Chapter 63). While these may be encountered as isolated lesions in the general population, multiple tumors are characteristic of NF1. Malignant transformation of neurofibromas into malignant peripheral nerve sheath tumors (MPNSTs) has been reported in 2% to 5% of NF1 patients with plexiform neuromas, compared with 0.001% of the general population (62). Lisch nodules (Fig. 5) occur in at least 80% of NF1 patients (129). These lesions are histologically indistinguishable from nevi and are

(A)

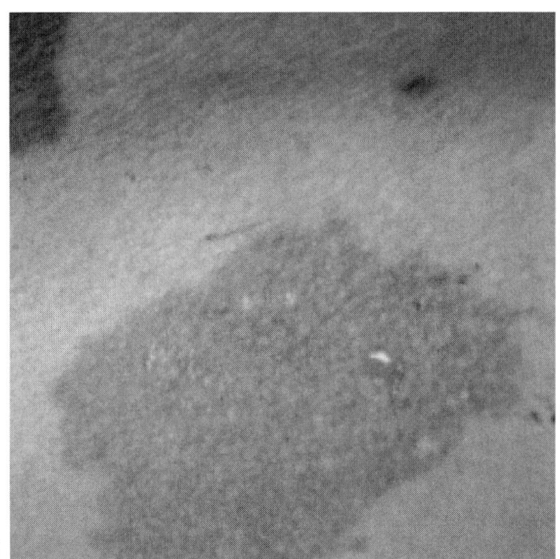

(B)

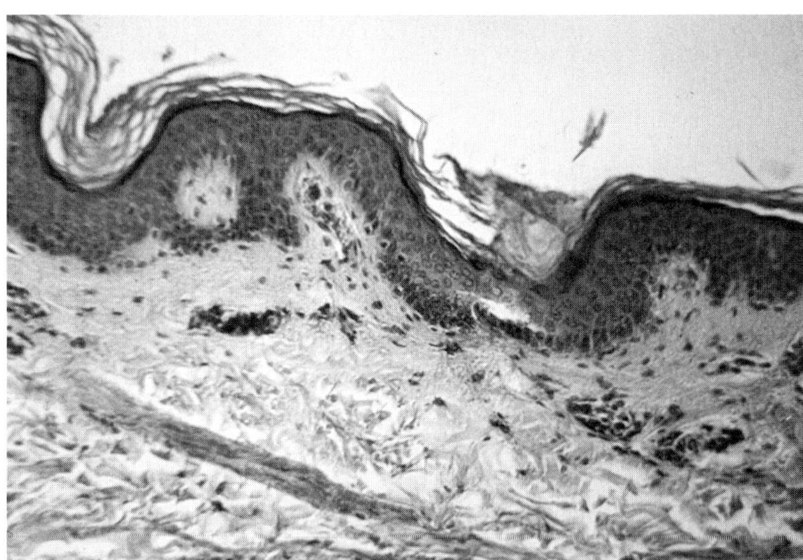

Figure 3 Histologic section of the skin at the site of *café au lait* spots, (**A**) showing hyper-pigmentation of the basal cell layer, with (**B**) increased number of melanocytes (hematoxylin and eosin, ×45).

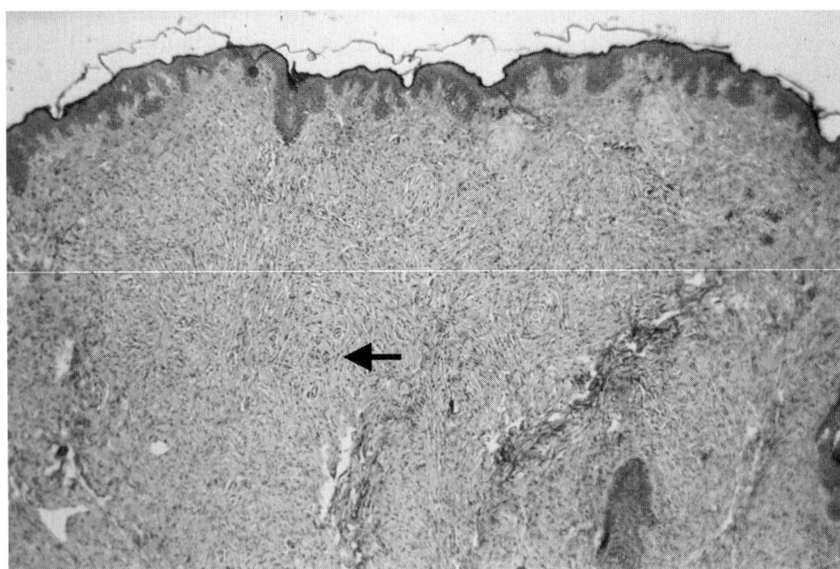

Figure 4 Cutaneous neurofibroma composed of enlarged cutaneous nerves with a proliferation of Schwann cells (*arrow*) and other connective tissue elements (hematoxylin and eosin, ×45; AFIP. Acc. 958185).

located on the anterior border of the iris or deeper in the stroma (25,72,248). Prominently thickened corneal and conjunctival nerves may also be seen (238). Additional ocular lesions include diffuse neurofibromas of the uvea, particularly of the choroid (Fig. 6); localized or diffuse uveal melanocytosis; and astrocytomas of the retina (Fig. 7). Approximately 10% to 15% of primary tumors of the optic nerve are associated with NF1 (72,242). Optic nerve gliomas (Fig. 8) occur in about 20% of NF1 patients (129,149,198). These are pilocytic astrocytomas, which cause expansion of the optic nerve and may extend posteriorly into the optic chiasm (197). Meningiomas do not appear to occur with greater frequency in NF1 (149,198). An increased incidence of uveal melanoma in NF1 patients has been reported (210). Retinal ischemia, due to retinal arterial occlusive disease, has also been described (135).

Hamartomas may occur in the trabecular meshwork, and Grant and Walton (92) observed unilateral congenital glaucoma in about 50% of patients with visible or palpable plexiform neuromas of the eyelid

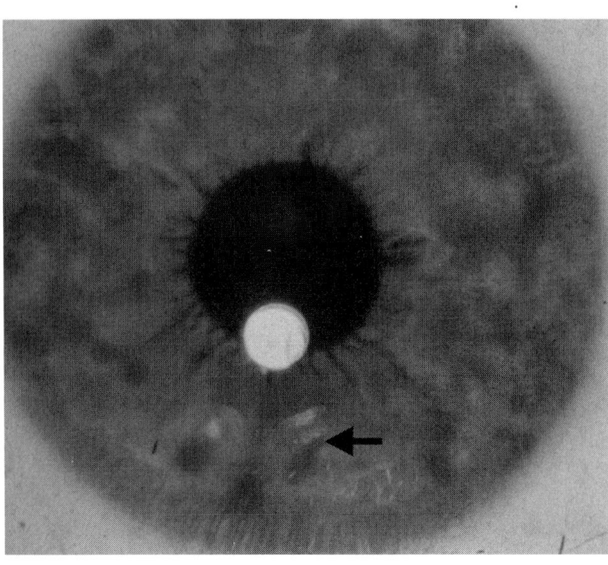

Figure 5 Tan or brown neurofibroma on the iris (*arrow*), usually less than 2 mm in diameter, consistent with Lisch nodules (AFIP. Acc. 776134).

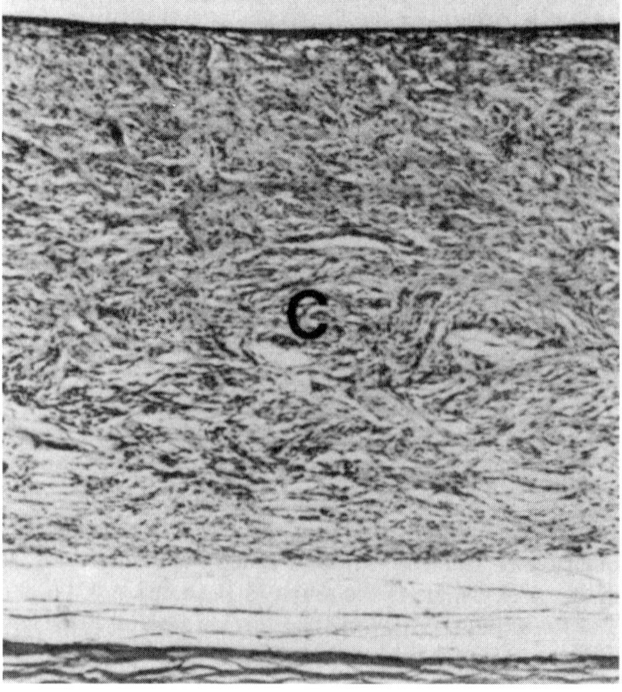

Figure 6 Diffuse choroidal lesion (C) from a patient with neurofibromatosis is composed of neural elements and melanocytes (hematoxylin and eosin, ×60).

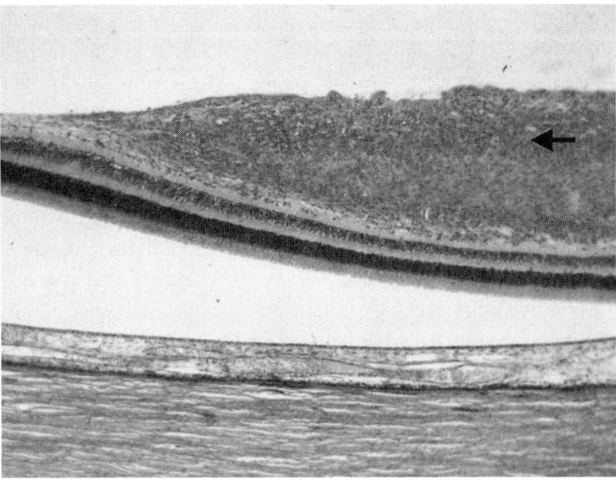

Figure 7 Retinal astrocytoma (*arrow*) in patient with neurofibromatosis (hematoxylin and eosin, ×45; AFIP. Acc. 958185).

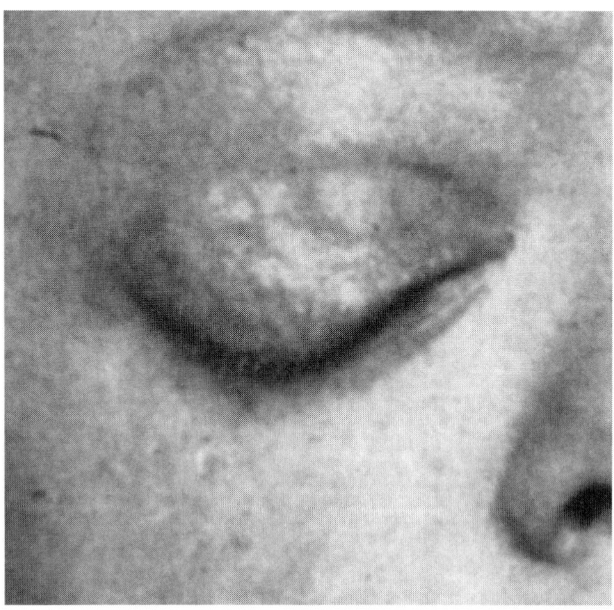

Figure 9 Plexiform neurofibroma of the eyelid.

(Fig. 9) and ipsilateral hemihypertrophy of the face. Three mechanisms have been postulated to explain the glaucoma that occurs in NF1 patients: (*i*) obstruction to the outflow of aqueous humor by neurofibromatous tissue or by a developmental anomaly in the anterior chamber angle, (*ii*) closure of the anterior chamber angle by a hamartoma involving the ciliary body and anterior choroid, and (*iii*) a secondary fibrovascular membrane in the anterior chamber angle and the formation of peripheral anterior synechiae secondary to iris neovascularization. The astrocytic hamartomas, which may occur in the retina, are localized to the ganglion cell and nerve fiber layer and do not extend beyond the internal limiting membrane. They are benign and identical to the tumors seen in this location in patients with tuberous sclerosis.

Orbital plexiform neurofibromas may cause unilateral exophthalmos, as well as enlargement of the orbit, and bony defects, such as an absence of the greater wing of the sphenoid or the orbital roof. Intracranial tissue herniating into the orbit through a bony defect may produce a pulsating exophthalmos.

The principal ophthalmological findings in NF2 are posterior capsular and/or cortical cataracts, which occur in about 80% of affected NF2 patients (96,181). Other eye findings include retinal hamartomas, epiretinal membranes, combined hamartomas of the retina and retinal pigment epithelium (RPE), and optic nerve gliomas (182,197).

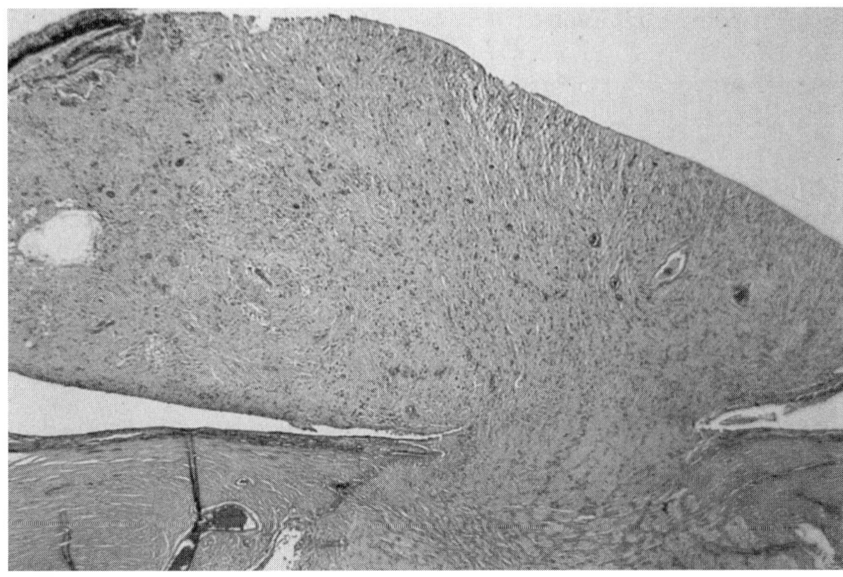

Figure 8 Optic nerve glioma protruding in the vitreous cavity in a case of neurofibromatosis (hematoxylln and eosln, ×45; AFIP. Acc. 862102).

Tuberous Sclerosis (Bourneville Disease)

In 1880, Bourneville, a French physician, drew attention to a 15-year-old cognitively impaired girl with epilepsy and cutaneous lesions thought to be adenoma sebaceum (actually angiofibromas). At postmortem examination, she was found to have multiple sclerotic nodules in the cerebral cortex and similar masses protruding into the ventricles. Noting the "potato-like" character of the lesions, Bourneville applied the term "tuberous sclerosis" to the disease (23).

Symptoms of tuberous sclerosis (MIM #191100) usually become manifest during the first 3 years of life and classically consist of a triad of cognitive impairment, seizures and angiofibromas of the face (59). However, in some case series not originating from institutions for the cognitively impaired, as many as 38% of patients are of normal intelligence (133). There is no gender or racial predilection, and approximately 25% of patients die within 35 years of diagnosis, usually due to involvement of the brain or kidney (208). Tuberous sclerosis is transmitted as an autosomal dominant trait with complete penetrance and a high sporadic case rate, leading to a reported prevalence as high as 1:6000 (130).

Two distinct genes are responsible for the disease, *TSC1* on human chromosome 9 (9q34) and *TSC2* on human chromosome 16 (16p13.3), that encode the proteins hamartin (236) and tuberin (67), respectively (10,116,130). Hamartin and tuberin form a heterodimeric complex within the cell that is involved in the control of cell division, and thus are classified as tumor suppressors, similar to the gene products of hereditary retinoblastoma (see Chapter 60), neurofibromatosis and VHLD (130). More specifically, the hamartin/tuberin complex regulates the activity of a particular enzyme, mTOR kinase, which in turn stimulates protein synthesis by phosphorylating other proteins involved in translation control (10,111). Of note, there are additional hamartomatous diseases with an established molecular link to the mTOR kinase pathway, e.g., Peutz–Jeghers syndrome (MIM #175200) and the phosphatase and tensin homolog (*PTEN*)-related disorders, and still others are postulated to involve dysregulation of this pathway (111).

Hamartomatous lesions of the brain are a hallmark of TSC, being present in >90% of patients and accounting for the seizure disorders and cognitive impairment often associated with this disease (117). The brain lesions are classified as cortical tubers, subependymal nodules (SEN) and subependymal giant cell astrocytomas (SEGA). Cortical tubers are benign, present at birth, usually located in the cortex or subcortical white matter, and commonly calcified. SENs are very common and are composed of elongated glial cells, multinucleated giant cells and, eventually, calcium deposits (117). SEGAs are similar to the associated nodules, except that they are larger and tend to grow, sometimes resulting in significant morbidity and mortality. It has been postulated that SENs have the potential to grow and differentiate into SEGAs (194), and that the giant cells found in tubers and SEGAs may be of the same cellular lineage (118,137). Outside the CNS, hamartomas and varied malformations can be found in a small subset of TSC patients, typically involving the heart, bones, thyroid and/or kidneys.

Cutaneous manifestations of TSC are numerous and important for the diagnosis. In the older literature, the symmetrically distributed, small, reddish angiofibromas of the face were incorrectly referred to as "adenoma sebaceum" of Pringle. Nickel and Reed (167) demonstrated that the sebaceous glands in these lesions are, in fact, generally atrophic, with the main histological finding being dermal fibrosis (owing to the large size and stellate shape of the fibroblasts) (Figs. 10A,B). In older lesions, perifollicular proliferation of collagen may be seen, leading to the compression of atrophic hair follicles. Elastic tissue is lacking in angiofibromas.

Additional cutaneous lesions in TSC include the shagreen patch, ash leaf spots, nevi, *café au lait* spots and periungual fibromas. The "shagreen patch" (Fig. 11) usually located in the lumbosacral region, is a thickened plaque of skin present in about 25% of cases. "Ash leaf spots" are congenital hypomelanotic macules that are located on the trunk and limbs of 86% of patients. They can be demonstrated with a Wood light and are an important early sign of TSC (71). Normal skin shows a uniform dark coloration under the Wood light because of the absorption of blue light by melanin. The ash leaf lesions show a lighter coloration, presumably because of the lesser degree of melanization.

Ocular involvement of tuberous sclerosis was initially recognized by van der Hoeve in 1921 (158). The ocular and periocular findings (16,72,73,170,257) include astrocytic hamartomas, white pedunculated tumors of the palpebral conjunctiva, yellowish-red thickenings of the bulbar conjunctiva and angiofibromas of the eyelids. The most common of these lesions is the astrocytic hamartoma, which occurs in >50% of patients (158). Astrocytic hamartomas are gray-white retinal tumors that develop a nodular appearance like a mulberry (150) over time, probably due to dystrophic calcification. On occasion, they can be aggressive, leading to enucleation in rare cases (211). Initially, when these lesions are smooth in appearance, they may resemble retinoblastomas. The tumors may be solitary or multiple, unilateral or bilateral, and, although usually located near the optic nerve head,

(A)

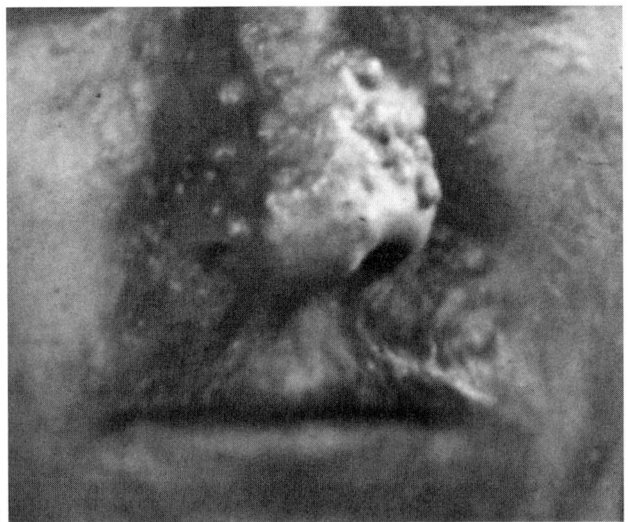

(B)

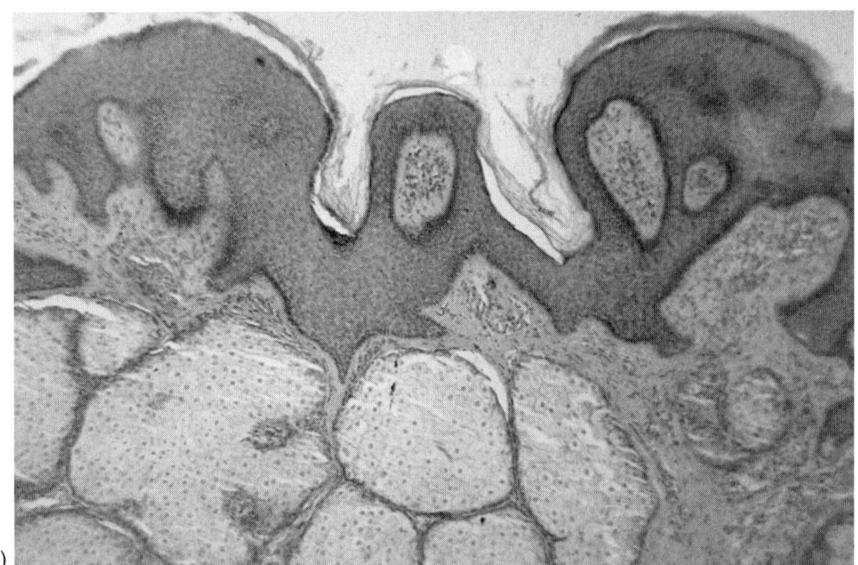

Figure 10 (**A**) Typical symmetrically distributed, small, reddish angiofibromas of the face are seen in a case of tuberous sclerosis. (**B**) Histologic evaluation of these lesions reveals atrophic sebaceous glands with dermal fibrosis (hematoxylin and eosin, ×45).

may occur anywhere in the retina (9,25,44,257). In addition, glial hamartomas of the optic nerve head may be visible anterior to the lamina cribrosa. Although referred to as giant drusen, these lesions should not be confused with ordinary drusen of the optic disc or Bruch membrane or with a true glioma (93,105,242).

The retinal and optic nerve astrocytic hamartomas are composed of elongated, fibrous astrocytes containing small, oval nuclei with fine, interlacing cytoplasmic processes. The retinal tumors are limited to the nerve fiber and ganglion cell layers and do not extend beyond the internal limiting membrane or infiltrate other structures (9,156,196). The astrocytomas arising from the optic nerve tend to calcify, and osseous metaplasia of the adjacent RPE often occurs (Figs. 12A–D). It should be noted that astrocytic hamartomas can occur as isolated lesions (9,44,93,105,108,113,156,174,185,193) and these may be difficult to differentiate from localized forms of "massive" retinal gliosis and from retinoblastomas (53,199,210,239,256).

Encephalotrigeminal Angiomatosis (Sturge–Weber Syndrome)

In 1879, Sturge (222) described a clinical syndrome consisting of unilateral buphthalmos, ipsilateral facial hemangioma, and contralateral focal epilepsy. He suspected the coexistence of an intracranial hemangioma in this disorder, which was later confirmed by Kalischer in 1897 (242), several years after choroidal hemangiomas became recognized by Jenning-Mills in 1884 (115). The currently recognized, complete syndrome of encephalotrigeminal angiomatosis was described by Weber in 1922 (244), and includes an intracranial hemangioma (characteristically an occipital or posterior parietal leptomeningeal angioma);

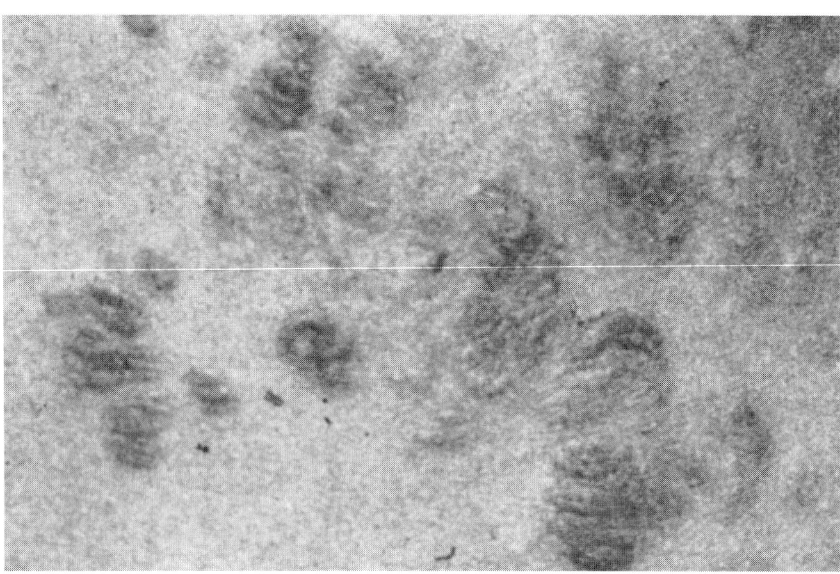

Figure 11 Lumbosacral region of a patient with tuberous sclerosis showing thickened plaque of skin consistent with shagreen patch.

facial hemangioma ("port-wine stain/nevus") in the ophthalmic distribution of the trigeminal nerve (Fig. 13); ipsilateral choroidal hemangioma (Fig. 14); and congenital glaucoma. In most cases, incomplete forms of the syndrome are present, but according to Reese (185), at least two of these lesions must be present to warrant the diagnosis. The inclusion of SWS (MIM 185300) within the group of phakomatoses is justified by the presence of hamartomas (hemangiomas) involving the CNS, retina, and skin.

SWS occurs sporadically, with a frequency of approximately 1 in 50,000 (13,230). However, there are reports of familial transmission of certain features of SWS (241), and some chromosomal abnormalities (particularly on the short arm of chromosome 17) have been associated with the syndrome (47). There does not appear to be a significant gender or race predilection for SWS (13,73), and there are no environmental or prenatal factors that are known to contribute to the disease. The peculiar constellation of hemangiomas found in SWS is postulated to arise from a failure of the primitive cephalic venous plexus to regress during the first trimester of development (46). At this embryologic time point, the ectoderm of the future upper face and the neuroectoderm of the future parietal-occipital cortex are in close proximity, and a somatic mutation occurring in this region could account for the findings in SWS. The somatic mutation hypothesis is bolstered by a report of a single monozygotic twin with classic bilateral SWS (175).

Systemic manifestations of SWS include disseminated angiomas and nevi, varices of the legs and arms, and *café au lait* spots (139). Ipsilateral angiomas of the meninges may be associated with neurological signs, the most common of which are seizures, which develop in up to 90% of patients, usually by the age of 2 years (230). Headaches, hemiplegia, hemiparesis, developmental delay, and progressive cognitive impairment have also been reported, the latter occurring in 50% of SWS patients (13). Intracranial, dystrophic calcifications may be observed on neuroimaging, along with vascular abnormalities and atrophic cortical changes (230).

Microscopic examination of the port-wine nevus of the skin reveals dilated, ectatic capillaries in the epidermis, dermis, and subcutaneous tissue (139). There is no increase in the number of blood vessels, and immunohistochemical analysis has not revealed any significant antigenic differences from normal blood vessels (166). It should be noted that although the facial angioma is present at birth, telangiectases first become apparent histologically in patients at about 10 years of age. This may result from congenital weakness of the capillary walls. Histologic analysis of intracranial hemangiomas demonstrates thickened leptomeninges and tortuous blood vessels, with underlying brain atrophy and extensive gliosis in some circumstances (55,168).

Ocular manifestations of SWS are common and numerous. In up to 71% of patients (224), a diffuse choroidal hemangioma occurs on the side of the facial angioma, appearing as a yellowish to red, flat to slightly elevated, circular area with indiscrete margins. These features often produce a classic "tomato ketchup" appearance on funduscopic examination (13,63,64,83). In contrast, choroidal hemangiomas not associated with SWS are characteristically discrete and raised. Of all reported choroidal hemangiomas, about 50% have been in patients with SWS (64,79). Episcleral hemangioma is suggestive of uveal involvement, while cavernous hemangioma or telangiectasis of the eyelids on the side of the facial angioma is

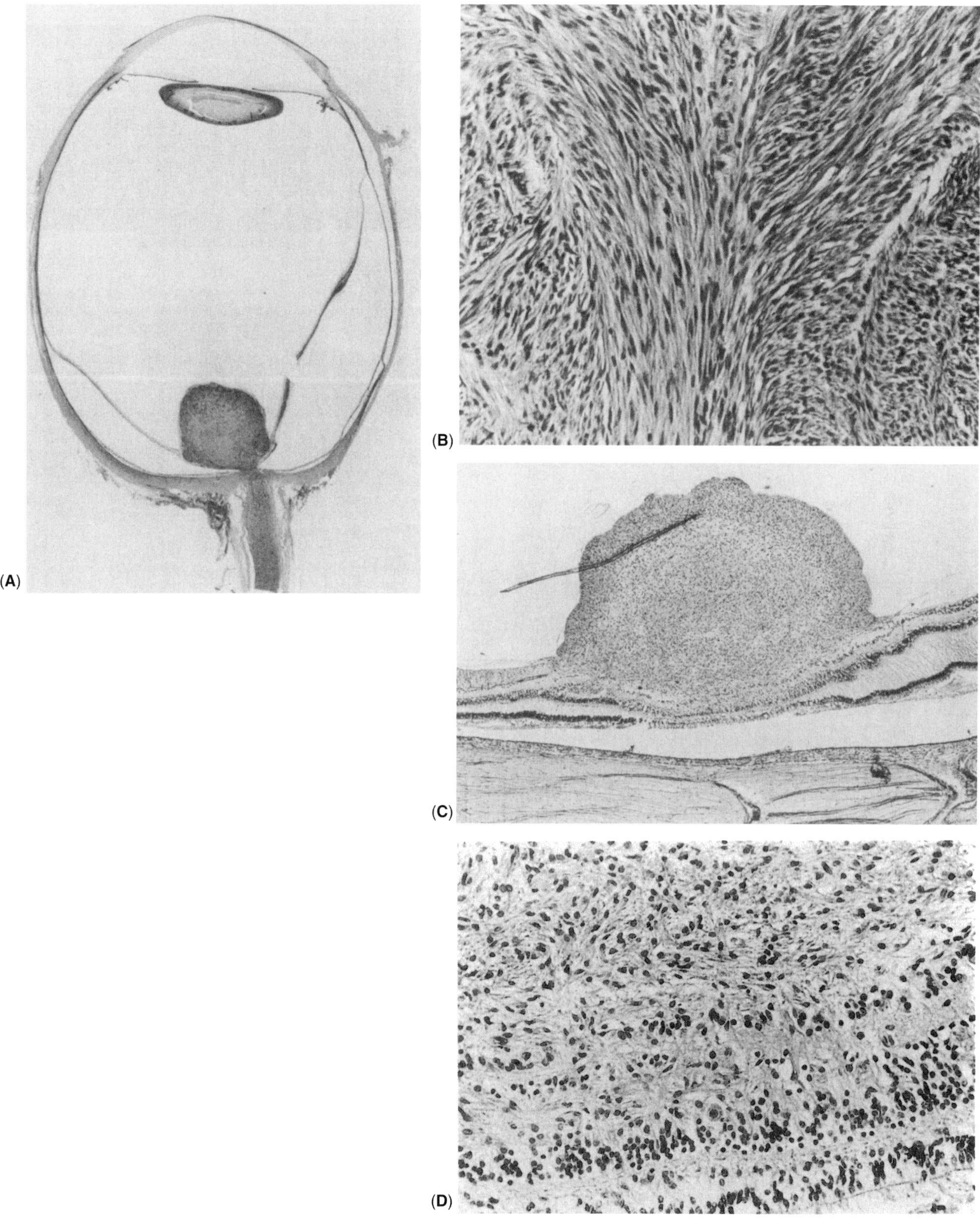

Figure 12 (**A**) Astrocytoma arising from the retina of a patient with tuberous sclerosis (hematoxylin and eosin, ×3). (**B**) Higher power view, showing pattern of growth of astrocytic hamartoma (hematoxylin and eosin, ×145). (**C**) Isolated astrocytoma of the retina. Note that the tumor is limited to the retina and remains within the confines of the internal limiting membrane (hematoxylin and eosin, ×30). (**D**) Higher power view showing elongated, fibrous astrocytes with small, oval nuclei, and a delicate meshwork of interlacing cytoplasmic processes merging with normal retina (hematoxylin and eosin, ×30).

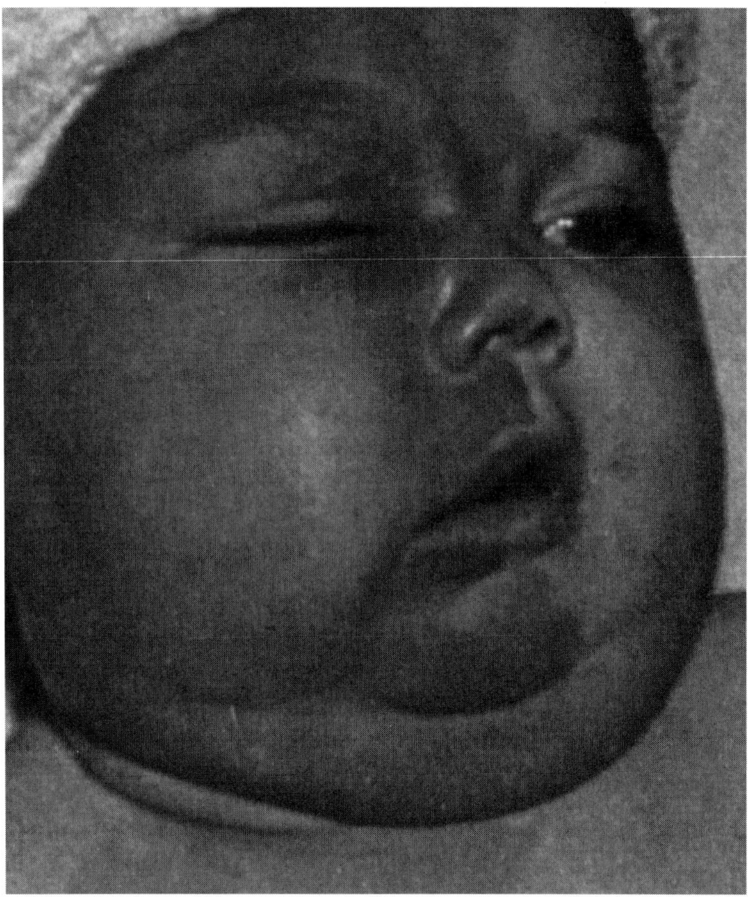

Figure 13 Port-wine stain in the ophthalmic distribution of trigeminal nerve in an infant with Sturge–Weber syndrome.

frequently associated with glaucoma (13). Buphthalmos, cataract, iris heterochromia, optic disc coloboma, and nevus of Ota have also been reported in SWS (13). Additional ocular changes found in enucleated eyes include microcystoid degeneration of the retina overlying a hemangioma, leakage of serous fluid into the subretinal space, and serous retinal detachment (13,72).

Glaucoma is a common ocular manifestation of SWS, occurring in as much as 30% to 60% of patients (13,223) with a median age of onset of 5 years (range: birth to 41 years) (223). The glaucoma is usually associated with ipsilateral hemangiomas of the facial skin, but bilateral glaucoma with unilateral port wine stains can occur (8). Leading theories to explain the development of glaucoma in SWS include increased episcleral pressure leading to decreased aqueous humor outflow and developmental anomalies of the anterior chamber angle (39,230). Histological studies of trabeculectomy specimens in SWS patients have demonstrated abnormalities of Schlemm canal, hemangiomas within the trabecular meshwork, and increased vascularization and abnormal collagen deposition within intra-trabecular spaces (4,42,246). The latter finding occurs exclusively in SWS-associated glaucoma (13).

Ataxia-Telangiectasia (Louis-Bar Syndrome)

In 1941, Louis-Bar described a 9-year-old boy with progressive cerebellar ataxia and bilateral oculocutaneous telangiectasia. Boder and Sedgewick subsequently studied additional cases of this entity, documenting the clinical features and establishing it as one of the phakomatoses (17,18). However, while ataxia-telangiectasia (MIM #208900) has neurological, cutaneous, and ocular manifestations similar to other neurocutaneous syndromes, it differs from other phakomatoses in that it is not associated with hamartomas. The incidence of AT varies from country to country. It occurs at a frequency of 1 in 40,000 live births in the United States, but it affects only 1 in 300,000 in the United Kingdom (12,41,228). AT is present in all races, but it is more prevalent among ethnic groups with high consanguinity, consistent with its autosomal recessive mode of inheritance (41).

In the decades following its initial description, the constellation, progression, and variability of symptoms and findings in AT have been more fully elucidated (30,176). Infants born with AT initially appear normal, but neurological symptoms usually begin by the age of one, and most children lose their ability to walk independently by 10 years of age (12,41,80). Immunodeficiency is also present to some degree, although the

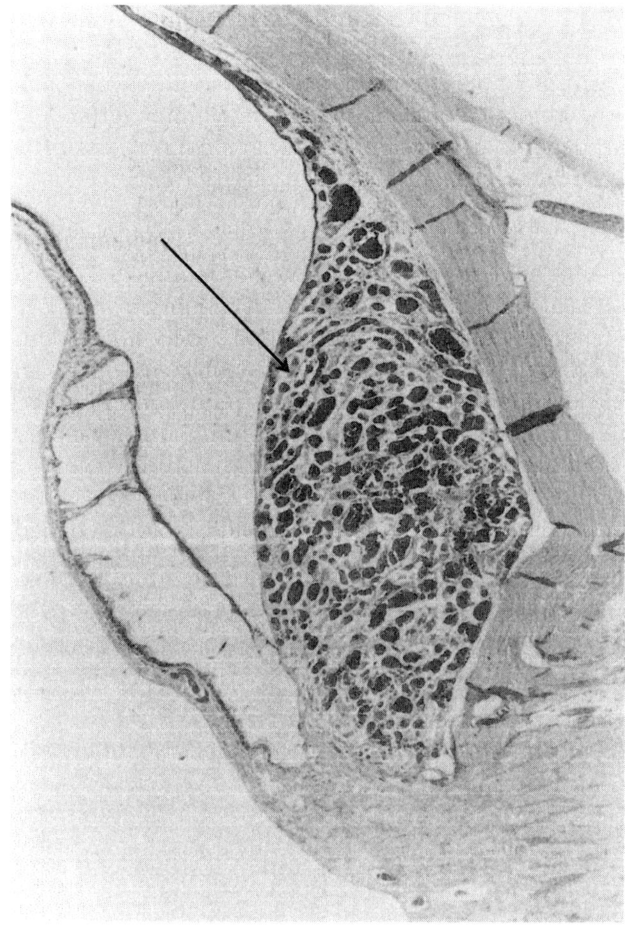

Figure 14 Juxtapapillary cavernous hemangioma arising in choroid (hematoxylin and eosin, ×45).

resulting susceptibility to infection varies considerably between patients (228). Telangiectatic blood vessels develop on the skin and conjunctiva many years after the neurological symptoms appear.

The list of nonocular findings in AT is long and includes: (*i*) progressive cerebellar ataxia; (*ii*) dysarthric speech; (*iii*) choreoathetosis; (*iv*) hypersensitivity of fibroblasts and lymphocytes to ionizing radiation; (*v*) an extremely high cancer incidence (usually non-Hodgkin lymphoma) affecting one-third of patients (225); (*vi*) a cell-mediated immune deficiency with variable humoral immune deficiencies, leading to frequent and often fatal sinopulmonary infections; (*vii*) thymic hypoplasia; and (*viii*) cutaneous telangiectasis of the ears, face, and extensor surfaces of both extremities (41,176,228). Laboratory and radiological findings include elevated alphafetoprotein; low serum immunoglobulin A (IgA), immunoglobulin E (IgE), and immunoglobulin G2 (IgG2); and cerebellar atrophy on magnetic resonance imaging (MRI) (41). Histological analysis of post-mortem specimens obtained from patients of various ages shows progressive loss of cerebellar Purkinje and granular cells with preservation of basket cells (82,177). This suggests that Purkinje cells develop and mature normally, only to degenerate early in childhood.

The most conspicuous ocular finding of AT is bilateral bulbar conjunctival telangiectasis (Fig. 15), which usually develops during childhood after the onset of ataxia. The telangiectasia on both the eyes and skin appear as dark red patches resulting from chronic dilated groups of capillaries (12,29). Various ocular motility disorders, including oculomotor apraxia, are also frequent in this disorder.

Like many of the phakomatoses, the molecular pathology of AT has become increasingly clear. The gene causing AT, *ATM*, was localized to chromosome 11 (11q22–23) in 1988 (81) and later cloned in 1995 (201,202). It encodes a 350 kDa protein kinase that is expressed in many tissues and plays a crucial role in the detection and repair of DNA double-strand breaks (98). Such breaks occur naturally during meiosis and other cellular events and also after exposure to ionizing radiation or other DNA damaging agents. Hundreds of distinct mutations have been found in the *ATM* gene, occurring in all 62 exons, which likely accounts for at least some of the phenotypic heterogeneity of the disease (41,176).

Wyburn–Mason Syndrome

In 1943, Wyburn–Mason described 27 patients with retinal arteriovenous malformations (AVMs), of which 81% were thought to have similar involvement of the midbrain (250). In a less comprehensive report six years earlier, Bonnet, Dechaume, and Blanc noted the combination of retinal and intracranial AVMs. This syndrome is thus also known as the Bonnet-Dechaume–Blanc syndrome. The type of retinal AVMs occurring in this syndrome were appreciated, however, long before either report (257).

Wyburn–Mason syndrome is a rare, sporadic phakomatosis characterized by congenital ipsilateral retinal and brain malformations. The disorder results from a disturbance in the embryologic development of the vascular mesoderm (206). Because of its rarity and the anecdotal information available in the literature, few conclusions can be drawn regarding the epidemiology or natural history of the intracranial AVMs. These are usually asymptomatic and only found after the observation of retinal AVMs (184).The original report by Wyburn–Mason antedated the general use of cerebral angiography. In a subsequent study, in which the diagnosis of intracranial hemangioma was accepted only when it could be demonstrated by angiography, surgery, or autopsy, Bech and Jensen found an intracranial intravenous aneurysm coexisting with similar lesions in the retina in only

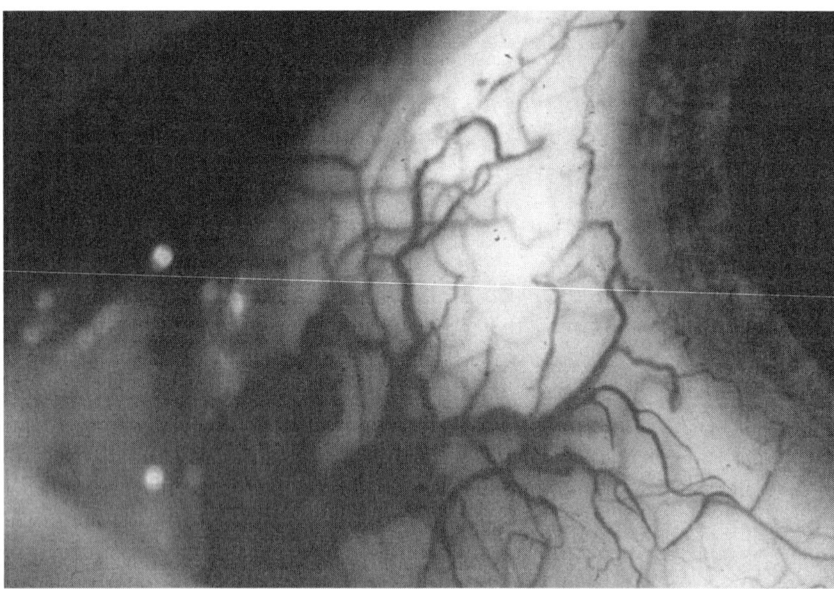

Figure 15 Bulbar conjunctival telangiectasis in a child with ataxia-telangiectasia.

17% of patients (14). Theron et al. (229) reported that of the 80 cases stated to have retinal AVMs before 1974, 25 also had intracranial AVMs (31%). In addition, 10 of the 25 cases with intracranial AVMs also had facial AVMs. Unlike retinal AVMs, the intracranial AVMs have a tendency to hemorrhage or become infarcted. Hydrocephalus may occur from compression of the Sylvian aqueduct. Complications of the brain lesions can result in visual impairment, strabismus, gaze palsies, diplopia, pulsating exophthalmos, and ptosis (251). Less frequently described manifestations include seizures, delirium, disorientation, hallucinations, somnolence, sleep inversion, and mental retardation (136).

The vascular lesion occurring in the retina and brain in this disorder has been termed both a racemose hemangioma (Fig. 16) and a cirsoid aneurysm (14). It is congenital and usually non-progressive. These lesions may, however, change their configuration over many years, becoming increasingly tortuous (11). Vascular occlusions may occur (14,229) causing retinal ischemia (229). The retinal AVMs usually do not leak or bleed and generally do not cause vision loss (27). Neovascular glaucoma has been reported,

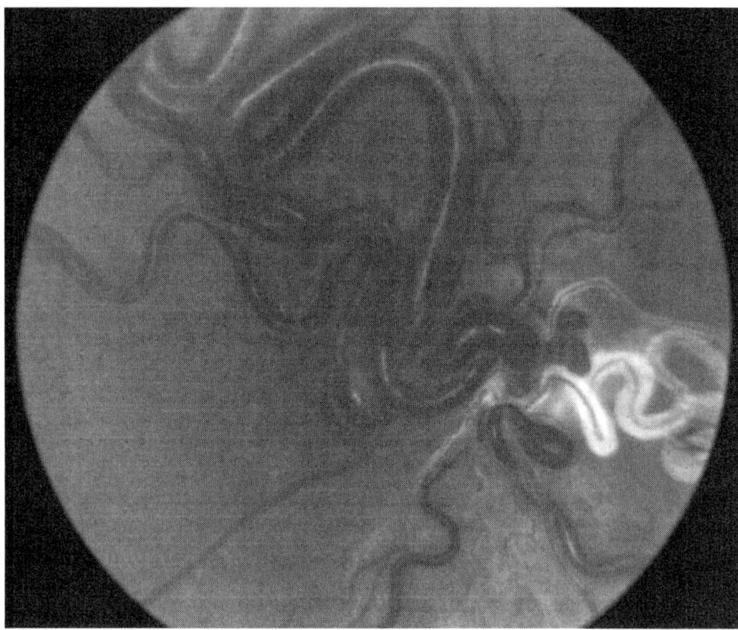

Figure 16 Retinal arteriovenous malformations in a case of Wyburn–Mason syndrome.

resulting from retinal ischemia (65). In addition, several patients have been described with progressive optic neuropathy caused by accompanying orbitocranial AVMs (11,26,51,65,123,162). FA demonstrates a dilated and tortuous arteriole, contiguous with a similar vein involving the optic disc and retina. There is rapid flow of dye through the lesion without leakage (27,206).

Nevus Sebaceus of Jadassohn

Patients with nevus sebaceus of Jadassohn (MIM 163200) manifest an organoid malformation of the sebaceous glands, apocrine glands, hair follicles, and epidermal layer of the skin. These individuals may also have systemic malformations involving the eyes and CNS, as well as skeletal deformities (192). The nevus sebaceus is a well-described dermatologic entity, but the full-blown syndrome is uncommon and the incidence is unknown (212).

The cardinal feature in this phakomatosis is the "nevus" itself, which characteristically is present on the face and scalp from early childhood. The individual lesions are yellow to orange and waxy in appearance, with a papillomatous surface (112). The nevi usually enlarge during adolescence and secondary tumors, including basal cell carcinoma, squamous cell carcinoma, nodular hidradenoma, and syringocystadenoma papilliferum may develop during adulthood (58,249).

The two most important ocular lesions are epibulbar complex choristomas (178) and posterior intrascleral cartilage and bone, which create a yellow discoloration of the ocular fundus (214). The epibulbar complex choristoma is a fleshy lesion of the conjunctiva, often extending onto the cornea, which appears histopathologically as a dermal lipoma with variable combinations of ectopic lacrimal gland and hyaline cartilage. In addition, optic nerve colobomas (247) and choroidal osteomas have been described. J.A. Shields and C.L. Shields maintain that these represent misinterpretations of the discoloration of the fundus in the area of the posterior scleral cartilage (213,214). An additional ophthalmic abnormality described in this condition is microphthalmos (57). Non-ophthalmic findings include epilepsy, mental retardation, and other neurologic disorders, as well as cardiovascular, urogenital, and skeletal anomalies.

Prophylactic excision of the benign nevus sebaceus has not been effective, but removal of suspected secondary neoplasms is indicated (40). The nevus sebaceus of Jadassohn and linear nevus are often difficult to differentiate both clinically and histologically. Distinguishing features are the linear configuration of the linear nevus, its flesh-colored and slightly raised appearance, and its location in the epidermis on histopathologic examination (57).

NEOPLASTIC ENDOCRINE SYNDROMES

Multiple Endocrine Neoplasia Syndromes

The multiple endocrine neoplasia (MEN) syndromes are autosomal dominant disorders that were recognized early in the 20th century. Their natural history and the causative genes have become clear only during the past 30 years (104). These constitute a rare group of diseases, but their importance is heightened by the fact that an understanding of their molecular bases has given important insights into human cancer. The genetic syndromes comprising the multiple endocrine neoplasias are listed in Table 2. The MEN syndromes

Table 2 Genetic Syndromes with Endocrine Neoplasms

Syndrome	MIM number	Gene	Sites of neoplasms
Multiple endocrine neoplasia type 1	+131100	*MEN1*	Pituitary gland, parathyroid glands, pancreatic islets, adrenal cortex, cutaneus angiofibromas, and lipomas
Multiple endocrine neoplasia type 2A	#171400	*RET*	C-cell of the thyroid (medullary thyroid carcinoma), adrenal medulla (pheochromocytoma), parathyroid glands
Multiple endocrine neoplasia type 2B	#162300	*RET*	C-cell of the thyroid (medullary thyroid carcinoma), adrenal medulla (pheochromocytoma), intestinal ganglioneuromatosis, marfanoid features
von Hippel–Lindau disease	#193300	*VHL*	Adrenal medulla (pheochromocytoma), pancreatic islets, hemangioblastomas of the CNS, retinal angiomas, renal cell carcinomas, visceral cysts
Neurofibromatosis type 1	+162200	*NF1*	Neurofibromas, variable development of endocrine tumors, adrenal medulla (pheochromocytomas), C-cell of thyroid gland (medullary thyroid carcinoma), parathyroid gland, somatostatin-producing carcinoid tumors
Carney complex type 1	#160980	*PRKARIA*	Pituitary gland, thyroid gland, testicles, adrenal cortex, heart, breast, and skin (myxomas), cutaneous spotty pigmentation
Carney complex type 2	%605244	Unknown	Pituitary gland, heart, skin (myxomas), adrenal cortex, thyroid gland, cutaneous spotty pigmentation

Source: Modified from Ref. 104.

are classified as either MEN type 1 (MIM +131100) or MEN2, with MEN2 being further differentiated into MEN2A (MIM #171400) and MEN2B (MIM #162300) (Table 2). Criteria for diagnosis of the MEN syndromes are not universally accepted. As a result of this, and because of the rarity and diversity of these syndromes, epidemiologic data is not available.

MEN2A, MEN2B, and familial medullary thyroid carcinoma are all caused by mutations in the *RET* proto-oncogene, which is located near the centromere on chromosome 10 (227). About half of MEN2B cases arise spontaneously, and half are inherited as an autosomal dominant disease, usually through the father (31). Greater than 95% of all patients with MEN2B show the same mutation in the *RET* gene (161). The mechanism of action of *RET* is being intensively studied (172). Most tumors in MEN2B patients can be related to functional changes in *RET* occurring in the embryonic thyroid C-cells, adrenal medulla, parathyroid gland, and autonomic nerve plexuses of the gut (171). Patients at risk for the MEN syndromes should have genetic analyses as early as possible, since regular screening and counseling are of paramount importance (142).

The neoplastic features of the various MEN syndromes are given in Table 2. MEN2A, in addition, is associated with cutaneous lichen amyloidosis (28,75,169) and with failure of normal colonic neural development (Hirschsprung disease) (MIM #142623) (237). In addition to the endocrine neoplasms, MEN2B is characterized by a marfanoid habitus and neuromas of the lips, tongue, and gastrointestinal tract (35,36,183). All patients with MEN2 develop medullary thyroid carcinoma, and 15% to 25% of those affected die from it (104).

The MEN syndromes of particular importance to ophthalmologists are MEN2A, MEN2B, and familial medullary thyroid carcinoma. Specific ocular findings include thickened corneal nerves, occurring in 57% of patients with MEN2A (126). These are also a prominent and consistent finding in MEN2B (163). Additional findings in the latter include thickening and eversion of the upper eyelid margin with the tarsal plates visible, as well as neuromas of the eyelids and large, prominent eyebrows. Cases of MEN2B with typical ocular findings, but without systemic malignancies, have been described (54).

Carney Complex

In 1985, Carney described 39 patients with a complex of myxomas, spotty pigmentation of the skin and mucosae, and endocrine overactivity (32,219). Carney complex (MIM #160980), as it was termed, also affects the adrenal cortex, thyroid glands, gonads, and ocular adnexa. Carney complex is considered a MEN syndrome and shares features in common with many phakomatoses, including involvement of the brain (pituitary gland), skin and eyes, the presence of tumors of mesenchymal and neural crest origin, and a presumed autosomal dominant inheritance (219). It is easily confused with "Carney syndrome," which consists of a triad of gastric leiomyosarcoma, pulmonary chondroma and extraadrenal paraganglioma (33). Carney complex is also included in the group of genetic disorders known as the lentiginoses, which includes Peutz–Jeghers syndrome (MIM #175200), LEOPARD (multiple Lentigines, Electrocardiographic conduction abnormalities, Ocular hypertelorism, Pulmonic stenosis, Abnormal genitalia, Retardation of growth, sensorineural Deafness) syndrome (MIM #151100); Bannayan–Riley–Ruvalcaba syndrome (MIM #153480); Laugier–Hunziker syndrome (a rare, benign, acquired hyperpigmentation of the oral mucosa and lips); along with Cowden disease (MIM #158350). The lentiginoses refers to the small, flat macules with variable pigmentation found on the skin, called "lentigines." On histologic examination, they demonstrate true melanocytic hyperplasia with prominent rete ridges and basal cell layer hyperpigmentation (186). Blue nevi (usual and epithelioid types); combined and common junctional, dermal and compound nevi; and *café au lait* spots are other examples of pathologic skin lesions found in Carney complex (34,219).

The myxomas (composed of mucoid connective tissue) can affect numerous organs, including the heart, skin, and breast (219). Unlike sporadic cardiac myxomas, those associated with Carney complex are usually multiple, have no gender predilection, occur in younger individuals, and affect all chambers of the heart (32). Cutaneous myxomas often occur in the eyelids and external ear canals. Other, non-myxoid tumors can also occur with the Carney complex, such as testicular tumors, growth hormone-secreting tumors, ductal adenoma of the breast, and psammomatous melanotic schwannoma (221).

The most common endocrine abnormality in Carney complex is Cushing syndrome, which affects one-third of patients and is due to unique adrenal nodules located within an atrophic adrenal cortex, referred to as primary pigmented nodular adrenal disease. These lesions are visible on computed tomography (CT) and MRI (60). Ten percent of patients also have acromegaly from a growth hormone-secreting pituitary adenoma (219,220). Other endocrine manifestations include three different types of testicular tumor: large-cell calcifying Sertoli cell tumor, adrenocortical rests, and Leydig cell tumor (179).

Ophthalmic findings in Carney complex are found in approximately three-quarters of affected individuals, and consist of the aforementioned eyelid myxomas and lentigines, pigmented lesions on the caruncle or conjunctival semilunar fold, and relative hypertelorism (122). The ocular features often precede the onset of the manifestations of cardiac myxomas by several years; therefore, their recognition should prompt a thorough medical evaluation to identify and treat these tumors early (121).

The genetics of Carney complex have not been fully elucidated. However, it is known to be transmitted in an autosomal dominant manner, and genetic loci for Carney complex have been identified by linkage analysis on chromosome 17 (17q23–24) (Carney complex type 1) and chromosome 2 (2p16) (Carney complex type 2) (37,220). Carney complex type I is due to mutations in the *PRKARIA* gene. The 2p16 locus is of particular interest since it includes genes known to be involved in regulating DNA stability and genomic instability is frequently found in the myxoid tumors of Carney complex patients (56,219). Like many other disorders, the ultimate identification of the genetic defect of Carney complex is expected to offer considerable insight into its pathogenesis.

McCune–Albright Syndrome

In the 1930s, McCune and Albright separately described a syndrome that included osteitis fibrosa disseminata, *café au lait* macules, and precocious puberty (6,155). The latter finding affects girls almost exclusively. The specific triad of McCune–Albright syndrome (MAS) (MIM #174800) has been refined to poly/monostotic fibrous dysplasia, *café au lait* pigmented skin lesions, and hyperfunctioning endocrinopathies (15,144). The presence of two of these three findings is sufficient to make the diagnosis. Specific endocrinopathies associated with MAS include hyperthyroidism, hypercortisolism, hypersomatotropism, and hypophosphatemic rickets (15).

MAS is a rare and sporadic disorder and, although it is associated with cutaneous and neurological (endocrine-related) manifestations, its ophthalmic findings (optic nerve compression and resultant vision loss) are secondary to hyperostosis of the skull, and overall the disorder only superficially resembles the phakomatoses. Like SWS, however, MAS is postulated to arise from a dominant somatic mutation that occurs early in development, leading to a mosaic distribution of defective cells (101,144). Because of the importance of the intracellular signal transduction molecule cAMP in the control of endocrine activity and the growth of melanocytes and osteoblasts, a defect leading to its overproduction in MAS was theorized in 1986 (152). Indeed, endocrine tissues from patients with MAS were later found to contain somatic mutations in the *GNAS1* gene on chromosome 20 (20q13.2) that codes for a particular G-protein ($G_S\alpha$), which leads to constitutive activation of adenyl cyclase and subsequent overproduction of cAMP (204,216,245). Thus, MAS constitutes yet another example of how molecular biology has contributed to our knowledge of the pathophysiology of complex clinical syndromes.

OTHER NEOPLASTIC SYNDROMES

Nevoid Basal Cell Carcinoma Syndrome (Gorlin–Goltz Syndrome)

The nevoid basal cell carcinoma syndrome (NBCCS) (MIM #109400) was initially described by Jarish in 1894 (114). In 1959, Howell and Caro reported a relationship of the basal cell nevus to other cutaneous disorders and anomalies (106). A year later, Gorlin and Goltz included multiple nevoid basal cell carcinomas as part of a syndrome with jaw keratocysts and skeletal anomalies, completing the characteristic triad (91). Since that time, additional ophthalmologic, neurologic, endocrine, and genital manifestations have been documented to occur in this syndrome (147).

NBCCS includes an autosomal dominant form of basal cell carcinoma (BCC), with a prevalence of about 1 per 60,000 in the population (87). Although most reports have been in Caucasians, this syndrome probably arises in all ethnic groups. The clinical features become manifest in the first, second, or third decades, with males and females equally affected (68,125). Sixty percent of new cases arise spontaneously in patients with no known affected family members, with an estimated 35% to 50% of these representing new mutations (88).

The underlying genetic defect responsible for the NBCCS syndrome is mutations in the human homologue of the *Drosophila patched* gene (*PTCH*) (148,218). The causative gene is on chromosome 9 (9q22.3–q31) (22,76). *PTCH* is a transmembrane protein that functions as a component of the Hedgehog signaling pathway (148,218). The gene also functions as a tumor suppressor (226), similar to genes responsible for other phakomatoses.

Systemically, the most frequent skin lesions occurring in NBCCS patients are cutaneous BCCs, which affect 80% of Caucasians and 38% of blacks (86,125). Ultraviolet B (UVB) radiation (290–320 nm) appears to be a strong risk factor for the formation of BCC (77). The lesions are variable in both number and size and affect primarily the thoracic and cervicofacial areas. The skin of the eyelids, periorbital areas, nose, and upper lip are the most commonly affected regions of the face (89). Odontogenic keratocysts occur in about 75% of patients with NBCCS (66). These have a strong tendency to recur following local resection (3) and may have some premalignant potential (160). Other, less common manifestations include dystrophia canthorum, skeletal abnormalities, hypogonadism, ovarian fibromas, medulloblastoma, and meningioma (89,107,132,147).

With regard to ocular findings, about a quarter of the patients with NBCCS develop eyelid tumors (100,253), with the tumors usually developing in adolescence, although they may also be seen in early childhood (91). On histologic examination, these tumors are generally superficial and resemble in all regards the noninherited form of BCC (140,151). In the advanced stages these tumors become more invasive and destructive and may involve the orbit. In addition to the eyelid lesions, hypertelorism affects 40% of patients with NBCCS and esotropia is noted in 15% (147). Other ophthalmic abnormalities reported with this syndrome are exotropia, congenital amaurosis, ptosis, glaucoma, colobomas of the choroid and optic nerve, cataract, and blindness (89,132,147).

Adenomatous Polyposis Coli

Adenomatous polyposis coli (APC) (MIM +175100) was described in 1861 (61). It is an autosomal dominant disorder characterized by the presence of multiple adenomatous polyps in the gastrointestinal tract. It occurs at a frequency of approximately 1 in 50,000 worldwide, and there is no gender predilection (61). Without colectomy, patients with APC invariably develop colon cancer, usually by the age of 40 years (61,231). Other polyposis syndromes are characterized by hamartomatous polyps, in that they are comprised of cells native to the tissue in which they reside (203). Gardner syndrome involves a subset of APC patients with extracolonic manifestations (78) such as osteomas, dental anomalies, polyps of the gastric fundus and duodenum, soft tissue cancers, desmoid tumors, thyroid and adrenal tumors, hepatoblastoma, and pigmented lesions of the ocular fundus. The term Turcot syndrome is applied when brain tumors are also present (99).

The most common ocular findings in APC (Gardner syndrome subtype) are multiple, congenital hamartomas of the retinal pigment epithelium (RPE) that resemble congenital hypertrophy of the retinal pigment epithelium (CHRPE) (120,173,232). Other, less common ophthalmologic findings in Gardner syndrome include orbital osteomas and soft tissue tumors of the eyebrows or eyelids (231). The pigmented lesions of the ocular fundus are present in 70% of patients with APC and do not increase in number or size with age (231). They are usually small, flat, round, deeply pigmented and found in the midperiphery of the fundus in both eyes, but larger lesions tend to be closer to the posterior pole and possess areas of hypopigmentation and lacunae formation. The presence of three or more of these ocular lesions predicts carrier status for the disease (231). Histopathologically, these lesions are most often comprised of a single layer of hypertrophied RPE cells with enlarged pigment granules, although some have multiple cell layers (231), which are not found in isolated CHRPE.

The genetic defect in APC occurs in the *APC* gene, which was mapped to chromosome 5 (5q21–22) and subsequently cloned (19,94,127,138). Most of the clinically significant mutations in the *APC* gene lead to truncation of the encoded protein (APC), which normally functions as a tumor suppressor protein and is particularly important in the regulation of colorectal epithelial and RPE cell proliferation and migration (61,141,207).

REFERENCES

1. Abbott M, Nathanson K, Nightingale S, et al. The von Hippel-Lindau (VHL) germline mutation V84L manifests as early-onset bilateral pheochromocytoma. Am J Med Genet A 2006; 140:685–690.
2. Adams R, Reed W. Neurocutaneous diseases. In: Fitzpatrick T, Arndt K, Clark W, Eisen A, van Scott E, Vaughan J, eds. Dermatology in General Medicine. New York: McGraw-Hill; 1971:1393–1396.
3. Ahlfors E, Larsson A, Sjogren S. The odontogenic keratocyst: a benign cystic tumor? J Oral Maxillofac Surg 1984; 42:10–19.
4. Akabane N, Hamanaka T. Histopathological study of a case with glaucoma due to Sturge-Weber syndrome. Jpn J Ophthalmol 2003; 47:151–157.
5. Albrecht-Munchen. Ueber Hamartome. Verh Dtsch Pathol Ges Jena 1904; 7:153–157.
6. Albright F, Butler A, Hamptom A, Smith P. Syndrome characterized by osteitis fibrosa disseminata, areas of pigmentation and endocrine dysfunction, with precocious puberty in females: reports of five cases. N Engl J Med 1937; 216:727–746.
7. Allen R, Webster A, Sui R, et al. Molecular characterization and ophthalmic investigation of a large family with type 2A von Hippel-Lindau disease. Arch Ophthalmol 2001; 119:1659–1665.
8. Amirikia A, Scott I, Murray T. Bilateral diffuse choroidal hemangiomas with unilateral facial nevus flammeus in Sturge-Weber syndrome. Am J Ophthalmol 2000; 130: 362–364.
9. Apple D, Boniuk M. Clinical pathological review: Solitary retinal astrocytoma. Surv Ophthalmol 1985; 30:173–191.
10. Astrinidis A, Henske E. Tuberous sclerosis complex: linking growth and energy signaling pathways with human disease. Oncogene 2005; 24:7475–7481.
11. Augsburger J, Goldberg R, Shields J, et al. Changing appearance of retinal arteriovenous malformation. Graefes Arch Klin Exp Ophthalmol 1980; 215:65–70.
12. Ball L, Xiao W. Molecular basis of ataxia telangiectasia and related diseases. Acta Pharmacol Sin 2005; 26: 897–907.
13. Baselga E. Sturge-Weber syndrome. Semin Cutan Med Surg 2004; 23:87–98.
14. Bech K, Jensen O. On the frequency of co-existing racemose haemangiomata of the retina and brain. Acta Psychiatr Scand 1961; 36:47–56.

15. Bhansali A, Sharma B, Sreenivasulu P, et al. Acromegaly with fibrous dysplasia: McCune-Albright syndrome-clinical studies in 3 cases and brief review of literature. Endocr J 2003; 50:793–799.
16. Binaghi M, Coscas G, Nucci T. Les phacomes retiniens. J Fr Ophtalmol 1983; 6:275–290.
17. Boder E, Sedgewick R. Ataxia telangiectasis. A familial syndrome of progressive cerebellar ataxia, oculocutaneous telangiectasia and frequent pulmonary infections. Pediatrics 1958; 21:525–554.
18. Boder E, Sedgewick R. Ataxia telangiectasis. Univ South Calif Med Bull 1957; 9:15–27.
19. Bodmer W, Bailey C, Bodmer J, et al. Localization of the gene for familial adenomatous polyposis on chromosome 5. Nature 1987; 328:614–616.
20. Bolande R. Neurocristopathy: Its growth and development in 20 years. Pediatr Pathol Lab Med 1997; 17:1–25.
21. Bolande R. The neurochristopathies. A unifying concept of disease arising in neural crest malformations. Hum Pathol 1974; 5:409–429.
22. Bonifas J, Bare J, Kerschmann R, et al. Parental origin of chromosome 9q22.3-q31 lost in basal cell carcinomas from basal cell nevus syndrome patients. Hum Mol Genet 1994; 3:447–448.
23. Bourneville D. Sclerose tubereuse des circonvolutions cerebrales: Idiotie et epilepsie hemiplegique. Arch Neurol 1980; 1:69–91.
24. Brauch H, Kishida T, Glavac D, et al. Von Hippel-Lindau disease with pheochromocytoma in the Black Forest region of Germany: evidence for a founder effect. Hum Genet 1995; 95:551–556.
25. Brini A, Dhermy P, Sahel J. Oncology of the Eye and Adnexa. Dordrecht NL: Kluwer; 1990.
26. Brown D, Hilal S, Tenner M. Wyburn-Mason syndrome. Report of two cases without retinal involvement. Arch Neurol 1973; 28:67–69.
27. Brown G. Congenital retinal arteriovenous communications (racemose hemangiomas). In: Guyer D, Yannuzzi L, Chang S, et al. eds. Retina-Vitreous-Macula. Philadelphia: W.B. Saunders Co; 1999:1172–1174.
28. Bugalho M, Limbert E, Sobrinho L, et al. A kindred with multiple endocrine neoplasia type 2A associated with pruritic skin lesions. Cancer 1992; 70:2664–2667.
29. Cabana M, Crawford T, Winkelstein J, et al. Consequences of the delayed diagnosis of ataxia-telangiectasia. Pediatrics 1998; 102:98–100.
30. Carbonari M, Cherchi M, Paganelli R, et al. Relative increase of T cells expressing the gamma/delta rather than the alpha/beta receptor in ataxia telangiectasia. N Engl J Med 1990; 322:73–76.
31. Carlson K, Bracamontes J, Jackson C, et al. Parent of origin effects in multiple endocrine neoplasia type 2B. Am J Hum Genet 1994; 55:1076–1082.
32. Carney J. Differences between nonfamilial and familial cardiac myxoma. Am J Surg Pathol 1985; 9:53–55.
33. Carney J. The triad of gastric epithelioid leiomyosarcoma, pulmonary chondroma, and functioning extra-adrenal paraganglioma: a five-year review. Medicine 1983; 62: 159–169.
34. Carney J, Ferreiro J. The epithelioid blue nevus. A multicentric familial tumor with important associations, including cardiac myxoma and psammomatous melanotic schwannoma. Am J Surg Pathol 1996; 20:259–272.
35. Carney J, Go V, Sizemore G, Hayles A. Alimentary-tract ganglioneuromatosis. A major component of the syndrome of multiple endocrine neoplasia type 2B. N Engl J Med 1976; 295:1287–1291.
36. Carney J, Sizemore G, Hayles A. Multiple endocrine neoplasia type 2B. Pathobiol Annu 1978; 8:105–153.
37. Casey M, Mah C, Merliss A, et al. Identification of a novel genetic locus for familial cardiac myxomas and Carney complex. Circulation 1998; 98:2560–2566.
38. Chen F, Kishida T, Yao M, et al. Germline mutations in the von Hippel-Lindau disease tumour suppressor gene: correlations with phenotype. Hum Mutat 1995; 5:66–75.
39. Cheng K. Ophthalmologic manifestations of Sturge-Weber syndrome. In: Bodensteiner J, Roach E, eds. Sturge-Weber Syndrome. Mount Freedom, NJ: The Sturge-Weber Foundation; 1999:17–26.
40. Chum K, Vasquez M, Sanchez J. Nevus sebaceus: clinical outcome and considerations for prophylactic excision. Int J Dermatol 1995; 34:538.
41. Chun H, Gatti R. Ataxia-telangiectasia, an evolving phenotype. DNA Repair 2004; 3:1187–1196.
42. Cibis G, Tripathi R, Tripathi B. Glaucoma in Sturge-Weber syndrome. Ophthalmology 1984; 91:1061–1071.
43. Cichowski K, Jacks T. NF1 tumor suppressor gene function: narrowing the GAP. Cell 2001; 104:593–604.
44. Cleasby G, Fung W, Shekter W. Astrocytoma of the retina: report of two cases. Am J Ophthalmol 1967; 64: 633–637.
45. Clifford S, Cockman M, Smallwood A, et al. Contrasting effects on HIF-1alpha regulation by disease-causing pVHL mutations correlate with patterns of tumourigenesis in von Hippel-Lindau disease. Hum Mol Genet 2001; 10:1029–1038.
46. Comi A. Pathophysiology of Sturge-Weber syndrome. J Child Neurol 2003; 18:509–516.
47. Comi A, Mehta P, Hatfield L, Dowling M. Sturge-Weber syndrome associated with other abnormalities. Arch Neurol 2005; 62:1924–1927.
48. Crossey P, Eng C, Ginalska-Malinowska M, et al. Molecular genetic diagnosis of von Hippel-Lindau disease in familial phaeochromocytoma. J Med Genet 1995; 32:885–886.
49. Crossey P, Richards F, Foster K, et al. Identification of intragenic mutations in the von Hippel-Lindau disease tumour suppressor gene and correlation with disease phenotype. Hum Mol Genet 1994; 3:1303–1308.
50. Cybulski C, Krzystolik K, Murgia A, et al. Germline mutations in the von Hippel-Lindau (VHL) gene in patients from Poland: disease presentation in patients with deletions of the entire VHL gene. J Med Genet 2002; 39:E38.
51. Danis R, Appen R. Optic atrophy and the Wyburn-Mason syndrome. J Clin Neuroophthalmol 1984; 4:91–95.
52. de Paulsen N, Brychzy A, Fournier M, et al. Role of transforming growth factor-alpha in von Hippel-Lindau $(VHL)^{-/-}$ clear cell renal carcinoma cell proliferation: a possible mechanism coupling VHL tumor suppressor inactivation and tumorigenesis. Proc Natl Acad Sci USA 2001; 98:1387–1392.
53. Dejean C. Le vrai gliome de la retine adulte. Arch Ophtalmol (Paris) 1934; 51:257–276.
54. Dennehy P, Feldman G, Kambouris M, et al. Relationship of familial prominent corneal nerves and lesions of the tongue resembling neuromas to multiple endocrine neoplasia type 2B. Am J Ophthalmol 1995; 120:456–461.
55. Di Trapani G, Di Rocco C, Abbamondi A, et al. Light microscopy and ultrastructural studies of Sturge-Weber disease. Childs Brain 1982; 9:23–36.
56. Dijkhuizen T, van der Derg E, Molenaar W, et al. Cytogenetics of a case of cardiac myxoma. Cancer Genet Cytogenet 1992; 63:73–75.

57. Diven D, Solomon A, McNelly M, Font R. Nevus sebaceus associated with major ophthalmic abnormalities. Arch Dermatol 1987; 123:383.
58. Domingo J, Helwig E. Malignant neoplasms associated with nevus sebaceus of Jadassohn. J Am Acad Dermatol 1979; 1:545–56.
59. Donegi G, Grattarola F, Wildie H. Tuberous sclerosis: Bourneville disease. In: Vinken P, Bruyn G, eds. Handbook of Clinical Neurology, Vol. 14. New York: Elsevier; 1972:340–349.
60. Doppman J, Travis W, Nieman L, et al. Cushing syndrome due to primary pigmented nodular adrenocortical disease: findings at CT and MR imaging. Radiology 1989; 172:415–420.
61. Doxey B, Kuwada S, Burt R. Inherited polyposis syndromes: molecular mechanisms, clinicopathology, and genetic testing. Clin Gastroenterol Hepatol 2005; 3: 633–641.
62. Ducatman B, Scheithauer B, Piepgras D, et al. Malignant peripheral nerve sheath tumours: a clinicopathologic study of 120 cases. Cancer 1986; 57:2006–2021.
63. Duke-Elder S. Diseases of the Lens and Vitreous: Glaucoma and Hypotony. System of Ophthalmology, Vol. 11. St. Louis: C.V. Mosby; 1969:637–640.
64. Duke-Elder S. Diseases of the uUveal tTract. System of Ophthalmology, Vol. 9. St. Louis: C.V. Mosby; 1966: 775–936.
65. Effron L, Zakov Z, Tomsak R. Neovascular glaucoma as a complication of the Wyburn-Mason syndrome. J Clin Neuroophthalmol 1985; 5:95–98.
66. Esposito S, Kast G, Bradrick J. Basal cell nevus syndrome: a clinical report. J Prosthet Dent 1995; 73:405–410.
67. European Chromosome 16 Tuberous Sclerosis Consortium. Identification and characterization of the tuberous sclerosis gene on chromosome 16. Cell 1993; 75: 1305–15.
68. Evans D, Farndon P, Burnell L, et al. The incidence of Gorlin syndrome in 173 consecutive cases of medulloblastoma. Br J Cancer 1991; 64:959–961.
69. Feldkamp M, Gutmann D, Guha A. Neurofibromatosis type 1: piecing the puzzle together. Can J Neurol Sci 1998; 25:181–191.
70. Fitz E, Newman S. Neuro-ophthalmology of von Hippel-Lindau. Curr Neurol Neurosci Rep 2004; 4:384–390.
71. Fitzpatrick T, Szabo G, Hori Y, et al. White-leaf shaped macules: Earliest sign of tuberous sclerosis. Arch Dermatol 1968; 98:1–6.
72. Font F, Ferry A. The phakomatoses. Int Ophthalmol Clin 1972; 12:1–50.
73. Francois J. Ocular aspects of the phakomatoses. In: Vinken P, Bruyn G, eds. Handbook of Clinical Neurology, Vol. 14. New York: Elsevier; 1972:689–732.
74. Friedman J, Birch P. Type 1 neurofibromatosis: a descriptive analysis of the disorder in 1,728 patients. Am J Med Genet 1997; 70:138–143.
75. Gagel R, Levy M, Donovan D, et al. Multiple endocrine neoplasia type 2A associated with cutaneous lichen amyloidosis. Ann Intern Med 1989; 111:802–806.
76. Gailani M, Bale A. Developmental genes and cancer: role of patched in basal cell carcinoma of the skin. N Natl Cancer Inst 1997; 89:1103–1109.
77. Gailani M, Bale S, Leffell D, et al. Developmental defects in Gorlin syndrome related to a putative tumor suppressor gene on chromosome 9. Cell 1992; 69:111–117.
78. Gardner E, Richards R. Multiple cutaneous and subcutaneous lesions occurring simultaneously with hereditary polyposis and osteomatosis. Am J Hum Genet 1953; 5:139–47.
79. Gass J, Braunstein R. Sessile and exophytic capillary angiomas of the juxtapapillary retina and optic nerve head. Arch Ophthalmol 1980; 98:1790–1797.
80. Gatti R. Ataxia-telangiectasia. In: Vogelstein B, Kinzler K, eds. The Genetic Basis of Human Cancer. New York: McGraw-Hill; 2002:239–266.
81. Gatti R, Berkel I, Boder E, et al. Localization of an ataxia-telangiectasia gene to chromosome 11q22-23. Nature 1988; 336:577–580.
82. Gatti R, Vinters H. Cerebellar pathology in ataxia-telangiectasia: the significance of basket cells. Kroc. Found Ser 1985; 19:225–232.
83. Giuffre G. Cavernous hemangioma of the retina and retinal telangiectasis. Distinct or related vascular malformations. Retina 1985; 5:221–224.
84. Glasker S. Central nervous system manifestations in VHL: genetics, pathology, and clinical phenotypic features. Fam Cancer 2005; 4:37–42.
85. Glenn G, Linehan W, Hosoe S et al. Screening for von Hippel-Lindau by DNA polymorphism analysis. J Am Med Asssoc 1992; 267:1226–1231.
86. Goldstein A, Pastakia B, Di Giovanna J, et al. Clinical findings in two African-American families with the nevoid basal cell carcinoma syndrome (NBCC). Am J Med Genet 1994; 50:272–281.
87. Gorlin R. Nevoid basal cell carcinoma (Gorlin) syndrome: unanswered issues. J Lab Clin Med 1999; 134:551–552.
88. Gorlin R. Nevoid basal cell carcinoma syndrome. Dermatol Clin 1995; 13:113–125.
89. Gorlin R. Nevoid basal cell carcinoma syndrome. Medicine 1987; 66:98.
90. Gorlin R, Cohen MJ, Levine M. The neurofibromatoses (Nf1 Recklinghausen type, Nf2 acoustic type, other types). In: Gorlin R, Cohen MJ, Levine M, eds. Syndromes of the head and neck. Oxford: Oxford University Press; 1992:392–399.
91. Gorlin R, Goltz R. Multiple nevoid basal cell epithelioma, jaw cysts, and bifid rib: a syndrome. N Engl J Med 1960; 262:908–912.
92. Grant W, Walton D. Distinctive findings in glaucoma due to neurofibromatosis. Arch Ophthalmol 1968; 79:127–134.
93. Green W. The Retina. In: Spencer W, ed. Ophthalmic Pathology: An Atlas and Textbook,. 3rd ed. Philadelphia: W.B. Saunders; 1986:589–1291.
94. Groden J, Thliveris A, Samowitz W et al. Identification and characterization of the familial adenomatous polyposis coli gene. Cell 1991; 66:589–600.
95. Gusella J, Ramesh V, MacCollin M, et al. Merlin: the neurofibromatosis 2 tumor suppressor. Biochim Biophys Acta 1999; 1423:M29–M36.
96. Gutmann D, Aylsworth A, Carey J, et al. The diagnostic evaluation and multidisciplinary management of neurofibromatosis 1 and neurofibromatosis 2. J Am Med Assoc 1997; 278:51–57.
97. Gutmann D, Collins F. The neurofibromatosis type 1 gene and its protein product, neurofibromin. Neuron 1993; 10: 335–343.
98. Hall J. The ataxia-telangiectasia mutated gene and breast cancer: gene expression profiles and sequence variants. Cancer Lett 2005; 227:105–114.
99. Hamilton S, Liu B, Parsons R, et al. The molecular basis of Turcot's syndrome. N Engl J Med 1995; 332:839–847.
100. Hammani H, Faggioni R, Streiff E, Daiker B. Le syndrome depitheliomatose naevobasocellulaire multiple. Ophthalmologica 1976; 172:382.

101. Happle R. The McCune-Albright syndrome: a lethal gene surviving by mosaicism. Clin Genet 1986; 29:321–324.
102. Hasselblatt M, Jeibmann A, Gerss J, et al. Cellular and reticular variants of haemangioblastoma revisited: a clinicopathologic study of 88 cases. Neuropathol Appl Neurobiol 2005; 31:618–622.
103. Hes F, Zewald R, Peeters T, et al. Genotype-phenotype correlations in families with deletions in the von Hippel-Lindau (VHL) gene. Hum Genet 2000; 106:425–431.
104. Hoff A, Cote G, Gagel R. Multiple endocrine neoplasias. Annu Rev Physiol 2000; 62:377–411.
105. Hogan M, Zimmerman L. Ophthalmic Pathology: An Atlas and Textbook, 2nd ed. Philadelphia: W.B. Saunders; 1962:433–607.
106. Howell J, Caro M. The basal cell nevus. Its relationship to multiple cutaneous cancer and associated anomalies of development. Arch Dermatol 1959; 79:67.
107. Howell J, Freeman R. Structure and significance of the pits with their tumors in the nevoid basal cell carcinoma syndrome. Am J Acad Dermatol 1980; 2:224.
108. Huggert A, Hultquist G. True glioma of the retina. Ophthalmology 1960; 113:193–202.
109. Husen S, Clark P, Compston D, et al. A genetic study of von Recklinghausen neurofibromatosis in South East Wales. 1: Prevalence, fitness, mutation rate, and effect of parental transmission on severity. J Med Genet 1991; 26: 704–711.
110. Husen S, Harper P, Compston D. Von Recklinghausen neurofibromatosis. Brain 1988; 111:1355–1381.
111. Inoki K, Corradetti M, Guan K. Dysregulation of the TSC-mTOR pathway in human disease. Nat Genet 2005; 37: 19–24.
112. Jadassohn J. Bemerkungen zur Histologie der systematisierten Naevi und uber "Talgdrusen-Naevi". Arch fur Derm Syph 1895; 33:355–372.
113. Jakobiec F, Brodie S, Haik B, Iwamoto T. Giant cell astrocytoma. A tumor of possible Mueller cell origin. Ophthalmology 1983; 90:1565–1575.
114. Jarish W. Zur lehre von den autgeschwulsten. Archiv Jur Dermatologic und Syphilogic 1894; 28:163–222.
115. Jenning-Milles W. Nevus of the right temporal and orbital region: Nevus of the choroid and detachment of the retina in the right eye. Trans Ophthalmol Soc UK 1884; 4: 168–171.
116. Jozwiak J. Hamartin and tuberin: working together for tumour suppression. Int J Cancer 2006; 118:1–5.
117. Jozwiak J, Jozwiak S. Giant cells: contradiction to two-hit model of tuber formation. Cell Mol Neurobiol 2005; 25: 795–805.
118. Jozwiak J, Jozwiak S, Skopinski P. Immunohistochemical and microscopic studies on giant cells in tuberous sclerosis. Histol Histopathol 2005; 20:1321–1326.
119. Kaelin WJ. Molecular basis of the VHL hereditary cancer syndrome. Nat Rev Cancer 2002; 2:673–682.
120. Kasner L, Traboulsi E, DeLaCruz Z, Green W. A histopathologic study of the pigmented fundus lesions in familial adenomatous polyposis. Retina 1992; 12:35–42.
121. Kennedy R, Flanagan J, Eagle RJ, Carney J. The Carney complex with ocular signs suggestive of cardiac myxoma. Am J Ophthalmol 1991; 111:699–702.
122. Kennedy R, Waller R, Carney J. Ocular pigmented spots and eyelid myxomas. Am J Ophthalmol 1987; 104:533.
123. Kim J, Kim O, Suh J, et al. Wyburn-Mason syndrome: an unusual presentation of bilateral orbital and unilateral brain arteriovenous malformation. Pediatr Radiol 1998; 28:161.
124. Kim W, Kaelin W. Role of VHL gene mutation in human cancer. J Clin Oncol 2004; 22:4991–5004.
125. Kimonis V, Goldstein A, Pastakia B, et al. Clinical manifestations in 105 persons with nevoid basal cell carcinoma syndrome. Am J Med Genet 1997; 69:299–308.
126. Kinoshita S, Tanaka F, Ohashi Y, et al. Incidence of prominent corneal nerves in multiple endocrine neoplasia type 2A. Am J Ophthalmol 1991; 111:311.
127. Kinzler K, Nilbert M, Su L, et al. Identification of FAP locus genes from chromosome 5q21. Science 1991; 253: 661–665.
128. Knudson AJ. Mutation and cancer: Statistical study of retinoblastoma. Proc Natl Acad Sci USA 1971; 68:820–823.
129. Kordic R, Sabol Z, Cerovski B, et al. Eye disorders in neurofibromatosis (NF1). Coll Antropol 2005; 29:29–31.
130. Korf B. The phakomatoses. Neuroimag Clin N Am 2004; 14:139–148.
131. Korf B. The phakomatoses. Clin Dermatol 2005; 23:78–84.
132. Kronish J, Tse D. Basal cell nevus syndrome. In: Gold D, Weingeist T, eds. The Eye in Systemic Disease. Philadelphia: JB Lippincott; 1990:583.
133. Lagos J, Gomez M. Tuberous sclerosis. Reappraisal of a clinical entity. Mayo Clin Proc 1967; 42:26–49.
134. Latif F, Kalman T, Gnarra J, et al. Identification of the von Hippel-Lindau disease tumor suppressor gene. Science 1993; 260:1317–1320.
135. Lecleire-Collet A, Cohen S, Vignal C, et al. Retinal ischaemia in type 1 neurofibromatosis. Br J Ophthalmol 2006; 90:117.
136. Lecuire J, Duchaume J, Bret P. Bonnet-Duchaume-Blanc syndrome. In: Vinken P, Bruyn G, eds. Handbook of Clinical Neurology,. Vol. 14. New York: Elsevier; 1978: 280–315.
137. Lee A, Maldonado M, Baybis M, et al. Markers of cellular proliferation are expressed in cortical tubers. Ann Neurol 2003; 53:668–673.
138. Leppert M, Dobbs M, Scambler P, et al. The gene for familial polyposis coli maps to the long arm of chromosome 5. Science 1987; 238:1411–1413.
139. Lever W, Schumburg-Lever G. Histopathology of the Skin, 5th ed. Philadelphia: J.B. Lippincott; 1975.
140. Lindeberg H, Jepsen F. The nevoid basal cell carcinoma syndrome: Hhistopathology of the basal cell tumors. J Cutan Pathol 1983; 10:68.
141. Liou G, Samuel S, Matragoon S, et al. Alternative splicing of the APC gene in the neural retina and retinal pigment epithelium. Mol Vis 2004; 10:383–391.
142. Lips C, Hoppener J, Van Nesselrooij B, Van der Luijt R. Counselling in multiple endocrine neoplasia syndromes: from individual experience to general guidelines. J Intern Med 2005; 257:69–77.
143. Lonser R, Glenn G, Walther M, et al. von Hippel-Lindau disease. The Lancet 2003; 361:2059–2067.
144. Lumbroso S, Paris F, Sultan C. McCune-Albright syndrome: molecular genetics. J Pediatr Endocrinol Metab 2002; 15:875–882.
145. MacDonald I, Bech-Hansen N, Britton WJ, et al. The phakomatoses: recent advances in genetics. Can J Ophthalmol 1997; 32:4–11.
146. Maher E, Webster A, Richards F, et al. Phenotypic expression in von Hippel-Lindau disease: correlations with germline VHL gene mutations. J Med Genet 1996; 33:328–332.
147. Manfredi M, Vescovi P, Bonanini M, Porter S. Nevoid basal cell carcinoma syndrome: a review of the literature. Int J Oral Maxillofac Surg 2004; 33:117–124.

148. Marigo V, Davey R, Zuo Y, et al. Biochemical evidence that patched is the Hedgehog receptor. Nature 1996; 384: 176–179.
149. Marshall D. Glioma of the optic nerve as a manifestation of von Recklinghausen''s disease. Trans Am Ophthalmol Soc 1953; 51:117–155.
150. Martyn L. Tuberous sclerosis of Bourneville. In: Tasman W, ed. Retinal Diseases of Children. New York: Harper and Row; 1971:98–101.
151. Mason J, Helwig E, Graham J. Pathology of the nevoid basal cell carcinoma syndrome. Arch Pathol 1965; 79:401.
152. Mauras N, Blizzard R. The McCune-Albright syndrome. Acta Endocrinol 1986; 279:207–217.
153. Mautner V, Lindenau M, Baser M, et al. The neuroimaging and clinical spectrum of neurofibromatosis type 2. Neurosurgery 1996; 38:880–886.
154. McCormick F. The superfamily of Ras-related GTPases. Jpn J Cancer Res 1997; 88:inside front cover.
155. McCune D. Osteitis fibrosa cystica: the case of nine year old girl who also exhibits precocious puberty, multiple pigmentation of the skin and hyperthyroidism. Am J Dis Child 1936; 52:743–747.
156. McLean J. Astrocytoma (true glioma) of the retina. Arch Ophthalmol 1937; 18:255–262.
157. Meng J, Lowrie D, Sun H, et al. Interaction between two isoforms of the NF2 tumor suppressor protein, merlin, and between merlin and esrin, suggests modulation of ERM proteins by merlin. J Neurosci Res 2000; 62:491–502.
158. Mennel S, Meyer C, Eggarter F, Peter S. Autofluorescence and angiographic findings of retinal astrocytic hamartomas in tuberous sclerosis. Ophthalmologica 2005; 219: 350–356.
159. Miyagami M, Katayama Y. Long-term prognosis of hemangioblastomas of the central nervous system: clinical and immunohistochemical study in relation to recurrence. Brain Tumor Pathol 2004; 21:75–82.
160. Moos K, Rennie J. Squamous cell carcinoma arising in a mandibular keratocyst in a patient with Gorlin''s syndrome. Br J Oral Maxillofac Surg 1987; 25:280–284.
161. Morrison P, Nevin N. Multiple endocrine neoplasia type 2B (mucosal neuroma syndrome, Wagenmann-Froboese syndrome). J Med Genet 1996; 33:779–782.
162. Muthukumar N, Sundaralingam M. Retinocephalic vascular malformation: case report. Br J Neurosurg 1998; 12: 458–460.
163. Nasir M, Yee R, Piest K, et al. Multiple endocrine neoplasia type III. Cornea 1991; 10:454–459.
164. National Institutes of Health. Consensus Development Conference Statement: Neurofibromatosis. Arch Neurol 1988; 45:575–578.
165. Neumann H, Eng C, Mulligan L, et al. Consequences of direct genetic testing for germline mutations in the clinical management of families with multiple endocrine neoplasia, type II. J Am Med Assoc 1995; 274:1149–1151.
166. Neumann R, Leonhartsberger H, Knobler R, et al. Immunohistochemistry of port-wine stains and normal skin with endothelium-specific antibodies PAL-E, anti-1CAM-1, anit-ELAM-1, and anti-factor VIIIrAg. Arch Dermatol 1994; 130:879–883.
167. Nickel W, Reed W. Tuberous sclerosis. Special reference to microscopic alterations in cutaneous hamartomas. Arch Dermatol 1962; 89:209–226.
168. Norman M, Schoene W. The ultrastructure of Sturge-Weber disease. Acta Neuropathol(Berl) 1977; 37:199–205.
169. Nunziata V, Giannattasio R, di Giovanni G, et al. Hereditary localized pruritus in affected members of a kindred with multiple endocrine neoplasia type 2A (Sipple''s syndrome). Clin Endocrinol 1989; 30:57–63.
170. Nyboer J, Robertson D, Gonney M. Retinal lesions in tuberous sclerosis. Arch Ophthalmol 1976; 94:1277–1280.
171. Pachnis V, Mankoo B, Costantini F. Expression of the *c-ret* proto-oncogene during mouse embryogenesis. Development 1993; 119:1005–1017.
172. Panta G, Du L, Nwariaku F, Kim L. Direct phosphorylation of proliferative and survival pathway proteins by RET. Surgery 2005; 138:269–274.
173. Parker J, Kalnins V, Deck J, et al. Histopathological features of congenital fundus lesions in familial adenomatous polyposis. Can J Ophthalmol 1990; 25:159–163.
174. Paufique L, Audibert J, Laurent C. Le gliome de la retine. Notions genetiques, anatomiques et cliniques. Etat actuel du traitment. J med Lyon 1960; 41:1555–15660.
175. Pedailles S, Martin N, Launay V, et al. Sturge-Weber syndrome. A severe form in a monozygote female twin. Ann Dermatol Venereol 1993; 120:379–382.
176. Perlman S, Becker-Catania S, Gatti R. Ataxia-telangiectasia: diagnosis and treatment. Semin Pediatr Neurol 2003; 10:173–183.
177. Perry T, Kish S, Hinton D, Hansen S, et al. Neurochemical abnormalities in a patient with ataxia-telangiectasia. Neurology 1984; 34:187–191.
178. Pokorny K, Hyman B, Jakobiec F, et al. Epibulbar choristomas containing lacrimal tissue: clinical distinction from dermoids and histologic evidence of an origin from palpebral lobe. Ophthalmology 1987; 94:1249.
179. Premkumar A, Stratakis C, Shawker T, et al. Testicular ultrasound in Carney complex. J Clin Ultrasound 1997; 25:211–214.
180. Qi H, Gervais M, Li W, et al. Molecular cloning and characterization of the von Hippel-Lindau-like protein. Mol Cancer Res 2004; 2:43–52.
181. Ragge N, Baser M, Klein J, et al. Ocular abnormalities in neurofibromatosis 2. Am J Ophthalmol 1995; 120:634–641.
182. Raimondi A. Pediatric Neurosurgery. Theoretical Principles—Art of Surgical Techniques, 2nd ed. Berlin, Heidelberg, New York: Springer; 1998.
183. Rashid M, Khairi M, Dexter R, et al. Mucosal neuroma, pheochromocytoma and medullary thyroid carcinoma: multiple endocrine neoplasia type 3. Medicine 1975; 54: 89–112.
184. Reck S, Zacks D, Eibschitz-Tsimhoni M. Retinal and intracranial arteriovenous malformations: Wyburn-Mason Syndrome. J Neuro-Ophthalmol 2005; 25: 205–208.
185. Reese A. Tumors of the Eyes, 3rd ed. New York: Harper and Row; 1976.
186. Rhodes A. Neoplasms: benign neoplasias, hyperplasias, and dysplasias of melanocytes. In: Fitzpatrick T, Eisen A, Wolff K, Freedberg I, Austen K, eds. Dermatology in General mMedicine. New York: McGraw Hill; 1993: 1078–1116.
187. Riccardi V. Neurofibromatosis: clinical heterogeneity. Curr Probl Cancer 1982; 7:1–34.
188. Riccardi V. Neurofibromatosis: Phenotype, Natural history and Pathogenesis. Baltimore: Johns Hopkins University Press; 1992.
189. Richard S, David P, Marsot-Dupuch K, et al. Central nervous system hemangioblastomas, endolymphatic sac tumors, and von Hippel-Lindau disease. Neurosurg Rev 2000; 23:1–22.
190. Richard S, Graff J, Lindau J, Resche F. Von Hippel-Lindau disease. The Lancet 2004; 363:1231–1234.

191. Ritter M, Frilling A, Crossey P, et al. Isolated familial pheochromocytoma as a variant of von Hippel-Lindau disease. J Clin Endocrinol Metab 1996; 81:1035–1037.
192. Rodgers I, Jakobiec F, Hidayat A. Eyelid tumors of apocrine, eccrine, and pilar origins. In: Albert D, Jakobiec F, eds. Principles and Practice of Ophthalmology, 2nd Editioned. Philadelphia: W.B. Saunders Company; 2000: 3405–3430.
193. Rosa D. Contributions to the study of so-called "glioma of the retina". Boll Ocul 1961; 40:492–505.
194. Roszkowski M, Drabik K, Barszcz S, Jozwiak S. Surgical treatment of intraventricular tumors associated with tuberous sclerosis. Child''s Nerv Syst 1995; 11:335–339.
195. Rouleau G, Merel P, Lutchman M, et al. Alteration in a new gene encoding a putative membrane-organizing protein causes neurofibromatosis type 2. Nature 1993; 363:515–521.
196. Rubinstein L. Embryonal central neuroepithelial tumors and their differentiating potential—a cytogenetic view of a complex neurooncological problem. J Neurosurg 1985; 62:795–805.
197. Ruggieri M. The different forms of neurofibromatosis. Child's Nerv Syst 1999; 15:295–308.
198. Russell D, Rubenstein L. Pathology of the Nervous System, 4th ed. Baltimore: Williams and Wilkins; 1977.
199. Sahel J, Frederick A, Pesavento R, Albert D. Idiopathic retinal gliosis mimicking a choroidal melanoma. Retina 1988; 8:282–287.
200. Sano T, Horiguchi H. Von Hippel-Lindau disease. Microsc Res Tech 2003; 60:159–164.
201. Savitsky K, Bar-Shira A, Gilad S, et al. A single ataxia-telangiectasia gene with a product similar to PI-3 kinase. Science 1955; 268:1749–1753.
202. Savitsky K, Sfez S, Tagle D, et al. The complete sequence of the coding region of the ATM gene reveals similarity to cell cycle regulators in different species. Hum Mol Genet 1995; 4:2025–2032.
203. Schreibman I, Baker M, Amos C, McGarrity T. The hamartomatous polyposis syndromes: a clinical and molecular review. Am J Gastroenterol 2005; 100:476–490.
204. Schwindinger W, Francomano C, Levine M. Identification of a mutation in the gene encoding the alpha subunit of the stimulatory G protein of adenylyl cyclase in McCune-Albright syndrome. Proc Natl Acad Sci USA 1992; 89: 5152–5156.
205. Seizinger B, Rouleau G, Ozelius L, et al. Common pathogenetic mechanism for three tumor types in bilateral acoustic neurofibromatosis. Science 1987; 236: 317–319.
206. Selhorst J. Phacomatoses. In: Miller N, Newman N, eds. Walsh and Hoyt Clinical Neuro-Ophthalmology, 5th ed. Baltimore: Williams and Wilkins; 1998.
207. Senda T, Shimomura A, Iizuka-Kogo A. Adenomatous polyposis coli (Apc) tumor suppressor gene as a multifunctional gene. Anat Sci Int 2005; 80:121–131.
208. Shepherd C, Gomez M. Mortality in the Mayo Clinic Tuberous Sclerosis Complex Study. Ann N Y Acad Sci 1991; 615:375–377.
209. Shiao Y. The von Hippel-Lindau gene and protein in tumorigenesis and angiogenesis: a potential target for therapeutic designs. Curr Med Chem 2003; 10:2461–2470.
210. Shields J. Diagnosis and Management of Intraocular Tumors. St. Louis: C.V. Mosby; 1983.
211. Shields J, Eagle RJ, Shields C, Marr B. Aggressive retinal astrocytomas in 4 patients with tuberous sclerosis complex. Arch Ophthalmol 2005; 123:856–863.
212. Shields J, Shields C. Other phakomatoses. In: Ryan S, Hinton D, Schachat A, eds. Retina,. Fourth Edition 4th ed. London: Elsevier Mosby;, 2006:633–640.
213. Shields J, Shields C, Eagle RJ, et al. Ophthalmic features of the organoid nevus syndrome. Trans Am Ophthalmol Soc 1996; 94:65–86.
214. Shields J, Shields C, Engle R, et al. Ocular manifestations of the organoid nevus syndrome. Ophthalmology 1997; 104:549.
215. Shuin T, Yamazaki I, Tamura K, et al. Recent advances in ideas on the molecular pathology and clinical aspects of Von Hippel-Lindau disease. Int J Clin Oncol 2004; 9: 283–287.
216. Spiegel A, Shenker A, Weinstein L. Receptor-effector coupling by G-proteins – implications for normal and abnormal signal transduction. Endocr Rev 1992; 13: 536–565.
217. Stebbins C, Kaelin W, Pavletich N. Structure of the VHL-ElonginC-ElonginB complex: implications for VHL tumor suppressor function. Science 1999; 284:455–461.
218. Stone D, Hynes M, Armanini M, et al. The tumour-suppressor gene patched encodes a candidate receptor for Sonic hedgehog. Nature 1996; 384:129–134.
219. Stratakis C. Genetics of Carney complex and related familial lentiginoses, and other multiple tumor syndromes. Front Biosci 2000; 5:D353–366.
220. Stratakis C, Carney J, Lin J, et al. Carney complex, a familial multiple neoplasia and lentiginosis syndrome: analysis of 11 kindreds and linkage to the short arm of chromosome 2. J Clin Invest 1996; 97:699–705.
221. Stratakis C, Kirschner L, Carney J. Carney complex: Diagnosis and management of the complex of spotty skin pigmentation, myxomas, endocrine overactivity, and schwannomas. Am J Med Genet 1998; 80:183–185.
222. Sturge W. A case of partial epilepsy, apparently due to a lesion of one of the vaso-motor centers of the brain. Trans Clin Soc Lond 1879; 12:162–167.
223. Sujansky E, Conradi S. Outcome of Sturge-Weber syndrome in 52 adults. Am J Med Genet 1995; 57:35–45.
224. Sullivan T, Clarke M, Morin J. The ocular manifestations of the Sturge-Weber syndrome. J Pediatr Ophthalmol 1992; 29:349–356.
225. Swift M, Reitnauer P, Morrell D, Chase C. Breast and other cancers in families with ataxia-telangiectasia. N Engl J Med 1987; 316:1289–1294.
226. Taipale J, Beachy P. The Hedgehog and Wnt signalling pathways in cancer. Nature 2001; 411:349–354.
227. Takahashi M, Ritz J, Cooper G. Activation of a novel human transforming gene, ret, by DNA rearrangement. Cell 1985; 42:581–588.
228. Taylor A, Byrd P. Molecular Ppathology of ataxia telangiectasia. J Clin Pathol 2005; 58:1009–1015.
229. Theron J, Newton T, Hoyt W. Unilateral retinocephalic vascular malformations. Neuroradiology 1974; 7:185–196.
230. Thomas-Sohl K, Vaslow D, Maria B. Sturge-Weber syndrome: a review. Pediatr Neurol 2004; 30:303–310.
231. Traboulsi E. Ocular manifestations of familial adenomatous polyposis (Gardner syndrome). Ophthalmol Clin N Am 2005; 18:163–166.
232. Traboulsi E, Murphy S, DeLaCruz Z, et al. A clinicopathologic study of the eyes in familial adenomatous polyposis with extracolonic manifestations (Gardner''s syndrome). Am J Ophthalmol 1990; 110:550–561.
233. Trofatter J, MacCollin M, Rutter J, et al. A novel moeisin-, ezrin-, radixin-like gene is a candidate for the neurofibromatosis 2 tumor suppressor. Cell 1993; 72:791–800.

234. Van der Hoeve T. The Doyne Memorial Lecture: eye symptoms in phakomatoses. Trans Ophthalmol Soc UK 1932; 52:380–401.
235. Van der Hoeve T. Eye disease in tuberose sclerosis of the brain and in Recklinghausen''s disease. Trans Ophthalmol Soc UK 1923; 43:534–541.
236. Van Slegtenhorst M, de Hoogt R, Hermans C, et al. Identification of the tuberous sclerosis gene TSC1 on chromosome 9q34. Science 1997; 277:805–808.
237. Verdy M, Weber A, Roy C, et al. Hirschsprung's disease in a family with multiple endocrine neoplasia type 2. J Pediatr Gastroenterol Nutr 1982; 1:603–607.
238. Verhoeff F. Discussion of Snell, S. and Collins, E.T. Plexiform neuroma (elephantiasis neuromatosis) of temporal region, orbit, eyelid and eyeball. Notes of three cases. Trans Ophthalmol Soc UK 1903; 23:176–177.
239. Verhoeff F. A rare tumor arising from the pars ciliaris retineas (teratoneuroma) of a nature hitherto unrecognized and its relation to the so-called glioma retinae. Trans Am Ophthalmol Soc 1904; 10:351–377.
240. Von Recklinghausen F. Uber die multiplin Fibrome der Haut und ihre Beziehung zu den multiplen Neuromen. Berlin: Hirschwald; 1882.
241. Waardenburg P, Franceschetti A, Klein D. Genetics and Ophthalmology, Vol. 2. Springfield, IL: Charles C. Thomas; 1963.
242. Walsh F, Hoyt W, Miller N. Clinical Neuro-Ophthalmology, 4th ed. Baltimore: Williams and Wilkins; 1989.
243. Wanebo J, Lonser R, Glenn G, Oldfield E. The natural history of hemangioblastomas of the central nervous system in patients with von Hippel-Lindau disease. J Neurosurg 2003; 98:82–94.
244. Weber F. Right-sided hemihypotrophy resulting from right sided congenital spastic hemiplagia, with a morbid condition of the brain revealed by radiograms. J Neurol Psychopathol 1922; 3:134–139.
245. Weinstein L, Shenker A, Gejman P, et al. Activating mutations of the stimulatory G protein in the McCune-Albright syndrome. N Engl J Med 1991; 325:1688–1695.
246. Weiss D. Dual origin of glaucoma in encephalotrigeminal haemangiomatosis. Trans Ophthalmol Soc UK 1973; 93: 477–493.
247. Wilkes S, Campbell R, Walker R. Ocular malformations in association with ipsilateral facial nevus of Jadassohn. Am J Ophthalmol 1981; 92:344.
248. Williamson T, Garner A, Moore A. Structure of Lisch nodules in neurofibromatosis type 1. Ophthal Pediatr Genet 1991; 12:11–17.
249. Wilson-Jones E, Heyl T. Naevus sebaceus: A report of 140 cases with special regard to the development of secondary malignant tumors. Br J Dermatol 1970; 82:99.
250. Wyburn-Mason R. Arteriovenous aneurysm of mid-brain and retina, facial naevi and mental changes. Brain 1943; 66:163–203.
251. Yanoff M, Fine B. Ocular Pathology: A Text and Atlas New York: Harper and Row; 1989:686–698.
252. Young T. Ophthalmic genetics/inherited eye disease. Curr Opin Ophthalmol 2003; 14:296–303.
253. Zackheim H, Loud A, Howell A. Nevoid basal cell carcinoma syndrome: Ssome histologic observations on the cutaneous lesions. Arch Dermatol 1996; 93:317.
254. Zaroff C, Isaacs K. Neurocutaneous syndromes: Behavioral features. Epilepsy Behav 2005; 7:133–142.
255. Zbar B, Kishida T, Chen F, et al. Germline mutations in the Von Hippel-Lindau disease (VHL) gene in families from North America, Europe, and Japan. Hum Mutat 1996; 8:348–357.
256. Zimmerman L. Retinoblastoma and retinocytoma. In: Spencer W, ed. Ophthalmic Pathology. Philadelphia: W.B. Saunders; 1985:1292–1351.
257. Zion V. Tuberous sclerosis, Bourneville's disease. In: Duane T, ed. Clinical Ophthalmology, Vol. 5. New York: Harper and Row; 1967.

56

Epithelial Tumors of the Eyelids

Diva R. Salomão
Department of Pathology, Mayo Clinic, Mayo Foundation, and Mayo Medical School, Rochester, Minnesota, U.S.A.

INTRODUCTION

A wide variety of neoplasms in the eyelid arise from different cell types. Many of these cells are present in other tissues of the eye and its adnexa. These tumors are covered elsewhere in chapters devoted specifically to tumors of melanocytes (Chapter 59), blood vessels (Chapter 62), nerves (Chapter 63), soft tissues (Chapter 64), and lymphoid tissue (Chapter 66). This chapter focuses on the epithelial tumors, particularly from the standpoint of their pathobiology. Excellent detailed histological descriptions of the neoplasms described in this chapter are found in the published books of ophthalmic and surgical pathology (73,100). The classification of tumors outlined here is adapted from the World Heath Organization (WHO) histological classification of tumors. The staging of cancer at specific anatomical sites is as outlined by the American Joint Committee on Cancer (6).

EPITHELIAL TUMORS AND RELATED LESIONS OF THE EYELID EPIDERMIS

Epithelial neoplasms and related lesions of the eyelid can be divided according to their origin from the epithelial cells of the epidermis or cutaneous adnexa. Benign neoplasms are approximately three times more frequent than malignant tumors (10).

Benign Lesions and Tumors of the Epidermis

Squamous Papilloma

This common benign tumor of the eyelid may be sessile or pedunculated. Fingerlike processes of vascularized connective tissue are covered by a squamous epithelium, often hyperplastic with parakeratosis and variable degrees of hyperkeratosis. The clinical appearance of this soft elevated flesh-colored lesion is similar to that of other benign lesions, such as seborrheic keratosis and verruca vulgaris.

Seborrheic Keratosis (Verruca Senilis, Basaloid Cell Papilloma)

Seborrheic keratosis is a well-demarcated, brownish lesion with a greasy appearance reflecting abundant surface keratin that develops most often on the face, trunk, and arms. Seborrheic keratosis usually occurs as multiple lesions in patients older than 40 years. On the eyelids, seborrheic keratosis is found most frequently along the line of the cilia. The degree of pigmentation varies and occasionally is sufficiently marked to simulate a malignant melanoma.

Microscopically, both squamous and basal cells proliferate above the plane of the dermis and do not extend into the dermis (Fig. 1). Hyperkeratosis, papillomatosis, and pseudohorn cysts are present in varying degrees and this has led to subclassification into hyperkeratotic (papillomatous), acanthotic (solid), and adenoid (reticulated) types (72). Seborrheic keratosis rarely undergoes malignant transformation. Chronic irritation of seborrheic keratoses may be associated with a lichenoid inflammatory infiltrate and pseudoepitheliomatous hyperplasia with numerous squamous eddies. Irritated seborrheic keratosis may be misinterpreted clinically as squamous cell carcinoma (SCC). The presence of apoptotic cells in the base of seborrheic keratosis and in areas of squamous differentiation (90) has been interpreted as a histological sign of immunological regression (12). Such an irritated seborrheic keratosis is sometimes referred to as an inverted follicular keratosis, a designation introduced by Helwig (54) in 1955 to describe a benign, usually solitary nodule or papule with a predilection for the face. Although the cheeks and upper lip are the sites of predilection, the eyelids may also be involved (105). Characteristically, there is an inverted (endophytic) configuration of the acanthotic epithelium, and the cells in the deepest portion resemble basal cells; squamous eddies or small keratin-containing cysts may be present in the fingerlike extensions of tumor. Edema with vesicle formation may be present but is not usually a prominent feature. The lesion is sharply delineated from the underlying dermis. Which may show a lymphohistiocytic infiltrate, and the surface of the lesion shows a variable degree of hyperkeratosis and parakeratosis, resembling keratoacanthoma both clinically and morphologically.

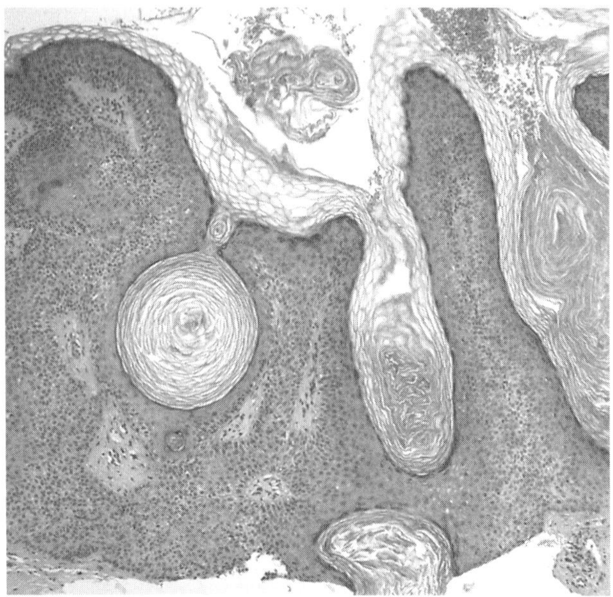

Figure 1 Seborrheic keratosis. Light micrograph showing acanthosis due to the proliferation of the basal layer epithelial cells, hyperkeratosis, and multiple pseudohorny cysts (hematoxylin and eosin, $\times$ 100).

Keratoacanthoma

A keratoacanthoma is a solitary elevated cutaneous lesion with a central keratin-filled crater, developing in exposed areas in elderly people (21), particularly in the sixth and seventh decade, with a male predominance (26). It also occurs following renal transplantation and in other immunosuppressed patients (121). Rarely, multiple contiguous lesions involve the face, including the eyelids, and the extremities; this predisposition to multiple keratoacanthomas may be familial (119).

The tumor arises from the upper portion of a hyperplastic hair follicle and has a squamous phenotype. In most instances, the lesion consists of a 1 to 2 cm dome-shaped nodule with a central keratin-filled crater. Maximal size is reached within a few months, and if the tumor is left untreated, spontaneous regression may occur within 6 months, leaving a minimal scar. This spontaneous involution is still poorly understood but an immunological process has been proposed (84). A study comparing SCC and keratoacanthoma found that keratoacanthomas have significantly higher number of CD3+ and activated CD4 positive T-lymphocytes infiltrating this lesion, and these activated T cells are responsible for the expression interleukin-2 receptor (IL2R). This study suggests that keratoacanthoma regression is immunologically mediated, with activated (IL2R+) CD4+ T cells and adhesion molecules playing an important role in the immune response (89). Expression of *OCL2*, a protooncogene, which inhibits apoptosis, is lost in regressing keratoacanthomas (115). Two unusual giant palpebral keratoacanthomas have been reported (39). None of these cases had evidence of spontaneous regression and both tumors were so large that skin grafts were required. Lesions on the nose and eyelid can be very destructive and difficult to excise (51).

The lesion must be distinguished from SCC, which it may resemble both clinically and histopathologically (16). Difficulties arise with the few keratoacanthomas that grow slowly for up to 12 months and reach a large size. In one report, a keratoacanthoma grew out of the eyelid margin and extended to the palpebral conjunctiva. The tumor disappeared 4 months after partial excision (80).

Microscopic features include a characteristic cup profile with bordering acanthotic epithelium and elongated rete ridges that can only be appreciated by complete excision of the lesion and a section through the center of the tumor. A central keratin plug is embraced by the acanthotic epithelium. Important histological guidelines in the differentiation from SCC include the absence of cellular atypia at the margin of the epidermis in keratoacanthoma and the marked keratinization of the tumor cells. Another feature favoring keratoacanthoma is a sharp outline between the tumor nests and stroma. This distinction may be difficult, however, because a keratoacanthoma may occur in actinically damaged skin. Although viral particles have been described within some lesions, these are not present in all (135).

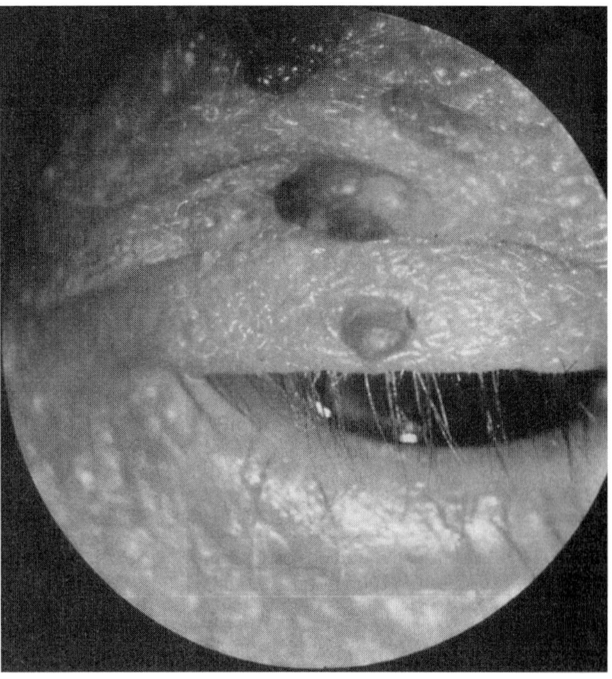

Figure 2 Actinic keratosis. Clinical photograph showing the presence in the upper eyelid multiple exophytic tan to brownish hyperkeratotic lesions.

Preneoplastic Dermatoses and Squamous Cell Carcinoma in Situ

The most common lesions in the eyelid that may, but do not necessarily, undergo malignant change include actinic keratosis, radiation dermatitis, and a genodermatologic condition, xeroderma pigmentosum (XP). Bowen disease is an in situ carcinoma of the epidermis (14).

Actinic Keratosis (Solar Keratosis)

Most often actinic keratosis occurs in the sun-exposed skin of elderly fair-skinned persons, relatively unprotected by melanin pigment. It is common on the dorsum of the hands but also develops on the eyelids. Multiple lesions commonly coexist and are frequently associated with other cutaneous neoplasms, such as squamous cell or basal cell carcinoma (BCC).

Clinically, the area is recognized as a flat hyperemic area of skin that is slightly elevated, brownish, scaly, and usually <1 cm in diameter (Fig. 2). Keratin production may be increased and a cutaneous horn sometimes develops on the surface. An essential component of the lesion is the dermal change, actinic elastosis [ultraviolet (UV) radiation-induced degeneration of collagenous components of the dermis]. Although cutaneous horns are associated with actinic keratosis, they are also occasionally associated with seborrheic keratosis, SCC in situ, and verruca vulgaris. Actinic keratoses may progress to SCC but, apart from sun-induced carcinomas of the lip (122), the lesions do not metastasize. SCC is reported to develop in 12% to 13% of untreated cases of actinic keratosis (46).

Microscopically, three types of actinic keratosis can be recognized: hypertrophic, atrophic, and Bowenoid. All three are associated with dermal actinic elastosis and a moderately dense, lymphocytic infiltrate. The most frequent histological type is the hypertrophic variety, in which hyperkeratosis and parakeratosis are present with acanthosis (Fig. 3), cellular pleomorphism, and disorderly maturation. The limitation of pleomorphic cells to the deep layers of the epithelium differentiates this lesion from in situ carcinoma (Bowen disease), in which the entire thickness of the epithelium is involved.

In the atrophic variety, the epidermis is atrophied and atypical basal cells proliferate into the dermis, forming buds and duct-like structures. Undifferentiated cells lose their intercellular bridges and as a result clefts form within the epidermis (67). The epidermis above such clefts often appears normal. The "Bowenoid" type of actinic keratosis is characterized by intraepithelial cellular atypia, that may be indistinguishable from that of SCC in situ, but as a rule there is less overall atypia in actinic keratosis.

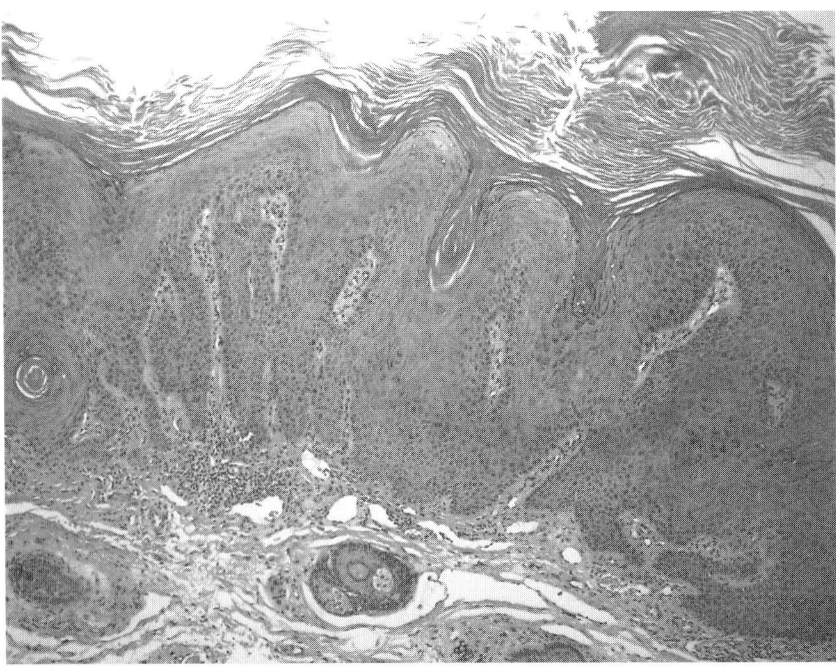

Figure 3 Actinic keratosis. Microscopic picture shows epithelial hyperplasia, hyperkeratiosis, mild atypia in the epithelial cells located in the Malpighian layers, and the presence of dermal inflammation (hematoxylin and eosin, ×115).

When actinic keratosis progresses to a SCC, the usual sharp demarcation line between the lesion and the adjacent normal skin disappears. Because this change can be localized and may not be evident in random sections through the lesion, it is difficult to exclude a SCC in the absence of serial sections. This distinction is neither practical nor necessarily critical because SCC arising in an actinic keratosis rarely metastasizes.

Premalignant Lesions of the Epidermis

In Situ Squamous Cell Carcinoma (Bowen Disease, Intraepidermal Carcinoma)

In 1912, Bowen (18) first described intraepithelial SCC. The condition may occur anywhere on the skin including nonexposed surfaces, such as the genital region (133). A high percentage (80%) of cases of Bowen disease occurring in nonexposed skin are associated with other cancers of the skin or viscera (49,91), although this is disputed by some authors (8).

Clinically, Bowen disease is usually a solitary lesion that appears as a flat, dark red, diffuse area with an irregular or indistinct outline. Growth occurs by slow, peripheral extension of the margins, leaving either a central ulcer or a fungating mass. Microscopically, Bowen disease is characterized by full thickness cellular atypia and disorderly maturation, associated with hyperkeratosis, parakeratosis, and acanthosis with loss of the granular layer and irregular elongation of the rete ridges. Pleomorphic epithelial cells with large hyperchromatic nuclei show loss of polarity. Multinucleated epidermal cells are occasionally present. Mitoses, instead of being limited to the basal layer, are seen at all levels of the epidermis. Individual cell keratinization is a frequent and characteristic finding. The dysplastic process occupies the full thickness of the epithelium but does not invade into the dermis (Fig. 4). As a rule, there is a sharp transition between the zone of atypical neoplastic epithelium and the adjacent normal epithelium. Approximately 5% of cases progress to an invasive SCC by breaking the integrity of the basement membrane at one or several points (49); metastasis may then occur.

Radiation Dermatitis

Acute radiation dermatitis of the eyelids sometimes follows therapeutic irradiation to the orbit, the globe, or the eyelids. Erythema occurs within a week of treatment, and telangiectasia, desquamation of surface epithelial cells, and eventually pigmentation develop. Less commonly blisters and ulcers may form, followed by healing with scarring (61). Chronic radiation dermatitis occurs months to years after treatment. Microscopically, an atrophic epithelium overlies a dermis with prominent actinic elastosis throughout its depth and numerous telangiectatic blood vessels with hyalinized walls. A dose of 40 Gy or more produces severe atrophic changes in the skin appendages, occlusion of blood vessels, and fibrosis. A small percentage of patients develop squamous or BCCs in the irradiated area after 15 years or more (71). In the first well-documented patient with bilateral retinoblastoma cured by radiation and

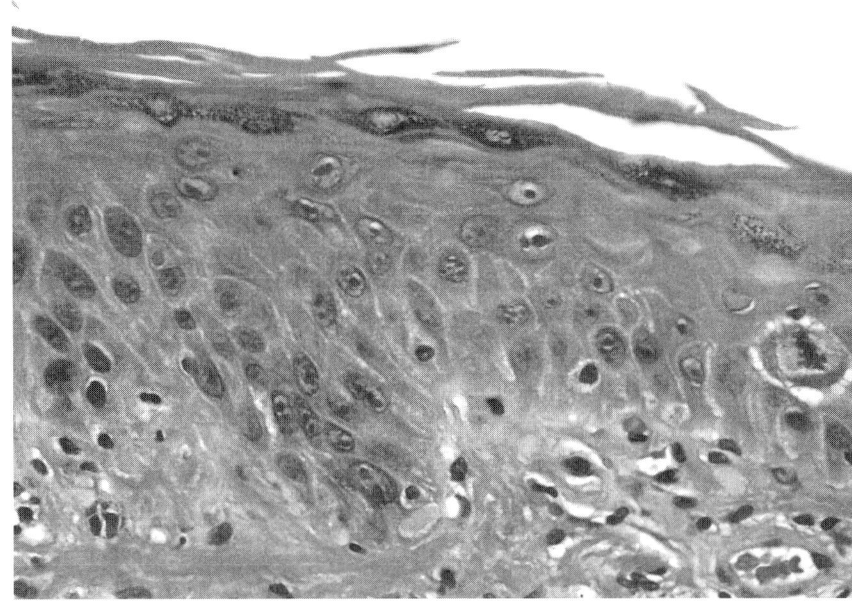

Figure 4 Carcinoma in situ. This microscopic picture shows epithelial atypia characterized by nuclear enlargement, prominent nucleoli, and mitosis involving the full thickness of the epithelium and resulting in architectural maturation disarray (hematoxylin and eosin, $\times$ 450).

cared for by Verhoeff, both BCC and SCC developed in the eyelid 60 years later (4).

Xeroderma Pigmentosum

Xeroderma Pigmentosum (XP) is a rare, autosomal recessive-inherited disease, belonging to a group of genetic abnormalities recognized as epidermal genodermatoses. It is characterized by deficient DNA repair, photophobia, severe solar sensitivity, cutaneous pigmentary changes, xerosis, and early development of cutaneous and ocular neoplasms. Many affected patients are the offspring of consanguineous marriages (28). Abnormalities affecting the eyelids, conjunctiva and cornea, which are areas exposed to UV radiation, have been reported in 40% of published cases (66). Heterogeneity of the molecular defect in XP has been recognized (34). Through somatic cell fusion studies, a heterokaryon (a cell with nuclei from different donors in a common cytoplasm) is formed by fusion of fibroblasts from one patient with those of another patient. Each cell supplies the other with what is lacking, the implication being that each cell has different defects so-called "complementation groups." Several of these groups (A to G) have deficient excision repair of UV radiation-induced DNA damage (nucleotide excision repair), while in one ("xP Variant") there is a defective ability to convert newly synthesized DNA from low to high-molecular weight after UV irradiation (62,92).

A defective gene locus has been identified in many of the individual complementation groups (78). In XP complementation group A (MIM +276700), the genetic determinant has been located on the long arm of chromosome 1 (63). Others have located the defect in group A to chromosome 9 (9q22). An increased frequency of chromatin breaks and gaps after irradiation of G_2 phase peripheral blood lymphocytes and fibroblasts has been detected in carriers of XP (88).

In XP there is a deficiency of an endonuclease that cleaves thymidine dimers. In consequence, there is a defect in the repair of DNA damaged by UV light and a pronounced predisposition to sun-induced cancers (98). Both the skin and the conjunctiva eventually develop many varieties of malignant tumor, including BCC and SCC, as well as malignant melanoma (67). The prevalence of cutaneous cancer in patients with XP is much higher than in the general population. The eyelids are frequently affected (Fig. 5) and may manifest degenerative changes with atrophy, ectropion, and secondary inflammation. Most patients die before the age of 21 years from metastatic carcinoma or melanoma.

Although the histological appearance is initially nonspecific, the combination of hyperkeratosis, atrophy of the stratum malpighii and rete ridges, and proliferation of adjacent rete ridges, accompanied by a chronic inflammatory infiltrate of the epidermis and accumulation of melanin in the basal layer, is suggestive of XP. A combination of atrophy and acanthosis marks the second stage; these features are superimposed on the existing changes of hyperkeratosis and hyperpigmentation, but the latter are more

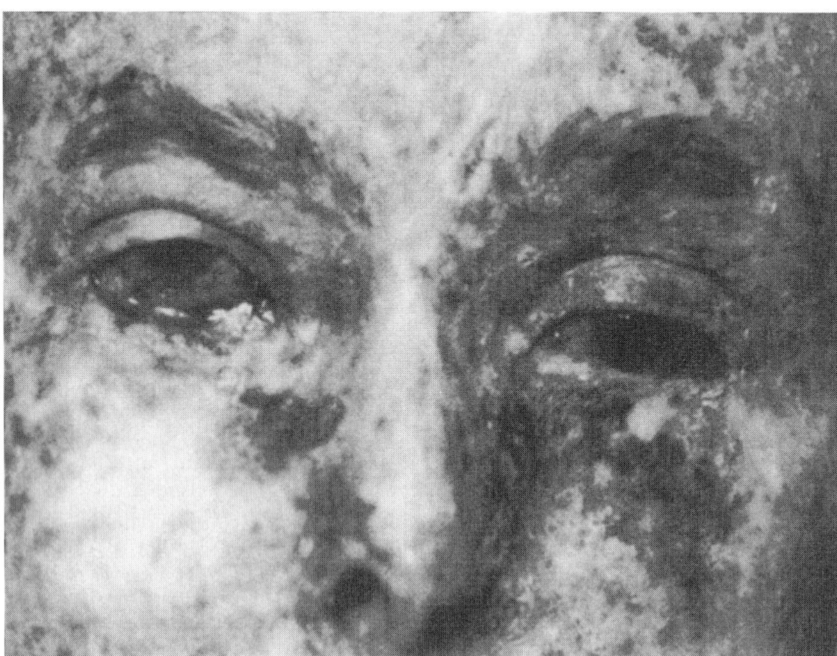

Figure 5 Xeroderma pigmentosum. Note the presence of multiple skin lesions and eyelid involvement.

pronounced. Finally, malignant transformation occurs.

Malignant Tumors of the Epidermis

Basal Cell Carcinoma

BCC arises from the basal epidermis and pilosebaceous units. It is thought to be differentiating into skin adnexal tumors but remains in a primitive basaloid state. Because of this attempt at differentiation there are many clinical phenotypes and histological patterns (100,131). BCC is the most common malignant neoplasm of the eyelid (more than 90%) and occurs mainly on the lower eyelid in fair-skinned adults. Prolonged exposure to sunlight commonly precedes the lesion (19). Immunohistochemical techniques have demonstrated an overexpression of a long-lived mutant form of p53 protein in BCC and this overexpression is also demonstrable in the adjacent keratinocytes but is not in skin protected from sunlight (107). Such findings suggest that the mutation of the tumor suppressor gene p53 on chromosome 17 (17p13) results from chronic exposure to UV light (107). The mutant protein results from a point mutation of the p53 gene. Usually, BCC is a tumor of later life, although it has been described in younger patients who are fair skinned or who have the nevoid basal cell syndrome (81). This syndrome, also known as Gorlin–Goltz syndrome (MIM #109400) (48), is inherited as an autosomal-dominant disorder. Chromosome studies have shown a normal karyotype (120). Patients present with cysts of the jaw, pitting of the palms and soles, frontal bossing, skeletal abnormalities, ectopic calcification, and multiple BCCs. The diagnosis can be made on the basis of the family history, clinical appearance, and radiographs (99). The skin tumors appear in childhood or early adolescence and usually affect the upper eyelid (40). This feature contrasts with the more common lower eyelid predilection in the elderly adult.

Clinically BCCs are initially firm but subsequently ulcerate in the center to impart a pearly appearance with a rolled edge (Fig. 6). Its various clinical appearances allow confusion with SCC and sebaceous carcinoma (68), as well as with keratoacanthoma (16), and it has also been reported to masquerade as an ectropion of the eyelid (14). When situated at the medial canthus, the tumor shows more aggressive behavior and the recurrence rate at this site is high. The tumor appears to invade early but this may reflect the anatomy of this region adjacent to the nasolacrimal drainage system.

Because the basal cell is pluripotential, the tumor has a propensity to differentiate toward a wide variety of cutaneous structures (32). Typically, the growth forms lobules that extend from the epidermis into the dermis. The cells, with hyperchromatic nuclei and scanty cytoplasm, cluster in solid nests with a palisade of nuclei around the periphery (Fig. 7) (104). Squamous differentiation or a cystic (adenocystic) pattern, as well as pigmentation, may develop, although the biological behavior is independent of such morphological variability (71).

The morpheiform BCC is particularly aggressive. Clinically, this variety forms a pale indurated plaque composed of compressed bands of basal cells

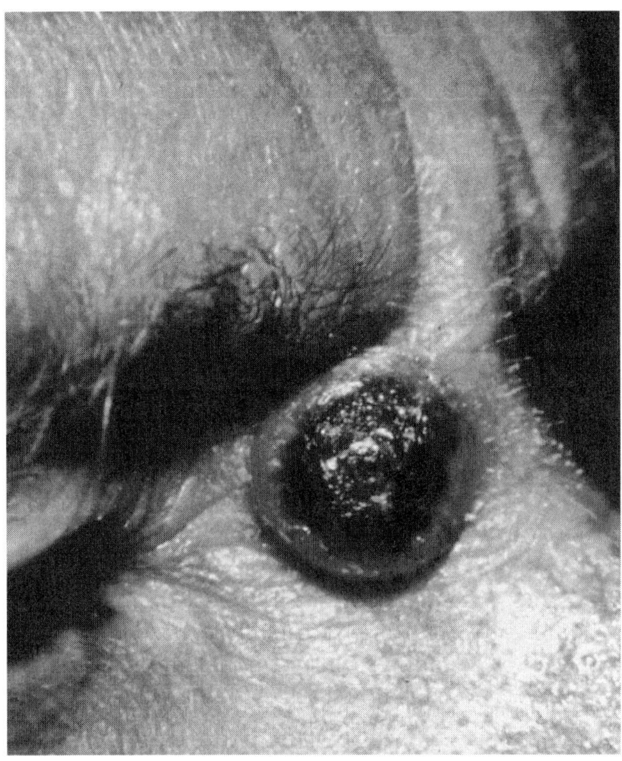

Figure 6 Basal cell carcinoma. This clinical photograph shows the presence of a nodular and centrally ulcerated lesion.

entrenched in a dense fibrous matrix. This type of tumor often extends beyond the margins observed clinically and is more likely to be incompletely excised. Multifocality has been reported in 60% of patients with BCC of the morpheiform type (128). It may invade the orbit or the superficial part of the sclera, but intraocular invasion is most unusual. Although invasive, BCCs rarely metastasize (31). The risk of metastasis correlates with tumor size (usually greater than 5 cm for significant risk). Meningeal carcinomatosis has followed a primary BCC of the upper eyelid (118). Of 17 cases of metastatic BCC studied by Farmer and Helwig (37), one tumor was of the lower eyelid and one of the infraorbital region. Metastasis occurs to the lymph nodes, lungs, bone, liver, spleen, and adrenal gland.

Squamous Cell Carcinoma

Several early studies indicated a high incidence of SCC of the eyelid because of misinterpretation of other cutaneous tumors (56). In the Western Hemisphere, SCC is an uncommon tumor of the palpebral tissue; it composes only 9% of all eyelid malignancies (96). At this site, the ratio of SCC to BCC is 1:39 (36,68). In Japan, SCC is reported as the most frequent malignancy of the eyelid (1).

The large majority of SCCs of the skin are sun-induced (3). One pathogenetic mechanism is the induction of p53 mutations by UV light (19). Elderly fair-skinned persons are particularly prone to SCC. SCC of the skin may be a complication of XP, epidermodysplasia verruciformis, chemical exposure to arsenic and other substances, organ transplantation (109), and human papillomavirus (HPV) infection. Its occurrence in an immunosuppressed patient with Graves disease (42) and after renal transplantation

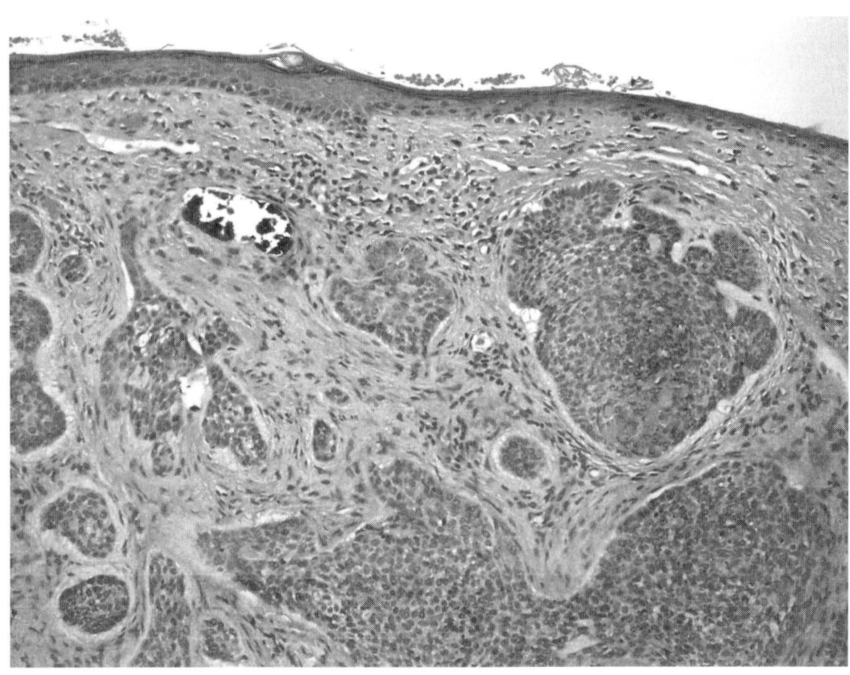

Figure 7 Basal cell carcinoma. Microscopic picture shows dermal invasion by nests of neoplastic cells with characteristic peripheral palisading (hematoxylin and eosin, ×200).

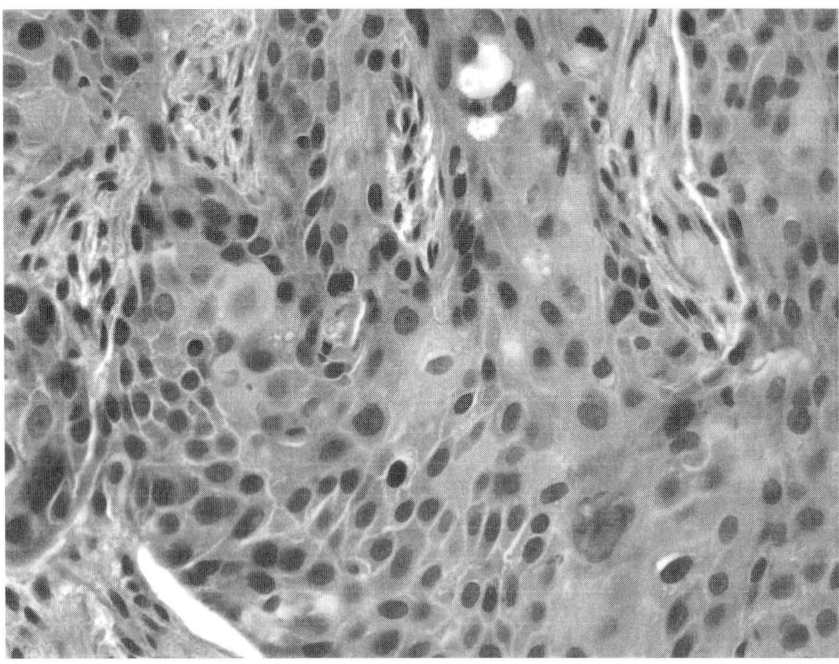

Figure 8 Squamous cell carcinoma. This microscopic picture shows deeply invasive moderately differentiated squamous cell carcinoma. The tumor nests are composed by allomorphic cells with keratohyaline granules. Intercellular bridges can also be seen (hematoxylin and eosin, ×450).

(121) suggests that immunosuppressive therapy may enhance the growth of a preexisting malignancy. SCC occurring after exposure to high doses of irradiation or associated with XP may occur at multiple sites (67,117).

The presence of HPV type 16 (HPV16) DNA has been demonstrated in a recurrent SCC of the lower eyelid with use of the polymerase chain reaction (PCR) to amplify specific target DNA sequences. With primers specific for HPV16 DNA, this procedure yielded a single band of amplified DNA product that was positive with radiolabeled HPV16 dot-blot analysis. The implications of these findings in regard to the causative role of these viruses in the development of neoplasia and their management and prognosis have been stressed by McDonnell and colleagues (77).

Microscopically, 80% of SCCs are well-differentiated and produce large amounts of keratin, seen as horn pearls or intracytoplasmic keratohyaline granules. Invasion of the dermis is a required feature (Fig. 8). Microscopic subtypes include spindle cell or metaplastic carcinoma, adenoid SCC, and verrucous

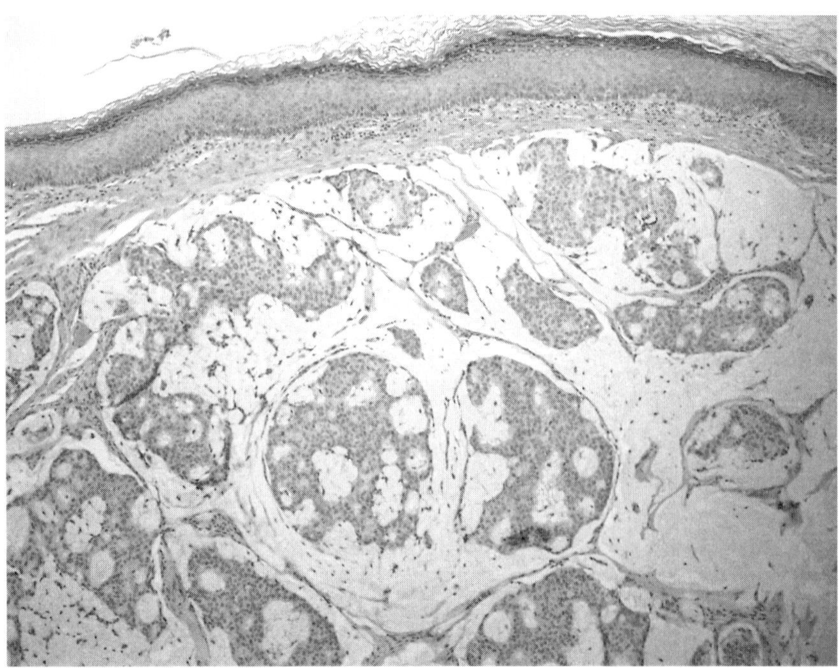

Figure 9 Mucinous eccrine adenocarcenoma. (hematoxylin and eosin, ×225).

SCC. The adenoid form is characterized histologically by acantholysis and a pseudoglandular pattern with alveolar and tubular structures.

In a report of 21 cases of SCCs of the eyelid in patients aged 43 to 85 years, local recurrence occurred in approximately one-third of patients, but there were no tumor-related deaths in an 8.8 year follow-up (23). The differential diagnosis of SCC, both clinically and histologically, includes actinic keratosis, keratoacanthoma, pseudoepitheliomatous hyperplasia, BCC, and sebaceous gland carcinoma.

Immunohistochemical studies reveal positivity for high-molecular keratins, epithelial membrane antigen (EMA) and often carcinoembryonic antigen (CEA). Poorly differentiated SCCs can also be immunoreactive for vimentin. Accumulation of p53 protein has been observed in 50% of the cases (53).

Late presentation allows metastasis to preauricular and submaxillary lymph nodes.

SWEAT GLAND TUMORS OF THE EYELID

Various tumors may arise from the sweat glands and their ducts (69,72). Among the more common neoplasms of these eccrine glands are the syringoma, the eccrine spiradenoma, and pleomorphic adenoma (benign mixed tumor). Tumors of the apocrine glands of Moll also occur (52,70,103).

Benign Tumors

Syringoma

Histochemical and transmission electron microscopic (TEM) studies have shown that this benign adenoma arises from eccrine sweat gland ducts. Enzymes of eccrine glands such as phosphorylase, leucine aminopeptidase, and succinic dehydrogenase, are present in abundance (72). The individual tumor cells have glandular characteristics such as numerous short microvilli, abundant lysosomes, and tonofilaments arranged in a periluminal band. The presence of keratin within such ducts adjacent to the epidermis is evidence of the keratin-forming capacity of the cells lining the intraepidermal eccrine sweat ducts.

Immunohistochemical studies support the theory that syringoma of the eyelids and eruptive syringoma of the neck and upper chest are similar tumors and are of eccrine duct origin (52). The monoclonal antikeratin antibody EKH4, which predominantly labels the basal epithelial cells, also labels the cordlike epithelial structures of the syringoma and the peripheral cells of the cyst walls. The antibody EKH6, which recognizes normal eccrine secretory and ductal structures, is positive along the luminal border of the cyst walls. The antibody EKH5, which labels the eccrine secretory portion of the gland, is negative.

The syringoma occurs predominantly in females at puberty or in later life. Single and multiple lesions of the axillae, abdomen, vulva, or cheeks fsorm, and in many patients the lower eyelids alone are involved. The tumor is a pink or yellowish, soft nodule measuring 1 to 2 mm in diameter. Familial cases that involve the eyelids as well as the neck and body have been reported (52).

Microscopically, small ducts lined by two rows of epithelial cells are embedded in a fibrous stroma. Many ducts have a tail-like extension of epithelial cells and amorphous eosinophilic debris within the lumen. Keratin horn cysts are a frequent finding. A clear cell variant rich in glycogen is frequently associated with diabetes mellitus and cannot be distinguished clinically from the conventional syringoma. TEM shows that intracytoplasmic and extracytoplasmic multivesicular bodies are present (5).

Eccrine Spiradenoma

The eyelids or other parts of the upper body may bear these solitary, benign, tender, flat pink lesions (2). Well-demarcated dermal lobules consist of two types of cells, one with a small hyperchromatic nucleus and the second with a large vesicular nucleus forming ductlike structures. TEM observations indicate differentiation toward dermal ducts as well as to the secretory segment of the gland (104). In an immunohistochemical and ultrastructural study of an eccrine acrospiroma, Grossniklaus and Knight (50) showed that the tumor cells stain for cytokeratins of high-molecular weight but are negative for those of low-molecular weight. EMA is also demonstrable. CEA and muscle-specific actin are focally positive. Negative staining is demonstrated with antibodies to S100 protein, glial fibrillary acidic protein (GFAP), and desmin. Ultrastructurally, tonofilaments are present in the polyhedral cells, clear cells contain glycogen granules, and microvilli are present on cells lining the lumen.

Pleomorphic Adenoma

The pleomorphic adenoma (benign mixed tumor, chondroid syringoma) is a benign subcutaneous nodule that frequently occurs in the skin of the eyelids, head, and neck. Microscopically, it is identical to the lacrimal gland or salivary gland tumors (Fig. 9).

APOCRINE TUMORS OF THE EYELID

Tumors of apocrine origin occur usually at the eyelid margin, where the apocrine glands of Moll are present. This group includes the hidrocystoma

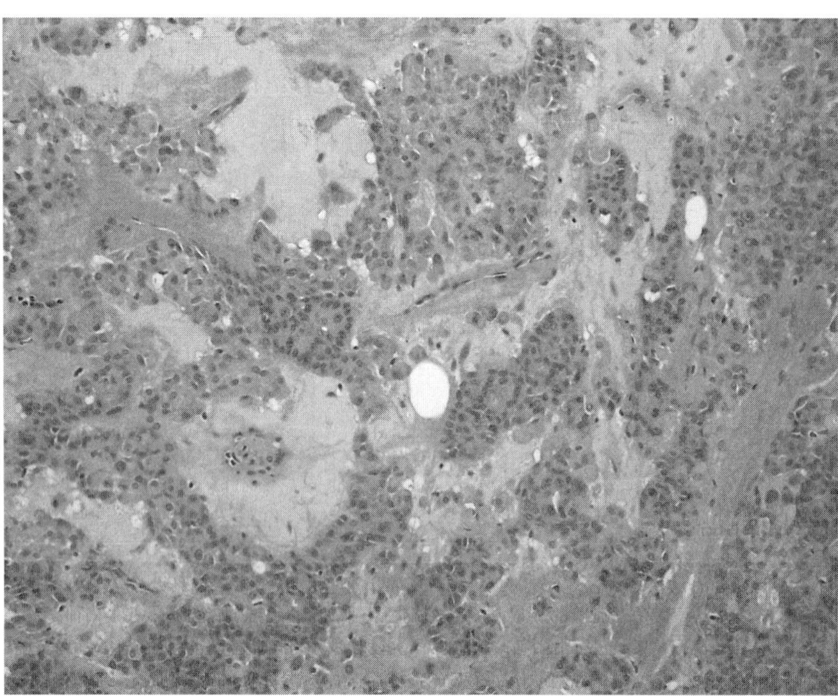

Figure 10 Benign mixed tumor. This microscopic picture shows clusters and cords of myoepithelial cells admixed in myxoid stroma (hematoxylin and eosin, × 225).

(83,103) and the syringocystadenoma papilliferum (59). The origin of these tumors from the apocrine glands is supported by TEM (59,103) and immunohistochemical studies (70). The tumor may be single (59) or multiple (70,103). Bilateral apocrine hidrocystomas occur as a feature of ectodermal dysplasia (41). Hidradenoma papilliferum can also derive from the glands of Moll but more commonly it originates from the apocrine glands of the anogenital region. It is a rare tumor of the eyelid (82,104). The smooth surface contrasts with the verrucous surface of the syringocystadenoma. In the two cases described, the tumor has shown a central feature of either umbilication (104) or an epidermal pore (82). It has been suggested that this opening represents an ectasia of the pilar canal of the cilia through which the secretions of the glands of Moll escape. Its identification may be of help in the diagnosis of tumors at this site. Histologically, the pattern is similar to that of intraductal papilloma of the breast, but the tumor cells have apical snouts. Ultrastructurally, there are apical secretory granules, and myofilaments are present in myoepithelial cells. The tumor is considered benign and has a low possibility of malignant progression.

MALIGNANT TUMORS OF THE CUTANEOUS ADNEXA

Malignant sweat gland tumors are rare, and each of the forms may be misinterpreted both clinically and histologically as SCC (30). The malignant form of the syringoma is rare. It is a slow-growing tumor of the lower or upper eyelid and has been reported in patients of 18, 20, and 70 years of age (47,64). TEM confirms the origin from the eccrine sweat gland (67). The large size and evidence of muscle and nerve invasion are indications of malignancy.

Mucinous Eccrine Adenocarcinoma

Mucinous adenocarcinoma is a rare neoplasm that arises from the eccrine secretory coil (129). Wright and Font (132) found that almost half of the cases reported (21 of 45) were located in the eyelid. The median age at presentation is 60 years (range 33–84 years), and the tumor is mostly found in males. Mucinous adenocarcinoma occurs on the upper and lower eyelids as well as the inner canthus, presenting as a bluish to red, papillomatous, pedunculated, or fungating lesion. Microscopically, mucinous eccrine adenocarcinomas are identical to metastatic mucinous carcinoma of the breast and gastrointestinal tract. The tumor is characterized by nests of neoplastic epithelial cells floating in pools of mucin (Fig. 9). These pools of nonsulfated sialic acid-containing mucosubstance are produced by the tumor cells and are periodic acid Schiff-positive, diastase-resistant, and also positive with alcian blue and the Hale colloidal iron method. Enzymatic and TEM studies have been used to confirm the diagnosis (75). The tumor is of low-grade malignancy and has a slightly better prognosis than sweat gland carcinomas; the duration of survival is at least 8 years.

TUMORS OF THE SEBACEOUS GLANDS

The eyelid contains several types of sebaceous glands: the Meibomian or tarsal glands; the glands of Zeis associated with the cilia, and sebaceous glands associated with the fine hair follicles that cover the cutaneous surfaces of the eyelids. Therefore, the eyelid is the most common location for tumors with sebaceous differentiation.

Torre (127) was the first to describe the association of sebaceous gland neoplasms with multiple visceral carcinomas. The Muir–Torre syndrome (MIM #158300) comprises coexpression of cutaneous neoplasms and carcinomas of the breast, ovary, gastrointestinal tract, and larynx (20,29,101). This syndrome is found in both sexes and presents between the fifth and sixth decades; the mean age at diagnosis is 46 years. The sebaceous gland tumors of the eyelid are usually benign sebaceous adenomas and may be single (57), but more commonly multiple tumors occur. Other associated eyelid tumors include adenomatoid sebaceous hyperplasia, BCC with foci of sebaceous differentiation (sebaceous epithelioma), keratoacanthoma, and less commonly SCC (60,127).

Most of the visceral carcinomas are adenocarcinomas of colonic or gastric origin (24,38,57,126,127), but malignancies may also occur in the larynx, endometrium, urogenital system, breast, and hematopoietic system (38). The visceral carcinoma is usually the first to present clinically and a family history of carcinoma is usually apparent (38).

The biologic basis of the visceral and sebaceous neoplasms in Muir–Torre syndrome is an aberrant mismatch repair gene (*MSH2*) and its coded protein can be assayed immunohistochemically and is absent in sebaceous neoplasms in this setting (126).

Benign Tumors of Sebaceous Glands

Sebaceous Adenoma

The solitary sebaceous adenoma is a pale yellow nodular lesion, less than 1 cm in diameter, and most reported examples have been situated on the scalp or face in patients more than 50 years old. Microscopically, sebaceous adenoma is characterized by a mixture of germinative and sebaceous cells in a nodular arrangement. Distinction between sebaceous adenoma and sebaceous gland hyperplasia may be difficult, as this latter lesion can also show a lobular arrangement around a hair follicle structure (Fig. 11).

Gardner syndrome (MIM +175100) (45) and Oldfield syndrome (85) are to be distinguished from Torre syndrome (97,116). Gardner syndrome consists of multiple epidermal and "sebaceous" cysts and occurs in association with intestinal polyps, osteomas, and tumors of soft tissue (45). In Oldfield syndrome (85), multiple cutaneous cysts are found in association with familial polyposis and colonic carcinoma.

Malignant Tumors of Sebaceous Glands

Sebaceous Carcinoma

Although sebaceous carcinoma can occur anywhere, ocular sebaceous carcinoma is far more common than the nonocular counterpart (130). The upper eyelid is the most frequent site of sebaceous carcinoma (35). Occasionally, both eyelids may be involved simultaneously, and the tumor may appear to be multicentric (94). In this case, the tumor may be misdiagnosed as ocular cicatricial pemphigoid, actinic keratosis, BCC, or SCC (130). Most sebaceous gland carcinomas arise from Meibomian glands but they may also arise from the glands of Zeis or other pilosebaceous units. Determining the exact site of origin may not always be possible by histological examination.

Sebaceous carcinoma is a disorder of middle-aged and elderly patients, mean age 62 to 72 years, with a female predominance (15,58,93,114). The incidence of sebaceous carcinoma varies from 1% to 5.5% of all malignant neoplasms of the eyelid (62). Sebaceous carcinoma of the eyelid is prevalent in Asian countries (87,124,134). Although uncommon in Western countries, it is important because it may

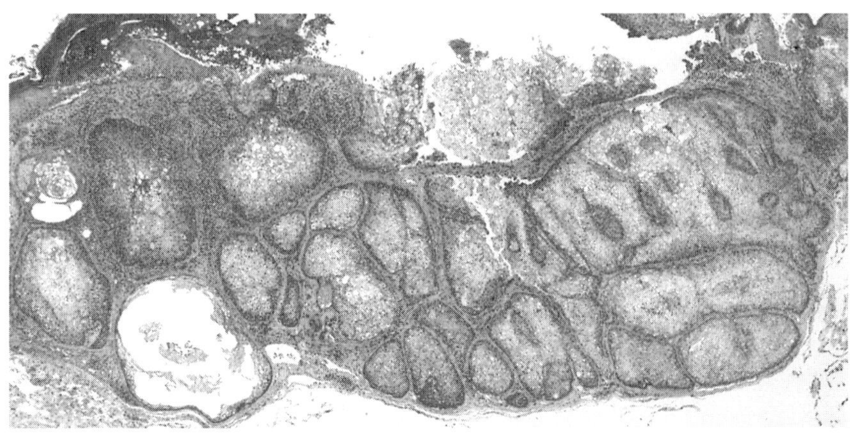

Figure 11 Sebaceous adenoma. The microscopic picture shows a distinct lobular architecture. The light and dark areas correspond to the sebaceous and the germinative cells (hematoxylin and eosin, ×115).

masquerade as a chalazion (foreign body granuloma of the eyelid due to rupture of a Meibomian gland) or as unilateral chronic blepharoconjunctivitis (62,130, 133). In a few instances, the tumor has presented as an orbital neoplasm, the primary site having been unrecognized clinically; rare cases have followed radiation treatment of retinoblastoma (17,57).

Due to the infrequency of sebaceous carcinoma and the variety of clinical presentations, delay in recognition has extended from 5 months to 7 years. Early case series reported a high mortality rate, 30% after 5 year follow-up in Boniuk and Zimmerman's series (17). There is initial spread of the tumor to parotid and submandibular lymph nodes. In general metastasis is a late event and when death occurs, metastases are widespread.

Clinically, the tumor usually presents as a circumscribed yellow nodule involving the tarsal plate when viewed from the tarsal conjunctival surface (Fig. 12). However, sebaceous carcinoma may also occur as a morpheic plaque (Fig. 13). When the origin is from the glands of Zeis, the margin of the eyelid is involved, with thickening and loss of cilia. Intraepithelial spread of tumor cells (Pagetoid invasion) may extend as far as the cornea without causing significant thickening of either the conjunctival or corneal epithelium. Occasionally, however, papillary fronds develop and cause confusion with SCC and BCC.

Histologically, sebaceous carcinomas are divided into low-, medium-, and high-grade according to the degree of differentiation. In low-grade tumors, a common pattern consists of lobules of various sizes and separated from the connective tissue by a basement membrane (Fig. 14). The individual polyhedral cells have vesicular nuclei with prominent nucleoli and foamy vacuolated cytoplasm as a result of the high lipid content, which is readily demonstrated in frozen sections by the oil red O stain. Higher grade tumors show scant cytoplasmic vacuolation with more prominent nucleoli, atypical mitoses, and abundant necrosis (Fig. 15). These lesions are more likely to show Pagetoid spread in the overlying epidermis, conjunctival epithelium, or corneal epithelium, which contain cells with abundant pale cytoplasm and hyperchromatic nuclei admixed within the nonneoplastic epithelium. These cells resemble those found in association with invasive ductal carcinomas of the breast (Paget disease of the breast), and this phenomenon may be a presenting manifestation of the sebaceous carcinoma (102,130). Pagetoid spread is associated with a worse prognosis, because of the widespread nature of the neoplasm (93). Histologically, confusion with BCC or a high-grade SCC is possible, but the cells of these tumors can be distinguished by the absence of fine intracellular droplets of fat.

TEM indicates that the neoplastic cell is of epidermoid origin in as much as tonofibrils and desmosomes are present. This pattern suggests an origin from the sebaceous duct rather than the secretory cells.

Immunohistochemical studies have proved very helpful in distinguishing sebaceous carcinoma from other epithelial neoplasms, in particular clear cell SCC and clear cell BCC. Sebaceous carcinomas are reactive with antibodies against EMA and low-molecular-weight cytokeratins such as CAM 5.2, a finding not observed in the other two neoplasms mentioned (113). Positivity with antibodies CU18, antibreast carcinoma-associated antigen 225, anti-CA 15.3, and anti-CD15 antibody has also been reported in sebaceous carcinoma (7).

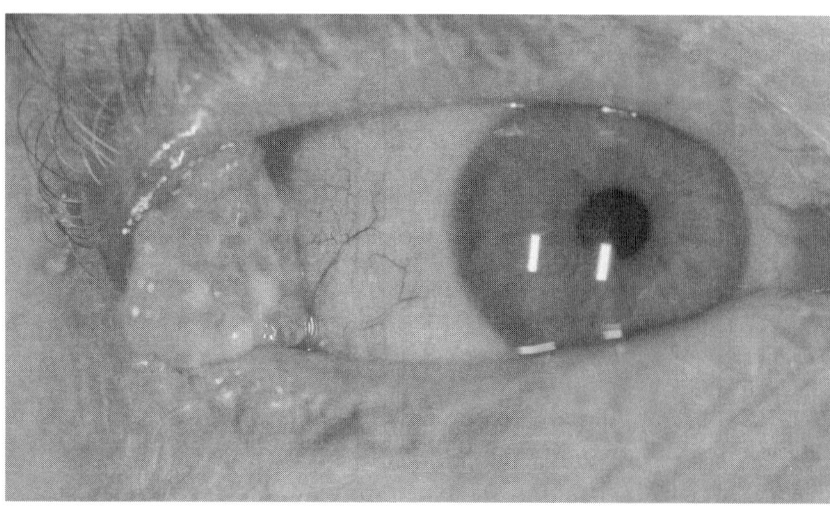

Figure 12 Sebaceous carcinoma. This clinical photograph shows a mass protruding from the lateral canthus.

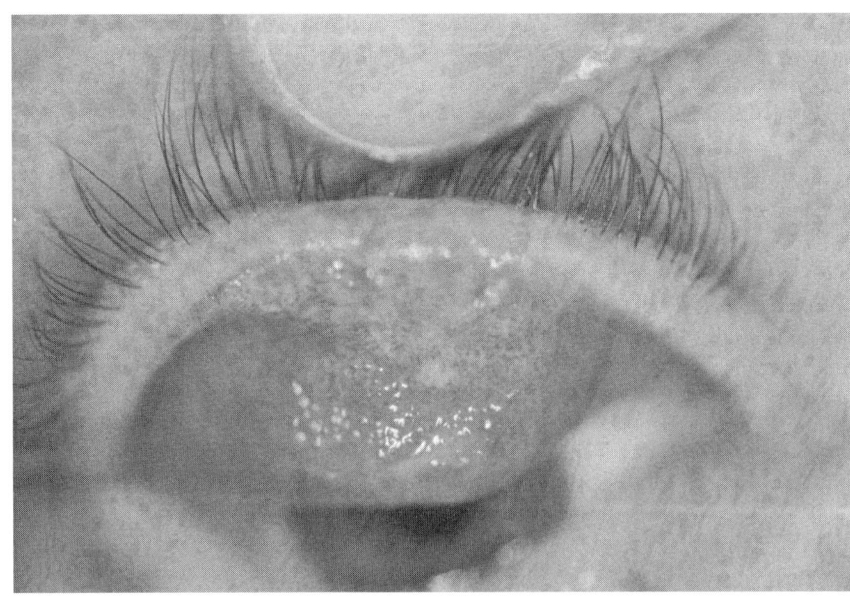

Figure 13 Sebaceous carcinoma—morpheic plaque. This clinical photograph shows an irregular lesion, flat, causing thickening of the upper eyelid.

NEOPLASMS ORIGINATING IN HAIR FOLLICLES OR SHOWING HAIR FOLLICLE DIFFERENTIATION

Benign eyelid tumors from hair follicles are rare. Frequently, they are misdiagnosed as BCC. Included in this group are trichoepithelioma, trichilemmoma, trichofolliculoma, and pilomatrixoma. In one large series, 117 such tumors were diagnosed over a 30-year period; in contrast, 2447 BCCs were removed during the same period (112). It is important to diagnose these benign tumors of hair follicles to avoid unnecessarily extensive surgical treatment.

Trichoepithelioma

This tumor occurs as a solitary lesion or as an inherited condition, when it is likely to be multiple (27). The solitary nodule is firm and elevated and appears in both men and women during the later decades of life. The multiple type (Spiegler–Brooke syndrome tumor, MIM %605041) is inherited in an autosomal-dominant pattern. Microscopically, basaloid cells are arranged in strands and nests with multiple horn cysts, which represent immature hair follicles. The main differential diagnosis is with BCC, which is closely related histogenetically.

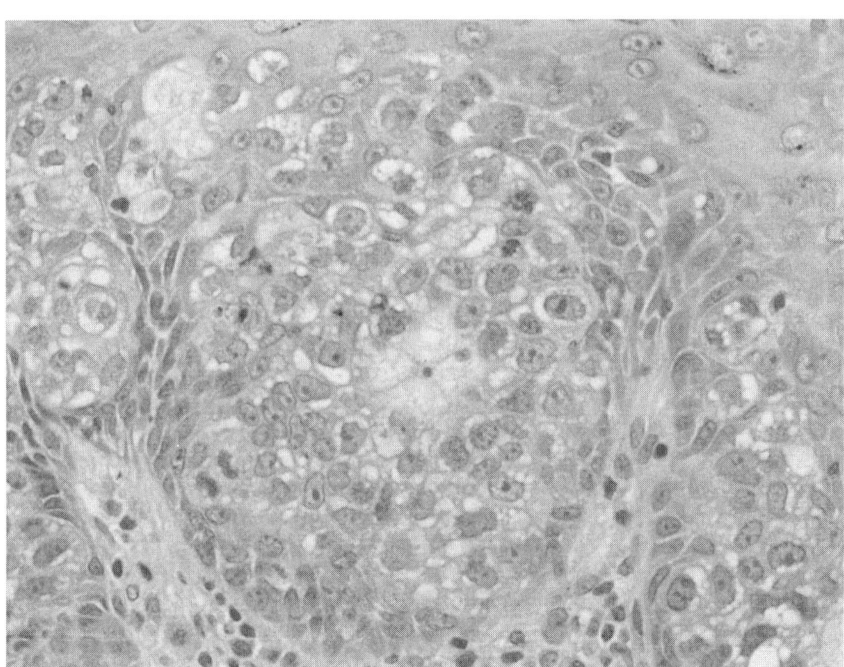

Figure 14 Sebaceous carcinoma. This photomicrograph shows a well-differentiated sebaceous carcinoma. The tumor nests are composed by pleomorphic cells with prominent nucleoli and vacuolated cytoplasm (hematoxylin and eosin, ×450).

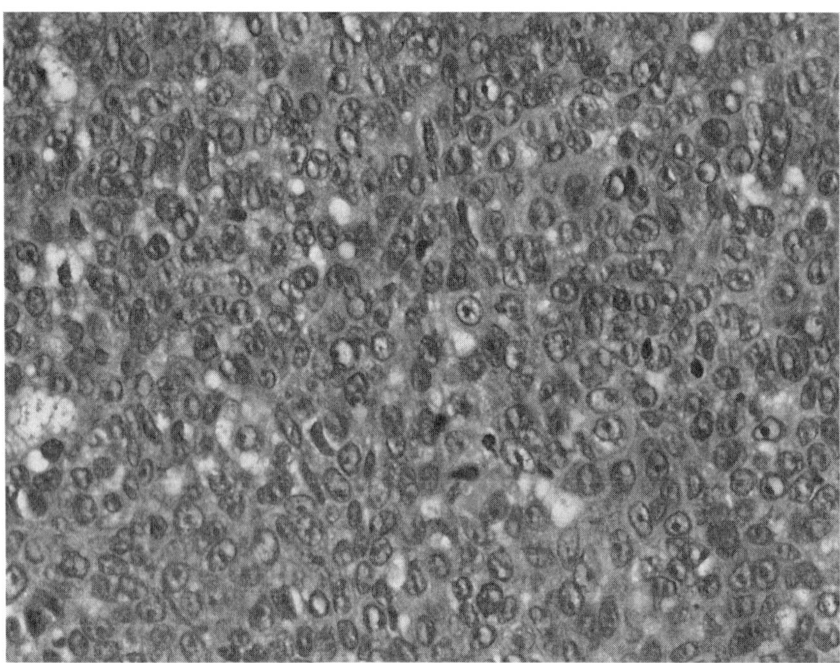

Figure 15 Sebaceous carcinoma. This photomicrograph shows a poorly differentiated sebaceous carcinoma. The tumor nests are composed of sheets of cells with enlarged nuclei, scant cytoplasm, and prominent nucleoli. Rare cells demonstrate the cytoplasmic vacuolation resembling sebaceous differentiation (hematoxylin and eosin, ×450).

Immunostaining for stromelysin-3 (a matrix metalloproteinase) is said to be helpful in the distinction (125).

Trichilemmoma

This benign tumor arises from the outer sheath of the hair follicle. The eyelid is the second most common site after the nose. In a study of 31 such tumors of the eyelid (28) and eyebrow (3), the age range of the patients was 22 to 88 years (mean 53 years) (55). Microscopically, glycogen-rich cells are arranged in lobules and show a palisade pattern at the periphery of the lobule, which may lead to confusion with BCC. Multiple facial trichilemmomas, which may include the eyelid, are pathognomonic of Cowden disease (MIM #158350), a rare genodermatosis (11) caused by mutations in the *PTEN* or *BMPRIA* genes.

Trichofolliculoma

A benign entity, the trichofollicutoma is a hamartoma that consists of a large cystic follicle that represents a dilated hair follicle and contains immature hair structures. The appearance of white hairs growing from the central core may be distinctive, but this feature is not seen in all cases (22).

Pilomatrixoma

The pilomatrixoma (calcifying epithelioma of Malherbe) is a benign, solitary, cystic tumor that favors the upper eyelid and eyebrow in children and young adults. In one study of 150 children 10 years of age or younger, 17% of these tumors were of the upper eyelid and brow (86). Ashton (9) was the first to record this tumor of the eyelids in the ophthalmic literature. Clinically, it resembles a pilar cyst and arises from the primitive hair matrix. Histologically, the basaloid cell proliferation includes "ghost cells," and foci of calcification and foreign body giant cells are common in the supporting stroma. Reported rare complications are corneal ulceration secondary to an ectopic lesion in the tarsal plate (33) and necrosis with malignant degeneration (44).

EPITHELIAL CYSTS OF THE EYELID

Milia

Milia are densely opaque, well-demarcated nodules that are 1 to 2 mm in diameter. They are retention cysts caused by occlusion of a pilosebaceous follicle. Histologically, they resemble epidermal cysts.

Pilar Cysts

In the past, the pilar cyst was called a sebaceous cyst. Once it became apparent that the differentiation within these cysts was toward hair keratin, the terminology was changed. The cyst has an epithelial cell lining in which the cells lack easily visible bridges and the basal layer is distinctly palisaded. In contrast to the epidermal cyst, the epithelial lining lacks a granular layer. The innermost cells have increased numbers of filaments and fibrils and these cells are shed into the lumen. As they are shed, they lose their nuclei and cytoplasmic organelles. The contents of the cysts form an amorphous eosinophilic mass, which becomes calcified in approximately 25% of cases. In most instances the cyst is single, but multiple cysts may occur and form part of Gardner or Oldfield syndrome (45,85).

Epidermal Cysts

Although clinically similar to the pilar cyst, the epidermal cyst lacks a palisade arrangement of the peripheral cells, and the luminal contents do not calcify. The epithelial wall contains a stratum granulosum, and the innermost cells are laminated. Growth is slow and is caused by the accumulation of keratin from the cornified cells of the epithelial lining. The lesion is round and firm and may enlarge to 3 cm in diameter. It is situated in the superficial or deep corium. On rupture, both pilar and epidermal cysts excite a foreign body giant cell reaction. Clinically, the lesion becomes red and indurated.

NEUROENDOCRINE TUMORS

Merkel Cell Carcinoma

Merkel, in 1875 (79), described the so-called Merkel tactile cell in the snout of the mole. The cell is oval and dendritic, with a round to oval nucleus that contains finely dispersed chromatin and one to three inconspicuous nucleoli. The cytoplasm is scanty.

The Merkel cell carcinoma has several synonyms, including trabecular carcinoma, small cell carcinoma, cutaneous APUDoma, and neuroendocrine carcinoma of the skin (110). These names reflect the appearance and the function of the cell, which is derived from the neural crest. It migrates to the deep layers of the epidermis, where it forms complexes with nerve endings to function as mechanoreceptors for the sensation of touch (*Tastzellen*).

This tumor is malignant, most commonly occurs in adults and elderly patients, and is found most frequently on the head and neck (95). The first Merkel cell tumor of the eyelid was described in 1983 (13). Since then, approximately 20 cases have been reported. In the series of Searl and colleagues (106), of 69 such patients, 7 (9%) had eyelid involvement. Six of the seven tumors affected the upper eyelid, and one was on the eyebrow. Predilection for the upper eyelid has been observed by others (65). Most of these tumors have occurred in women. The median age of patients reported is 71 years (106), but a Merkel cell tumor of the eyelid has been described in a 15-year-old girl with ectodermal dysplasia (46).

Clinically, the tumor appears as a nontender, reddish blue nodule with telangiectatic vessels on its surface. One case manifested as a recurrent chalazion (76).

Microscopically, the neoplasm is centered in the dermis or sometimes subcutaneous tissue, with the overlying epidermis being usually uninvolved. The neoplastic cells are characterized by scant cytoplasm and round and vesicular nuclei with fine ("dusty") granular chromatin. Therefore, Merkel cell carcinoma may be confused with small cell neoplasms, such as small cell carcinoma of the lung and large cell lymphoma. Immunohistochemical and ultrastructural studies help to characterize the cell (74,108). Ultrastructurally, the neoplastic cells contain dense-core neurosecretory granules and tightly packed perinuclear intermediate filaments (43,109).

The tumor cells are argyrophilic with the Grimelius reaction, especially if the tissue has been fixed in Bouin solution. Immunohistochemically, positivity for low-molecular-weight keratin, neurofilaments, and neuron-specific enolase is usually seen. Cytokeratin 20 positivity in a distinct perinuclear dot-like pattern, in association with negativity for thyroid transcription factor-1 (TTF-1) and cytokeratin 7 are important to distinguish from metastatic pulmonary small cell carcinoma (25). Other immunostains that also might be positive in Merkel cell carcinoma are chromogranin, synaptophysin, calcitonin, vasoactive intestinal peptide, somatostatin, CD117, and adrenocorticotrophin (111,132).

Merkel cell carcinoma is an aggressive neoplasm with rapid growth. Regional lymph node metastases are common and distant metastases may occur, particularly in lungs, liver, and bones. Fine-needle biopsy with immunohistochemical studies has established the nature of such metastases in the parotid gland (46). In the series of Searl and colleagues (106), death due to metastasis occurred in approximately 20% of patients.

REFERENCES

1. Abe M, Ohnishi Y, Hara Y, Shinoda Y, Jingu K. Malignant tumor of the eyelid—clinical survey during 22-year period. Jpn J Ophthalmol 1983; 27:175–84.
2. Ahluwalia BK, Khurana AK, Chugh AD, Mehtani VG. Eccrine spiradenoma of eyelid: case report. Br J Ophthalmol 1986; 70:580–3.
3. Alam M, Ratner D. Cutaneous squamous-cell carcinoma. N Engl J Med 2001; 344:975–83.
4. Albert DM, McGhee CNJ, Seddon JM, Weichselbaum RR. Development of additional primary tumors after 62 years in the first patient with retinoblastoma cured by radiation therapy. Am J Ophthalmol 1984; 97:189–96.
5. Ambrojo P, Requena Caballero L, Aguilar Martinez A, et al. Clear-cell syringoma: immunohistochemistry and electron microscopy study. Dermatologica 1989; 178: 164–6.
6. American Joint Committee on Cancer. Staging of cancer at specific anatomic sites: ophthalmic tumors. In: Fleming ID, Fleming JS, Cooper D, et al. eds. Manual for Staging of Cancer. 5th ed. Philadelphia, PA: JB Lippincott, 1997: 251–77.
7. Ansai S, Mitsuhashi Y, Kondo S, et al. Immunohistochemical differentiation of extra-ocular carcinoma from other skin cancers. J Dermatol 2004; 31:998–1008.

8. Arbesman H, Ransohoff DF. FS Bowen's disease a predictor for the development of internal malignancy? A methodological critique of the literature. JAMA 1987; 257:516–8.
9. Ashton N. Benign calcined epithelioma of eyelid. Trans Ophthalmol Soc UK 1951; 71:301–7.
10. Aurora AL, Blodi FC. Lesions of the eyelids: a clinicopathological study. Surv Ophthalmol 1970; 15:94–104.
11. Bardenstein DS, McLean IW, Nerney J, Boatwright RS. Cowden's disease. Ophthalmology 1988; 95:1038–41.
12. Berman A, Winkelmann RK. Inflammatory seborrheic keratoses with mononuclear cell infiltration. J Cutan Pathol 1978; 5:353–60.
13. Beyer CK, Goodman M, Dickersin GR, Dougherty M. Merkel cell tumor of the eyelid: a clinico-pathologic case report. Arch Ophthalmol 1983; 101:1098–101.
14. Beyer TL, Dryden RM. Basal cell carcinoma masquerading as ectropion (case report). Arch Ophthalmol 1988; 106:170–1.
15. Bhalla JS, Vashisht S, Gupta VK, Sen AK. Meibomian gland carcinoma in a 20-year-old patient (letter). Am J Ophthalmol 1991; 711:114–5.
16. Boniuk M, Zimmerman LE. Eyelid tumors with reference to lesions confused with squamous cell carcinoma III. Keratoacanthoma. Arch Ophthalmol 1967; 77:29–40.
17. Boniuk M, Zimmerman LE. Sebaceous carcinoma of the eyelid, eyebrow, caruncle, and orbit. Trans Am Acad Ophthalmol Otolaryngol 1968; 72:619–42.
18. Bowen IT. Precancerous dermatoses: a study of two cases of chronic atypical epithelial proliferation. J Cutan Dis 1912; 30:251–5.
19. Brash DE, Rudolph JA, Simon JA, et al. A role for sunlight in skin cancer: UV-induced p53 mutations in squamous cell carcinoma. Proc Natl Acad USA 1991; 88:10124–8.
20. Burgdorf WHC, Schosser RH, et al. Muir–Torre syndrome. Histologic spectrum of sebaceous proliferations. Am J Dermatopathol 1986; 8:202–8.
21. Burkhart CG. Looking at eyelid lesions—a clinical roundup. Geriatrics 1981; 36:91–3.
22. Carreras B Jr, Lopez-Marin I Jr, Mellado VG, Gutierrez MT. Trichofolliculoma of the eyelid. Br J Ophthalmol 1981; 65:214–5.
23. Caya JG, Hidayat AA, Weiner JM. A clinicopathologic study of 21 cases of adenoid squamous cell carcinoma of the eyelid and periorbital region. Am J Ophthalmol 1985; 99:291–7.
24. Charpentier P, Bloch-Michel E, Caillou B, Soussaline M, Boudier V, Offret H. A proposd'uncasde syndrome de Torre: association d'un adenocarcinome meibomien et d'une tumeur caecale. J Fr Ophtalmol 1985; 8:479–85.
25. Cheuk K, Kwan MY, Suster S, Chan JK. Immunostaining for thyroid transcription factor 1 and cytokeratin 20 aids the distinction of small cell carcinoma from Merkel cell carcinoma, but not pulmonary from extrapulmonary small cell carcinomas. Arch Pathol Lab Med 2001; 125:228–31.
26. Chuang T-Y, Reizner G-T, Elpern DJ, et al. Keratocanthoma in Kauai, Hawaii. The first documented incidence in a defined population. Arch Dermatol 1993; 129:317–9.
27. Clarke J, Ioffreda M, Helm KF. Multiple familial trichoepitheliomas: a folliculoebaceous-apocrine genodermatosis. Am J Dermatopathol 2002; 24:402–5.
28. Cleaver JE, Bootsma D. Xeroderma pigmentosum: biochemical and genetic characteristics. Ann Rev Genet 1975; 9:19–38.
29. Cohen PR, Khon SR. Association of sebaceous gland tumors and internal malignancy: the Muir–Torre syndrome. Am J Med 1991; 90:606–13.
30. Cooper PH. Carcinomas of sweat glands. Pathol Ann 1987; 22:83–124.
31. Costanza ME, Dayal Y, Binder S, Nathanson L. Metastatic basal cell carcinoma: review, report of a case, and chemotherapy. Cancer 1974; 34:230–5.
32. Crowson AN. Basal cell carcinoma: biology, morphology and clinical implications. Mod Pathol 2006; 19:S127–47.
33. de Azevedo ML, Milani JAA, de Souza EC, Nemer RS. Pilomatrixoma: an unusual case with secondary corneal ulcer. Arch Ophthalmol 1985; 103:553–4.
34. de Weerd-Kastelein EA, Keijzer W, Bootsma D. Genetic heterogeneity of xeroderma pigmentosum demonstrated by somatic cell hybridization. Nat New Biol 1972; 238: 80–1.
35. Doxanas MT, Green WR. Sebaceous gland carcinoma: review of 40 cases. Arch Ophthalmol 1984; 102:245–9.
36. Doxanas MT, Iliff WJ, Iliff NT, Green WR. Squamous cell carcinoma of the eyelids. Ophthalmology 1987; 94:538–41.
37. Farmer ER, Helwig EB. Metastatic basal cell carcinoma: a clinicopathologic study of seventeen cases. Cancer 1980; 46:748–57.
38. Finan MC, Connolly SM. Sebaceous gland tumors and systemic disease: a clinicopathologic analysis. Medicine (Baltimore) 1984; 63:232–42.
39. Flament J, Kouhil M, Amiar MK, Boukoffa OS, Forest M. Giant keratoacanthoma of the palpebral region (diagnostic and therapeutic problems). Bull Soc Ophthalmol Fr 1981; 81:611–5.
40. Font RL. Eyelids and lacrimal drainage system: nevoid basal cell carcinoma syndrome. In: Spencer WJ, ed. Ophthalmic Pathology: An Atlas and Textbook, vol. 3. Philadelphia, PA: WB Saunders, 1986:2177–8.
41. Font RL, Stone MS, Schanzer MC, Lewis RA. Apocrine hidrocystomas of the lids, hypodontia, palmar-plantar hyperkeratosis, and onychodystrophy: a new variant of ectodermal dysplasia. Arch Ophthalmol 1986; 104:1811–3.
42. Ford HC, Delahunt JW, Teague CA. Squamous cell carcinoma of the eyelid masquerading as "malignant" ophthalmopathy of Graves's disease. Br J Ophthalmol 1983; 67:596–9.
43. Frigerio B, Capella C, Eusebi V, Tenti P, Azzopardi JG. Merkel cell carcinoma of the skin. The structure and origin of normal Merkel cells. Histopathology 1983; 7: 229–49.
44. Galimova RZ, Bastimieva BE. Malherbe's necrotizing epithelioma of the eyelid without malignant degeneration. Vestn Oftalmol 1990; 106:62–4 [in Russian].
45. Gardner EJ. Follow-up study of a family group exhibiting dominant inheritance for a syndrome including intestinal polyps, osteomas, fibromas and epidermal cysts. Am J Hum Genet 1962; 14:376–90.
46. Gherardi G, Marveggio C, Stiglich E. Parotid metastasis of Merkel cell carcinoma in a young patient with ectodermal dysplasia: diagnosis by fine needle aspiration cytology and immunocytochemistry. Ada Cytol 1990; 34: 831–6.
47. Glatt HJ, Proia AD, Tsoy EA, et al. Malignant syringoma of the eyelid. Ophthalmology 1984; 91:987–90.
48. Gorlin RJ, Goltz RW. Multiple nevoid basal-cell epithelioma, jaw cysts and bifid rib: a syndrome. TV. Engl J Med 1960; 262:908–12.
49. Graham JH, Helwig EB. Premalignant cutaneous and mucocutaneous diseases. In: Graham JH, Johnson WC, Helwig EB, eds. Dermal Pathology. Hagerstown, MD: Harper & Row, 1972:561–624.
50. Grossniklaus HE, Knight SH. Eccrine acrospiroma (clear cell hidradenoma) of the eyelid: immuno histochemical

and ultrastructural features. Ophthalmology 1991; 98: 347–52.
51. Grossniklaus HE, Wojno TH, Yanoff M, Font RL. Invasive keratoacanthoma of the eyelid and ocular adnexa. Ophthalmology 1996; 103:937–41.
52. Hashimoto K, Blum D, Fukaya T, Eto H. Familial syringoma: case history and application of monoclonal anti-eccrine gland antibodies. Arch Dermatol 1985; 121:756–60.
53. Helander SD, Peters MS, Pittelkow MR. Expression of p53 protein in benign and malignant epidermal pathologic conditions. J Am Acad Dermatol 1993; 29:741–8.
54. Helwig EB. Inverted follicular keratosis. In: Seminar on the Skin: Neoplasms and Dermatoses, Proceedings of 20th Seminar, American Society of Clinical Pathology, Washington, D.C., American Society of Clinical Pathology, Indianapolis, IN, 1955:38.
55. Hidayat AA, Font RL. Trichilemmoma of eyelid and eyebrow: a clinicopathologic study of 31 cases. Arch Ophthalmol 1980; 98:844–7.
56. Homblass A, Stefano JA. Pigmented basal cell carcinoma of the eyelids. Am J Ophthalmol 1981; 92:193–7.
57. Howrey RP, Lipham WJ, Scultz WH, et al. Sebaceous gland carcinoma: a subtle second malignancy following radiation therapy in patients with bilateral retinoblastoma. Cancer 1998; 83:767–71.
58. Jakobiec FA. Sebaceous adenoma of the eyelid and visceral malignancy. Am J Ophthalmol 1974; 78:952–60.
59. Jakobiec FA, Austin P, Iwamoto T, et al. Primary infiltrating signet ring carcinoma of the eyelids. Ophthalmology 1983; 90:291–9.
60. Jakobiec FA, Streeten BW, Iwamoto T, et al. Syringocystadenoma papilliferum of the eyelid. Ophthalmology 1981; 88:1175–81.
61. Jakobiec FA, Zimmerman LE, La Piana F, et al. Unusual eyelid tumors with sebaceous differentiation in the Muir–Torre syndrome: rapid clinical regrowth and frank squamous transformation after biopsy. Ophthalmology 1988; 95:1543–8.
62. James WD, Odom RB. Late subcutaneous fibrosis following megavoltage radiotherapy. Jam Acad Dermatol 1980; 3:616–8.
63. Kass LG, Hornblass A. Sebaceous carcinoma of the ocular adnexa. Surv Ophthalmol 1989; 33:477–90.
64. Keijzer W, Stepanini M, Bootsma D, et al. Localization of a gene involved in complementation of the defect in xeroderma pigmentosum group A cells on human chromosome 1. Exp Cell Res 1987; 169:490–501.
65. Khalil M, Brownstein S, Codere F, Nicolle D. Eccrine sweat gland carcinoma of the eyelid with orbital involvement. Arch Ophthalmol 1980; 98:2210–4.
66. Kivela T, Tarkkanen A. The Merkel cell and associated neoplasms in the eyelids and periocular region. Surv Ophthalmol 1990; 35:171–87.
67. Kraemer KH, Myung ML, Scotto J. Xeroderma pigmentosum: cutaneous, ocular, and neurologic abnormalities in 830 published cases. Arch Dermatol 1987; 123:241–50.
68. Kunnert C, Boukoffa W, Forest M, et al. Xeroderma pigmentosum: a propos des localisations conjonctivales et palpebrales dans 2 cas. Bull Soc Ophtalmol Fr 1988; 88: 1145–6.
69. Kwitko ML, Boniuk M, Zimmerman LE. Eyelid tumors with reference to lesions confused with squamous cell carcinoma. I. Incidence and errors in diagnosis. Arch Ophthalmol 1963; 69:693–7.
70. Lahav M, Albert DM, Bahr R, Craft J. Eyelid tumors of sweat gland origin. Graefes Arch Clln Exp Ophthalmol 1981; 216:301–11.
71. Langer K, Konrad K, Smolle J. Multiple apocrine hidrocystomas on the eyelids. Am J Dermatopathol 1989; 11:570–3.
72. Lazar P, Culleu SI. Basal cell epithelioma and chronic radiodermatitis. Arch Dermatol 1963; 88:172–5.
73. Lever WF, Schaumburg-Lever G. Histopathology of the Skin. 7th ed. Philadelphia, PA: JB Lippincott, 1990.
74. Li S, Brownstein S, Addison DJ, et al. Merkel cell carcinoma of the eyelid. Can J Ophthalmol 1997; 32: 455–61.
75. Liszauer AD, Brownstein S, Codere E. Mucinous eccrine sweat gland adenocarcinoma of the eyelid. Can J Ophthalmol 1988; 23:17–21.
76. Mamalis N, Medlock RD, Holds IB, et al. Merkel cell tumor of the eyelid: a review and report of an unusual case. Ophthal Surg 1989; 20:410–4.
77. McDonnell JM, McDonnell PI, Stout WC, Martin WJ. Human papillomavirus DNA in a recurrent squamous carcinoma of the eyelid. Arch Ophthalmol 1989; 107: 1631–4.
78. McKusick VA. Mendelian inheritance in man: catalogs of autosomal dominant, autosomal recessive, and X-linked phenotypes. 9th ed. Baltimore, MD: Johns Hopkins University Press, 1990.
79. Merkel E. Tastzellen und Taskorkorperchen bei den Hausthieren und beim Menschen. Arch Mikrost Anal 1875; 11:636.
80. Mert M, Wozniewicz B. Keratoacanthoma. Klin Oczna 1979; 81:537–8.
81. Nerad JA, Whitaker DC. Periocular basal cell carcinoma in adults 35 years of age and younger. Am J Ophthalmol 1988; 106:723–9.
82. Netland PA, Townsend DJ, Albert DM, Jakobiec EA. Hidradenoma papilliferum of the upper eyelid arising from the apocrine gland of Moll. Ophthalmology 1990; 97:1593–8.
83. Ni C, Wagoner M, Kieval S, Albert DM. Tumours of the Moll's glands. Br J Ophthalmol 1984; 68:502–6.
84. Nicolau SG, Badanoiu A, Balus L. Untersuchungen iiber spezifische antitumorale Reaktionen bei an Keratoakanthom leidenden Kranken mit einigen Betrachtungen beziiglich des Eingreifens von Immunitatsprozessen bei der spontanen Heilung dieserGeschwulst. Arch Klin Exp Dermatol 1963; 217: 308–20.
85. Oldfield MC. The association of familial polyposis of the colon with multiple sebaceous cysts. Br J Surg 1954; 41: 534–41.
86. Orlando RG, Rogers GL, Bremer DL. Pilomatricoma in a pediatric hospital. Arch Ophthalmol 1983; 101:1209–10.
87. Parsa ED. Sebaceous gland carcinoma of the eyelids in Hawaii. Hawaii Med J 1989; 48:165–6.
88. Parshad R, Sanford KK, Kraemer KH, et al. Carrier detection in xeroderma pigmentosum. J Clin Invest 1990; 8:135–8.
89. Patel A, Halliday GM, Cooke BE, Barnetson RS-C. Evidence suggests that regression in keratoacanthoma is immunologically mediated: a comparison with squamous cell carcinoma. Br J Dermatol 1994; 131:789–98.
90. Pesce C, Scalora S. Apoptosis in the areas of squamous differentiation of irritated seborrheic keratosis. J Cutan Pathol 2000; 27:121–3.
91. Peterka ES, Lynch EW, Goltz RW. An association between Bowen's disease and internal cancer. Arch Dermatol 1961; 84:623–9.
92. Petit-frere C, Capulas E, Lowe JE, et al. Ultraviolet-B-induced apoptosis and cytokine release in xeroderma

pigmentosum keratinocytes. J Invest Dermatol 2000; 115: 687–93.
93. Rao NA, Hidayat AA, McLean IW, Zimmerman LE. Sebaceous carcinomas of the ocular adnexa: a clinicopathologic study of 104 cases, with five-year follow-up data. Hum Pathol 1982; 13:113–22.
94. Rao NA, McLean IW, Zimmerman LE. Sebaceous carcinoma of eyelids and caruncle: correlation of clinicopathologic features with prognosis. In: Jakobiec EA, ed. Ocular and Adnexal Tumors. Birmingham, AL: Aesculapius Publishing, 1978:461–76.
95. Ratner D, Nelson BR, Brown MD, Johnson TM. J Am Acad Dermatol 1993; 29:143–56.
96. Reifler DM, Hornblass A. Squamous cell carcinoma of the eyelid. Surv Ophthalmol 1986; 30:349–65 (published erratum appears in Surv Ophthalmol 1986; 31:77).
97. Rishi K, Font RL. Sebaceous gland tumors of the eyelids and the conjunctiva in the Muir–Torre syndrome: a clinicopathological study of five cases and literature review. Ophthal Plast Reconstr Surg 2004; 20:30–6.
98. Robbins HH, Kraemer KH, Andrews AD. Inherited DNA repair defects in *H. sapiens*: their relation to UV-associated processes in xeroderma pigmentosum. In: Yuhas JM, Tennani RW, Regan JD, eds. Biology of Radiation Carcinogenesis. New York, NY: Raven Press, 1976:115.
99. Rogers PA. The ophthalmological significance of the basal cell naevus syndrome. Aust NZ J Ophthalmol 1983; 11: 275–9.
100. Rosai J. Skin. Dermatoses. Tumors and tumorlike conditions. In: Rosa and Ackerman's Surgical Pathology. Edinburgh, Mosby, 2004:90–245 [chap 4].
101. Rulon DB, Helwig EB. Multiple sebaceous neoplasms of the skin: in association with multiple visceral carcinomas, especially of the colon. Am J Clin Pathol 1973; 60: 745.
102. Russell WG, Page DL, Hough AI, Rogers LW. Sebaceous carcinoma of Meibomian gland origin: the diagnostic importance of Pagetoid spread of neoplastic cells. Am J Clin Pathol 1980; 73:504–11.
103. Sacks E, Jakobiec FA, McMillan R, et al. Multiple bilateral apocrine cyst-adenomas of the lower eyelids: light and electron microscopic studies. Ophthalmology 1987; 94: 65–71.
104. Santa Cruz DJ, Prioleau PG, Smith ME. Hidradenoma papilliferum of the eyelid. Arch Dermatol 1981; 117:55–6.
105. Sassani JW, Yanoff M. Inverted follicular keratosis. Am J Ophthalmol 1979; 87:810–3.
106. Searl SS, Boynton JR, Markowitch W, diSant'Agnese PA. Malignant Merkel cell neoplasm of the eyelid. Arch Ophthalmol 1984; 102:907–11.
107. Shea CR, McNutt NS, Volkenandt M, et al. Overexpression of p53 protein in basal cell carcinomas of human skin. Am J Pathol 1992; 141:25–9.
108. Sidhu GS, Feiner H, Flotte TJ, et al. Merkel cell neoplasms: histology, electron microscopy, biology, and histogenesis. Am J Dermatopathol 1980; 2:101–19.
109. Silva A, Mackay B. Neuroendocrine (Merkel cell) carcinomas of the skin. An ultrastructural study of nine cases. Ultrastruct Pathol 1981; 2:101–19.
110. Silva EG, Mackay B, Goepfert H, Burgess MA, Fields RS. Endocrine carcinoma of the skin (Merkel cell carcinomas). Pathol Ann 1984, 19(Pt 2):1–30.
111. Silva EG, Ordonez NG, Lechago J. Immunohistochemical studies in endocrine carcinoma of the skin. Am J Clin Pathol 1984; 81:558–61.
112. Simpson W, Garner A, Collin JRO. Benign hair-follicle derived tumours in the differential diagnosis of basal-cell carcinoma of the eyelids: a clinicopathological comparison. Br J Ophthalmol 1989; 73:347–53.
113. Sinard JH. Immunohistochemical distinction of sebaceous carcinoma from basal cell carcinoma and squamous cell carcinoma. Arch Ophthalmol 1999; 117: 776–83.
114. Shields JA, Demirci H, Marr BP, et al. Sebaceous carcinoma of the eyelids: personal experience with 60 cases. Ophthalmology 2004; 111:2151–7.
115. Slater JP, Beers BB, Stephens CA, Hendrichs JB. Keratoacanthoma: a deficient squamous cell carcinoma? Study of bcl-2 expression. J Cutan Pathol 1994; 21: 514–9.
116. Smoller BR, Crowson AN. Epidermal neoplasms. USCAP Long Course 2005. Mod Pathol 2006; 19 (Suppl. 2):S1–163.
117. Smoller BR, Krueger J, McNutt NS, Hsu A. "Activated" keratinocyte phenotype is unifying feature in conditions which predispose to squamous cell carcinoma of the skin. Mod Pathol 1990; 3:171–5.
118. Soffer D, Kaplan H, Weshler Z. Meningeal carcinomatosis due to basal cell carcinoma. Hum Pathol 1985; 16:530–2.
119. Sommerville J, Milne JA. Familial primary self-healing squamous epithelioma of the skin (Ferguson Smith type). Br J Dermatol 1950; 62:485–90.
120. Southwick GJ, Schwartz RA. The basal cell nevus syndrome: disasters occurring among a series of 36 patients. Cancer 1979; 44:2294–305.
121. Stewart WB, Nicholson DH, Hamilton G, et al. Eyelid tumors and renal transplantation. Arch Ophthalmol 1980; 98:1771–2.
122. Stoll HL Jr. Squamous cell carcinoma. In: Fitzpatrick TB, Arndt KA, Clark WH, et al. eds. Dermatology in General Medicine. New York, NY: McGraw-Hill, 1971: 407–25.
123. Su LD, Fullen DR, Lowe L, et al. CD117 (Kit receptor) expression in Merkel cell carcinoma. Am J Dermatopathol 2002; 24:289–93.
124. Sun W, Yao Y, Yi G. Clinicopathological analysis of 30 cases of Meibomian gland carcinoma. Chung Hua Yen Ko Tsa Chih 1982; 18:363–5.
125. Thewes M, Worret WI, Engst R, Ring J. Stromelysin-3: a potent marker of histopathologic differentiation between desmoplastic trichoepithelioma and morphea-like basal cell carcinoma. Am J Dermatopathol 1998; 20: 140–2.
126. Tillawi I, Katz R, Pellettiere EV. Solitary tumors of Meibomian gland origin and Torre's syndrome. Am J Ophthalmol 1987; 104:179–82.
127. Torre D. Multiple sebaceous tumors. Arch Dermatol 1968; 98:549–51.
128. Wesley RE, Collins JW. Basal cell carcinoma of the eyelid as an indicator of multifocal malignancy. Am J Ophthalmol 1982; 94:591–3.
129. Wick MR, Swanson PE, Barnhill RL. Sweat gland tumors. In: Barnhill RL, Crowson AN, eds. Textbook of Dermatopathology. 2nd ed. New York, NY: McGraw-Hill 2004:745–84.
130. Wolfe JT III, Yeatts RP, Wick MR, Campbell RJ, Waller RR. Sebaceous carcinoma of the eyelid: Errors in clinical and pathologic diagnosis. Am J Surg Pathol 1984; 8:597–606.
131. Wong CS, Strange RC, Lear JT. Clinical review. Basal cell carcinoma. BMJ 2003; 327:794–8.

132. Wright JD, Font RL. Mucinous sweat gland adenocarcinoma of eyelid: a clinicopathologic study of 21 cases with histochemical and electron microscopic observations. Cancer 1979; 44:1757–68.
133. Wright P, Collin RJO, Garner A. The masquerade syndrome. Trans Ophthalmol Soc UK 1981; 101:244–50.
134. Yaun NF. Meibomian gland adenocarcinoma with regional lymph node metastasis. Chung Hua Yen Ko Tsa Chih 1989; 25:144–5.
135. Zelickson AS, Lynch FW. Electron microscopy of virus-like particles in a keratoacanthoma. Invest Dermatol 1961; 37:79–83.

57

Tumors of the Ocular Surface

Diva R. Salomão
Department of Pathology, Mayo Clinic, Mayo Foundation, and Mayo Medical School, Rochester, Minnesota, U.S.A.

INTRODUCTION

The conjunctiva extends from the eyelid margin to the corneoscleral limbus, and its morphology varies in the different regions. The palpebral conjunctiva covers the inner eyelid surface, and is represented by a non-keratinized pseudo-stratified columnar epithelium with interspersed goblet cells (mucin-producing), over a thin layer of substantia propria that is firmly attached to the tarsus. In the fornices, the epithelium becomes stratified cuboidal with an increased number of goblet cells. The substantia propria in this region is more abundant, and it may contain lymphoid follicles and accessory lacrimal gland tissue. Over the ocular surface, the bulbar conjunctiva is characterized by non-keratinized stratified squamous epithelium without goblet cells, lying over a layer of fibrous vascular connective tissue, firmly attached to the sclera.

The conjunctiva has several anatomic variations; the plica semilunaris, the caruncle, and the corneoscleral limbus where histologic peculiarities characterize each location. For example, the substantia propria underlying the mucosa of the caruncle contains cutaneous adnexa.

Tumors of the conjunctiva comprise a spectrum of benign and malignant neoplasms that can be divided by their origin in the surface epithelium or in the substantia propria, and further more according to the differentiation into epithelial, melanocytic, mesenchymal or lymphoid neoplasms. Any lesion with a hydrated keratin covering of appreciable thickness appears white (leukoplakia), whether it is benign or malignant; therefore, the term "leukoplakia" is without clinicopathological correlation.

Primary neoplasms of the cornea are exceedingly rare (16,37,56) and the cornea is most commonly involved by direct extension of conjunctival neoplasms.

EPITHELIAL TUMORS

Benign

Papilloma

Squamous papilloma of the conjunctiva is a benign neoplasm associated with human papilloma virus infection of the conjunctival mucosa (17,36,60,67). It occurs most commonly in children and young adults and has a soft consistency. The surface is irregular, cauliflower-like, and a peduncle is frequently present. In dark-skinned individuals, the presence of melanin within the lesion may lead the clinician to suspect a melanoma. Microscopically, finger-like projections are characterized by a vascularized connective tissue stalk covered by squamous epithelium containing a variable number of goblet cells (Fig. 1).

In a few patients, conjunctival papilloma tends to be multiple and recurrent, but despite the common recurrences, malignant potential is low. On occasion, recurrent conjunctival papilloma can cause nasolacrimal duct obstruction (24,36).

An unusual subtype is the inverted papilloma (15,63). The juxtalimbal area, the plica semilunaris, the caruncle, or the tarsal conjunctiva may be involved. The squamous epithelium undergoes acanthosis and invaginates in the underlying connective tissue without evidence of keratinization or inflammation. Initially the invaginations appear cystic, but solid lobules develop secondarily and mucus-producing goblet cells are scattered throughout. The lesion is benign, does not exhibit local aggressive growth, and does not involve extensive segments of the conjunctival epithelium. Thus, it is distinct from its counterpart in the nasal cavity and paranasal sinuses, where it frequently recurs and rarely might develop invasive carcinoma.

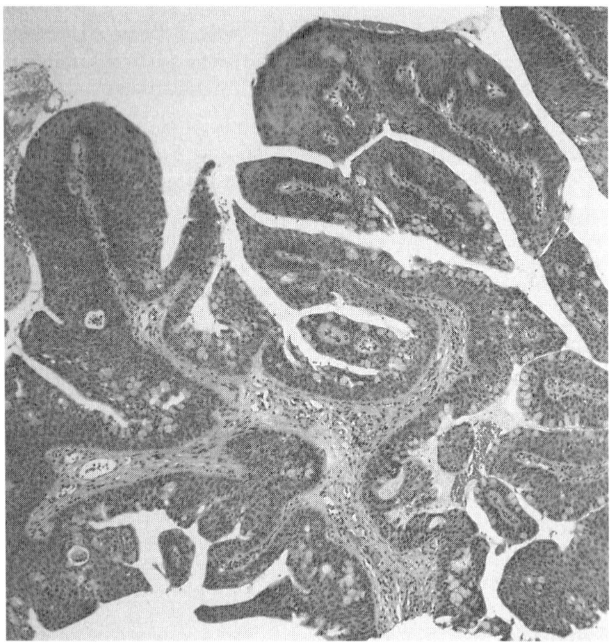

Figure 1 Squamous Papilloma. Finger-like projections lined by conjunctival squamous epithelium with interspersed goblet cells (hematoxylin and eosin, ×115).

Human papillomavirus subtypes 6, 11, 16, and 18 have been detected in association with conjunctival squamous papillomas (17,21,22,23). Immunohistochemical methods have allowed identification of papillomavirus common antigen within the epithelial cell nuclei (21,22,30,41,42,51). In situ hybridization studies have demonstrated several types of papillomavirus (9,33–35). Human papillomavirus type 6 is apparently responsible for most of the conjunctival papillomas of children and young adults (34). Human papillomavirus type 6 has also been demonstrated in a caruncular papilloma of a patient who suffered from genital warts and in the conjunctiva of a child born of a mother with genital warts (38).

Oncocytoma

Oncocytoma is a benign neoplasm that may develop in caruncle, canthal conjunctiva, and also in the lacrimal gland or lacrimal sac. It is more commonly located in the caruncle as demonstrated by Biggs and Font in a review of oncocytic lesions of the ocular adnexa (3,10). It grows slowly, and the most common clinical presentation is the presence of a mass, although epiphora has also been described in tumors involving the lacrimal sac. It occurs in middle-aged and elderly persons and is slightly more common in women (3,10,11,57).

The tumor may be solid or cystic or a combination of the two patterns. Histologically the cells are polyhedral with well-demarcated cell membranes. The nuclei are small, and the cytoplasm is deeply eosinophilic (Fig. 2). It is believed that the tumor arises from oncocytic metaplasia of ductal and acinar cells in the ocular adnexa.

Oncocytic carcinomas have been documented in the lacrimal drainage system but not in the conjunctiva (10,44,45,66). These tumors are usually locally aggressive, manifesting by multiple local recurrences. Histologically, these neoplasms are characterized by oncocytic cells with cellular pleomorphism, increased mitotic activity, and infiltrating borders. The distinction between the benign and malignant counterparts is not always easy based on morphological criteria alone.

An ultrastructural study by Freddo and Leibowitz (11) of a benign oncocytoma showed that the cells are packed with two types of mitochondria resulting in the eosinophilic granular appearance of the cytoplasm. Most of the mitochondria are very large, and the cristae show a wide variation in pattern. Transmission electron microscopic (TEM) examination used to be the only definitive diagnostic procedure until just recently, when an anti-mitochondrial anti-serum was developed by

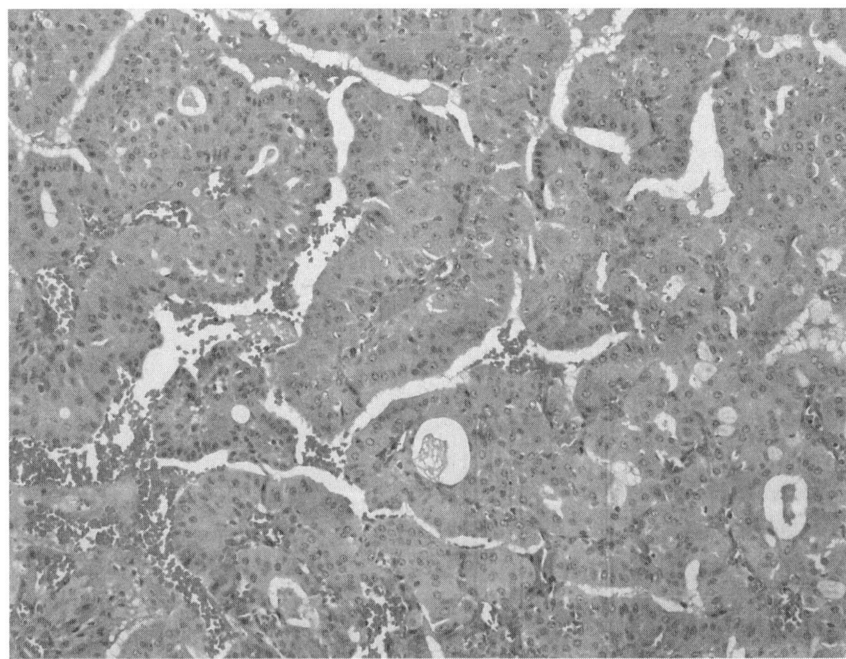

Figure 2 Oncocytoma of the caruncle. Polyhedrical cells with abundant finely granular cytoplasm, centrally placed nuclei with no atypia (hematoxylin and eosin, ×225).

Papotti and collaborators, which has allowed the demonstration of cytoplasmic mitochondria by means of immunohistochemistry (42).

Hereditary Benign Intraepithelial Dyskeratosis

Dyskeratosis refers to individual cell keratinization seen as eosinophilic intracytoplasmic bodies measuring 10 μm in diameter, and it may occur in benign keratoses, precancerous lesions, and squamous cell carcinoma (28). It is also the predominant abnormality in a rare inherited disease (autosomal dominant) known as hereditary benign intraepithelial dyskeratosis (HBID). This disorder, with lesions of the bulbar and oral mucosa, was first recognized in North Carolina and affects descendants of a triracial isolate called the Haliwa-Saponi Indians (50,58). Bilateral horseshoe-shaped plaques at the nasal and temporal aspects of the limbus are conspicuous abnormalities in HBID. The plaques, which are typified morphologically by a dyskeratotic hyperplastic epithelium, become apparent from birth or early infancy and persist throughout life, with fluctuations in thickness. These perfectly benign lesions recur after excision and may give the clinician a false impression of malignancy (50). The responsible gene has been mapped to chromosome 4 (4q35) (see Chapter 31).

Premalignant

Conjunctival Intraepithelial Neoplasia

The term conjunctival intraepithelial neoplasia (CIN) encompasses a spectrum of morphologic changes that vary from mild dysplasia to squamous cell carcinoma in situ (47,48). Because the corneal epithelium might be involved by the same process, the term ocular surface squamous neoplasia has been proposed recently (43).

Clinically lesions arise within the interpalbebral fissure, preferentially at the corneoscleral limbus, and occur most commonly in adult patients, with a male predominance (Fig. 3) (8,25,39). The incidence is higher in countries located closer to the Equator, where solar exposure is high. Solar ultraviolet radiation has been identified in many studies as a major etiologic factor (26,27,39). Human papilloma virus 16 has been demonstrated in biopsies of conjunctival intraepithelial neoplasia and it may also play an etiologic role in this process (23,34).

Similar to dysplasia described in the uterine cervix, loss of polarity and disordered maturation are observed. The degree of severity is determined by the proportional thickness of the epithelium involved; mild dysplasia (<30%), moderate dysplasia (up to 50% of the thickness) and severe dysplasia (>50%). The epithelial basal membrane remains intact. The substantia propria usually shows actinic changes (elastotic degeneration) and chronic inflammation, as changes of CIN are seen most commonly in the interpalpebral conjunctiva.

Microscopically, there is a sharp demarcation between the dysplastic and uninvolved epithelium (Fig. 4). Nuclear enlargement, pleomorphism, and mitosis are seen in the dysplastic epithelium.

The clinical appearance and degree of dysplasia do not necessarily correlate with the recurrence rate as much as does involvement of the margins of the initial

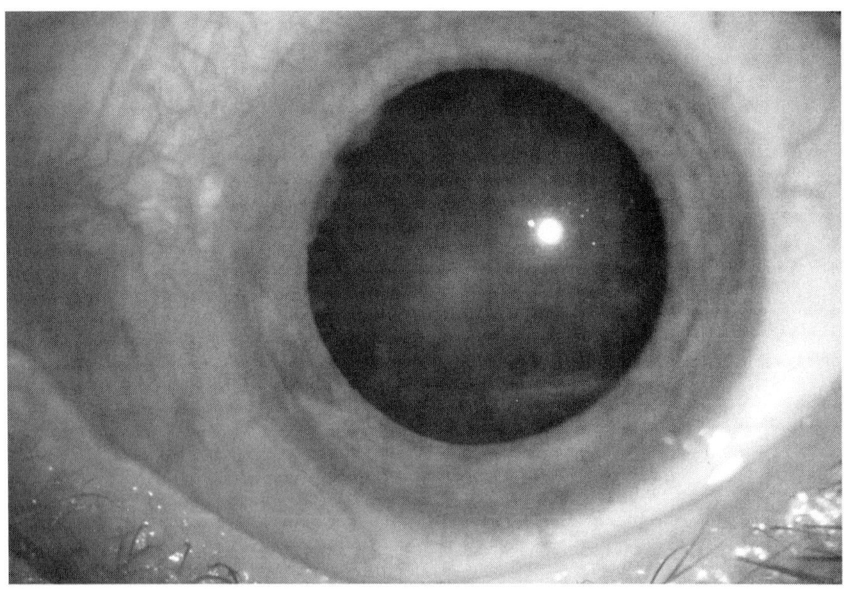

Figure 3 Conjunctival intraepithelial neoplasia. Lesion observed at the corneoscleral limbus from approximately the 9 to 11 o'clock positions.

excision (8). Erie et al. reported a 24% recurrence rate after surgical excision. Most lesions tend to recur within 2 years (8,26).

Malignant

Despite the histological similarity of malignant cutaneous and conjunctival epithelial neoplasms, their biological behavior is often different. Local recurrence is common, but metastasis is rare. The histological features of the recurrent tumor may differ from the initial growth pattern.

Epibulbar epithelial tumors tend to lie in a horizontal position in the interpalpebral fissure, the area relatively unprotected by the eyelids. They occur most often as a papillary growth with a broad base at the corneoscleral limbus, but sometimes as a single plaque of acanthotic epithelium. The tendency is toward exophytic growth, and even when the basal lamina is disrupted the tumor remains superficial, in contrast to cutaneous lesions.

An epidemiological survey imputes exposure to UV radiation as the main influence in the

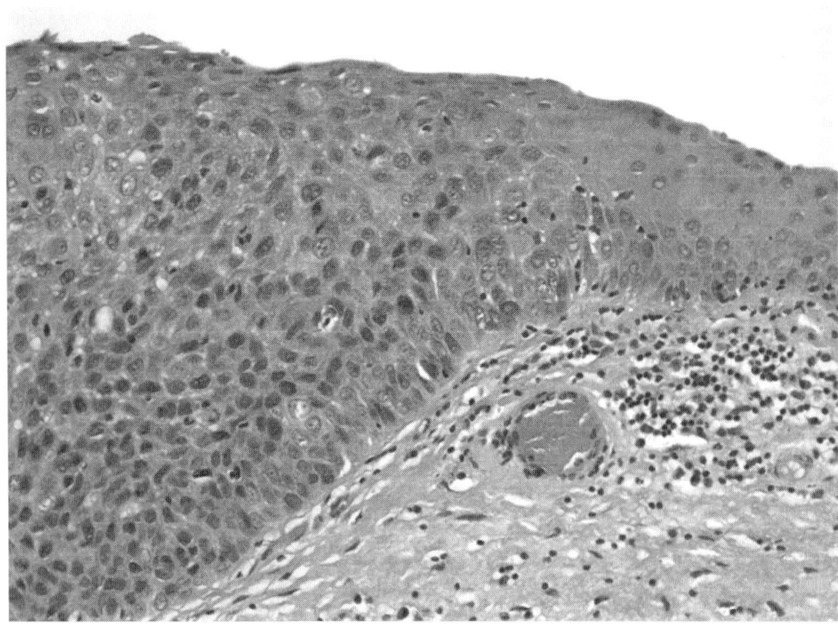

Figure 4 Conjunctival intraepithelial neoplasia. There is a sharp demarcation between the benign and the dysplastic epithelium. The epithelial basal membrane is intact (hematoxylin and eosin, ×450).

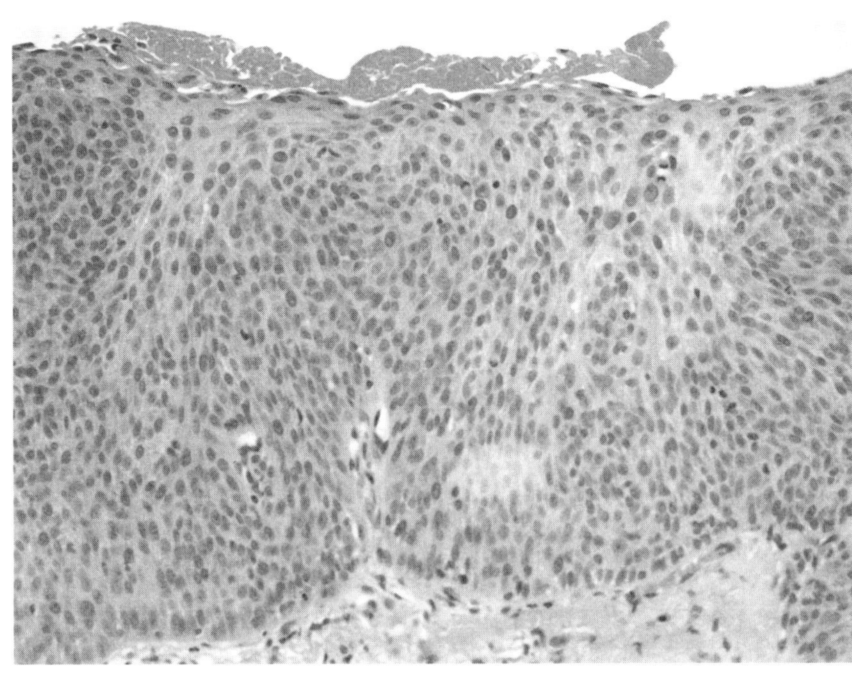

Figure 5 Squamous cell carcinoma in situ. The dysplastic cells replace the full thickness of the epithelium. The epithelial basal membrane is intact. A sharp demarcation is usually observed between the normal and dysplastic epithelium (hematoxylin and eosin, $\times$ 450).

development of squamous cell carcinoma of the conjunctiva (4,27,60,64).

In situ squamous cell carcinoma. In situ squamous cell carcinoma (SCC) of the conjunctiva occurs at the corneoscleral limbus as a firm white plaque or fleshy mass. Atypical pleomorphic squamous cells replace the entire thickness of the epithelium; with lack of maturation towards the surface. Usually the neoplastic area is sharply demarcated from the adjacent normal epithelium. The basal epithelial membrane remains intact (Fig. 5).

Invasive squamous cell carcinoma. Conjunctival SCC commonly appears exophytic, with a tendency to spread superficially onto the cornea (Fig. 6). It is often preceded by *in situ* SCC, and despite the malignant cells breaking through the basement membrane, growth usually remains superficial. The sclera and Bowman layer of the cornea are excellent barriers to invasion, and only rarely are these structures directly penetrated (6,20). This is a tumor of the later decades of life, and growth is slow and indolent. Microscopically, conjunctival SCC are usually well differentiated with keratinized areas. It is one of the least malignant forms of SCC particularly if treated early. In some countries such as Saudi Arabia, SCC of the conjunctiva appears to follow a more

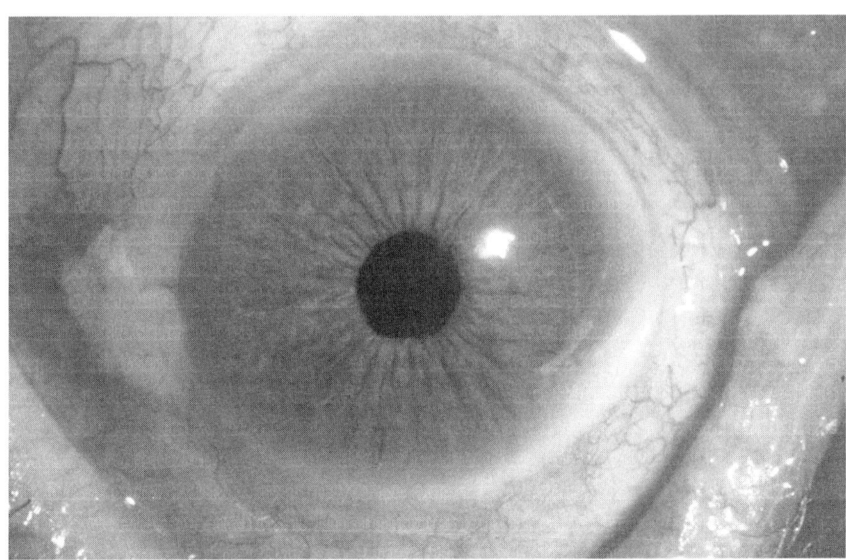

Figure 6 Invasive squamous cell carcinoma. A white, leukoplastic, lesion located at the corneoscleral limbus at the 9 o'clock position.

aggressive course and metastasizes widely (65). Rarely this tumor may masquerade as orbital cellulitis (52) or necrotizing scleritis (18,29).

Pigmentation may be a feature and cause confusion with malignant melanoma, both clinically and histologically. Such cases have been reported in patients of color, who normally have conjunctival melanocytes, but dark-skinned Caucasians can also be affected. Ultrastructural studies have demonstrated the presence of melanosomes within squamous cells as well as Langerhans cells, melanocytes, and macrophages (53). It is important to distinguish pigmented SCC from melanoma, a neoplasm with a more ominous prognosis (16,19,61).

Metastasis of conjunctival SCC is extremely unusual (2,14,65). The pre-auricular and cervical lymph nodes are sites initially involved, followed by lungs and bones. Intra-ocular invasion, although rare, may also occur (6,54).

Spindle cell carcinoma. Spindle cell carcinoma is a variant of SCC well-known in many locations such as the larynx and the lung, but rather rare in the conjunctiva (5,13,40,68). It may appear as a single nodule or a diffuse growth; a few cases have presented in phthisical or atrophic eyes (13,40). This tumor is characterized by spindle-shaped cells in continuity with an overlying normal or dysplastic epithelium. The epithelial origin of the tumor can be readily established by TEM and by immunohistochemical positivity with anti-keratin antibodies (13,39).

As in other sites, this neoplasm has an aggressive behavior and invades early the adjacent ocular tissues, eventually requiring enucleation. Metastatic spread to regional lymph nodes may also occur.

Mucoepidermoid carcinoma. As an entity, the mucoepidermoid carcinoma is most common in the salivary glands of both children and adults. Its occurrence in the conjunctiva is rare. It was first described at this site in a review of five patients by Rao and Font (49) and since then an additional nine cases have since been recorded (7,12,31,32,55).

Clinically, mucoepidermoid carcinoma may be indistinguishable from SCC (12). The tumor usually occurs in elderly persons in the seventh decade of life, but it may present as early as the fourth decade (7,31). The most common presenting manifestations are a conjunctival mass arising at the corneoscleral limbus accompanied by redness and irritation, but tumor may also occur in the lower fornix (49) and caruncle (32). In addition, it may present as a diffuse limbal thickening or as a quiescent corneoscleral ulcer (7). Histologically, the appearance is distinctive and the mucus-secreting cells can be demonstrated with the appropriate stains. Mucin production may be confined to a small portion of the tumor, and in one patient this feature was seen for the first time in the recurrent lesion (55). Stains such as mucicarmine, alcian-blue, and the Hale colloidal iron technique may be needed to highlight the mucin-producing cells (12,31,49,55).

Tumor growth is aggressive, and recurrence following excision is common. Distinction from SCC is of practical importance because of the marked difference in behavior between these two tumors.

EPITHELIAL CYSTS

Epithelial cysts of the conjunctiva are common and although they can be congenital, these are usually acquired, as a result of epithelial implantation due to trauma, inflammation or previous surgical procedures in the area. These implantation cysts are lined by conjunctival epithelium and contain clear fluid from the goblet cell secretion. Intrastromal cysts rarely occur in the cornea (1,51), but intra-epithelial microcysts are common (see Chapter 32). Corneal cysts mainly occur in childhood and are congenital or traumatic in origin. Corneal cysts have been documented after cataract surgery, lamellar keratoplasty, and squint surgery. Regardless of the cause all stromal cyst in the cornea seem to result from a displacement of epithelial cells into the corneal stroma (1).

REFERENCES

1. Bhatt PR, Ramaesh K. Intrastromal corneal limbal epithelial implantation cyst. Eye 2007; 21:133–5.
2. Bhattacharyya N, Wenokur RK, Rubin PAD. Metastasis of squamous cell carcinoma of the conjunctiva: case report and review of the literature. Am J Otolaryngol 1997; 18: 217–9.
3. Biggs SL, Font RL. Oncocytic lesions of the caruncle and other ocular adnexae. Arch Ophthalmol 1977; 95:474–8.
4. Clear AS, Chirambo MC, Hutt MSR. Solar keratosis, pterygium, and squamous cell carcinoma in Malawi. Br J Ophthalmol 1979; 63:102–9.
5. Cohen BH, Green WR, Iliff NT, et al. Spindle cell carcinoma of the conjunctiva. Arch Ophthalmol 1980; 98: 1809–13.
6. De Felice GP, Viale G, Caroli R. Deeply invasive squamous cell carcinoma of the conjunctiva: case report. Int Ophthalmol 1990; 74:241–4.
7. Dhermy P, Pouliquen Y, Haye C, Parent A. Carcinome muco-epidermoide de la conjunctive: etude clinique, histologique et ultrastructurale. J Fr Ophthalmol 1983; 6: 553–63.
8. Erie JC, Campbell RJ, Leisegang TJ. Conjunctival and corneal intraepithelial and invasive neoplasia. Ophthalmology 1986; 93:176–83.
9. Fierlbeck G, Rassner G, Thiel HJ, Pfister H. Virusinduziertes Papillom der Bindehaut. Nachweis von HPA 6a DNA. Z Hautkr 1990; 65:497–9.

10. Font RL. Eyelids and lacrimal drainage system. In: Ophthalmic Pathology. An Atlas and Textbook. 4th ed, Vol. 4, Chapter 11, 1996; 241–2420.
11. Freddo TF, Leibowitz HM. Oncocytoma of the caruncle: a case report and ultrastructural study. Cornea 1991; 10:175–82.
12. Gamel JW, Eiferman RA, Guibor P. Mucoepidermoid carcinoma of the conjunctiva. Arch Ophthalmol 1984; 102:730–1.
13. Huntington AC, Langloss JM, Hidayat AA. Spindle cell carcinoma of the conjunctiva: an immuno-histochemical and ultrastructural study of six cases. Ophthalmology 1990; 97:711–7.
14. Illif WJ, Marback R, Green WR. Invasive squamous cell carcinoma of the conjunctiva. Arch Ophthalmol 1975; 93: 119–22.
15. Jakobiec FA, Harrison W, Aronian D. Inverted mucoepidermoid papillomas of the epibulbar conjunctiva. Ophthalmology 1987; 94:283–7.
16. Jauregui HO, Klintworth GK. Pigmented squamous cell carcinoma of the cornea and conjunctiva: a light microscopic, histochemical and ultrastructural study. Cancer 1976; 38:778–88.
17. Karcioglu ZA, Issa TM. Human papilloma virus in neoplastic and non-neoplastic conditions of the external eye. Br J Ophthalmol 1997; 81:595–8.
18. Kim RY, Seiff SR, Howes EL, Jr, O'Donnell JJ. Necrotizing scleritis secondary to conjunctival squamous cell carcinoma in acquired immunodeficiency syndrome. Am J Ophthalmol 1990; 109:231–3.
19. Kremer I, Sandback J, Weinberger D, et al. Pigmented epithelial tumors of the conjunctiva. Br J Ophthalmol 1992; 76:294–6.
20. Ku E, Avendano J. Intraocular extension of a squamous cell carcinoma of the conjunctiva. Rev Oftalmol 1986; 7: 35–9.
21. Lass JH, Grove AS, Papale JJ, Albert, DM. Detection of human papillomavirus DNA sequences in conjunctival papilloma. Am J Ophthalmol 1983; 96:670–4.
22. Lass JH, Jenson AB, Papale JJ, Albert DM. Papillomavirus in human conjunctival papillomas. Am J Ophthalmol 1983; 95:364–8.
23. Lauer SA. Recurrent conjunctival papilloma causing nasolacrimal duct obstruction (letter). Am J Ophthalmol 1990; 110:580–1.
24. Lauer SA, Malter JS, Meier, JR. Human papillomavirus type 18 in conjunctival intraepithelial neoplasia. Am J Ophthalmol 1990; 110:23–7.
25. Lee GA, Hirst LW. Incidence of ocular surface epithelial dysplasia in metropolitan Brisbane: a ten-year survey. Arch Ophthalmol 1992; 110:525–7.
26. Lee GA, Hirst LW. Retrospective study of ocular surface squamous neoplasia. Aust N Z J Ophthalmol 1997; 25: 269–76.
27. Lee GA, Williams G, Hirst LW Green AC. Risk factors in the development of ocular surface epithelial dysplasia. Ophthalmology 1994; 110:525–7.
28. Lever WF, Schaumburg-Lever G. Histopathology of the Skin. 7th ed. Philadelphia: J.B. Lippincott, 1990.
29. Lindenmuth KA, Sugar A, Kincaid MC, et al. Invasive squamous cell carcinoma of the conjunctiva presenting as necrotizing scleritis with scleral perforation and uveal prolapse. Surv Ophthalmol 1988; 33:50–4.
30. Mantyjarvi J, Syrjanen S, Kaipiainen S, et al. Detection of human papillomavirus type 11 DNA in a conjunctival squamous cell papilloma by in situ hybridization with biotinylated probes. Ada Ophthalmol (Copenh.) 1989; 67: 425–9.
31. Margo CE, Groden LR. Intraepithelial neoplasia of the conjunctiva with mucoepidermoid differentiation. Am J Ophthalmol 1989; 108:600–1.
32. Margo CE, Weitzenkorn DE. Mucoepidermoid carcinoma of the conjunctiva: report of a case in a 36-year-old with paranasal sinus invasion. Ophthalmic Surg 1986; 17: 151–4.
33. McDonnell JM, Mayr AJ, Martin WJ. DNA of human papillomavirus type 16 in dysplastic and malignant lesions of the conjunctiva and cornea. N Engl J Med 1989; 320: 1442–6.
34. McDonnell JM, McDonnell PJ, Mounts P, et al. Demonstration of papillomavirus capsid antigen in human conjunctival neoplasia. Arch Ophthalmol 1986; 104: 1801–5.
35. McDonnell PJ, McDonnell JM, Kessis T, et al. Detection of human papillomavirus type 6/11 DNA in conjunctival papillomas by in situ hybridization with radioactive probes. Hum Pathol 1987; 18:1115–9.
36. Migliori ME, Putterman AM. Recurrent conjunctival papilloma causing nasolacrimal duct obstruction. Am J Ophthalmol 1990; 110:17–22.
37. Mizuno K. Squamous cell carcinoma of cornea. Arch Ophthalmol 165; 74;807–8.
38. Naghashfar Z, McDonnell PJ, McDonnell JM, et al. Genital tract papillomavirus type 6 in recurrent conjunctival papilloma. Arch Ophthalmol 1986; 104:1814–5.
39. Newton R, Ferlay J, Reeves G, et al. Effect of ambient solar ultraviolet radiation on incidence of squamous cell carcinoma of the eye. Lancet 1996; 347:1450–1.
40. Ni C, Guo B-K. Histological types of spindle cell carcinoma of the cornea and conjunctiva: A clinicopathologic report of 8 patients with ultrastructural and immunohistochemical findings in three tumors. Clin Med J 1990; 103:915–20.
41. Odrich MG, Jakobiec FA, Lancaster WD, et al. A spectrum of bilateral squamous conjunctival tumors associated with human papillomavirus type 16. Ophthalmology 1991; 98: 628–35.
42. Papotti M, Gigliotta P, Forte G, Bussolati G. Immunocytochemical identification of oxyphilic mitochondrion-rich cells. Appl Immunohist 1994; 2:261–7.
43. Pe'er J. Ocular surface squamous neoplasia. Ophthalmol Clin N Am 2005; 18:1–13.
44. Peretz WL, Ettinghausen SE, Gray GF. Oncocytic adenocarcinoma of the lacrimal sac. Arch Ophthalmol 1978; 96:303–4.
45. Perlam JI, Specht CS, McLean IW, Wolfe SA. Oncocytic adenocarcinoma of the lacrimal sac: report of a case with paranasal sinus and orbital extension. Ophthalmic Surg 1995; 26:377–37.
46. Pfister H, Fuchs RG, Volcker HE. Human papillomavirus DNA in conjunctival papilloma. Graefes Arch Clin Exp Ophthalmol 1985; 223:164–7.
47. Pierse D, Steele AD McG, Garner A, Tripathi RC. Intraepithelial carcinoma ("Bowen's disease") of the cornea. Br J Ophthalmol 1971; 55:664–70.
48. Pizzarello LD, Jakobiec EA. Bowen's disease of the conjunctiva: a misnomer. In: Jakobiec EA ed. Ocular and Adnexal Tumors. Birmingham, AL: Aesculapius Publishing, 1978:553–71.
49. Rao NA, Font RL. Mucoepidermoid carcinoma of the conjunctiva: a clinicopathologic study of five cases. Cancer 1976; 38:1699–709.
50. Reed JW, Cashwell LF, Klintworth GK. Corneal manifestations of hereditary benign intraepithelial dyskeratosis. Arch Ophthalmol 1979; 97:297–300.
51. Reed JW, Dohlman CH. Corneal cysts: a report of eight cases. Arch Ophthalmol 1971; 86:648–52.

52. Rootman J, Roth AM, Crawford JB, Fox LP, Patel S. Extensive squamous cell carcinoma of the conjunctiva presenting as orbital cellulitis: the hermit syndrome. Can J Ophthalmol 1987; 22:40–4.
53. Salisbury JA, Szpak CA, Klintworth GK. Pigmented squamous cell carcinoma of the conjunctiva: a clinicopathologic ultrastructural study. Ophthalmology 1983; 90: 1477–81.
54. Schlote T, Mielke J, Rohrback JM. Massive intraocular invasion of the conjunctiva by squamous cell carcinoma: a case report. Klin Monasbl Augenheilkd 2001; 218: 518–21.
55. Searl SS, Krigstein HJ, Albert DM, Grove AS Jr. Invasive squamous cell carcinoma with intraocular mucoepidermoid features: conjunctival carcinoma with intraocular invasion and diphasic morphology. Arch Ophthalmol 1982; 100:109–11.
56. Shields CL, Shields JA. Tumors of the conjunctiva and cornea. Survey of Ophthalmology 2004; 49:3–24.
57. Shields CL, Shields JA, Arbizo V. Oncocytoma of the caruncle. Am J Ophthalmol 1986; 102:315–9.
58. Shields CL, Shields JA, Eagle RC. Hereditary benign intraepithelial dyskeratosis. Arch Ophthalmol 1987; 105: 422–3.
59. Shields JA, Shields CL. Pediatric ocular and periocular tumors. Pediatr Ann 2001; 30:491–501.
60. Shields JA, Shields CL. Tumors and pseudotumors of the conjunctiva. In: Shields JA, Shields CL, eds. Atlas of Eyelid and Conjunctival Tumors. Philadelphia: Lippincott Williams and Wilkins Co., 1999:199–334.
61. Shields JA, Shields CL, Eagle RC Jr et al. Pigmented conjunctival squamous cell carcinoma simulating a conjunctival melanoma. Am J Ophthalmol 2001; 132:104–6.
62. Sjo NC, Heegaard S, Prause JU et al. Human papilloma virus in conjunctival papilloma. Br J Ophthalmol 2001; 85: 785–7.
63. Streeten BW, Carrillo R, Jamison R, et al. L.E. Inverted papilloma of the conjunctiva. Am J Ophthalmol 1979; 88: 1062–6.
64. Sun EC, Fears TR, Goedert JJ. Epidemiology of squamous cell conjunctival cancer. Cancer Epidemiol Biomarkers Prev 1997; 6:73–7.
65. Tabbara KF, Kersten R, Daouk N, Blodi EC. Metastatic squamous cell carcinoma of the conjunctiva. Ophthalmology 1988; 95:318–21.
66. Tomic S, Warner TF, Brandenburg JH. Malignant oncocytoma of the lacrimal sac: ultrastructure and immunocytochemistry. Ear Nose Throat J 1995; 74:717–20.
67. Vadot E, Merignargues G. Papillomes conjonctivaux et papillomavirus. Bull Soc Ophthalmol Fr 1990; 90:789–90.
68. Wise AC. A limbal spindle-cell carcinoma. Surv Ophthalmol 1967; 12:244–6.

58

Intraocular Epithelial Tumors and Cysts

Thomas J. Cummings
Departments of Pathology and Ophthalmology, Duke University, Durham, North Carolina, U.S.A.

INTRODUCTION

Neuroepithelial tumors of the eye are rare and typically occur in the ciliary body but can also involve the iris and retina. They may be congenital or acquired. Congenital tumors include medulloepitheliomas and glioneuromas, while acquired tumors include adenomas and adenocarcinomas. The congenital tumors typically involve the nonpigment ciliary epithelium (NPCE), whereas the acquired tumors involve the ciliary pigment epithelium (CPE), the NPCE, the retinal pigment epithelium (RPE), and the iris pigment epithelium (IPE).

Embryologically, the outer layer of the optic cup gives rise to the IPE, CPE, and RPE. Lesions of these pigment epithelia are capable of being misdiagnosed as melanocytomas or uveal melanomas. Although the pigment epithelia of the retina, ciliary body, and iris share a common embryological origin and are prone to considerable hyperplastic reactions in response to various stimuli, their neoplastic proclivities are surprisingly limited, and in some cases the histological distinction between a hyperplastic reaction and a neoplastic proliferation is not always possible. Anterior to the ora serrata of the retina the neuroepithelium of the developing eye gives rise to the NPCE.

TUMORS OF THE NONPIGMENTED CILIARY EPITHELIUM

Medulloepithelioma

Overview

Medulloepitheliomas are uncommon neuroepithelial tumors believed to arise during embryonic development of the immature (primitive medullary) NPCE (3,12,125). Two types of medulloepithelioma are recognized: teratoid and nonteratoid. Rarely they arise from remaining embryonic retina in the posterior part of the sensory retina or in the optic nerve (28,34,37,69,71,113). In contrast to medulloepithelioma, the hyperplastic and the neoplastic ciliary epithelial lesions of adults often include the participation of the pigment epithelial elements, although in some cases it may be difficult to ascertain from which layer the tumor has originated.

The first description of a medulloepithelioma of the ciliary body is believed to have been by Badal and Lagrange in 1892 using the name *carcinome primitif* (6). In 1904 Verhoeff proposed the term "teratoneuroma" for a case which he described histologically and differentiated from retinoblastoma (117). The alternative designation "diktyoma" (Greek: diktyon, a net) was suggested by Fuchs because of the net-like character of the neuroepithelial bands that extend into the adjacent cavities of the eye (31). The designation "medulloepithelioma" was preferred by the World Health Organization (WHO) ocular tumor panel (126). They are further classified as teratoid if they contain heterologous elements such as skeletal muscle or cartilage, and nonteratoid if they are devoid of such elements.

Clinical Features

Medulloepitheliomas of the ciliary body usually occur in young children with a median age of approximately 5-years (4,12,17,106,114) Medulloepitheliomas in adults are exceptional (18,28,39,46,54). Generally, both eyes are equally affected, with no apparent gender or racial predilection, and the majority of cases are unilateral (4,64,80,114). Cases that present in adults may give rise to diagnostic confusion with malignant melanoma (18,26,39). These tumors frequently recur after surgery as the tumor cells may grow as a thin sheet on the surface of ocular structures including the retina (28) and associated fibrovascular cyclitic membranes (49,88).

Patients may experience pain, poor vision, hemorrhage or scleral perforation (12,55). Glaucoma and cataract are frequently associated. Irregularity and dilatation of the pupil are recorded in some cases, but colobomas of the iris have not been documented in a true medulloepithelioma (49).

A rare medulloepithelioma has been noted in the ciliary body many years after a retinoblastoma (68). Iris neovascularization, especially in children, may be an early manifestation of medulloepithelioma (12,98). Rare cases have apparently arisen in a persistent Bergmeister papilla, and persistent hyperplastic primary vitreous is reported as concomitant in 20% of cases (69). No relationship with neoplasms or malformations of other tissues or organs is usually demonstrated although, because of the well-established association of pineal tumors with retinoblastomas, it is noteworthy that a benign teratoid medulloepithelioma has been documented with a pineoblastoma (60).

Histopathology

Gross Appearance

Grossly, medulloepitheliomas may appear as flat white or gray masses in the ciliary body or retina. Rare cases are pigment (33,88). They tend to spread over the iris, crystalline lens, and posterior surface of the cornea. Although of slowly progressive growth, they may ultimately fill the eye with net-like extensions and infiltrate the iris and even perforate the globe through the sclera.

Microscopic Appearance

When examined by light microscopy, medulloepitheliomas are characterized architecturally by convoluted cords and ribbons of multilayered undifferentiated neoplastic cells that enclose lumina of variable shape and size mimicking the primitive neural tube (Fig. 1). The cells resemble the primitive medullary epithelium of the brain, early embryonic retina, and immature ciliary epithelium (117). The inner free surface is bounded by a limiting membrane, but at the opposite side the cells rest on a tenuous supporting stroma. Multilayered sheets of poorly differentiated neuroepithelial cells resembling the primary medullary epithelium of the optic cup are the most noticeable component of the nonteratoid form, presenting in two-thirds of cases (14,38,39,87,113). Tubular and papillary structures composed of a single-layer of cuboidal cells resembling more differentiated ciliary epithelium are also formed, often with gradual transitions between these two components (Fig. 2). The sheets of medullary epithelium are polarized, forming along one surface tissue that resembles the myxoid connective tissue of the primary vitreous and along the opposite surface a structure analogous to the external limiting membrane of the retina. When the multilayered tubular structures are cut transversely, they may appear as rosettes resembling to a certain extent Flexner–Wintersteiner rosettes of retinoblastoma, or Homer-Wright pseudorosettes similar to retinal anlage and neuroectodermal tumors elsewhere (4). When the single-layered tubules are cut transversely, they may also resemble the adenoid structures of the adult-type tumors of the differentiated ciliary epithelium. The proliferating medullary epithelium may form anastomosing cords and sheets separated by loose tissue, giving these tumors a net-like appearance, hence the old term "diktyoma." Heterologous elements that define the teratoid medulloepithelioma are lacking.

Usually, the folding of the medullary epithelium occurs in such a way that the lumen of the resulting rosette or tubule is empty, lined by a surface with zonulae adherentes corresponding to the external limiting membrane, and it is here that the mitotic

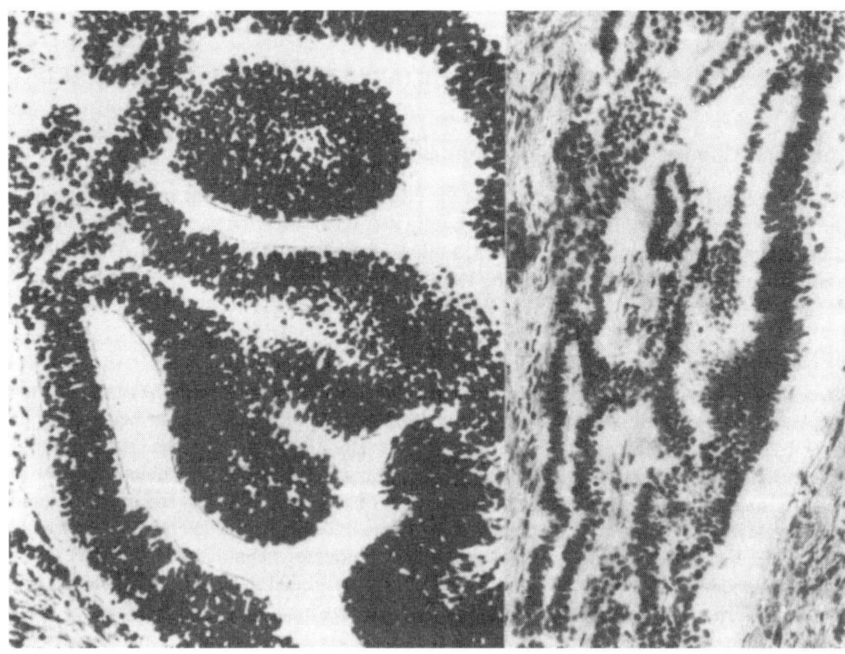

Figure 1 Nonteratoid medulloepithelioma from posterior retina and optic nerve. Multilayered membranes on left, single-layered on the right (hematoxylin and eosin, × 130). *Source*: Courtesy of the late Dr. S. Ry Anderson.

activity is most marked. This mitotic activity may be entirely appropriate, since in the developing retina, which this tumor mimics, mitoses of all cells of the neuroblastic retina occurs adjacent to the external (outer) limiting membrane. Confusion with the rosettes of retinoblastoma is usually avoidable since in medulloepithelioma a stromal component is almost always found, whereas in retinoblastoma there is no true stroma, the connective tissue being confined to the perivascular supporting tissues (12). The loose tissue surrounding the rosettes and tubules resembles primitive vitreous and stains intensely for glycosaminoglycans (GAGs) sensitive to bovine testicular and streptococcal hyaluronidase (127).

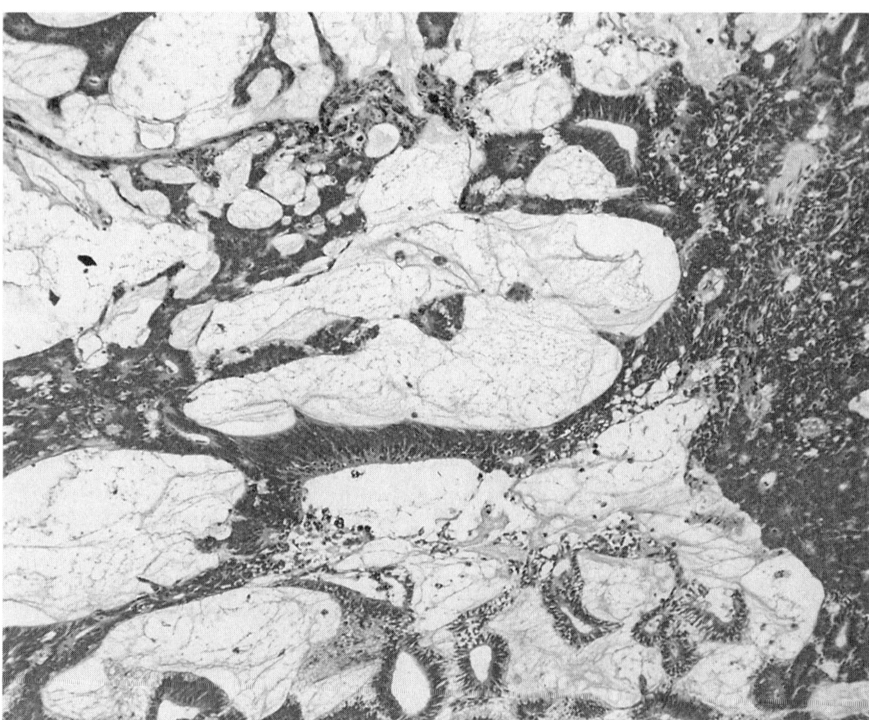

Figure 2 Nonteratoid medulloepithelioma showing a net-like appearance of epithelium including rosettes and tubules (hematoxylin and eosin, ×11).

In a few cases, free-floating cysts filled with hyaluronic acid occur in the anterior or posterior chambers. Differentiation into astrocytes and some formation of pigment epithelium is commonly observed.

The multilayered tubular structures, which have been described as neuroepithelial sheaths, stain positively for neuron-specific enolase, vimentin, S100 protein, glial fibrillary acid protein (GFAP), neurofilament protein and cytokeratins AE1/AE3 and CAM5.2 (39,49,113). In some cases photoreceptor differentiation has been detected (21). Transmission electron microscopy (TEM) studies support the primitive character of this neoplasm and attributes of embryonal retinal and ciliary epithelium, with the development, in places, of structures akin to neurons, nerve fibers, and primitive neuroepithelium (43,113). Cilia remnants and three types of rosettes have been described (41,43), and in another case the lumina of the rosettes were shown to contain microvilli (72).

The teratoid medulloepithelioma is a tumor with all the foregoing characteristics but in addition contains heteroplastic tissues not normally found during either embryonic or postnatal development of the eye: mature hyaline cartilage or chondroblasts (Fig. 3), rhabdomyoblasts, and cerebral tissue, including specialized central nervous system (CNS) structures such as ganglion cells (Figs. 4 and 5), ependyma or choroid plexus (12,55,87,102,124–127). Ganglion cells are normal constituents of the retina, however, and as such probably should not be regarded as unusual within a medulloepithelioma. The heteroplastic elements may be inconspicuous, with only tiny islands of hyaline cartilage or occasional rhabdomyoblasts, sometimes in the form of strap cells with cross-striations (Fig. 6). Rarely, the tumor may resemble a rhabdomyosarcoma (128).

In other cases the tumors are composed largely of mesenchymal tissue elements, such as chondroblastic or rhabdomyosarcomatous tissue. In the teratoid medulloepitheliomas the mature mesenchymal heteroplastic tissues, such as hyaline cartilage and well-differentiated cross-striated rhabdomyoblasts, may be explained as metaplasia of the stromal elements of these tumors. Hyaline cartilage is often present in trisomy 13 and other chromosomal disorders and has been described in microphthalmic eyes with persistent hyperplastic primary vitreous (122). The chondroblastic and rhabdomyoblastic elements with features of malignancy in some of the teratoid forms are more difficult to explain but may reflect malignant change within mesenchymal components, ostensibly derived from neuroectoderm (18).

Since the neural crest is capable of evolving mesenchymal components, other parts of the developing neuroectoderm may retain this potential pathway of development, or alternatively the neural crest itself may contribute. Neural crest mesenchymal differentiation is postulated to give rise to other

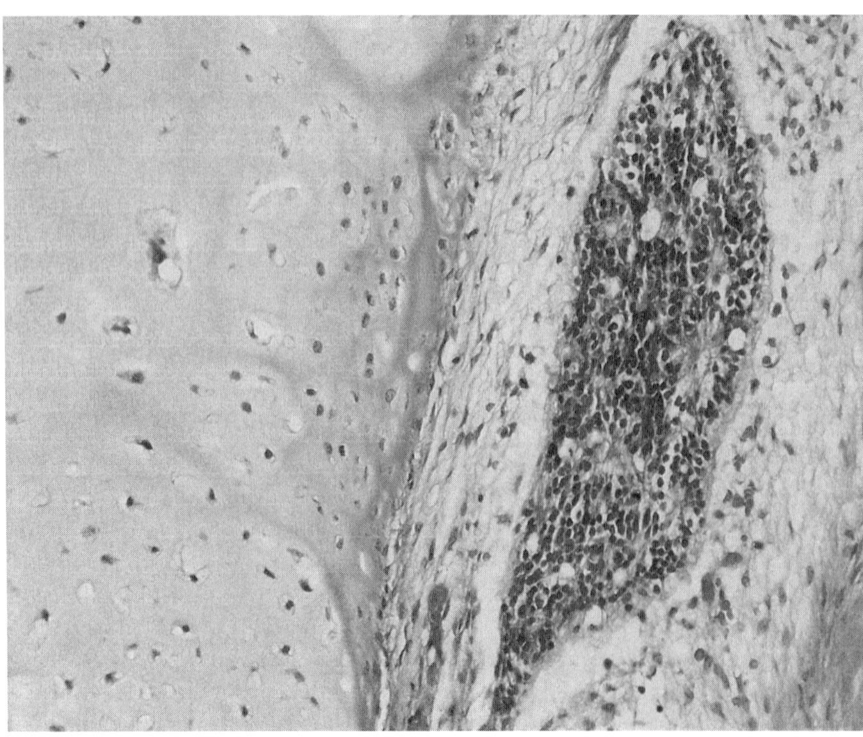

Figure 3 Teratoid medulloepithelioma containing hyaline cartilage (hematoxylin and eosin, $\times$ 23).

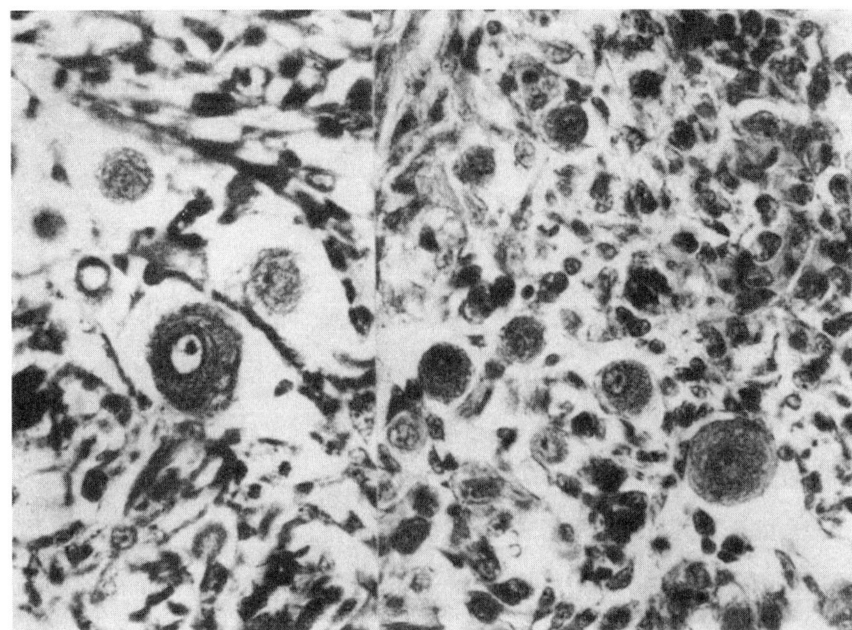

Figure 4 Ganglion cells within medulloepithelioma (hematoxylin and eosin, × 135). *Source*: Courtesy of the late Dr. S. Ry Anderson.

tumors, including smooth muscle tumors of the orbit (42), and such disorders as the neurocristopathies (11).

Histopathological Criteria for Malignancy

Distinction between benign and malignant medulloepitheliomas is difficult. Malignancy may be inferred by the presence of overtly sarcomatous or carcinomatous tissues (34), but in some reports the designation malignant has been used for tumors that are locally aggressive with an invasion of adjacent tissues. With numerous tumors elsewhere in the body this is not an absolute criterion for malignancy, and most "malignant" medulloepitheliomas have not metastasized, the "gold standard" for malignancy. An extensive literature review demonstrated only four cases with lymph node metastasis, two with parotid gland metastasis, and a single case of lung metastasis (49).

Malignant medulloepitheliomas produce solid aggregates of undifferentiated cells resembling a retinoblastoma. Sectioning through the tumor results in variations of pattern, and complex folding may produce rosettes which superficially resemble those of a retinoblastoma (64). In malignant tumors the tubules and rosettes are usually retained, but they may be only an inconspicuous component of a largely undifferentiated neuroblastic tumor with some resemblance to a retinoblastoma.

Criteria for malignancy have included numerous mitotic figures, pronounced pleomorphism, and extraocular extension and, although only one-quarter of the cases satisfied these requirements, such medulloepitheliomas should be considered potentially malignant (4,81). Broughton and Zimmerman classified two-thirds of their cases as malignant, and in addition to the criteria for malignancy just listed, they included areas of poorly differentiated neuroblastic, chondroblastic and rhabdomyoblastic cells, and invasion of the uvea, cornea, sclera, and or optic nerve (12). In their malignant group 46% of tumors were teratoid, compared to 21% in the benign group. It is noteworthy that in both these series and in a later series (17) the mortality, which was due to invasion of the brain or to distant metastases, was very low. Deaths were recorded in <10% of the combined groups, when they were usually due to local aggressive growth, including growth into the orbit and brain; some patients were lost to follow-up, however. Intractable iris neovascularization may affect the eye (17,88).

Comparison with Medulloepitheliomas of the Brain

Medulloepitheliomas of the brain are thought to derive from primitive subependymal cells. Abnormal re-expression of genes for early neural tube determinants, or neoplastic transformation at some stage of fetal or early postnatal development, are theories for their development (9,47). Clinically, they typically affect children between 6 months and 5 years of age. They occur both supratentorially and infratentorially, and are most commonly seen in a periventricular location within the cerebral hemispheres.

The clinical course is often rapid, usually causing death within 1 year. There is often cerebrospinal fluid (CSF) dissemination, but rarely systemic metastases (9). The apparently greater morbidity in the intracerebral tumors may reflect their mass effect

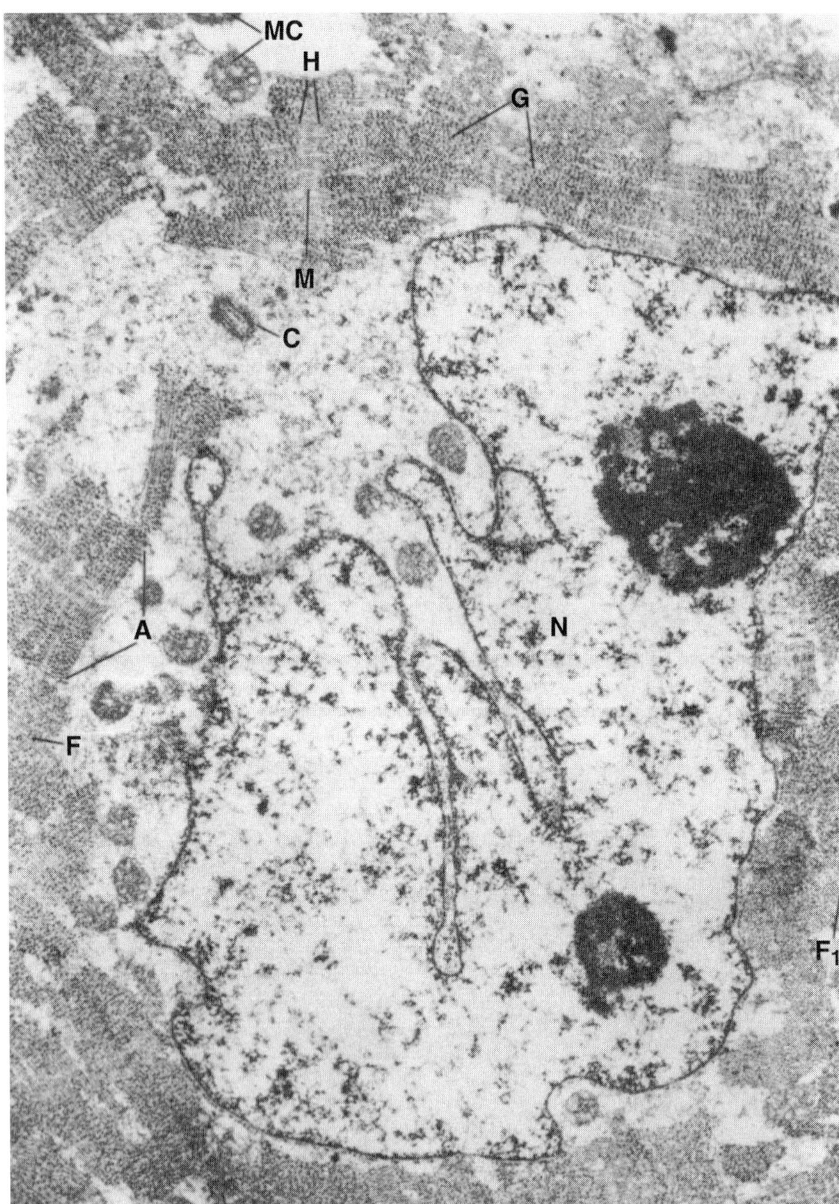

Figure 5 Ganglion-like cells in medulloepithelioma. Ganglion-like cells with numerous bundles of myofilaments, some of which are cut longitudinally (F), whereas others are seen in cross section (F_1) arranged concentrically about the nucleus (N). Several A bands (A) containing light H bands (H) with their dark central M lines (M) are present. Mitochondria (MC) are also present (transmission electron microscopy, × 16,300). *Source*: Adapted from Ref. 40. Courtesy of the late Dr. S. Ry Anderson.

within the cranial cavity and their propensity to seed along the spinal canal.

The histologic features resemble those of the primitive neural tube. Light microscopy reveals a malignant embryonal neoplasm with a distinctive pseudostratified appearance of neuroepithelium arranged in papillary, trabecular or tubular formations. There is a distinctive external limiting basement membrane on which the outer surface of the epithelium rests, and which stains with periodic acid Schiff (PAS) and a collagen type IV immunostain. These tumors may manifest a wide range of differentiation including glial, neural and mesenchymal elements. The mesenchymal components may include areas of cartilage, bone, striated muscle and vascular or fibrous connective tissue stroma. Histologically, both cerebral and intraocular medulloepitheliomas seem to mimic the primitive neural tube. Rhabdomyosarcomatous and chondroblastic elements associated with neuroepithelial elements have sometimes been described in brain tumors, and Rubinstein interpreted this as evidence of a teratomatous nature (79,116).

The four-tiered grading scheme recommended by the WHO for grading intracranial medulloepitheliomas does not include the rare intraocular and optic nerve medulloepitheliomas. Noteworthy in this regard is the generally better prognosis and less malignant behavior associated with intraocular tumors compared to the highly

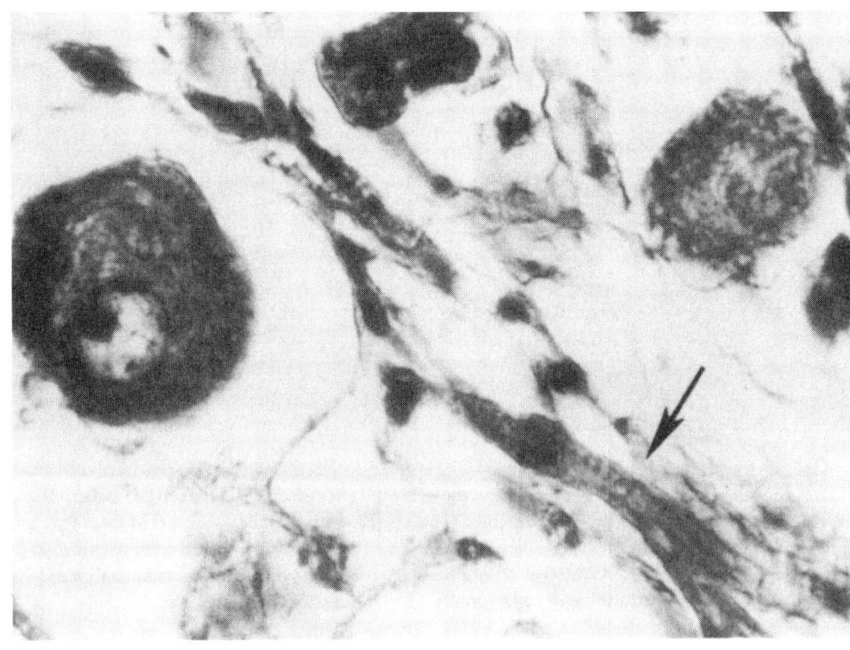

Figure 6 Malignant teratoid medulloepithelioma. Arrow points to rhabdomyoblast with cross-striations (Wilder reticulin stain, × 1,070). *Source*: Courtesy of the late Dr. S. Ry Anderson.

malignant WHO grade IV intracerebral counterparts of the same name (9).

Histogenesis

At about week 7 of human embryonic development (20 mm stage), the iridic, ciliary, and sensory part of the inner wall of the optic cup are similar in appearance, although the development of the central retina is slightly advanced relative to the periphery (see Chapter 51). The cells are arranged in ranks or rows, with an overall appearance that might be called the embryonal retina stage (5) (Fig. 7), which still resembles the medullary epithelium (Fig. 8) of the brain of which it is an outgrowth with a direct connection. In the embryo the outer layer of the optic cup at 20 mm is still partly multilayered, but melanin granules have become visible in the pigment epithelial portions of the iridic and ciliary parts as well as in the RPE. The "embryonal retina" stage disappears completely after the third embryonal month (about 60 mm) (120).

Morphologically, all ocular medulloepitheliomas seem to reflect to some extent this early embryonal retina. Even when the rosettes and tubules in these

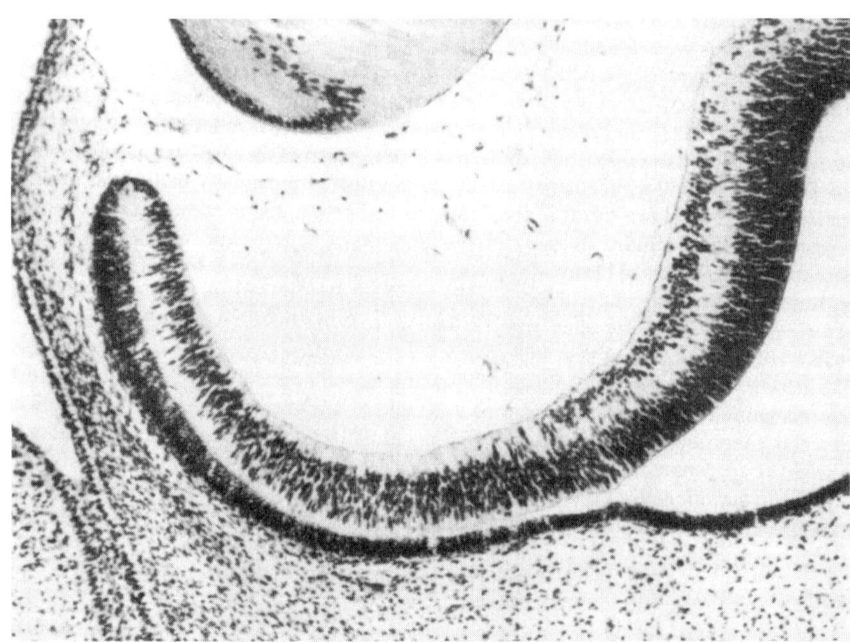

Figure 7 Anterior part of the optic cup in human fetus of 22 mm in week 7, showing multilayered undifferentiated epithelium resembling the medullary epithelium of the brain as the inner layer of the cup and pigment formation in the outer layer (hematoxylin and eosin, × 135). *Source*: Courtesy of the late Dr. S. Ry Anderson.

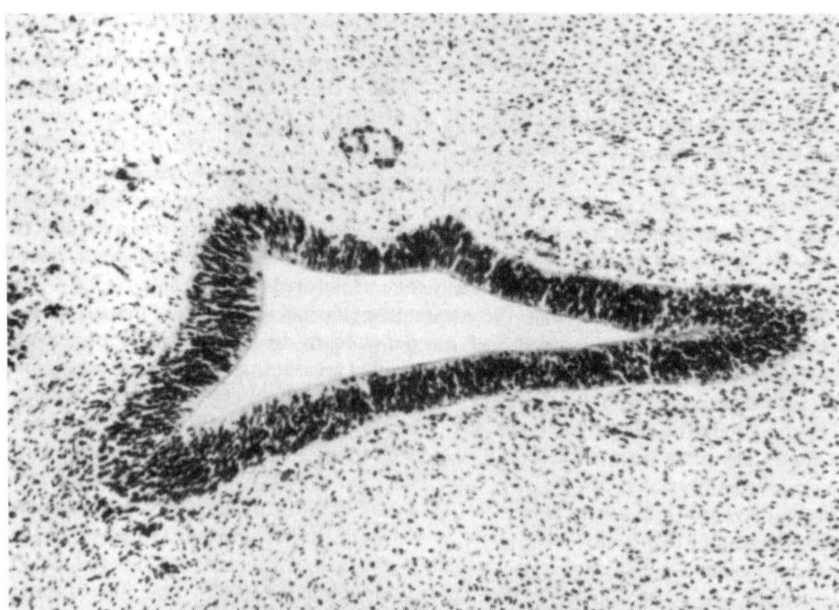

Figure 8 Undifferentiated medullary epithelium within the lateral ventricular wall of the brain of the same fetus (hematoxylin and eosin, × 135). *Source*: Courtesy of the late Dr. S. Ry Anderson.

tumors have ostensibly neoplastic features, they resemble the mitotic and developmental stages of the medullary tube. Folding and displacement of premature retinal tissue may give rise to structures that are analogous to the rosettes in other types of dysplastic retinal tissue (5), which might perhaps be more accurately described as dystrophic or distorted. In the rare cases of medulloepitheliomas presenting in adults, it is unclear whether they have been present since birth, have arisen from residual embryonic retina, or have emerged as a result of dedifferentiation. The single-layered tubules, which are almost ubiquitous in medulloepitheliomas, resemble more differentiated ciliary epithelium rather than the mature ependymal layer.

The medullary neuroectodermal epithelium of the optic vesicle gives rise to a remarkable variety of tissues, including photoreceptors, neurons, neuroglia, pigment and nonpigment epithelia, the vitreous body, and the involuntary smooth muscles of the iris and ciliary body. The medulloepitheliomas of the eye are further evidence of the pluripotentiality of this epithelium.

Glioneuroma

Glioneuroma is an extremely rare benign tumor resembling brain tissue and containing ganglion cells and axons as well as neuroglia arising in a malformed sector of the optic cup (2,48,61,100). Glioneuromas are usually discovered during childhood and typically involve the iris and ciliary body (2,48).

Histologically, they are characterized by a loose aggregate of well-differentiated glial and neuronal elements. Adenoid nonpigment tubules seem to imitate the single-layered adult ependymal lining of the cerebral ventricles. Structures resembling the embryonic retina or ciliary epithelium are not observed in glioneuroma. A rare glioneuroma involving the anterior retina, temporal iris, and ciliary body clinically resembling a medulloepithelioma was associated with colobomatous dysplasia of the anterior uvea and retina (48).

The glial component of these tumors exhibit immunoreactivity for GFAP, vimentin, and S100 protein, and the neuronal component displays immunoreactivity for neuron-specific enolase, synaptophysin, and neurofilaments (48).

ADENOMAS AND ADENOCARCINOMAS OF THE NONPIGMENTED CILIARY EPITHELIUM

Overview

The NPCE is rarely the site of the acquired neoplastic entities of adenoma and adenocarcinoma. Patients are usually in the fifth decade. In one study (5) the mean age was 43 years with a range of 1.5–82 years and with no difference in incidence between the sexes. Tumors are usually solitary and unilateral, and without associated tumors or malformations in other tissues. There is no apparent racial or genetic predisposition.

Clinical Features

Frequent presenting manifestations are recognition of a mass arising from the iris or ciliary body, decreased visual acuity, signs of intraocular inflammation, secondary cataract and lens subluxation (65,85,86). Less frequently cases present with glaucoma or a congenital coloboma of the iris. Some tumors develop in eyes that have been blind for many years as a result of traumatic injury. They transmit light well during transillumination, and with ultrasonography they demonstrate high internal reflectivity (86). Clinically they rarely mimic malignant melanoma of the iris (104). They portend a fair visual prognosis and exhibit a very low rate or recurrence and metastasis (86).

Histopathology

On gross examination, adenomas most often present as a variably pigment, circumscribed, round or oval solid tumor of the ciliary body and iris root, often encroaching on the lens, which may contain a localized cataract. The upper and temporal quadrants are the preferred regions. A rather uniform proliferation of cuboidal and columnar epithelial cells, similar cytologically to those of the NPCE, is seen. Larger adenomas of the NPCE display cytologic pleomorphism (5,32,35,66,112) and their histological features include mosaic, solid, tubular, and papillary patterns (112). Papillary structures or adenoid-like tubules often dominate. Adenomas do not imitate embryonal retina or show spongioblastic or neuroblastic differentiation.

The stroma is loosely organized, with many reticulin fibers in a netlike pattern and a rich content of GAGs mostly sensitive to bovine testicular hyaluronidase (in contrast to most metastatic tumors, in which the GAGs are resistant to degradation with this enzyme). The tumor cells may manifest some pleomorphism and most often some mitoses and/or invasion of adjacent structures. The pleomorphism and the delicate stroma help to distinguish the adenomas from localized hyperplasias. Invasion of the iris root, ciliary muscle, or anterior chamber-angle structures is not necessarily an indication of malignancy, because it is noticed sometimes in such nonneoplastic lesions as unequivocal hyperplasias, melanocytomas, and juvenile nevoxanthogranulomas. With immunohistochemistry, tumor cells react with antibodies to cytokeratin (such as AE1/AE3), S100 protein and vimentin, and are nonreactive to HMB45 (105).

The presence of a prominent basement membrane around the tumor cells, immunopositivity for epithelial markers, and the identification ultrastructural junctional complexes by TEM, are useful in distinguishing these tumors from sarcomas or an amelanotic melanoma, but not necessarily from metastatic carcinomas (20,36,45,51,66,70,105). In contrast to melanoma, adenoma and adenocarcinomas of the NPCE are more likely to have an irregular surface and exhibit inflammatory signs.

Histopathological Criteria for Malignancy

Differentiation between a benign adenoma and a malignant adenocarcinoma can be difficult. Andersen classified only 3 of 23 tumors as malignant, using stricter criteria of malignancy than most other investigators, including many mitoses, pronounced pleomorphism and marked invasion of the choroid, optic nerve, orbit, or facial bones (5). One of Andersen's cases metastasized to the mandible. The good prognosis in almost all published cases seems to justify the use of these strict criteria. The tumors usually follow a very slow course over many years but may in extremely rare instances become malignant and run a lethal course, especially in eyes with phthisis bulbi, in which symptoms are late and adequate examination of the eye may be impossible. The designation adenocarcinoma is applied to tumors of the NPCE that usually arise in eyes previously subjected to trauma or having longstanding inflammation. The tumors are thought to result from the neoplastic transformation of reactive ciliary epithelium (62). They can span a spectrum of well-differentiated neoplasms that resemble the ciliary epithelium to poorly differentiated sarcoma-like pleomorphic adenocarcinomas. Histologically, they are characterized by cellular pleomorphism and prominent mitotic activity. Adenocarcinomas of the ciliary epithelium can recur following excision and, widespread metastases have rarely been documented (66). They may also extend into the CNS.

Fuchs Adenoma

First described by Fuchs, this is a small, discrete, hyperplastic nodule within the nonpigment epithelium of the pars plicata of the ciliary body (31). It is observed almost exclusively as an incidental finding in eyes enucleated for other reasons. It is also a common finding in post-mortem eyes, increasing in incidence with age. They can be bilateral and multiple. Fuchs adenoma is sometimes observed in both eyes and multiple lesions may be present. Fuchs adenomas measure <1 mm in diameter and are characterized histologically by sheets and tubules of NPCE within a PAS positive matrix of basement membrane-like material (66).

ADENOMAS AND ADENOCARCINOMAS OF THE CILIARY PIGMENTED EPITHELIUM

Overview

Similar to those of the NPCE, adenomas and adenocarcinomas of the CPE are rare tumors often confused clinically with uveal melanoma (22,76,93).

Clinical Features

Adenomas and adenocarcinomas of the CPE are typically seen in adults as solitary and unilateral tumors without predilection for laterality. Patients may be asymptomatic, or may experience decreased visual acuity due to secondary cataract or lens subluxation. Clinically, these tumors exhibit abruptly elevated margins but not with a mushroom-shaped appearance. They show high internal reflectivity with A-scan ultrasonography and are acoustically solid with B-scan ultrasonography (93).

Histopathology

Histologically, the tumor appears dome shaped or pedunculated, arises from the CPE on a small base, and does not involve the ciliary body stroma. The pigmentation varies considerably, but the melanosomes are larger than those derived from the neural crest, being of the size seen in the neuroectodermally derived iris, ciliary body, and retinal pigment epithelia (63,65,93). The large pigment cells contain large, spherical melanosomes, and exhibit characteristic round or oval clear vacuoles. Tumor cells may be arranged in nodules, lobules and sheets or have a cystic appearance (53). The vacuoles contain hyaluronidase-resistant GAGs and are lined by cells with microvilli and occasional cilia (66,93). Immunoreactivity for low molecular cytokeratin, vimentin and S100 protein has been demonstrated (53).

As with tumors of the NPCE, the term adenocarcinoma has been used when worrisome histologic features such as cellular anaplasia and increased mitotic activity are present (23). A rare adenocarcinoma arising from the CPE in a child has been reported (73). Although tumors can exhibit growth, they are not thought to have metastatic potential.

ADENOMAS AND ADENOCARCINOMAS OF THE RETINAL PIGMENT EPITHELIUM

Overview

Neoplasms of the RPE tend to occur in previously normal eyes and in patients who are usually women in the fifth decade of life. These uncommon tumors are black masses similar to those found in the pigment epithelium of the ciliary body. They are usually located in the peripheral retina and rarely grow over and obscure the optic disc (89). Most tumors of the RPE are adenomas rather than adenocarcinomas (32).

Clinical Features

In one series of adenomas of the RPE the most common presenting symptom was a decrease in visual acuity, and the average duration of symptoms was 2.5 years before enucleation, the latter taking place at a mean age of 45.8 years (112). In some instances there is a history of inflammation, which raises the possibility of a preceding hyperplastic proliferation. Most neoplasms arise in otherwise normal eyes with clear media.

Histopathology

RPE neoplasms often contain abundant nonsulfated GAGs within intracytoplasmic vacuoles, which compress the melanosomes of the pigment epithelial cells (13,29). The enlarging vacuoles displace the melanosomes to the periphery, which may account in part for their dark appearance. Histological types of these tumors include regular mosaic or tubular or papillary patterns, and in addition patternless variants containing vacuolated and anaplastic cells may occur. Although reactive hyperplasia of the RPE may simulate malignancy, neoplastic RPE lesions lose their cellular polarity, manifest greater atypia, and usually form less basement membrane.

Adenomas may be difficult to distinguish histologically from the far more common reactive hyperplasia of the RPE, and the distinction between adenoma and adenocarcinoma has not been well-defined. As with tumors of the ciliary epithelium, the distinction of adenocarcinoma from adenoma of the RPE is based on degree of nuclear atypia and local invasiveness (94). Although they can exhibit aggressive clinical behavior characterized by tumor growth and visual loss, they seem to lack a tendency to metastasize (94).

Adenocarcinomas of the RPE commonly present as a melanotic intraocular tumor in women with uveitis that can be misinterpreted clinically as a choroidal melanoma. Local invasion of the retina and choroid may occur, but deaths from distant metastases have been reported (25). Compared to reactive hyperplasia and adenomas of the RPE, adenocarcinomas can be expected to display greater cytological anaplasia and increased mitotic counts (67). They can display tubular, papillary, and pleomorphic histologic patterns (Fig. 9). Melanin bleaching techniques with potassium permanganate to extinguish the melanin granules may be necessary to evaluate cytologic detail to diagnose some cases. Ultrastructural analyses disclose melanosomes, microvilli, and the presence of a basal lamina confirming the identity of the RPE as the cell of origin.

Metastatic (8) and astrocytic (24) lesions must also be excluded in the differential diagnosis of tumors of the RPE.

ADENOMAS AND ADENOCARCINOMA OF THE IRIS PIGMENT EPITHELIUM

Overview

Adenomas and adenocarcinomas of the iris pigment epithelium (IPE) are rare. They are usually diagnosed in adulthood, with a mean age at diagnosis of 60 years.

Clinical Features

Patients tend to be asymptomatic, and without visual impairment. These tumors are less aggressive clinically than pigment neuroepithelial tumors of the

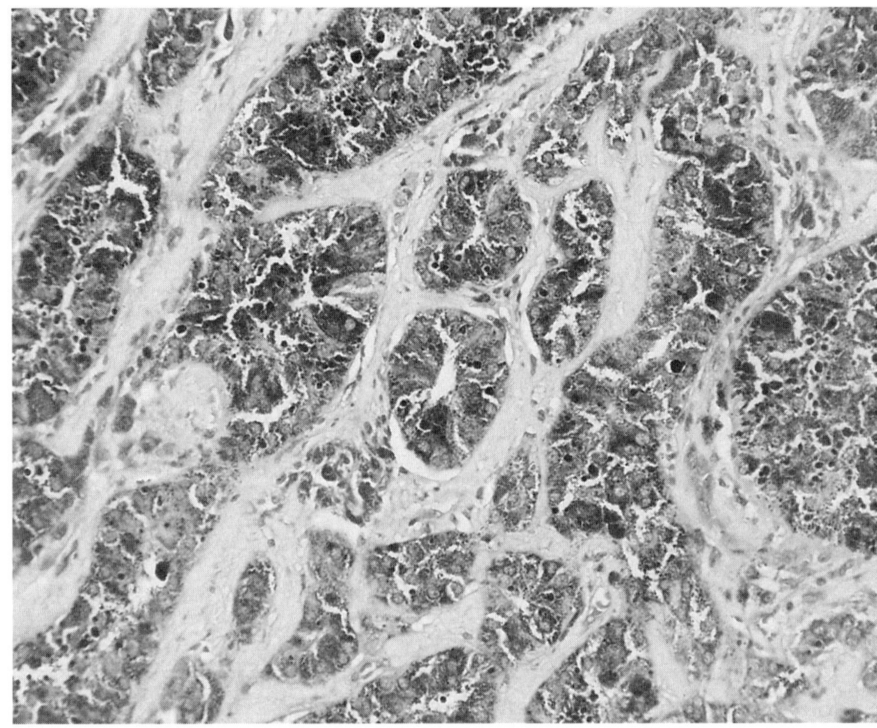

Figure 9 Adenocarcinoma of the retinal pigment epithelium exhibiting adenoid structures (hematoxylin and eosin, × 23).

ciliary body and retina (96). They tend to compress or completely efface the overlying iris stroma, but they do not infiltrate the stroma. This distinguishes them from the iris nevus, melanocytoma and malignant melanoma, which typically arise from and blend with the iris stroma (96,99).

Histopathology

Histologically, adenomas of the IPE arise from the posterior pigment epithelial layer of the iris, and an origin from adjacent normal IPE can sometimes be seen. Architecturally the tumor cells are arranged in acini, cords and tubules, and cystoid spaces containing melanophages are occasionally present (96). The distinction between adenoma and low-grade adenocarcinoma is based upon the degree of cellular pleomorphism and local invasiveness (101).

IRIS AND CILIARY CYSTS

Separation of the anterior and posterior layers of iridic or ciliary epithelium may produce a black cyst that fills the posterior chamber or becomes prolapsed through the pupil. Pieces of epithelium may become detached and be carried into the anterior chamber, where they may give rise to cysts that may be mistaken clinically for melanomas (95).

Iris cysts are classified as primary or secondary. Primary cysts of the iris can be divided into those that involve the IPE and those that involve the iris stroma. Primary cysts of the IPE are further categorized as peripheral (iridociliary), mid-zonal, central (papillary), or dislodged (95). Dislodged cysts can either be fixed or free-floating in aqueous humor or vitreous. Primary iris stromal cysts are congenital or acquired and often present in childhood (56,57,95).

Secondary acquired iris cysts may arise secondary to epithelial ingrowth or implantation following trauma or surgery, parasitic infection, or be tumor induced (95,119). Acquired cysts usually give rise to more complications, such as secondary glaucoma, corneal edema, and iridocyclitis, than congenital cysts (95,106).

Spontaneously occurring cysts are uncommon and usually present in the first few months of life, appearing as thin-walled vesicles that project into the anterior chamber (103). Clinically and histologically, they can be difficult to distinguish from acquired posttraumatic cysts, which may also be lined by epithelium resembling that of the conjunctiva. Spontaneous iris stromal cysts are lined by stratified squamous epithelium or cuboidal epithelium, with subjacent melanocytes and occasionally other structures, such as accessory lacrimal gland (78). Immunohistochemical staining for cytokeratins within the epithelium suggests that the cysts arise from ectopic surface ectoderm rather than neuroectoderm, probably at the time of lens vesicle formation (74).

CONGENITAL, REACTIVE, AND HAMARTOMATOUS LESIONS OF THE PIGMENTED AND NONPIGMENTED CILIARY AND RETINAL EPITHELIUM

Congenital Anomalies of Pigment Epithelium

Congenital hypertrophy of the retinal pigment epithelium (CHRPE) is traditionally regarded as a solitary, unilateral and benign nonproliferative pigmentary disturbance of the RPE (15,16). Histologically, the lesions exhibit tall epithelial cells tightly packed with numerous large pigment granules that obscure nuclear detail (16,19). The bilateral diffuse uveal melanocytic hyperplasia associated with occult malignancy, especially intra-abdominal (77), may also be confused with these lesions (see Chapter 59).

CHRPE lesions occur typically in otherwise normal individuals and in association with Gardner syndrome (MIM +175100). Gardner syndrome is an autosomal dominant form of familial adenomatous polyposis of the intestine, and is associted with heightened potential for colonic adenocarcinoma and skeletal and soft tissue hamartomas (7,58,59,107–110,115) (see Chapter 55). Pigmented ocular fundus lesions have been reported in a case of familial polyposis coli associated with hepatoblastoma (50), but not in those of hereditary nonpolyposis-associated colorectal neoplasia or Peutz–Jeghers syndrome (intestinal polyposis with excessive melanin pigmentation of the skin and mucous membranes) (MIM #175200) (110). However, CHRPE-like anomalies have been recorded in microcephalic children without mental retardation or Gardner syndrome (1).

Although originally described as a nonproliferative lesion, CHRPE has been uncommonly documented to enlarge and, as well as to give rise to adenocarcinomas. They present as elevated, solid low-grade adenocarcinomas of the RPE located between the retinal equator and ora serrata. Localized exudative retinal detachments, cystoid macular edema, and surface-wrinkling retinopathy may be associated findings (83,92,97,111).

Reactive Hyperplasia

The pigment epithelia of the eye are highly reactive and exhibit an exuberant hyperplasia in response to a variety of insults, including old injury, chronic inflammation in adjacent structures, or longstanding retinal detachment with traction (118). Reactive hyperplasia of nonpigment (and pigment) ciliary epithelium occurs typically in eyes that previously suffered injury or long-standing inflammation. Clinically and histologically, it is easily confused with neoplasia, but evidence of active inflammation, scarring, and an excessive production of basement membrane material by the hyperplastic ciliary epithelium helps to differentiate the lesion from a benign adenoma.

Reactive hyperplasia of the pigment epithelium is often accompanied by abundant basement membrane material. Migration and invasion of the uvea, retina and sclera can occur but pleomorphism and mitoses are absent or inconspicuous. Differentiation from a neoplasm may be difficult (32). Proliferation and migration can be accompanied by a metaplastic fibrous and osseous response with or without calcification (30). Reactive hyperplasia of the RPE occurs mainly in older adults at the ora serrata in eyes with chronic retinal detachment and is referred to as *Ringschwiele*. It also occurs at other sites in previously diseased or traumatized eyes.

Combined Hamartomas

Combined hamartomas of the sensory retina and RPE are rare, benign, congenital lesions of the ocular fundus typified as pigment, elevated juxtapapillary lesions with epiretinal membrane formation (27,82,84). A retinal vascular tortuosity results in a characteristic hyperfluorescent appearance on fluorescein angiography (FA). Rarely they enlarge and mimic a melanoma. A few enucleated globes with this condition have been examined histologically, disclosing disorganized retinal tissue intermixed with vascular elements, glial tissue, and tubules of proliferating RPE (27).

RARE INTRAOCULAR TUMORS OF NEUROECTODERMAL ORIGIN

Leiomyomas are benign smooth muscle tumors (see Chapter 64). Special morphologic attributes are present when they arise from neuroectodermally derived smooth muscle of the sphincter and dilator muscles of the iris (52). The designation mesectodermal leiomyoma has been coined for these tumors, which may also occur in the ciliary body (10,40,42,44,90,91,121,123). A rare low-grade mesectodermal leiomyosarcoma of the ciliary body has been documented (75).

ACKNOWLEDGMENTS

Portions of the material included in this chapter were originally presented in the two previous editions authored by Drs. S. Ry Andersen and A.C.E. McCartney.

REFERENCES

1. Abdel-Salam GM, Vogt G, Halasz A, et al. Microcephaly with normal intelligence, and chorioretinopathy. Ophthalmic Genet 1999; 20:259–64.
2. Addison DJ, Font RL. Glioneuroma of iris and ciliary body. Arch Ophthalmol 1984; 102:419–21.
3. al Torbak A, Abboud EB, al Sharif A, et al. Medulloepithelioma of the ciliary body. Indian J Ophthalmol 2002; 50:138–40.
4. Andersen SR. Medulloepithelioma of the retina. Int Ophthalmol Clin 1962; 2:483–506.
5. Andersen SR. Differentiation features in some retinal tumors and in dysplastic retinal conditions. Am J Ophthalmol 1971; 1:231–41.
6. Badal J, Lagrange F. Carcinome primitif des proceset du corps ciliare. Arch Ophthalmol (Paris) 1892; 12:143–8.
7. Ballhausen WG. Genetic testing for familial adenomatous polyposis. Ann NY Acad Sci 2000; 910:36–47.
8. Bardenstein DS, Char DH, Jones C, et al. Metastatic ciliary body carcinoid tumor. Arch Ophthalmol 1990; 108: 1590–4.
9. Becker LE, Sharma MC, Rorke LB. Medulloepithelioma. In Kleihues P, Cavenee WK, eds. World Health Organization Classification of Tumours, Pathology and Genetics, Tumours of the Nervous System Lyon. France: IARC Press, 2000:124–6.
10. Biswas J, Kumar SK, Gopal L, et al. Leiomyoma of the ciliary body extending to the anterior chamber: clinicopathologic and ultrasound biomicroscopic correlation. Surv Ophthalmol 2000; 44:336–42.
11. Bolande RP. Neurocristopathy: its growth and development in 20 years. Pediatr Pathol Lab Med 1997; 17:1–25.
12. Broughton WL, Zimmerman LE. A clinicopathologic study of 56 cases of intraocular medulloepitheliomas. Am J Ophthalmol 1978; 85:407–18.
13. Brown HH, Glasgow BJ, Foos RY. Ultrastructural and immunohistochemical features of coronal adenomas. Am J Ophthalmol 1991; 112: 34–0.
14. Brownstein S, Barsoum-Homsy M, Conway VH, et al. Nonteratoid medulloepithelioma of the ciliary body. Ophthalmology 1984; 91:1118–22.
15. Buettner H. Congenital hypertrophy of the retinal pigment epithelium (RPE). A nontumorous lesion. Mod Probl Ophthalmol 1974; 12:528–35.
16. Buettner H. Congenital hypertrophy of the retinal pigment epithelium. Am J Ophthalmol 1975; 79:177–89.
17. Canning CR, McCartney AC, Hungerford J. Medulloepithelioma (diktyoma). Br J Ophthalmol 1988; 72:764–7.
18. Carrillo R, Streeten BW. Malignant teratoid medulloepithelioma in an adult. Arch Ophthalmol 1979; 97:695–9.
19. Champion R Daicker BC. Congenital hypertrophy of the pigment epithelium: light microscopic and ultrastructural findings in young children. Retina 1989; 9:44–8.
20. Cursiefen C, Schlotzer-Schrehardt U, Holbach LM, et al. Adenoma of the nonpigment ciliary epithelium mimicking a malignant melanoma of the iris. Arch Ophthalmol 1999; 117:113–6.
21. Desai VN, Lieb WE, Donoso LA, et al. Photoreceptor cell differentiation in intraocular medulloepithelioma: an immunohistopathologic study. Arch Ophthalmol 1990; 108:481–2.
22. Dinakaran S, Rundle PA, Parsons MA, et al. Adenoma of ciliary pigment epithelium: a case series. Br J Ophthalmol 2003; 87:504–5.
23. Dryja TP, Albert DM, and Horns D. Adenocarcinoma arising from the epithelium of the ciliary body. Ophthalmology 1981; 88:1290–2.
24. Farber MG, Smith ME, Gans LA. Astrocytoma of the ciliary body. Arch Ophthalmol 1987; 105:536–7.
25. Finger PT, McCormick SA, Davidian M, et al. Adenocarcinoma of the retinal pigment epithelium: a diagnostic and therapeutic challenge. Graefes Arch Clin Exp Ophthalmol 1996; 234:S22–7.
26. Floyd BB, Minckler DS, Valentin L. Intraocular medulloepithelioma in a 79-year-old man. Ophthalmology 1982; 89:1088–94.
27. Font RL, Moura RA, Shetlar DJ, et al. Combined hamartoma of sensory retina and retinal pigment epithelium. Retina 1989; 9:302–11.
28. Font RL, Rishi K. Diffuse retinal involvement in malignant nonteratoid medulloepithelioma of ciliary body in an adult. Arch Ophthalmol 2005; 123:1136–8.
29. Font RL, Zimmerman LE, Fine BS. Adenoma of the retinal pigment epithelium: histochemical and electron microscopic observations. Am J Ophthalmol 1972; 73:544–54.
30. Frayer WC. Reactivity of the retinal pigment epithelium: an experimental and histopathologic study. Trans Am Ophthalmol Soc 1966; 64:586–643.
31. Fuchs EW. Geschwulste des Ciliarepithels. Graefes Arch Clin Exp Ophthalmol 1908; 68:534–87.
32. Garner A. Tumours of the retinal pigment epithelium. Br J Ophthalmol 1970; 54:715–23.
33. Gopal L, Babu EK, Gupta S, et al. Pigmented malignant medulloepithelioma of the ciliary body. J Pediatr Ophthalmol Strabismus 2004; 41:364–6.
34. Green WR, Iliff WJ, Trotter RR. Malignant teratoid medulloepithelioma of the optic nerve. Arch Ophthalmol 1974; 91:451–4.
35. Grossniklaus HE and Lim JI. Adenoma of the nonpigment ciliary epithelium. Retina 1994; 14:452–6.
36. Grossniklaus HE, Zimmerman LE, Kachmer ML. Pleomorphic adenocarcinoma of the ciliary body. Immunohistochemical and electron microscopic features. Ophthalmology 1990; 97:763–8.
37. Hamburg A. Medulloepithelioma arising from the posterior pole. Ophthalmologica 1980; 181:152–9.
38. Hausmann N, Stefani FH. Medulloepithelioma of the ciliary body. Acta Ophthalmol (Copenh) 1991; 69:398–401.
39. Husain SE, Husain N, Boniuk M, et al. Malignant nonteratoid medulloepithelioma of the ciliary body in an adult. Ophthalmology 1998; 105:596–9.
40. Ishigooka H, Yamabe H, Kobashi Y, et al. Clinical and pathological status of mesectodermal leiomyoma of the ciliary body. A case report and review of the literature. Graefes Arch Clin Exp Ophthalmol 1989; 227:101–5.
41. Iwamoto T, Witmer R, Landolt E. Diktyoma, a clinical histological and electron-microscopical observation. Albrecht Von Graefes Arch Klin Exp Ophthalmol 1967; 172:293–316.
42. Jakobiec FA, Font RL, Tso MO, et al. Mesectodermal leiomyoma of the ciliary body: a tumor of presumed neural crest origin. Cancer 1977; 39:2102–13.
43. Jakobiec FA, Howard GM, Ellsworth RM, et al. Electron microscopic diagnosis of medulloepithelioma. Am J Ophthalmol 1975; 79:321–9.
44. Jakobiec FA, Iwamoto T. Mesectodermal leiomyoma of the ciliary body associated with a nevus. Arch Ophthalmol 1978; 96:692–5.
45. Jakobiec FA, Zimmerman LE, Spencer WH, et al. Metastatic colloid carcinoma versus primary carcinoma

of the ciliary epithelium. Ophthalmology 1987; 94: 1469–80.
46. Jumper MJ, Char DH, Howes EL Jr, et al. Neglected malignant medulloepithelioma of the eye. Orbit 1999; 18: 37–43.
47. Karch SB, Urich H. Medulloepithelioma: definition of an entity. J Neuropathol Exp Neurol 1972; 31:27–53.
48. Kivela T, Kauniskangas L, Miettinen P, et al. Glioneuroma associated with colobomatous dysplasia of the anterior uvea and retina. A case simulating medulloepithelioma. Ophthalmology 1989; 96:1799–808.
49. Kivela T, Tarkkanen A. Recurrent medulloepithelioma of the ciliary body. Immunohistochemical characteristics. Ophthalmology 1988; 95:1565–75.
50. Krush AJ, Traboulsi EI, Offerhaus JA, et al. Hepatoblastoma, pigment ocular fundus lesions and jaw lesions in Gardner syndrome. Am J Med Genet 1988; 29:323–32.
51. Laver NM, Hidayat AA, Croxatto JO. Pleomorphic adenocarcinomas of the ciliary epithelium. Immunohistochemical and ultrastructural features of 12 cases. Ophthalmology 1999; 106:103–10.
52. Li ZY, Tso MO, Sugar J. Leiomyoepithelioma of iris pigment epithelium. Arch Ophthalmol 1987; 105:819–24.
53. Lieb WE, Shields JA, Eagle RC Jr, et al. Cystic adenoma of the pigment ciliary epithelium. Clinical, pathologic, and immunohistopathologic findings. Ophthalmology 1990; 97:1489–93.
54. Litricin O, Latkovic Z. Malignant teratoid medulloepithelioma in an adult. Ophthalmologica 1985; 191:17–21.
55. Lloyd WC III, O'Hara M. Malignant teratoid medulloepithelioma: clinical–echographic–histopathologic correlation. J AAPOS 2001; 5:395–7.
56. Lois N, Shields CL, Shields JA, et al. Primary cysts of the iris pigment epithelium. Clinical features and natural course in 234 patients. Ophthalmology 1998; 105:1879–85.
57. Lois N, Shields CL, Shields JA, et al. Primary iris stromal cysts. A report of 17 cases. Ophthalmology 1998; 105: 1317–22.
58. Lynch HT, Priluck I, Fitzsimmons ML. CHRPE in non-Gardner's familial polyposis coli patients. Ophthalmology 1989; 96:399–400.
59. Lyons LA, Lewis RA, Strong LC, et al. A genetic study of Gardner syndrome and congenital hypertrophy of the retinal pigment epithelium. Am J Hum Genet 1988; 42: 290–6.
60. Mamalis N, Font RL, Anderson CW, et al. Concurrent benign teratoid medulloepithelioma and pineoblastoma. Ophthalmic Surg 1992; 23:403–408.
61. Manz HJ, Rosen DA, Macklin RD, et al. Neuroectodermal tumor of anterior lip of the optic cup. Glioneuroma transitional to teratoid medullo-epithelioma. Arch Ophthalmol 1973; 89:382–6.
62. Margo CE, Brooks HL Jr. Adenocarcinoma of the ciliary epithelium in a 12-year-old black child. J Pediatr Ophthalmol Strabismus 1991; 28:232–5.
63. McCartney AC, Bull TB, Spalton DJ. Fuchs' heterochromic cyclitis: an electron microscopy study. Trans Ophthalmol Soc UK 1986; 105:324–9.
64. McCartney ACE. Intraocular epithelial tumors and cysts. In Garner A, Klintworth GK, eds. Pathobiology of Ocular Disease. A Dynamic Approach, 2nd ed. New York: Marcel Dekker, Inc., 1994:1405–21.
65. McGowan HD, Simpson ER, Hunter WS, et al. Adenoma of the nonpigment epithelium of the ciliary body. Can J Ophthalmol 1991; 26:328–33.
66. McLean IW, Burnier MN, Zimmerman LE, et al. Tumors of the retina. In: McLean IW, Burnier MN, Zimmerman LE, Jakobiec FA, eds. Atlas of Tumor Pathology. Tumors of the Eye and Ocular Adnexa. Washington D.C.: Armed Forces Institute of Pathology, 1993:97–154.
67. Minckler D, Allen AW Jr. Adenocarcinoma of the retinal pigment epithelium. Arch Ophthalmol 1978; 96:2252–4.
68. Minoda K, Hirose Y, Sugano I, et al. Occurrence of sequential intraocular tumors: malignant medulloepithelioma subsequent to retinoblastoma. Jpn J Ophthalmol 1993; 37:293–300.
69. Mullaney J. Primary malignant medulloepithelioma of the retinal stalk. Am J Ophthalmol 1974; 77:499–504.
70. Nicolo M, Nicolo G, Zingirian M. Pleomorphic adenocarcinoma of the ciliary epithelium: a clinicopathological, immunohistochemical, ultrastructural, DNA-ploidy and comparative genomic hybridization analysis of an unusual case. Eur J Ophthalmol 2002; 12:319–23.
71. O'Keefe M, Fulcher T, Kelly P, et al. Medulloepithelioma of the optic nerve head. Arch Ophthalmol 1997; 115: 1325–7.
72. Orellana J, Moura RA, Font RL, et al. Medulloepithelioma diagnosed by ultrasound and vitreous aspirate. Electron microscopic observations. Ophthalmology 1983; 90: 1531–9.
73. Papale JJ, Akiwama K, Hirose T, et al. Adenocarcinoma of the ciliary body pigment epithelium in a child. Arch Ophthalmol 1984; 102:100–3.
74. Paridaens AD, Deuble K, McCartney AC. Spontaneous congenital non-pigment epithelial cysts of the iris stroma. Br J Ophthalmol 1992; 76:39–42.
75. Park SW, Kim HJ, Chin HS, et al. Mesectodermal leiomyosarcoma of the ciliary body. Am J Neuroradiol 2003; 24:1765–8.
76. Rennie IG, Faulkner MK, Parsons MA. Adenoma of the pigment ciliary epithelium. Br J Ophthalmol 1994; 78: 484–5.
77. Rohrbach JM, Roggendorf W, Thanos S, et al. Simultaneous bilateral diffuse melanocytic uveal hyperplasia. Am J Ophthalmol 1990; 110:49–56.
78. Roy FH, Hanna C. Spontaneous congenital iris cyst. Am J Ophthalmol 1971; 72:97–108.
79. Rubinstein LJ. Embryonal central neuroepithelial tumors and their differentiating potential. A cytogenetic view of a complex neuro-oncological problem. J Neurosurg 1985; 62:795–805.
80. Sahel JA, Albert DM. Tumors of the retina. In: Garner A, Klintworth GK, eds. Pathobiology of Ocular Diseases, A Dynamic Approach. 2nd ed. New York: Marcel Dekker, 1994:1405–13.
81. Sawa H, Takeshita I, Kuramitsu M, et al. Immunohistochemistry of retinoblastomas. J Neurooncol 1987; 5:351–5.
82. Schachat AP, Shields JA, Fine SL, et al. Combined hamartomas of the retina and retinal pigment epithelium. Ophthalmology 1984; 91:1609–15.
83. Shields CL, Mashayekhi A, Ho T, et al. Solitary congenital hypertrophy of the retinal pigment epithelium: clinical features and frequency of enlargement in 330 patients. Ophthalmology 2003; 110:1968–76.
84. Shields CL, Shields JA, Marr BP, et al. Congenital simple hamartoma of the retinal pigment epithelium: a study of five cases. Ophthalmology 2003; 110:1005–11.
85. Shields JA, Augsburger JJ, Wallar PH, et al. Adenoma of the nonpigment epithelium of the ciliary body. Ophthalmology 1983; 90:1528–30.

86. Shields JA, Eagle RC Jr, Shields CL, et al. Acquired neoplasms of the nonpigment ciliary epithelium (adenoma and adenocarcinoma). Ophthalmology 1996; 103: 2007–16.
87. Shields JA, Eagle RC Jr, Shields CL, et al. Congenital neoplasms of the nonpigment ciliary epithelium (medulloepithelioma). Ophthalmology 1996; 103:1998–2006.
88. Shields JA, Eagle RC Jr, Shields CL, et al. Pigmented medulloepithelioma of the ciliary body. Arch Ophthalmol 2002; 120:207–10.
89. Shields JA, Melki T, Shields CL, et al. Epipapillary adenoma of retinal pigment epithelium. Retina 2001; 21:76–8.
90. Shields JA, Shields CL, Eagle RC Jr. Mesectodermal leiomyoma of the ciliary body managed by partial lamellar iridocyclochoroidectomy. Ophthalmology 1989; 96:1369–76.
91. Shields JA, Shields CL, Eagle RC Jr, et al. Observations on seven cases of intraocular leiomyoma. The 1993 Byron Demorest Lecture. Arch Ophthalmol 1994; 112:521–8.
92. Shields JA, Shields CL, Eagle RC Jr, et al. Adenocarcinoma arising from congenital hypertrophy of retinal pigment epithelium. Arch Ophthalmol 2001; 119:597–602.
93. Shields JA, Shields CL, Gunduz K, et al. Adenoma of the ciliary body pigment epithelium: the 1998 Albert Ruedemann, Sr, memorial lecture, Part 1. Arch Ophthalmol 1999; 117:592–7.
94. Shields JA, Shields CL, Gunduz K, et al. Neoplasms of the retinal pigment epithelium: the 1998 Albert Ruedemann, Sr, memorial lecture, Part 2. Arch Ophthalmol 1999; 117: 601–8.
95. Shields JA, Shields CL, Lois N, et al. Iris cysts in children: classification, incidence, and management. The 1998 Torrence A. Makley Jr. Lecture. Br J Ophthalmol 1999; 83:334–8.
96. Shields JA, Shields CL, Mercado G, et al. Adenoma of the iris pigment epithelium: a report of 20 cases: the 1998 Pan-American Lecture. Arch Ophthalmol 1999; 117: 736–41.
97. Shields JA, Shields CL, Singh AD. Acquired tumors arising from congenital hypertrophy of the retinal pigment epithelium. Arch Ophthalmol 2000; 118:637–41.
98. Singh A, Singh AD, Shields CL, et al. Iris neovascularization in children as a manifestation of underlying medulloepithelioma. J Pediatr Ophthalmol Strabismus 2001; 38:224–8.
99. Singh AD, Rundle PA, Longstaff S, et al. Iris pigment epithelial adenoma: resection and repair. Eye 2005; 20: 385–6.
100. Spencer WH, Jesberg DO. Glioneuroma (choristomatous malformation of the optic cup margin). A report of two cases. Arch Ophthalmol 1973; 89:387–91.
101. Spraul CW, d'Heurle D, Grossniklaus HE. Adenocarcinoma of the iris pigment epithelium. Arch Ophthalmol 1996; 114:1512–7.
102. Steinkuller PG, Font RL. Congenital malignant teratoid neoplasm of the eye and orbit: a case report and review of the literature. Ophthalmology 1997; 104:38–42.
103. Sugar HS Nathan LE. Congenital epithelial cysts of the iris stroma. Ann Ophthalmol 1982; 14:483–5.
104. Tarkkanen A, Tervo T, Tervo K, et al. Immunohistochemical evidence for preproenkephalin A synthesis in human retinoblastoma. Invest Ophthalmol Vis Sci 1984; 25:1210–2.
105. Terasaki H, Nagasaka T, Arai M, et al. Adenocarcinoma of the nonpigment ciliary epithelium: report of two cases with immunohistochemical findings. Graefes Arch Clin Exp Ophthalmol 2001; 239:876–81.
106. Torczynski E, Jacobiec FA, Johnston MC, et al. Synophthalmia and cyclopia: a histopathologic, radiographic, and organogenetic analysis. Doc Ophthalmol 1977; 44:311–78.
107. Tourino R, Conde-Freire R, Cabezas-Agricola JM, et al. Value of the congenital hypertrophy of the retinal pigment epithelium in the diagnosis of familial adenomatous polyposis. Int Ophthalmol 2004; 25: 101–12.
108. Traboulsi EI. Ocular manifestations of familial adenomatous polyposis (Gardner syndrome). Ophthalmol Clin North Am 2005; 18:163–6.
109. Traboulsi EI, Krush AJ, Gardner EJ, et al. Prevalence and importance of pigment ocular fundus lesions in Gardner's syndrome. N Engl J Med 1987; 316:661–7.
110. Traboulsi EI, Maumenee IH, Krush AJ, et al. Pigmented ocular fundus lesions in the inherited gastrointestinal polyposis syndromes and in hereditary nonpolyposis colorectal cancer. Ophthalmology 1988; 95:964–9.
111. Trichopoulos N, Augsburger JJ, Schneider S. Adenocarcinoma arising from congenital hypertrophy of the retinal pigment epithelium. Graefes Arch Clin Exp Ophthalmol 2006; 244:125–8.
112. Tso MO, Albert DM. Pathological condition of the retinal pigment epithelium. Neoplasms and nodular non-neoplastic lesions. Arch Ophthalmol 1972; 88:27–38.
113. Vadmal M, Kahn E, Finger P, et al. Nonteratoid medulloepithelioma of the retina with electron microscopic and immunohistochemical characterization. Pediatr Pathol Lab Med 1996; 16:663–72.
114. Vajaranant TS, Mafee MF, Kapur R, et al. Medulloepithelioma of the ciliary body and optic nerve: clinicopathologic, CT, and MR imaging features. Neuroimaging Clin N Am 2005; 15:69–83.
115. Valanzano R, Cama A, Volpe R, et al. Congenital hypertrophy of the retinal pigment epithelium in familial adenomatous polyposis. Novel criteria of assessment and correlations with constitutional adenomatous polyposis coli gene mutations. Cancer 1996; 78:2400–10.
116. VandenBerg SR, Herman MM, Rubinstein LJ. Embryonal central neuroepithelial tumors: current concepts and future challenges. Cancer Metastasis Rev 1987; 5:343–65.
117. Verhoeff FH. A rare tumor arising from the pars ciliaris retinae (terato-neuroma), of a nature hitherto unrecognized, and its relation to the so-called glioma retinae. Trans Am Ophthalmol Soc 1904; 10:351–77.
118. Vogel MH, Zimmerman LE, Gass JD. Proliferation of the juxtapapillary retinal pigment epithelium simulating malignant melanoma. Doc Ophthalmol 1969; 26: 461–81.
119. Wearne MJ, Buckley RJ, Cree IA, et al. Cystic epithelial ingrowth as a late complication of penetrating keratoplasty. Arch Ophthalmol 1999; 117:1444–5.
120. Weston JA. The migration and differentiation of neural crest cells. Adv Morphog 1970; 8:41–114.
121. White V, Stevenson K, Garner A, et al. Mesectodermal leiomyoma of the ciliary body: case report. Br J Ophthalmol 1989; 73:12–8.
122. Yanoff M, Font RL. Intraocular cartilage in a microphthalmic eye of an otherwise healthy girl. Arch Ophthalmol 1969; 81:238–40.
123. Yu DY, Cohen SB, Peyman G, et al. Mesectodermal leiomyoma of the ciliary body: new evidence for neural crest origin. J Pediatr Ophthalmol Strabismus 1990; 27: 317–21.

124. Zimmerman LE. The remarkable polymorphism of tumours of the ciliary epithelium. Trans Aust Coll Ophthalmol 1970; 2:114–25.
125. Zimmerman LE. Verhoeff's "terato-neuroma" A critical reappraisal in light of new observations and current concepts of embryonic tumors. Am J Ophthalmol 1971; 72:1039–57.
126. Zimmerman LE. Histological typing of tumours of the eye and its adnexa. In: Zimmerman LE, Sobin L, eds. International Histological Classification of Tumours, Vol. 21. Geneva: World Health Organization, 1980.
127. Zimmerman LE, Fine BS. Production of hyaluronic acid by cysts and tumors of the ciliary body. Arch Ophthalmol 1964; 72:365–79.
128. Zimmerman LE, Font RL, Andersen SR. Rhabdomyosarcomatous differentiation in malignant intraocular medulloepitheliomas. Cancer 1972; 30: 817–35.

59

Tumors of Melanocytes

Bryan J. Schwent
Department of Ophthalmology, Emory University, Atlanta, Georgia, U.S.A.

Hans E. Grossniklaus
Departments of Ophthalmology and Pathology, Emory University, Atlanta, Georgia, U.S.A.

INTRODUCTION

There are approximately 41,000 new cases of melanoma in the United States each year and approximately 7200 patients die from the disease (47). Although the vast majority of melanomas affect the skin, a large number of people are affected by melanoma involving the eye and its surrounding tissues. Ocular melanoma represents 5.3% of all cases in the United States while cutaneous melanoma accounts for 91% of cases (47).

Malignant melanoma is a neoplasm of melanocytes that are embryologically derived from the neural crest and are responsible for producing pigment in the skin and other structures. During development, the progenitors of melanocytes migrate to either the basal epithelium of the skin or mucous membranes like the conjunctiva or to connective tissues such as the dermis, the choroid, or the sclera/episclera of the eye. Melanocytes produce melanin in organelles called melanosomes through the activity of the enzyme tyrosinase. Melanosomes are then transferred from melanocytes to keratinocytes through dendritic processes. A single melanocyte will link to as many as 36 keratinocytes by such processes. The distribution of the melanosomes in keratinocytes is responsible for the normal differential pigmentation of skin: in Caucasians the melanosomes are clustered inside the keratinocytes whereas in persons of color they are dispersed within the cells. Melanocytes in connective tissue differ from those in epithelia in that they do not have dendritic processes connecting them to adjacent cells. Instead they release melanin into the surrounding extracellular space. Melanocytes are typically separated from each other in the epithelium but can be found in aggregates in melanocytic nevi. These nevi have been described both as hamartomas and as benign tumors and they are thought to play some role in the development of malignant melanoma (96,168,329).

Ocular melanoma is a generic term referring to several distinct entities and has caused some confusion in the literature. In this chapter, we divide ocular melanoma into four categories: (*i*) cutaneous melanoma of the eyelid, (*ii*) conjunctival melanoma, (*iii*) melanoma of the orbit, and (*iv*) uveal melanoma. They are considered in the context of melanocytic tumors as a whole.

MELANOCYTIC PROLIFERATIONS OF THE EYELID

Although cutaneous melanoma accounts for only 4% of all skin cancers, it causes the greatest number of deaths of all cutaneous neoplasms (115). Periorbital malignant melanomas constitute <1% of all cutaneous melanomas (319). In addition, they represent <1% of malignant tumors of the eyelid, being far less common than basal cell carcinoma (BCC) or squamous cell carcinoma (SCC) (58). Because of their rarity the literature contains only case reports and small series discussing the etiology, histopathology, management and prognosis. Their importance lies in the possibly dire outcome for patients whose diagnosis and/or management is delayed. To understand melanomas of the eyelid other pigmented lesions that may precede or masquerade as melanoma must be understood.

Melanocytes and Nevus Cells of the Skin

Melanocytes of the eyelid skin are generally located in the basal layer of the epidermis, but some reside in the dermis. Normal melanocytes are not found next to one another. In nevi, on the other hand, melanocytes do not exhibit the same type of dendritic processes and form nests (96,329).

Ephelides

Ephelides (freckles) are pigmented macules that appear in sun-exposed areas and tend to darken after sun exposure. They are often found in lightly pigmented individuals and are characterized histologically by hyperpigmentation of the basilar epidermis without hyperplasia of the melanocytes (96).

Solar Lentigo

Lentigines are also pigmented macules, but they tend to occur in older individuals in areas of sun exposure and are typically uniformly pigmented with sharp borders (329). Histologically, there is hyperpigmentation of the basal layer of the epidermis with an increased number of individual melanocytes (96,329).

Lentigo Maligna

Lentigo maligna is a special type of lentigo that is usually large and flat with variable pigmentation and irregular borders. It appears in elderly individuals in areas of high sun exposure and carries a significant risk of malignant transformation (55).

Nevi

Congenital Melanocytic Nevi

Common Nevus

Congenital common nevi are hamartomatous collections of melanocytes that are present at birth and usually become clinically apparent in the first year of life. They are present much earlier than the more common acquired nevi and may become much larger. They consist of nests of melanocytes within and immediately beneath the epithelium (junctional nevus), above and below the basement membrane (compound nevus), or completely beneath the basement membrane (subepithelial nevus). Nevus cells are found in the lower 2/3 of the dermis and may extend around nerves, blood vessels, and dermal appendages (196,248).

A special type of congenital melanocytic nevus of the eyelid skin is the divided or "kissing" nevus (Figs. 1 and 2) which gives important clues to the timing and location of the embryologic development of congenital nevi. During development, the eyelids are fused at the epidermis between the ninth and the 20th week of gestation and the "kissing" nevus represents a pigmented lesion on both the upper and lower eyelids that has split into two separate nevi with the formation of the palpebral fissure. Congenital nevi that are localized entirely within the epithelium at one point probably later migrate into the deeper locations (132). This maturation process from junctional to compound to subepithelial nevus has been noted with acquired nevi and clinically relates to some of the changes in the color of nevi that occur with age (329).

Congenital melanocytic nevi are associated with an increased risk of melanoma, ranging from 2% to 31%, with higher risks associated with the larger giant congenital nevi (329), as many as 8% of which reach a diameter of 40 mm or larger (44). A large congenital melanocytic nevus of the eyelid would be unusual because of anatomical constraints in this area.

Blue Nevus

Blue nevi are composed of melanocytes located in the dermis. They are believed to result from a failure of melanocytes to reach the epidermis during their developmental migration. These nevi, which contain brown melanin pigment, appear blue in the skin because of the filtering effect of the overlying

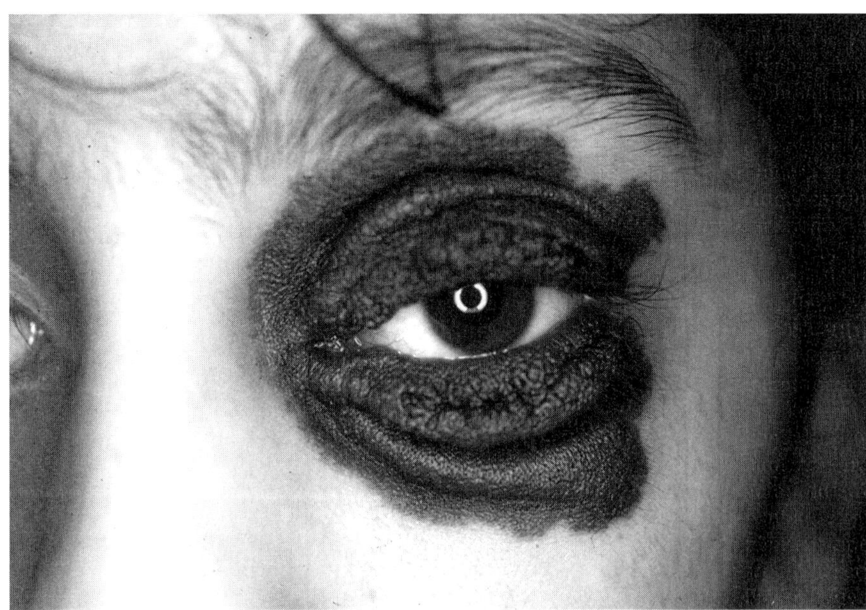

Figure 1 Congenital melanocytic nevus of the eyelids (a "kissing nevus") of a 12-year-old girl.

epidermis and dermis (the Tyndall effect). Two main types of blue nevi exist, the common blue nevus and the cellular blue nevus. The common blue nevus is smaller and consists of elongated, branching melanocytes that are interspersed between collagen bundles within the mid to upper dermis. The melanocytes are uniformly pigmented and interspersed melanophages may be present. The cellular blue nevus is similar but additionally has nests of pale epithelioid to plump spindle cells arranged in tight nodules that may bulge into the subcutaneous fat (96,329). Malignant change can occur.

Oculodermal Melanocytosis

Oculodermal melanocytosis (also known as nevus of Ota) represents a congenital hamartoma consisting of dendritic melanocytes within the dermis or ocular structures. Clinically, it appears as a blue to slate-gray discoloration of the periocular skin and sclera/episclera (Fig. 3). This lesion is histologically similar to the common blue nevus, but clinically it covers a much larger area. Typically it occurs along the first and second divisions of the trigeminal nerve and can affect the skin, sclera, episclera, choroid, and meninges. It is most common in Asians, with an incidence in

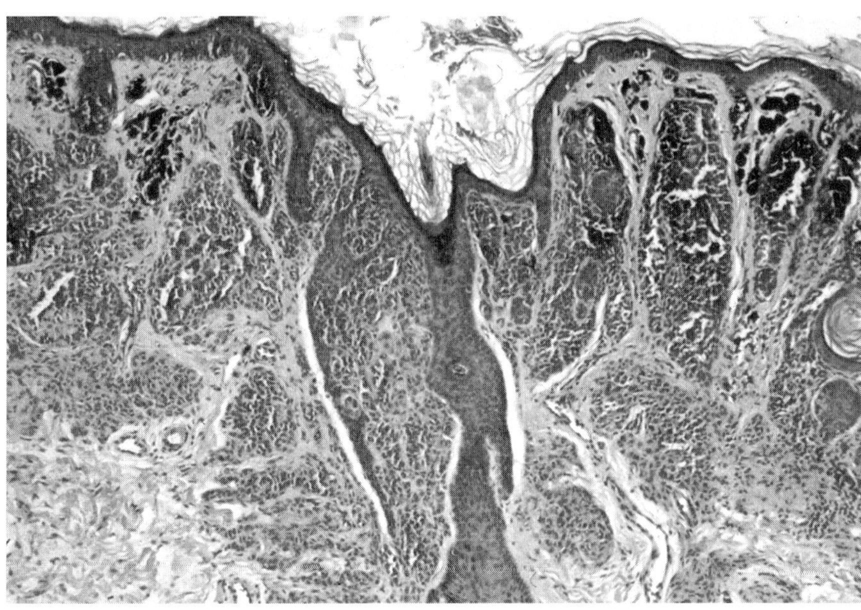

Figure 2 Histopathology of the congenital melanocytic nevus of the eyelid from Figure 1 showing a proliferation of melanocytes within the basal epithelium and tightly coherent nests of pigmented cells within the dermis. The lesion shows maturation from its superficial to its deepest aspect (hematoxylin and eosin, $\times$ 28).

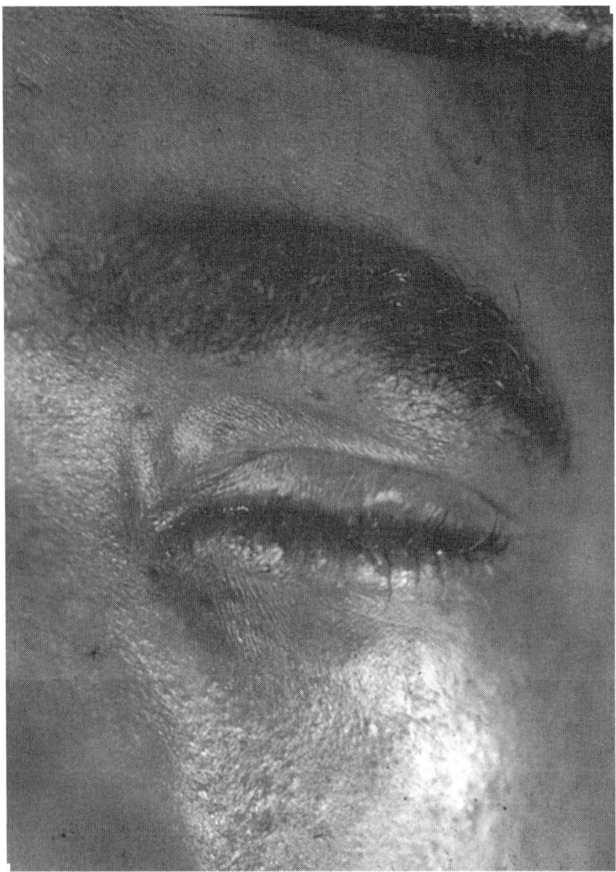

Figure 3 Oculodermal melanocytosis of the left eye showing the slate-gray coloration of the periocular skin.

Japan of 0.1% to 0.2% (60), while the incidence is estimated to be 0.014% in black persons and 0.038% in Caucasians (118). More than 90% of cases are unilateral and it is more common in females than males (60). Involvement of the skin but not the eye is seen in approximately one-third of patients, whereas eye involvement without the skin being affected is reported in 6% of cases (315). Ocular involvement is associated with glaucoma in approximately 10% of cases (315). Several cases of malignant change have been reported, involving the skin (226), choroid (119), orbit (207,289), and brain (86).

"Acquired" Nevi

Common Nevus

Acquired common nevi, like congenital common nevi, are classified histologically into three distinct types: junctional, compound, and subepithelial. They are extremely prevalent and most individuals have between 15 and 40 such nevi (85,120,186). They usually become apparent within the first two decades of life, though they may represent congenital aggregates of melanocytes that become clinically evident after a period of growth. The three types of common nevi are thought to represent different stages of nevus development. Nevi are believed to mature over many years by the migration of nevus cells originally localized to the basal epithelium (junctional) into the deeper tissues (compound and then dermal/subepithelial) (Figs. 4 and 5). Some epithelial components migrate with the nevus cells into the deeper tissues and form clinically detectable cysts. As nevi mature, they lose some pigmentation and the cells become smaller and more "neuroid" as they travel into deeper tissues (329). Evidence of this maturation of benign

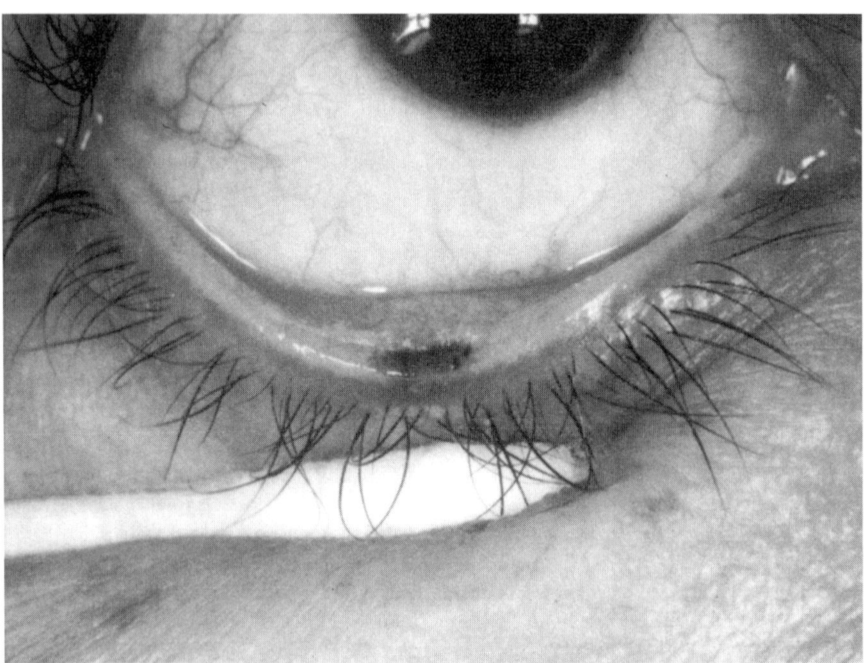

Figure 4 Compound nevus of the lower eyelid margin in a 50-year-old woman. Note the characteristic location of this lesion. The patient had noticed growth of the lesion over the last several months prior to excision.

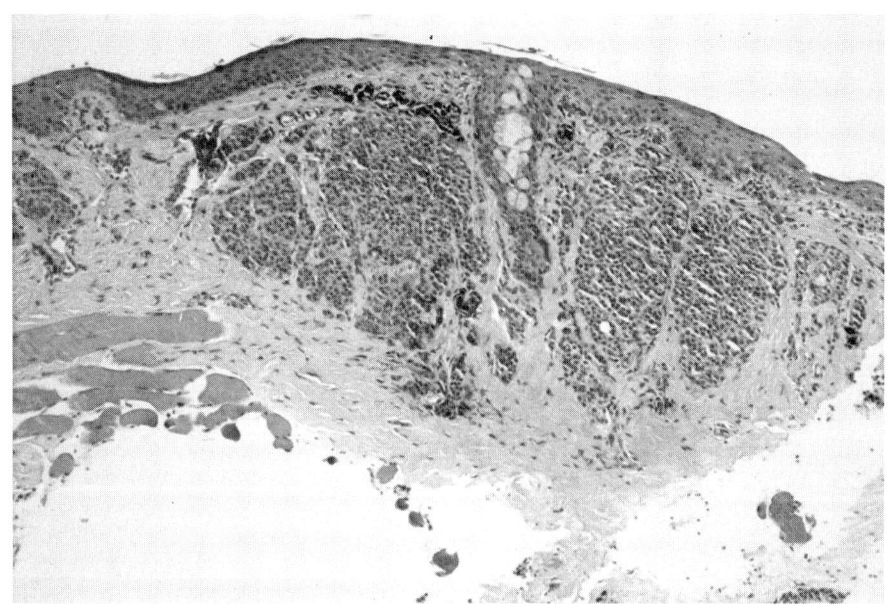

Figure 5 Histopathology of the compound nevus of the eyelid seen in Figure 4. It is composed of tightly coherent nests of cells with bland nuclei. Some of the cells contain melanin pigment granules in their cytoplasm. There is maturation from the surface to the base of the lesion (hematoxylin and eosin, ×28).

nevi may be used to differentiate them from other melanocytic lesions (96,329).

Recurrent Nevus

Occasionally, previously excised nevi recur, often as a result of incomplete excision. Such a recurrence suggests the possibility of melanoma, but this may be rare (329).

Spitz or Epithelioid Cell Nevus

A Spitz nevus usually appears as a flesh colored nodule in Caucasian children or young adults, but it may be pigmented and occur in other ethnic groups. Spitz nevi may manifest significant growth over time and may clinically be mistaken for melanoma. The lesions consist of nevus cells arranged in groups, usually as a compound nevus. Histologically, the Spitz nevus is symmetric and characterized by epithelioid or spindle cells that display maturation through the depth of the lesion. It does not exhibit pagetoid spread, but is often difficult to differentiate histologically from melanoma (329).

The Spitz nevus may contain characteristic eosinophilic globules (Kamino bodies) composed of fibronectin and degenerating components of melanocytes and keratinocytes (166).

Dysplastic Nevus

Dysplastic nevi (otherwise known as atypical or Clark nevi) are usually larger than common nevi and often have a variable color and texture (121). They are characterized histologically by the presence of cytologic atypia (Fig. 6) (84). The dysplastic nevus syndrome (MIM %155600) is characterized by multiple (up to 80 or more) dysplastic or atypical nevi with an increased risk for development of malignant melanoma, almost 20 times that of individuals without dysplastic nevi (329).

Cutaneous Eyelid Melanoma

Clinical Features

Melanoma of the eyelid should be suspected in any patient with a new pigmented lesion or one that shows documented growth and/or ulceration or hemorrhage (128). Larger lesions with asymmetry, irregular borders and variable color should also raise suspicion of melanoma (329). Other symptoms that may be reported by patients include irritation or crusting (326). The lower eyelid appears to be affected most often (Fig. 7) (128,326), followed by the upper eyelid and then the medial and lateral canthi (326), similar to the distribution of BCC and SCC of the eyelid (58). The eyelid margin may be involved in 17–22% of cases (111,128) and contiguous conjunctival melanoma can occur at the same time.

The average age of a patient presenting with eyelid melanoma ranges from 60 to 68 years (47,128,326), somewhat older than the 55.3 years reported for cutaneous melanoma in general (47). More than 90% of patients are Caucasian, and there appears to be no significant sex predilection (326). Cutaneous melanoma has shown an increasing incidence over the last 25 years (69) raising the possibility of a corresponding increase in eyelid melanoma.

Risk Factors

The rarity of eyelid melanoma makes it difficult to determine which factors place patients at risk. However, given the similarity of eyelid and other

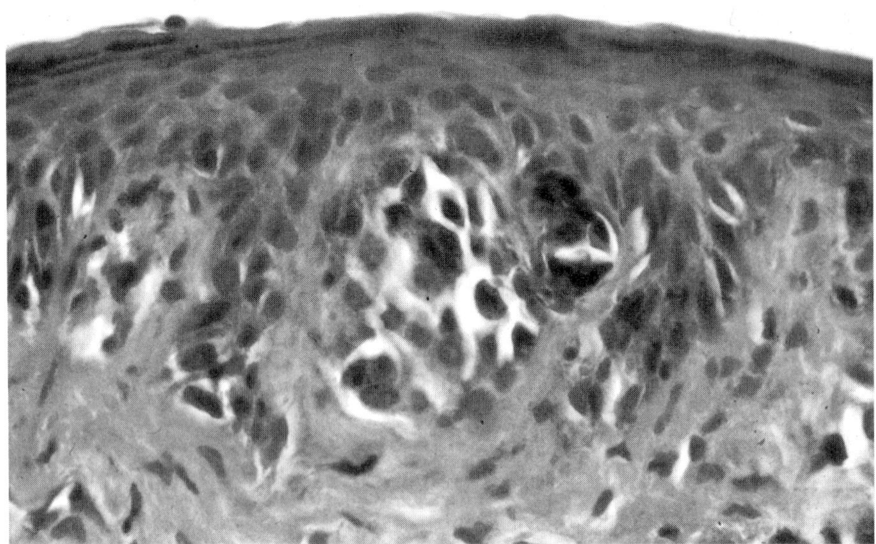

Figure 6 Histopathology of a dysplastic nevus of the eyelid. The lesion located at the subepithelial junction is composed of cells arranged in loosely coherent nests and display mildly pleomorphic nuclei and eosinophilic cytoplasm that contains melanin pigment granules. There is maturation of the lesion from the surface to the base and no mitotic figures are seen (hematoxylin and eosin, × 185).

cutaneous melanomas, information on risk factors for the one may be applicable to the other. These factors include light skin and hair color, freckles, a tendency to sunburn, a history of blistering sunburns, use of tanning salons, the presence of nevi, immunosuppression, and certain genetic disorders including xeroderma pigmentosum (MIM #278700 and others) (329). In addition dysplastic nevi (167) and certain congenital melanocytic nevi (80) have been associated with a higher incidence of melanoma.

Histopathology

The histological features of cutaneous melanoma (Fig. 8) include nuclear pleomorphism, nucleolar variability, mitoses (both deep and atypical), and increased apoptosis. The tumor may also be characterized by asymmetric growth and poor circumscription; epidermal and dermal nests of melanocytes showing confluence, variability in size and shape, as well as lack of maturation; and solitary epidermal melanocytes showing pagetoid spread and random arrangement (329).

Primary cutaneous melanoma has traditionally been classified into four types: nodular melanoma, superficial spreading melanoma, lentigo maligna melanoma and acral lentiginous melanoma. A recent report has questioned the validity of this classification system, citing several studies that failed to show any prognostic difference between the types, once thickness of the lesion is taken into account. In

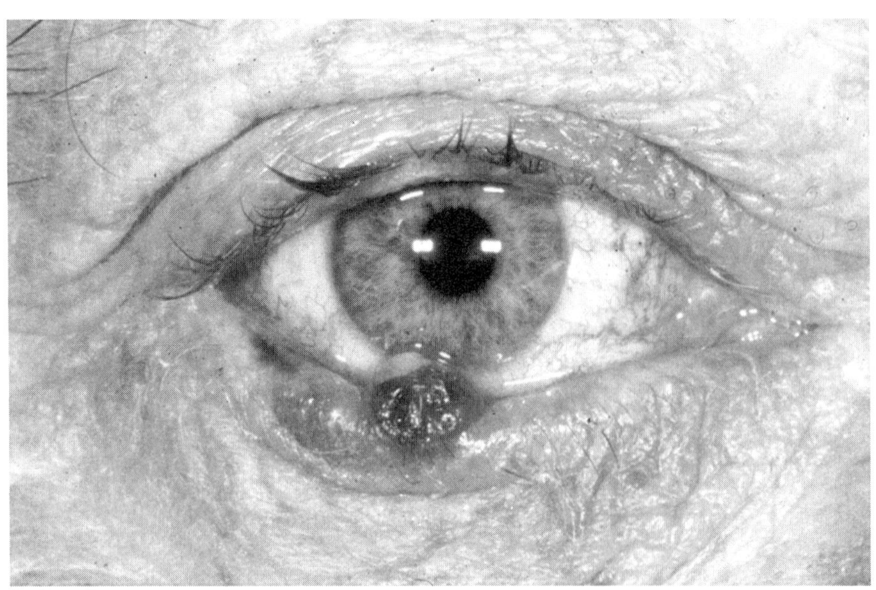

Figure 7 Eyelid melanoma located at the lower eyelid margin. There was an area of conjunctival melanosis adjacent to this cutaneous melanoma.

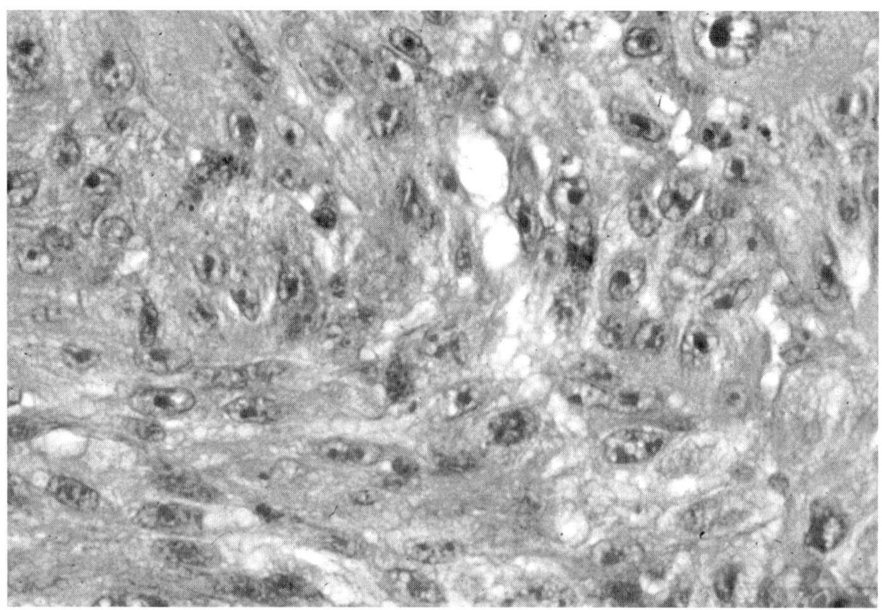

Figure 8 Histopathology of the eyelid melanoma from Figure 7. The lesion consists of cells forming swirling cords and nodules with scattered vascular channels present. The cells contain pleomorphic nuclei with prominent nucleoli and clumped chromatin (hematoxylin and eosin, ×185).

addition, no single set of criteria in the literature can reproducibly differentiate between these four types (331). Acral lentiginous melanoma affects only the palms and soles and superficial spreading melanoma is the most common form elsewhere. It is characterized by a pronounced radial growth phase (i.e., epidermal spread beyond the horizontal extent of the dermal invasion) and may be present for a prolonged period prior to becoming invasive. Nodular melanoma, in contrast, is described as having vertical growth throughout the lesion, with coexistent dermal invasion wherever there is intraepithelial disease. This type is thought to become invasive shortly after its appearance. Lentigo maligna melanoma arises in lentigo maligna (Figs. 9 and 10) and displays basilar palisading of atypical melanocytes within the epidermis and dermal appendages. This type of melanoma was originally thought to be less invasive than the other forms (128,329).

Several studies have looked at the relative frequency of the various histologic types of cutaneous melanoma found in the eyelid. Nodular melanoma was found in 13% to 59%, superficial spreading in 22% to 38%, and lentigo maligna in 19% to 61% (87,111,128,326). The wide ranges may reflect interobserver variability in diagnosis and the relatively small number of patients in most of these series.

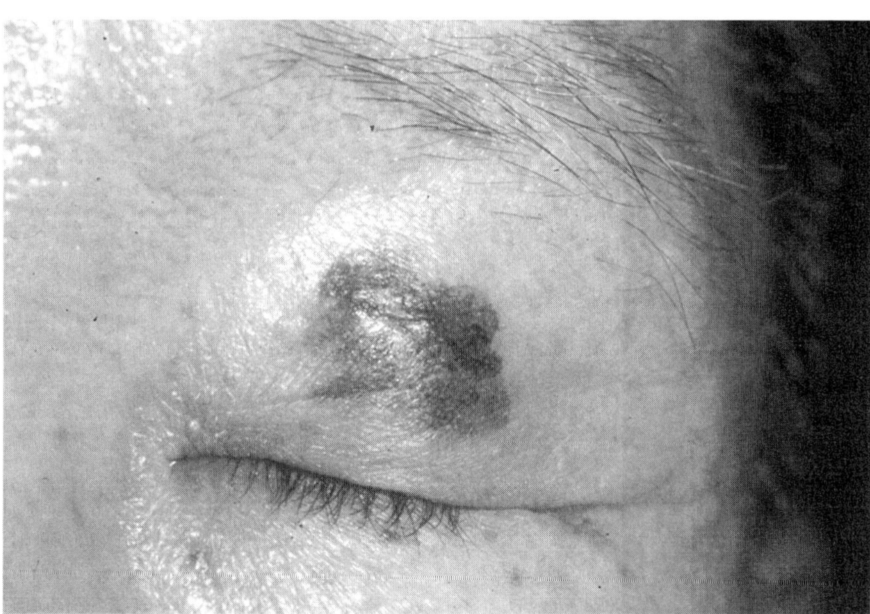

Figure 9 Lentigo maligna melanoma of the eyelid in a 55-year-old man. The lesion had been present for 7 years before showing significant growth over the last year. Note the irregular shape and variable pigmentation of the lesion.

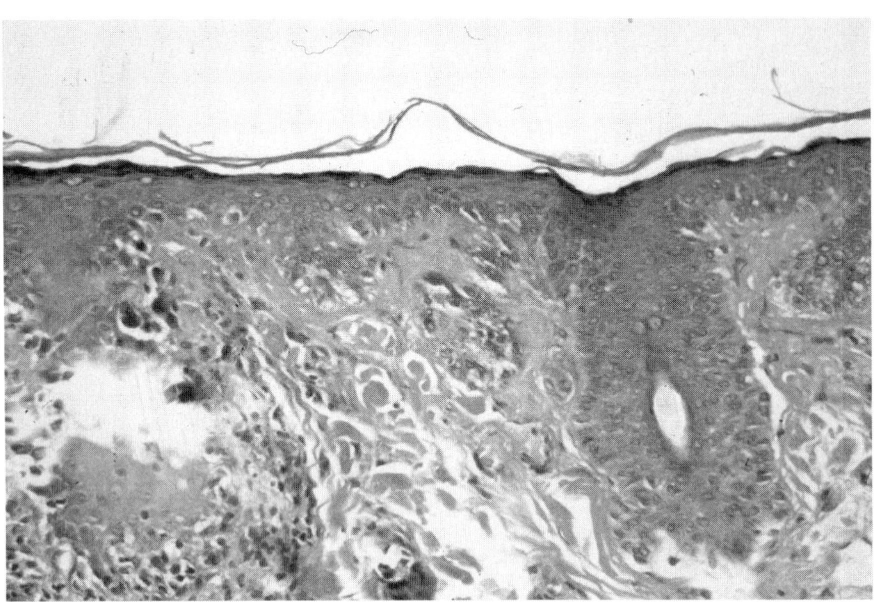

Figure 10 Histopathology of the lentigo maligna melanoma from Figure 9. There is a proliferation of atypical melanocytes present at the epidermal–dermal junction that show atypical cytologic features including nuclear pleomorphisim, high nuclear to cytoplasmic ratios, and prominent nucleoli. These cells invade the superficial dermis (hematoxylin and eosin, × 72).

Nonetheless, the histological type did not influence survival in any of these studies.

Depth of Invasion

The depth of invasion of a given melanoma can be described in two different ways: the histological tissue level at the deepest point of invasion (Clark level) or the measured depth of invasion in millimeters (Breslow thickness).

Clark levels

Level I: Confined to epidermis

Level II: Invasion into papillary dermis, past the basement membrane

Level III: Tumor filling papillary dermis, compressing, but not invading, reticular dermis

Level IV: Invasion of the reticular dermis

Level V: Invasion of the subcutaneous tissue

Often both measures are given in pathologic reports because they have been shown to have prognostic implications (87).

Metastases

Malignant melanoma of the eyelid has been reported to metastasize to regional lymph nodes in 11% of cases, with distant metastases in 7% of cases (128). Another review of 24 cases showed a metastatic rate of 54% with longer follow-up (87). The technique of sentinel lymph node biopsy to aid in staging and determination of treatment protocols is under investigation (87,90).

Prognosis

A large retrospective study of cutaneous melanoma in Sweden examined the prognosis for patients with skin melanoma at various body sites (319). It found that eyelid melanomas (66 out of 12,353 cutaneous melanomas) had the best prognosis, with a 5-year Relative Survival Rate of 97.6% for men and 75.3% for women, a reduction in mortality of approximately 40% compared to melanoma in the upper extremity (the control in the study) (319). Another study of eyelid melanoma with a follow-up of 3 to 18 years found a death rate of 58% (50% related to melanoma) and a metastatic rate of 54% (87). Because of the rarity of eyelid melanomas and the limited follow-up in many retrospective studies, the prognosis for eyelid skin melanoma is difficult to pinpoint, but in general it seems to be equal to or better than cutaneous melanoma at other body sites.

Several case series have considered factors that may affect the prognosis in cutaneous melanoma of the eyelid. One study of 24 patients determined that age, sex, location, and histological type were not significant prognostic indicators, whereas Clark level >IV and Breslow thickness >1.5 mm conferred a worse prognosis (87). Another study found no statistical benefit with clear surgical margins >5 mm compared to those less <5 mm, but confirmed the poor prognosis related to increased Breslow thickness (89). One retrospective study suggested that an eyelid margin location carried a worse prognosis (111).

MELANOCYTIC PROLIFERATIONS OF THE CONJUNCTIVA

Nevi

Nevi of the conjunctiva are similar to those of the skin and are classified in a similar way. The major difference anatomically relates to the absence of a dermis in the conjunctiva.

Congenital Melanocytic Nevi

Common Nevus

Congenital and acquired common conjunctival nevi exhibit similar clinical and histopathologic characteristics, but the common congenital melanocytic nevi are typically larger than the acquired type and present at an earlier age. Large congenital nevi of the skin have shown an increased risk of malignant change (compared to acquired forms) but this is not repeated in conjunctival congenital melanocytic nevi. The nests of nevus cells that make up common conjunctival nevi may be located in a junctional, compound, or subepithelial location. They are more common on the bulbar conjunctiva but when present on the palpebral conjunctiva, their cells may penetrate deep into the tarsus. The cells display maturation from dendritic to neuroid as they reach deeper tissue planes (96).

Oculodermal and Ocular Melanosis

A clinical variant of oculodermal melanosis that only involves ocular structures, and not the periocular skin, does occur and is called congenital ocular melanosis. This presents as a blue to slate-gray coloration of the globe and with a dark fundus secondary to increased pigmentation of the sclera, episclera, and uvea. The melanocytes in this condition are uniformly pigmented and are located at the level of the sclera/episclera, rather than the substantia propria of the conjunctiva. For this reason, the lesion is not mobile when tested with a cotton tip applicator at the slit lamp. No relationship between this condition and conjunctival melanoma has been found (96).

Blue Nevus

Blue nevi of the conjunctiva (Fig. 11) are similar to those of the skin, although they often appear brown because the non-keratinized epithelium of the conjunctiva does not cause the Tyndall effect (96).

Melanocytoma

Melanocytomas typically occur in the uveal tract and optic nerve head, but can be found within the deep substantia propria and episclera. They are very darkly pigmented, almost black in color. Microscopically, they consist of large polyhedral melanocytes that are filled with melanin (96).

"Acquired" Conjunctival Melanocytic Nevi

Common Nevus

Common acquired conjunctival nevi typically develop during the first decade of life. Initially, they appear as flat pigmented lesions, but with maturation they thicken and display cysts. They typically have sharp margins and are most often found along the corneoscleral limbus followed by other bulbar sites, the plica, caruncle, and eyelid margin. Very rarely, they occur in the conjunctival fornix or on the palpebral conjunctiva and pigmented lesions in these locations should be suspected of malignancy. They are found superficially in the conjunctiva and are therefore freely mobile when manipulated by a cotton tip applicator. With very rare exceptions, they do not extend onto the cornea. Feeder vessels may be present with these lesions and are therefore not necessarily indicative of melanoma. Compound nevi often contain cysts that can be seen by slit lamp biomicroscopy (Figs. 12 and 13). Common nevi may increase in size or change pigmentation, especially during puberty or pregnancy (96). One study showed a gradual change in size in 8% of patients, with an alteration in pigmentation in 13% (276). Less than 1% of these conjunctival nevi were found to transform into

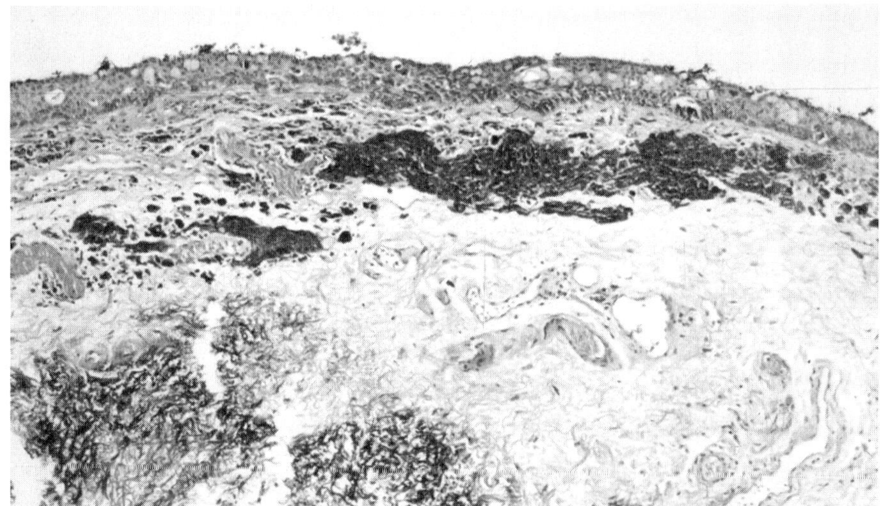

Figure 11 Histopathology of a conjunctival blue nevus. The lesion is composed of heavily pigmented spindle-shaped cells with bland nuclei. Scattered melanophages are also present within the lesion (hematoxylin and eosin, ×28).

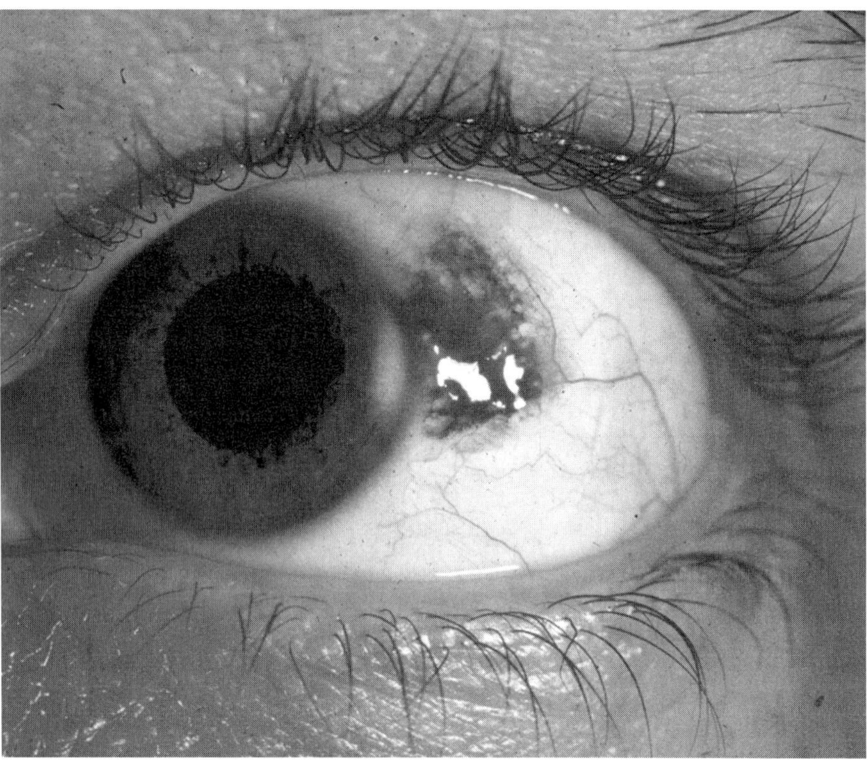

Figure 12 Conjunctival compound nevus near the temporal limbus. Note the small cysts that can be seen clinically in this picture.

malignant melanoma (276), and it is noteworthy that 16–30% of conjunctival nevi are non-pigmented (96, 276).

Microscopically, congenital and acquired melanocytic conjunctival nevi are similar, but the acquired lesions may be less cellular. In histopathologic studies 70% to 77% of specimens were compound, 4% to 16% subepithelial, and only 2% to 3% were junctional (126,276). A junctional nevus in a young individual may appear histologically identical to an area of primary acquired melanosis (PAM, discussed below). Often the only distinguishing feature between the two conditions is the patient's age, with junctional nevi being a lesion of children and young adults, whereas PAM affects individuals >30 years of age (96).

Combined Nevus

A nevocellular nevus is sometimes associated with a blue nevus. In a review of 30 patients with this so-called combined nevus, Crawford suggested that this

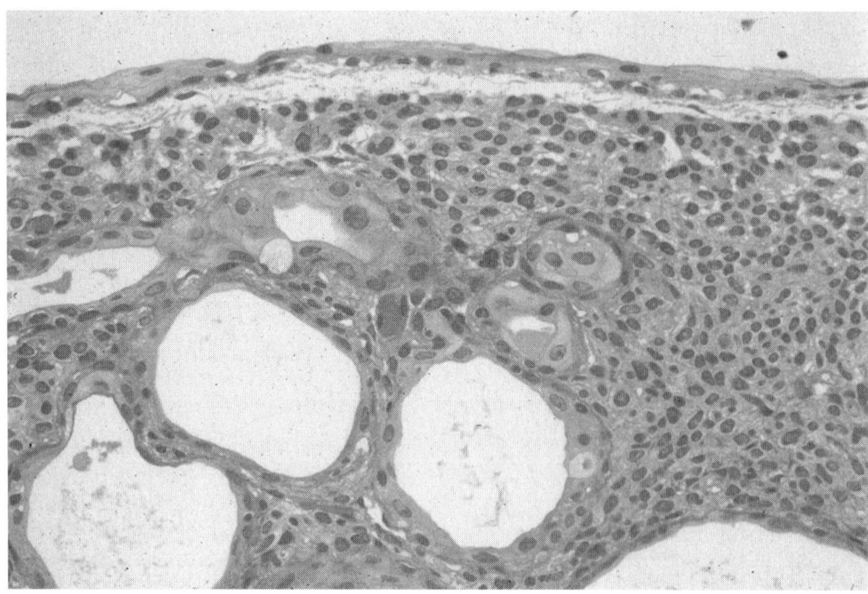

Figure 13 Histopathology of the conjunctival compound nevus from Figure 12. The lesion is composed of tightly coherent nests of cells with bland nuclei. Numerous cysts are contained within the lesion (hematoxylin and eosin, ×72).

combination is fairly common despite the paucity of reported cases. Clinically, it may be suggested by a history of a pigmented conjunctival lesion since birth that develops cysts or has both a blue-gray and a brown color. They are thought to have a benign behavior (61).

Spitz Nevus

Spitz nevi of the conjunctiva appear similar to those of the skin. They often are lightly pigmented and may display rapid growth. Microscopically they are composed of spindle cells arranged in fascicles oriented perpendicular to the overlying epithelium and unlike Spitz nevi of the skin do not include epithelioid cells. They may have Kamino bodies and show mitoses in the subepithelial nevus cells (96).

Recurrent Nevus

A pigmented lesion may recur at the site of a previously excised nevus and raise the possibility of a malignant melanoma. The distinction between a recurrent nevus and a melanoma cannot be determined without histopathologic evaluation (96).

Inflamed Nevus

Despite the fact that conjunctival melanoma is extremely rare in adolescents and young adults, the rapid growth of pigmented lesions in the conjunctiva in this age group may lead to suspicion of malignant melanoma and the need for an excisional biopsy. Microscopically, these lesions appear to be common nevocellular nevi with an impressive inflammatory infiltrate that is usually predominantly lymphocytic, though plasma cells and eosinophils may be present. The cause of the inflammation remains uncertain, but the inflammatory reaction does not appear to destroy the nevi. Pathologically, inflamed nevi may be difficult to differentiate from a lymphoid tumor if a lymphocytic infiltrate predominates and nevocellular nests are extremely sparse (96).

Dysplastic Nevus

While the histological characteristics of cutaneous dysplastic nevi have been described earlier, there are no specific criteria for the diagnosis in the conjunctiva. If they do exist as a separate clinical entity, they may lack the typical maturation of common conjunctival nevi (96). A conjunctival melanoma has been documented in a patient with the dysplastic nevus syndrome (109).

Racial Melanosis

Individuals with dark complexions can develop brown conjunctival pigmentation, commonly termed racial melanosis. This pigmentation, consisting of uniform hyperpigmentation of the basal epithelium, is bilateral but may be somewhat asymmetric and often becomes more apparent with age. It is often darker near the corneoscleral limbus and typically involves the interpalpebral area, becoming less obvious further from the limbus. The pigment, which occasionally extends into the peripheral cornea is superficial and therefore easily moved over the deeper scleral tissue. Hyperactive melanocytes are often difficult to identify because of the deep pigmentation of the surrounding epithelial cells. Racial melanosis lacks cellular atypia and has no malignant potential (96).

Primary Acquired Melanosis

Clinical Characteristics

Primary acquired melanosis (PAM) is a variably pigmented, clinically flat, unilateral, acquired conjunctival lesion that may involve all areas of the conjunctiva, including the fornices and palpebral conjunctiva. It usually occurs in middle-aged to elderly Caucasians, though it may be seen in persons of color. It arises in an area that previously lacked pigmentation, hence the designation acquired. It has been estimated to occur to some degree in up to 36% of Caucasian populations (117), though this is likely an overestimate of the true prevalence because some lesions that were really nevi were histologically classified as PAM in this study. The pigmentation of these lesions is variable, ranging from being absent (PAM *sine pigmento*) to dark brown, and the lesions are often not uniformly pigmented. They are typically flat but may vary in thickness and contain cystic areas and have irregular borders without sharp margins. The lesions may change in color and size with time. PAM can involve a major part of the conjunctiva or multiple regions of a single eye, which can make complete excision impossible (157).

In contrast to racial melanosis the vast majority of cases of PAM occur in Caucasians and the condition is unilateral as opposed to bilateral. PAM tends to have more irregular borders and pigmentation than conjunctival nevi, and its changing shape and pigmentation over time may help to differentiate it from a simple nevus. Congenital ocular melanosis may mimic PAM by being unilateral and having irregular patchy borders. However, the blue to slate-gray coloration of ocular melanosis is atypical for PAM and PAM moves with conjunctival manipulation while ocular melanosis does not.

Histopathology

Microscopically PAM exists with and without atypia. This distinction cannot be made clinically, so PAM must be excised and examined by a pathologist to make this determination and guide therapy. PAM *sine pigmento* may be very difficult to diagnose clinically (123).

PAM without atypia occurs when there is an overabundance of melanin in a conjunctival epithelial lesion in the absence of melanocytic hyperplasia or when melanocytic hyperplasia occurs only along the basilar epithelium and does not show signs of cellular atypia. Four types of atypical melanocytes are recognized in PAM with atypia: (*i*) small polyhedral, (*ii*) spindle shaped, (*iii*) large with complex arborizing dendrites, and (*iv*) round epithelioid (Fig. 14). PAM with atypia can have one of several growth patterns: (*i*) basilar hyperplasia, (*ii*) basilar nests, (*iii*) intraepithelial nests, (*iv*) pagetoid spread, and (*v*) complete replacement of the epithelium (melanoma in situ) (98,157). Microscopic evidence of melanocytes invading the substantia propria indicates a malignant melanoma, rather than PAM (157).

Prognosis

A histopathologically confirmed diagnosis of PAM without atypia with a benign follow-up of 10 years is thought to carry a minimal risk of melanoma progression (97). PAM with atypia, on the other hand, has shown progression to melanoma in 46% of patients (97). The presence of epithelioid cells within the lesion increases the risk of progression to melanoma to 75%. Any growth pattern other than basilar hyperplasia carries a 90% risk of malignant transformation, compared to approximately 20% for lesions without either of these characteristics (97,98). The progression to melanoma typically occurs within 6 years of the diagnosis of PAM with atypia (157).

Secondary Acquired Melanosis

Secondary acquired melanosis refers to conjunctival pigmentation resulting from an increased production of melanin in response to a systemic or external cause without melanocytic hyperplasia. This may be unilateral or bilateral depending on the cause. The causes include pregnancy, chronic inflammation, irradiation, chemical irritation, medications, and systemic disorders such as Addison disease (174).

Conjunctival Melanoma

Clinical Characteristics

Conjunctival melanoma presents clinically as a unilateral pigmented lesion of the conjunctiva that may have a variable color and irregular borders. It may be indistinguishable from PAM by slit lamp biomicroscopy. A physical finding suggestive of melanoma rather than PAM is the presence of nodules within the pigmented lesion. Conjunctival melanoma most commonly occurs on the epibulbar conjunctiva, more specifically in the perilimbal area (211,322). Less commonly it will invade the palpebral conjunctiva, superficial cornea and caruncle (Fig. 15) (211,322). Conjunctival melanoma arises in three clinical settings: in apparently normal conjunctiva (de novo), associated with a nevus, or associated with PAM (Figs. 16 and 17). Conjunctival melanoma arises de novo in about 12% of patients (97). Approximately 75% of conjunctival melanomas arise in an area of PAM and the rest have evidence of a preexisting conjunctival nevus (97). The occurrence of malignant progression of benign pigmented lesions is the reason why conjunctival nevi and PAM must be followed for evidence of clinical change. As mentioned earlier, nevi transform into melanoma at a rate of <1% (276), while PAM with atypia progresses to melanoma in

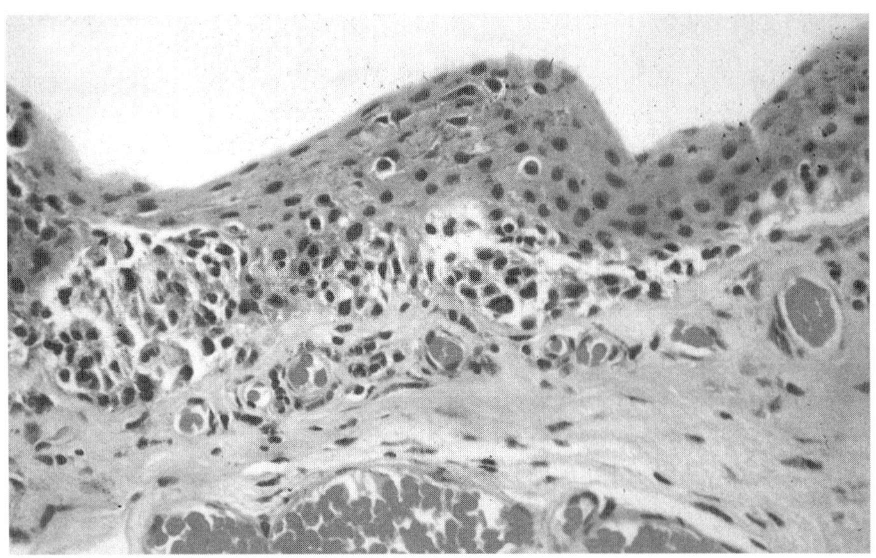

Figure 14 Primary acquired melanosis with atypia of the conjunctiva. The lesion is composed of a junctional proliferation of atypical pleomorphic cells with high nuclear to cytoplasmic ratios and hyperchromatic nuclei. These nests of cells are loosely coherent. Occasional cells contain melanin pigment (hematoxylin and eosin, × 72).

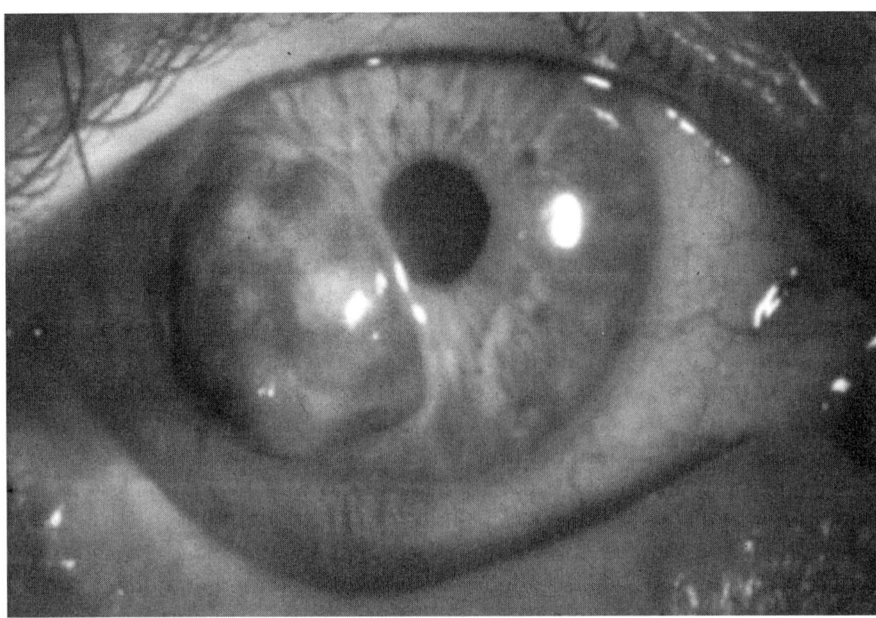

Figure 15 Conjunctival melanoma extending onto the surface of the cornea.

approximately 50% of cases (98). Any significant change in size of a pigmented lesion or the development of new nodules within the lesion should prompt a biopsy.

From the standpoint of metastases, conjunctival melanoma behaves more like cutaneous melanoma than uveal melanoma. Because the conjunctiva contains lymphatic vessels, lymphatic spread to regional lymph nodes occurs, in contrast to uveal melanoma, which very rarely spreads via the lymphatics due to a lack of intraocular lymphatic channels (270). In addition, conjunctival melanoma may be present in multiple areas within the conjunctiva due to local spread within the subepithelial lymph channels (Fig. 18) (155). In one study with an average follow-up of 6 years, metastases to regional lymph nodes occurred in 41% of patients, most commonly to the preauricular lymph nodes, followed by the deep cervical and submandibular nodes. Approximately 26% had distant metastases without evidence of regional lymph node metastasis (88). Another study found a 10-year incidence of regional lymph node

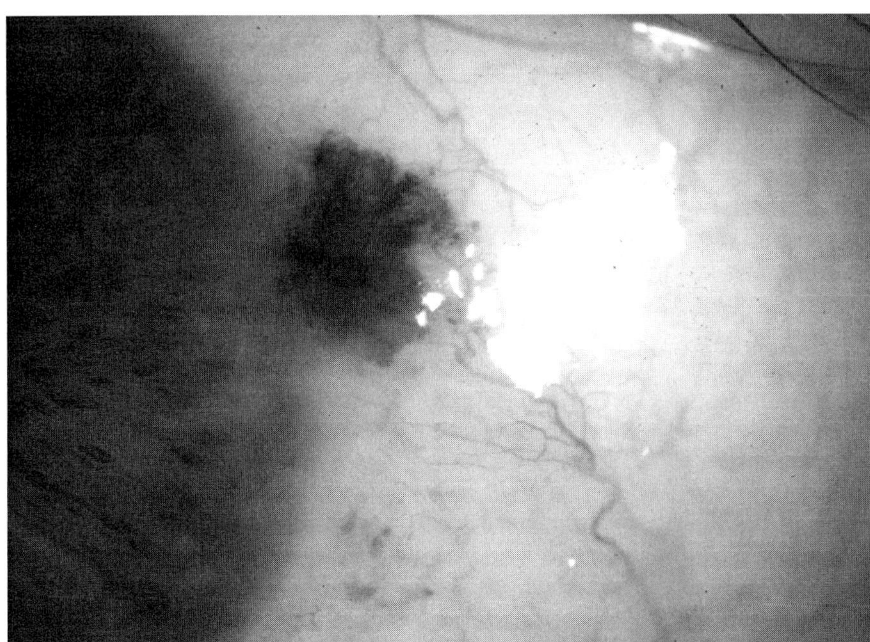

Figure 16 Conjunctival melanoma arising in primary acuquired melanosis with atypia. Note the perilimbal location and the similarity with the clinical appearance of the conjunctival compound nevus seen in Figure 12.

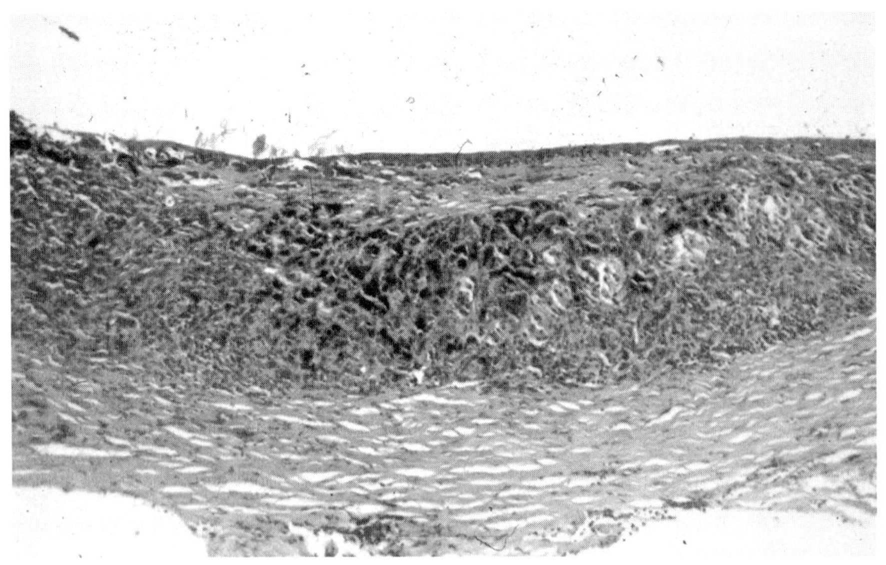

Figure 17 Histopathology for the conjunctival melanoma from Figure 16. The lesion consists of loosely coherent nests of cells with melanin pigment, pleomorphic hyperchromatic nuclei, prominent nucleoli, and variable amounts of cytoplasm. It invades the lymphatic channels and is surrounded by a lymphocytic infiltrate (hematoxylin and eosin, × 28).

metastasis of 11% and of systemic metastasis of 18% (323). An analysis of 194 patients over 52 years found regional metastases in 21% and distant metastases in 25% (211).

Epidemiology

Primary conjunctival melanoma is rare and accounts for <5% of ocular melanomas (47). It occurs in less than 1 per million Caucasians individuals (270), and appears to be increasing in frequency in recent years, specifically in white males >60 years of age (339). This follows the trend in cutaneous melanoma (69), possibly reflecting common risk factors. Over 93% of cases in the United States are found in Caucasians, with >87% of patients being over the age of 40 years (339). The average age at diagnosis is approximately 60 years (322). Some studies suggest a greater prevalence in men than in women (339) whereas others show no sex predilection (268) and yet others find a female predominance (224). It is the second most common form of melanoma affecting the eye and adnexa, representing approximately 5% of all ocular melanomas (47). Previously considered with uveal melanoma as a single entity, ocular melanoma, conjunctival melanoma is now recognized as having significant differences in clinical behavior, particularly in its mode of metastasis. Regarded as one of the most malignant forms of cancer, it was treated with

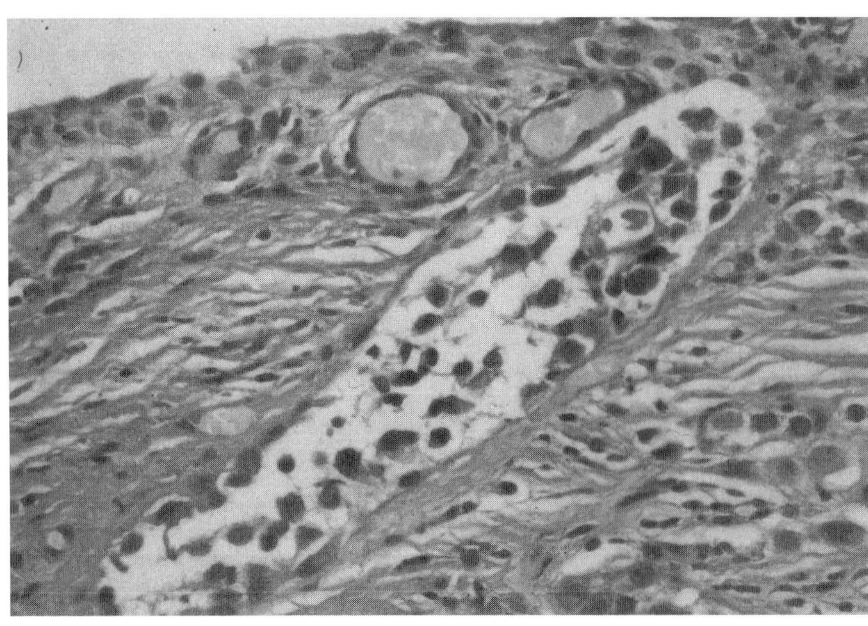

Figure 18 Conjunctival melanoma with invasion of the lymphatic channels. Note the tumor cells within the large lymph duct in the center of the figure (hematoxylin and eosin, × 115).

exenteration of the affected orbit in the majority of cases. Several lesions may clinically mimic conjunctival melanoma.

Risk Factors

Because of the rarity of conjunctival melanoma, specific risk factors for its development are difficult to determine. Ultraviolet (UV) radiation has been evaluated as a possible risk factor, but with inconclusive results (270). Conjunctival nevi and PAM without atypia impose a small risk, but PAM with atypia has a much larger risk of conjunctival melanoma (97). It is unclear whether patients with the dysplastic nevus syndrome or neurofibromatosis have an increased risk of conjunctival melanoma (270).

Histopathology

Four types of atypical cells have been noted in conjunctival melanoma: (*i*) small polyhedral cells, (*ii*) large epithelioid cells, (*iii*) spindle cells, and (*iv*) balloon cells (97). By themselves the small polyhedral cells are not indicative of a melanoma as they resemble nevus cells. However, additional architectural characteristics suggestive of melanoma should be sought, such as lack of maturation as the lesion invades the deeper tissues, the presence of mitoses in the melanocytes in the substantia propria, and an epithelial component that extends laterally beyond the area of deeper invasion (157).

Occasionally when the microscopic findings are equivocal immunohistochemical staining may be helpful, specifically in differentiating melanocytic from non-melanocytic lesions. S-100 protein, tyrosinase, melan-A, HMB45/50, and MiTF have all been shown to have high expression in conjunctival melanomas (151). HMB45 has also been helpful in distinguishing benign from malignant melanocytic lesions (274).

Prognosis

The 5- and 10-year mortality rates for patients with conjunctival melanoma range from 12% to 20% and 23% to 30%, respectively (183,211,224,268,322,330). Local recurrence rates of 26%, 51%, and 65% at 5, 10, and 15 years, respectively, have been seen in a cohort of patients with extensive follow-up (278). Multiple studies have evaluated clinical and histological factors that may affect prognosis. These are summarized below.

Age

A slightly worse prognosis may relate to increased age according to one small case series (62), but subsequent studies have not found this to be a strong prognostic indicator.

Location

Multiple studies have found that melanomas in a perilimbal location have a better prognosis than those in other locations (62,97,158,183,211,224,278,322,330). Patients with solitary tumors also do better than those with multifocal lesions (224).

Tumor Thickness

In general, tumors of increasing thickness tend to have a worse prognosis (9,97,158,183,211,224). Specifically, several studies have shown this to be true with tumors >2 mm in depth compared to those <2 mm (158,183). Another case series study found a worse prognosis with tumor invasion into the deeper substantia propria, without limiting the evaluation to a precise measurement (9).

Histological Features

Multiple histological factors have been investigated for their effect on prognosis. The presence of epithelioid cells (9), mixed cell types (224), and the absence of small polyhedral cells in the lesion (97) have all been associated with worse outcomes. Architectural characteristics such as lack of associated PAM (278), presence of pagetoid spread in associated PAM (97), and presence of PAM *sine pigmento* (158) also carry an unfavorable prognosis. Higher numbers of mitoses within the lesion (62,97) and microscopic evidence of lymphatic invasion (224) are also negative prognostic factors.

Clinical Staging

Higher tumor staging based on the tumor, nodes, metastases (TNM) system of the American Joint Committee on Cancer, although not discussed much in the literature, was associated with a worse prognosis in one study (330).

Management

Incomplete surgical excision has an adverse effect on outcome (9,278). Simple surgical excision without adjuvant therapy was found to have a negative prognosis, regardless of surgical margins (68,224,330).

Indeterminate Melanocytic Proliferations of the Conjunctiva

Some melanocytic lesions of the conjunctiva do not clearly fall into one of the above categories and experienced ocular pathologists have been shown to have difficulty coming to a consensus on these lesions in randomized studies (127). The prognostic significance of an indeterminate melanocytic proliferation is uncertain.

MELANOCYTIC PROLIFERATIONS OF THE ORBIT

Melanocytoma

Melanocytomas (magnocellular nevi) are benign heavily pigmented tumors that are most commonly found on the optic nerve, but which may arise wherever uveal melanocytes are present. They are typically asymptomatic and are often found in dark-complexioned individuals (343). They are often jet black and typically remain stable in size, but may enlarge over time. Histologically, they are composed of plump, round to polyhedral melanocytes with distinct cellular borders, small circular nuclei, and a low nuclear:cytoplasmic ratio. Because of their dark pigmentation, histologic specimens often must be bleached to allow demonstration of the cellular morphology (Figs. 19 and 20). The overall rate of malignant transformation is thought to be very low, but a few reports document malignant change in patients followed regularly by fundoscopy (67,207,285). Characteristics of malignant change include increased size and decrease in visual acuity. Because melanocytoma and melanoma of the optic nerve can be difficult to distinguish clinically, patients must be followed closely.

Primary Orbital Melanoma

Although one series of orbital tumors including secondary and metastatic neoplasms reported orbital involvement by a melanoma in 7% (288), primary orbital melanoma is extremely rare and probably the rarest form of ocular melanoma. J.A. Shields and C.L. Shields classified orbital melanoma into four distinct categories: (*i*) primary orbital melanoma, (*ii*) secondary orbital melanoma, (*iii*) metastatic orbital melanoma, and (*iv*) radiation-induced orbital melanoma (289). This classification system provides a framework in which to discuss orbital melanoma.

Primary orbital melanoma represents <1% of orbital masses (284) and 12% of all melanomas involving the orbital tissues (289). Of those determined to be primary tumors, a large percentage (90%) are thought to arise from a predisposing pigmentary lesion: either congenital melanosis or an intraorbital blue nevus (316). The mean age at diagnosis is 42 years old (316), 18 years younger than reported for uveal melanoma (301). Some studies suggest a male predominance, while others do not. The vast majority of patients are Caucasians, with only two African-American cases documented (316). Histologically, these tumors have been classified using the modified Callender classification (see the section entitled Primary Melanoma of the Uvea). Approximately 50% of primary orbital melanomas have a spindle cell morphology and the other 50% are of mixed spindle and epithelioid cell type (316). A poor prognosis is associated with older age at diagnosis, underlying congenital melanosis, tumors of mixed cell type, and tumors with a high-mitotic rate (316). In the small series of Tellada et al. tumor size and lymphocytic response did not have any prognostic significance (316) and mortality rate from metastasis was 38% (with a 1- to 13-year follow-up), with the majority involving the liver (88%) (316).

Schultz et al. compared primary orbital melanomas and central nervous system (CNS) melanocytomas and proposed that the two entities represent a single-disease process (262). They reached this conclusion because the tumors tend to present in patients of similar age and behave in a similar manner. In

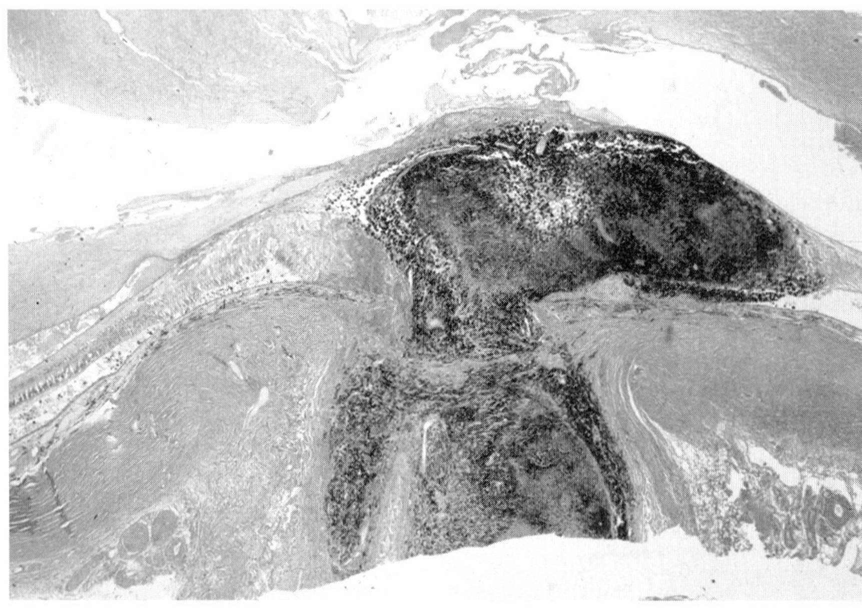

Figure 19 Melanocytoma of the optic nerve. Note the heavily pigmented, necrotic tumor that invades into the peripapillary retina (hematoxylin and eosin, ×6).

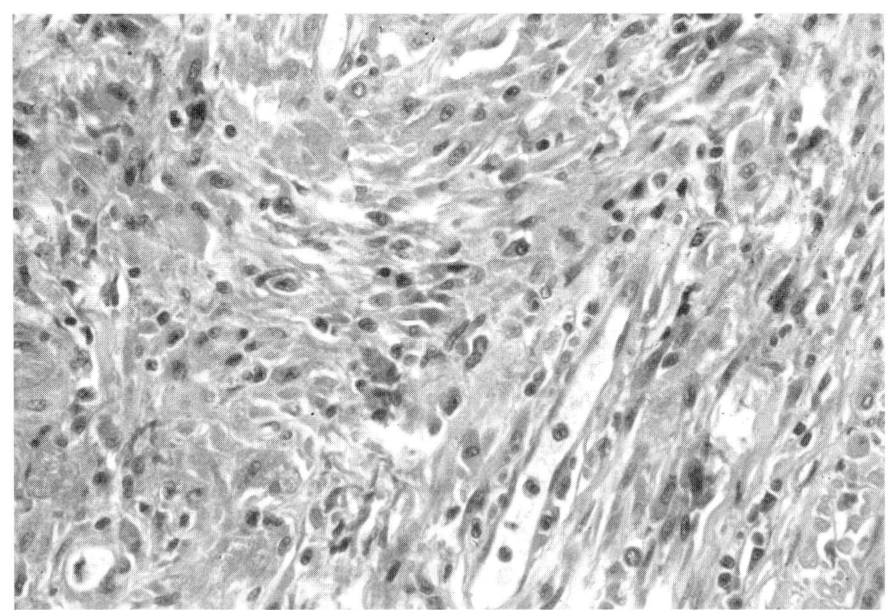

Figure 20 Higher magnification of a bleached section of the melanocytoma from Figure 19. This staining process allows identification of the plump polyhedral cells with small nuclei and numerous melanophages (hematoxylin and eosin, ×115).

addition, the gross and microscopic appearances of the two tumor types are almost identical and both are derived from neural crest cells. They proposed using the term melanocytic tumors of the CNS and orbit for all of these cases (262).

Secondary Orbital Melanoma

Secondary orbital melanomas represent approximately 75% of orbital melanomas (289). This category consists of invasive uveal, conjunctival, or eyelid melanomas that have extended into the orbit. The most common form of secondary orbital melanoma, representing 66% of cases in one series, comes from extrascleral extension of uveal melanomas (289), which has been detected clinically in 8–10% of all uveal melanomas prior to enucleation (223,271). The usual route for extraocular extension is alongside the scleral emissaries and vortex veins. Less commonly, uveal melanoma may extend into the orbit along the optic nerve or by direct scleral penetration.

Orbital extension from a primary conjunctival melanoma is less common but it accounted for 29% of secondary orbital melanomas in the Shields series (289). Because of the superficial location of the primary tumor, these melanomas are often diagnosed at an earlier stage than uveal melanomas.

The least common (approximately 5%) form of secondary orbital melanoma represents extension of a cutaneous eyelid melanoma (289). As with conjunctival melanomas, cutaneous melanomas of the eyelid are often detected and treated at an early stage because of their conspicuous location. Given that depth of invasion is thought to be a major prognostic factor for cutaneous melanoma of the eyelid, the prognosis may be worse in these tumors with orbital extension (87).

Metastatic Orbital Melanoma

Metastatic melanoma to the orbit is relatively uncommon, representing 13% of all orbital melanomas (289) and <1% of all orbital masses (288). Most commonly, the metastases come from a primary cutaneous site (Figs. 21 and 22) and these patients often have other metastases at the time of diagnosis. Metastasis from a primary uveal melanoma is somewhat less common, but does occur (289). Often these patients have already undergone treatment for the primary tumor and the metastasis is discovered later. Prognosis for metastatic tumors to the orbit is much worse than for primary and secondary tumors, with an average survival of 1.3 years, and a 2-year survival rate of 27% (49).

Radiation-Induced Orbital Melanoma

There have been reports of an orbital melanoma developing in patients treated with radiation for orbital rhabdomyosarcoma at a young age (178,184). Because of the rarity of these cases, it is difficult to establish a causal link between the radiation and subsequent development of the melanoma.

MELANOCYTIC PROLIFERATIONS OF THE UVEA

Uveal melanoma is much more common than the other forms of ocular melanoma, representing approximately 85% of all cases (47). The uvea normally contains melanocytes that are derived from neural crest cells, as are the melanocytes of skin and

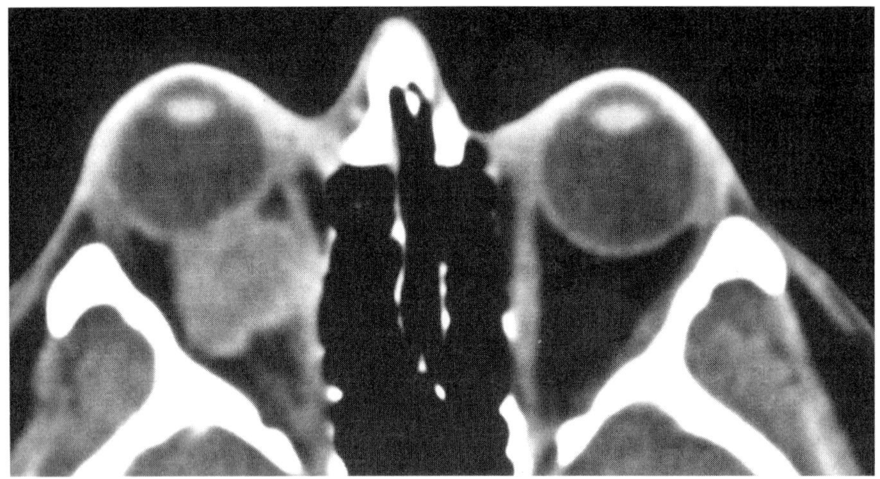

Figure 21 Axial computed tomography CT scan of the orbits of a patient with metastatic melanoma to the orbit from a primary cutaneous site.

conjunctiva. They differ from pigmented epithelium of the iris, ciliary body and retinal pigment epithelium (RPE). Melanocytic proliferations of the uvea fall into the same broad categories as those found in other areas of the body but key differences will be discussed in the relevant sections.

Common Uveal Melanocytic Nevi

Iris Nevus

Iris nevi appear as pigmented nodules on the surface of the iris and are visible in approximately 50% of adults (209). They may be single or multiple and may affect both eyes. Microscopically, they appear as aggregates of variably pigmented melanocytes with distortion or replacement of normal iris architecture (243). The melanocytes are usually located within the anterior stroma of the iris (124). Iris freckles may appear similar clinically, but they lack melanocytic hyperplasia and do not disrupt the iris architecture (124). The incidence of iris nevi has been reported to be increased in eyes with choroidal melanomas (241,333), although not all agree (209). Rarely, lesions suspected of being iris nevi may show evidence of growth suggesting transformation into an iris melanoma and such lesions are often excised for pathological evaluation.

Iris Nevus Syndrome

The iris nevus syndrome is a curious condition with a predilection for middle-aged women, characterized by whorls and/or nodules of nevi, atrophy of the iris stroma, heterochromia iridis, ectropion uveae, and

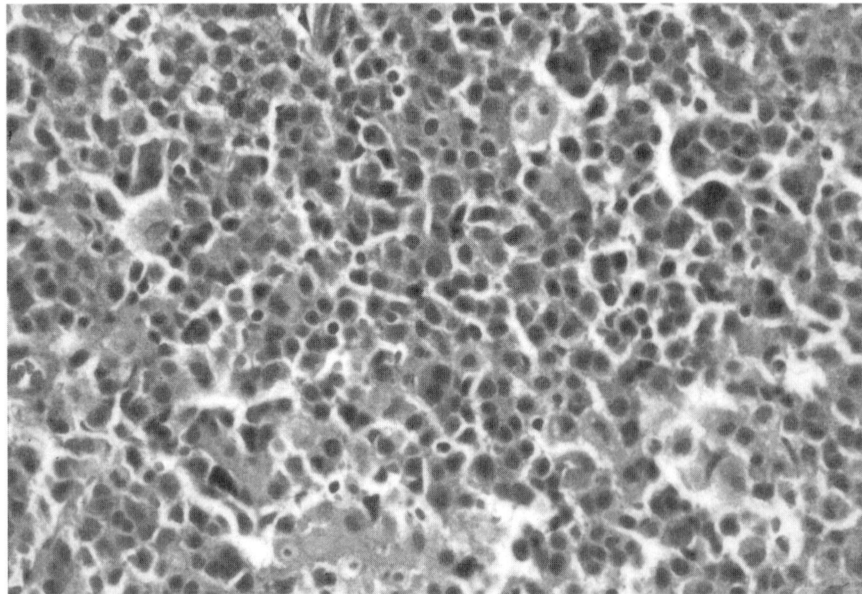

Figure 22 Histopathology of the melanoma from Figure 21. Note the nests and sheets of cells with pleomorphic, hyperchromatic nuclei, occasional prominent nucleoli, and eosinophilic cytoplasm. Immunohistochemical stains were positive for S100, HMB45, and MITF in this specimen (hematoxylin and eosin, $\times$ 115).

peripheral anterior synechiae (54). Histopathological studies have shown a diffuse nevus involving the anterior surface of the iris and overgrowth of endothelium, with descemetization of the anterior chamber angle and the anterior iris surface (79,160,260). Eagle and colleagues (79) postulate that some cases lack nevi and that what appear to be nevi are defects in the corneal endothelium and basement membrane extending over the anterior iris surface. The condition has features in common with Chandler syndrome and essential iris atrophy, and all are part of the iridocorneal endothelial syndrome (see chapter 30).

Choroidal/Ciliary Body Nevus

Because of their location and size, ciliary body nevi do not ordinarily become clinically evident. One histopathological study of 400 eyes postmortem found a 2% prevalence of ciliary body nevi (130). Choroidal nevi are more common clinically and a recent report estimated a prevalence of 4.6, 7.9% in the Caucasian population of the United States (297). Most nevi are <4.5 mm in diameter, slightly thicker than the adjacent normal choroid, and occur predominantly in the posterior choroid (218). Their degree of pigmentation ranges from homogeneous black to yellow-white with only scattered pigmentation.

The types of cells comprising a choroidal/ciliary body nevus vary and are generally classified as plump polyhedral, slender spindle, plump spindle or fusiform, dendritic, or balloon cells (Figs. 23–26) (217). Large round cells with abundant densely pigmented cytoplasm (magnocellular nevus cells) may also be found and the entire spectrum of cells may be present in a single nevus.

Subretinal fluid associated with a pigmented choroidal lesion strongly suggests a melanoma rather than a nevus (180,245,249). In a study of 933 choroidal nevi examined by fluorescein angiography (FA), however, approximately 2% had subretinal fluid in the foveal area (234). The ophthalmoscopic appearance and clinical course over a 10-year period suggested that all nevi except one were benign. One nevus enlarged after remaining stable for 4 years and, following enucleation, was found to be a melanoma. Serous retinal detachment associated with SubRPE neovascularization over a choroidal nevus has also been observed (308).

Since it has been estimated that only one in 8845 choroidal nevi in Caucacians transforms into a malignant melanoma each year (297), there is a need to identify high-risk nevi. In this regard, four features have been identified by Mims and Shields as indicating special risk (210): (*i*) nevi with dimensions of two to five disc diameters, (*ii*) nevi with an apparent elevation on clinical examination or stereoscopic fundus photographs of >3 mm, (*iii*) nevi with a significant disruption of the RPE, and (*iv*) nevi associated with subretinal fluid. Mims and Shields (210) followed 50 suspicious choroidal nevi with these criteria and 194 non-suspicious nevi over a 4-year period: Five (10%) of the suspicious nevi manifested photographic evidence of enlargement over a 4- to 30-month period. The eyes containing these lesions were enucleated, and all were found to contain melanomas. None of the apparently innocuous nevi demonstrated growth. However, enlargement has been documented in at least one histopathologically confirmed choroidal nevus (185).

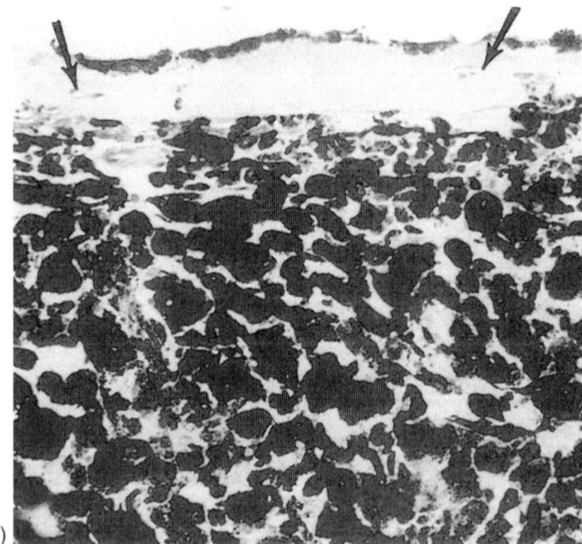

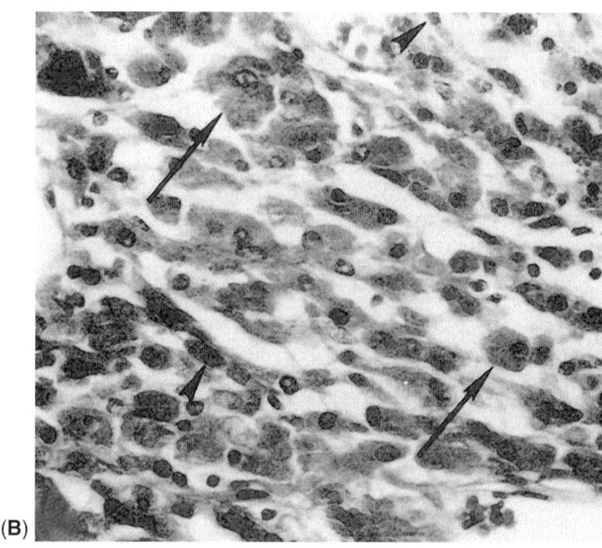

Figure 23 (**A**) Choroidal nevus composed of plump polyhedral and plump spindle-shaped nevus cells. Subretinal pigment epithelium neovascularization (*arrows*) is present over the lesion (hematoxylin and eosin, × 210). (**B**) Bleaching of pigment with potassium permanganate shows the plump polyhedral (*arrows*) and plump spindle-shaped nevus cells (*arrowheads*) more clearly (hematoxylin and eosin, × 330).

(A)
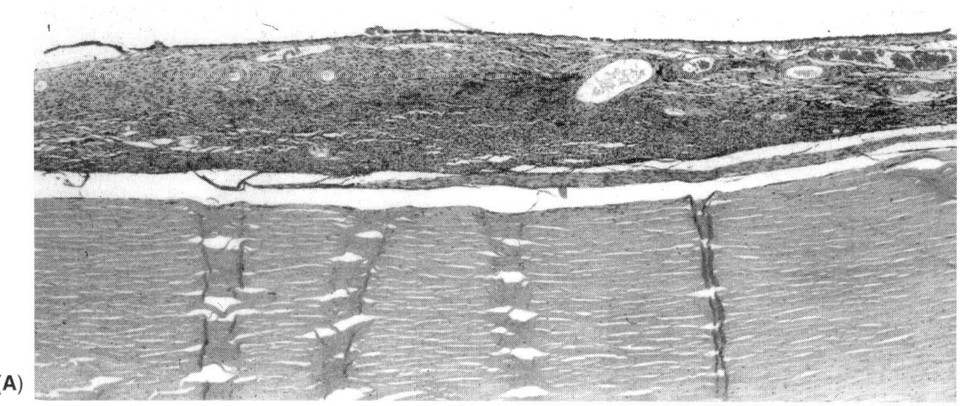

(B)
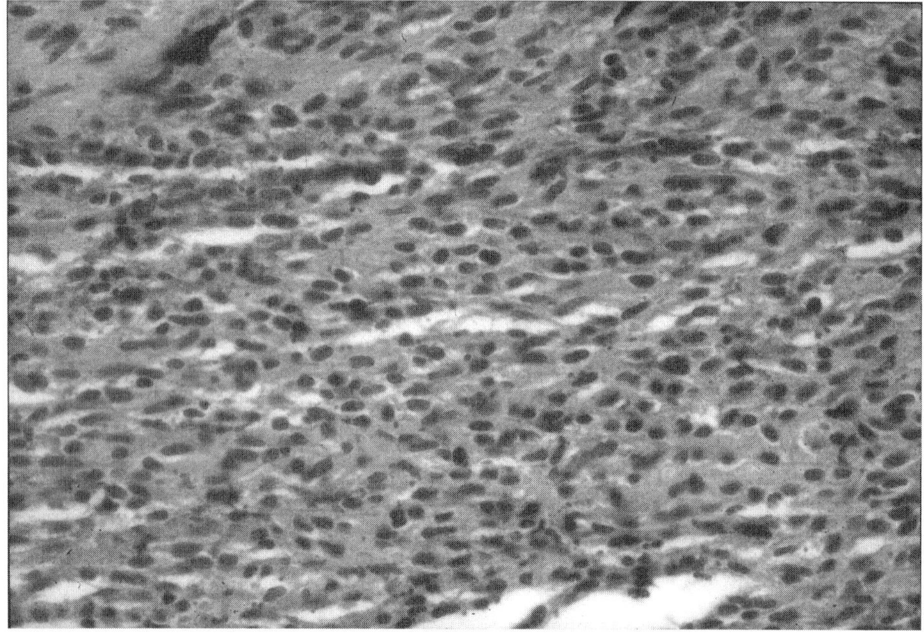

Figure 24 (**A**) Low magnification shows choroidal nevus between Bruch membrane and the sclera (hematoxylin and eosin, ×11). (**B**) The nevus is composed of slender, spindle-shaped, and slightly plump spindle-shaped cells (hematoxylin and eosin, × 115).

Melanocytoma

As described under melanocytic proliferations of the orbit, a melanocytoma is a densely pigmented tumor composed of relatively uniform, plump, round or polyhedral cells with abundant deeply pigmented cytoplasm and small round or oval nuclei without conspicuous nucleoli (Figs. 25 and 26). This distinctive nevus, which was originally described in the optic nerve head, is deeply and usually uniformly pigmented (292,343). It may be located anywhere in the uveal tract (107,146,343) and may be difficult to distinguish clinically from a melanoma (35,261,286). Ciliary body melanocytomas are usually unilateral, may extend into contiguous structures, and slowly enlarge with time (107). Rarely iris and ciliary body melanocytomas undergo partial necrosis with liberation of pigment (107,281). Melanin-laden macrophages can block the trabecular meshwork leading to secondary open-angle glaucoma. A melanocytoma of the ciliary body may extend anteriorly into the base of the iris and lead to a clinical misdiagnosis of a primary iris melanoma (35). Hemorrhage under the RPE overlying

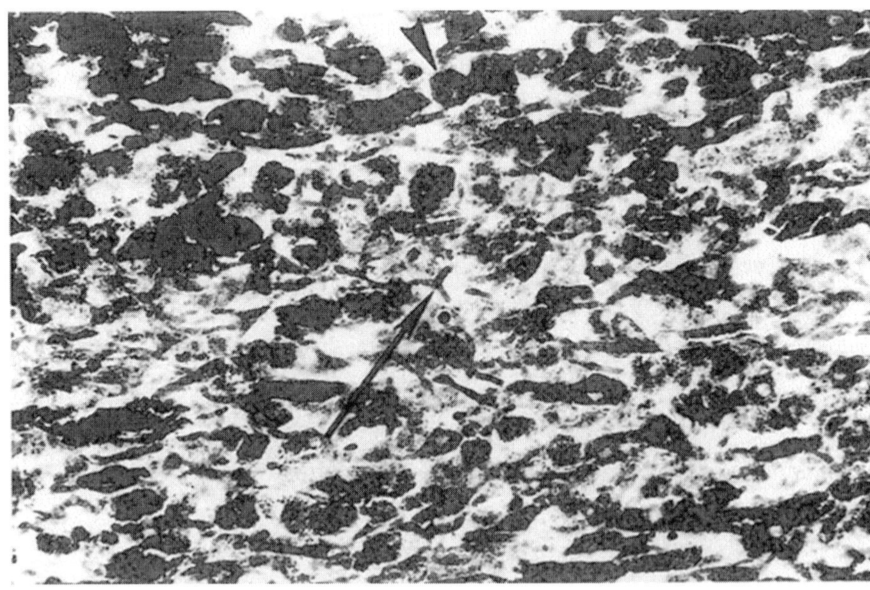

Figure 25 Unbleached section of choroidal nevus composed of dendritic (*arrow*) and plump polyhedral (*arrowhead*) nevus cells (hematoxylin and eosin, × 340).

a melanocytoma may simulate growth (146), but they very rarely affect vision or undergo malignant transformation (22,83,254,318).

Congenital Ocular Melanocytosis

Congenital ocular melanocytosis (melanosis oculi) is due to increased pigmentation of part or all of the uvea and it may be associated with ipsilateral dermal melanocytosis (nevus of Ota). Clinical features include heterochromia iridis, grayish episcleral pigmentation, and a dark fundus (Figs. 27–29). The melanocytes are identical to those normally found in the uveal tract.

According to Reese, eyes with melanocytosis have a propensity to develop melanoma (240). Blodi disagreed and found no statistical difference in the incidence of uveal melanoma between the general population and patients with ocular melanocytosis (30). However, more recent reports have supported Reese's theory (296,300) and there have been several

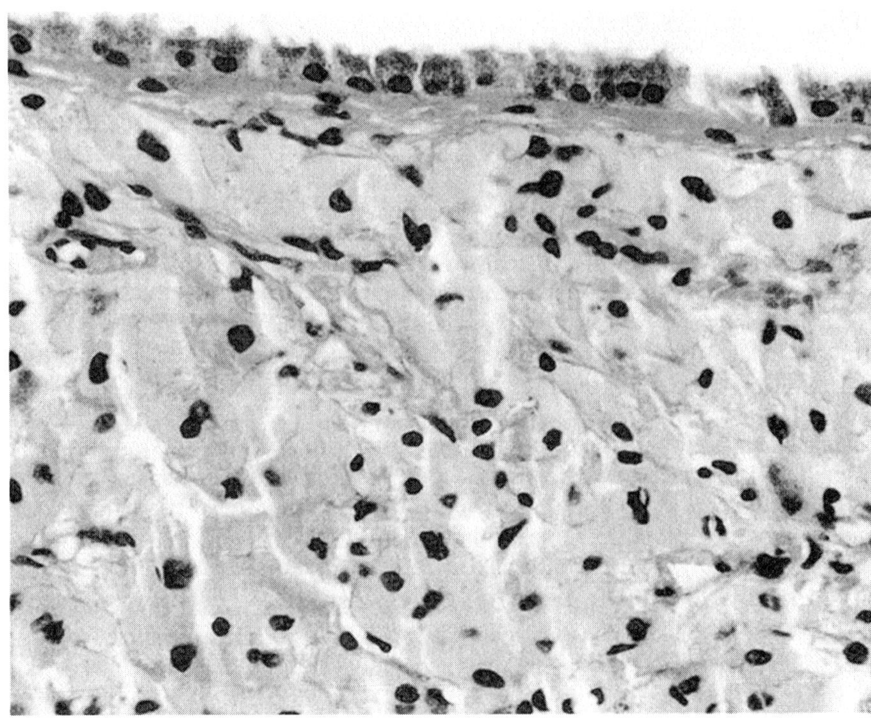

Figure 26 Melanocytoma of choroid. Bleached section disclosed plump nevus cells (hematoxylin and eosin, × 600).

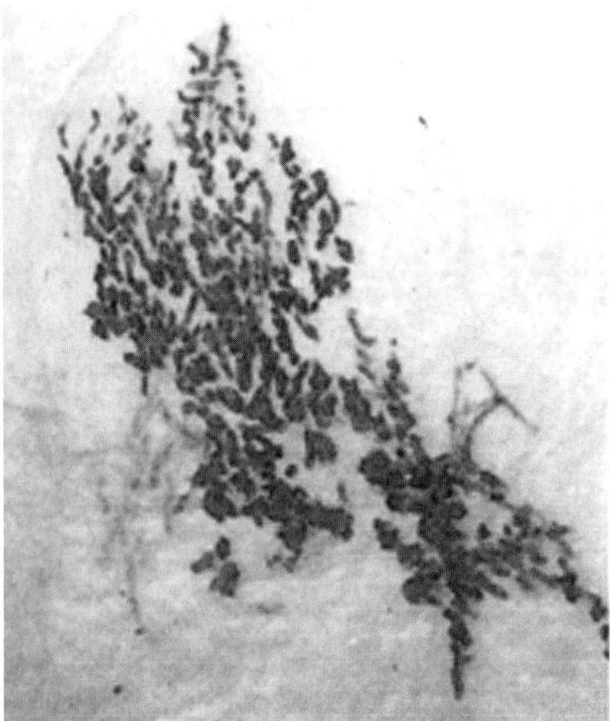

Figure 27 Gross appearance of episcleral pigmentation in eye with melanosis oculi (ocular melanocytosis) (× 14).

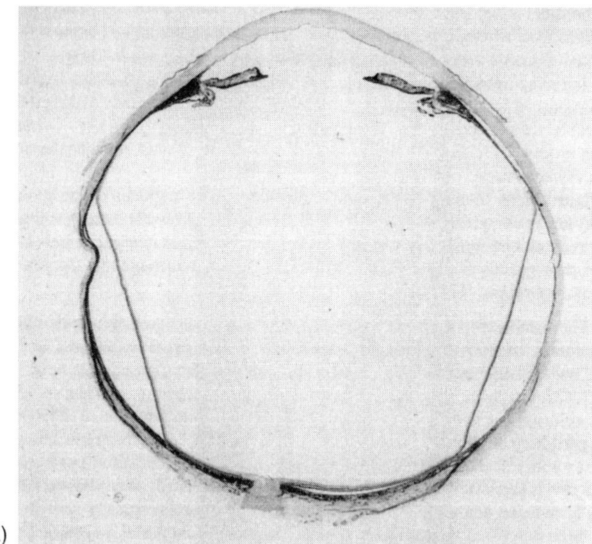

(A)

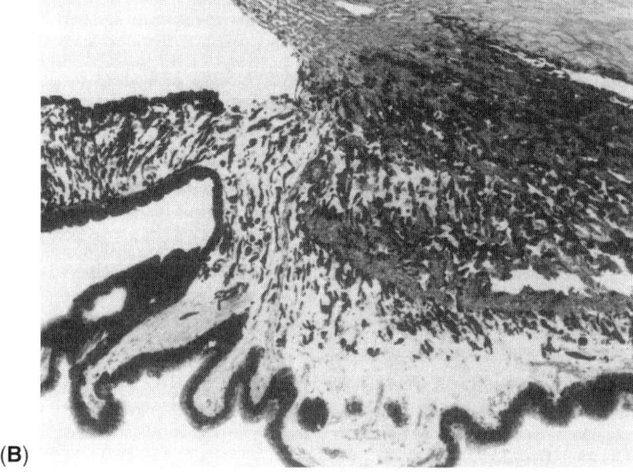

(B)

Figure 28 (**A**) Melanosis oculi with diffuse hyperpigmentation of iris, ciliary body, choroid, and scleral canals (hematoxylin and eosin, ×3). (**B**) Higher power, showing hyperpigmentation of iris and ciliary body due to increased number of melanocytes (hematoxylin and eosin, × 180).

reported cases of multiple independent choroidal melanomas (230,257) and bilateral uveal melanomas (300) occurring in patients with ocular melanocytosis. The increased number of uveal melanocytes in this condition is thought to account for the tendency to develop uveal melanoma (296).

Bilateral Diffuse Uveal Melanocytic Proliferation

Bilateral diffuse uveal melanocytic proliferation (BDUMP, supernevus syndrome) is a condition characterized by multiple patchy uveal tumors giving a "giraffe skin" appearance, diffuse uveal thickening, cataract, and exudative retinal detachment (112). This paraneoplastic syndrome is associated with visceral malignancies, in particular ovarian carcinoma (23,112, 195).

Primary Melanoma of the Uvea

Choroidal Melanomas

Because choroidal melanomas account for the vast majority of uveal melanomas, this section will consider uveal melanomas in general. Specific information on ciliary body and iris melanomas will be discussed later.

Epidemiology

Melanoma is the most common primary malignant intraocular tumor in adults (342). The incidence rate ranges from 4.3 to 10.9 per million population based on country of origin, inclusion criteria, and methods of calculation (294). The incidence of uveal melanoma does not appear to have significantly increased in the United States over the last 50 years (301).

The average age of patients with uveal melanomas in a large U.S. study is about 60 years, with a range of 6 to 100 years (301), but a choroidal melanoma has been reported in a 2.5-year-old girl (50). The incidence of uveal melanomas at specific ages increases steeply from the age of 30 to 70 years, after which the tumor decreases in frequency (301). A slightly higher rate of uveal melanoma has been reported in males than females (294,301). Although heredity does not apparently predispose individuals to uveal melanoma, several reports document familial examples (299). A relationship between the dysplastic nevus syndrome and uveal melanoma may exist (2,24,327).

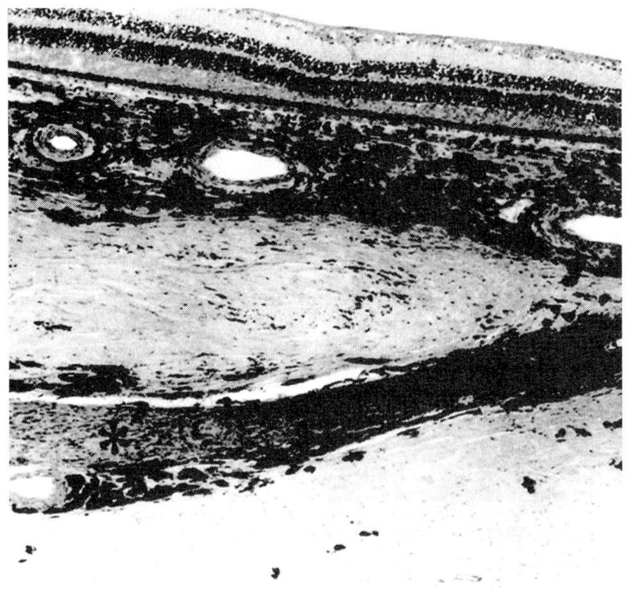

Figure 29 Higher power of choroid posteriorly and scleral canal with ciliary nerve (*asterisk*) due to an increased number of melanocytes (hematoxylin and eosin, × 180).

Uveal melanomas are much more prevalent in non-Hispanic white individuals than in the general population and in one study in the United States the incidence per million population was 0.31 (black persons), 0.38 (Asians), 1.67 (Hispanics) to 6.02 (non-Hispanic white persons) (148). Black patients with choroidal melanoma are more prone to tumor necrosis and darkly pigmented tumors than white patients (193). Uveal melanomas are extremely rare in non-whites living in Asia (63,313) and Africa (317). Persons of Northern European ancestry and greater than 5 years residence below latitude N-40° are at increased risk for uveal melanoma (267). Patients with ocular melanocytosis (296) and neurofibromatosis (335) may also have an increased risk.

Bilateral choroidal melanomas are rare (273,300) and in a population of 50 million whites, one person would be expected to develop choroidal melanomas in both eyes. Hence bilateral uveal melanomas are likely to occur about once every 18 years in the United States (273).

Clinical Features

The usual presenting symptom of posterior-pole choroidal melanomas is increasing hyperopia. At first this may be correctable by refractive lenses but eventually leads to uncorrectable blurred vision. Of all patients with choroidal melanomas, 65% give a history of visual symptoms of 6 months duration or less (165). The patient may be asymptomatic if the tumor is not near the macula.

Anterior segment abnormalities may aid in the clinical diagnosis of choroidal melanomas (245). These include dilated episcleral blood vessels corresponding to the site of the tumor, which are seen in about one-third of cases. These may be nutrient vessels of the tumor (244,245) or reflections of poor venous drainage (33).

Abnormalities of the Iris. Choroidal melanomas rarely spread to the iris, although tumor implants were reported in one case by Reese (246). Numerous iris nevi have been noted histopathologically in eyes with choroidal melanomas (241,333) and Reese initially believed that this would be a clinically useful sign (244). However, these nevi are situated deep in the iris and are not appreciated clinically. A significant increase in iris nevi was not detected in a clinical study of 50 patients with unilateral choroidal or ciliary body melanomas compared to age-matched controls without melanomas (209).

Iris neovascularization may occur and in one series was present in 46 of 308 eyes enucleated for melanoma (42). Neovascular glaucoma was the reason for the enucleation of 18 eyes in 59 patients (31%) following plaque radiotherapy for posterior uveal melanoma (279).

Glaucoma. A unilateral elevation of intraocular pressure (IOP) may be a sign of a choroidal melanoma (293) and at one time about one-third of eyes enucleated for this tumor were glaucomatous (246). Secondary glaucoma usually develops in eyes harboring large melanomas, but the IOP may actually be decreased in a high percentage of eyes with melanomas (78). In one series of 96 eyes with uveal melanomas, 19 (20%) presented with secondary glaucoma, and many of these melanomas were not recognized clinically, especially in eyes with opaque media and no diagnostic ultrasonography (338). The glaucoma is most often caused by angle closure secondary to peripheral anterior synechiae or cellular obstruction of the trabecular meshwork in the presence of an open angle. With a partially necrotic choroidal melanoma the glaucoma may be caused by macrophages containing phagocytosed melanin (melanomalytic cells) in the trabecular meshwork (83).

Pigmentation. Choroidal melanomas appear as gray, light tan, brown, or black lesions (Fig. 30). On FA, these pigmented lesions block the normal background fluorescence of the choroid. The tumor surface has an abnormal vascular pattern in 20% of cases and a yellow-orange pigment is sometimes evident (244). This yellow-orange pigment is lipofuscin (see Chapter 1) (102). While lipofuscin granules are normally found in RPE cells and increase with age (311), numbers in RPE cells and macrophages overlying choroidal melanomas

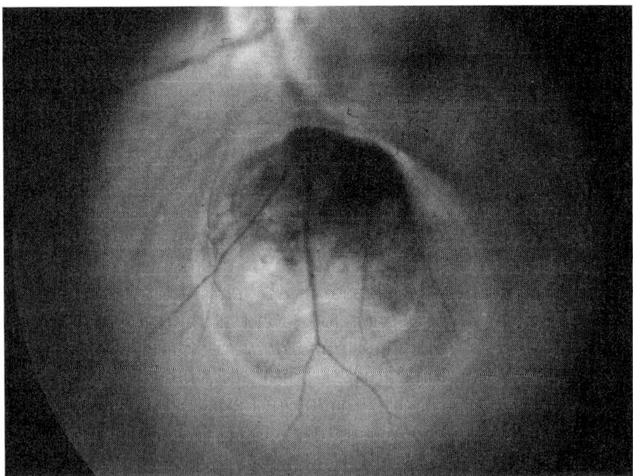

Figure 30 Fundus photograph of a choroidal melanoma in a 26-year-old female who presented with a one month history of photopsias and blurred vision in the affected eye. The elevated pigmented lesion was found adjacent to the optic nerve. A portion of the tumor broke through Bruch membrane and was associated with a serous retinal detachment inferiorly.

are markedly increased. This pigment has some diagnostic significance. Although often observed over choroidal melanomas, it is rarely seen over nevi, metastatic carcinomas, or hemangiomas in this part of the eye (304).

Retinal Detachment. A serous retinal detachment often overlies a choroidal melanoma (Fig. 30). In an analysis of the clinicopathological features of 57 eyes with choroidal melanomas from patients who were operated on for retinal detachment, Boniuk and Zimmerman (32) found that 2% of the cases had one or more operations for retinal detachment before enucleation. Retinal detachments associated with uveal melanomas are often accompanied by retinal tears (33) and many cases of rhegmatogenous retinal detachments in the setting of a choroidal melanoma have been documented (25,26,191,199). A retinal tear sometimes overlies the tumor (191), but it may be located away from the tumor (25). Detachment may follow the development of a hole in an area of cystic degeneration in the retina overlying the tumor.

Retinal exudates are not usually a feature of choroidal melanomas, but they have been documented in some cases (31). Subretinal exudates are common at the edges of choroidal melanomas and are frequent in the inferior part of the eye when the tumor is superiorly located. Subretinal exudation may follow treatment of choroidal melanomas with irradiation (194).

Visual Fields. A dense visual field defect may be present if the function of the retinal photoreceptors overlying the melanomas is compromised (265). If the tumor is surrounded by an area of serous retinal detachment, there may be a surrounding partial field defect.

Cystoid Macular Edema. Cystoid macular edema without serous detachment of the macula may be the initial presentation in a patient with a peripherally located choroidal melanoma (39). This may be coincidental, but the possibility of a causal relationship has been raised (39).

Inflammation. Necrotic melanomas can cause considerable inflammation and result in a florid uveitis, and rarely severe panophthalmitis with exophthalmos. Granulomatous inflammation has been reported in an eye treated with proton beam irradiation for a choroidal melanoma (194).

Hemorrhage. Most uveal melanomas grow slowly and a rapidly expanding, relatively flat, pigmented lesion at the posterior pole should suggest a hemorrhagic rather than a neoplastic lesion (239). Hemorrhage into the vitreous may prevent visualization of the ocular fundus. Because of the presence of hemosiderin, vitreous hemorrhages often impart a brownish discoloration to the vitreous and can lead to the clinical impression of melanoma. In Ferry's series, 5% of eyes that were mistakenly enucleated for choroidal melanomas had vitreous hemorrhage (94).

Vitreous hemorrhages occasionally arise from the dilated vascular channels in choroidal melanomas that have ruptured through Bruch membrane. Necrosis of the tumor may contribute to vitreous hemorrhage (244).

Shape. Although most choroidal melanomas present as localized, mushroom-shaped or globular (Figs. 31–34) masses with growth toward the interior of the eye, 5% have a flat or diffuse type of growth and remain external to Bruch membrane (138,237,253, 277).

Special Variant: Diffuse Choroidal Melanoma. On fundoscopic examination a diffuse choroidal melanoma may resemble chorioretinitis (43) or choroidal sclerosis (21). A conspicuous feature of diffuse uveal melanomas is the long duration of visual symptoms and sometimes pain, ranging from 7 months to 10 years, before the diagnosis becomes established (165). Delayed diagnosis is frequent and thus the tendency to extraocular extension is greater and the prognosis is worse than in the usual type of choroidal melanoma (101,277). A unique, diffuse uveal melanoma with extrascleral extension presented clinically as a ring-shaped amelanotic limbal tumor, suggestive of a diffuse SCC (309).

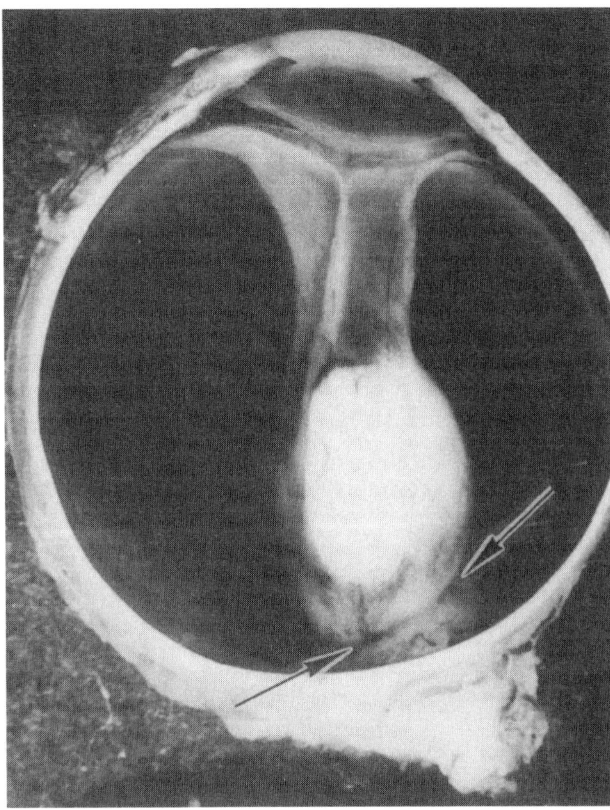

Figure 31 Melanoma of choroid with an elongated, mushroom configuration and total retinal detachment. The narrowed area (*between the arrows*) of the tumor is the point at which the tumor has broken through Bruch membrane.

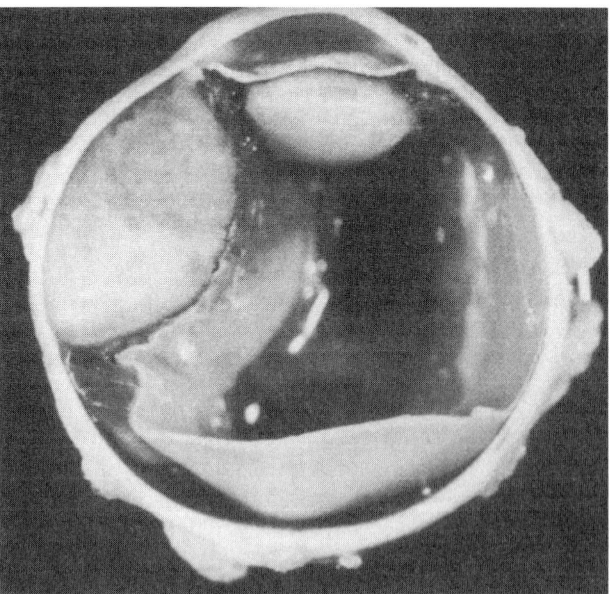

Figure 32 Melanoma of ciliary body and anterior choroid of a 56-year-old man who presented with visual complaints that were attributed to pressure on the lens. Two family members had also had choroidal melanomas.

Diagnosis and Differential Diagnosis. Numerous lesions simulate choroidal melanomas clinically (Table 1), and a variety of benign lesions may lead to enucleation (244). Benign lesions accounted for about 20% of enucleations for suspected melanoma in eyes with clear media and ophthalmoscopically visible lesions reported in 1964 (94) and 1973 (291). Clinical misdiagnoses of uveal melanomas have occurred less frequently from teaching institutions to which numerous patients are referred. Blodi and Roy documented a misdiagnosis rate of 10.2% for 82 enucleated eyes sent from outside sources to their pathology laboratory, but only 5.6% among the eyes enucleated at their hospital (29). More recently, the Collaborative Ocular Melanoma Study (COMS) reported a very low misdiagnosis rate (0.48%) for choroidal melanoma (10). Lower rates of misdiagnosis in patients have been attributed to a greater clinical awareness of lesions that simulate melanomas, use of indirect ophthalmoscopy, serial fundus photography, FA, trans-illumination of the globe (Fig. 33), and multiple ophthalmological consultations. Computed tomography (CT), ultrasonography, and magnetic resonance imaging (MRI) (45,187) also aid in the diagnosis of choroidal melanoma. Fine-needle aspiration has been utilized successfully to identify choroidal melanoma (18,116).

Spread. Extrascleral extension has been noted in 8–10% of enucleated eyes with choroidal melanomas.

Table 1 Differential Diagnosis of Choroidal Melanoma

Condition	Refs.
Retinal lesions	
Retinal detachment (rhegmatogenous, serous, or hemorrhagic)	291
Disciform macular degeneration	244
Senile retinoschisis	94,291
Chorioretinitis	94,291
Hyperplasia or hypertrophy of retinal pigment epithelium	328
Hemorrhage from macroaneurysm of retinal arteries	229
Solitary retinal cyst with hemorrhage	265
Subretinal pigment epithelial hematoma	320
Congenital pits of optic nerve head with serous macular degeneration	95
Choroidal lesions	
Detachment	21
Nevi (including melanocytoma)	94,291
Hemorrhage	65,165,250
Hemangioma	94,291
Metastatic carcinoma	92
Lymphoid hyperplasia	256
Osteoma	113
Scleral lesions	
Cellular blue nevus	306

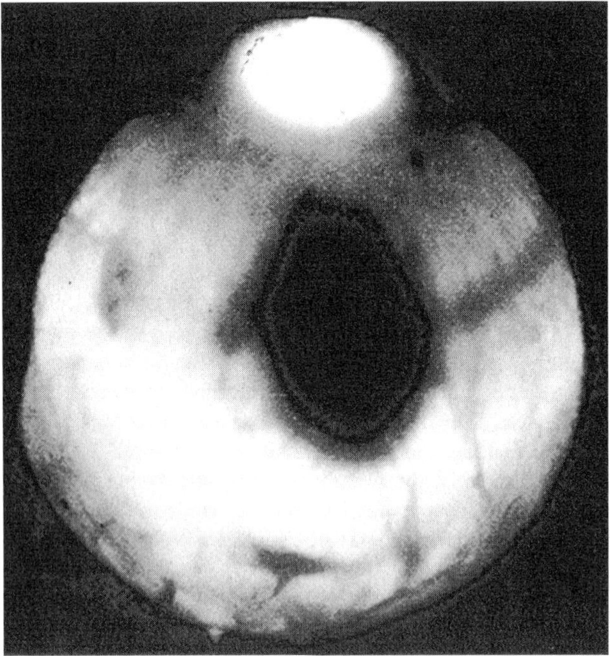

Figure 33 Melanoma of choroid and ciliary body demonstrated by transillumination.

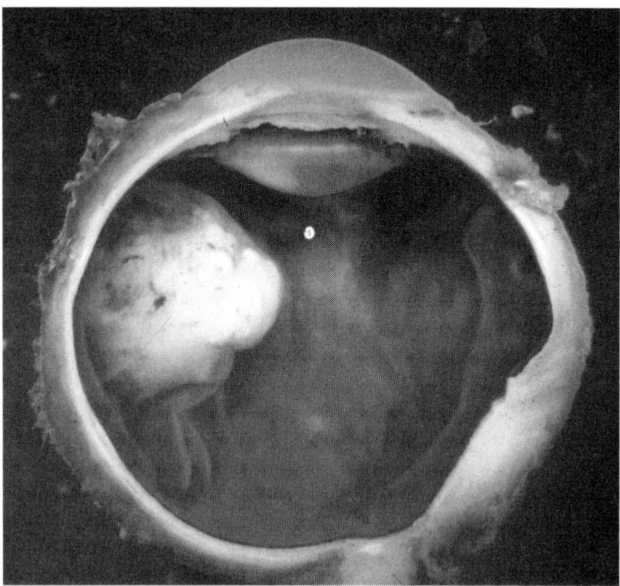

Figure 34 Gross photograph of a choroidal and ciliary body melanoma found in a 53-year-old woman.

This occurs almost invariably through emissary canals (223,271). Unlike retinoblastoma, extension of choroidal melanomas into the optic nerve is uncommon, occurring in only 5% of cases in one series (165). However, approximately 80% of peripapillary choroidal melanomas extend along the optic nerve and its sheaths (272). Most melanomas that invade the optic nerve are necrotic or of mixed or epithelioid cell type and they almost invariably occur in eyes with secondary glaucoma (310). Choroidal melanomas may also break through the retina and seed within the vitreous (77).

Metastases from choroidal melanoma primarily spread via blood vessels. Metastasis has been observed in 31%, 45%, and 50% of patients at 5, 15, and 25 years after initial diagnosis, respectively (173). At the time of initial diagnosis, only 2% of patients with large melanomas (12), and 0.4% with medium-sized melanomas (72) have clinically detectable metastases. In the past, enucleation was thought to possibly increase the rate of metastasis because the mortality rate increases significantly in the first 2 years after surgery (340). Since then, studies evaluating tumor doubling times suggest that clinically undetectable micrometastases occur before the primary tumor is diagnosed in most cases (298). The most common sites of metastases are the liver (93%) (Fig. 35), lung (24%), and bone (16%) and up to 87% of patients with metastasic disease have multiple sites involved (280).

Biological Behavior. It has long been suspected that the development and dissemination of a malignant melanoma may depend largely on the immune competence of the host (see Chapter 7) and several case reports document the spontaneous regression of uveal melanomas (164,176,246). It is possible that the long delays in the appearance of metastases after enucleation in some patients reflect immunological resistance to tumor cells (220) but this theory has yet to be substantiated.

Association of Uveal Melanomas with Other Tumors. Multiple primary malignant neoplasms sometimes occur in the same patient, and at least 39 patients with nonocular malignant tumors have had independent primary intraocular neoplasms, especially choroidal melanomas (16,139,216). Therefore, from a clinical standpoint an intraocular mass in a patient with a history of known cancer should not be dismissed simply as a metastatic tumor.

Multicentric Melanomas. Multicentric melanomas of the choroid are rare, but several case reports document more than one melanoma in a single eye or bilateral uveal melanomas (75,143,182,273,300,321). Bilateral melanomas need to be differentiated from BDUMP because of the different clinical implications.

Histopathology

Callender (41,200) originally classified uveal melanomas based on three basic types of tumor cells: (*i*) small

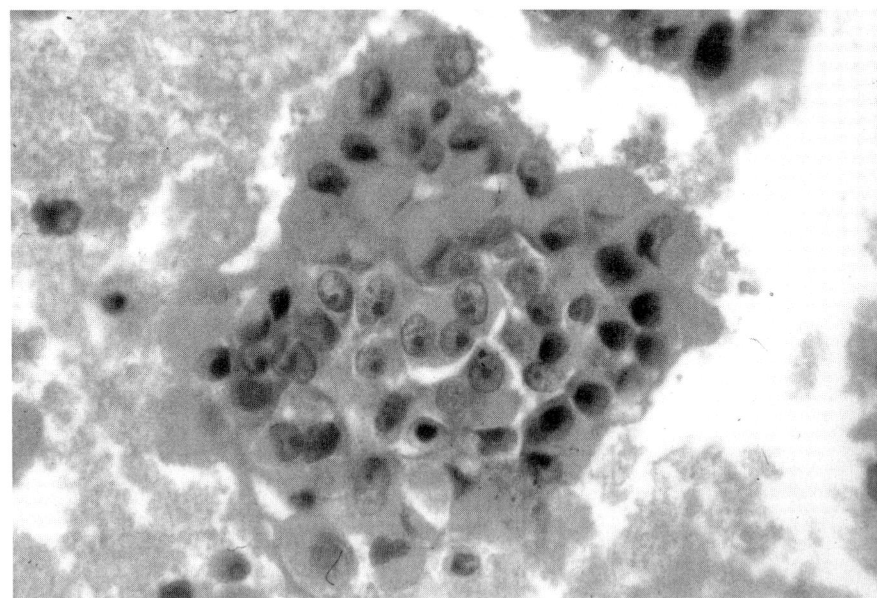

Figure 35 Histopathology of a liver metastasis found in the same patient from Figure 34 six years after the enucleation. The lesion contained clumps and individual cells with round to oval nuclei, prominent nucleoli, and high nuclear to cytoplasmic ratios. Scattered cells displayed melanin pigment (hematoxylin and eosin, × 170).

spindle-shaped cohesive cells with hyperchromatic, spindle-shaped nuclei without distinct nucleoli but often with a central dark stripe produced by a nuclear fold (spindle A cells) (Fig. 36). The cytoplasm of these cells is indistinct without well-defined borders, and mitotic figures are almost never seen. Melanomas composed entirely of these cells (spindle A melanomas) account for 5% of all choroidal and ciliary body melanomas and 90% of iris melanomas. It is now thought that spindle A cells are actually nevus cells. (*ii*) Spindle cells that are similar, but with distinct nucleoli (spindle B cells) (Fig. 36) are found in about 39% of choroidal and ciliary body melanomas (spindle B melanomas). In about 6% of spindle B melanomas, the cells have a palisaded arrangement creating a fascicular pattern (227). (*iii*) The third cell type is non-cohesive with large, round nuclei, prominent nucleoli, abundant eosinophilic cytoplasm, distinct cell borders, and frequent mitoses (epithelioid cell) (Fig. 37). A fourth cell type that is similar to epithelioid cells, but smaller with indistinct cell borders, became recognized by the Pathology

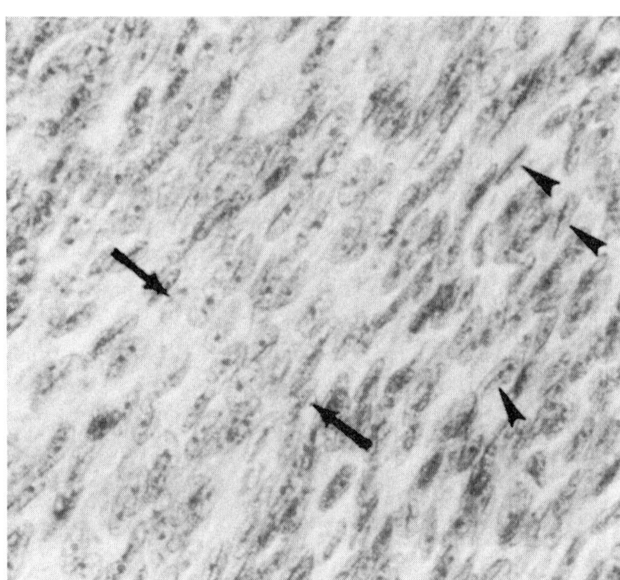

Figure 36 Choroidal melanoma with spindle A (*arrowheads*) and spindle B (*between arrows*) cells (hematoxylin and eosin, × 630).

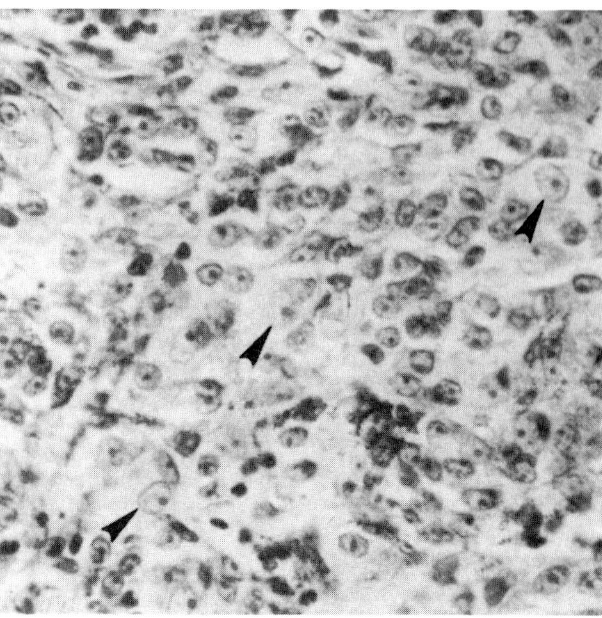

Figure 37 Choroidal melanoma with epithelioid cells (*arrowheads*) (hematoxylin and eosin, × 630).

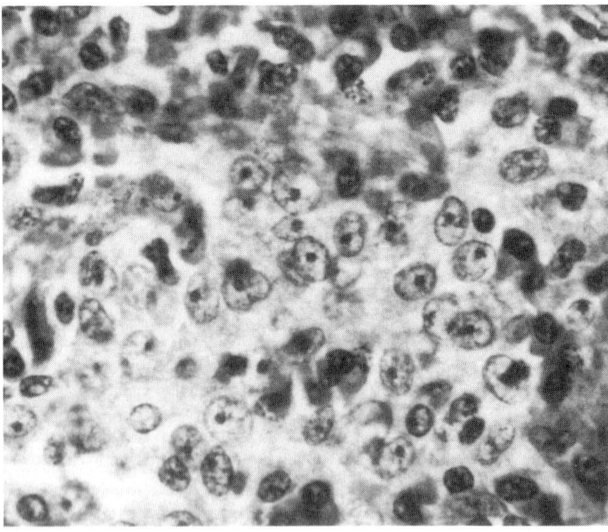

Figure 38 Choroidal melanoma with intermediate epithelioid cells (hematoxylin and eosin, × 1,030).

Committee of the Collaborative Ocular Melanoma Study (COMS) (intermediate epithelioid cells) (Fig. 38). Pure epithelioid cell tumors are the rarest of uveal melanomas, accounting for only 3% of choroidal and ciliary body melanomas.

Melanomas may be composed almost entirely of one of the foregoing cell types, but more often they consist of mixtures of these cell types. According to the original Callender classification a melanoma of the mixed cell type consists of spindle cells (usually spindle B cells) and epithelioid cells. This mixed tumor is the most common type of uveal melanoma accounting for 45% of these tumors. The designation "necrotic melanoma" refers to those melanomas in which the cell type cannot be identified because of necrosis. About 7% of choroidal melanomas are of this variety (227). The cause of necrosis in melanomas is uncertain but ischemia and autoimmunity may play roles (235,246).

Immunophenotype

Specific antigenic determinants have been demonstrated in uveal melanoma cells by immunohistochemistry. In one study all uveal meanomas were immunolabelled with microphthalmia transcription factor (MITF), HMB45, HMB50, tyrosinase, and melan-A but not with p75ntr (152). MIB-1 positivity has been used to estimate proliferative activity in uveal melanomas because it stains cells containing a proliferation associated nuclear antigen (52,212). Matrix metalloproteinase-2 (MMP-2), one of a class of enzymes involved in the breakdown of extracellular matrix (ECM) (20), has been demonstrated by immunohistochemistry in almost half of uveal melanomas and may have prognostic importance, especially in respect of their metastatic potential (324).

Transmission Electron Microscopy

Examination of uveal melanomas by transmission electron microscopy (TEM) (27,153,171) reveals the following characteristics: the size and reticulation of nucleoli and the number of free ribosomes and mitochondria increases from spindle A to spindle B and epithelioid cells, which corresponds with the growth potential of the different cell types. Nuclear membrane infolding is seen in spindle A cells. Rough-surfaced endoplasmic reticulum (RER) is most prominent in the spindle B cell type. Cytoplasmic filaments are most numerous in the spindle A cells and least common in epithelioid cells.

Origin

It is widely believed that many uveal melanomas originate from preexisting nevi and histopathological studies have suggested that this occurred in about 70% of uveal melanomas (101,217,335,336). However, this conclusion is based on the interpretation of the cells at the base and periphery of choroidal melanomas as "nevus cells" (4). Albert and colleagues have argued that these nevus-like cells actually reflect local, mechanical compression of the cells of the choroid and have found morphologically similar cells at the base of experimentally induced ocular melanomas in hamsters (5,336).

Clinical observations of choroidal nevi suggest that malignant transformation to melanoma is a rare event (246). Few reports document the malignant transformation of a choroidal nevus (141,246,307) and in these instances the possibility of the original lesion being a low-grade malignant melanoma, rather than a nevus, cannot be excluded. In one large clinical study of choroidal nevi, malignant transformation was not observed during follow-up periods of 6 months to 16 years (210). Since in clinical (141,297) and postmortem studies (130) the incidence of choroidal nevi ranges from 4.6 to 11.0% in the general population, the rate of malignant transformation, should it occur, has been estimated to be <1 in 8000 (297).

Uveal melanomas have been reported after ocular trauma (82,181), which may be a "promoter" of tumor neoplasia after initiation of oncogenesis. Virus particles have been found in isolated uveal melanomas (8), but the probability of a causal relationship is slim. Chemicals, such as methylcholanthrene, *N*-*Z*-fluorenylacetamide, ethiorine, radium, nickel subsulfide, and polychorinated biphenyls, have been linked to uveal melanoma in a few studies looking at occupational exposure (6,7,81).

Genetics

Recent studies have provided evidence for genetic involvement in the development of uveal melanoma. Cytogenetic studies identified several chromosomal abnormalities in some uveal melanomas, suggesting chromosomal locations of possible genes related to melanomagenesis. Loss of part or all of chromosome 3 has been found in >50% of uveal melanomas (1,145,232,303), while gain of an extra copy of chromosome 8 or material on the long arm of chromosome 8 has also been found in approximately 50% of melanomas (145,231,303). Abnormalities involving chromosome 6 have frequently been found (1,231,295) and occasionally chromosomes 1, 9, 17, or 21 have been defective (1,219,231,295).

Specific genes involved in oncogenesis have also been studied for possible roles in uveal melanoma formation. One of the most intriguing is the double minute 2 gene (*MDM2*) (also known as *HDM2*), which can inhibit the activity of p53, the product of the tumor suppressor gene *TP53* (135,233). Strong immunohistochemical expression of the protein product of *MDM2* has been detected in up to 95% of untreated uveal melanomas (36), and inhibition of *MDM2* causes apoptosis in tumor cells (134). *MDM2* may serve as a potential therapeutic target in the future.

The *TP53* gene has also been investigated extensively in uveal melanomas and in one study an increased expression was noted (161). This study, however, involved previously irradiated tumors (161), and irradiation is known to increase the expression of p53 (38). Increased levels of *MDM2* may lead to a functional loss of p53 activity resulting in tumor progression.

Bcl-2, an anti-apoptotic factor, is the product of the *BCL2* gene that has been under investigation for its possible role in uveal melanomas. Immunohistochemical studies have shown overexpression of Bcl-2 in a high percentage of uveal melanomas (36,46,163). As with the protein product of *MDM2*, inhibition of Bcl-2 activity causes apoptosis in uveal melanoma tumor cells (134).

The complicated pathway involving RB, the product of the *RB1* gene (see Chapter 60), cyclin D1 and CDK4 that controls cell cycle progression has been investigated in uveal melanoma (133). While mutations and or underexpression of *RBI* have not been found in any uveal melanomas (36), RB has been shown to be hyperphosphorylated (and its actions possibly modified) in many primary uveal melanomas (37). The kinase responsible for this hyperphosphorylation is CDK4, which in turn is activated by cyclin D1. The latter has been found to have strong expression in many uveal melanomas (37). An inhibitor of cyclin D1 (p16Ink4a) may be modified in some tumor lines (206,325).

MYC, an oncogene located on the long arm of chromosome 8 (140), appears to be overrepresented in many uveal melanomas. Immunohistochemical studies have shown that the protein product of this gene is overexpressed in 70% of uveal melanomas (46,225,255). Additional investigation has focused on telomerase expression (137) and the genes *BRCA2* (264), *NF1* (106), and *TGFBI* (215). While much information has been elicited recently on the genetic factors involved in the development of uveal melanoma, the process is complicated and may involve multiple oncogenic pathways.

Prognosis

Despite significant research and changes in the therapeutic armamentarium for uveal melanoma, prognosis has remained relatively stable in the United States over the last 25 years. Singh showed that 5-year survival rates have ranged from 77% to 84% without any statistically significant change between 1973 and 1997 (302).

Age. Older patients have a worse prognosis than those diagnosed at a younger age (13,73,150).

Tumor Size. Large tumors are associated with a worse prognosis than small tumors. Diener-West et al. performed a meta-analysis of eight studies and found a 5-year mortality rate of 16%, 32%, and 53% for small, medium, and large sized uveal melanomas, respectively (74). The COMS data showed a similar trend, with 6% (11), 18% to 19% (73), and 38% to 43% (13). Five-year mortality rates for small-, medium-, and large-sized uveal melanomas, respectively.

Tumor Location. Iris melanomas have a relatively favorable prognosis, with a mortality rate 10 times less than other uveal melanomas (201). Uveal melanomas involving the ciliary body on the other hand have a relatively poor prognosis, with a mortality rate over three times greater than choroidal melanomas in one study (266).

Tumor Growth Pattern. Choroidal melanomas are characterized by different patterns of growth. Those exhibiting the diffuse growth pattern, with predominantly horizontal rather than vertical growth, have been associated with a worse prognosis than those with a vertical growth pattern, with a 5-year risk of metastasis of 24% (277).

Extraocular Extension. Transscleral extension is associated with a significantly increased mortality rate (3), estimated at 75% at 10 years, double that seen with melanomas confined within the eye (266). The 5-year survival rate of patients without orbital extension of the uveal melanoma is 78% compared with 27% with orbital extension (271).

Cell Type. Traditionally, the histological cell type of the melanoma, as first proposed by Callender (41), has been useful in predicting death after enucleation (227). Statistical analysis has shown cell type to be a prognostic indicator superior to other factors, including tumor size, mitotic activity, pigmentation, and extrascleral extension (204,341,342). The subjective nature of the Callender and the modified Callender classifications (200) is demonstrated by a 12% to 17% interobserver variability (48,204). The 15-year actuarial survival rates based on a study of 2652 cases by Paul and colleagues using the original Callender classification were 81.2% for patients with spindle A melanoma, 73.6% for patients with spindle B and fascicular tumors, 40.6% for patients with mixed epithelioid and spindle B cell and necrotic melanomas, and 28% for patients with purely epithelioid tumors (227). The malignant potential of spindle A type cells has been questioned (203) and the modified Callender classification defines essentially three types of uveal melanoma: spindle, mixed cell, and epithelioid (200). Although a transitional cell type that is difficult to classify within these three categories appears to exist, significant prognostic information is gained from the presence of epithelioid cells. The prognosis is better with spindle cell melanomas and progressively worse with increasing percentages of epithelioid cells (200–202,266).

Morphometry. Because assigning individual melanomas into specific categories within the modified Callender classification is subjective, morphometric analysis has been used to obtain objective prognostic indicators for uveal melanomas. In some studies the prognosis has been proportional to the standard deviation of the nucleolar area, a measure of nucleolar pleomorphism (56,110,149). A simpler and less expensive method determining the mean diameter of the 10 largest nucleoli has prognostic significance in some studies (149,198), but a larger study failed to confirm this observation and noted significant interobserver variability in measurement.

Mitoses. Progressively increasing mitotic activity, as measured by the number of mitoses identified per high-power field (HPF) by light microscopy, has been shown to have a progressively worsening prognosis for uveal melanomas (204,213). The 6-year mortality rate for tumors with <1 mitosis per HPF was 15% compared to 56% for tumors with 9 to 48 mitoses per HPF (204).

Proliferation Markers. Immunohistochemical studies using antibodies to markers of cell proliferation have been performed on uveal melanomas to determine if a correlation between high expression of these markers and poor prognosis exists. Mooy et al. found the Mib-1 index (a marker for cell cycle proliferation) to be a significant independent predictive factor for mortality. In addition it was related to a higher percentage of epithelioid cells and apoptosis (213). Immunoexpression of the PC-10 antibody to the proliferating cell nuclear antigen in uveal melanoma cells was also associated with a worse prognosis. Patients with tumors below the median PC-10 cell count had a 10-year survival rate of 84% while those above the median had a 40% survival rate (269).

Microvascular Density. Because uveal melanomas metastasize through a hematogenous route, tumor vasculature has been thought to play an important role in metastasis and therefore survival. A commonly used measure of tumor vasculature is microvascular density (MVD), employing antibodies to CD34 or factor VIII to highlight the blood vessels, which are then counted within those areas with the highest vascularization. Foss et al. evaluated 116 patients and found that increasing MVD was a strong predictor of survival (105), and this observation was confirmed by one large study (188), but not in another investigation (177).

Microvascular Patterns. Folberg and colleagues examined tumor vasculature in tissue sections of uveal melanomas stained with the periodic acid Schiff (PAS) reagent. They identified nine different vascular architectural patterns (Fig. 39): (*i*) normal, (*ii*) silent, (*iii*) straight, (*iv*) parallel, (*v*) parallel with cross-linking, (*vi*) arcs, (*vii*) arcs with branching, (*viii*) loops, and (*ix*) networks (99,100). They found networks to be the strongest predictor of metastatic death in a regression analysis, ahead of largest tumor dimension, mitoses, age, and high numbers of tumor-infiltrating lymphocytes (TIL). The 10-year mortality rate for patients with networks was close to 50% while tumors without networks carried a mortality rate of about 10% (100). Others have found loops in uveal melanomas to have prognostic significance (202). Foss et al. have suggested that the PAS staining patterns reflect fibrovascular septa and not a true microvasculature. They attribute the patterns to disoriented tumor growth, emergence of subclones, and section orientation and found those associated with disoriented tumor growth to carry prognostic significance (104).

While there is no general agreement about the causes and significance of microvascular architectural patterns in uveal melanoma, a clinical study has identified some of these complex microcirculation patterns in vivo in patients with small choroidal melanocytic tumors with confocal indocyanine green angiography (214). A significant prognostic relationship between the rate of tumor growth and the

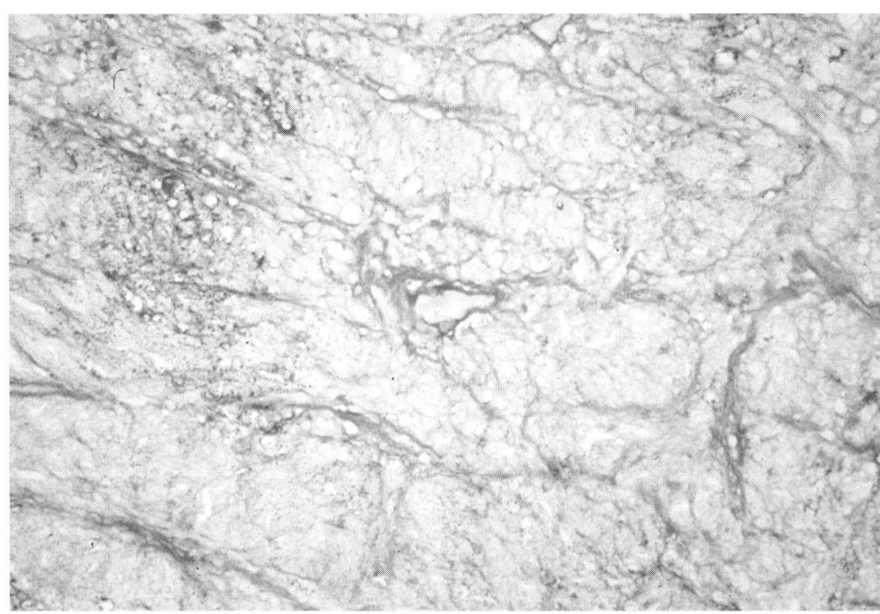

Figure 39 Choroidal melanoma displaying characteristic microvascular channels (periodic acid Schiff, ×25).

microvascular patterns of parallel with cross-linking, arcs with branching, loops, and networks was found. If these observations are confirmed in a larger population, this non-invasive technique may allow clinically relevant prognostic information to be obtained without biopsy or enucleation (214).

Tumor-Infiltrating Lymphocytes. Some uveal melanomas contain numerous lymphocytes. The presence of >100 lymphocytes per 20 HPFs is associated with an unfavorable prognosis in uveal melanoma (66,100). The 15-year survival rate was 36.7% for patients with tumors in the high-lymphocytic group compared to 69.6% for those with tumors in the low-lymphocytic group (66). The reason for this is not clear and different studies have reported favorable and unfavorable associations between TIL and prognosis (see Chapter 7).

Aneuploidy. Flow cytometric analysis has been used to determine DNA content (ploidy) in uveal melanoma cells. Tumors with hyperploidy were associated with a worse outcome than those with aneuploidy. Tumors with the highest DNA indices had an 88% mortality compared to 34% with diploid tumors (205).

Cytogenetics. Of the chromosomal abnormalities found in uveal melanomas some have significant prognostic implications. Monosomy 3 has prognostic significance for both metastasis and survival. In one study of 54 patients chromosome 3 monosomy was found in 30 patients (232), and 17 (57%) of them experienced an orbital or distant metastasis, yielding a 3-year tumor-free survival rate of 50%. None of the patients with chromosome 3 disomy developed metastases. Another study found that 66% of 71 patients who died from metastatic melanoma had tumors with monosomy 3, while 0 of 40 patients without metastases had monosomy 3 (259). Yet another study found that abnormalities of chromosome 3 and 8 tended to occur together and were associated with a poor prognosis while chromosome 6 abnormalities were associated with a better prognosis (332).

p53, Cyclin D1, and HDM2. In a study of the prognostic significance of p53, cyclin D1, and MDM2 in 96 uveal melanomas, expression of cyclin D1 and p53 was associated with an unfavorable outcome, while MDM2 was not. Cyclin D1 also showed an association with extraocular extension and epithelioid cell type (59).

C-myc. Using flow cytometry Chana et al. detected MYC expression in 70% of 71 uveal melanomas and found that expression was associated with an improved survival (46).

Matrix Metalloproteinases. Matrix metalloproteinase 2 (MMP-2, collagenase type IV) was detected in an immunohistochemical study of 29 human uveal melanomas. Its expression was associated with a 5-year mortality rate of 51% versus 14% in MMP-2 negative tumors (324).

Gene Microarray Analysis. Using microarray analysis to characterize gene expression profiles for in uveal melanoma cells, Onken and colleagues were able to demonstrate two distinct molecular classes of uveal melanoma with different clinical behavior, based on the identification of three genes, *PHLDA1*, *FZD6*, and *ENPP2* (222). They could reproducibly place tumors into either class 1 melanomas, which were considered low-grade and correlated strongly with spindle cell melanomas, or class 2 melanomas, which were more strongly associated with epithelioid cell melanomas. This molecular classification system was the strongest predictor of survival showing 92-month survival rates of 95% and 31% for class 1 and class 2 tumors, respectively (222).

Melanoma Inhibitory Activity. Serum levels of melanoma inhibitory activity (MIA), a protein first isolated from cultured cutaneous melanoma cells (28), correlates with the clinical stage of cutaneous melanomas (34). A study of 305 patients with uveal melanoma found the serum concentration of this marker significantly higher in patients with metastatic disease than in those without known metastases (247). In addition, the MIA serum level in individuals who develop metastases is greater than their pre-metastasis levels, indicating that serum MIA may be of value in screening patients for metastases (247).

Ciliary Body Melanomas

Clinical Features

The earliest and most consistent symptom is a progressive decrease in vision not correctable with refractive lenses (103,275). Reduction in vision, generally in the range 20/40–20/70 (144), is usually due to tumor encroachment on the lens (Fig. 40) with displacement and changes in lens shape. Melanomas of the ciliary body have at times been discovered only after cataract extraction (51). Hence preoperative ultrasonography is essential on eyes in which dense cataracts preclude internal examination (51,283).

An early but subtle sign of a ciliary body melanoma is a slightly lower (2–3 mmHg) IOP in the involved eye compared with its fellow eye (103). Although the mechanism responsible for this relative hypotony is incompletely understood, it may reflect diminished aqueous humor secretion because of the tumor in the ciliary body.

Spread. Ciliary body melanomas may spread to distant sites via the bloodstream or they may spread to surrounding structures by one of four routes (144). (*i*) The tumor may spread anteriorly to the iris root, sometimes giving the appearance of an iridodialysis. As with melanomas of the iris, those in the ciliary body may extend circumferentially along the major arterial circle to produce a "ring melanoma" (342). A ring melanoma may also arise from the coalescence of tumors arising at multiple sites, as suggested by a melanoma of the ciliary body and iris that was manifested in two locations in the same eye (175). (*ii*) The tumor may extend centrally into the posterior chamber and vitreous resulting in lenticular

(A)

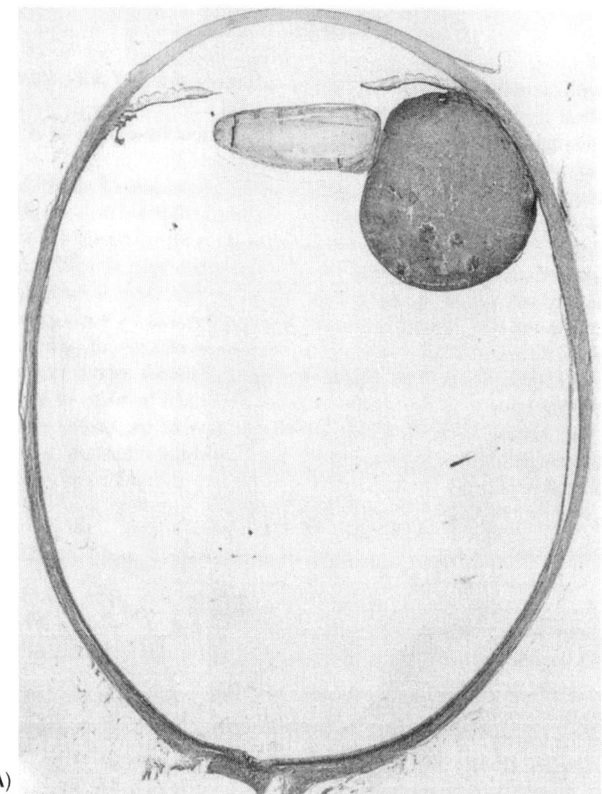

(B)

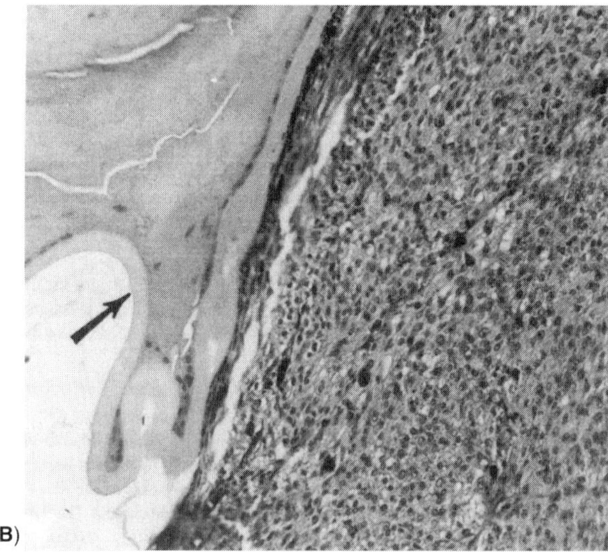

Figure 40 (**A**) Melanoma of ciliary body with compression of lens from a 27-year-old woman who presented because of visual complaints and the appearance of a pigmented area in the periphery of the iris (partially bleached; hematoxylin and eosin, ×4.5). (**B**) Higher power, showing distortion of the lens (*arrow*) by ciliary body malignant melanoma (partially bleached; hematoxylin and eosin, × 220).

astigmatism, lens subluxation, and cataract formation. Initially, the lens opacity is restricted to the portion contiguous with the tumor, but eventually the entire lens becomes opaque. (*iii*) Posterior extension of the tumor tends to be relatively late, and when the melanoma arises in the posterior part of the pars plana, choroidal invasion may suggest a primary choroidal melanoma. A visual field defect accompanies choroidal extension that produces secondary retinal detachment. (*iv*) Extrabulbar extension may occur along the scleral emissaries of the ciliary nerves and vessels, producing an episcleral pigmented lesion, but it is unusual for this to be the presenting sign (Fig. 41) (197).

Glaucoma. Pain is infrequent with ciliary body melanomas but occurs when the tumor causes glaucoma. Glaucoma may occur by one or more of three methods (144): (*i*) most commonly, the tumor infiltrates the iris root, the trabecular meshwork and Schlemm canal; (*ii*) the tumor may displace the iris root against the trabecular meshwork and mechanically obstruct aqueous humor outflow; or (*iii*) less commonly, tumor cells exfoliate and are carried by the aqueous humor circulation into the anterior chamber, where they may block the trabecular outflow channels.

Secondary glaucoma is one of the earliest findings in diffuse melanomas of the anterior uvea and is usually due to a circumferential infiltration of the chamber angle. Before or after the glaucoma becomes evident, the clinical picture may resemble iridocyclitis with pigmented keratic precipitates. If a ciliary body melanoma becomes necrotic, unilateral acute open-angle glaucoma may result from obstruction to the trabecular meshwork by macrophages containing melanin pigment and other cellular debris liberated from necrotic tumor cells (melanomalytic glaucoma) (334).

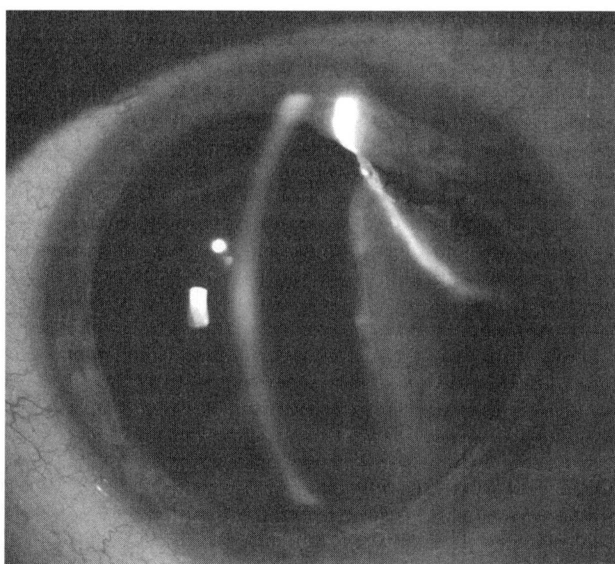

Figure 41 Clinical photograph of a ciliary body melanoma seen through the dilated pupil.

Diagnosis and Differential Diagnosis. A variety of benign lesions arising in the ciliary body can simulate malignant melanomas (Table 2) and benign solid tumors may be difficult to differentiate from malignant melanomas by clinical appearance. Ultrasound biomicroscopy helps to determine the size and extent of ciliary body melanomas providing useful information relevant to the treatment and prognosis prior to surgical intervention (57). When flare and cells are present in the anterior chamber of an eye with a suspected ciliary body melanoma, cytological study of an aqueous humor aspiration may differentiate inflammatory cells from neoplastic cells (142).

Epidemiology

Circumscribed ciliary body melanomas constitute 2% to 9% of uveal melanomas (76) and the peak age of occurrence is in the sixth decade of life, with an equal incidence in males and females. Like other uveal melanomas, they predominate in Caucasians (144).

Histopathology

The morphological features of ciliary body melanomas are indistinguishable from those of choroidal melanomas.

Prognosis

Ciliary body melanomas have a less favorable prognosis than choroidal melanomas with a mortality rate approximately three times higher in one study (266).

Table 2 Differential Diagnosis of Ciliary Body Melanoma

Condition	Refs.
Cysts	
Ciliary body cyst	189,242,337
Inflammatory lesions	
Juvenile xanthogranuloma	305
Inflammatory pseudotumor	256
Granulomatous inflammation	192,194
Nevi	
Ciliary body nevus	130
Melanocytoma of ciliary body with extrascleral extension	35
Neoplasms	
Medulloepithelioma	190
Leiomyoma	190
Metastatic carcinoma	91,190
Hyperplastic lesions	
Hyperplasia of pigmented ciliary epithelium	190

Prognostic factors are also thought to be identical to those for choroidal melanomas.

Iris Melanomas

Clinical Features

The first description of an iris melanoma was by Tay in 1866 (314). They are relatively uncommon but, based on clinical observations, are thought to arise from iris nevi (208,333). Since the iris is easily observed, changes in color, distortion of the pupil, and other abnormalities related to neoplastic growth can be detected earlier than melanomas of the posterior uveal tract.

Iris melanomas are usually present in the stroma and anterior border layer of the iris but they may break through the surface or extend out from the iris crypts to grow on the surface. They may have a nodular appearance and bulge into the anterior chamber. They may spread as a relatively flat mass on the iris surface to infiltrate the anterior chamber angle and be inapparent for some time. Iris melanomas are usually densely pigmented, but when the tumor lacks pigment, prominent, dilated blood vessels occur on the fleshy tumor surface. These newly formed vessels are seen in 7% to 20% of cases (15,252), and sometimes the blood vessels are sufficiently prominent to cause confusion with hemangiomas (19,131,190).

Most iris melanomas are located inferiorly, and the majority involves the midzone and periphery of the iris (15,252). A melanoma of the superior iris is most unusual (290). The tumors grow more slowly than choroidal melanomas but may suddenly enlarge. An increase in pigmentation alone should not be considered definite evidence of tumor growth, since it may occur at puberty or during pregnancy. Indicators of tumor growth include enlargement of the lesion and neovascularization, and incomplete dilation of the pupil in the area of the tumor signifies stromal invasion. The pupil is often distorted, being elongated toward the lesion, and this appearance may be accentuated by ectropion uveae. A melanoma in the extreme periphery of the iris may not be detected during a routine clinical examination. Episcleral hyperemia corresponding to the location of the iris tumor is generally indicative of ciliary body involvement (103).

Although visual symptoms are frequently denied, the patient may have noted a pigmented spot on the iris that recently enlarged or became darker (Fig. 42). In the presence of a diffuse iris melanoma, the patient may comment on the gradual development of heterochromia iridis, the involved eye having the darker iris. The hyperpigmentation in a diffuse iris melanoma is often irregular and blotchy, and tumor growth obscures the iris architecture and causes stromal thickening. While heterochromia iridis is a relatively rare finding in iris melanomas (108,208,246), the diagnosis of melanoma needs to be considered in the differential for patients with this clinical finding. Other associated preoperative clinical features of iris melanomas include spontaneous hyphema (7–13%) (252), secondary glaucoma (14%) (15), and a cataract (10%) (15). Hyphema may also be a first indication of tumor recurrence after the excision of an iris melanoma (175). Conjunctival hyperpigmentation in the vicinity of the iris tumor has been noted in

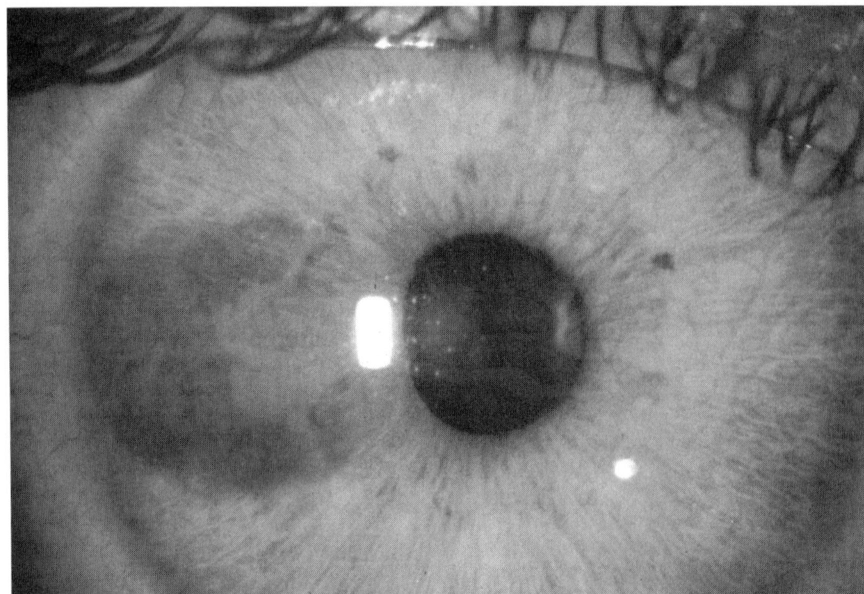

Figure 42 Iris melanoma disrupting the normal architecture of the iris and displaying large irregular blood vessels on its surface.

one study (236), but it was not observed in one large series (15).

Spread. Iris melanomas may extend around the anterior chamber angle and obstruct enough trabecular meshwork to cause secondary glaucoma, which can be the initial cause of symptoms (190). The combination of increased pigmentation of one iris (heterochromia iridis) and ipsilateral glaucoma should arouse suspicion of a diffuse melanoma of the iris (251). The glaucoma associated with diffuse melanomas is relentless, does not respond to treatment, and eventually leads to visual loss. Occasionally, an iris melanoma extends circumferentially in the anterior chamber angle and anterior aspect of ciliary body and produces a so-called ring melanoma (144).

Fine granular pigment over the trabecular meshwork in the dependent part of the filtration angle is an almost constant finding during gonioscopy of an eye with an iris melanoma. This pigment differs from implantations of tumor cells, which are larger and tend to grow over the iris surface. Seeding of tumor cells is an important mode of intraocular spread to the angle structures and eventual extrabulbar extension.

If an iris melanoma becomes necrotic, cells and a flare appear in the anterior chamber. Rarely, an iris melanoma simulates granulomatous uveitis clinically, with iris nodules, aqueous flare, and glaucoma (162). The neoplastic cells of an iris melanoma are reported to have implanted on the surface of the optic nerve head and inner surface of the retina (258). Extraocular extension of iris melanomas presents clinically as an extrabulbar pigmented mass and, as with those of the ciliary body, usually occurs via scleral vascular and neural channels.

Variants of Iris Melanomas. An unusual clinical variant of iris melanoma (tapioca melanoma) is characterized by lightly pigmented and translucent nodules, resembling tapioca pudding (162,238). Reese and colleagues documented this entity in nine patients and noted that the tapioca melanoma of the iris presents as a large irregular segmental nodule or as multifocal nodules, and the individual masses are sometimes pedunculated (238). Even when the nodules are multifocal, they are thought to represent separate primary growths rather than secondary implantations, because they have been shown histopathologically to lie within the iris stroma rather than on the iris surface. The average age of presentation of tapioca melanomas is about 30 years (younger than with the usual type of iris melanoma) (15). They have histopathological features and prognosis similar to those of other iris melanomas (154).

Diagnosis and Differential Diagnosis. In one review of 69 eyes enucleated with a clinical diagnosis of iris melanoma, the clinical impression was not confirmed in 24 eyes (35%) (93). This surprisingly high rate of misdiagnosis was partly because one-fourth of the patients in this series were not Caucasians (iris melanomas being very uncommon in non-white ethnic groups). In another series of 48 cases examined at a single-teaching center, incorrect clinical diagnoses were made in only 2% of the cases (147). A study of 200 patients referred to a major center with a clinical diagnosis of melanoma found that only 42 patients (24%) had melanoma (287).

Iris FA is helpful in distinguishing benign from malignant melanocytic tumors (156). In clinically obvious melanomas of the iris that are non-pigmented or lightly pigmented, angiograms of the anterior segment can disclose an abnormal pattern of disorderly interconnected vascular channels that leak fluorescein to permit pooling of dye in and around the tumor. In heavily pigmented lesions the vascular pattern may be obscured. Disorganized vasculature and leakage are more apt to be associated with melanomas and tumors of intermediate cytology than with nevi (64), although iris FA may be normal in histopathologically proven melanomas (170).

Ultrasound biomicroscopy is also being used in the diagnosis of iris melanomas to help delineate the location and extent of invasion of the tumors and is thought to be superior to conventional B-scan (57,221). Fine-needle aspiration biopsy has been shown to provide an adequate specimen for cytological diagnosis, although the experience of the pathologist examining the specimen is important (129). Many lesions need to be considered in the clinical differential diagnosis of iris melanomas (Table 3) (189).

An anterior staphyloma and sudden prolapse of hemorrhagic intraocular contents through the site of a corneal or scleral perforation may simulate extrabulbar extension of an iris melanoma (236).

Epidemiology

Iris melanomas account for 0.5–8% of uveal melanomas in adults and occurred in only 0.9–1.3% of eyes enucleated before the introduction of conservative treatment of these lesions (17,40,172). Rarely, iris melanomas may be bilateral (71).

The average age of patients with iris melanomas is in the fifth decade of life (15,17,40,172), 10 to 20 years younger than for ciliary body or choroidal melanomas (108). Iris melanomas are uncommon in young patients, but Lerner reported 16 examples in patients under the age of 10 years and 25 cases between the ages of 10 and 19 years (179). Apt described 19 juvenile iris melanomas (14 in patients older than 11 years) and noted an increased incidence

Table 3 Differential Diagnosis of Iris Melanoma

Conditions	Refs.
Conditions with diffuse pigmentation of iris	
Congenital ocular melanosis	30,93
Herpes zoster ophthalmicus	169
Cysts	
Cysts of the iris pigment epithelium	337
Neoplasms	
Leiomyoma	190
Metastatic carcinoma	91,190
Inflammatory lesions	
Syphilis	263
Inflammatory pseudotumor	282
Sarcoidosis	190
Tuberculosis	93,190
Juvenile xanthogranuloma	93
Abscess	114
Vascular lesions	
Pigmented iris and retrocorneal membrane secondary to old central retinal vein occulsion	136
Ectropion uveae associated with iris neovascularization	236
Hemangioma	19,131,190
Nevi	
Iris nevus (Cogan–Reese) syndrome	54,160
Necrotic melanocytoma of iris, producing secondary glaucoma	281
Ciliary body melanocytoma with anterior extension into the base of the iris	35
Miscellaneous	
Stromal atrophy of the iris with baring of iris pigment epithelium	93
Metallic foreign bodies embedded in the iris	93
Anterior staphyloma	93,236

after puberty (14). Arentsen and Green, in a series of 72 iris melanomas, found 10% in patients <20 years old (15). An iris melanoma has been reported in a 7-month-old infant (40) and a congenital melanoma of the iris has also been documented (122). Despite being much less common in children than adults, iris melanomas represent 41% of uveal melanomas in childhood (14). There is probably no significant difference in the incidence of iris melanomas between the sexes (17), but some studies have reported a slightly higher incidence in females (15,40), whereas others have described an excess of males (252). As with other uveal melanomas, those in the iris are rare in non-whites and of 169 patients in one series, all were Caucasian (280).

Histopathology

The histopathological classification of iris melanomas is similar to that for other uveal melanomas: spindle cells, epithelioid cells, or mixed cell tumors. In one series, 55% of cases of iris melanoma contained spindle cells only, 5% were epithelioid cell melanomas, and the rest were of mixed cell type (280). Diffuse iris melanomas have been shown to have a higher likelihood of containing epithelioid cells, up to 88% in one series (70).

Prognosis

Diffuse iris melanomas are thought to have a worse prognosis than circumscribed iris melanomas, and are often treated with more aggressive surgical management (enucleation). Their rate of metastasis is 13% at approximately 6 years follow-up (70).

Even mixed and epithelioid cell types of iris melanomas are relatively benign compared with posterior uveal tumors of similar cell type. Iris melanomas have a mortality rate 10 times less than that of other uveal melanomas (201). Of approximately 800 reported iris melanomas, only 37 deaths have been attributed to metastases, but the nature of the metastases was only confirmed histologically in seven patients who died (14,15,30,40,53,125, 159,165,236,252,290,312). The length of time that an iris melanoma is present does not seem to affect longevity (252). In a series of 22 cases observed for 1 to 20 years, no tumor-related metastatic deaths were reported (236). Morphological features of iris melanomas that relate to the benign behavior include the predominance of spindle-shaped cells and the cohesion of these cells. The tumor cells in one series of 92 iris melanomas were compact and cohesive in 92% of the tumors (15). It is also possible that many tumors historically classified as melanomas were nevi. The favorable outcome of patients with iris melanomas may also reflect their early diagnosis and small size.

A recent study found that the method of management (resection, enucleation, or radiation) had no impact on the likelihood of metastasis, but that increasing age, elevated IOP, posterior tumor margin at the anterior chamber angle or iris root, extraocular extension, and prior surgical treatment were associated with an unfavorable prognosis (280).

REFERENCES

1. Aalto Y, Eriksson L, Seregard S, et al. Concomitant loss of chromosome 3 and whole arm losses and gains of chromosome 1, 6, or 8 in metastasizing primary uveal melanoma. Invest Ophthalmol Vis Sci 2001; 42(2):313–7.
2. Abramson DH, Rodriguez-Sains RS, Rubman R. B-K mole syndrome. Cutaneous and ocular malignant melanoma. Arch Ophthalmol 1980; 98(8):1397–9.
3. Affeldt JC, Minckler DS, Azen SP, Yeh L. Prognosis in uveal melanoma with extrascleral extension. Arch Ophthalmol 1980; 98(11):1975–9.
4. Albert DM, Gaasterland DE, Caldwell JB, et al. Bilateral metastatic choroidal melanoma, nevi, and cavernous degeneration. Involvement of the optic nervehead. Arch Ophthalmol 1972; 87(1):39–47.

5. Albert DM, Lahav M, Packer S, Yimoyines D. Histogenesis of malignant melanomas of the uvea. Occurrence of nevus-like structures in experimental choroidal tumors. Arch Ophthalmol 1974; 92(4):318–23.
6. Albert DM, Puliafito CA, Fulton AB, et al. Increased incidence of choroidal malignant melanoma occurring in a single population of chemical workers. Am J Ophthalmol 1980; 89(3):323–37.
7. Albert DM, Puliafito CA. Choroidal melanoma: possible exposure to industrial toxins. N Engl J Med 1977; 296(11): 634–5.
8. Albert DM. The association of viruses with uveal melanoma. Trans Am Ophthalmol Soc 1979; 77:367–421.
9. Anastassiou G, Heiligenhaus A, Bechrakis N, et al. Prognostic value of clinical and histopathological parameters in conjunctival melanomas: a retrospective study. Br J Ophthalmol 2002; 86(2):163–7.
10. Anonymous. Accuracy of diagnosis of choroidal melanomas in the Collaborative Ocular Melanoma Study. COMS report no. 1. Arch Ophthalmol 1990; 108(9):1268–73.
11. Anonymous. Mortality in patients with small choroidal melanoma. COMS report no. 4. The Collaborative Ocular Melanoma Study Group. Arch Ophthalmol 1997; 115(7): 886–93.
12. Anonymous. The Collaborative Ocular Melanoma Study (COMS) randomized trial of pre-enucleation radiation of large choroidal melanoma I: characteristics of patients enrolled and not enrolled. COMS report no. 9. Am J Ophthalmol 1998; 125(6):767–78.
13. Anonymous. The Collaborative Ocular Melanoma Study (COMS) randomized trial of pre-enucleation radiation of large choroidal melanoma II: initial mortality findings. COMS report no. 10. Am J Ophthalmol 1998; 125(6): 779–96.
14. Apt L. Uveal melanomas in children and adolescents. Int Ophthalmol Clin 1962; 2:403–10.
15. Arentsen JJ, Green WR. Melanoma of the iris: report of 72 cases treated surgically. Ophthalmic Surg 1975; 6(2): 23–37.
16. Ashbury MK, Vail D. Multiple primary malignant neoplasms: Report of a case of malignant melanoma of the choroid and glioblastoma multiforme of the right cerebral hemisphere. Am J Ophthalmol 1943; 26:688–93.
17. Ashton N. Primary tumours of the iris. Br J Ophthalmol 1964; 48:650–68.
18. Augsburger JJ, Shields JA, Folberg R, et al. Fine needle aspiration biopsy in the diagnosis of intraocular cancer. Cytologic-histologic correlations. Ophthalmology 1985; 92(1):39–49.
19. Baghdassarian SA, Spencer WH. Pseudoangioma of the iris—its association with melanoma. Report of a case. Arch Ophthalmol 1969; 82(1):69–71.
20. Baker JK, Elshaw SR, Mathewman GE, et al. Expression of integrins, degradative enzymes and their inhibitors in uveal melanoma: differences between in vitro and in vivo expression. Melanoma Res 2001; 11(3):265–73.
21. Bard LA. Eyes With choroidal detachments removed for suspected melanoma. Arch Ophthalmol 1965; 73:320–3.
22. Barker-Griffith AE, McDonald PR, Green WR. Malignant melanoma arising in a choroidal magnacellular nevus (melanocytoma). Can J Ophthalmol 1976; 11(2):140–6.
23. Barr CC, Zimmerman LE, Curtin VT, Font RL. Bilateral diffuse melanocytic uveal tumors associated with systemic malignant neoplasms. A recently recognized syndrome. Arch Ophthalmol 1982; 100(2):249–55.
24. Bellet RE, Shields JA, Soll DB, Bernardino EA. Primary choroidal and cutaneous melanomas occurring in a patient with the B-K mole syndrome phenotype. Am J Ophthalmol 1980; 89(4):567–70.
25. Berson E, Bigger JF, Smith ME. Malignant melanoma, retinal hole, and retinal detachment. Arch Ophthalmol 1967; 77(2):223–5.
26. Bierman EO. Retinal tears associated with tumors. Am J Ophthalmol 1958; 46(1):74–5.
27. Bierring F, Jensen OA. Electron microscopy of melanomas of the human uveal tract: the ultrastructure of four malignant melanomas of the mixed cell type. Acta Ophthalmol (Copenh) 1964; 42:665–71.
28. Blesch A, Bosserhoff AK, Apfel R, et al. Cloning of a novel malignant melanoma-derived growth-regulatory protein, MIA. Cancer Res 1994; 54(21):5695–701.
29. Blodi FC, Roy PE. The misdiagnosed choroidal melanoma. Can J Ophthalmol 1967; 2(3):209–11.
30. Blodi FC. Ocular melanocytosis and melanoma. Am J Ophthalmol 1975; 80(3):389–95.
31. Blodi FC. The difficult diagnosis of choroidal melanoma. Arch Ophthalmol 1963; 69:253–6.
32. Boniuk M, Zimmerman LE. Occurrence and behavior of choroidal melanomas in eyes subjected to operations for retinal detachment. Trans Am Acad Ophthalmol Otolaryngol 1962; 66:642–58.
33. Boniuk M, Zimmerman LE. Problems in differentiating idiopathic serous detachments from solid retinal detachments. Int Ophthalmol Clin 1962; 2:411–30.
34. Bosserhoff AK, Lederer M, Kaufmann M, et al. MIA, a novel serum marker for progression of malignant melanoma. Anticancer Res 1999; 19(4A):2691–3.
35. Bowers JF. Melanocytoma of the ciliary body. Arch Ophthalmol 1964; 71:649–52.
36. Brantley MA Jr, Harbour JW. Deregulation of the Rb and p53 pathways in uveal melanoma. Am J Pathol 2000; 157 (6):1795–801.
37. Brantley MA Jr, Harbour JW. Inactivation of retinoblastoma protein in uveal melanoma by phosphorylation of sites in the COOH-terminal region. Cancer Res 2000; 60 (16):4320–3.
38. Brantley MA Jr, Worley L, Harbour JW. Altered expression of Rb and p53 in uveal melanomas following plaque radiotherapy. Am J Ophthalmol 2002; 133(2):242–8.
39. Brownstein S, Orton R, Jackson B. Cystoid macular edema with equatorial choroidal melanoma. Arch Ophthalmol 1978; 96(11):2105–7.
40. Burki E. Uber ein Sarkom der Iris im Sauglingsalter. Ophthalmologica 1961; 142:487–99.
41. Callender GR. Malignant melanotic tumors of the eye. A study of histologic types in 111 cases. Trans Am Acad Ophthalmol Otolaryngol 1931; 36:131.
42. Cappin JM. Malignant melanoma and rubeosis iridis. Histopathological and statistical study. Br J Ophthalmol 1973; 57(11):815–24.
43. Cargill LV, Mayou S. A case of flat sarcoma of the choroid. Trans Ophthalmol Soc UK 1907; 27:149–55.
44. Castilla EE, da Graca Dutra M, Orioli-Parreiras IM. Epidemiology of congenital pigmented naevi: I. Incidence rates and relative frequencies. Br J Dermatol 1981; 104(3):307–15.
45. Chambers RB, Davidorf FH, McAdoo JF, Chakeres DW. Magnetic resonance imaging of uveal melanomas. Arch Ophthalmol 1987; 105(7):917–21.
46. Chana JS, Wilson GD, Cree IA, et al. c-myc, p53, and Bcl-2 expression and clinical outcome in uveal melanoma. Br J Ophthalmol 1999; 83(1):110–4.
47. Chang AE, Karnell LH, Menck HR. The National Cancer Data Base report on cutaneous and noncutaneous

melanoma: a summary of 84,836 cases from the past decade. The American College of Surgeons Commission on Cancer and the American Cancer Society. Cancer 1998; 83(8):1664–78.
48. Char DH, Crawford JB, Irvine AR, et al. Correlation between degree of malignancy and the radioactive phosphorus uptake test in ocular melanomas. Am J Ophthalmol 1976; 81(1):71–5.
49. Char DH, Miller T, Kroll S. Orbital metastases: diagnosis and course. Br J Ophthalmol 1997; 81(5):386–90.
50. Chaves E, Granville R. Choroidal malignant melanoma in a two-and-one-half-year-old girl. Am J Ophthalmol 1972; 74(1):20–3.
51. Chess J, Henkind P, Albert DM, et al. Uveal melanoma presenting after cataract extraction with intraocular lens implantation. Ophthalmology 1985; 92(6):827–30.
52. Chowers I, Amer R, Pe'er J. The correlation among different immunostaining evaluation methods for the assessment of proliferative activity in uveal melanoma. Curr Eye Res 2002; 25(6):369–72.
53. Cleasby GW. Malignant melanoma of the iris. AMA Arch Ophthalmol 1958; 60(3):403–17.
54. Cogan DG, Reese AB. A syndrome of iris nodules, ectopic Descemet's membrane, and unilateral glaucoma. Doc Ophthalmol 1969; 26:424–33.
55. Cohen LM. Lentigo maligna and lentigo maligna melanoma. J Am Acad Dermatol 1995; 33(6):923–36; quiz 37–40.
56. Coleman K, Baak JP, van Diest PJ, Mullaney J. Prognostic value of morphometric features and the callender classification in uveal melanomas. Ophthalmology 1996; 103(10):1634–41.
57. Conway RM, Chew T, Golchet P, et al. Ultrasound biomicroscopy: role in diagnosis and management in 130 consecutive patients evaluated for anterior segment tumours. Br J Ophthalmol 2005; 89(8):950–5.
58. Cook BE Jr, Bartley GB. Treatment options and future prospects for the management of eyelid malignancies: an evidence-based update. Ophthalmology 2001; 108(11): 2088–98; quiz 99, 100, 121.
59. Coupland SE, Anastassiou G, Stang A, et al. The prognostic value of cyclin D1, p53, and MDM2 protein expression in uveal melanoma. J Pathol 2000; 191(2): 120–6.
60. Cowan TH, Balistocky M. The nevus of Ota or oculodermal melanocytosis. The ocular changes. Arch Ophthalmol 1961; 65:483–92.
61. Crawford JB, Howes EL Jr, Char DH. Combined nevi of the conjunctiva. Arch Ophthalmol 1999; 117(9):1121–7.
62. Crawford JB. Conjunctival melanomas: prognostic factors a review and an analysis of a series. Trans Am Ophthalmol Soc 1980; 78:467–502.
63. Cunningham ER. Ocular tumors of west China, a statistical and clinical study. Trans Can Ophthalmol Soc 1952; 5:102–21.
64. Dart JK, Marsh RJ, Garner A, Cooling RJ. Fluorescein angiography of anterior uveal melanocytic tumours. Br J Ophthalmol 1988; 72(5):326–37.
65. Davies WS. Malignant melanomas of the choroid and ciliary body. A clinicopathologic study. Am J Ophthalmol 1963; 55:541–6.
66. de la Cruz PO Jr, Specht CS, McLean IW. Lymphocytic infiltration in uveal malignant melanoma. Cancer 1990; 65(1):112–5.
67. De Potter P, Shields CL, Eagle RC Jr, et al. Malignant melanoma of the optic nerve. Arch Ophthalmol 1996; 114(5):608–12.
68. De Potter P, Shields CL, Shields JA, Menduke H. Clinical predictive factors for development of recurrence and metastasis in conjunctival melanoma: a review of 68 cases. Br J Ophthalmol 1993; 77(10):624–30.
69. de Vries E, Bray FI, Coebergh JW, Parkin DM. Changing epidemiology of malignant cutaneous melanoma in Europe 1953–1997: rising trends in incidence and mortality but recent stabilizations in western Europe and decreases in Scandinavia. Int J Cancer 2003; 107(1): 119–26.
70. Demirci H, Shields CL, Shields JA, et al. Diffuse iris melanoma: a report of 25 cases. Ophthalmology 2002; 109(8):1553–60.
71. Diamond S, Borley WE, Miller WW. Partial iridocyclectomy for chamber angle tumors. Am J Ophthalmol 1964; 57:88–94.
72. Diener-West M, Earle JD, Fine SL, et al. The COMS randomized trial of iodine 125 brachytherapy for choroidal melanoma, II: characteristics of patients enrolled and not enrolled. COMS Report No. 17. Arch Ophthalmol 2001; 119(7):951–65.
73. Diener-West M, Earle JD, Fine SL, et al. The COMS randomized trial of iodine 125 brachytherapy for choroidal melanoma, III: initial mortality findings. COMS report no. 18. Arch Ophthalmol 2001; 119(7):969–82.
74. Diener-West M, Hawkins BS, Markowitz JA, Schachat AP. A review of mortality from choroidal melanoma. II. A meta-analysis of 5-year mortality rates following enucleation, 1966 through 1988. Arch Ophthalmol 1992; 110(2):245–50.
75. Dithmar S, Volcker HE, Grossniklaus HE. Multifocal intraocular malignant melanoma: report of two cases and review of the literature. Ophthalmology 1999; 106(7): 1345–8.
76. Duke-Elder S, Perkins ES. Malignant melanoma. In: Duke-Elder S, ed. System of Ophthalmology. Vol. 9. St. Louis, MO: Mosby, 1967.
77. Dunn WJ, Lambert HM, Kincaid MC, et al. Choroidal malignant melanoma with early vitreous seeding. Retina 1988; 8(3):188–92.
78. Dunnington JH. Intraocular tension in cases of sarcoma of the choroid and ciliary body. Arch Ophthalmol 1938; 20: 359–63.
79. Eagle RC Jr, Font RL, Yanoff M, Fine BS. Proliferative endotheliopathy with iris abnormalities. The iridocorneal endothelial syndrome. Arch Ophthalmol 1979; 97(11): 2104–11.
80. Egan CL, Oliveria SA, Elenitsas R, et al. Cutaneous melanoma risk and phenotypic changes in large congenital nevi: a follow-up study of 46 patients. J Am Acad Dermatol 1998; 39(6):923–32.
81. Egan KM, Seddon JM, Glynn RJ, et al. Epidemiologic aspects of uveal melanoma. Surv Ophthalmol 1988; 32(4): 239–51.
82. el Baba F, Blumenkranz M. Malignant melanoma at the site of penetrating ocular trauma. Arch Ophthalmol 1986; 104(3):405–9.
83. el Baba F, Hagler WS, De la Cruz A, Green WR. Choroidal melanoma with pigment dispersion in vitreous and melanomalytic glaucoma. Ophthalmology 1988; 95(3): 370–7.
84. Elder DE, Green MH, Guerry Dt, et al. The dysplastic nevus syndrome: our definition. Am J Dermatopathol 1982; 4(5):455–60.
85. English JS, Swerdlow AJ, Mackie RM, et al. Site-specific melanocytic naevus counts as predictors of whole body naevi. Br J Dermatol 1988; 118(5):641–4.

86. Enriquez R, Egbert B, Bullock J. Primary malignant melanoma of central nervous system. Pineal involvement in a patient with nevus of ota and multiple pigmented skin nevi. Arch Pathol 1973; 95(6):392–5.
87. Esmaeli B, Wang B, Deavers M, et al. Prognostic factors for survival in malignant melanoma of the eyelid skin. Ophthal Plast Reconstr Surg 2000; 16(4):250–7.
88. Esmaeli B, Wang X, Youssef A, Gershenwald JE. Patterns of regional and distant metastasis in patients with conjunctival melanoma: experience at a cancer center over four decades. Ophthalmology 2001; 108(11):2101–5.
89. Esmaeli B, Youssef A, Naderi A, et al. Margins of excision for cutaneous melanoma of the eyelid skin: the Collaborative Eyelid Skin Melanoma Group Report. Ophthal Plast Reconstr Surg 2003; 19(2):96–101.
90. Esmaeli B. Sentinel node biopsy as a tool for accurate staging of eyelid and conjunctival malignancies. Curr Opin Ophthalmol 2002; 13(5):317–23.
91. Ferry AP, Font RL. Carcinoma metastatic to the eye and orbit II. A clinicopathological study of 26 patients with carcinoma metastatic to the anterior segment of the eye. Arch Ophthalmol 1975; 93(7):472–82.
92. Ferry AP, Font RL. Carcinoma metastatic to the eye and orbit. I. A clinicopathologic study of 227 cases. Arch Ophthalmol 1974; 92(4):276–86.
93. Ferry AP. Lesions mistaken for malignant melanoma of the iris. Arch Ophthalmol 1965; 74:9–18.
94. Ferry AP. Lesions mistaken for malignant melanoma of the posterior uvea. A clinicopathologic analysis of 100 cases with ophthalmoscopically visible lesions. Arch Ophthalmol 1964; 72:463–9.
95. Ferry AP. Macular detachment associated with congenital pit of the optic nerve head. Pathologic findings in two cases simulating malignant melanoma of the choroid. Arch Ophthalmol 1963; 70:346–57.
96. Folberg R, Jakobiec FA, Bernardino VB, Iwamoto T. Benign conjunctival melanocytic lesions. Clinicopathologic features. Ophthalmology 1989; 96(4):436–61.
97. Folberg R, McLean IW, Zimmerman LE. Malignant melanoma of the conjunctiva. Hum Pathol 1985; 16(2): 136–43.
98. Folberg R, McLean IW, Zimmerman LE. Primary acquired melanosis of the conjunctiva. Hum Pathol 1985; 16(2):129–35.
99. Folberg R, Pe'er J, Gruman LM, et al. The morphologic characteristics of tumor blood vessels as a marker of tumor progression in primary human uveal melanoma: a matched case-control study. Hum Pathol 1992; 23(11): 1298–305.
100. Folberg R, Rummelt V, Parys-Van Ginderdeuren R, et al. The prognostic value of tumor blood vessel morphology in primary uveal melanoma. Ophthalmology 1993; 100(9): 1389–98.
101. Font RL, Spaulding AG, Zimmerman LDM. Diffuse malignant melanoma of the uveal tract: a clinicopathologic report of 54 cases. Trans Am Acad Ophthalmol Otolaryngol 1968; 72(6):877–95.
102. Font RL, Zimmerman LE, Armaly MF. The nature of the orange pigment over a choroidal melanoma. Histochemical and electron microscopical observations. Arch Ophthalmol 1974; 91(5):359–62.
103. Foos RY, Hull SN, Straatsma BR. Early diagnosis of ciliary body melanomas. Arch Ophthalmol 1969; 81(3): 336–44.
104. Foss AJ, Alexander RA, Hungerford JL, et al. Reassessment of the PAS patterns in uveal melanoma. Br J Ophthalmol 1997; 81(3):240–6; discussion 7, 8.
105. Foss AJ, Alexander RA, Jefferies LW, et al. Microvessel count predicts survival in uveal melanoma. Cancer Res 1996; 56(13):2900–3.
106. Foster WJ, Fuller CE, Perry A, Harbour JW. Status of the NF1 tumor suppressor locus in uveal melanoma. Arch Ophthalmol 2003; 121(9):1311–5.
107. Frangieh GT, el Baba F, Traboulsi EI, Green WR. Melanocytoma of the ciliary body: presentation of four cases and review of nineteen reports. Surv Ophthalmol 1985; 29(5):328–34.
108. Friedenwald JS, Wilder HC, Maumanee AE, et al. Ophthalmic Pathology: An Atlas and Textbook. Philadelphia: W. B. Saunders, 1952:398.
109. Friedman RJ, Rodriguez-Sains R, Jakobiec F. Ophthalmo-logic oncology: conjunctival malignant melanoma in association with sporadic dysplastic nevus syndrome. J Dermatol Surg Oncol 1987; 13(1): 31–4.
110. Gamel JW, McCurdy JB, McLean IW. A comparison of prognostic covariates for uveal melanoma. Invest Ophthalmol Vis Sci 1992; 33(6):1919–22.
111. Garner A, Koornneef L, Levene A, Collin JR. Malignant melanoma of the eyelid skin: histopathology and behaviour. Br J Ophthalmol 1985; 69(3):180–6.
112. Gass JD, Gieser RG, Wilkinson CP, et al. Bilateral diffuse uveal melanocytic proliferation in patients with occult carcinoma. Arch Ophthalmol 1990; 108(4): 527–33.
113. Gass JD, Guerry RK, Jack RL, Harris G. Choroidal osteoma. Arch Ophthalmol 1978; 96(3):428–35.
114. Gass JD. Iris abscess simulating malignant melanoma. Arch Ophthalmol 1973; 90(4):300–2.
115. Geller AC, Annas GD. Epidemiology of melanoma and nonmelanoma skin cancer. Semin Oncol Nurs 2003; 19(1): 2–11.
116. Glasgow BJ, Brown HH, Zargoza AM, Foos RY. Quantitation of tumor seeding from fine needle aspiration of ocular melanomas. Am J Ophthalmol 1988; 105(5): 538–46.
117. Gloor P, Alexandrakis G. Clinical characterization of primary acquired melanosis. Invest Ophthalmol Vis Sci 1995; 36(8):1721–9.
118. Gonder JR, Ezell PC, Shields JA, Augsburger JJ. Ocular melanocytosis. A study to determine the prevalence rate of ocular melanocytosis. Ophthalmology 1982; 89(8): 950–2.
119. Gonder JR, Shields JA, Albert DM, et al. Uveal malignant melanoma associated with ocular and oculodermal melanocytosis. Ophthalmology 1982; 89(8):953–60.
120. Green A, Siskind V, Hansen ME, et al. Melanocytic nevi in schoolchildren in Queensland. J Am Acad Dermatol 1989; 20(6):1054–60.
121. Greene MH, Clark WH Jr, Tucker MA, et al. Acquired precursors of cutaneous malignant melanoma. The familial dysplastic nevus syndrome. N Engl J Med 1985; 312(2):91–7.
122. Greer CH. Congenital melanoma of the anterior uvea. Arch Ophthalmol 1966; 76(1):77–8.
123. Griffith WR, Green WR, Weinstein GW. Conjunctival malignant melanoma originating in acquired melanosis sine pigmento. Am J Ophthalmol 1971; 72(3):595–9.
124. Grin JM, Grant-Kels JM, Grin CM, et al. Ocular melanomas and melanocytic lesions of the eye. J Am Acad Dermatol 1998; 38(5):716–30.
125. Grossniklaus HE, Brown RH, Stulting RD, Blasberg RD. Iris melanoma seeding through a trabeculectomy site. Arch Ophthalmol 1990; 108(9):1287–90.

126. Grossniklaus HE, Green WR, Luckenbach M, Chan CC. Conjunctival lesions in adults. A clinical and histopathologic review. Cornea 1987; 6(2):78–116.
127. Grossniklaus HE, Margo CE, Solomon AR. Indeterminate melanocytic proliferations of the conjunctiva. Arch Ophthalmol 1999; 117(9):1131–6.
128. Grossniklaus HE, McLean IW. Cutaneous melanoma of the eyelid. Clinicopathologic features. Ophthalmology 1991; 98(12):1867–73.
129. Grossniklaus HE. Fine-needle aspiration biopsy of the iris. Arch Ophthalmol 1992; 110(7):969–76.
130. Hale PN, Allen RA, Straatsma BR. Benign melanomas (nevi) of the choroid and ciliary body. Arch Ophthalmol 1965; 74(4):532–8.
131. Hamburg A. Iris melanoma; with vascular proliferation simulating a hemangioma. Arch Ophthalmol 1969; 82(1): 72–6.
132. Hamming N. Anatomy and embryology of the eyelids: a review with special reference to the development of divided nevi. Pediatr Dermatol 1983; 1(1):51–8.
133. Harbour JW, Dean DC. The Rb/E2F pathway: expanding roles and emerging paradigms. Genes Dev 2000; 14(19): 2393–409.
134. Harbour JW, Worley L, Ma D, Cohen M. Transducible peptide therapy for uveal melanoma and retinoblastoma. Arch Ophthalmol 2002; 120(10):1341–6.
135. Haupt Y, Maya R, Kazaz A, Oren M. Mdm2 promotes the rapid degradation of p53. Nature 1997; 387(6630):296–9.
136. Haver RP. Pigmented iris and retrocorneal membrane simulating an iris melanoma. Arch Ophthalmol 1967; 78(1):55–7.
137. Heine B, Coupland SE, Kneiff S, et al. Telomerase expression in uveal melanoma. Br J Ophthalmol 2000; 84(2):217–23.
138. Heitman KF, Kincaid MC, Steahly L. Diffuse malignant change in a ciliochoroidal melanocytoma in a patient of mixed racial background. Retina 1988; 8(1):67–72.
139. Henkind P, Roth MS. Breast carcinoma and concurrent uveal melanoma. Am J Ophthalmol 1971; 1(1):198–203.
140. Henriksson M, Luscher B. Proteins of the Myc network: essential regulators of cell growth and differentiation. Adv Cancer Res 1996; 68:109–82.
141. Hogan M. Melanomas of the uvea and optic nerve: clinical aspects, management and prognosis. Highlights Ophthalmol 1963; 6(2):146–66.
142. Hogan MJ. Pigmented intraocular tumors: clinical aspects, management, and prognosis of melanomas of the uvea and optic nerve. In: Boniuk M, ed. Ocular and Adnexal Tumors: New and Controversial Aspects. St. Louis, MO: Mosby, 1964.
143. Honavar SG, Shields CL, Singh AD, et al. Two discrete choroidal melanomas in an eye with ocular melanocytosis. Surv Ophthalmol 2002; 47(1):36–41.
144. Hopkins RE, Carriker FR. Malignant melanoma of the ciliary body. Am J Ophthalmol 1958; 45(6):835–43.
145. Horsthemke B, Prescher G, Bornfeld N, Becher R. Loss of chromosome 3 alleles and multiplication of chromosome 8 alleles in uveal melanoma. Genes Chromosomes Cancer 1992; 4(3):217–21.
146. Howard GM, Forrest AW. Incidence and location of melanocytomas. Arch Ophthalmol 1967; 77(1):61–6.
147. Howard GM. Erroneous clinical diagnoses of retinoblastoma and uveal melanoma. Trans Am Acad Ophthalmol Otolaryngol 1969; 73(2):199–203.
148. Hu DN, Yu GP, McCormick SA, et al. Population-based incidence of uveal melanoma in various races and ethnic groups. Am J Ophthalmol 2005; 140(4):612–7.
149. Huntington A, Haugan P, Gamel J, McLean I. A simple cytologic method for predicting the malignant potential of intraocular melanoma. Pathol Res Pract 1989; 185(5): 631–4.
150. Isager P, Ehlers N, Overgaard J. Prognostic factors for survival after enucleation for choroidal and ciliary body melanomas. Acta Ophthalmol Scand 2004; 82(5): 517–25.
151. Iwamoto S, Burrows RC, Grossniklaus HE, et al. Immunophenotype of conjunctival melanomas: comparisons with uveal and cutaneous melanomas. Arch Ophthalmol 2002; 120(12):1625–9.
152. Iwamoto S, Burrows RC, Kalina RE, et al. Immunophenotypic differences between uveal and cutaneous melanomas. Arch Ophthalmol 2002; 120(4):466–70.
153. Iwamoto T, Jones IS, Howard GM. Ultrastructural comparison of spindle A, spindle B, and epithelioid-type cells in uveal malignant melanoma. Invest Ophthalmol 1972; 11(11):873–89.
154. Iwamoto T, Reese AB, Mund ML. Tapioca melanoma of the iris. 2. Electron microscopy of the melanoma cells compared with normal iris melanocytes. Am J Ophthalmol 1972; 74(5):851–61.
155. Jakobiec FA, Buckman G, Zimmerman LE, et al. Metastatic melanoma within and to the conjunctiva. Ophthalmology 1989; 96(7):999–1005.
156. Jakobiec FA, Depot MJ, Henkind P, Spencer WH. Fluorescein angiographic patterns of iris melanocytic tumors. Arch Ophthalmol 1982; 100(8):1288–99.
157. Jakobiec FA, Folberg R, Iwamoto T. Clinicopathologic characteristics of premalignant and malignant melanocytic lesions of the conjunctiva. Ophthalmology 1989; 96(2): 147–66.
158. Jakobiec FA, Rini FJ, Fraunfelder FT, Brownstein S. Cryotherapy for conjunctival primary acquired melanosis and malignant melanoma. Experience with 62 cases. Ophthalmology 1988; 95(8):1058–70.
159. Jakobiec FA, Silbert G. Are most iris "melanomas" really nevi? A clinicopathologic study of 189 lesions. Arch Ophthalmol 1981; 99(12):2117–32.
160. Jakobiec FA, Yanoff M, Mottow L, et al. Solitary iris nevus associated with peripheral anterior synechiae and iris endothelialization. Am J Ophthalmol 1977; 83(6): 884–91.
161. Janssen K, Kuntze J, Busse H, Schmid KW. p53 oncoprotein overexpression in choroidal melanoma. Mod Pathol 1996; 9(3):267–72.
162. Jarrett WH, Goldberg MF, Schulze RR. An unusual iris melanoma. Associated with atrophy of iris pigment epithelium, heterochromia, and multicentric tumor foci. Arch Ophthalmol 1966; 75(4):469–74.
163. Jay V, Yi Q, Hunter WS, Zielenska M. Expression of bcl-2 in uveal malignant melanoma. Arch Pathol Lab Med 1996; 120(5):497–8.
164. Jensen OA, Andersen SR. Spontaneous regression of a malignant melanoma of the choroid. Acta Ophthalmol (Copenh) 1974; 52(2):173–82.
165. Jensen OA. Malignant melanomas of the uvea in Denmark 1943–1952. A clinical, histopathological, and prognostic study. Acta Ophthalmol (Copenh) 1963; 43(Suppl.), 75:1–220.
166. Kamino H, Flotte TJ, Misheloff E, et al. Eosinophilic globules in Spitz's nevi. New findings and a diagnostic sign. Am J Dermatopathol 1979; 1(4):319–24.
167. Kang S, Barnhill RL, Mihm MC Jr, et al. Melanoma risk in individuals with clinically atypical nevi. Arch Dermatol 1994; 130(8):999–1001.

168. Kincannon J, Boutzale C. The physiology of pigmented nevi. Pediatrics 1999; 104(4):1042–5.
169. Klien BA, Farkas TG. Pseudomelanoma of the Iris after Herpes Zoster Ophthalmicus. Am J Ophthalmol 1964; 57: 392–7.
170. Kottow M. Fluorescein angiographic behaviour of iris masses. Ophthalmologica 1977; 174(4):217–23.
171. Kroll AJ, Kuwabara T. Electron microscopy of uveal melanoma: a comparison of spindle and epithelioid cells. Arch Ophthalmol 1965; 73:378–86.
172. Kronenberg B. Topography and frequency of complications of uveal sarcoma. Arch Ophthalmol 1938; 59:917–21.
173. Kujala E, Makitie T, Kivela T. Very long-term prognosis of patients with malignant uveal melanoma. Invest Ophthalmol Vis Sci 2003; 44(11):4651–9.
174. Kurli M, Finger PT. Melanocytic conjunctival tumors. Ophthalmol Clin North Am 2005; 18(1):15–24, vii.
175. Kurz GH. Malignant melanoma of ciliary body and iris manifested in two locations. Am J Ophthalmol 1965; 59: 917–21.
176. Lambert SR, Char DH, Howes E Jr, et al. Spontaneous regression of a choroidal melanoma. Arch Ophthalmol 1986; 104(5):732–4.
177. Lane AM, Egan KM, Yang J, et al. An evaluation of tumour vascularity as a prognostic indicator in uveal melanoma. Melanoma Res 1997; 7(3):237–42.
178. Leff SR, Henkind P. Rhabdomyosarcoma and late malignant melanoma of the orbit. Ophthalmology 1983; 90(10):1258–60.
179. Lerner HA. Malignant melanoma of the iris in children. A report of a case in a 9-year-old girl. Arch Ophthalmol 1970; 84(6):754–7.
180. Lincoff H, Kreissig I. Patterns of non-rhegmatogenous elevations of the retina. Br J Ophthalmol 1974; 58(11): 899–906.
181. Litricin O. Unsuspected uveal melanomas. Am J Ophthalmol 1973; 76(5):734–8.
182. Lois N, Shields CL, Shields JA, et al. Trifocal uveal melanoma. Am J Ophthalmol 1997; 124(6):848–50.
183. Lommatzsch PK, Lommatzsch RE, Kirsch I, Fuhrmann P. Therapeutic outcome of patients suffering from malignant melanomas of the conjunctiva. Br J Ophthalmol 1990; 74(10):615–9.
184. Lumbroso L, Sigal-Zafrani B, Jouffroy T, et al. Late malignant melanoma after treatment of rhabdomyosarcoma of the orbit during childhood. Arch Ophthalmol 2002; 120(8):1087–90.
185. MacIlwaine WAt, Anderson B Jr, Klintworth GK. Enlargement of a histologically documented choroidal nevus. Am J Ophthalmol 1979; 87(4):480–6.
186. MacKie RM, English J, Aitchison TC, et al. The number and distribution of benign pigmented moles (melanocytic naevi) in a healthy British population. Br J Dermatol 1985; 113(2):167–74.
187. Mafee MF, Peyman GA, Peace JH, et al. Magnetic resonance imaging in the evaluation and differentiation of uveal melanoma. Ophthalmology 1987; 94(4): 341–8.
188. Makitie T, Summanen P, Tarkkanen A, Kivela T. Microvascular density in predicting survival of patients with choroidal and ciliary body melanoma. Invest Ophthalmol Vis Sci 1999; 40(11):2471–80.
189. Makley TA Jr, King GL. Multiple cysts of the iris and ciliary body simulating a malignant melanoma. Trans Am Acad Ophthalmol Otolaryngol 1958; 62(3):441–3.
190. Makley TA Jr. Management of melanomas of the anterior segment. Surv Ophthalmol 1974; 19(3):135–53.
191. Manschot WA. Retinal hole in a case of choroidal melanoma. Arch Ophthalmol 1965; 73:666–8.
192. Margo CE, Hidayat AA, Polack H. Ciliary body granuloma. Simulating malignant melanoma after herpes zoster ophthalmicus. Cornea 1982; 1:147–53.
193. Margo CE, McLean IW. Malignant melanoma of the choroid and ciliary body in black patients. Arch Ophthalmol 1984; 102(1):77–9.
194. Margo CE, Pautler SE. Granulomatous uveitis after treatment of a choroidal melanoma with proton-beam irradiation. Retina 1990; 10(2):140–3.
195. Margo CE, Pavan PR, Gendelman D, Gragoudas E. Bilateral melanocytic uveal tumors associated with systemic non-ocular malignancy. Malignant melanomas or benign paraneoplastic syndrome? Retina 1987; 7(3):137–41.
196. Mark GJ, Mihm MC, Liteplo MG, et al. Congenital melanocytic nevi of the small and garment type. Clinical, histologic, and ultrastructural studies. Hum Pathol 1973; 4(3):395–418.
197. Matas BR. Unusual course of a ciliary body melanoma. Am J Ophthalmol 1971; 72(3):592–4.
198. McCurdy J, Gamel J, McLean I. A simple, efficient, and reproducible method for estimating the malignant potential of uveal melanoma from routine H & E slides. Pathol Res Pract 1991; 187(8):1025–7.
199. McGraw Jl. Malignant melanoma associated with retinal hole. AMA Arch Ophthalmol 1951; 46(6):666–7.
200. McLean IW, Foster WD, Zimmerman LE, Gamel JW. Modifications of Callender's classification of uveal melanoma at the Armed Forces Institute of Pathology. Am J Ophthalmol 1983; 96(4):502–9.
201. McLean IW, Foster WD, Zimmerman LE. Uveal melanoma: location, size, cell type, and enucleation as risk factors in metastasis. Hum Pathol 1982; 13(2): 123–32.
202. McLean IW, Keefe KS, Burnier MN. Uveal melanoma. Comparison of the prognostic value of fibrovascular loops, mean of the ten largest nucleoli, cell type, and tumor size. Ophthalmology 1997; 104(5):777–80.
203. McLean IW, Zimmerman LE, Evans RM. Reappraisal of Callender's spindle a type of malignant melanoma of choroid and ciliary body. Am J Ophthalmol 1978; 86(4): 557–64.
204. McLean MJ, Foster WD, Zimmerman LE. Prognostic factors in small malignant melanomas of choroid and ciliary body. Arch Ophthalmol 1977; 95(1):48–58.
205. Meecham WJ, Char DH. DNA content abnormalities and prognosis in uveal melanoma. Arch Ophthalmol 1986; 104(11):1626–9.
206. Merbs SL, Sidransky D. Analysis of p16 (CDKN2/MTS-1/INK4A) alterations in primary sporadic uveal melanoma. Invest Ophthalmol Vis Sci 1999; 40(3):779–83.
207. Meyer D, Ge J, Blinder KJ, et al. Malignant transformation of an optic disk melanocytoma. Am J Ophthalmol 1999; 127(6):710–4.
208. Meyer-Schwickerath G. The preservation of vision by treatment of intraocular tumors with light coagulation. Arch Ophthalmol 1961; 66:458–66.
209. Michelson JB, Shields JA. Relationship of iris nevi to malignant melanoma of the uvea. Am J Ophthalmol 1977; 83(5):694–6.
210. Mims JL III, Shields JA. Follow-up studies of suspicious choroidal nevi. Ophthalmology 1978; 85(9):929–43.
211. Missotten GS, Keijser S, De Keizer RJ, De Wolff-Rouendaal D. Conjunctival melanoma in the Netherlands: a nationwide study. Invest Ophthalmol Vis Sci 2005; 46(1):75–82.

212. Mooy CM, de Jong PT, Van der Kwast TH, et al. Ki-67 immunostaining in uveal melanoma. The effect of pre-enucleation radiotherapy. Ophthalmology 1990; 97(10): 1275–80.
213. Mooy CM, Luyten GP, de Jong PT, et al. Immunohistochemical and prognostic analysis of apoptosis and proliferation in uveal melanoma. Am J Pathol 1995; 147(4):1097–104.
214. Mueller AJ, Freeman WR, Schaller UC, et al. Complex microcirculation patterns detected by confocal indocyanine green angiography predict time to growth of small choroidal melanocytic tumors: MuSIC Report II. Ophthalmology 2002; 109(12):2207–14.
215. Myatt N, Aristodemou P, Neale MH, et al. Abnormalities of the transforming growth factor-beta pathway in ocular melanoma. J Pathol 2000; 192(4):511–8.
216. Nadbath RP, Bullwinkel HG. Coexistence of intraocular melanoma and lymphatic leukemia. AMA Arch Ophthalmol 1952; 48(3):349–51.
217. Naumann G, Yanoff M, Zimmerman LE. Histogenesis of malignant melanomas of the uvea. I. Histopathologic characteristics of nevi of the choroid and ciliary body. Arch Ophthalmol 1966; 76(6):784–96.
218. Naumann GOH, Hellner K, Naumann LR. Pigmented nevi of the choroid. Clinical study of secondary changes in the overlying tissues. Trans Am Acad Ophthalmol Otolaryngol 1971; 75:110–23.
219. Naus NC, van Drunen E, de Klein A, et al. Characterization of complex chromosomal abnormalities in uveal melanoma by fluorescence in situ hybridization, spectral karyotyping, and comparative genomic hybridization. Genes Chromosomes Cancer 2001; 30(3): 267–73.
220. Newton FH. Malignant melanoma of choroid. Report of a case with clinical history of 36 years and follow up of 32 years. Arch Ophthalmol 1965; 73:198–9.
221. Nordlund JR, Robertson DM, Herman DC. Ultrasound biomicroscopy in management of malignant iris melanoma. Arch Ophthalmol 2003; 121(5):725–7.
222. Onken MD, Worley LA, Ehlers JP, Harbour JW. Gene expression profiling in uveal melanoma reveals two molecular classes and predicts metastatic death. Cancer Res 2004; 64(20):7205–9.
223. Pach JM, Robertson DM, Taney BS, et al. Prognostic factors in choroidal and ciliary body melanomas with extrascleral extension. Am J Ophthalmol 1986; 101(3):325–31.
224. Paridaens AD, Minassian DC, McCartney AC, Hungerford JL. Prognostic factors in primary malignant melanoma of the conjunctiva: a clinicopathological study of 256 cases. Br J Ophthalmol 1994; 78(4):252–9.
225. Parrella P, Caballero OL, Sidransky D, Merbs SL. Detection of c-myc amplification in uveal melanoma by fluorescent in situ hybridization. Invest Ophthalmol Vis Sci 2001; 42(8):1679–84.
226. Patel BC, Egan CA, Lucius RW, et al. Cutaneous malignant melanoma and oculodermal melanocytosis (nevus of Ota): report of a case and review of the literature. J Am Acad Dermatol 1998; 38(5):862–5.
227. Paul EV, Pamell BL, Fraker M. Prognosis of malignant melanomas of the choroid and ciliary body. Int Ophthalmol Clin 1962; 2:387–402.
228. Pe'er J, Rummelt V, Mawn L, et al. Mean of the ten largest nucleoli, microcirculation architecture, and prognosis of ciliochoroidal melanomas. Ophthalmology 1994; 101(7): 1227–35.
229. Perry HD, Zimerman LE, Benson WE. Hemorrhage from isolated aneurysm of a retinal artery: report of two cases simulating malignant melanoma. Arch Ophthalmol 1977; 95(2):281–3.
230. Pomeranz GA, Bunt AH, Kalina RE. Multifocal choroidal melanoma in ocular melanocytosis. Arch Ophthalmol 1981; 99(5):857–63.
231. Prescher G, Bornfeld N, Friedrichs W, et al. Cytogenetics of twelve cases of uveal melanoma and patterns of nonrandom anomalies and isochromosome formation. Cancer Genet Cytogenet 1995; 80(1):40–6.
232. Prescher G, Bornfeld N, Hirche H, et al. Prognostic implications of monosomy 3 in uveal melanoma. Lancet 1996; 347(9010):1222–5.
233. Prives C, Hall PA. The p53 pathway. J Pathol 1999; 187(1): 112–26.
234. Pro M, Shields JA, Tomer TL. Serous detachment of the macular associated with presumed choroidal nevi. Arch Ophthalmol 1978; 96(8):1374–7.
235. Reese AB, Archila EA, Jones IS, Cooper WC. Necrosis of malignant melanoma of the choroid. Am J Ophthalmol 1970; 69(1):91–104.
236. Reese AB, Cleasby GW. The treatment of iris melanoma. Am J Ophthalmol 1959; 47(5):118–25.
237. Reese AB, Howard GM. Flat uveal melanomas. Am J Ophthalmol 1967; 64(6):1021–8.
238. Reese AB, Mund ML, Iwamoto T. Tapioca melanoma of the iris. 1. Clinical and light microscopy studies. Am J Ophthalmol 1972; 74(5):840–50.
239. Reese AB. Hematomas under the retinal pigment epithelium. Trans Am Ophthalmol Soc 1961; 59:43–79.
240. Reese AB. Melanosis oculi: a case with microscopic findings. Am J Ophthalmol 1925; 8:865–70.
241. Reese AB. Pigment freckles of the iris (benign melanomas): their significance in relation to malignant melanoma of the uvea. Am J Ophthalmol 1944; 27:217–26.
242. Reese AB. Spontaneous cysts of the ciliary body simulating neoplasms. Am J Ophthalmol 1950; 33(11):1738–46.
243. Reese AB. The association of uveal nevi with skin nevi. Trans Am Ophthalmol Soc 1951; 49:47–57.
244. Reese AB. The differential diagnosis of malignant melanoma of the choroid. AMA Arch Ophthalmol 1957; 58(4):477–82.
245. Reese AB. Tumors of the Eye. 3rd ed. New York: Harper & Row, 1976.
246. Reese AB. Tumors of the Eye. New York: Harper & Row, 1976, 174–262.
247. Reiniger IW, Schaller UC, Haritoglou C, et al. "Melanoma inhibitory activity" (MIA): a promising serological tumour marker in metastatic uveal melanoma. Graefes Arch Clin Exp Ophthalmol 2005.
248. Rhodes AR. Congenital nevomelanocytic nevi. Histologic patterns in the first year of life and evolution during childhood. Arch Dermatol 1986; 122(11):1257–62.
249. Rones B, Linger HT. Early malignant melanoma of the choroid. Am J Ophthalmol 1954; 38(2):163–70.
250. Rones B, Zimmerman LE. An unusual choroidal hemorrhage simulating malignant melanoma. Arch Ophthalmol 1963; 70:30–2.
251. Rones B, Zimmerman LE. The production of heterochromia and glaucoma by diffuse malignant melanoma of the iris. Trans Am Acad Ophthalmol Otolaryngol 1957; 61(4): 447–63.
252. Rones B, Zimmerman LE. The prognosis of primary tumors of the iris treated by iridectomy. Arch Ophthalmol 1958; 60:193–205.
253. Rosenbaum PS, Boniuk M, Font RL. Diffuse uveal melanoma in a 5-year-old child. Am J Ophthalmol 1988; 106(5):601–6.

254. Roth AM. Malignant change in melanocytomas of the uveal tract. Surv Ophthalmol 1978; 22(6):404–12.
255. Royds JA, Sharrard RM, Parsons MA, et al. C-myc oncogene expression in ocular melanomas. Graefes Arch Clin Exp Ophthalmol 1992; 230(4):366–71.
256. Ryan SJ, Zimmerman LE, King FM. Reactive lymphoid hyperplasia. An unusual form of intraocular pseudotumor. Trans Am Acad Ophthalmol Otolaryngol 1972; 76(3): 652–71.
257. Sabates FN, Yamashita T. Congenital melanosis oculi complicated by two independent malignant melanomas of the choroid. Arch Ophthalmol 1967; 77(6):801–3.
258. Samuels SL, Payne BF. Malignant melanoma of the iris. Mode of extension and dissemination. Am J Ophthalmol 1963; 55:629–31.
259. Sandinha MT, Farquharson MA, McKay IC, Roberts F. Monosomy 3 predicts death but not time until death in choroidal melanoma. Invest Ophthalmol Vis Sci 2005; 46(10):3497–501.
260. Scheie HG, Yanoff M. Iris nevus (Cogan-Reese) syndrome. A cause of unilateral glaucoma. Arch Ophthalmol 1975; 93(10):963–70.
261. Scheie HG, Yanoff M. Pseudomelanoma of the ciliary body. Report of a patient. Arch Ophthalmol 1967; 77(1): 81–3.
262. Schultz AB, Hunter S, Grossniklaus HE. Primary melanocytic tumor of the orbit and central nervous system. Ophthalmol Clin North Am 1996; 9(4):705–20.
263. Schwartz LK, O'Connor GR. Secondary syphilis with iris papules. Am J Ophthalmol 1980; 90(3):380–4.
264. Scott RJ, Vajdic CM, Armstrong BK, et al. BRCA2 mutations in a population-based series of patients with ocular melanoma. Int J Cancer 2002; 102(2):188–91.
265. Scruggs JH. Malignant melanoma of the uvea. Am J Ophthalmol 1960; 49:594–605.
266. Seddon JM, Albert DM, Lavin PT, Robinson N. A prognostic factor study of disease-free interval and survival following enucleation for uveal melanoma. Arch Ophthalmol 1983; 101(12):1894–9.
267. Seddon JM, Gragoudas ES, Glynn RJ, et al. Host factors, UV radiation, and risk of uveal melanoma. A case-control study. Arch Ophthalmol 1990; 108(9):1274–80.
268. Seregard S, Kock E. Conjunctival malignant melanoma in Sweden 1969–91 Acta Ophthalmol (Copenh) 1992; 70(3): 289–96.
269. Seregard S, Oskarsson M, Spangberg B. PC-10 as a predictor of prognosis after antigen retrieval in posterior uveal melanoma. Invest Ophthalmol Vis Sci 1996; 37(7): 1451–8.
270. Seregard S. Conjunctival melanoma. Surv Ophthalmol 1998; 42(4):321–50.
271. Shammas HF, Blodi FC. Orbital extension of Choroidal and ciliary body melanomas. Arch Ophthalmol 1977; 95 (11):2002–5.
272. Shammas HF, Blodi FC. Peripapillary choroidal melanomas. Extension along the optic nerve and its sheaths. Arch Ophthalmol 1978; 96(3):440–5.
273. Shammas HF, Watzke RC. Bilateral choroidal melanomas. Case report and incidence. Arch Ophthalmol 1977; 95(4): 617–23.
274. Sharara NA, Alexander RA, Luthert PJ, et al. Differential immunoreactivity of melanocytic lesions of the conjunctiva. Histopathology 2001; 39(4):426–31.
275. Shaw H. Melanoma of ciliary body. Am J Ophthalmol 1954; 38:104–5.
276. Shields CL, Fasiudden A, Mashayekhi A, Shields JA. Conjunctival nevi: clinical features and natural course in 410 consecutive patients. Arch Ophthalmol 2004; 122(2): 167–75.
277. Shields CL, Shields JA, De Potter P, et al. Diffuse choroidal melanoma. Clinical features predictive of metastasis. Arch Ophthalmol 1996; 114(8):956–63.
278. Shields CL, Shields JA, Gunduz K, et al. Conjunctival melanoma: risk factors for recurrence, exenteration, metastasis, and death in 150 consecutive patients. Arch Ophthalmol 2000; 118(11):1497–507.
279. Shields CL, Shields JA, Karlsson U, et al. Enucleation after plaque radiotherapy for posterior uveal melanoma. Histopathologic findings. Ophthalmology 1990; 97(12): 1665–70.
280. Shields CL, Shields JA, Materin M, et al. Iris melanoma: risk factors for metastasis in 169 consecutive patients. Ophthalmology 2001; 108(1):172–8.
281. Shields JA, Annesley WH Jr, Spaeth GL. Necrotic melanocytoma of iris with secondary glaucoma. Am J Ophthalmol 1977; 84(6):826–9.
282. Shields JA, Augsburger JJ, Gonder JR, MacLeod D. Localized benign lymphoid tumor of the iris. Arch Ophthalmol 1981; 99(12):2147–8.
283. Shields JA, Augsburger JJ. Cataract surgery and intraocular lenses in patients with unsuspected malignant melanoma of the ciliary body and choroid. Ophthalmology 1985; 92(6):823–6.
284. Shields JA, Bakewell B, Augsburger JJ, Flanagan JC. Classification and incidence of space-occupying lesions of the orbit. A survey of 645 biopsies. Arch Ophthalmol 1984; 102(11):1606–11.
285. Shields JA, Demirci H, Mashayekhi A, Shields CL. Melanocytoma of optic disc in 115 cases: the 2004 Samuel Johnson Memorial Lecture, part 1. Ophthalmology 2004; 111(9):1739–46.
286. Shields JA, Font RL. Melanocytoma of the choroid clinically simulating a malignant melanoma. Arch Ophthalmol 1972; 87(4):396–400.
287. Shields JA, Sanborn GE, Augsburger JJ. The differential diagnosis of malignant melanoma of the iris. A clinical study of 200 patients. Ophthalmology 1983; 90(6):716–20.
288. Shields JA, Shields CL, Scartozzi R. Survey of 1264 patients with orbital tumors and simulating lesions: the 2002 Montgomery Lecture, part 1. Ophthalmology 2004; 111(5):997–1008.
289. Shields JA, Shields CL. Orbital malignant melanoma: the 2002 Sean B Murphy lecture. Ophthal Plast Reconstr Surg 2003; 19(4):262–9.
290. Shields JA. Diagnosis and Management of Intraocular Tumors. St. Louis, MO: Mosby, 1983.
291. Shields JA. Lesions simulating malignant melanoma of the posterior uvea. Arch Ophthalmol 1973; 89(6):466–71.
292. Shields JA. Melanocytoma of the optic nerve head: a review. Int Ophthalmol 1978; 1(1):31–7.
293. Shields MB, Klintworth GK. Anterior uveal melanomas and intraocular pressure. Ophthalmology 1980; 87(6):503–17.
294. Singh AD, Bergman L, Seregard S. Uveal melanoma: epidemiologic aspects. Ophthalmol Clin North Am 2005; 18(1):75–84, viii.
295. Singh AD, Boghosian-Sell L, Wary KK, et al. Cytogenetic findings in primary uveal melanoma. Cancer Genet Cytogenet 1994; 72(2):109–15.
296. Singh AD, De Potter P, Fijal BA, et al. Lifetime prevalence of uveal melanoma in white patients with oculo(dermal) melanocytosis. Ophthalmology 1998; 105(1):195–8.
297. Singh AD, Kalyani P, Topham A. Estimating the risk of malignant transformation of a choroidal nevus. Ophthalmology 2005; 112(10):1784–9.

298. Singh AD, Rennie IG, Kivela T, et al. The Zimmerman–McLean–Foster hypothesis: 25 years later. Br J Ophthalmol 2004; 88(7):962–7.
299. Singh AD, Shields CL, De Potter P, et al. Familial uveal melanoma. Clinical observations on 56 patients. Arch Ophthalmol 1996; 114(4):392–9.
300. Singh AD, Shields CL, Shields JA, De Potter P. Bilateral primary uveal melanoma. Bad luck or bad genes? Ophthalmology 1996; 103(2):256–62.
301. Singh AD, Topham A. Incidence of uveal melanoma in the United States: 1973–1997. Ophthalmology 2003; 110(5):956–61.
302. Singh AD, Topham A. Survival rates with uveal melanoma in the United States: 1973–1997. Ophthalmology 2003; 110(5):962–5.
303. Sisley K, Rennie IG, Parsons MA, et al. Abnormalities of chromosomes 3 and 8 in posterior uveal melanoma correlate with prognosis. Genes Chromosomes Cancer 1997; 19(1):22–8.
304. Smith LT, Irvine AR. Diagnostic significance of orange pigment accumulation over choroidal tumors. Am J Ophthalmol 1973; 76(2):212–6.
305. Smith ME, Sanders TE, Bresnick GH. Juvenile xanthogranuloma of the ciliary body in an adult. Arch Ophthalmol 1969; 81(6):813–4.
306. Smith TR, Brockhurst RJ. Cellular blue nevus of the sclera. Arch Ophthalmol 1976; 94(4):618–20.
307. Smolin G. Malignant change of a benign melanoma. Report of a case. Am J Ophthalmol 1966; 61(1):174–7.
308. Snip RC, Green WR, Jaegers KR. Choroidal nevus with subretinal pigment epithelial neovascular membrane and a positive P-32 test. Ophthalmic Surg 1978; 9(5): 35–42.
309. Spaulding AG, Green WR, Font RL. Ring-shaped limbal tumor. Secondary to unrecognized diffuse malignant melanoma of the uvea. Arch Ophthalmol 1967; 77(1): 76–80.
310. Spencer WH. Optic nerve extension of intraocular neoplasms. Am J Ophthalmol 1975; 80(3 Pt 1):465–71.
311. Streeten BW. The sudanophilic granules of the human retinal pigment epithelium. Arch Ophthalmol 1961; 66: 391–8.
312. Sunba MS, Rahi AH, Morgan G. Tumors of the anterior uvea. I. Metastasizing malignant melanoma of the iris. Arch Ophthalmol 1980; 98(1):82–5.
313. Takahashi K, Hattori H, Ieb Q, et al. Statistical observation on ocular tumors (Japanese). Rinsho Ganka 1969; 23: 295–300.
314. Tay W. Primary cancer of the iris. R Lond Ophthalmol Hosp Rep 1866; 5:230.
315. Teekhasaenee C, Ritch R, Rutnin U, Leelawongs N. Ocular findings in oculodermal melanocytosis. Arch Ophthalmol 1990; 108(8):1114–20.
316. Tellada M, Specht CS, McLean IW, et al. Primary orbital melanomas. Ophthalmology 1996; 103(6):929–32.
317. Templeton AC. Tumors of the eye and adnexa in Africans of Uganda. Cancer 1967; 20:1689–98.
318. Thomas CI, Purnell EW. Ocular melanocytoma. Am J Ophthalmol 1969; 67(1):79–86.
319. Thorn M, Adami HO, Ringborg U, et al. The association between anatomic site and survival in malignant melanoma. An analysis of 12,353 cases from the Swedish Cancer Registry. Eur J Cancer Clin Oncol 1989; 25(3): 483–91.
320. Tredici TJ, Fenton RH. Hematoma beneath the retinal pigment epithelium. Report of a case mistaken clinically for a malignant melanoma of the choroid. Arch Ophthalmol 1964; 72:796–9.
321. Tsukahara S, Wakui K, Ohzeki S. Simultaneous bilateral primary diffuse malignant uveal melanoma: case report with pathological examination. Br J Ophthalmol 1986; 70(1):33–8.
322. Tuomaala S, Eskelin S, Tarkkanen A, Kivela T. Population-based assessment of clinical characteristics predicting outcome of conjunctival melanoma in whites. Invest Ophthalmol Vis Sci 2002; 43(11):3399–408.
323. Tuomaala S, Kivela T. Metastatic pattern and survival in disseminated conjunctival melanoma: implications for sentinel lymph node biopsy. Ophthalmology 2004; 111(4): 816–21.
324. Vaisanen A, Kallioinen M, von Dickhoff K, et al. Matrix metalloproteinase-2 (MMP-2) immunoreactive protein—a new prognostic marker in uveal melanoma? J Pathol 1999; 188(1):56–62.
325. van der Velden PA, Metzelaar-Blok JA, Bergman W, et al. Promoter hypermethylation: a common cause of reduced p16(INK4a) expression in uveal melanoma. Cancer Res 2001; 61(13):5303–6.
326. Vaziri M, Buffam FV, Martinka M, et al. Clinicopathologic features and behavior of cutaneous eyelid melanoma. Ophthalmology 2002; 109(5):901–8.
327. Vink J, Crijns MB, Mooy CM, et al. Ocular melanoma in families with dysplastic nevus syndrome. J Am Acad Dermatol 1990; 23(5):858–62.
328. Vogel MH, Zimmerman LE, Gass JD. Proliferation of the juxtapapillary retinal pigment epithelium simulating malignant melanoma. Doc Ophthalmol 1969; 26:461–81.
329. Weedon D. Lentigines, nevi, and melanomas. In: Skin Pathology. 2nd ed. New York: Churchill Livingstone, 2002.
330. Werschnik C, Lommatzsch PK. Long-term follow-up of patients with conjunctival melanoma. Am J Clin Oncol 2002; 25(3):248–55.
331. Weyers W, Euler M, Diaz-Cascajo C, et al. Classification of cutaneous malignant melanoma: a reassessment of histopathologic criteria for the distinction of different types. Cancer 1999; 86(2):288–99.
332. White VA, Chambers JD, Courtright PD, et al. Correlation of cytogenetic abnormalities with the outcome of patients with uveal melanoma. Cancer 1998; 83(2):354–9.
333. Wilder HC. Relationship of pigment cell clusters in the iris to malignant melanoma of the uveal tract. In: The Biology of Melanomas, Vol. 4. New York: New York Academy of Sciences, 1948.
334. Yanoff M, Scheie HG. Melanomalytic glaucoma. Report of a case. Arch Ophthalmol 1970; 84(4):471–3.
335. Yanoff M, Zimmerman LE. Histogenesis of malignant melanomas of the uvea. 3. The relationship of congenital ocular melanocytosis and neurofibromatosis in uveal melanomas. Arch Ophthalmol 1967; 77(3):331–6.
336. Yanoff M, Zimmerman LE. Histogenesis of malignant melanomas of the uvea. II. Relationship of uveal nevi to malignant melanomas. Cancer 1967; 20(4):493–507.
337. Yanoff M, Zimmerman LE. Pseudomelanoma of anterior chamber caused by implantation of iris pigment epithelium. Arch Ophthalmol 1965; 74:302–5.
338. Yanoff M. Glaucoma mechanisms in ocular malignant melanomas. Am J Ophthalmol 1970; 70(6):898–904.
339. Yu GP, Hu DN, McCormick S, Finger PT. Conjunctival melanoma: is it increasing in the United States? Am J Ophthalmol 2003; 135(6):800–6.
340. Zimmerman LE, McLean IW, Foster WD. Does enucleation of the eye containing a malignant melanoma prevent

or accelerate the dissemination of tumour cells. Br J Ophthalmol 1978; 62(6):420–5.

341. Zimmerman LE, McLean IW. Montgomery Lecture, 1975. Changing concepts of the prognosis and management of small malignant melanomas of the choroid. Trans Ophthalmol Soc UK 1975; 95(4):487–94.

342. Zimmerman LE. Malignant melanoma of the uveal tract. In Spencer WH, ed. Ophthalmic Pathology: An Atlas and Textbook. Philadelphia: W. B. Saunders, 1986.

343. Zimmerman LE. Melanocytes, melanocytic nevi, and melanocytomas. Invest Ophthalmol 1965; 34:11–41.

60

Retinoblastoma

David M. Gamm, Amol D. Kulkarni, and Daniel M. Albert
Department of Ophthalmology and Visual Sciences, University of Wisconsin, Madison, Wisconsin, U.S.A.

INTRODUCTION

Retinoblastoma is the most common and important malignant eye tumor of childhood, and after malignant melanoma it is the most common primary intraocular malignancy of the eye. This tumor was established as an entity by the Scotsman James Wardrop (1782–1869) in his *Observations on the Fungus Haematodes*. Wardrop appreciated that the tumor originated in the retina, and he was the first to advocate early enucleation in its treatment (12). The tumor, although accounting for only approximately 1% of deaths from cancer under 15 years of age (85), has attracted wide interest from a variety of disciplines, including epidemiology, genetics, and molecular biology. The seminal observation that retinoblastoma arises in susceptible developing retinal cells when both alleles of the retinoblastoma gene (*RB1*) are mutated, and the isolation and cloning of *RB1* gene (56,115,124), have established this tumor as a model of oncogenesis. The literature on the tumor and the causative gene has grown dramatically. These advances have been accompanied by a more complete understanding of the histogenesis, growth, and differentiation of the tumor (219), as well as a more complete elucidation of its molecular genetics (21). Improvement in the treatment of retinoblastoma has led to reports of 5-year survival rates of 90% and 98% in Europe and the United States, respectively (255,300).

EPIDEMIOLOGY

Incidence

An accurate determination of the incidence of retinoblastoma is difficult to achieve. Even in the United States and Western Europe, differences in methods of study, sample size, and stage of diagnosis result in variations in reported data (85,156). Nevertheless, useful estimates have been derived from population-based studies. Since 1970, the incidence is estimated at 11 cases per 1 million children under 5 years of age or 1 case per 18,000 live births (85) and 3.58 cases per

1 million children under the age of 15 (13,85,261). Recent data from the Surveillance, Epidemiology, and End Results (SEER) Study from 1974 to 1984 has established an average incidence of 10.9 per 1 million for children under 5 years of age and 5.8 per 1 million children younger than 10 years (336). These findings are consistent with more recent reports as well (130,165). A British study (1969–1980) provides a registration rate of 1 per 23,000 births (297). Other studies from Australia, Sweden, New Zealand, the Netherlands, Saudi Arabia, Oman, Singapore, and Namibia report similar rates (11,145,166,188,235,256, 302,331,367).

An increased incidence of retinoblastoma in Finland and Holland between 1915 and 1965 has been reported (29,137,303,341). It seems likely that improvements in methods of diagnosis may account for this apparent increase (392). Schipper, after a thorough analysis of the Dutch registry, demonstrated stabilization at around 1 per 15,560 births since 1950 (304). Seregard et al. (309) reviewed data from Swedish and Finnish cancer registries and corresponding national referral centers for retinoblastoma. The pooled incidence by birth cohort was 6.0 per 100,000 live births and corresponded to 1 in 16,642 live births. From these, the authors concluded that the incidence of retinoblastoma is stable in Northern Europe.

Age at Diagnosis, Sex, Race, and Laterality and Tumor Numbers

The mean age at diagnosis and the median age at diagnosis are both approximately 18 months (22,23). Many reports (8,179) have found that the mean age at diagnosis for the hereditary type, which is characteristically bilateral, is earlier (between 12 and 14 months of age), than for the sporadic (usually unilateral) variety. In the latter, the diagnosis is made at about 24 to 30 months of age (179,186). Retinoblastoma is occasionally detected at birth, in premature babies, or even as an intrauterine disorder (267,295). In a study by Plotsky et al. (267) of 220 cases, 95% were diagnosed before 5 years of age and 40% before 1 year. On the other end of the spectrum, retinoblastoma is occasionally diagnosed after the age of 10 years and rarely after 20 years (226,333). Many retinoblastomas first diagnosed in juveniles or adults are thought to arise from retinocytomas (spontaneously arrested retinoblastomas) that have transformed to viable retinoblastomas (22). The SEER study (336) as well as earlier studies (2) shows worsening survival with increasing age at diagnosis. However, beyond 2 years of age, this relationship becomes less clear (2,3).

In almost all studies, retinoblastoma affects males and females approximately equally. Retinoblastoma is seen in all ethnic and racial groups, with a similar cumulative lifetime incidence (235). In lower socioeconomic groups, particularly in developing countries, the diagnosis tends to be made when the disease is more advanced and at a higher median age (22).

Most large series find approximately 70% of cases to be unilateral and 30% bilateral. Individuals with unilateral disease usually have a single discrete tumor, whereas individuals with bilateral disease more frequently have multifocal involvement in either one or both eyes.

GENETICS AND MOLECULAR BIOLOGY

Despite its infrequency, retinoblastoma has played a leading role in our understanding of tumor-suppressor genes and the molecular pathways involved in cell cycle control and oncogenesis.

Historical Background

Familial transmission of a retinoblastoma from an enucleated survivor to an offspring was apparently first reported in 1886 by DeGouveia (13). Despite a few reports of families with tumors in sibships, it was not until the beginning of the 20th century that the role of heredity was really appreciated, when survivors and their offspring became more numerous (13).

Between 60% and 70% of retinoblastomas cases appear sporadically and are not transmitted to offspring, and 30% to 40% of cases (13,114,123,207,274,392) appear clinically to be transmitted as an autosomal-dominant trait with 80% to 90% penetrance (hereditary retinoblastomas) (13,108,123,250,274). Sporadic cases develop unilateral and unifocal tumors at a later age than the inherited retinoblastomas. Hereditary retinoblastomas appear in about 85% of cases as familial, bilateral, or unilateral multifocal lesions (13,299,361).

Knudson Hypothesis

The original theory of retinoblastoma as an inherited, irregular autosomal-dominant trait was widely recognized as unsatisfactory until Knudson proposed an alternative model in 1971 (181). From an epidemiological and statistical study of the ages at diagnosis and the laterality of tumors, Knudson and colleagues derived a "two-hit" model involving a double mutational event (178–185). Patients with nonhereditary retinoblastoma develop two mutations in the same postzygotic somatic cell, giving rise to a single unilateral tumor. Since both mutations have to occur de novo in the same cell independently, the likelihood of multifocal tumors in nonhereditary retinoblastoma is essentially nonexistent and tumors take longer to appear.

In contrast, in hereditary retinoblastoma the first mutation occurs in germinal cells either as a result of inheritance of a predisposing mutation from a carrier parent (accounting for one-third of cases, according to Vogel) (359) or through a new germ-line mutation which, although not present in either parent, can be transmitted to the affected person's offspring (247). The second mutation occurs in a postzygotic retinal cell (or cells). Consequently, every retinal cell contains the first mutation. Should the second mutational event occur, which is likely among the many developing retinal cells, tumors will appear. Comings, suggesting a general model of oncogenesis, proposed that inactivation of the two alleles of a single regulatory locus could release the cell from normal growth control (71).

Chromosomal Studies

The well-recognized hereditary nature of retinoblastoma, together with the occasional occurrence of congenital malformations in some of these patients (79,229,335), stimulated a search for causative chromosomal abnormalities (114,299). In 1962, Stallard investigated a female infant with retinoblastoma and noted the presence of a deletion in the D group of chromosomes (13,155). Subsequently, similar findings were reported, and improvement in cytogenetic techniques in the 1970s allowed assignment of the chromosome abnormality to chromosome 13 (150). Retinoblastoma later came to be included within the 13q– syndromes (184,243,365), and Yunis and Ramsay and others specifically observed that all deletions in the long arm of chromosome 13 in patients with retinoblastomas involved the 13q14 band (150,389). Moreover, if the 13q14 was not deleted, retinoblastoma was not encountered; consequently, this became the possible locus for the candidate gene (183,389). In 1980, Sparkes and colleagues demonstrated that the polymorphic marker enzyme esterase D locus also maps to chromosome band 13q14 (76,325). In patients with no cytogenetic abnormality of 13q14, esterase D levels were normal but, in all patients with retinoblastoma and 13q14 deletion, low esterase D levels were found. Despite the finding of such a 13q14 deletion in only 5% of patients with retinoblastoma, these data directed attention to this locus as the site of the "retinoblastoma gene" (58,96,241,325,327).

Molecular Genetics: Identifying the *RB1 Gene*

By comparing constitutional and tumor genotypes through the use of restriction fragment-length polymorphisms, the Benedict (35), Cavenee (55,57), and Dryja groups (95,96,98) provided evidence that in some retinoblastomas the tumor cells had become homozygous for loci on chromosome 13. In inherited retinoblastoma, it was shown that the chromosome 13 homolog present in tumors was derived from the affected parent. Using a DNA probe (H3–8) previously assigned to the region 13q14–l, analysis of 37 retinoblastomas showed that these tumors displayed hybridization patterns consistent with homologous deletions (55,95). These data, taken together with various other studies, confirmed that loss of heterozygosity for chromosome 13 in tumors was a key factor for a recessive mechanism at the molecular level (34–36,96,98). The mutations of the RB1 locus responsible for cancer result in a loss of function, but only one copy of the normal allele is needed to prevent malignant transformation. In nonheritable retinoblastoma, both alleles of the RB1 locus are normal in the germinal cells. A mutation at both loci (equating the two hits of Knudson) is therefore necessary to induce tumorigenesis in a retinal cell. In contrast, in heritable retinoblastoma, one copy of the gene is altered in all cells. A second mutational event in a retinal cell is sufficient to produce the retinoblastoma (13,77). This event appears more commonly to be a conspicuous abnormality of chromosome 13 rather than a point mutation.

Starting from the H3–8 probe, chromosome walking techniques allowed identification of a cDNA sequence coding for a 4.7 kb mRNA representing the *RB1* transcript (115). Friend and colleagues detected this RNA transcript in adenovirus 12-immortalized retinal cells, normal human adult retina, and many tumor types, but no transcript was found in retinoblastomas or osteosarcomas (115). These investigators found partial and internal deletions of the gene in the retinoblastoma tumors. Others demonstrated structural changes within 16 of 40 retinoblastomas, but among the other tumors the RB1 transcript was absent or truncated (116,198). Methods of amplification and sequencing of the *RB1* gene allowed identification of mutations within the *RB1* gene (144,383). Shortly after identification of the RB1 transcript, the sequence of the cDNA was established. The *RB1* gene was found to have a complex organization spanning over 200 kb of DNA that includes 27 exons (44,141,198,218). The isolation of the *RB1* gene in 1986 (115), the first tumor-suppressor gene to be cloned, established retinoblastoma as a monogenetic disease and provided the basis for advances in many areas of basic and clinical sciences, including:

1. Determining the causes of *RB1* gene inactivation (53,74,139,144,196,197,199).
2. Understanding the function of the RB1 protein and its role in tumorigenesis (119,132,221,245,381, 385,390).
3. Insight into other tumor-suppressor genes (119,132,221,245,381,385).
4. Development of animal models of retinoblastoma (374).
5. Establishment of techniques for genetic diagnosis (74,75,127,247).
6. Interest in gene therapy applications (208,220,380).

The *RB1* gene product has been characterized as a 928 amino acid, 110 kDa nuclear phosphoprotein that has two other family members, p107 and p130. These latter proteins, however, are rarely mutated in human cancers (271). RB1, p107, and p130 are collectively referred to as "pocket proteins," since they share a common sequence for oncoprotein binding termed the "pocket" (390). In the resting (G0) and early G1 phases of the cell cycle, RB1 remains hypophosphorylated, allowing it to associate with and suppress the activity of several genes belonging to E2F transcription factor family (271).

With the activation of cyclin-dependent kinases during the G1 to S phase transition, RB1 becomes hyperphosphorylated and loses its ability to repress the activity of the E2F transcription factor complex. The E2Fs are then free to exert their effects through a host of E2F-responsive genes involved in cell cycle progression, DNA replication, apoptosis, and differentiation. The ability of RB1 to influence differentiation of particular cell types may explain the tissue-specific patterns of tumor formation in RB1-associated cancer (390). For example, *RB1* gene loss has been demonstrated in osteosarcomas (97,112,133), small cell lung cancer (135), bladder carcinoma, and breast cancer (337), and its loss is widely seen as a factor in the initiation of several tumor types (143). However, loss of RB1 function alone is not sufficient to precipitate tumor formation. Secondary genetic and epigenetic changes in other gene(s) (yet to be identified) are also necessary (66–68,108,151,202).

The mechanisms by which RB1 suppresses E2F-mediated gene transcription are more complicated than originally anticipated (390). In addition to binding directly to the transactivation domain of E2F and blocking its ability to interact with basic transcriptional machinery, *RB1* can promote covalent modification of chromatin by recruiting histone deacetylases to the promoters of E2F-responsive genes, contributing to their repression (46,110,205,210). Furthermore, long-term silencing of E2F-responsive genes can be brought about by *RB1* through the recruitment of histone methyltransferases (126,249,252). It is important to mention that, while the importance of the RB1:E2F interaction is well-established, at least 70 other transcription factors are also bound by *RB1*, suggesting that *RB1* can act through E2F-independent mechanisms as well (238,390). Attempts have been made to reintroduce the *RB1* gene into cultured retinoblastoma cell lines (the WERI-27 line) using a retrovirus containing the full-length cDNA (208). Such treated cells produced p105–RB1, with an associated decrease in the growth rate and reduced tumorigenicity in nude mice (208).

Although *RB1* gene therapy has clinical promise, a more immediate application of the *RB1* gene discovery is in determining whether a given retinoblastoma is heritable (49,75,85,127,371,372). This is critical, since germ-line mutations show near complete penetrance and place the patient at risk of secondary tumors (up to 30% at 40 years) (108,234). Wiggs and colleagues identified restriction fragment-length polymorphisms within the *RB1* gene and tested their usefulness in predicting the risk of retinoblastoma in families with a positive history of familial retinoblastoma (372). They were successful in 19 of 20 kindreds. The use of enzymatic amplification and DNA sequence analysis has allowed Yandell and colleagues to identify oncogenic mutations in seven retinoblastoma patients with a negative family history (383). Using this technique, they showed that four of these were sporadic cases and three others had new germ cell mutations. Techniques to detect gene mutations in patients have advanced considerably; however, DNA sequence analysis remains the most common direct approach (108). Genetic testing on individuals with bilateral or familial retinoblastoma can be performed on peripheral blood and tumor samples (7,108). The 27 known coding exons, splice boundaries, and the promoter of the *RB1* gene can be amplified by the polymerase chain reaction (PCR) and subjected to direct sequencing. This approach reveals detectable germ-line mutations (typically truncations) in almost all cases of bilateral or familial retinoblastoma (134,202). Occasionally, patients with bilateral, nonfamilial retinoblastoma will possess mutational mosaicism with no detectable oncogenic mutations in the peripheral blood. Patients with unilateral, nonfamilial retinoblastoma can undergo genetic testing on tumor samples to identify the mutations that inactivated each *RB1* allele (108). Such techniques have made possible a major improvement in genetic counseling accuracy (7,50,127).

HISTOPATHOLOGY

Historical Aspects

Wardrop's astute observations, based on dissections made without the benefit of the microscope, that retinoblastoma arose from the retina were subsequently confirmed by various pathologists of the 19th century, including Robin and Langenbeck (100). Virchow concluded that the tumor arose from the glial cells and named it a glioma of the retina (357). Flexner and later Wintersteiner described the characteristic rosettes named after them. Both suggested the use of the term "neuroepithelioma," believing that the tumor was of neuroepithelial origin, and regarded rosettes as an attempt to form photoreceptors (112,347,375). This led to the use of the term "retinoblastoma" suggested by Verhoeff, who concluded that the tumor was derived from undifferentiated embryonic retinal cells, called "retinoblasts," comparable to the neuroblasts originating from the medullary epithelium (138,353,373). Ts'o et al. in 1969 described cytologically benign cells in retinoblastoma that exhibited photoreceptor differentiation (348–350). These cells appear in small bouquet-like clusters that these authors termed "fleurettes." Ts'o and colleagues recognized that rare tumors existed that were composed entirely of cells with benign cytological features (350). In 1983, Margo et al. proposed the term "retinocytoma" for this benign counterpart of retinoblastoma (216). Gallie and coworkers (118), based on long-term clinical observations, proposed a different name, "retinoma."

Pathologic Features

Gross Examination and Growth Patterns

Several patterns of tumor growth can be appreciated on gross examination of the eye. These correlate with variations in clinical presentation and with differences in intra- and extraocular spread. The major growth patterns of retinoblastoma are *exophytic*, *endophytic*, *mixed*, and *diffuse*. Occasionally, spontaneous regression of the tumor may be observed.

Exophytic retinoblastomas grow primarily in the subretinal space, giving rise initially to a solid elevation of the retina. On ophthalmic examination, the tumor is seen through the retina, and the retinal vessels are observed to course over the tumor. With subsequent tumor growth, a total retinal detachment may occur (Fig. 1), with tumor cells spreading into the subretinal exudate and forming secondary implants on the outer retinal surface and on the retinal pigment epithelium (RPE). These implants may infiltrate through the Bruch membrane into the choroid (378) and subsequently invade blood vessels in the choroid, as well as ciliary nerves and vessels.

Endophytic retinoblastomas grow from the inner surface of the retina into the vitreous space (Fig. 2). The tumor is seen ophthalmoscopically as one or more masses on the surface of the retina. In contrast to the exophytic pattern, retinal vessels are not visible above the tumor. With further growth, the tumors become large and friable, and tumor cells may be seen as round masses floating in the vitreous or anterior chamber. It is important to distinguish retinal seeding from true multicentric retinoblastoma, since the presence of multiple primary tumors indicates a germinal mutation and the heritable form of retinoblastoma.

Mixed exophytic–endophytic retinoblastomas are probably more common than the pure endophytic or exophytic types and are often demonstrable on histopathologic examination (219). An unusual growth pattern is seen in *diffuse infiltrating retinoblastomas*, which grow diffusely within the retina without exhibiting marked thickening. Consequently, these may escape clinical recognition and likewise be overlooked on gross examination of the eye. Tumor cells, however, may spread into the vitreous and anterior chamber and simulate an inflammation. Complete spontaneous regression is a well-described phenomenon and is believed to occur more frequently in retinoblastoma than in any other malignant neoplasm (41). The significance of spontaneous regression is discussed below (see section entitled Natural History).

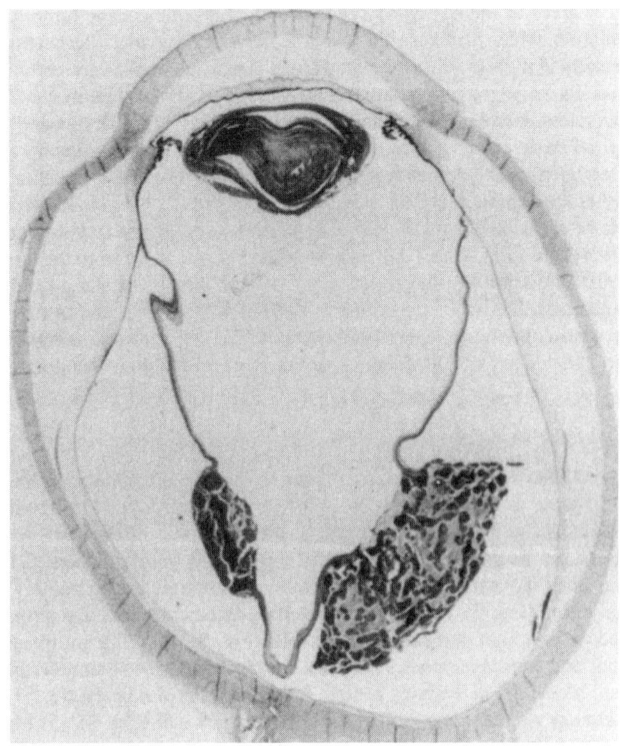

Figure 1 Exophytic pattern of growth in retinoblastoma with tumor growing beneath the retina. The retina is entirely detached (hematoxylin and eosin, ×4.8).

Histologic Features

Retinoblastomas are considered to be variably differentiated, malignant, neuroblastic tumors. Their cell of origin is disputed and is discussed below. By light microscopy, undifferentiated areas of retinoblastoma are composed of small round cells with large, variably shaped, hyperchromatic nuclei, and scanty cytoplasm (Fig. 3). Differentiated areas are present within many retinoblastomas, the most characteristic of these being the Flexner–Wintersteiner rosettes (112,375). These structures consist of clusters of cuboidal or short columnar cells arranged around a central lumen (Fig. 4). The nuclei are displaced away from the lumen, which by light microscopy appears to have a limiting membrane, resembling the external limiting membrane of the retina. Photoreceptor-like elements protrude through the membrane, and some taper into

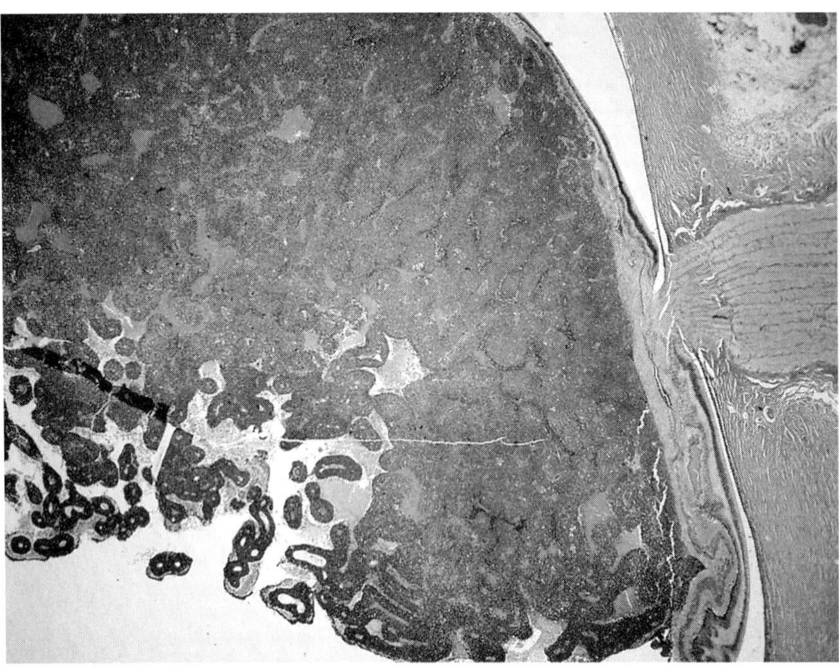

Figure 2 Endophytic retinoblastoma arising from the surface of the retina (hematoxylin and eosin, ×230).

fine filaments (347,392). The lumina of these rosettes contain hyaluronidase-resistant glycosaminoglycans (GAGs) similar to those found between normal photoreceptors and the RPE. It is similar to the material that normally surrounds photoreceptors (391). The only other neoplasms in which Flexner–Wintersteiner rosettes have been observed are pineoblastoma and medulloepithelioma; thus, these rosettes are highly characteristic of retinoblastoma. Less commonly found in retinoblastoma are rosettes of the Homer-Wright type, composed of radial arrangements of cells around a central tangle of fibrils (379). These are identical to rosettes found in neuroblastomas and medulloblastomas. Transmission electron microscopic (TEM) studies confirm that the cells composing the Flexner–Wintersteiner rosettes share many characteristics of photoreceptors. An additional differentiated structure is the fleurette, which represents a higher degree of photoreceptor differentiation (391). Fleurettes are seen by light microscopy in areas having larger cells with abundant eosinophilic cytoplasm and fewer hyperchromatic nuclei than the surrounding areas. The term "fleurette" was applied to denote the arrangement like a "fleur-de-lis" of the apparently abortive photoreceptor structures. In our experience, fleurettes can be found in approximately one-quarter of retinoblastomas if serial sectioning is undertaken. Ts'o and colleagues suggested that tumors containing such differentiated components are less radioresponsive (346). Tumors composed entirely of benign-appearing cells are now designated "retinomas" or "retinocytomas" (216). In addition to fleurettes, these tumors also contain cells resembling bipolar neurons, astrocytes, and Müller cells (216). The presence of glia is thought to represent reactive gliosis (216). Malignant transformations of retinomas and retinocytomas have been reported.

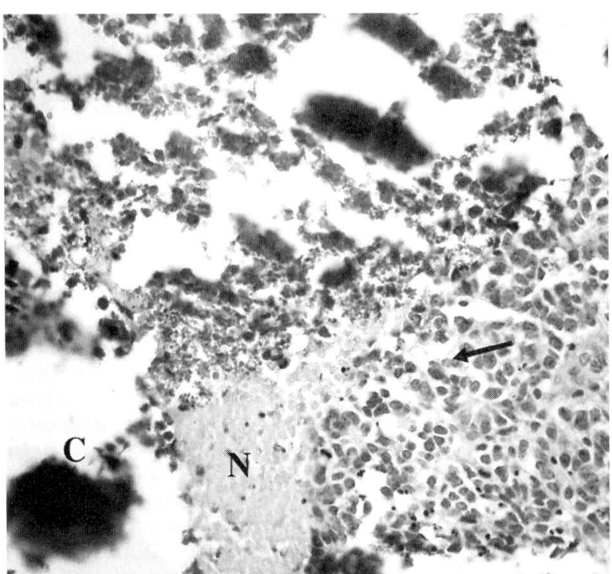

Figure 3 High-power light microscopic view of undifferentiated retinoblastoma showing small round cells (*arrow*) with large, variably shaped, hyperchromatic nuclei, and scanty cytoplasm. Note the area of necrosis (N), and focus of calcium deposition (C) (hematoxylin and eosin, ×455).

In recent years, there have been several reports of the histopathologic findings in eyes with

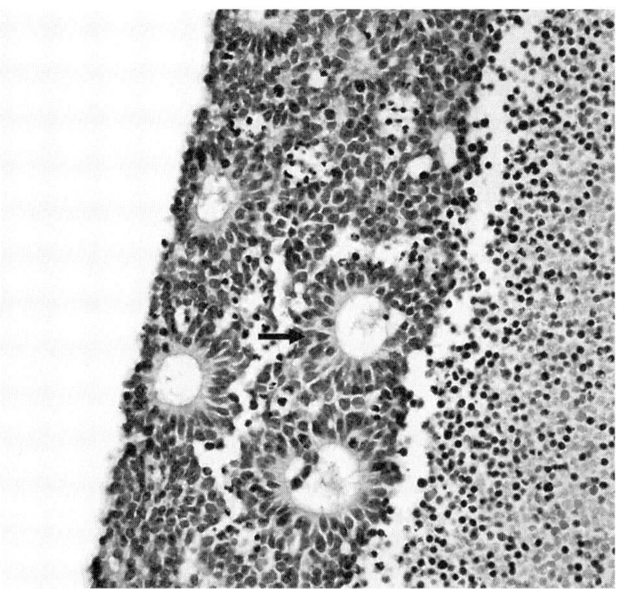

Figure 4 High-power light microscopic view of the Flexner–Wintersteiner rosette (*arrow*) in a retinoblastoma (hematoxylin and eosin, ×455).

retinoblastoma treated with chemoreduction (30,81,88). Although these reports indicate that chemoreduction has somewhat variable effects on retinoblastoma, the specific findings depend on the regression pattern observed and the presence of well-differentiated components with retinoma-like or retinocytoma-like features. In general, there is regression of the retinoblastoma with the presence of reactive gliosis, calcification (Fig. 3), and necrosis. In some eyes, although an area of posttherapeutic regression is present, foci of mitotically active, viable malignant cells are observed. Eyes with well-differentiated components show less shrinkage from chemoreduction.

Progress with regard to the histopathology of retinoblastoma with aniline dye stains was essentially complete by the last decade of the 20th century. Transmission electron microscopy (TEM) (Figs. 5–7), scanning electron microscopy (SEM) (Figs. 8 and 9), tissue culture of retinoblastoma cells, and xenograft models of these tumors have also provided valuable information regarding the nature and behavior of retinoblastoma. These earlier technologies still provide useful information in translational research aimed at developing more effective treatments for retinoblastoma patients. Findings from these earlier techniques have been well summarized (64,72,292).

IMMUNOCYTOCHEMISTRY AND CELL OF ORIGIN

Retinoblastoma cells typically express a restricted group of markers predominantly indicative of photoreceptors (308). In particular, the cone phenotype appears favored, and cone production may represent a default pathway of retinal development (38,125). However, a large number of antibodies recognizing many immuncytochemical markers have been used to identify the protein expression characteristics of retinoblastoma cells. These studies are valuable in the search for the retinoblastoma cell of origin, a pursuit that may yield insight into mechanisms of tumorigenesis and suggest novel treatment approaches for the disease (101,254). Information obtained from selected immunocytochemical markers

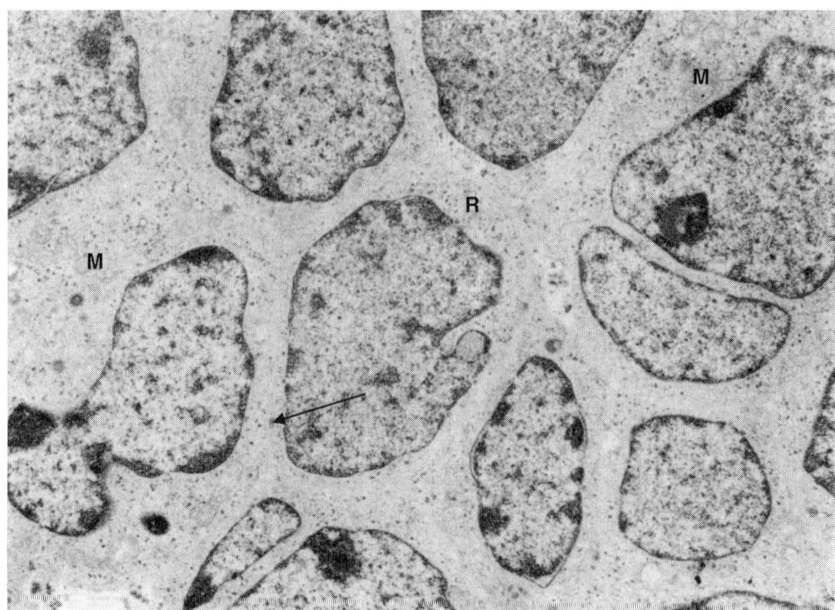

Figure 5 Undifferentiated retinoblastoma by transmission electron microscopy, showing cellular attachment (*arrow*), mitochondria (M), and aggregates of ribosomes (R) throughout the cytoplasm. Note the infoldings of some nuclear membranes (× 2,500).

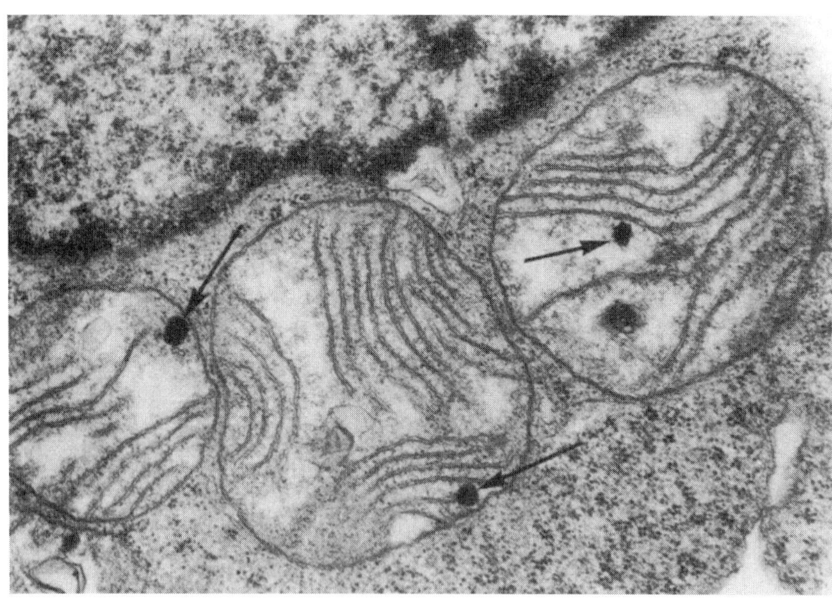

Figure 6 Giant mitochondria within a retinoblastoma cell. The dark material within the mitochondria (*arrows*) is calcium. This appears to be one of the earliest stages in the calcification of retinoblastoma cells (× 23,000).

and theories regarding the cell of origin in retinoblastoma are discussed in this section.

Immunocytochemistry

Neuron-Specific Enolase

"Neuron-specific" enolase (NSE) is a glycolytic isoenzyme of 2-phosphoglycerate and phosphoenolpyruvate (212,279). This dimeric protein, composed of two γ subunits, is present in most neurons of the retina and central nervous system (CNS) and in neuroendocrine cells, but also in neuroectodermal malignant tumors and in some reactive glia (43,86,122,129,217,257, 287–289,291,305,338,354,356,369). In the retina, NSE is detected in neuronal perikarya, but not in the glia (167,169). Many reports have demonstrated NSE in retinoblastoma and in tumor cell lines (5,162,167,169,187,382). The NSE has been detected both in undifferentiated areas and in well-differentiated Flexner–Wintersteiner rosettes and fleurettes (162,167,169,334,382). Its presence is evidence that the retinoblastoma cell of origin is capable of neuronal differentiation, but does not specify the type of neuron.

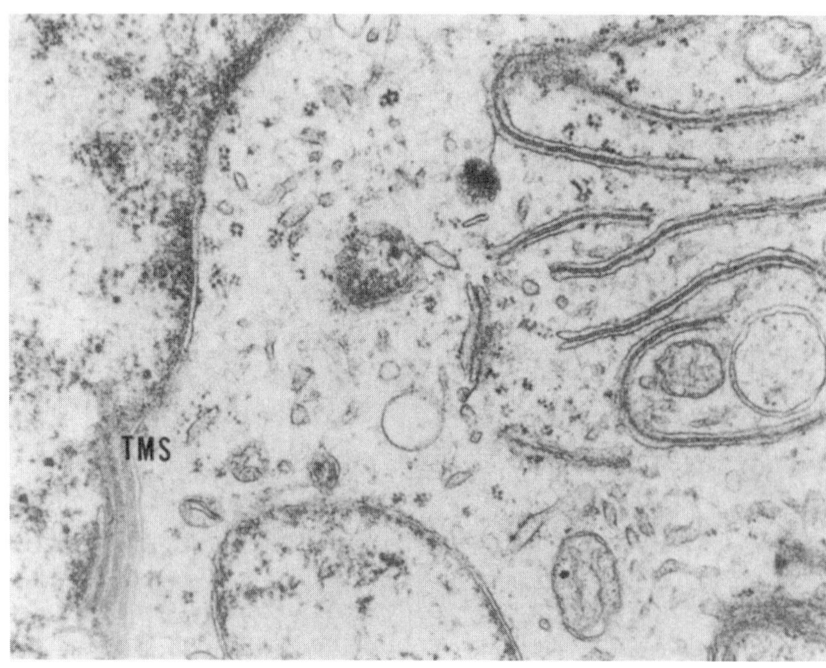

Figure 7 Retinoblastoma cell containing triple-membrane structures (TMS) involving the nuclear membrane. Note that triple-membrane infoldings are also present in the cytoplasm (× 27,400).

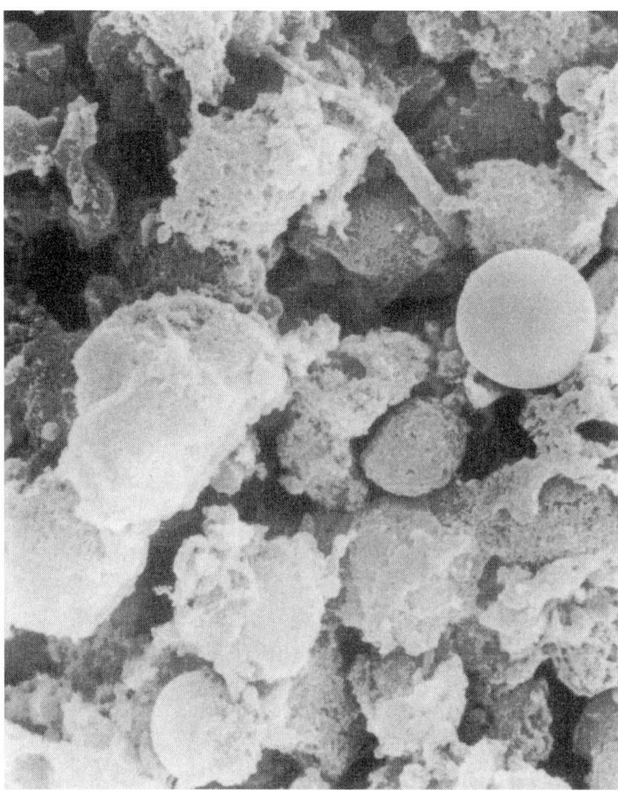

Figure 8 Scanning electron microscopy of retinoblastoma cells, showing two general types: the smooth, sphere-like cell and the more numerous cells with profuse surface features (× 1,900).

Synaptophysin

Synaptophysin, a neuron-associated membrane glycoprotein of presynaptic vesicles, was detected immunohistochemically in 45 of 54 formalin-fixed and paraffin-embedded retinoblastoma specimens (175,358).

Neurofilaments

Neurofilaments (NF) are intermediate filaments composed of three triplet polypeptides of 68, 145, and 200 kDa, respectively, which may be phosphorylated (344). Since malignant transformation is seldom reputed to alter cell intermediate filaments, these are seen as good markers of tumor cell origin and differentiation (258,301,345). Kivela and colleagues have demonstrated NF (200 kDa) in rare processes in the nerve fiber and inner plexiform layers in normal retinas; on the other hand, retinoblastoma cells were not stained (167,174,358). Perentes and colleagues, however, detected 200 kDa NF in three of seven retinoblastomas (262). Tarlton and Easty, using antibodies against two different NF antigens (155 and 210 kDa), found mild or no reactivity in retinoblastoma cells (342). Thus, the evidence on NF expression in retinoblastoma is unclear, and further studies using phosphorylated and nonphosphorylated epitopes of the 68 and 145 kDa NF polypeptides are needed (120).

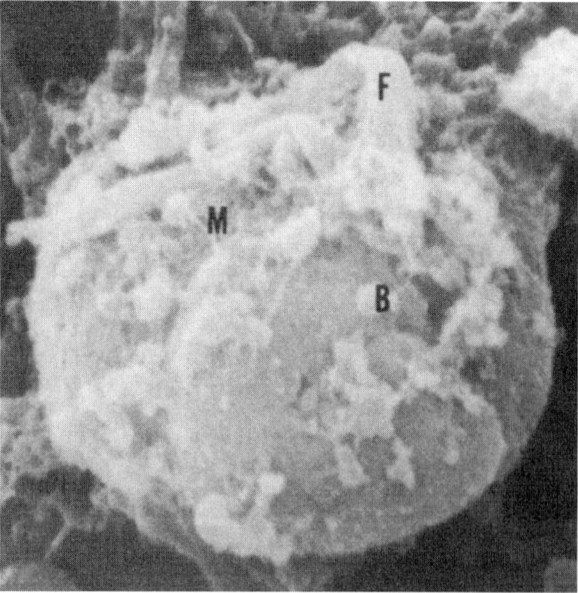

Figure 9 Retinoblastoma cells by Scanning electron microscopy showing zeiotic blebs (B), microvilli (M), and thick filopodia (F) (×4,200).

Miscellaneous Biologically Active Peptides

Biologically active peptides, such as substance P and proenkephalon A, have been demonstrated in a few retinoblastoma cells. These markers are usually attributed to amacrine cells (339,340), although another marker of amacrine cells, parvalbumin, was not detected in retinoblastoma samples (170). Somatostatin- and insulin-like immunoreactivity has also been detected in both retinoblastoma specimens and cultured Y-79 retinoblastoma cells (94,167). Tetanus toxin receptor, as well as dopamine β-hydroxylase, has been demonstrated in tumor cell lines (94,167). The latter could be linked to the occasional ultrastructural finding of dense-core neurosecretory granules and of small amounts of catecholamines within retinoblastoma cells detected by fluorescent and histochemical techniques (193,298). Nevertheless, neurotransmitters and their receptors are not reliable markers of retinoblastoma.

Photoreceptor Cell-Associated Antigens

Strong evidence exists for the presence of photoreceptor cell elements in retinoblastoma, suggesting that the retinoblastoma cell of origin has the potential to give rise to these highly specialized cells. After preliminary studies by Felberg and Donoso (109), many antigens attributed to photoreceptors have been scrutinized (360). Rhodopsin has been demonstrated in fleurettes and Flexner–Wintersteiner rosettes using monoclonal

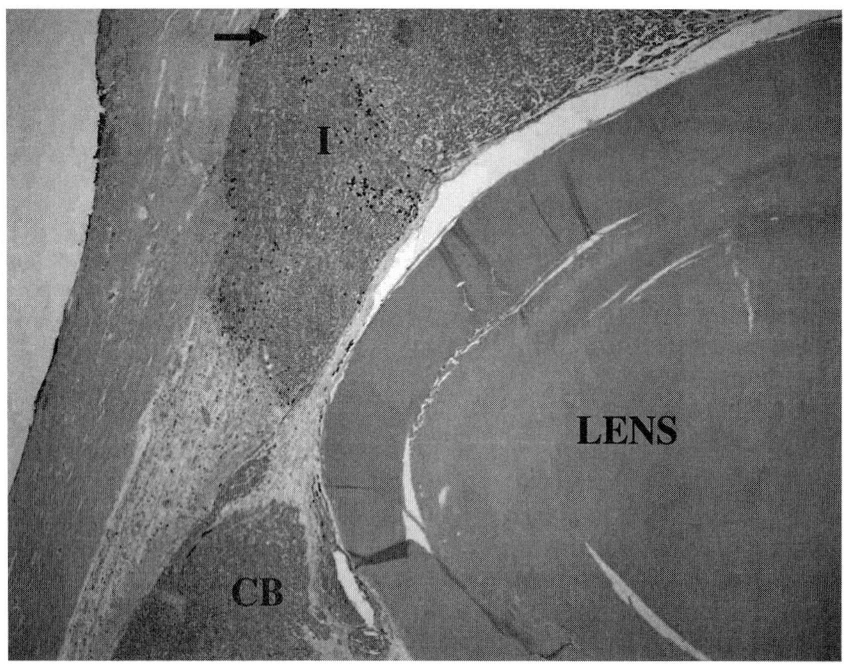

Figure 10 Massive invasion of the anterior chamber angle (*arrow*), iris (I), and ciliary body (CB) by retinoblastoma (hematoxylin and eosin, ×45).

antibodies (92), while photoreceptor proteins consisting of either rod or cone opsins were found in 16 of 22 retinoblastoma samples by Gonzalez-Fernandez et al. (125). Nork and colleagues further noted that retinoblastoma fleurettes stained predominantly for red and green cone-specific antibodies, while features of blue cones and rods were present in areas with high cytoplasm-to-nuclear ratios but no fleurettes (254). Recoverin, a calcium-binding protein expressed in photoreceptors and some cone bipolar cells, was demonstrated in the Y-79 human retinoblastoma cell line and upregulated following induced differentiation (370). Arrestin (a regulator of photoactivated rhodopsin signaling formerly known as S-antigen) was detected in different patterns by the use of both monoclonal and polyclonal antibodies (90,91,93,231,253,352) in differentiated retinoblastoma, trilateral retinoblastoma (TRB), and various retinoblastoma cell lines. Donoso and colleagues further demonstrated that monoclonal antibodies to rhodopsin and arrestin bound to the same areas (92). These results suggest that arrestin expression may be used to assess the degree of tumor differentiation in retinoblastoma. Donoso and colleagues (94) also mentioned a personal observation of retinoblastoma staining positively for α-transducin. This can be related to the finding of transcripts for L-transducin, as well as for the red or green cone cell photopigment, in all of seven low-passage retinoblastoma cell lines (39). No marker genes for rod cells were expressed, and it is conceivable from this study that retinoblastoma has a predominantly cone lineage. Lastly, Tsuji and colleagues detected mucin-like glycoprotein associated with photoreceptor cells (MLGAPC), a glycoprotein specific for photoreceptor cells and analogous to interphotoreceptor matrix proteoglycan-1, in 17 of 21 retinoblastoma cases, including undifferentiated tumors (351). As such, these authors suggest that MLGAPC is yet another useful marker of retinoblastoma.

Interphotoreceptor Cell-Binding Protein

Interphotoreceptor cell-binding protein (IRBP), which is secreted by the rod photoreceptor cells into the extracellular matrix, has been detected in the lumen of Flexner–Wintersteiner rosettes (282,284) and fleurettes (125). The amount of IRBP in tumor samples correlated with the degree of tumor differentiation (283). Using Western and Northern blots and radiolabeled ligand-binding techniques, Fong and colleagues investigated retinoid-binding proteins in fresh tumors and cell lines (47,113). They concluded that: (*i*) the expression of retinoid-binding proteins is variable in tumor cells; (*ii*) the only retinoid-binding protein consistently expressed by both types of cells is IRBP at a level similar to that in the normal retina at 22 weeks gestation; and (*iii*) these findings are consistent with an embryonic origin for the cells. Fong and colleagues further speculated that the tumor does not arise earlier than the 22-week stage.

Tarlton and Easty tested a panel of 18 monoclonal antibodies against six retinoblastomas and compared the reactivity of the tumors with adult and fetal retina. They concluded that the closest normal cell type is a 13- to 16-week outer retinal cell.

The antigens expressed in the tumor could be detected in both the inner and outer nuclear layers of the retina (342). Because of the potential of the precursor cell to differentiate into photoreceptor cells as well as "inner" retinal cells, Tarlton and Easty propose that the tumor arises from a primitive multipotential cell type that predominates before week 8 of gestation and declines in parallel with later retinal development. The variability of findings between studies implies phenotypic heterogeneity in retinoblastoma tumors and underscores the obstacles in defining the cell of origin.

Glia-Associated Antigens

A few studies have provided support for glial differentiation in retinoblastomas. Shuangshoti and colleagues (323) detected glial markers in 23 of 39 retinoblastomas, whereas 18 contained neuronal markers. These findings are consistent with those of Molnar and colleagues (236) and of Messmer and colleagues (223), who observed glial fibrillary acidic protein (GFAP), an intermediate filament typical of astrocytes, in 1 of 7 and 2 of 50 tumors, respectively. Cellular retinaldehyde-binding protein (CRALBP), a Müller glia cell marker, was used to identify neoplastic Müller cell differentiation in 12 of 16 cases in one study (125). Most reports, however, interpret GFAP as well as S100 and vimentin staining as markers of reactive astrocytes in retinoblastoma, since positive cells are located around blood vessels and in reactive areas of the tumor or radiating into the tumor from the bordering retina and optic nerve (125,161,162,173,174,194,293,343,392). Most cell culture experiments demonstrate exclusively neuronal differentiation, but a few document coexpression of neuronal and glial markers in tumor cell lines and fresh tumor tissue (51,52,167,192,254,382). In tissue studies, a glial component has been demonstrated in Flexner–Wintersteiner rosettes and is suspected of being neoplastic (78). As emphasized by several authors, the hypothesis that a multipotential neuroectodermal precursor of both neurons and glia exists has not been ruled out (84,192,254).

HNK-1 Epitope

HNK-1 is a carbohydrate epitope that is shared by human natural killer cells and many neuronal, glial, and neuroectodermal cells, and is present in myelin-associated glycoproteins, neuroendocrine secretory granules (167,263), and neural cell adhesion molecules (167,169,263). The HNK-1 epitope is expressed in the embryonic retina on putative precursor cells of both neuronal and glial cells (168). This epitope is detected in ganglion cell bodies near the inner limiting membrane and neuronal processes in both plexiform layers (168).

The monoclonal anti-Leu-7 antibody, directed against HNK-1, has not been detected in retinoblastoma cells (168,262,263). Carcinoembryonic antigen (CEA), which is elevated in the plasma of some patients with retinoblastoma, was not detected by immunohistochemistry in the tumors either (172). In 10 retinoblastomas, Kivela demonstrated lectin-binding properties similar to those of photoreceptor cells (concanavalin A conjugates) (167,168). Kivela's findings, as well as those of others (28,109) using cell lines, demonstrate similarities between photoreceptors and both differentiated and undifferentiated retinoblastoma cells. Questions of specificity suggest that lectin binding should be interpreted with caution.

Stem Cell Markers

The observation that not every cell within a tumor can maintain tumor growth suggested the existence of a group of stem-like cells (cancer stem cells) that contribute to chemoresistance and tumor progression (259,278). Cancer stem cells have since been identified in a number of malignancies (10,42,189,195,324). In mouse and human retinoblastoma, Seigel and colleagues (308) found subpopulations of cells that displayed a stem cell-like phenotype and expressed the stem cell markers ABCG2 (ATP-binding cassette reporter, G2 subfamily), aldehyde dehydrogenase 1, minichromosome maintenance marker 2 (MCM2), stem cell antigen-1, and p63. The existence of ABCG2 was particularly interesting, since it can confer resistance to over 20 different chemotherapeutic agents. In independent experiments, Mohan and colleagues also identified ABCG2 and MCM2 expression in human retinoblastoma tumors and further noted that their expression was higher in invasive tumors (233).

Cell of Origin

Determination of the cell of origin in retinoblastoma would greatly improve our clinical and scientific understanding of the disease. For example, it may provide insight into why *RB1* mutations lead to tumors in some tissues but not others, and reveal epigenetic, nongenetic, and secondary genetic features of certain cells that influence the progression of preneoplastic lesions to frank tumors. Childhood cancers like retinoblastoma arise from a constantly changing pool of immature progenitor and/or transition cells (101). Retinal progenitor cells are multipotent and undergo proliferation and differentiation in a precise temporospatial manner to produce the highly structured retina with its seven main classes of cells (386,387). Postmitotic transition cells arise from progenitor cells and are either committed or biased toward a particular cell fate, yet are not fully differentiated themselves. The normal, tumor-like properties of progenitor and transition cells, with their proliferative or immediately postproliferative cellular environment, likely contribute to their propensity to form tumors (101).

The initial mutations that inactivate *RB1* occur during mitosis due to errors in DNA replication or mitotic recombination, but do not immediately give rise to tumors (101). It is not until an affected cell requires the services of the RB1 protein that its absence is felt, and this may occur at different stages of retinal maturation. During development, the competency of multipotent retinal progenitor cells to yield particular cell types changes in a unidirectional manner, although extrinsic factors can influence cell fate choices to some degree (59,201). This knowledge, along with other available data, has been used to develop models of the cell of origin in retinoblastoma (101). The progenitor cell model states that *RB1* inactivation inhibits retinal progenitor cells from exiting the cell cycle at G1, whereas the transition cell model argues that loss of *RB1* function allows newly postmitotic, transition cells to reenter the cell cycle (101). These models are not mutually exclusive, and both offer explanations for the variation in the expression of retinal cell type markers in retinoblastomas.

In either model, the cell environment and gene expression profile is important in determining whether a tumor will develop following *RB1* inactivation (101). For instance, epigenetic features present in an early progenitor cell or a transition cell biased toward an amacrine cell fate may provide a more or less conducive environment for retinoblastoma formation than a late progenitor cell or a transition cell committed to become a cone photoreceptor. The same could be true for nonretinal cells that give rise to secondary tumors commonly found in retinoblastoma survivors. Knowledge of the cell of origin of retinoblastoma and the predisposing cellular factors leading to tumor formation (or, conversely, the tumor-resistant factors present in cells oblivious to *RB1* inactivation) will hopefully lead to novel avenues of treatment for afflicted patients.

NATURAL HISTORY

Spontaneous Regression

Complete spontaneous regression of retinoblastoma is an unusual but well-documented occurrence. It is usually characterized by a severe inflammatory reaction followed by phthisis bulbi, and numerous histopathological reports of such tumors have been published (16,40,41,163,200,239,251,274,330). Most authors have incriminated infarction of the tumor after a central vessel obstruction (16,301). Histopathological reports of these cases demonstrate dense calcification, necrotic tissue, fossilized tumor cells, massive proliferation of the RPE, inflammatory reaction, and variable degrees of ossification. Marcus and colleagues emphasize that a reliable distinction between such spontaneous necrosis and retinomas–retinocytomas in nonphthisical eyes has not been made (215) and these authors concur with Zimmerman in viewing such tumors as benign variants of retinoblastoma (392). Reports of a malignant transformation of a retinoma–retinocytoma variant support this concept (102). Both completely regressed retinoblastomas and retinocytomas differ from regression patterns observed after irradiation, where there is formation of a glial scar, complete destruction of the tumor and associated atrophy of surrounding choroid and blood vessels (215).

Intraocular Spread

The pattern of retinoblastoma spread both within and outside the eye is well-recognized and documented (140,274,306,384,392). Retinoblastoma is generally a poorly cohesive neoplasm that may grow in all directions. This poor cohesion may be related to the apparently defective or absent zonulae adherentes and/or filopodia, which normally contribute to cell–cell attachment. Tumor cells commonly seed anteriorly in the vitreous and aqueous humor. Cells may be deposited on the surface of the iris and in the anterior chamber angle, giving rise to a secondary glaucoma and/or pseudohypopyon (131,315). As previously noted, clusters of tumor cells may collect on the inner surface of the retina and grow as separate foci, particularly in the peripheral retina and at the ora serrata. These secondary lesions may be mistaken for additional primary sites of retinoblastoma development. The presence of intravitreal clusters of cells and of the major portion of the tumor at the inner retinal surface is helpful in distinguishing secondary deposits from additional primary foci (392). Another common pattern of spread is posteriorly into the subretinal space (Fig. 11). The significance of minimal choroidal invasion is still disputed. Massive choroidal invasion, however, usually correlates with a high risk of scleral, orbital, and hematogenous spread. Invasion of the optic nerve may occur at the base of the optic cup, in the area of the central vessels, or into the subarachnoid space adjacent to the optic nerve (Fig. 12).

Extraocular Spread

Tumor cells may disseminate hematogenously through choroidal or other blood vessels in proximity to the subarachnoid space (20,384,392) and dissemination into the choroid and optic nerve has been correlated with the tumor's relative vascular area

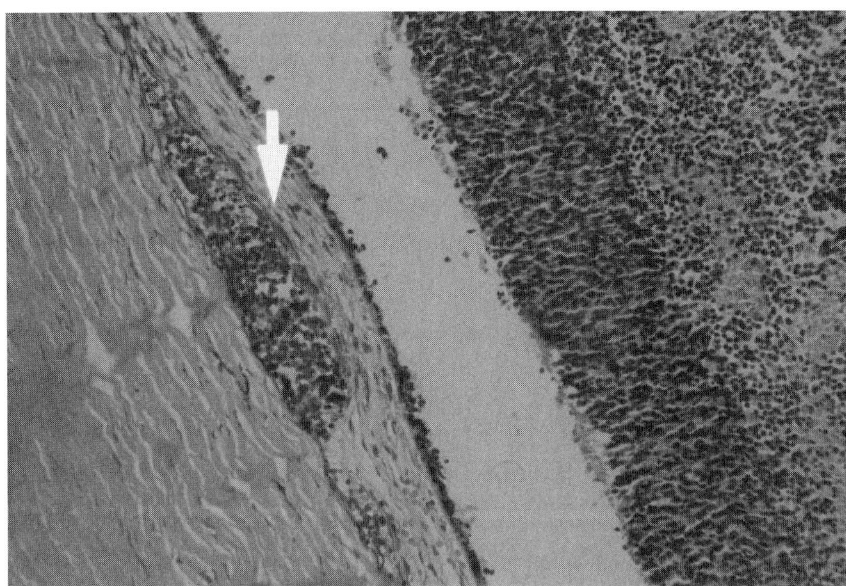

Figure 11 Extension of tumor cells in the subretinal space with minimal choroidal invasion (*arrow*) (hematoxylin and eosin, ×23).

and degree of angiogenesis (213). Infiltrative spread through the optic nerve (211) or subarachnoid space gives access to orbital tissues and the brain (363). Retinoblastoma may also reach the orbit through the emissaria and tumor growth through paracentesis sites and spread subconjunctivally (329). In advanced cases, retinoblastoma may massively penetrate through the sclera and grow extensively into the orbit (104). Metastases to the preauricular and cervical lymph nodes usually follow such massive extraocular metastases (54). Recurrence of retinoblastoma in the orbit following enucleation is suspected of being the consequence of subclinical orbital involvement escaping recognition or from residual tumor in the remaining optic nerve. Extraocular spread of tumor has also been documented following intraocular surgery on eyes with retinoblastoma (329).

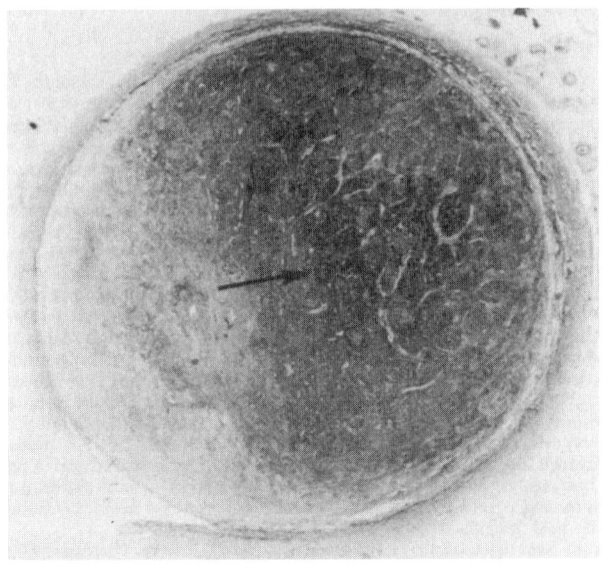

Figure 12 Massive invasion of the optic nerve by retinoblastoma (*arrow*) (hematoxylin and eosin, ×13).

Metastases

The most common sites of distant metastasis of retinoblastoma are the CNS, skull, distal bones, lymph nodes, and spinal cord (222), with spread to bones beyond the skull noted in about 50% of patients dying from the neoplasm. Wang and colleagues found clinical features such as exophthalmos, cataract, and pseudohypopyon to be significantly correlated with tumor invasion and metastasis (364). Bilaterality and delay in diagnosis are also important factors (111). Although most metastases are detected within the first 2 years after diagnosis, some may become apparent many years after the last evidence of tumor activity in the retina is noted (153,388). In such cases, a new primary tumor should be considered. Usually, metastases to bone and brain from retinoblastoma do not show evidence of rosette and fleurette formation and may resemble Ewing sarcoma, neuroblastoma, or other small round cell tumors of childhood. In such cases, immunohistochemistry and tissue culture, as well as TEM, may be of diagnostic value (14,73,392). This lack of differentiation is helpful to distinguish such lesions from midbrain tumors in TRB.

CLINICAL DIAGNOSIS

The presenting signs and symptoms in over 65% of retinoblastomas are, in order of decreasing frequency: leukocoria or "cat's eye" reflex (31,32,120,148), strabismus, and a red and painful eye with or without glaucoma and poor vision (48,62,245,274,317,318). Less frequent modes of presentation include ocular inflammation (granulomatous iridocyclitis), hyphema, glaucoma, or, in neglected cases, suspected trauma to the eye, or metastatic disease (136,326,366). Ocular inflammation is often a misdiagnosed presentation and is a poor prognostic sign (131,328). A child <3 years of age with any of these signs and symptoms should be suspected of retinoblastoma. Lueder found that the prognosis was greatly improved when physicians initially detected abnormalities rather than the parents (203).

The differential diagnosis for retinoblastoma is long (313,315), and nearly 50% of patients initially suspected of having retinoblastoma are ultimately diagnosed with a simulating condition (315). Shields and colleagues found that the four most common conditions simulating retinoblastoma in patients referred to their institution were persistent hyperplastic primary vitreous, Coats disease, ocular toxocariasis, and retinopathy of prematurity (313).

The finding of multiple tumors arising from the retina of variable color and appearance is almost diagnostic, as well as a large unilateral calcified tumor (149). Retinoblastoma is diagnosed occasionally in the first weeks of life. This occurs particularly when there is a family history of the disease and ocular examination is carried out under general anesthesia with indentation of the peripheral retina (149). Multiple tumor nodules can reflect either a truly multifocal origin or vitreous seeding of the tumor.

Computed tomography (CT) is sometimes a useful ancillary test in the diagnosis of retinoblastoma, since more than 90% of these tumors contain calcium. Roentgenography is far less sensitive (177,227,266,362). High-resolution CT can also detect retrobulbar and intracranial tumor growth (227), but retrolaminar spread is less reliably demonstrated (227). Ultrasonography is also able to detect calcifications (320) within the tumor and orbit. Optic nerve invasion is less accurately visualized with this latter diagnostic procedure, and intracranial metastases or pinealomas are beyond its scope. Measurement of the axial length of the globe can be helpful, since eyes with retinoblastoma are almost never microphthalmic, except for regressed tumors with phthisis bulbi (99). Magnetic resonance imaging (MRI) does not usually detect calcium but is useful in the assessment of the optic nerve, orbit, and brain (209,265,307,315). The pattern observed may also prove useful in discriminating retinoblastoma from Coats disease, toxocariasis, or persistent hyperplastic primary vitreous (209,265,393) and in the determination of tumor differentiation. Assays of aqueous humor lactic dehydrogenase (87,159,248,285,332) or NSE (33,37) and serum levels of α-fetoprotein, CEA, and catecholamines (128,225,230,242,272,276,277,299) have been inconsistent and unreliable in the diagnosis of retinoblastoma. Despite the availability of fine-needle aspiration biopsy to diagnose retinoblastoma (24,62,63), this technique has not been generally accepted as safe by the ophthalmic community. The usefulness of bone marrow aspirations and lumbar punctures in the initial metastatic work-up (17,296) has been called into question in view of the very infrequent positivity of those tests in children without clinical or histological evidence of extraocular tumor dissemination (270).

NONOCULAR TUMORS AND TRILATERAL RETINOBLASTOMA

Trilateral Retinoblastoma

The association of bilateral retinoblastoma with a midline intracranial malignancy located in the pineal or parasellar region was first reported in 1971 by Jensen and Miller (157), and thereafter became increasingly recognized (25,26,254,240,260,264,321). Although such intracranial tumors had been reported prior to 1971, they were considered either metastases or unrelated to retinoblastoma. Jakobiec and colleagues (154) recorded two indisputable cases in detail in 1977, and in 1980, the term TRB was introduced by Bader and colleagues (25,26). These intracranial tumors are most often suprasellar or parasellar primitive neuroectodermal tumors (PNET) and undifferentiated neuroblastic pineal tumors (pinealoblastomas). The mammalian pineal gland is involved in the regulation of circadian rhythms, while in certain lower animals, the pineal functions as a photoreceptor organ and histologically resembles the retina (25,206). These observations offer a natural link between these midline tumors and intraocular retinoblastoma.

Over 100 cases of TRB have now been reported (264,321). The average percentage of retinoblastoma patients that are diagnosed with TRB is 2.6% based upon a meta-analysis of publications spanning a period between 1957 and 2002 (240). There is no clear gender preference, and the median age at diagnosis is 26 to 31 months (median time from retinoblastoma diagnosis to TRB diagnosis = 21–22 months). In 11% to 12% of TRB patients, a midline intracranial neoplasm occurred with unilateral retinoblastoma (154,171,214,392). Patients with TRB can be asymptomatic or present with signs and symptoms related to increased intracranial pressure (214,240). Neuroimaging (CT and MRI) is used to confirm a suspicion of TRB. Some advocate its use for routine screening, but this practice is controversial and many view it as impractical (152,214,240). CT is valuable since calcification may be the only evidence for the existence of an intracranial neoplasm (27). Unfortunately, TRB is usually fatal, with an average survival time of 11.2 months, although combination chemotherapy can prolong survival (214).

Histological examinations of intracranial tumors in TRB patients have revealed PNET in approximately 60% of patients (214) and various degrees of neuronal and photoreceptor differentiation in the remaining cases. Primitive or undifferentiated tumors containing unique rosette clusters and possible fleurettes, along with occasional Flexner–Wintersteiner and Homer-Wright rosettes, have been documented (65,214,224). Pathologically, pineal tumors in TRB are indistinguishable from retinoblastoma in the eye (158,240). Together, case reports on TRB, along with histological data and descriptions of retinoblastoma-like differentiation in pineal tumors associated with TRB, suggest that the midline intracranial malignancies represent a third site of expression of the genetic predisposition to retinoblastoma. This suggestion is further supported by evidence from a transgenic mouse model (374).

Nonintracranial Second Primary Tumors After Retinoblastoma

Many children who have germline *RB1* mutations survive to adulthood and are prone to subsequent cancers. A comprehensive recent study analyzed the risk of new cancers in 1601 retinoblastoma survivors diagnosed from 1914 to 1984 at two medical centers in New York and Boston (176). The standardized incidence ratio (i.e., the ratio of the observed number of cancers to the expected number from the Connecticut Tumor Registry) was 19 for hereditary retinoblastoma patients and 1.2 for nonhereditary retinoblastoma patients. Radiation further increased the risk of another cancer in hereditary patients by 3.1-fold. This is consistent with earlier findings regarding the risk of new cancers in survivors of hereditary retinoblastoma or in their relatives (4,15,69,70,83,133,204,232,269,376). Further, the study by Kleinerman et al. (176) showed that the cumulative incidence for developing a new cancer by 50 years of age after diagnosis of retinoblastoma was 36% for hereditary and 5.7% for nonhereditary patients. The authors concluded that hereditary retinoblastoma predisposes to a variety of new cancers over time, with radiotherapy further enhancing the risk of tumors developing in the field of radiation. Although there was a wide range of tumor types and sites, sarcomas, melanoma, and cancer of the brain and nasal cavities were among the most common. It seems likely that an increased risk for second primary tumors also exists in patients with retinoma or retinocytoma who have a germline *RB1* mutation (191). Abramson and Schefler have provided extensive reviews regarding second cancers in retinoblastoma (1,6). In bilateral retinoblastoma, the incidence of second cancer in the field of irradiation is 35% compared to 6% for those patients who do not receive external beam radiation (281).

STAGING AND PROGNOSIS

Retinoblastoma is relatively unique among pediatric tumors in that it does not have a widely accepted, worldwide classification system that takes into account the entire spectrum of disease and its response to modern forms of treatment. The Reese–Elsworth classification was developed in the 1960s based on knowledge of the disease, examination techniques, and treatment options available at that time (105,244,275). Since then, globe-sparing (e.g., chemoreduction) treatment options have become more commonplace, as has our understanding of the genetics and pathophysiology of the disease. Thus, researchers have striven to develop an updated grouping and staging system to address the constantly advancing research on retinoblastoma. Such a system would be used to assess prognosis, guide initial therapy, predict treatment morbidity, and allow efficient communication between clinicians and researchers involved in individual patient care and multicenter trials. The past and present classifications and staging systems as well as proposals for updated schemes are discussed in this section. Of note, the terms "group" and "stage" are often misused by authors, as pointed out by Murphree (244). Groupings are based on observations of the intraocular tumor itself, whereas staging focuses on the patient and is concerned primarily with the spread of the disease.

Two clinical staging systems have traditionally been available to predict the local outcome of eye-saving conservative treatment. As mentioned previously, both are intended to provide information within the context of treatment regimens present at the time they were developed. The Reese–Ellsworth classification (Table 1) was developed to predict the chance of survival of the eye after external beam radiotherapy. It has been widely used for decades, but many ocular oncologists believe it requires significant changes (61,103,105,106,244,268). Thus, alternative working classifications were proposed in the 1980s by Hopping (142) and De Sutter and colleagues (80) (Essen Classification), and Rosengren and colleagues (based on the tumor, node, and metastasis [TNM] classification commonly employed in oncology) (80,142,286). The former found favor in several oncology centers (80,142), while the latter was not widely adopted (244). However, as clinical and scientific knowledge of retinoblastoma has evolved, treatment centers have felt the need to adapt these older classification systems independently, underscoring the need for further system modifications.

Table 1 Reese–Ellsworth Classification of Retinoblastomas

Group 1: Very favorable
- Solitary tumor <4 disc diameters, at or behind the equator
- Multiple tumors, none >4 disc diameters, all at or behind the equator

Group 2: Favorable
- Solitary tumor 4–10 disc diameters in size, at or behind the equator
- Multiple tumors 4–10 disc diameters in size, all behind the equator

Group 3: Doubtful
- Any lesion anterior to the equator
- Solitary tumor >10 disc diameters, behind the equator

Group 4: Unfavorable
- Multiple tumors, some >10 disc diameters
- Any lesion extending anterior to the ora serrata

Group 5: Very unfavorable
- Massive tumors involving >half the retina
- Vitreous seeding

In 1997, Pratt and colleagues proposed the modified St. Jude Children's Research Hospital staging and grouping scheme for intraocular and extraocular retinoblastoma based on an analysis of 103 globes from 73 patients (Table 2) (268). This system contained four broad stages based on tumor location (confined to retina, confined to globe, extrachoroidal extension, and distant disease) with three to five subgroups in each category. While this system was not superior to Reese–Ellsworth groupings in predicting progression-free survival, it was felt that it better facilitated the assignment of appropriate

Table 2 Modified St. Jude Staging Schema

Stage I: Tumor confined to the retina
- A. Solitary: <6 disc diameters
- B. Multiple: all <6 disc diameters
- C. Solitary or multiple lesions involving <50% of retinal surface behind equator
- D. >50% retinal involvement, behind equator
- E. >50% involvement, or involvement anterior to equator

Stage II: Tumor confined to globe/extraretinal
- A. Extends to optic nerve head
- B. Extends to choroid
- C. Anterior chamber involvement
- D. Extends to choroid and optic nerve

Stage III: Extrachoroidal extension
- A. Extends to emissaries
- B. Extends beyond cut end of optic nerve (includes subarachnoid)
- C. Extends through sclera into orbit
- D. Extends to choroid and beyond cut end of optic nerve (includes subarachnoid)
- E. Extends through sclera and cut end of optic nerve

Stage IV: Distant disease
- A. Extends through optic nerve into the brain (includes positive cerebrospinal fluid studies)
- B. Blood-borne metastases to soft tissue, nodes, or bone
- C. Bone marrow metastases

Source: From Ref. 268.

Table 3 Practical Grouping System of Retinoblastoma

Group 1: Presence of tumor only, regardless of number, size, or location

Group 2: Tumor plus subretinal fluid

Group 3: Tumor plus focal seeds
- a. Subretinal seeds ≤3 mm from tumor
- b. Vitreous seeds ≤3 mm from tumor

Group 4: Tumor plus diffuse seeds
- a. Subretinal seeds >3 mm from tumor
- b. Vitreous seeds >3 mm from tumor

Group 5: Tumor plus any one of the following: neovascular glaucoma, opaque media from hemorrhage in anterior chamber, vitreous or subretinal space, or invasion of postlaminar optic nerve, choroid (>2 mm), sclera, orbit, or anterior chamber

Source: From Ref. 311.

treatment modalities. In 2004, Shields and colleagues described a practical approach to management of retinoblastoma based on a five-group classification system emphasizing general clinical features, such as the presence of subretinal fluid, seeding, invasion, and secondary findings (Table 3) (311).

In 2001, the Children's Oncology Group (COG) developed a standing Retinoblastoma Disease Committee to develop protocols for clinical trials and a new group classification for intraocular retinoblastoma. With this challenge in mind, the International Intraocular Retinoblastoma Classification (IIRC) was formed based on observations of the natural history and outcome data analysis of patients treated for intraocular retinoblastoma (60,117,244). Several centers worldwide have evaluated the IIRC system, and the COG has adopted it for the development of numerous retinoblastoma protocols. The IIRC is designed to predict outcomes from current treatment modalities, most notably chemotherapy and focal therapy (117), and relies on presurgical information gathered about the tumor as opposed to information obtained from biopsy specimens. There are five IIRC groups that rank intraocular retinoblastoma tumors based upon their risk of treatment failure and subsequent need for enucleation or external beam radiation. The groups follow the natural history of the tumor from early (group A) to late (group E) disease, and are defined by morphologic features of the tumor(s) and the extent of intraocular disease at the time of diagnosis (Table 4). The system addresses risk of eye loss and is not a staging system to assess risk to the whole child. Importantly, preliminary evaluation of the IIRC has shown it to be superior to the Reese–Ellsworth classification in predicting the outcome of modern retinoblastoma treatment (60,117).

Another international staging system was proposed in 2005 by Chantada and colleagues to address the entire spectrum of disease that occurs with

Table 4 International Intraocular Retinoblastoma Classification (IIRC)

Group A: Very low risk—Eyes with small discrete tumors away from critical structures. (All tumors are 3 mm or smaller, confined to the retina, and located at least 3 mm from the foveola and 1.5 mm from the optic nerve. No vitreous or subretinal seeding is allowed.)
Group B: Low risk—Eyes with no vitreous seeding or subretinal seeding and discrete retinal tumor of any size or location. (Retinal tumors may be of any size or location not in Group A. A small cuff of subretinal fluid extending not more than 5 mm from the tumor base is allowed.)
Group C: Moderate risk—Eyes with only focal vitreous or subretinal seeding and discrete retinal tumors of any size and location. (Any seeding must be local, fine, and theoretically treatable with a radioactive plaque. Up to one quadrant of subretinal fluid may be present.)
Group D: High risk—Eyes with diffuse vitreous or subretinal seeding and/or massive, nondiscrete endophytic or exophytic disease. (Includes exophytic disease and more than one quadrant of retinal detachment.)
Group E: Very high risk—Eyes that have been destroyed anatomically or functionally by the tumor. (Eyes with one or more of the following: irreversible neovascular glaucoma, massive intraocular hemorrhage, aseptic orbital cellulitis, tumor anterior to anterior vitreous face, tumor touching the lens, diffuse infiltrating retinoblastoma, phthisis, or prephthisis.)

Source: From Refs. 117 and 244.

retinoblastoma, including advanced intraocular disease requiring enucleation and extraocular disease (61). This system takes into account histopathological features of enucleated specimens when available, and consists of five stages (0–IV) classified according to extent of disease and the presence of extraocular involvement (Table 5).

With regard to prognosis, the following considerations are important (190): (*i*) professional experience of the therapeutic team; (*ii*) patient's age at diagnosis; (*iii*) age at which diagnosis is made; (*iv*) grouping or staging; and (*v*) whether the tumor is unilateral or bilateral. Newer classification schemes await formal analyses prior to determining their prognostic value, although preliminary data obtained using the IIRC classifications purportedly reveal excellent segregation of outcome by group (60,244).

Table 5 Proposed International Retinoblastoma Staging System

Stage 0: Patients treated conservatively (presurgical)
Stage I[a]: Eye enucleated, completely resected histologically
Stage II[a]: Eye enucleated, microscopic residual tumor
Stage III: Regional extension
- a. Overt orbital disease
- b. Preauricular or cervical lymph node extension

Stage IV: Metastatic disease.
- a. Hematogenous metastasis (without CNS involvement)
  1. Single lesion
  2. Multiple lesions
- a. CNS extension (with or without any other site of regional or metastatic disease)
  1. Prechiasmatic lesion
  2. CNS mass
  3. Leptomeningeal and CSF disease

[a]Subclassifications exist for Stage I and II retinoblastoma based on additional histopathological features of enucleated specimens.
Source: From Ref. 61.
Abbreviations: CNS, central nervous system; CSF, cerebrospinal fluid.

Without treatment, retinoblastoma is almost always fatal. Mortality from retinoblastoma stems from metastases (typically via the optic nerve, although other routes are possible); from intracranial neuroblastic malignancy (TRB); and from second primary tumors (315). With multidisciplinary management, survival rates over 95% have been achieved, although these numbers can be misleading since many different clinical situations are lumped together (228). Patients with CNS dissemination and distant metastatic disease have a poor prognosis. Antoneli and colleagues documented a 5-year overall survival of 55% to 60% in patients with extraocular disease treated with chemotherapy (20).

In the era prior to modern chemoreduction protocols, a multivariate statistical analysis of tumors in Reese–Ellsworth group V tumors (290) showed that all prognostic factors are related to "histological" features; namely, insufficient optic nerve length removed at enucleation (<5 mm; $p = 0.001$), optic nerve involvement ($p = 0.004$), and large tumor size ($p = 0.01$). It seemed that histological features are the best survival predictors (80), with the degree of optic nerve involvement generally considered the most reliable single prognostic indicator (384,392). The mortality rate varies with the extent of optic nerve involvement, and it is essential that the surgeon excise a section of the optic nerve of at least 10 mm at enucleation. Some authors advocate the use of frozen sections at the time of surgery to check the adequacy of optic nerve resection (160). Magramm and colleagues (211), in a review of 814 patients, found 240 cases of optic nerve invasion (29.5%). These were classified as follows:

Grade I. Superficial invasion of the optic nerve head only (mortality rate 10%).
Grade II. Involvement up to and including the lamina cribrosa (mortality rate 29%).
Grade III. Involvement beyond the lamina cribrosa (mortality rate 42%).
Grade IV. Involvement up to and including the surgical margin (mortality rate 78%).

These investigators did not find choroidal involvement, scleral extension, or laterality to be significant covariants. The only other significant association was age at diagnosis. Other authors have found massive choroidal extension and iris neovascularization to be associated with poor prognosis (37,273).

Recently, the majority of patients with unilateral retinoblastoma classified as Reese–Ellsworth groups I to IV have undergone chemoreduction or other focal, globe-sparing treatments (7,60,315,316). Similarly, patients with bilateral tumors are usually treated with chemoreduction for at least one of the involved eyes. Thus, increasingly, studies evaluating retinoblastoma prognosis examine not only patient mortality but also ocular salvage rates. Such rates have improved with the addition of chemoreduction protocols, with 85% of Reese–Ellsworth group I to IV eyes and 47% of group V eyes avoiding enucleation (although some advanced tumors required external beam radiation in addition to chemoreduction) (310). However, 24% of patients (mostly those presenting as infants with a family history of retinoblastoma) developed new tumor foci during or after their chemotherapy (314). Recurrence of tumor following chemoreduction can be reduced from 45% to 22% with the addition of focal tumor consolidation techniques such as cryotherapy, laser photocoagulation, plaque radiotherapy, and thermotherapy (312). The presence of subretinal tumor seeds at diagnosis was most predictive of tumor recurrence (82). Of note, despite the strong trend toward eye preservation in the management of retinoblastoma, an adverse effect on overall survival has not been observed (89,121). With more eyes with retinoblastoma being salvaged, Demirci and colleagues (82) performed a retrospective analysis to examine the long-term visual outcome following chemoreduction for retinoblastoma. They found over 50% of eyes maintained visual acuity of 20/40 or better, with predictors for good visual acuity being a tumor margin at least 3 mm from the foveola and optic disc and the absence of subretinal fluid.

REFERENCES

1. Abramson D. Retinoblastoma in the 20th century: past success and future challenges the Weisenfeld lecture. Invest Ophthalmol Vis Sci 2005; 46:2683–91.
2. Abramson D, Ellsworth R, Grumbach N, Kitchin F. Retinoblastoma: survival, age at detection and comparison 1914–1983. J Pediatr Ophthalmol Strabismus 1985; 22:246–50.
3. Abramson D, Ellsworth R, Grumbach N, Sturgis-Buckhout L, Haik B. Retinoblastoma: correlation between age at diagnosis and survival . J Pediatr Ophthalmol Strabismus 1986; 23:174–7.
4. Abramson D, Ellsworth R, Kitchin F, Tung G. Second nonocular tumors in retinoblastoma survivors. Are they radiation induced? Ophthalmology 1984; 91: 1351–5.
5. Abramson D, Greenfield D, Ellsworth R, et al. Neuron-specific enolase and retinoblastoma: clinicopathological correlations. Retina 1989; 9:148–52.
6. Abramson D, Schefler A. The Treatment of Retinoblastoma. In: Albert D, Polans A, eds. Ocular Oncology. New York, NY: Marcel Dekker, 2003:353–76.
7. Abramson D, Schefler A. Update on retinoblastoma. Retina 2004; 24:828–48.
8. Aherne G, Roberts DF. Retinoblastoma. A clinical survey and its genetic implications. Clin Genet 1975; 8:275–90.
9. Akiyama K, Iwasaki M, Amemiya T, Yanai M. Chemotherapy for retinoblastoma. Ophthalmic Pediatr Genet 1989; 10:111–6.
10. Al-Hajj M, Wicha M, Benito-Hernandez A, Morrison S, Clarke M. Prospective identification of tumorigenic breast cancer cells. Proc Natl Acad Sci USA 2003; 100: 3983–8.
11. Al-Idrissi I, Al-Kaff A, Senft S. Cumulative incidence of retinoblastoma in Riyadh, Saudi Arabia. Ophthalmic Pediatr Genet 1992; 13:9–12.
12. Albert D. The development of ophthalmic pathology. In: Albert D, Edwards D, eds. The History of Ophthalmology. Cambridge, MA: Blackwell Science, 1996:65–106.
13. Albert D. Historic review of retinoblastoma. Ophthalmology 1987; 94:654–62.
14. Albert D, Lahav M, Lesser R, Craft J. Recent observations regarding retinoblastoma. I. Ultrastructure, tissue culture growth, incidence and animal models. Trans Ophthalmol Soc UK 1974; 94:909–28.
15. Albert D, McGee C, Seddon J, Weichselbaum R. Development of additional primary tumors after 62 years in the first patient with retinoblastoma cured by radiation therapy. Am J Ophthalmol 1984; 97:189–96.
16. Albert D, Sang D, Craft J. Clinical and histopathologic observations regarding cell death and tumor necrosis in retinoblastoma. Jpn J Ophthalmol 1978; 22:358–74.
17. Alexander R, Spriggs A. The differential diagnosis of tumor cells in circulating blood. J Clin Pathol 1960; 13: 414–24.
18. Allen R, Latta H, Straatsma B. Retinoblastoma. Invest Ophthalmol Vis Sci 1962; 1:728–44.
19. Amendola B, Markoe A, Augsburger J, et al. Analysis of treatment results in 36 children with retinoblastoma treated by scleral plaque irradiation. Int J Radiat Oncol Biol Phys 1898; 17:63–70.
20. Antoneli C, Steinhorst F, Ribeiro K, et al. Extraocular retinoblastoma: a 13-year experience. Cancer 2003; 98: 1292–8.
21. Audo I, Sahel J. Molecular genetics of retinoblastoma. In: Albert D, Polans A, eds. Ocular Oncology. New York, NY: Marcel Dekker, 2003:449–63.
22. Augsburger J. Epidemiology of retinoblastoma. In: Albert D, Polans A, eds. Ocular Oncology. New York, NY: Marcel Dekker, 2003:47–61.
23. Augsburger J, Oehlschlager U, Manzitti J, RICS Group. Multinational clinical and pathologic registry of retinoblastoma. Retinoblastoma international collaborative study report 2. Graefes Arch Clin Exp Ophthalmol 1995; 233:469–75.
24. Augsburger J, Shields J, Goldberg R. Classification and management of hereditary retinal angiomas. Int Ophthalmol Clin 1985; 30:173–81.
25. Bader J, Meadows A, Zimmerman L, et al. Bilateral retinoblastoma with ectopic intracranial retinoblastoma: trilateral retinoblastoma. Cancer Genet Cytogenet 1982; 5: 203–13.
26. Bader J, Miller R, Meadows A, et al. Trilateral retinoblastoma. Lancet 1980; 2:582–3.

27. Bagley L, Hurst R, Zimmerman R, et al. Imaging in the trilateral retinoblastoma syndrome. Neuroradiology 1996; 38:166–70.
28. Bardenstein D, Rodrigues M, Alroy J, Brownstein S. Lectin binding in retinoblastoma. Curr Eye Res 1987; 6: 1141–50.
29. Barry G, Mullaney J. Retinoblastoma in the Republic of Ireland. Trans Ophthalmol Soc UK 1971; 91:839–55.
30. Bechrakis N, Bornfeld N, Schueler A, et al. Clinicopathologic features of retinoblastoma after primary chemoreduction. Arch Ophthalmol 1998; 116:887–93.
31. Bedford M. Treatment of retinoblastoma. Adv Ophthalmol 1975; 31:2–32.
32. Bedford M, Bedotto C, MacFaul P. Retinoblastoma: a study of 139 cases. Br J Ophthalmol 1971; 55:19–27.
33. Beemer J, Vlug A, van Veelen C, et al. Isoenzyme pattern of enolase of childhood tumors. Cancer 1984; 54:293–6.
34. Benedict W, Fung Y, Murphree A. The gene responsible for the development of retinoblastoma and osteosarcoma. Cancer 1988; 62(Suppl.):1691–4.
35. Benedict W, Murphree A, Banerjee A, et al. Patient with 13 chromosome deletion: evidence that the retinoblastoma gene is a recessive cancer gene. Science 1983; 219:973–5.
36. Benedict W, Xu H, Hu S, Takahashi T. Role of the retinoblastoma gene in the initiation and progression of human cancer. J Clin Invest 1990; 85:988–93.
37. Berkow R, Fleshman J. Retinoblastoma in Navajo Indian children. Am J Dis Child 1983; 137:137–8.
38. Bernstein S, Kutty G, Wiggert B, et al. Expression of retina-specific genes by mouse retinoblastoma cells. Invest Ophthalmol Vis Sci 1994; 35:3931–7.
39. Bogenmann E, Lochrie M, Simon M. Cone cell specific genes expressed in retinoblastoma. Science 1988; 240:76–8.
40. Boniuk M, Girard L. Spontaneous regression of bilateral retinoblastoma. Trans Am Acad Ophthalmol Otolaryngol 1969; 73:194–8.
41. Boniuk M, Zimmerman L. Spontaneous regression of retinoblastoma. Int Ophthalmol Clin 1962; 2:525–42.
42. Bonnet D, Dick J. Human acute myeloid leukemia is organized as a hierarchy that originates from a primitive hematopoietic cell. Nat Med 1997; 3:730–7.
43. Bonnin J, Rubenstein L. Immunohistochemistry of central nervous system tumors: its contributions to neurosurgical diagnosis. J Neurosurg 1984; 60:1121–33.
44. Bookstein R, Lee E, To H, et al. Human retinoblastoma susceptibility gene: genomic organization and analysis of heterozygous intragenic deletion mutants. Proc Natl Acad Sci USA 1988; 85:2210–4.
45. Brady L, Markoe A, Amendola B, et al. The treatment of primary intraocular malignancy. Int J Radiat Oncol Biol Phys 1988; 15:1355–61.
46. Brehm A, Miska E, McCance D, et al. Retinoblastoma protein recruits histone deacetylase to repress transcription. Nature 1998; 391:597–601.
47. Bridges C, Fong S, Landers R, et al. Interstitial retinobinding protein (IRBP) in retinoblastoma. Neurochem Int 1985; 7:875–81.
48. Brini A, Dhermy P, Sahel J. Oncology of the Eye and Adnexa. Dordrecht: Kluwer, 1990.
49. Bunin G, Emanuel B, Meadows A, et al. Frequency of 13q abnormalities among 203 patients with retinoblastoma. J Natl Cancer Inst 1989; 81:370–4.
50. Bunin G, Emanuel B, Meadows A, et al. Pre- and postconception factors associated with sporadic heritable and nonheritable retinoblastoma. Cancer Res 1989; 49: 5730–5.
51. Campbell M, Chader G. Retinoblastoma cells in tissue culture. Ophthalmic Pediatr Genet 1988; 9:171–99.
52. Campbell M, Karras P, Chader G. Y-79 retinoblastoma cells—isolation and characterization of clonal lineages. Exp Eye Res 1989; 48:75–85.
53. Canning S, Dryja T. Short, direct repeats at the breakpoints of deletions of the retinoblastoma gene. Proc Natl Acad Sci USA 1989; 86:5044–8.
54. Carbajal U. Metastasis in retinoblastoma. Am J Ophthalmol 1959; 48:47–69.
55. Cavenee W, Dryja T, Phillips R, et al. Expression of recessive alleles by chromosomal mechanisms in retinoblastoma. Nature 1983; 305:779–84.
56. Cavenee W, Hansen M, Nordenskjold M, et al. Genetic origin of mutations predisposing to retinoblastoma. Science 1985; 228:501–3.
57. Cavenee W, Koufos A, Hansen M. Recessive mutant genes predisposing to human cancer. Mutat Res 1986; 168:3–14.
58. Cavenee W, Murphree A, Shull M, et al. Prediction of familial predisposition to retinoblastoma. N Engl J Med 1986; 314:1201–7.
59. Cepko C, Austin C, Yang X, Alexiades M, Ezzeddine D. Cell fate determination in the vertebrate retina. Proc Natl Acad Sci USA 1996; 93:589–95.
60. Chan H, Gallie B, Munier F, Popovic M. Chemotherapy for retinoblastoma. Ophthalmol Clin North Am 2005; 18: 55–63.
61. Chantada G, Doz F, Antoneli C, et al. A proposal for an international retinoblastoma staging system. Pediatr Blood Cancer 2006; 47:801–5.
62. Char D. Clinical Ocular Oncology. New York, NY: Churchill-Livingstone, 1989.
63. Char D, Miller T. Fine needle biopsy in retinoblastoma. Am J Ophthalmol 1984; 97:686–90.
64. Chevez-Barrios P, Hurwitz M, Louie K, et al. Metastatic and nonmetastatic models of retinoblastoma. Am J Pathol 2000; 157:1405–12.
65. Cho E, Suh Y, Shin H. Trilateral retinoblastoma: a case report. J Korean Med Sci 2002; 17:137–40.
66. Choy K, Lee T, Cheung K, et al. Clinical implications of promoter hypermethylation in RASSF1A and MGMT in retinoblastoma. Neoplasia 2005; 7:200–6.
67. Choy K, Pang C, Wang J, et al. Microsatellite instability and MLH1 promoter methylation in human retinoblastoma. Invest Ophthalmol Vis Sci 2004; 45: 3404–9.
68. Choy K, Pang C, Yu C, et al. Loss of heterozygosity and mutations are the major mechanisms of Rb1 gene inactivation in Chinese with sporadic retinoblastoma. Hum Mutat 2002; 20:408.
69. Cohen M, Augsburger J, Shields J, et al. Cancer in relatives of retinoblastoma patients. Jpn J Ophthalmol 1989; 33:173–6.
70. Cohen R. Metachronous sarcomas in a patient with bilateral retinoblastomas—a case report. S Afr Med J 1989; 76:117–8.
71. Comings D. A general theory of carcinogenesis. Proc Natl Acad Sci USA 1973; 70:3324–8.
72. Conway R, Wheeler S, Murray T, et al. Retinoblastoma: animal models. Ophthalmol Clin North Am 2005; 18:25–39.
73. Cooper E, Riker J. Malignant lymphoma of the uveal tract. Am J Ophthalmol 1951; 34:1153–8.
74. Cowell J. One hundred years of retinoblastoma research from clinic to the gene and back again. Ophthalmic Pediatr Genet 1989; 10:75–88.
75. Cowell J. Should all patients with retinoblastoma be screened for chromosome deletions? Lancet 1987; 2:544–5.

76. Cowell J, Hungerford J, Rutland P, Jay M. Genetic and cytogenetic analysis of patients showing reduced esterase D levels and mental retardation from a survey of 500 individuals with retinoblastoma. Ophthalmic Pediatr Genet 1989; 10:117–28.
77. Cowell J, Rutland P, Hungerford J, Jay M. Deletion of chromosome 13q14 is transmissible and does not always predispose to retinoblastoma. Hum Genet 1988; 80:43–5.
78. Craft J, Sang D, Dryja T, et al. Glial cell component in retinoblastoma. Exp Eye Res 1985; 40:647–59.
79. Day R, Wright S, Koons A, Quigley M. XXX 21-trisomy and retinoblastoma. Lancet 1963; 2:154–5.
80. de Sutter E, Havers W, Hopping W, et al. The prognosis of retinoblastoma in terms of globe saving treatment: a computer assisted study, part 1. Ophthal Pediatr Genet 1987; 8:77–84.
81. Demirci H, Eagle R, Shields C, Shields J. Histopathologic findings in eyes with retinoblastoma treated only with chemoreduction. Arch Ophthalmol 2003; 121:1125–31.
82. Demirci H, Shields C, Meadows A, Shields J. Long-term visual outcome following chemoreduction for retinoblastoma. Arch Ophthalmol 2005; 123:1525–30.
83. DerKinderen D, Koten J, Nagelkerke N, et al. Nonocular cancer in patients with hereditary retinoblastoma and their relatives. Int J Cancer 1988; 41:499–504.
84. Detrick B, Chader G, Rodrigues M, et al. Coexpression of neuronal, glial, and major histocompatibility complex class I antigens on retinoblastoma cells. Cancer Res 1988; 48:1633–41.
85. Devesa S. The incidence of retinoblastoma. Am J Ophthalmol 1975; 80:263–5.
86. Dhillon A, Rode J. Patterns of staining for neuron specific enolase in benign and malignant melanocytic lesions of the skin. Diagn Histopathol 1982; 5:169–74.
87. Dias P, Shanmuganathan S, Rajartham M. Lactic dehydrogenase activity of aqueous humor in retinoblastoma. Am J Ophthalmol 1975; 79:697–8.
88. Dithmar S, Aaberg T, Grossniklaus H. Histopathologic changes in retinoblastoma after chemoreduction. Retina 2000; 20:33–6.
89. Dondey J, Staffieri S, McKenzie J, et al. Retinoblastoma in Victoria, 1976–2000: changing management trends and outcomes. Clin Experiment Ophthalmol 2004; 32: 354–9.
90. Donoso L, Folberg N, Arbizo V. Retinal S-antigen and retinoblastoma. A monoclonal antibody histopathologic study. Arch Ophthalmol 1985; 103:855–7.
91. Donoso L, Folberg N, Augsburger J, Shields J. Retinal S-antigen and retinoblastoma: a monoclonal antibody and flow cytometry study. Invest Ophthalmol Vis Sci 1985; 26: 568–71.
92. Donoso L, Hamm H, Dietzschold B, et al. Rhodopsin and retinoblastoma. Arch Ophthalmol 1986; 104:111–3.
93. Donoso L, Rorke L, Shields J, et al. S-antigen immunoreactivity in trilateral retinoblastoma. Am J Ophthalmol 1987; 103:57–62.
94. Donoso L, Shields C, Lee E. Immunohistochemistry of retinoblastoma. Ophthalmic Pediatr Genet 1989; 10:3–32.
95. Dryja T, Cavenee W, White R, et al. Homozygosity of chromosome 13 in retinoblastoma. N Engl J Med 1984; 310:550–3.
96. Dryja T, Friend S, Weinberg R. Genetic sequence that predisposes to retinoblastoma and osteosarcoma. Symp Fund Cancer Res 1986; 39:115–9.
97. Dryja T, Rapaport J, Epstein J, et al. Chromosome homozygosity in osteosarcoma without retinoblastoma. Am J Hum Genet 1986; 38:59–66.
98. Dryja T, Rapaport J, Joyce J, Petersen R. Molecular detection of deletions involving band q14 of chromosome 13 in retinoblastoma. Proc Natl Acad Sci USA 1986; 83:7391–4.
99. Duke-Elder S. System of Ophthalmology, vol. XII, Diseases of the Lens and Vitreous: Glaucoma and Hypotony. St. Louis, MO: C.V. Mosby, 1969:637–40.
100. Dunphy E. The story of retinoblastoma. Trans Am Acad Ophthalmol Otolaryngol 1964; 68:249–64.
101. Dyer M, Bremner R. The search for the retinoblastoma cell of origin. Nat Rev Cancer 2005; 5:91–101.
102. Eagle R, Shields J, Donoso L, Milner R. Malignant transformation of spontaneously regressed retinoblastoma, retinoma/retinocytoma variant. Ophthalmology 1989; 96:1389–95.
103. Ellsworth R. Current concepts in the treatment of retinoblastoma. In: Peyman G, Apple D, Sanders D, eds. Intraocular Tumors. New York, NY: Appleton-Century-Crofts, 1977:335–55.
104. Ellsworth R. Orbital retinoblastoma. Trans Am Ophthalmol Soc 1974; 72:79–88.
105. Ellsworth R. The practical management of retinoblastoma. Trans Am Ophthalmol Soc 1969; 67:463–534.
106. Ellsworth R. Treatment of retinoblastoma. Am J Ophthalmol 1968; 66:49–51.
107. Epstein J, Shields C, Shields J. Trends in the management of retinoblastoma: evaluation of 1,196 consecutive eyes during 1974–2001. J Paediatr Ophthalmol Strabismus 2003; 40:196–203.
108. Fan B, Tam P, Choy K, et al. Molecular diagnostics of genetic eye diseases. Clin Biochem 2006; 39:231–9.
109. Felberg N, Donoso L. Surface cytoplasmic antigens in retinoblastoma. Invest Ophthalmol Vis Sci 1980; 19: 1242–5.
110. Ferreira R, Magnaghi-Jaulin L, Robin P, et al. The three members of the pocket proteins family share the ability to repress E2F activity through recruitment of a histone deacetylase. Proc Natl Acad Sci USA 1998; 95:10493–8.
111. Finger P, Harbour J, Karcioglu Z. Risk factors for metastasis in retinoblastoma. Surv Ophthalmol 2002; 47: 1–16.
112. Flexner S. A peculiar glioma (neuroepithelioma) of the retina. Bull Johns Hopkins Hosp 1891; 2:115–9.
113. Fong S, Balakier H, Canton M, et al. Retinoid binding proteins in retinoblastoma tumors. Cancer Res 1988; 48: 1124–8.
114. Francois J, Matton M, Debie S, et al. Genesis and genetics of retinoblastoma. Ophthalmologica 1975; 170:405–25.
115. Friend S, Bernards R, Rogelj S, et al. A human DNA segment with properties of the gene that predisposes to retinoblastoma and osteosarcoma. Nature 1986; 323:643–6.
116. Fung Y, Murphree A, Tang A, et al. Structural evidence for the authenticity of the human retinoblastoma gene. Science 1987; 236:1657–61.
117. Gallie B, Erraguntla V, Heon E, et al. Retinoblastoma. In: Taylor D, Hoyt C, eds. Pediatric Ophthalmology and Strabismus. New York, NY: Elsevier, 2005:486–505.
118. Gallie B, Phillips R, Ellsworth R, et al. Significance of retinoma and phthisis bulbi for retinoblastoma. Ophthalmology 1982; 89:1393–9.
119. Gallie B, Squire J, Goddard J, et al. Mechanisms of oncogenesis in retinoblastoma. Lab Invest 1990; 62: 394–408.
120. Gass J. Stereoscopic Atlas of Macular Disease. 3rd ed. St. Louis, MO: C.V. Mosby, 1987:654–7.
121. Gatta C, Capocaccia R, Stiller C, et al. Childhood cancer survival trends in Europe: a EUROCARE Working Group study. J Clin Oncol 2005; 23:3742–51.

122. Ghandour M, Langley O, Keller A. A comparative immunohistological study of cerebellar enolases. Double labelling technique and immunoelectronmicroscopy. Exp Brain Res 1981; 41:271–9.
123. Gifford A, Sorsby A. The genetics of retinoblastoma. Br J Ophthalmol 1944; 28:279–93.
124. Godbout R, Dryja T, Squire J, et al. Somatic inactivation of genes on chromosome 13 is a common event in retinoblastoma. Nature 1983; 304:451–3.
125. Gonzalez-Fernandez F, Lopes M, Garcia-Fernandez J, et al. Expression of developmentally defined retinal phenotypes in the histogenesis of retinoblastoma. Am J Pathol 1992; 141:363–75.
126. Gonzalo S, Garcia-Cao M, Fraga M, et al. Role of the RB1 family in stabilizing histone methylation at constitutive heterochromatin. Nat Cell Biol 2005; 7:420–8.
127. Greger V, Kerst S, Messmer E, et al. Application of linkage analysis to genetic counselling in families with hereditary retinoblastoma. J Med Genet 1988; 25:217–21.
128. Groover J, Rogers A. Immunologic tests for the detection of gastrointestinal cancers: status report on carcinoembryonic antigen (CEA) and alpha-fetoprotein (AFP). South Med J 1973; 66:1218–21.
129. Gu J, Polak J, Noorden V, et al. Immunostaining of neuron specific enolase as a diagnostic tool for Merckel cell tumors. Cancer 1983; 52:1039–43.
130. Gurney J, Severson R, Davis S, Robison L. Incidence of cancer in children in the United States. Sex-, race- and 1-year age-specific rates by histologic type. Cancer 1995; 75:2186–95.
131. Haik B, Dunleavy S, Cooke C, et al. Retinoblastoma with anterior chamber extension. Ophthalmology 1987; 94: 367–70.
132. Hansen M, Cavenee W. Retinoblastoma and the progression of tumor genetics. Trends Genet 1988; 4:123–9.
133. Hansen M, Koufos A, Gallie B, et al. Osteosarcoma and retinoblastoma: a shared chromosomal mechanism recessive predisposition. Proc Natl Acad Sci USA 1985; 82: 6216–20.
134. Harbour J. Overview of RB gene mutations in patients with retinoblastoma, implications for clinical genetic screening. Ophthalmology 1998; 105:1442–7.
135. Harbour J, Lai S, Whang-Peng J, et al. Abnormalities in the structure and expression of human retinoblastoma gene in SCLC. Science 1988; 241:353–7.
136. Helveston E, Knuth K, Ellis F. Retinoblastoma. J Paediatr Ophthalmol Strabismus 1987; 24:296–300.
137. Hemmes G. Untersuchung nach dem Vorkommen von Glioma retinae bei Verwandten von mit dieser Krankheit Behafteten. Klin Montasbl Augenheilkd 1931; 86:331–5.
138. Herm R, Heath P. A study of retinoblastoma. Am J Ophthalmol 1956; 41:22–30.
139. Higgins M, Hansen M, Cavenee W, Lalande M. Molecular detection of chromosomal translocations that disrupt the putative retinoblastoma susceptibility locus. Mol Cell Biol 1989; 9:1–5.
140. Hogan M, Zimmerman L. Ophthalmic Pathology: An Atlas and Textbook. 2nd ed. Philadelphia, PA: W.B. Saunders, 1962:516–34.
141. Hong F, Huang H, To H, et al. Structure of the retinoblastoma gene. Proc Natl Acad Sci USA 1989; 86:5502–6.
142. Hopping W. The new Essen prognosis classification for conservative sight-saving treatment of retinoblastoma. In: Lommatzsch P, Blodi F, eds. Intraocular Tumors: International Symposium under the Auspices of the European Ophthalmological Society. Berlin: Springer-Verlag, 1983:497–505.
143. Horowitz J, Park S, Bogenmann E, et al. Frequent inactivation of the retinoblastoma anit-oncogene is restricted to a subset of human tumor cells. Proc Natl Acad Sci USA 1990; 87:2775–9.
144. Horowitz J, Yandell D, Park S, et al. Point mutational inactivation of the retinoblastoma anti-oncogene. Science 1989; 243:937–40.
145. Horven I. Retinoblastoma in Norway. Acta Ophthalmol 1973; 6:103–9.
146. Horwarth C, Meyer D, Husto H, et al. Stage-related combined modality treatment of retinoblastoma: results of a prospective study. Cancer 1980; 45:851–8.
147. Howard G. Ocular effects of radiation and photocoagulation. Arch Ophthalmol 1966; 76:7–10.
148. Howard R, Ellsworth R. Differential diagnosis of retinoblastoma: a statistical survey of 500 children. II. Factors relating to the diagnosis of retinoblastoma. Am J Ophthalmol 1965; 60:618–21.
149. Howard R, Ellsworth R. Findings in the peripheral fundi of patients with retinoblastoma. Am J Ophthalmol 1966; 62:243–51.
150. Howard R, Warburton D, Breg W, et al. Retinoblastoma and partial deletion of the long arm of chromosome 13. Trans Am Ophthalmol Soc 1978; 76:172–83.
151. Huang Q, Choy K, Cheung K, et al. Genetic alterations on Chromosome 19, 20, 21, 22, and X detected by loss of heterozygosity analysis in retinoblastoma. Mol Vis 2003; 9:502–7.
152. Ibarra M, O'Brien J. Is screening for primitive neuroectodermal tumours in patients with unilateral retinoblastoma necessary? AAPOS 2000; 4:54–6.
153. Jafek B, Lindford R, Foos R. Late recurrent retinoblastoma in the nasal vestibule. Arch Otolaryngol 1971; 94:264–7.
154. Jakobiec F, Ts'o M, Zimmerman L, Danis P. Retinoblastoma and intracranial malignancy. Cancer 1977; 39:2048–58.
155. Jay M. Deficiencies of group D chromosome. The Eye in Chromosomal Duplications and Deficiencies. New York, NY: Marcel Dekker, 1977:77–100.
156. Jay M, Cowell J, Kingston J, Hungerford J. Demonstration of bias in an early series of retinoblastoma. Ophthalmic Pediatr Genet 1989; 10:89–92.
157. Jensen R, Miller R. Retinoblastoma: epidemiologic characteristics. N Engl J Med 1971; 285:307–11.
158. Johnson D, Chandra R, Fisher W, et al. Trilateral retinoblastoma: ocular and pineal retinoblastomas. J Neurosurg 1985; 63:367–70.
159. Kabak J, Romano P. Aqueous humor lactic dehydrogenase isoenzyme in retinoblastoma. Br J Ophthalmol 1975; 59:268–9.
160. Karcioglu Z, Haik B, Gordon R. Frozen section of the optic nerve in retinoblastoma surgery. Ophthalmology 1988; 95:674–6.
161. Karim M, Itoh H. Demonstration of S-100 protein immunoreactivity in normal human retina and retinoblastoma. Ophthalmologica 1997; 211:351–3.
162. Karim M, Yamamoto M, Itoh H. Retinoblastoma: clinical and immunocytochemical observations. Kobe J Med Sci 1996; 42:151–61.
163. Karsgaard A. Spontaneous regression of retinoblastoma: a report of two cases. Can J Ophthalmol 1971; 6: 218–22.
164. Keith C. Chemotherapy in retinoblastoma management. Ophthalmic Pediatr Genet 1989; 10:93–8.
165. Kenney L, Miller B, Gloeckler RL, et al. Increased incidence of cancer in infants in the US: 1980–1990. Cancer 1998; 82:1396–400.

166. Khandekar R, Ganesh A, Al Lawati J. A 12-year epidemiological review of retinoblastoma in Omani children. Ophthalmic Epidemiol 2004; 11:151–9.
167. Kivela T. Antigenic Properties of Retinoblastoma Tissue. Finland: University of Helsinki, 1987.
168. Kivela T. Expression of the HNK-1 carbohydrate epitope in human retina and retinoblastoma. An immunohistochemical study with the anti-Leu-7 monoclonal antibody. Virchows Arch A Pathol Anat Histopathol 1986; 410:139–46.
169. Kivela T. Neuron-specific enolase in retinoblastoma. An immunohistochemical study. Acta Ophthalmol (Copenh.) 1986; 64:19–25.
170. Kivela T. Parvalbumin, a horizontal cell-associated calcium-binding protein in retinoblastoma eyes. Invest Ophthalmol Vis Sci 1998; 39:1044–8.
171. Kivela T. Trilateral retinoblastoma: a meta-analysis of hereditary retinoblastoma associated with primary ectopic intracranial retinoblastoma. J Clin Oncol 1999; 17: 1829–37.
172. Kivela T, Tarkkanen A. Carcinoembryonic antigen in retinoblastoma. An immunohistochemical study. Graefes Arch Clin Exp Ophthalmol 1983; 221:8–11.
173. Kivela T, Tarkkanen A. S-100 protein in retinoblastoma revisited. Acta Ophthalmol (Copenh.) 1986; 64:664–73.
174. Kivela T, Tarkkanen A, Virtanen I. Intermediate filaments in the human retina and retinocytoma: an immunohistochemical study of vimentin, glial fibrillary acidic protein, and neurofilaments. Invest Ophthalmol Vis Sci 1986; 27: 1075–84.
175. Kivela T, Tarkkanen A, Virtanen I. Synaptophysin in the human retina and retinoblastoma: an immunohistochemical and western blotting study. Invest Ophthalmol Vis Sci 1989; 30:212–9.
176. Kleinerman R, Tucker M, Tarone R, et al. Risk of new cancers after radiotherapy in long-term survivors of retinoblastoma: an extended follow-up. J Clin Oncol 2005; 23:2272–9.
177. Klintworth G. Radiographic abnormalities in eyes with retinoblastoma and other disorders. Br J Ophthalmol 1978; 62:365–72.
178. Knudson A. Genetics and the etiology of childhood cancer. Pediatr Res 1976; 10:513–7.
179. Knudson A. The genetics of childhood cancer. Cancer 1975; 35:1022–6.
180. Knudson A. Hereditary cancer, oncogenes, and antioncogenes. Cancer Res 1985; 45:1437–43.
181. Knudson A. Mutation and cancer: statistical study of retinoblastoma. Proc Natl Acad Sci USA 1971; 68:820–3.
182. Knudson A. Persons at high risk of cancer. N Engl J Med 1979; 301:606–7.
183. Knudson A, Hethcote H, Brown B. Mutation and childhood cancer. A probabilistic model for the incidence of retinoblastoma. Proc Natl Acad Sci USA 1975; 72:5116–20.
184. Knudson A, Meadows A, Nichols W, Hill R. Chromosomal deletion and retinoblastoma. N Engl J Med 1976; 295: 1120–3.
185. Knudson A, Strong L. Mutation and cancer: a model for Wilms' tumor of the kidney. J Natl Cancer Inst 1973; 48: 313–24.
186. Knudson AJ. Mutation and cancer: statistical study of retinoblastoma. Proc Natl Acad Sci USA 1971; 68:820–3.
187. Kobayashi S, Sawada T, Mukai S. Immunohistochemical evidence of neuron specific enolase (NSE) in human adenovirus 12 induced retinoblastoma-like tumor cells in vitro. Acta Histochem Cytol 1985; 18: 551–6.
188. Kock E, Naeser P. Retinoblastoma in Sweden 1958–1971: a clinical and histopathological study. Acta Ophthalmol 1979; 57:344–350.
189. Kondo T, Setoguchi T, Taga T. Persistence of a small subpopulation of cancer stem-like cells in the C6 glioma cell line. Proc Natl Acad Sci USA 2004; 101:781–6.
190. Kopelman J, McLean I, Rosenberg S. Multivariate analysis of risk factors for metastasis in retinoblastoma treated by enucleation. Ophthalmology 1987; 94: 371–7.
191. Korswagen L, Moll A, Imhof S, et al. A second primary tumor in a patient with retinoma. Ophthal Genet 2004; 25: 45–8.
192. Kyritsis A, Tsokos M, Triche T, Chader G. Retinoblastoma—origin from a primitive neuroectodermal cell? Nature 1984; 307:471–3.
193. Kyritsis A, Weichman A, Bok D, Chader G. Hydroxyindole-*O*-methyltranserase in Y-79 human retinoblastoma cells: effect of cell attachment. J Neurochem 1987; 48:1612–6.
194. Lane J, Klintworth G. A study of astrocytes in retinoblastomas using the immunoperoxidase technique and antibodies to glial fibrillary acidic protein. Am J Ophthalmol 1982; 95:197–207.
195. Lapidot T, Sirard C, Vormoor J, et al. A cell initiating huma acute myeloid leukaemia after transplantation into SCID mice. Nature 1994; 367:645–8.
196. Lee E, Bookstein R, Young L, et al. Molecular mechanisms of retinoblastoma gene inactivation in retinoblastoma cell line Y-79. Proc Natl Acad Sci USA 1988; 85: 6017–21.
197. Lee E, To H, Shew J, et al. Inactivation of the retinoblastoma susceptibility gene. Science 1988; 241:218–22.
198. Lee W, Bookstein R, Hong F, et al. Human retinoblastoma susceptibility gene: cloning, identification, and sequence. Science 1987; 235:1395–7.
199. Lee W, Bookstein R, Lee E. Studies of the human retinoblastoma susceptibility gene. J Cell Biochem 1988; 38:213–27.
200. Lindley-Smith J. Histology and spontaneous regression of retinoblastoma. Trans Ophthalmol Soc UK 1974; 94: 953–67.
201. Livesey F, Cepko C. Vertebrate neural cell-fate determination: lessons from the retina. Nat Rev Neurosci 2001; 2: 109–18.
202. Lohmann D. RB1 gene mutations in retinoblastoma. Hum Mutat 1999; 14:283–8.
203. Lueder G. The effect of initial recognition of abnormalities by physicians on outcome of retinoblastoma. J AAPOS 2005; 9:383–5.
204. Lueder G, Judisch F, O'Gorman T. Second nonocular tumors in survivors of heritable retinoblastoma. Arch Ophthalmol 1986; 104:372–3.
205. Luo R, Postigo A, Dean D. Rb interacts with histone deacetylase to repress transcription. Cell 1998; 92:463–73.
206. Macchi M, Bruce J. Human pineal physiology and functional significance of melatonin. Front Neuroendocrinol 2004; 25:177–95.
207. Macklin M. A study of retinoblastoma in Ohio. Am J Hum Genet 1960; 12:1–43.
208. Madreperla S, Whittum-Hudson J, Prendergast R, et al. Suppression of intraocular retinoblastoma xenograft growth by the retinoblastoma gene. Invest Ophthalmol Vis Sci 1991; 32(Suppl.):981.
209. Mafee M, Goldberg M, Cohen S, et al. Magnetic resonance imaging versus computed tomography of leukocoric eyes and use of in vitro proton magnetic resonance spectroscopy of retinoblastoma. Ophthalmology 1989; 96:965–76.

210. Magnaghi-Jaulin L, Groisman R, Naguibneva I, et al. Retinoblastoma protein represses transcription by recruiting a histone deacetylase. Nature 1998; 391:601–5.
211. Magramm I, Abramson D, Ellsworth R. Optic nerve involvement in retinoblastoma. Ophthalmology 1989; 96: 217–22.
212. Marangos P, Schmechel D, Zis A, Goodwin F. The existence and neurobiological significance of neuronal and glial forms of the glycolytic enzyme enolase. Biol Psychiatry 1979; 14:563–79.
213. Marback E, Arias V, Paranhos A, et al. Tumour angiogenesis as a prognostic factor for disease dissemination in retinoblastoma. Br J Ophthalmol 2003; 87:1224–8.
214. Marcus D, Brooks S, Leff G, et al. Trilateral retinoblastoma: insights into histogenesis and management. Surv Ophthalmol 1998; 43:59–70.
215. Marcus D, Craft J, Albert D. Histopathologic verification of Verhoeff's 1918 irradiation cure of retinoblastoma. Ophthalmology 1990; 97:221–4.
216. Margo C, Hidayat A, Kopelman J, Zimmerman L. Retinocytoma. A benign variant of retinoblastoma. Arch Ophthalmol 1983; 101:1519–31.
217. Margo C, Lavellee M. Gamma-enolase activity in choroidal melanoma. Graefes Arch Clin Exp Ophthalmol 1986; 224:374–6.
218. McGee T, Yandell D, Dryja T. Structure and partial genomic sequence of the human retinoblastoma susceptibility gene. Gene 1989; 80:119–28.
219. McLean I. Retinoblastoma: pathology and prognosis. In: Albert D, Polans A, eds. Ocular Oncology. New York, NY: Marcel Dekker, 2003:427–47.
220. McNeish I, Bell S, Lemoine N. Gene therapy progress and prospects: cancer gene therapy using tumour suppressor genes. Gene Ther 2004; 11:497–503.
221. Meadows A. Risk factors for second malignant neoplasms: report from the late effects study group. Bull Cancer 1988; 75:125–30.
222. Merriam G. Retinoblastoma, analysis of 17 autopsies. Arch Ophthalmol 1950; 44:71–108.
223. Messmer E, Font R, Kirkpatrick J, Hopping W. Immunohistochemical demonstration of neuronal and astrocytic differentiation in retinoblastoma. Ophthalmology 1985; 92:167–73.
224. Meur G, Flament-Durand J, Denis R, Verougstraete C. Tumeur retinienne et tumeur cerebrale: a propos d'un cas. Bull Soc Belge Ophtalmol 1971; 159:661–70.
225. Michelson J, Felberg N, Shields J. Fetal antigens in retinoblastoma. Cancer 1976; 37:719–23.
226. Mietz H, Hutton W, Font R. Unilateral retinoblastoma in an adult. Report of a case and review of the literature. Ophthalmology 1997; 104:43–7.
227. Mikolajewski V, Messmer E, Sauerwain W, Freundlieb O. Orbital computed tomography. Does it help in diagnosing the infiltration of choroid, sclera, and/or optic nerve in retinoblastoma. Ophthalmic Pediatr Genet 1987; 8:101–4.
228. Miller R. Fifty-two forms of childhood cancer: United States mortality experience 1960–1966. J Pediatr 1969; 75: 685–9.
229. Miller R. Neoplasia and Down's syndrome. Ann NY Acad Sci 1970; 171:637–45.
230. Minei M, Yamana Y, Ohnishi Y. Carcinoembryonic antigens and alpha foeto-protein levels in retinoblastoma. Jpn J Ophthalmol 1983; 27:185–92.
231. Misrhahi M, Boucheix C, Dhermy P, et al. Expression of photoreceptor-specific S-antigen in human retinoblastoma. Cancer 1986; 57:1497–500.
232. Mitchell C. Second malignant neoplasms in retinoblastoma. Ophthalmic Pediatr Genet 1988; 9:161–5.
233. Mohan A, Kandalam M, Ramkumar H, et al. Stem cell markers: ABCG2 and MCM2 expression in retinoblastoma. Br J Ophthalmol 2006; 90:889–93.
234. Mohney B, Robertson D, Schomberg P, Hodge D. Second nonocular tumors in survivors of heritable retinoblastoma and prior radiation therapy. Am J Ophthalmol 1998; 126:269–77.
235. Moll A, Kuik D, Bouter L, et al. Incidence and survival of retinoblastoma in the Netherlands: a register based study 1862–1995. Br J Ophthalmol 1997; 81:559–62.
236. Molnar M, Stefansson K, Marton L, et al. Immunohistochemistry of retinoblastoma in humans. Am J Ophthalmol 1984; 97:301–7.
237. Moro F, Secchi A, Moschini G, et al. Retinoblastoma. Combined treatment of 21 cases. Critical review of the results. Ophthalmic Pediatr Genet 1989; 10:107–10.
238. Morris E, Dyson N. Retinoblastoma protein partners. Adv Cancer Res 2001; 82:1–54.
239. Morris E, LaPiana F. Spontaneous regression of bilateral retinoblastoma with preservation of normal visual acuity. Ann Ophthalmol 1974; 6:1192–94.
240. Mouratova T. Trilateral retinoblastoma: a literature review, 1971–2004. Bull Soc Belge Ophtalmol 2005; 297: 25–35.
241. Mukai S, Rapaport J, Shields J, et al. Linkage of genes for human esterase D and hereditary retinoblastoma. Am J Ophthalmol 1984; 97:681–5.
242. Mullaney J. DNA in retinoblastoma. Lancet 1968; 2:918.
243. Munier F, Pescia G, Jotterand-Bellomo M, et al. Constitutional karyotype in retinoblastoma. Case report and review of literature. Ophthalmic Pediatr Genet 1989; 10:129.
244. Murphree A. Intraocular retinoblastoma: the case for a new group classification. Ophthalmol Clin North Am 2005; 18:41–53.
245. Murphree A, Benedict W. Retinoblastoma: clues to human oncogenesis. Science 1984; 223:1028–33.
246. Murphree A, Rother C. Retinoblastoma. In: Ryan J, ed. Retina. St. Louis: C.V. Mosby, 1989:517–56.
247. Musarella M, Gallie B. A simplified scheme for genetic counseling in retinoblastoma. J Pediatr Ophthalmol 1987; 24:124–5.
248. Nakajima T, Kato K, Kaneko A, et al. High concentration of enolase, alpha and Y-subunits in the aqueous humor in cases of retinoblastoma. Am J Ophthalmol 1986; 101: 102–6.
249. Narita M, Nunez S, Heard E, et al. Rb-mediated heterochromatin formation and silencing of E2F target genes during cellular senescence. Cell 2003; 113:703–16.
250. Naumova A, Sapienza C. The genetics of retinoblastoma, revisited. Am J Hum Genet 1994; 54:264–73.
251. Nehen J. Spontaneous regression of retinoblastoma. Acta Ophthalmol (Copenh.) 1975; 53:647–51.
252. Nielsen S, Schneider R, Bauer U, et al. Rb targets histone H3 methylation and HP1 to promoters. Nature 2001; 412: 561–5.
253. Nork T, Millecchia L, de Venecia G, et al. Immunocytochemical features of retinoblastoma in an adult. Arch Ophthalmol 1996; 114:1402–6.
254. Nork T, Schwartz T, Doshi H, Millecchia L. Retinoblastoma: cell of origin. Arch Ophthalmol 1995; 113:791–802.
255. Novakovic B. U.S. childhood cancer survival, 1973–1987. Med Pediatr Oncol 1994; 23:480–6.

256. O'Day J, Billson F, Hoyt C. Retinoblastoma in Victoria. Med J Aust 1977; 2:428–32.
257. Odelstad L, Pahlman S, Bilsson K, et al. Neuron-specific enolase in relation to differentiation in human neuroblastoma. Brain Res 1981; 224:69–82.
258. Osborn M, Weber K. Tumor diagnosis by intermediate filament typing: a novel tool for surgical pathology. Lab Invest 1983; 48:372–94.
259. Pardal R, Clarke M, Morrison S. Applying the principles of stem-cell biology to cancer. Nat Rev Cancer 2003; 3: 895–902.
260. Paulino A. Trilateral retinoblastoma: is the location of the intracranial tumor important? Cancer 1999; 86:135–41.
261. Pendergrass T, Davis S. Incidence of retinoblastoma in the United States. Arch Ophthalmol 1980; 98:1204–10.
262. Perentes E, Herbort C, Rubinstein L, et al. Immunohistochemical characterization of human retinoblastoma in situ with multiple markers. Am J Ophthalmol 1987; 103: 647–58.
263. Perentes E, Rubinstein L. Immunohistochemical recognition of human neuroepithelial tumors by anti-leu 7 (HNK-1) monoclonal antibody. Acta Neuropathol (Berl.) 1986; 69:227–33.
264. Pesin S, Shields J. Seven cases of trilateral retinoblastoma. Am J Ophthalmol 1989; 107:121–6.
265. Peyster R, Augsburger J, Shields J, et al. Intraocular tumors: evaluation with MR imaging. Radiology 1988; 168:773–9.
266. Pfeiffer R. Roentgenographic diagnosis of retinoblastoma. Arch Ophthalmol 1936; 15: 811–21.
267. Plotsky D, Quinn G, Eagle R, et al. Congenital retinoblastoma: a case report. J Pediatr Ophthalmol Strabismus 1987; 24:120–3.
268. Pratt C, Fontanesi J, Lu X, et al. Proposal for a new staging scheme for intraocular and extraocular retinoblastoma based on an analysis of 103 globes. Oncologist 1997; 2:1–5.
269. Pratt C, George S. Second malignant neoplasms among children and adolescents treated for cancer. Proc Am Assoc Cancer Res 1981; 22:151.
270. Pratt C, Meyer D, Chenaille P, Crom D. The use of bone marrow aspirations and lumbar punctures at the time of diagnosis of retinoblastoma. J Clin Oncol 1989; 7: 140–3.
271. Prochownik E. Functional and physical communication between oncoproteins and tumor suppressors. Cell Mol Life Sci 2005; 62:2438–59.
272. Rapin A, Burger M. Tumor cell surfaces. Adv Cancer Res 1974; 20:1–91.
273. Redler L, Ellsworth R. Prognostic importance of choroidal invasion in retinoblastoma. Arch Ophthalmol 1973; 90: 294–6.
274. Reese A. Tumors of the Eye. 3rd ed. New York, NY: Harper & Row, 1976:89–132.
275. Reese A, Ellsworth R. The evaluation and current concept of retinoblastoma therapy. Trans Am Acad Ophthalmol Otolaryngol 1963; 67:164–72.
276. Reid T, Russell P. Recent observations regarding retinoblastoma. II. An enzyme study of retinoblastoma. Trans Ophthalmol Soc UK 1974; 94:929–37.
277. Renelt P, Trieschmann W. Vanilmandelic acid urinary excretion in the diagnostic of retinoblastoma. Graefes Arch Clin Exp Ophthalmol 1973; 188:281–3.
278. Reya T, Morrison S, Clarke M, Weissman I. Stem cells, cancer, and cancer stem cells. Nature 2001; 414:105–11.
279. Rider C, Taylor C. Enolase isoenzymes in rat tissues. Electrophoretic, chromatographic, immunological and kinetic properties. Biochim Biophys Acta 1974; 365: 285–300.
280. Riedel K. Hypertherme Therapieverfahren in Erganzung zur Strahlenbehandlung maligner intraokularer Tumoren. Klin Montasbl Augenheilkd 1988; 193:131–7.
281. Roarty J, McLean I, Zimmerman L. Incidence of second neoplasms in patients with retinoblastoma. Ophthalmology 1988; 95:1583–7.
282. Rodrigues M, Bardenstein D, Donoso L, et al. An immunohistopathologic study of trilateral retinoblastoma. Am J Ophthalmol 1987; 103:776–81.
283. Rodrigues M, Wiggert B, Shields J, et al. Retinoblastoma. Immunohistochemistry and cell differentiation. Ophthalmology 1987; 94:378–87.
284. Rodrigues M, Wilson M, Wiggert B, et al. Retinoblastoma. A clinical, immunohistochemical, and electron microscopic case report. Ophthalmology 1986; 93:1010–5.
285. Romano P, Kabak J. Aqueous humor lactic acid dehydrogenase in retinoblastoma. Am J Ophthalmol 1975; 79: 697–8.
286. Rosengren B, Monge O, Flage T. Proposal of a new pretreatment clinical TNM-classification of retinoblastoma. Acta Oncol 1989; 28:547–8.
287. Royds J, Parsons M, Rennie I, et al. Enolase isoenzymes in benign and malignant melanocytic lesions. Diagn Histopathol 1982; 5:175–81.
288. Royds J, Parsons M, Taylor C, Timperley W. Enolase isoenzyme distribution in the human brain and its tumors. J Pathol 1982; 137:37–49.
289. Rubenstein L. Embryonal central neuroepithelial tumors and their differentiating potential: a cytogenetic view of a complex neuro-oncological problem. J Neurosurg 1985; 62:795–805.
290. Rubin C, Robinson L, Camerson J, et al. Intraocular retinoblastoma group V: an analysis of prognostic factors. J Clin Oncol 1985; 3:680–5.
291. Russell D, Rubinstein L. Pathology of the Nervous System. 4th ed. Baltimore, MD: Williams and Wilkins, 1977:299–330.
292. Sahel J, Brini A, Albert D. Pathology of the retina and vitreous: retinoblastoma. In: Albert D, Jakobiec F, eds. Principles and Practice of Ophthalmology, vol. 6. 2nd ed. Philadelphia, PA: W.B. Saunders, 2000:3750–92.
293. Sahel J, Frederick A, Pesavento R, Albert D. Idiopathic retinal gliosis mimicking a choroidal melanoma. Retina 1988; 8:282–7.
294. Sahel R, Gross S, Cassano W, Gee A. Metastatic retinoblastoma successfully treated with immunomagnetically purged autologous bone marrow transplantation. Cancer 1988; 62:2301–3.
295. Salim A, Wiknjosastro G, Danukusumo D, et al. Fetal retinoblastoma. J Ultrasound Med 1998; 17:717–20.
296. Salsbury A, Bedford M, Dobree H. Bone marrow appearances in children suffering from retinoblastoma. Br J Ophthalmol 1968; 52:388–95.
297. Sanders B, Draper G, Kingston J. Retinoblastoma in Great Britain 1969–80: incidence, treatment, and survival. Br J Ophthalmol 1988; 72:576–83.
298. Sang D, Albert D. Catecholamine levels in retinoblastoma. In: Jakobiec F, ed. Ocular and Adnexal Tumors. Birmingham, AL: Aesculapius, 1978:172–80.
299. Sang D, Albert D. Recent advances in the study of retinoblastoma. In: Peyman G, Apple D, Sanders D, eds. Intraocular Tumors. New York, NY: Appleton-Century-Crofts, 1977:285–329.
300. Sant M, Capocaccia R, Badioni V. Survival for retinoblastoma in Europe. Eur J Cancer 2001; 37:730–5.

301. Sasaki A, Ogawa A, Nakazato Y, Ishida Y. Distribution of neuro-filament protein and neuron-specific enolase in peripheral tumors. Virchows Arch A Pathol Anat Histopathol 1985; 407:33–41.
302. Saw S, Tan N, Lee S, et al. Incidence and survival characteristics of retinoblastoma in Singapore from 1968–1995. J Paediatr Ophthalmol Strabismus 2000; 37:87–93.
303. Schappert-Kimmijser J, Hemmes G, Nijland R. The heredity of retinoblastoma. Ophthalmologica 1966; 151: 197–213.
304. Schipper J. Retinoblastoma: A Medical and Experimental Study. PhD thesis. The Netherlands: University of Utrecht, 1980.
305. Schmechel D, Marangos P, Zis A, et al. Brain enolases as specific markers of neuronal and glial cells. Science 1978; 199:313–5.
306. Schouten van Meeteren A, van der Valk P, van der Linden H, et al. Histopathologic features of retinoblastoma and its relation with in vitro drug resistance measured by means of the MTT assay. Cancer 2001; 92: 2933–40.
307. Schulman J, Peyman G, Mafee M, et al. The use of magnetic resonance imaging in the evaluation of retinoblastoma. J Pediatr Ophthalmol Strabismus 1986; 23:144–7.
308. Seigel G, Campbell L, Narayan M, et al. Cancer stem cell characteristics in retinoblastoma. Mol Vis 2005; 11: 729–37.
309. Seregard S, Lundell G, Svedberg H, Kivel T. Incidence of retinoblastoma from 1958 to 1998 in Northern Europe: advantages of birth cohort analysis. Ophthalmology 2004; 111:1228–32.
310. Shields C, Honavar S, Meadows A, et al. Chemoreduction plus focal therapy for retinoblastoma: factors predictive of need for treatment with external beam radiotherapy or enucleation. Am J Ophthalmol 2002; 133:657–64.
311. Shields C, Mashayckhi A, Demirci H, et al. Practical approach to management of retinoblastoma. Arch Ophthalmol 2004; 122:729–35.
312. Shields C, Mashayekhi A, Cater J, et al. Chemoreduction for retinoblastoma: analysis of tumor control and risks for recurrence in 457 tumors. Am J Ophthalmol 2004; 138: 329–37.
313. Shields C, Parsons H, Shields J. Lesions simulating retinoblastoma. J Pediatr Ophthalmol Strabismus 1991; 28:338–40.
314. Shields C, Shelil A, Cater J, et al. Development of new retinoblastomas after 6 cycles of chemoreduction for retinoblastoma in 162 eyes of 106 consecutive patients. Arch Ophthalmol 2003; 121:1571–6.
315. Shields C, Shields J. Diagnosis and management of retinoblastoma. Cancer Control 2004; 11:317–27.
316. Shields C, Shields J. Recent developments in the management of retinoblastoma. J Pediatr Ophthalmol Strabismus 1999; 36:8–18.
317. Shields J. Diagnosis and Management of Intraocular Tumors. St. Louis, MO: C.V. Mosby, 1983.
318. Shields J, Augsburger J. Current approaches to the diagnosis and management of retinoblastoma. Surv Ophthalmol 1981; 25:347–71.
319. Shields J, Giblin M, Shields C, et al. Episclera plaque radiotherapy for retinoblastoma. Ophthalmology 1989; 96:530–7.
320. Shields J, Leonard B, Michelson J, Sarin L. B-scan ultrasonography in the diagnosis of atypical retinoblastoma. Can J Ophthalmol 1976; 11:42–51.
321. Shields J, Pesin S, Shields C. Trilateral retinoblastoma—feature photo. J Clin Neuro Ophthalmol 1989; 9:222–3.
322. Shields J, Shields C, Sivalingam V. Decreasing frequency of enucleation in patients with retinoblastoma. Am J Ophthalmol 1989; 108:185–8.
323. Shuangshoti S, Chaiwun B, Kasantikul V. A study of 39 retinoblastomas with particular reference to morphology, cellular differentiation, and tumor origin. Histopathology 1989; 15:113–24.
324. Singh S, Clarke I, Terasaki M, et al. Identification of a cancer stem cell in human brain tumors. Cancer Res 2003; 63:5821–8.
325. Sparkes R, Murphree A, Lingua R, et al. Gene for hereditary retinoblastoma assigned to human chromosome 13 by linkage to esterase D. Science 1983; 219: 971–3.
326. Spaulding A, Naumann G. Unsuspected retinoblastoma. Arch Ophthalmol 1966; 76:575–9.
327. Squire J, Dryja T, Dunn J, et al. A polymorphic gene probe closely linked to the retinoblastoma locus on chromosome 13. Proc Natl Acad Sci USA 1986; 83: 6573–7.
328. Stafford W, Yanoff M, Parnell B. Retinoblastoma initially misdiagnosed as primary ocular inflammation. Arch Ophthalmol 1969; 82:771–3.
329. Stevenson K, Hungerford J, Garner A. Local extraocular extension of retinoblastoma following intraocular surgery. Br J Ophthalmol 1989; 73:739–42.
330. Stewart J, Smith J, Arnold E. Spontaneous regression of retinoblastoma. Br J Ophthalmol 1956; 40:449–61.
331. Suckling R, Fitzgerald P, Wells E. The incidence and epidemiology of retinoblastoma in New Zealand: a 30 year study. Br J Cancer 1982; 46:729–36.
332. Swartz M. Aqueous humor lactic acid dehydrogenase in retinoblastoma. In: Peyman G, Apple D, Sanders D, eds. Intraocular Tumors. New York, NY: Appleton-Century-Crofts, 1977:331–5.
333. Takahashi T, Tamura S, Inoue M, et al. Retinoblastoma in a 26 year old adult. Ophthalmology 1983; 90:179–83.
334. Takayama S, Yamamoto M, Ito H. Cases of retinoblastoma-pathological and immunohistological studies. Nippon Ganka Gakkai Zasshi 1985; 89:797–803.
335. Taktikos A. Association of retinoblastoma with mental defect and other pathological manifestations. Br J Ophthalmol 1964; 48:495–8.
336. Tamboli A, Podgor M, Horm J. The incidence of retinoblastoma in the United States: 1974–1985. Arch Ophthalmol 1990; 108:128–32.
337. Tang A, Varley J, Chakraborty S, et al. Structural arrangement of the retinoblastoma gene in human breast carcinoma. Science 1988; 242:263–6.
338. Tapia F, Polak J, Barbosa A, et al. Neuro-specific enolase is produced by neuroendocrine tumors. Lancet 1981; 1: 808–11.
339. Tarkkanen A, Tervo K, Eranko L, et al. Substance P immunoreactivity in normal human retina and in retinoblastoma. Ophthal Res 1983; 15:300–6.
340. Tarkkanen A, Tervo T, Tervo K, Panula P. Immunohistochemical evidence for preproenkephalin. A synthesis in human retinoblastoma. Invest Ophthalmol Vis Sci 1984; 25:1210–2.
341. Tarkkanen A, Tuovinen E. Retinoblastoma in Finland 1912–1964. Acta Ophthalmol 1971; 49:293–300.
342. Tarlton J, Easty D. Immunohistochemical characterization of retinoblastoma and related ocular tissue. Br J Ophthalmol 1990; 74:144–9.
343. Terenghi G, Polak J, Ballesta J, et al. Immunocytochemistry of neuronal and glial markers in retinoblastoma. Virchows Arch A Pathol Anat Histopathol 1984; 404:61–73.

344. Trojanowksi J, Obrocka M, Lee V. Distribution of neurofilament subunits in neurons and neuronal processes: immunohistochemical studies of bovine cerebellum with subunit-specific monoclonal antibodies. J Histochem Cytochem 1985; 33:557–63.
345. Trojanowksi J, Walkenstein N, Lee V. Expression of neurofilament subunits in neurons of the central and peripheral nervous system: an immunohistochemical study with monoclonal antibodies. J Neurosci 1986; 6:650–60.
346. Ts'o M, Zimmerman L, Fine B. A cause of radioresistance in retinoblastoma: photoreceptor differentiation. Trans Am Acad Ophthalmol Otolaryngol 1970; 74:959–69.
347. Ts'o M, Fine B, Zimmerman L. The Flexner–Wintersteiner rosette in retinoblastoma. Arch Pathol 1969; 88:664–71.
348. Ts'o M, Fine B, Zimmerman L. The nature of retinoblastoma: II. Photoreceptor differentiation: an electron microscopic study. Am J Ophthalmol 1970; 69:350–9.
349. Ts'o M, Fine B, Zimmerman L. Photoreceptor elements in retinoblastoma. A preliminary report. Arch Ophthalmol 1969; 82:57–9.
350. Ts'o M, Zimmerman L, Fine B. The nature of retinoblastoma: I. Photoreceptor differentiation: a clinical and histologic study. Am J Ophthalmol 1970; 69:339–649.
351. Tsuji M, Goto M, Uehara F, et al. Photoreceptor cell differentiation in retinoblastoma demonstrated by a new immunohistochemical marker mucin-like glycoprotein associated with photoreceptor cells. Histopathology 2002; 40:180–6.
352. Uusitalo H, Lehtosalo J, Gregerson D, et al. Ultrastructural localization of retinal S-antigen in the rat. Graefes Arch Clin Exp Ophthalmol 1985; 222:118–22.
353. Verhoeff F, Jackson E. Minutes of the proceedings. Sixty-second annual meeting. Trans Am Ophthalmol Soc 1926; 24:38–9.
354. Vinores S, Bonnin J, Rubinstein L, et al. Immunohistochemical demonstration of neuron-specific enonase in neoplasms of the CNS and other tissues. Arch Pathol Lab Med 1984; 108:536–40.
355. Vinores S, Herman M, Rubinstein L, et al. Electron microscopic localization of nueron-specific enolase in rat and mouse brain. J Histochem Cytochem 1984; 32: 1295–302.
356. Vinores S, Rubinstein L. Simultaneous expression of glial fibrillary acidic (GFA) protein and neuron-specific enolase (NSE) by the same reactive or neoplastic astrocytes. Neuropathol Appl Neurobiol 1985; 11:349–59.
357. Virchow R. Die kranklaften Gesschwuelste, vol. 2. Berlin: August Hirschwald, 1864.
358. Virtanen I, Kivela T, Bugnoli M, et al. Expression of intermediate filaments and synaptophysin show neuronal properties and lack of glial characteristics in Y79 retinoblastoma cells. Lab Invest 1988; 59:649–55.
359. Vogel F. Genetics of retinoblastoma. Hum Genet 1979; 52: 1–54.
360. Vrabec T, Arbizo V, Adamus G. Rod cell-specific antigens in retinoblastoma. Arch Ophthalmol 1989; 107:1061–3.
361. Waardenburg P, Franceschetti A, Klein D. Genetics and Ophthalmology, vol. 2. Springfield, IL: Charles C. Thomas, 1963.
362. Wackenheim A, van Damme W, Kosmann P, Bittighoffer B. Computed tomography in ophthalmology. Neuroradiology 1977; 13:135–8.
363. Walsh F, Hoyt W, Miller N. Clinical Neuro-ophthalmology. 4th ed. Baltimore, MD: Williams and Wilkins, 1989.
364. Wang A, Lai C, Hsu W, et al. Clinicopathologic factors related to apoptosis in retinoblastoma. J Paediatr Ophthalmol Strabismus 2001; 38:295–301.
365. Weichselbaum R, Zakov Z, Albert D, et al. New findings in the chromosome 13 long are deletion syndrome and retinoblastoma. Ophthalmology 1979; 86:1191–8.
366. Weizenblatt S. Differential diagnostic difficulties in atypical retinoblastoma. Arch Ophthalmol 1957; 58:699–709.
367. Wessels G, Hesseling P. Incidence and frequency rates of childhood cancer in Namibia. S Afr Med J 1997; 87:885–9.
368. Whyte P, Buchkovich K, Horowitz J, et al. Association between an oncogene and an anti-oncogene: the adenovirus E1A proteins bind to the retinoblastoma gene product. Nature 1988; 334:124–9.
369. Wick M, Scheithauer B, Kovacs K. Neuron-specific enolase in neuroendocrine tumors of the thymus, bronchus, and skin. Am J Clin Pathol 1988; 79:703–7.
370. Wiechmann A. Recoverin in cultured human retinoblastoma cells: enhanced expression during morphological differentiation. J Neurochem 1996; 67:105–10.
371. Wiggs J, Dryja T. Predicting the risk of hereditary retinoblastoma. Am J Ophthalmol 1988; 106:346–51.
372. Wiggs J, Nordenskjold M, Yandell D, et al. Prediction of the risk of hereditary retinoblastoma using DNA polymorphisms within the retinoblastoma gene. N Engl J Med 1988; 318:151–7.
373. Willis R. Pathology of Tumors. 3rd ed. Washington, D.C.: Butterworths, 1960.
374. Windle J, Albert D, O'Brien J, et al. Retinoblastoma in transgenic mice. Nature 1990; 343:665–9.
375. Wintersteiner H. Die Neuroepithelioma retinae. Eine anatomische und klinische Studie. Leipzig: Dentisae, 1897.
376. Winther J, Olsen J, De Nully Brown P. Risk of nonocular cancer among retinoblastoma patients and their parents: a population based study in Denmark, 1943–1984. Cancer 1988; 62:1458–62.
377. Winther J, Overgaard J. Photodynamic therapy of experimental intraocular retinoblastomas–dose response relationships to light energy and photofrin II. Acta Ophthalmol (Copenh.) 1989; 67:44–50.
378. Wolter J. Retinoblastoma extension into the choroid. Pathological study of the neoplastic process and thoughts about its prognostic significance. Ophthalmic Pediatr Genet 1987; 8:151–7.
379. Wright J. Neurocytoma or neuroblastoma, a kind of tumor not generally recognized. J Exp Med 1910; 12: 556–61.
380. Xu H. Retinoblastoma and tumor-suppressor gene therapy. Ophthalmol Clin North Am 2003; 16:621–9.
381. Xu H, Hu S, Hashimoto T, et al. The retinoblastoma susceptibility gene product: a characteristic pattern in normal cells and abnormal expression in malignant cells. Oncogene 1989; 4:807–12.
382. Xu K, Liu S, Ni C. Immunohistochemical evidence of neuronal and glial differentiation in retinoblastoma. Br J Ophthalmol 1995; 79:771–6.
383. Yandell D, Campbell T, Dayton S, et al. Oncogenic point mutations in the human retinoblastoma gene: their application to genetic counseling. N Engl J Med 1989; 321:1689–95.
384. Yanoff M, Fine B. Ocular Pathology: A Text and Atlas. New York, NY: Harper & Row, 1989:686–98.
385. Yokoyama T, Tsukahara T, Nakagawa C, et al. The N-myc gene product in primary retinoblastomas. Cancer 1989; 63:2134–8.
386. Young R. Cell differentiation in the retina of the mouse. Anat Rec 1985; 212:199–205.
387. Young R. Cell proliferation during postnatal development of the retina in the mouse. Brain Res 1985; 353:229–39.

388. Yttebsorg J, Arnesen K. Late recurrence of retinoblastoma. Acta Ophthalmol (Copenh.) 1972; 50:367–74.
389. Yunis J, Ramsay N. Retinoblastoma and subband deletion of chromosome 13. Am J Dis Child 1978; 132:161–3.
390. Zhu L. Tumour suppressor retinoblastoma protein Rb: a transcriptional regulator. Eur J Cancer 2005; 41:2415–27.
391. Zimmerman L. Application of histochemical methods for the demonstration of acid mucopolysaccharides to ophthalmic pathology. Trans Am Acad Ophthalmol Otolaryngol 1958; 62:697–703.
392. Zimmerman L. Retinoblastoma and retinocytoma. In: Spencer W, ed. Ophthalmic Pathology: An Atlas and Textbook. Philadelphia, PA: W.B. Saunders, 1985: 1292–351.
393. Zimmerman L, Bilaniuk L. Ocular MR imaging (editorial). Radiology 1988; 168:875–6.

61

Tumors of the Lacrimal Gland and Lacrimal Drainage Apparatus

J. Oscar Croxatto
Departments of Teaching and Research and Laboratory of Ophthalmic Pathology, Fundación Oftalmológica Argentina Jorge Malbran, Buenos Aires, Argentina

INTRODUCTION

The lacrimal gland is a nonencapsulated, multilobulated, secretory structure located in the lacrimal gland fossa behind the superotemporal orbital rim. The lateral edge of the levator palpebrae aponeurosis divides the lacrimal gland into a superficial, palpebral, subconjunctival lobe, and a deeper orbital lobe.

Histologically, the lacrimal gland is divided into acini and ducts (Fig. 1). The secretory acini consist of cuboidal zymogen-bearing cells, surrounded externally by myoepithelial cells. The acini are separated from each other and between lobules by intralobular and interlobular connective tissue. Mucus-secreting cells are not present. The interlobular ducts converge into main ducts that open into the superotemporal fornix of the conjunctiva. Plasma cells and lymphocytes are lightly dispersed among the secretory acini of the lacrimal gland. Occasionally, small lymphoid aggregates without well-defined germinal centers may be observed. The plasma cells of the lacrimal gland secrete monomeric immunoglobulin A (IgA). The secretory IgA is a dimer binded to a polypeptide chain (secretory piece) produced by epithelial cells. The secretory component binds to the Fc portion of the IgA dimer protecting the antibody from cleavage. Approximately 40% of the lymphocytes present in the normal lacrimal gland are T cells.

The lacrimal drainage system is composed of the puncta, the lacrimal canaliculi, the lacrimal sac, and the nasolacrimal duct. The lacrimal sac is lined by a stratified columnar epithelium containing scattered goblet cells.

The types of lacrimal gland tumors are more limited than those of the salivary glands. Currently, epithelial tumors represent approximately one-thirds of biopsied lacrimal gland masses (29,49,64). The cellular classification disclosed in Table 1, parallels that of salivary gland tumors in essence (9,66). In different series (18,64,73), the reported incidence of true primary epithelial tumors ranged from 21% to 39%, among which 29% to 55% were

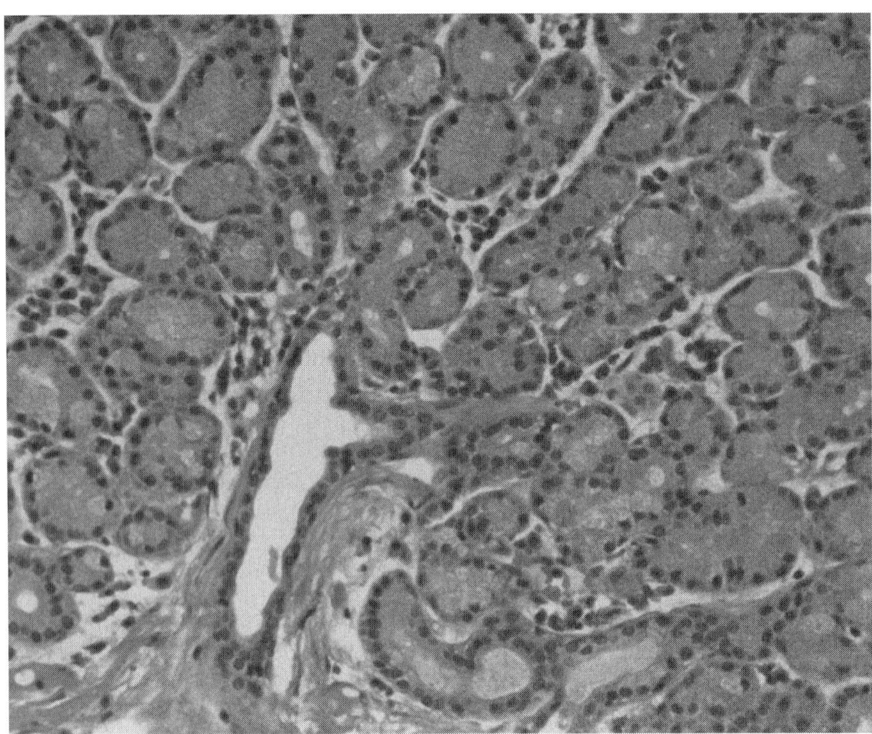

Figure 1 Normal lacrimal gland. Large duct is surrounded by acini composed of basophilic secretory epithelial cells (hematoxylin and eosin, × 68).

carcinomas (15,73). Malignant neoplasms of the lacrimal gland appear to be more common in some oriental populations (47,48). The simultaneous (synchronous) or "temporally displaced" (metachronous) presentation of epithelial tumors of the lacrimal and salivary gland is rare (35).

TUMORS OF THE LACRIMAL GLAND

Benign Tumors

Pleomorphic Adenoma

Accounting for slightly more than half of all lacrimal gland tumors (1,64,72), pleomorphic adenoma most often presents during the fourth decade with proptosis or displacement of the eye (Figs. 2 and 3). A common but less appropriate name for pleomorphic adenoma is benign mixed tumor since, according to evidence originally drawn from its counterpart in the parotid salivary gland, there is reason to regard the stromal components as being like the acinar and ductal tissue, of epithelial origin. This view was initially based on the character of the mucinous elements of the tumors but has recently been supported by immunohistochemical evidence, which suggests that the more obviously glandular elements derive from ductal epithelium while the "stromal" components are of myoepithelial origin (44,67). It is, moreover, possible that the tumor represents neoplastic transformation of a single stem cell of myoepithelial type (67). Direct evidence derived from an immunohistochemical study of lacrimal gland tumors points similarly to a pure epithelial histogenesis (21). Theoretically, it is conceivable that, as in the case of the salivary glands, there should be a spectrum of adenomatous tumors ranging from those with a pure ductal element to those composed exclusively of myoepithelium. As yet instances of such monomorphic adenomas in the lacrimal gland are limited to rare cases of myoepithelioma (25), but it seems sensible to consider the pleomorphic adenoma as occupying an intermediate position in a continuous spectrum of neoplastic development.

Histologically, the tumor is composed predominantly of a double cell layer of epithelium arranged in interlacing ducts and solid strands surrounded by a matrix of myxoid epithelial secretion in which islands of chondroid differentiation are common (Figs. 4–6). The overtly epithelial component is distinguished by a conspicuous keratin content whereas the myoepithelial stromal cells stain for smooth muscle actin and, less consistently, glial fibrillary acid protein (GFAP) and vimentin (21). Transmission electron microscopy (TEM) shows that the epithelial cell lining of the ducts resembles that of the normal ducts, but with fewer secretory granules (28). The outer, darker, myoepithelial cells retain epithelial features, with focal myofilament bundles at the cell periphery, attachment plaques, and intercellular junctions.

Despite being encapsulated (Figs. 5 and 7), it is not uncommon for histopathological examination of a pleomorphic adenoma to disclose small groups of

Table 1 Classification of Lacrimal Gland Tumors

Benign epithelial tumors
Pleomorphic adenoma (mixed tumor)
Oncocytoma (oxyphilic adenoma)
Warthin tumor (papillary cystadenoma lymphomatosum)
Myoepithelioma
Malignant epithelial tumors
Adenoid cystic carcinoma
Malignant mixed tumor (carcinoma in pleomorphic adenoma)
Adenocarcinoma (not otherwise specified)
Basal cell adenocarcinoma
Acinic cell carcinoma
Ductal adenocarcinoma
Cystadenocarcinoma
Polymorphous low-grade carcinoma
Mucinous adenocarcinoma
Mucoepidermoid carcinoma
Squamous cell carcinoma
Spindle cell carcinoma
Carcinosarcoma
Sebaceous carcinoma
Epithelial-myoepithelial carcinoma
Lymphoepithelioma-like carcinoma
Oncocytic carcinoma
Lymphoid tumors
Reactive lymphoid hyperplasia
Malignant lymphomas
Mesenchymal tumors
Hemangioma
Hemangiopericytoma
Neurofibroma and schwannoma
Solitary fibrous tumor
Lipoma
Secondary and mestastatic tumors
Tumor-like conditions
Chronic dacryoadenitis
Benign lymphoepithelial lesion
Inflammatory pseudotumor
Lacrimal duct cyst (dacryops)
Ectopic lacrimal gland

tumor cells extending through the capsule (bosselations). This is likely to contribute to a tendency to recur after surgical excision. It is also to be noted that the tumor may be surrounded by a marked lymphocytic infiltrate, which, in cases where biopsy specimens are taken from the edge of the lesion, may lead to a mistaken diagnosis of inflammatory pseudotumor.

Pleomorphic adenomas are DNA diploid tumors with low expression of p53 the product of the *TP53* gene (75). P21ras expression is apparently related to promotion and progression of pleomorphic adenomas (76). The actuarial estimate of malignant transformation is 10% by 20 years after initial treatment and 20% by 30 years (15).

Oncocytoma (Oncocytic Adenoma, Oxyphilic Adenoma)

Oncocytomas are epithelial tumors composed of large cells with finely granular acidophilic cytoplasm that, by TEM and immunohistochemical studies, are extremely rich in mitochondria. Based on histological features these lesions have been designated oncocytic hyperplasia, oncocytic adenoma, and oncocytic carcinoma. Oxyphilic cells may be present as part of other epithelial tumors. Oncocytic adenoma and carcinoma of the main and accessory lacrimal glands are exceedingly rare (53).

Myoepithelioma

Myoepitheliomas are rare tumors composed almost exclusively of myoepithelial cells and characterized by several growth patterns. As mentioned before, some authors suggest that pleomorphic adenomas, pure epithelial adenomas, and myoepitheliomas originate from a common cell precursor (21,28). By definition, predominantly myoepithelial tumors with prominent epithelial duct proliferation (more than 10%) are considered myoepithelial adenomas, a subset of pleomorphic adenomas. The tumors are mainly composed of spindle cells with scanty eosinophilic cytoplasm (17). Myoepithelial cells are immunoreactive for α-actin, specific muscle actin, cytokeratin, GFAP, vimentin, and S100 protein. Most myoepitheliomas of the lacrimal gland are benign and the prognosis is not different from pleomorphic adenomas. Depending on the predominant cell type myoepitheliomas are subdivided into epithelial or epithelioid, plasmacytoid or polygonal, and clear cell myoepitheliomas.

Malignant Tumors

Pleomorphic Adenocarcinoma

Malignant mixed lacrimal tumors carry a moderately poor prognosis and account for 10% to 20% of all epithelial lacrimal gland tumors (18,64,72). They develop within a preexisting benign adenoma, and a typical history is a prior removal of a pleomorphic adenoma followed by one or more recurrences and evidence of a more aggressive behavior in the form of local invasion or at least one distant metastasis (Fig. 8). Malignant transformation may develop initially as in situ adenocarcinoma in recurrent pleomorphic adenomas (43). The histological types of carcinoma include adenocarcinoma, adenoid cystic carcinoma, squamous cell carcinoma, and undifferentiated carcinoma. Rare involvement of the "stromal" element can result in a pseudosarcomatous spindle cell histology. Tumors composed of carcinomatous and sarcomatous elements are classified as carcinosarcomas.

Adenoid Cystic Carcinoma

Adenoid cystic carcinomas are infiltrative, highly malignant epithelial tumors that originate from

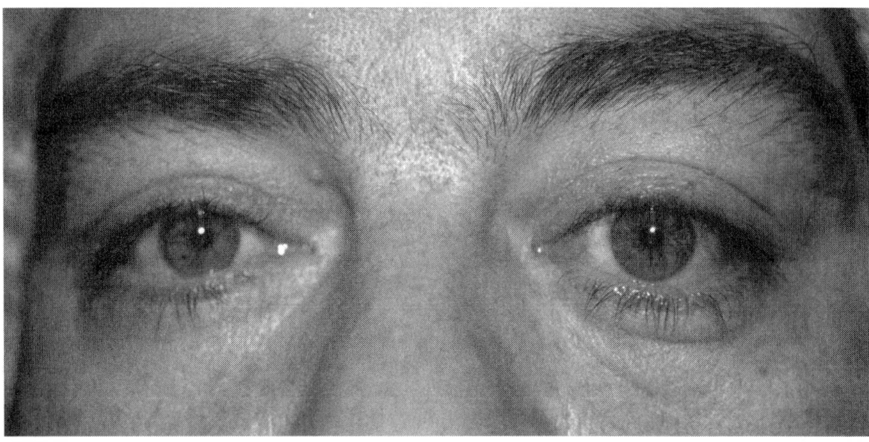

Figure 2 Pleomorphic adenoma of the lacrimal gland. A mass is protruding on the superior temporal area of the left orbit.

intralobular duct cells at the transition zone between the acini and the ducts (21). Adenoid cystic carcinoma accounts for approximately 25% of primary epithelial neoplasms of the lacrimal gland (16). It is the second most common epithelial lacrimal gland tumor and the most frequent malignant epithelial tumor in this structure (Fig. 9 and Fig. 10). In the series reported from the Armed Forces Institute of Pathology in the United States, about 1 in 9 adenoid cystic carcinomas developed within a pleomorphic adenoma (15).

Adenoid cystic carcinomas display a variety of architectural patterns (16). The histology of the usual cribiform tumor is one of anastomosing cords of small cells with hyperchromatic nuclei and sparse cytoplasm within a hyalinized or hypocellular fibrous stroma. The individual cords are perforated by multiple cystic spaces, which create a Swiss-cheese cylindromatous pattern (Fig. 11). The basaloid variant, which is formed by solid lobules of densely compacted cells with basophilic nuclei and scanty cytoplasm (Fig. 12), is particularly noteworthy because it carries a decidedly worse prognosis than the other types (20,73). The characteristic cytological features facilitate the diagnosis by fine needle aspiration biopsy (69).

TEM shows that adenoid cystic carcinomas of the lacrimal gland consist of four different cell types: small cuboidal cells containing either small duct-like granules (type 1A cells), or large acinus-like granules (type 1B cells); cells showing bundles of tonofilaments (type 2 cells); and cells that display features of myoepithelium (type 3 cells) (28). Adenoid spaces are surrounded by multilaminar basement membrane.

DNA analysis of salivary gland adenoid cystic carcinoma demonstrated that this tumor is aneuploid (19). The expression of p53 may be correlated with prognosis (74).

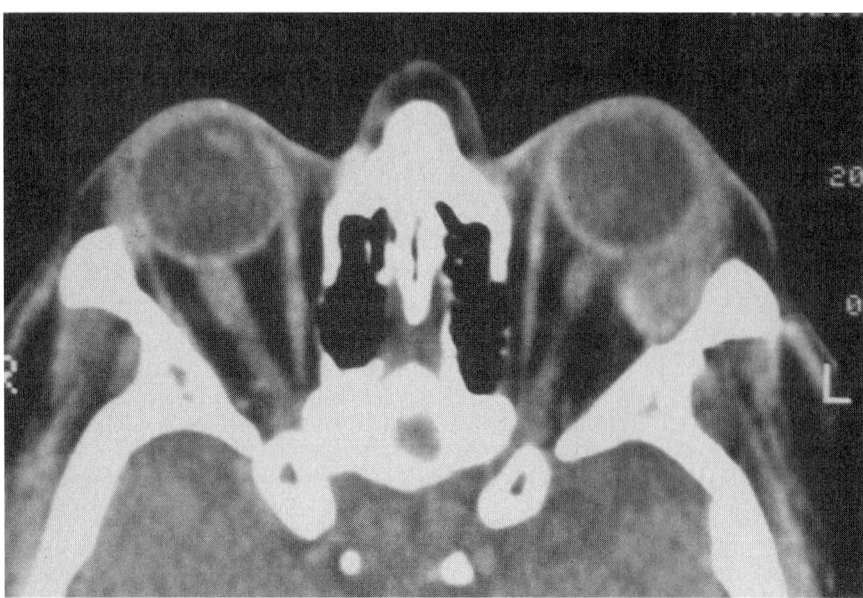

Figure 3 Computed tomography scan of the patient in Figure 2 revealed a well-circumscribed mass in the lacrimal fossa.

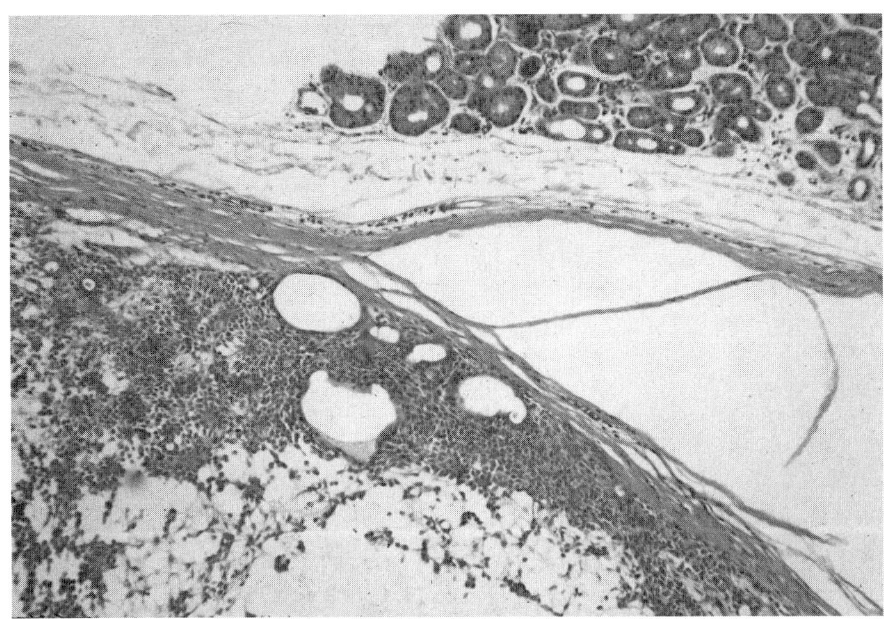

Figure 4 Low-power microscopic view of a pleomorphic adenoma with a thin connective tissue capsule and adjacent lacrimal gland (*upper right corner*) (hematoxylin and eosin, ×28).

A proclivity to infiltrate along nerves and blood vessels is the likely explanation for the rapidity with which adenoid cystic carcinoma invades adjacent structures, including the brain. Distant metastasis may also occur and the overall prognosis is poor (12), with a 10-year survival rate following surgery being 10% to 25% (20,73).

Primary Adenocarcinoma

Primary adenocarcinomas (otherwise unclassified) of the lacrimal gland that do not arise in association with a preexisting pleomorphic adenoma account for 5% to 10% of epithelial tumors of the lacrimal gland (Fig. 13) (15,24,51,52). The prognosis for such carcinomas that develop de novo is considerably worse than for malignant transformation within pleomorphic adenomas, with median survival rates of 3.5 and 12.0 years, respectively (24).

Mucoepidermoid Tumors

In the salivary gland a tumor characterized by the proliferation of intimately related squamous and mucus-secreting epithelium is not uncommon, but in the lacrimal gland it is a rarity (Fig. 14) (57). However, unless sufficient sections are examined to exclude other kinds of tissue differentiation, which would establish a diagnosis of pleomorphic adenoma (or carcinoma), recognition of mucoepidermoid tumor is

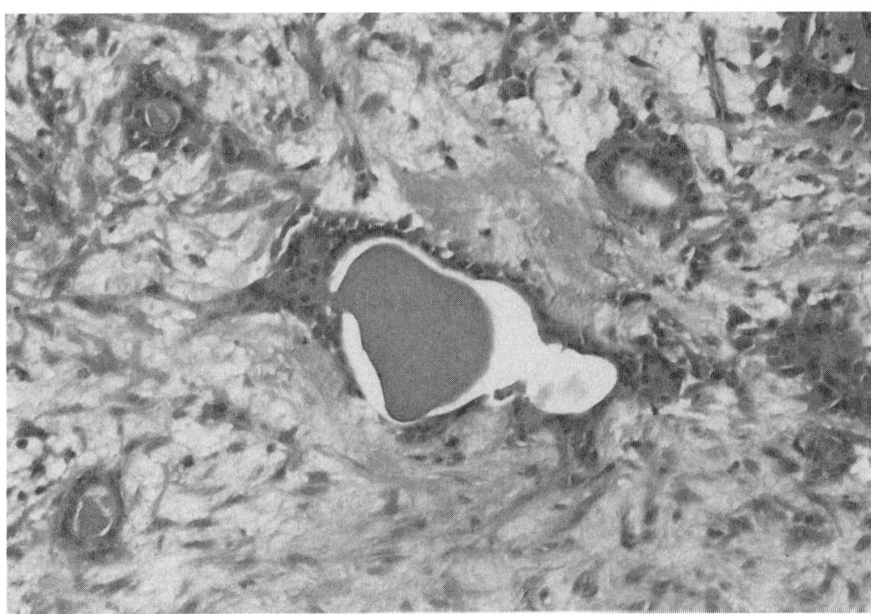

Figure 5 Pleomorphic adenoma. Proliferating ducts with prominent proliferation of myoepithelial cells and loose extracellular matrix (hematoxylin and eosin, ×68).

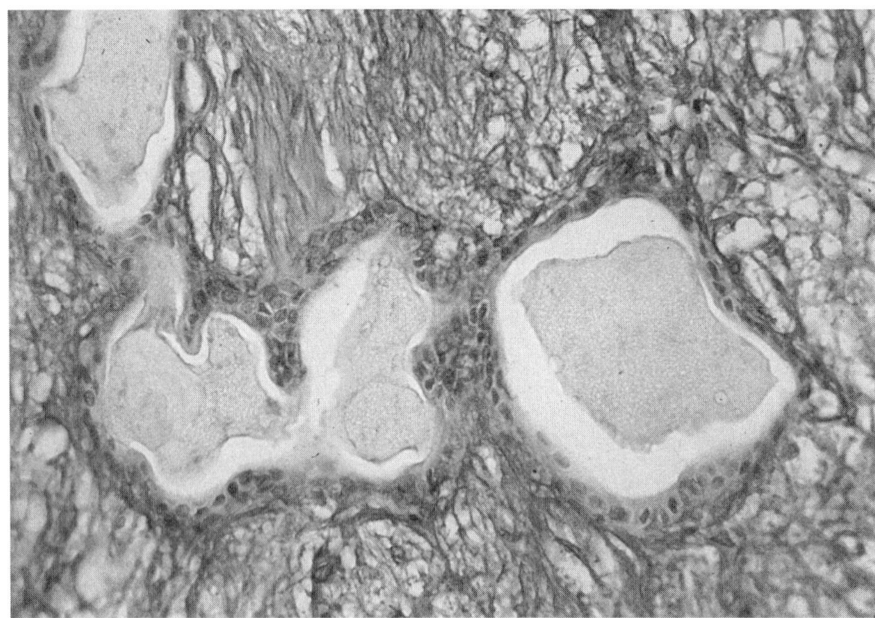

Figure 6 Pleomorphic adenoma. Connective tissue stromal between proliferating duct structures (trichrome stain, ×285).

tenuous, and Ashton (1) found only one acceptable case in his review of the published cases. This tumor is considered to stem from the duct epithelium and can show a variable degree of malignancy, which is not always reflected in the histological appearance. Correspondingly, some pathologists prefer not to define mucoepidermoid tumors in terms of adenoma or carcinoma.

Primary Ductal Adenocarcinoma

Primary ductal adenocarcinoma originates from the excretory portion of the lacrimal duct (33,45,51). Although, the tumors may appear circumscribed grossly, they are highly infiltrative, usually solid with occasional cystic areas. The cells are cuboidal or polygonal with eosinophilic cytoplasm and apocrine features. The duct-like structures are embedded in a collagenous matrix. Comedonecrosis and a high rate of mitoses are characteristic.

Miscellaneous Malignant Epithelial Tumors

Specific subtypes of adenocarcinomas and carcinomas have been reported in reviews of series of cases from single institutions or in single case reports. They include acinic cell carcinoma (8,30,46), basal cell adenocarcinoma (34), squamous cell carcinoma (26,73), polymorphous low-grade carcinoma (62,72),

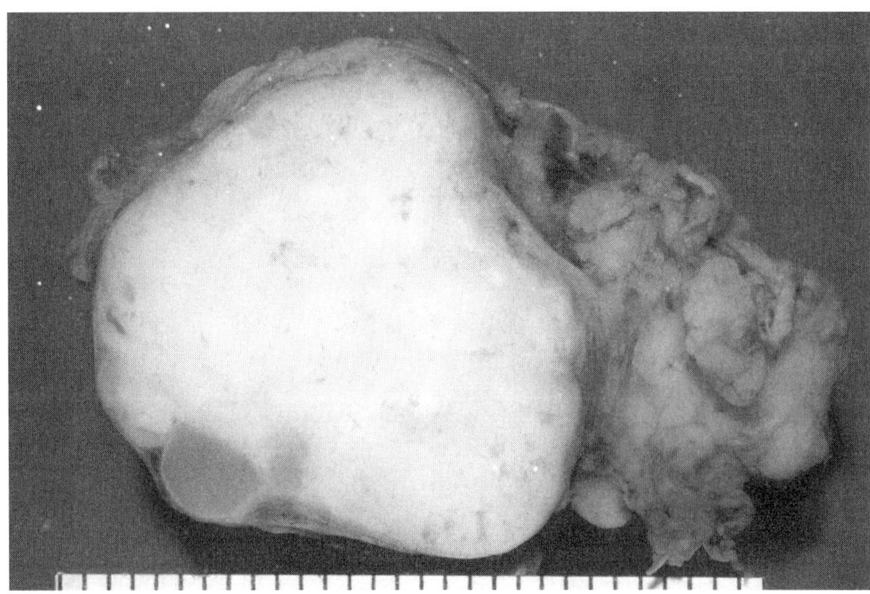

Figure 7 Gross appearance of a resected pleomorphic adenoma. The tumor is well-circumscribed and the cut surface shows a few cysts containing mucoid material.

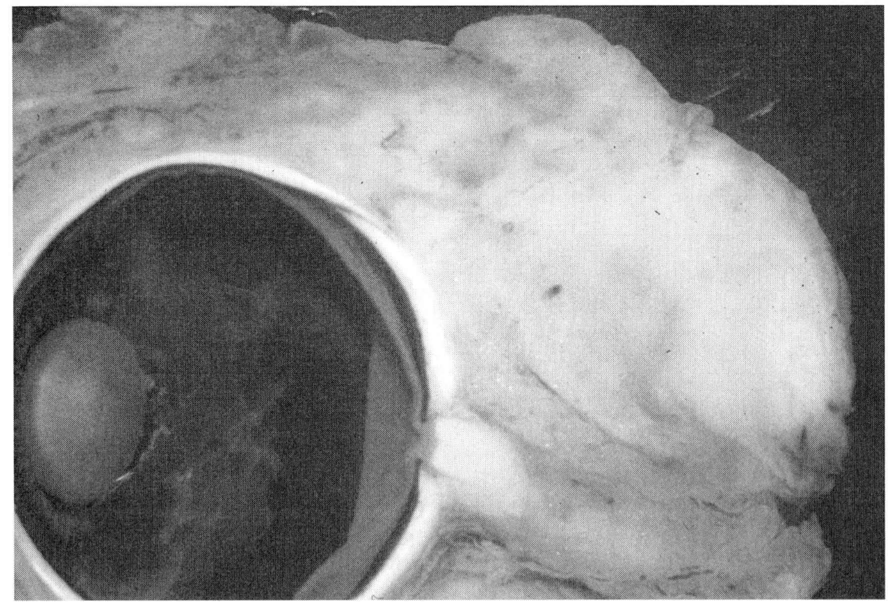

Figure 8 Exenteration specimen of a patient with malignant pleomorphic adenocarcinoma with orbital invasion.

cystadenocarcinoma (9), mucinous adenocarcinoma, spindle cell carcinoma (51), sebaceous carcinoma (5,23,38,59,65), carcinosarcoma, and lymphoepithelioma-like carcinoma (4,58). Since these tumors are extremely rare in the lacrimal gland, prognosis is predicted on the behavior of similar tumors of the salivary glands.

TUMORS OF THE LACRIMAL SAC

Neoplasms originating within the lacrimal sac reflect their histogenesis from ectodermal epithelium continuous with the Schneiderian membrane of the nasal passages and usually present with epiphora, swelling, and inflammation due to obstructed outflow (27,39). Pain is a feature of the malignant lesions. In the series of 13 tumors of the lacrimal sac collected between 1948 and 1967 by Harry and Ashton (22), eight were of epithelial origin. They subclassified their eight epithelial tumors into three types: type I as a transitional papilloma, type II as an intermediate transitional cell tumor, and type III as a transitional cell carcinoma. More than one half of epithelial tumors are malignant (68). In another series from China (46), most epithelial tumors were malignant perhaps reflecting race or exposure to environmental factors. Local and lymphatic dissemination are more common that distant metastasis but they can be fatal. Tumors of the lacrimal sac require long-term follow-up for recurrence and metastasis (50).

Human papillomavirus (HPV) is implicated in benign and malignant neoplasia of several tissues including the conjunctiva (41,42). HPV types 6 or 11 are found in benign papillomas and HPV 16 or 18 among others are present in dysplastic and malignant lesions. In a series of primary epithelial tumors of the lacrimal sac, all six cases studies contained HPV sequences (40). Papillomas were positive for HPV type 11, and one carcinoma was characterized as HPV type 18 (40). These findings suggest that HPV infection may

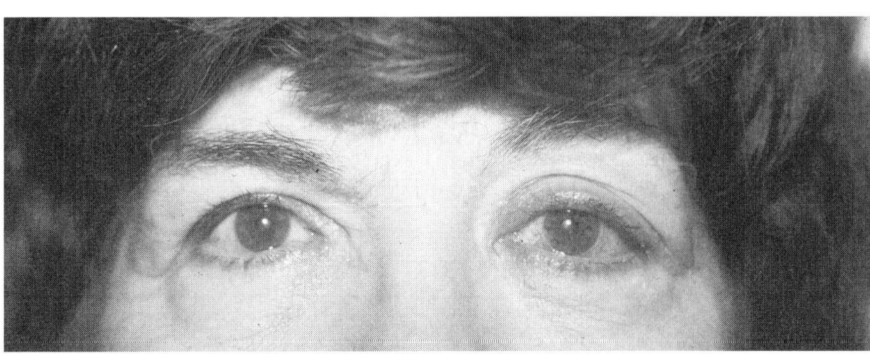

Figure 9 Adenoid cystic carcinoma. Clinical appearance of a patient with a painful tumor of the right lacrimal gland.

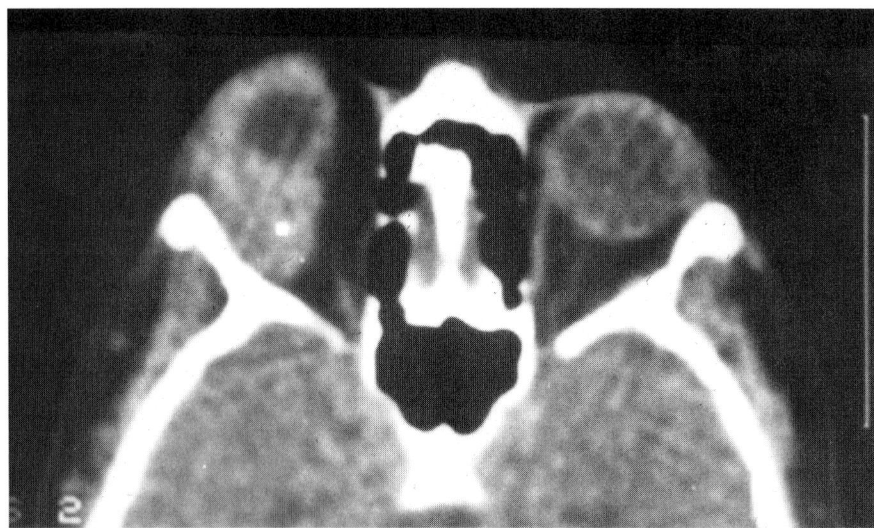

Figure 10 Computed tomography scan of the patient in Figure 9 shows an irregular tumor arising from the lacrimal fossa and infiltrating the adjacent soft tissues of the orbit and bone.

be involved in the pathogenesis of benign and malignant epithelial proliferations of the lacrimal sac.

Benign Tumors

Transitional Cell Papilloma

According to two studies covering 35 epithelial neoplasms of the lacrimal sac (22,61), transitional cell papillomas are the most common type of benign neoplasm in this tissue. These tumors are composed of columnar cells, commonly with evidence of early squamous differentiation and growing toward the wall of the sac as a result of infolding. Mitotic activity is slight, differentiation is good, and the basement membrane of the proliferating epithelium is intact. Lacrimal sac papillomas may contain a conspicuous number of neutrophils and nuclear debris within the proliferated epithelium. Some papillomas are composed of oncocytes displaying large eosinophilic cytoplasm containing numerous mitochondria.

While the prognosis for a well-differentiated papilloma is excellent if completely excised, recurrences are common because of surgical difficulties in achieving this goal, and some of these tumors undergo malignant transformation (22,61). Papillomas can be subdivided into three groups according to their growth pattern: exophytic, inverted, and mixed (61). In the forgoing series reported by Ryan and Font none of the six purely exophytic papillomas evolved into carcinoma. In contrast, 7 of the 12

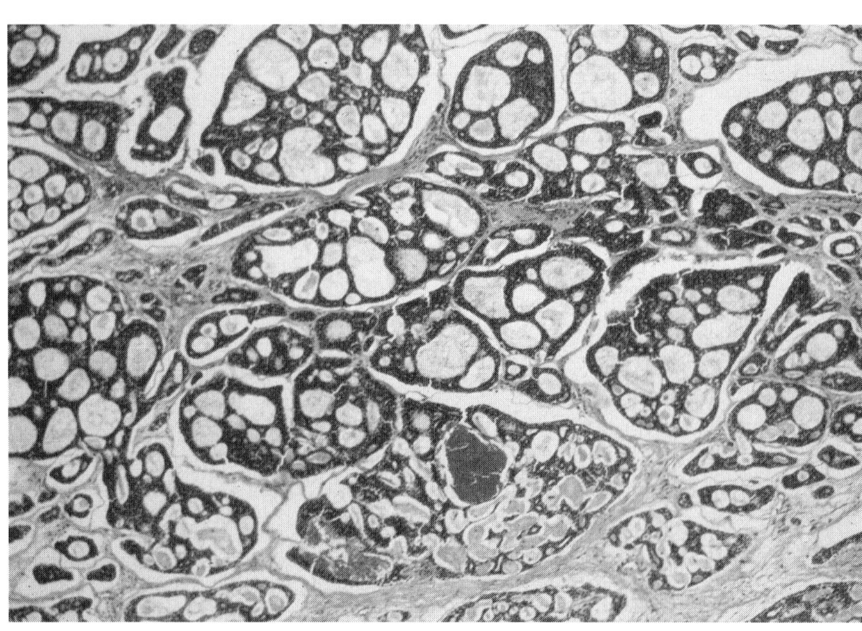

Figure 11 Adenoid cystic carcinoma. Cribiform pattern of the epithelial tumor (hematoxylin and eosin, ×28).

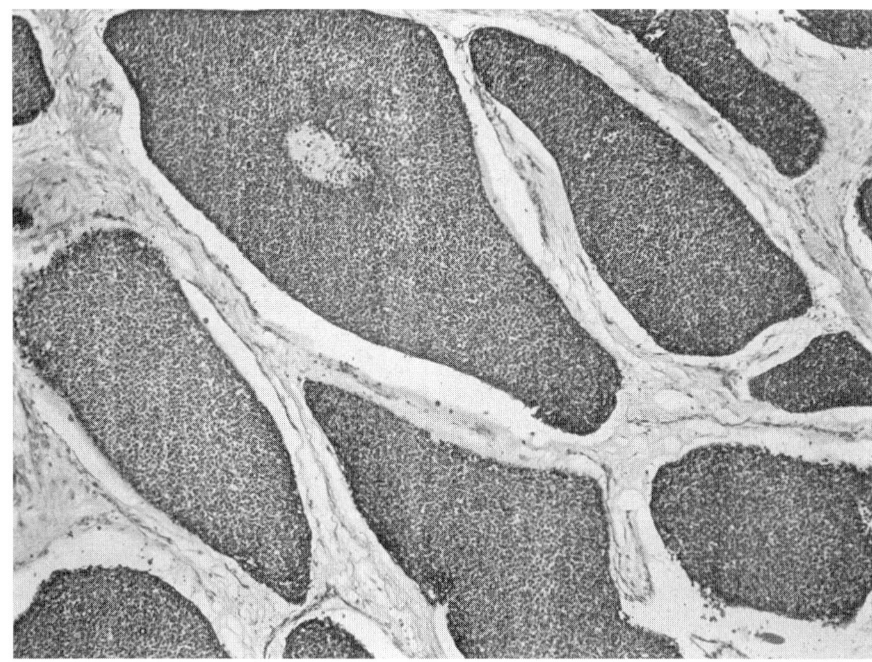

Figure 12 Adenoid cystic carcinoma. Solid pattern composed of basaloid-like epithelial cells (hematoxylin and eosin, ×28).

papillomas with an inverted or mixed growth pattern contained foci of carcinoma or evolved into carcinoma.

Squamous Cell Papilloma

A minority of lacrimal sac tumors consists entirely of differentiated squamous epithelium and, while such papillomas may have a preference for proliferation within the cavity of the lacrimal sac, as opposed to "transitional" cell papillomas, which grow mainly into the supporting stroma, there is no practical reason to regard them separately. The designation Schneiderian papilloma has been proposed as a convenient inclusive term (32).

Malignant Tumors

Transitional Cell Carcinoma

Malignant tumors with recognizable stratified columnar epithelium may arise de novo or complicate a papilloma. Diagnosis is based on a conspicuous level of mitotic activity, cellular pleomorphism with nuclear irregularity, and ultimately, evidence of extension into the wall of the lacrimal sac with penetration of

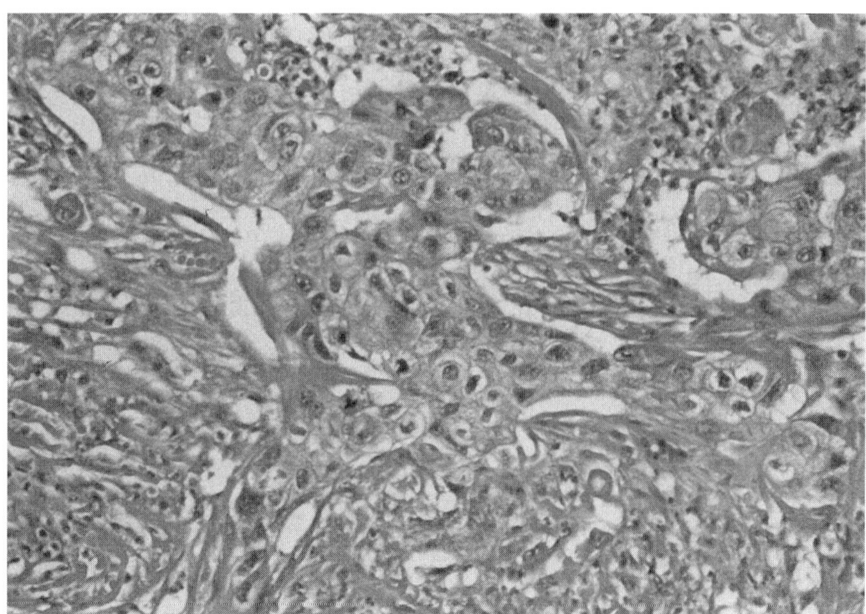

Figure 13 Primary adenocarcinoma. This tumor was composed of pleomorphic neoplastic epithelial cells (hematoxylin and eosin, ×135).

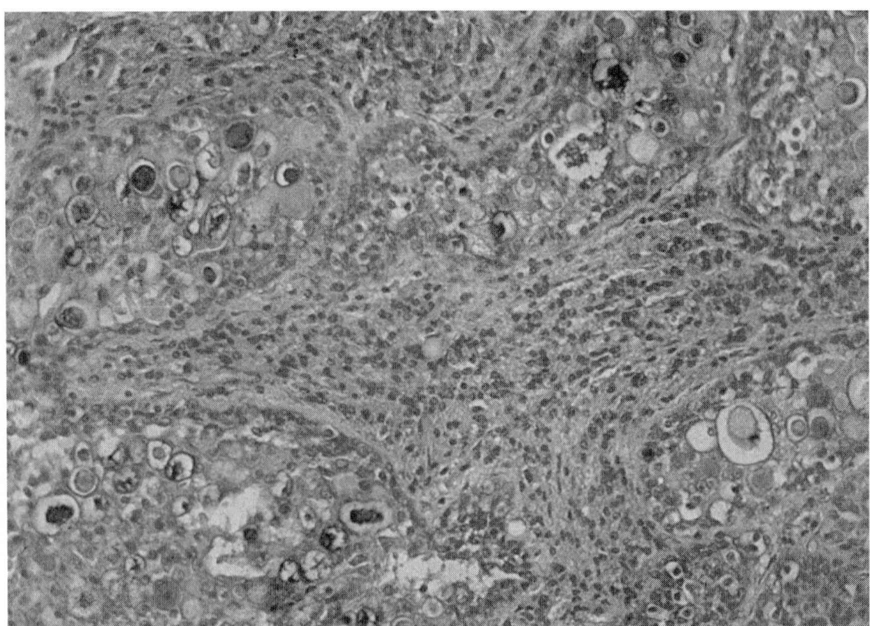

Figure 14 Mucoepidermoid carcinoma. The neoplastic epithelial cells show multiple vacuoles and spaces containing mucin (Alcian blue stain, × 68).

the epithelial basal lamina. Local recurrence after surgery with spread into the orbit has complicated about one-half of the cases in two reported series and, exceptionally, widespread carcinomatosis has been recorded (22).

In addition to frank carcinoma, Ryan and Font (61) have described instances of focal malignant change within transitional cell papillomas. Harry and Ashton (22) also recognized a state intermediate between benignity and unequivocal malignancy, and there appears to be a correlation between repeated recurrence and increasing histological evidence of malignancy. Histological distinction between benign and malignant epithelial tumors can be very difficult and is sometimes impossible; hence, the initial surgery should aim for complete excision in all cases (13). The prognosis for histologically malignant lesions is not encouraging (22). Ni and coworkers classify lacrimal sac tumors into four clinical stages: stage I (incipient stage) characterized by nonspecific signs and symptoms with no palpable mass in the lacrimal sac region. Stage II is obvious tumor in the lacrimal sac. In stage III the tumor extended into adjacent structures. Stage IV tumors show evidence of metastates (46). Most cases were diagnosed at stage III. Although most tumors of the lacrimal drainage apparatus arise within the lacrimal sac the tumor apparently originate in the canaliculus and extend into the lacrimal sac (37,52).

Squamous Cell Carcinoma

In the experience of Ryan and Font (61), squamous cell carcinoma is the most frequent lacrimal sac malignancy, arising de novo or complicating benign transitional cell or squamous cell papillomas.

Other Tumors

Isolated examples of fibrous histiocytoma (7,35), benign and malignant oncocytic tumors (2,55), lymphoma (71), angiosarcoma (22,31), schwannoma (63), malignant melanoma (10,11,22,70), hemangiopericytoma (6), adenoid cystic carcinoma (36), adenocarcinoma ex-pleomorphic adenoma, and mucoepidermoid carcinoma (3) have also been reported in the lacrimal sac (14). A series of 35 nonepithelial tumors of the lacrimal sac contained 13 fibrous histiocytomas, 10 lymphoid lesions, 8 malignant melanomas, and 1 example of hemangiopericytoma, lipoma, granulocytic sarcoma, and neurofibroma (54).

REFERENCES

1. Ashton N. Epithelial tumours of the lacrimal gland. Mod Probl Ophthalmol 1975; 14:306–23.
2. Aurora AL. Oncocytic metasplasia in a lacrimal sac papilloma. Am J Ophthalmol 1973; 75:466–8.
3. Blake J, Mullaney J, Gillan J. Lacrimal sac mucoepidermoid carcinoma. Br J Ophthalmol 1986; 70:681–5.
4. Bloching M, Hinze R, Berghaus A. Lymphoepithelioma-like carcinoma of the lacrimal gland. Eur Arch Otorhinolaryngol 2000; 257:399–401.
5. Briscoe D, Mahmood S, Bonshek R, et al. Primary sebaceous carcinoma of the lacrimal gland. Br J Ophthalmol 2001; 85:625–6.
6. Carnevali L, Trimarchi F, Rosso R, Stringa M. Haemangiopericytoma of the lacrimal sac: a case report. Br J Ophthalmol 1988; 72:782–5.

7. Cole SH, Ferry AP. Fibrous histiocytoma (fibrous xanthoma) of the lacrimal sac. Arch Ophthalmol 1978; 96:1647–9.
8. De Rosa G, Zeppa P, Tranfa F, Bovolonta G. Acinic cell carcinoma arising in a lacrimal gland: firs case report. Cancer 1986; 57:1988–91.
9. Devoto MH, Croxatto JO. Primary cystadenocarcinoma of the lacrimal gland. Ophthalmology 2003; 110:2006–10.
10. Duguid IM. Malignant melanoma of the lacrimal sac. Br J Ophthalmol 1964; 48:394–8.
11. Farkas TG, Lamberson RE. Malignant melanoma of the lacrimal sac. Am J Ophthalmol 1968; 66:45–8.
12. Esmaeli B, Ahmadi MA, Youssef A, et al. Outcomes in patients with adenoid cystic carcinoma of the lacrimal gland. Ophthal Plast Reconstr Surg 2004; 20:22–6.
13. Flanagan JC, Mauriello JA Jr, Stefanyszyn J. Lacrimal sac tumors and inflammations. In: Mauriello JA Jr, Flanagan JC, eds. Management of Orbital and Ocular Adnexal Tumors and Inflammations. Berlin: Springer-Verlag, 1990: 187–96.
14. Mauriello JA Jr, Flanagan JC. Eds. Management of Orbital and Ocular Adnexal Tumors and Inflammations. Berlin: Springer-Verlag, 1990.
15. Font RL, Gamel JW. Epithelial tumors of the lacrimal gland: an analysis of 265 cases. In: Jakobiec FA, ed. Ocular and Adnexal Tumors. Birmingham, AL: Aesculapius Publishing Co., 1978:787–805.
16. Font RL, Gamel JW. Adenoid cystic carcinoma of the lacrimal gland: a clinicopathologic study of 79 cases. In: Nicholson D, ed. Ocular Pathology Update, New York: Masson Publishing USA, 1980:277–83.
17. Font RL, Garner A. Myoepithelioma of the lacrimal gland: report of a case with spindle cell morphology. Br J Ophthalmol 1992; 76:634–6.
18. Font RL, Smith SL, Bryan RG. Malignant epithelial tumors of the lacrimal gland: a clinicopathologic study of 21 cases. Arch Ophthalmol 1998; 116:613–6.
19. Franzen G, Nordgard S, Boysen M, Larsen PL, Halvorsen TB, Clausen OP. DNA content in adenoid cystic carcinomas. Head Neck 1995; 17:49–55.
20. Gamel JW, Font RL. Adenoid cystic carcinoma of the lacrimal gland: the clinical significance of a basaloid histologic pattern. Hum Pathol 1982; 13:219–25.
21. Grossniklaus HE, Abbuhl MF, McLean IW. Immunohistologic properties of benign and malignant mixed tumor of the lacrimal gland. Am J Ophthalmol 1990; 110:540–9.
22. Harry J, Ashton N. The pathology of tumours of the lacrimal sac. Trans Ophthalmol Soc UK 1968; 88:19–35.
23. Harvey P A, Parsons A, Rennie I. Primary sebaceous carcinoma of lacrimal gland: a previously unreported primary neoplasm. Eye 1994; 8:592–5.
24. Heaps RS, Miller NR, Albert DM, et al. Primary adenocarcinoma of the lacrimal gland. A retrospective study. Ophthalmology 1993; 100:1856–60.
25. Heathcote JG, Hurwitz JJ, Dardick I. A spindle-cell myoepithelioma of the lacrimal gland. Arch Ophthalmol 1990; 108:1135–9.
26. Henderson JW. Orbital Tumors. 3rd ed. New York: Raven Press, 1994.
27. Hornblass A, Jakobiec FA, Bosniak S, Flanagan J. The diagnosis and management of epithelial tumors of the lacrimal sac. Ophthalmology 1980; 87:476–90.
28. Iwamoto T, Jakobiec FA. A comparative ultrastructural study of the normal lacrimal gland and its epithelial tumors. Hum Pathol 1982; 13:236–62.
29. Jakobiec FA, Bilyk JR, Font RL. Orbit. In: Spencer WH, ed. Ophthalmic Pathology. An Atlas and Textbook. 4th ed. Philadelphia, PA: WB Saunders, 1996:2485–525.
30. Jang J, Kie JH, Lee SY, et al. Acinic cell carcinoma of the lacrimal gland with intracranial extension: a case report. Ophthal Plast Reconstr Surg 2001; 17:454–7.
31. Jones IS. Tumors of the lacrimal sac. Am J Ophthalmol 1956; 42:561–6.
32. Karcioglu ZA, Caldwell DR, Reed HT. Papillomas of lacrimal drainage system: a clinicopathologic study. Ophthalmic Surg 1984; 15:670–6.
33. Katz SE, Rootman J, Dolman PJ, et al. Primary ductal adenocarcinoma of the lacrimal gland. Ophthalmology 1996; 103:157–62.
34. Khalil M, Arthurs B. Basal cell adenocarcinoma of the lacrimal gland. Ophthalmology 2000; 107:164–8.
35. Klijanienko J, El-Naggar AK, Servios V, et al. Histologically similar, synchronous or metachronous, lacrimal salivary-type and parotid gland tumors: a series of II cases. Head Neck 1999; 21:512–6.
36. Kincaid MC, Green R, Iliff WJ. Fibrous histiocytoma of the lacrimal sac. Am J Ophthalmol 1982; 93:511–7.
37. Kincaid MC, Meis JM, Lee MW. Adenoid cystic carcinoma of the lacrimal sac. Ophthalmology 1989; 96:1655–8.
38. Kohn R, Nofsinger K, Freedman SI. Rapid recurrence of papillary squamous cell carcinoma of the canaliculus. Am J Ophthalmol 1981; 92:363–7.
39. Konrad EA, Thiel HJ. Adenocarcinoma of the lacrimal gland with sebaceous differentiation: a clinical study using light and electron microscopy. Graefes Arch Chin Exp Ophthalmol 1983; 221:81–5.
40. Lacrimal Gland Tumor Study Group. An epidemiological survey of lacrimal fossa lesions in Japan: number of patients and their sex ratio by pathological diagnosis. Jpn J Ophthalmol 2005; 49:343–8.
41. Madreperla SA, Green WR, Daniel R, Shah KW. Human papillomavirus in primary epithelial tumors of the lacrimal sac. Ophthalmology 1993; 100:569–73.
42. McDonnell PJ, McDonnell JM, Kessis T, et al. Detection of human papillomavirus type 6/11 DNA in conjunctival papillomas by in situ hybridization with radioactive probes. Hum Pathol 1987; 18:1115–9.
43. McDonnell JM, Mayr AJ, Martin WJ. DNA of human papillomavirus type 16 in dysplastic and malignant lesions of the conjunctiva and cornea. N Engl J Med 1989; 320:1442–6.
44. Mensink HW, Mooy CM, Paridaens D. In situ adenocarcinoma of the lacrimal gland. Clin Exp Ophthalmol 2005; 33: 669–71.
45. Morinaga S, Nakajima T, Shimosato Y. Normal and neoplastic myoepithelial cells in salivary glands: an immunohistochemical study. Hum Pathol 1987; 18:1218–26.
46. Nasu M, Haisa T, Kondo T, Matsubara O. Primary ductal adenocarcinoma of the lacrimal gland. Pathol Int 1998; 48: 981–4.
47. Ni C, D'Amico DJ, Fan CQ, Kuo PK. Tumors of the lacrimal sac: a clinicopathological analysis of 82 cases. Int Ophthalmol Clin 1982; 22:121–40.
48. Ni C, Kuo PK, Dryja TP. Histopathological classification of 272 primary epithelial tumors of the lacrimal gland. Chin Med J (Engl) 1992; 105:481–5.
49. Ni C. Primary epithelial lacrimal gland tumors: the pathologic classification of 272 cases Yan Ke Xue Bao 1994; 10:201–5.
50. Ni C, Ma X. Histopathologic classification of 1921 orbital tumors Yan Ke Xue Bao 1995; 11:101–4.
51. Parmar DN, Rose GE. Management of lacrimal sac tumours. Eye. 2003; 17:599–606.
52. Paulino AF, Huvos AG. Epithelial tumors of the lacrimal glands: a clinicopathologic study. Ann Diagn Pathol 1999; 3:199–204.

53. Paxton BR, Davidorf FH, Makley TA. Carcinoma of lacrimal canaliculi and lacrimal sac. Arch Ophthalmol 1970; 84:749–53.
54. Pecorella I, Garner A. Ostensible oncocytoma of accessory lacrimal glands. Histopathology 1997; 30:264–70.
55. Pe'er JJ, Stefanyszyn M, Hidayat AA. Nonepithelial tumors of the lacrimal sac. Am J Ophthalmol 1994; 118: 650–8.
56. Peretz WL, Ettinghausen SE, Gray GF. Oncocytic adenocarcinoma of the lacrimal sac. Arch Ophthalmol 1978; 96: 304–4.
57. Perzin KH, Jakobiec FA, Livolsi VA, Desjardins L. Lacrimal gland malignant mixed tumors (carcinomas arising in benign mixed tumors): a clinico-pathologic study. Cancer 1980; 45:2593–606.
58. Pulitzer DR, Eckert ER. Mucoepidermoid carcinoma of the lacrimal gland: an oxyphilic variant. Arch Ophthalmol 1987; 105:1406–9.
59. Rao NA, Kaiser E, Quiros PA, et al. Lymphoepithelial carcinoma of the lacrimal gland. Arch Ophthalmol 2002; 120:1745–8.
60. Rodgers IR, Jakobiec FA, Gingold MP, et al. Anaplastic carcinoma of the lacrimal gland presenting with recurrent subconjunctival hemorrhages and displaying incipient sebaceous differentiation. Ophthal Plast Reconstr Surg 1991; 7:229–37.
61. Rosembaum PS, Mahadevia PS, Goodman LA, Kress Y. Acinic cell carcinoma of the lacrimal gland. Arch Ophthalmol 1995; 113:781–5.
62. Ryan SJ, Font RL. Primary epithelial neoplasms of the lacrimal sac. Am J Ophthalmol 1973; 76:73–88.
63. Selva D, Davis GJ, Dodd T, Rootman J. Polymorphous low-grade adenocarcinoma of the lacrimal gland. Arch Ophthalmol 2004; 122:915–7.
64. Sen DK, Mohan H, Chatterjee PK. Neurilemmoma of the lacrimal sac. Eye Ear Nose Throat Mon 1971; 50:179–80.
65. Shields CL, Shields JA, Eagle RC, Rathmell JP. Clinicopathologic review of 142 cases of lacrimal gland lesions. Ophthalmology 1989; 96:431–5.
66. Shields JA, Font RL. Meibomian gland carcinoma presenting as a lacrimal gland tumor. Arch Ophthalmol 1974; 92: 304–6.
67. Shields JA, Shields CL, Epstein JA, et al. Review: primary epithelial malignancies of the lacrimal gland: the 2003 Ramon L. Font lecture. Ophthal Plast Reconstr Surg 2004; 20:10–21.
68. Stead RH, Qizilbash AH, Kontozoglou T, et al. An immunohistochemical study of pleomorphic adenomas of the salivary gland: glial fibrillary acidic protein- like immunoreactivity identifies a major myoepithelial component. Hum Pathol 1988; 19:32–40.
69. Stefanyszyn MA, Hidayat AA, Pe'er JJ, Flanagan JC. Lacrimal sac tumors. Ophthal Plast Reconstr Surg 1994; 10:169–84.
70. Sturgis CD, Silverman JF, Kennerdell JS, Raab SS. Fine-needle aspiration for the diagnosis of primary epithelial tumors of the lacrimal gland and ocular adnexa. Diagn Cytopathol 2001; 24:86–9.
71. Thomas A, Sujatha S, Ramakrishnan PM, Sudarsanam D. Malignant melanoma of the lacrimal sac. Arch Ophthalmol 1975; 3:84–6.
72. Wolpiuk M. Przypadek obutronnego chloniaka zloshiwego workow Izowych. Klin Oczna 1975; 45:61–4.
73. Wright JE, Rose GE, Garner A. Primary malignant neoplasms of the lacrimal gland. Br J Ophthalmol 1992; 76:401–7.
74. Wright JE. Lacrimal gland tumours. Trans Ophthalmol Soc NZ 1983; 35:101–6.
75. Yamamoto Y, Wistuba II, Kishimoto Y, et al. DNA analysis at p53 locus in adenoid cystic carcinoma: comparison of molecular study and p53 immunostaining. Pathol Int 1998; 48:273–80.
76. Zhao P, Sun X. Quantitative analyses of DNA content and p53 gene product expression from epithelial lacrimal gland tumors. Chung Hua Yen Ko Tsa Chih 1996; 32:424–8.
77. Zheng L, He S, Fan Z, Han C. Relationship between expression of P21ras and cellular DNA in pleomorphic adenoma of lacrimal gland Yan Ke Xue Bao 1996; 12:54–7.

62

Vascular Tumors

Harry H. Brown
Harvey and Bernice Jones Eye Institute, University of Arkansas for Medical Sciences, Little Rock, Arkansas, U.S.A.

INTRODUCTION

Vascular neoplasms and malformations account for a significant number of ocular adnexal disorders, but are rare within the eye. Vascular lesions can be subdivided according to whether they represent true hyperplasia of vascular endothelium, either reactive or neoplastic, or are nonproliferative and enlarge only as a function of the growth of the individual or due to an accumulation of intraluminal or extravasated fluids. However, vascular proliferative processes such as infantile hemangioma have an involutional phase such that the term proliferative may not always apply, and certain entities may have both proliferative and nonproliferative features, defying exact categorization. Vascular proliferations with potentially aggressive clinical behavior, such as local recurrence following their excision and/or metastasis are exceedingly rare in the eye and ocular adnexae.

The understanding, and consequently the terminology, of these processes continues to evolve, but not without controversy. The terminology introduced in this chapter is based on modifications of the recommendations proposed in 1996 by the International Society for the Study of Vascular Anomalies (ISSVA) (Table 1). The ISSVA nomenclature attempts to expunge entrenched terms from the literature, and therefore may take considerable time and effort to attain acceptance. For instance, certain terms, like pyogenic granuloma, are so embedded in the fabric of clinical practice despite their obvious inaccuracies, that they may not be discarded readily.

VASCULAR PROLIFERATIONS

Reactive Vascular Proliferations

Pyogenic Granuloma

Pyogenic granuloma (polypoid granulation tissue, granulation tissue-type hemangioma) is an exuberant reactive lobular proliferation of capillaries within a loose, edematous stroma, often containing an inflammatory infiltrate of polymorphonuclear leukocytes (PMNs), lymphocytes, and plasma cells. Pedunculated

Table 1 Vascular Proliferations and Malformations

Proposed terminology (ISSVA)	Current terminology (where different)
Proliferative	
Reactive	
Polypoid (exuberant) granulation tissue	Pyogenic granuloma, lobular capillary hemangioma, granulation tissue-type hemangioma
Intravascular papillary endothelial hyperplasia	
Bacillary angiomatosis	
Neoplastic	
Benign	
Infantile hemangioma	Capillary hemangioma
Intermediate (low malignant potential)	
Hemangioendothelioma	
Malignant	
Angiosarcoma	
Kaposi sarcoma	
Nonproliferative	
Arteriovenous malformation	
Venous malformation	Cavernous hemangioma
Mixed venous–lymphatic malformation	
Lymphatic malformation	Lymphangioma

masses have a fibrovascular stalk, with the capillary proliferation assuming an arborizing pattern from the central trunk. The vascular proliferation is likely a reactive process and often occurs at sites of irritation or trauma, such as in association with foreign bodies or sutures. Mucous membranes are common sites of occurrence, and the conjunctiva is the most common ocular adnexal location, particularly the palpebral conjunctiva or eyelid margins (11). Rapid but finite enlargement up to a centimeter is the typical clinical course. The proliferation assumes a polypoid configuration, with surface ulceration the rule, and a collarette of epithelium at the base of the polyp (Fig. 1). Capillary endothelium may appear more "plump" than usual, with reactive atypia in the form of nuclear enlargement and presence of nucleoli (Fig. 2). Occasional mitotic figures may be observed; atypical mitotic figures are not. The pathogenesis of such an exuberant granulation tissue-type proliferative response is not understood. Some but not all cases are associated with previous trauma, surgical or otherwise, at the site. Those occurring in pregnant women have been shown to be responsive to estrogen stimulation, perhaps related to its enhancement of vascular endothelial growth factor (VEGF) by macrophages (21). VEGF and another angiogenic stimulator, basic fibroblast growth factor, have been demonstrated by immunohistochemistry to be increased in oral pyogenic granuloma (46). Complete excision is curative, but recurrences and satellite lesions may develop (11).

Intravascular Papillary Endothelial Hyperplasia

Intravascular papillary endothelial hyperplasia (Masson tumor) is a proliferation of vascular endothelium, predominantly within veins, that may be one pattern of an organizing thrombus. It may also be seen in vascular anomalies in which there is sluggish blood flow or stasis. This process may attain tumoral dimensions of up to a few centimeters in diameter, and retains a circumscribed nature due to its intravascular location. The eyelid and orbit have been the reported ocular sites affected, albeit rarely (12). The well-developed lesions are characterized histopathologically by collagenous spherules or trabeculae lined by a single layer of plump endothelial cells lacking nuclear hyperchromasia, pleomorphism, or

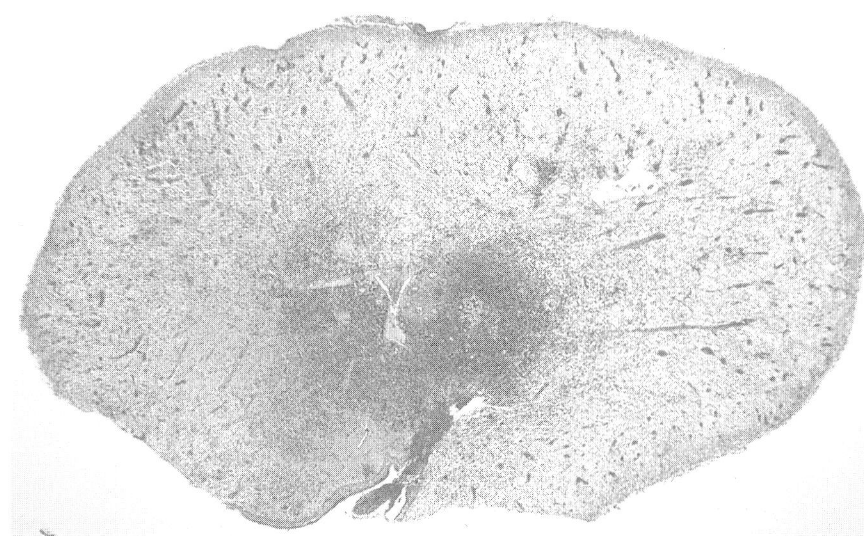

Figure 1 Low-power photomicrograph of pyogenic granuloma (polypoid granulation tissue). Note the surface ulceration, edematous stroma, and collarette of epithelium at the base (hematoxylin and eosin, ×2.3).

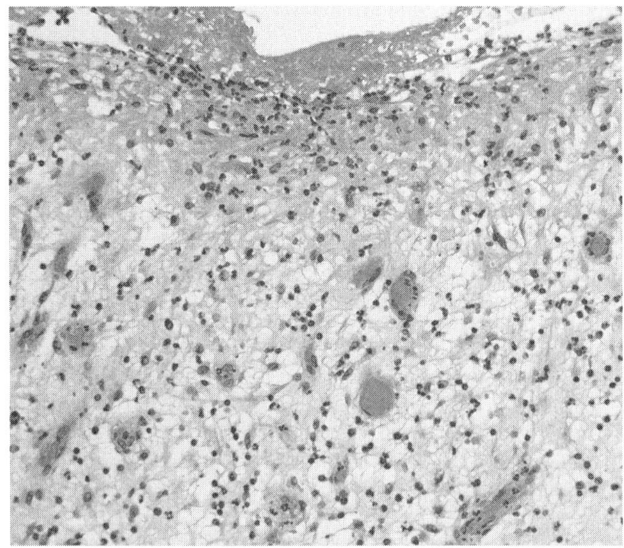

Figure 2 Acute inflammatory cells are increased at the surface of the granulation tissue. Endothelial cells are variably flattened to rounded, but without overt nuclear atypia (hematoxylin and eosin, ×23).

mitotic activity (Fig. 3). The irregular luminal pattern formed may simulate that of an angiosarcoma, but the circumscription of the mass and the lack of nuclear features of malignancy in papillary endothelial hyperplasia should obviate any concern of malignancy (41).

Bacillary Angiomatosis

Bacillary angiomatosis is a reactive vascular proliferation to infection by *Bartonella* sp. Both *B. henselae* and *B. quintana* have been documented as causative microorganisms (39). It occurs almost exclusively in immunocompromised patients, most commonly as a complication of the acquired immunodeficiency syndrome (AIDS). The typical ophthalmic clinical appearance is one of a polypoid vascular lesion of the conjunctiva, simulating a pyogenic granuloma. Rare cases of eyelid, retinal and presumed choroidal involvement have been reported. Histo-pathologically, the lobular vascular endothelial proliferation with an inflammatory infiltrate of PMNS seen in bacillary angiomatosis again may mimic a pyogenic granuloma, but the endothelial cells have abundant clear cytoplasm, containing numer-ous bacillary forms that can be identified in Warthin–Starry or Dieterle silver-stained preparations (Fig. 4). Antibiotic treatment effects complete resolution (22).

Angiolymphoid Hyperplasia with Eosinophilia

One entity which is not well understood as to pathogenesis, and therefore difficult to classify is angiolymphoid hyperplasia with eosinophilia, also called epithelioid hemangioma or histiocytoid hemangioma (23). Angiolymphoid hyperplasia with eosinophilia has been reported in the eyelid and orbit (18). Most examples have occurred in young- to middle-aged adults, presenting as gradually progressive ptosis or proptosis, depending on the location of the mass. On gross examination the lesions are circumscribed and firm. Histopathological examination reveals a lobular proliferation of capillaries, often surrounding a larger blood vessel. An associated stromal inflammatory infiltrate of lymphocytes,

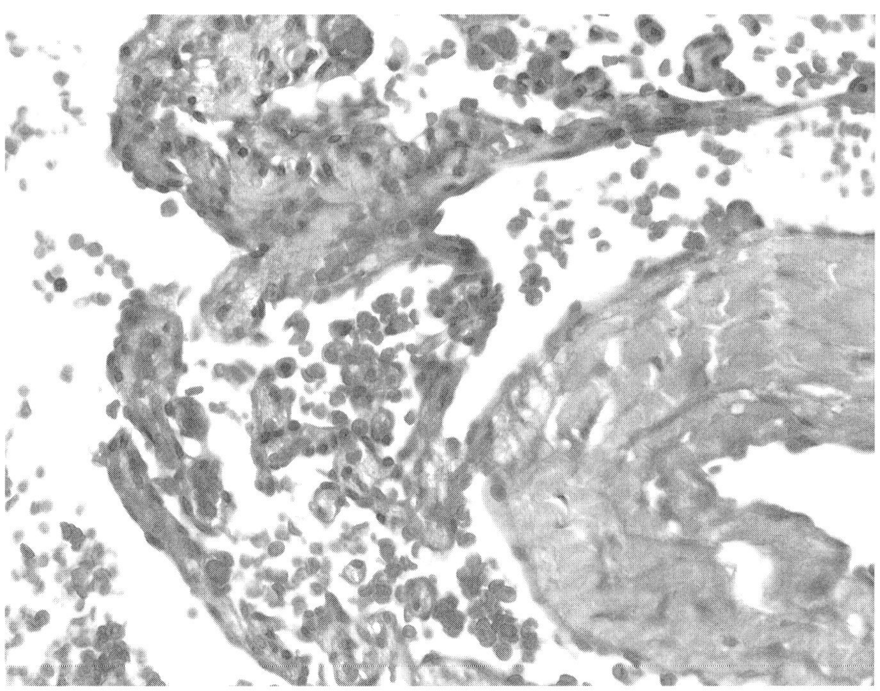

Figure 3 Intravascular papillary endothelial hyperplasia involving venous malformation. Note the complex papillary projections lined by a single layer of plump endothelial cells lacking nuclear atypia (hematoxylin and eosin, ×46).

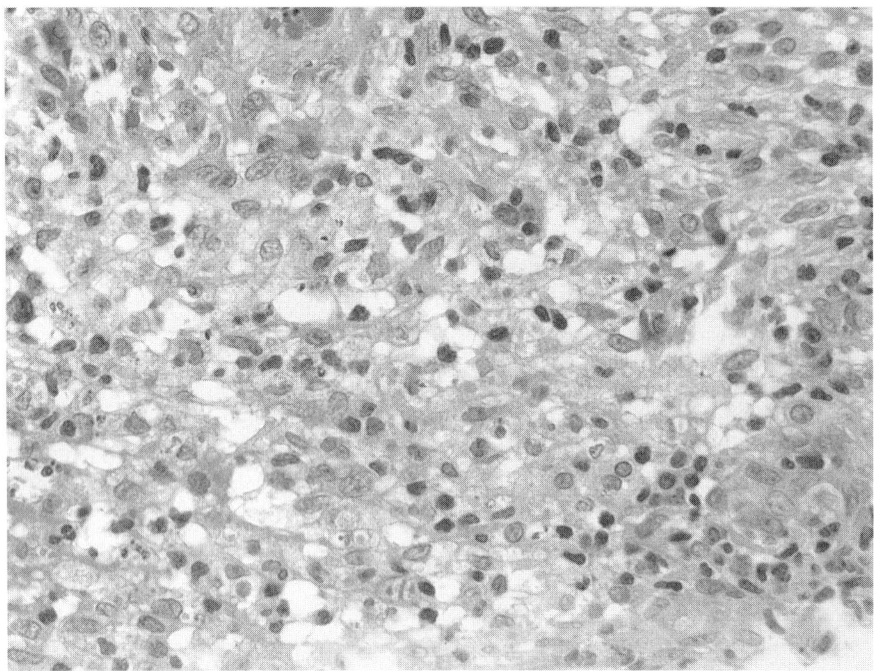

Figure 4 Bacillary angiomatosis is characterized by endothelial cells with vacuolated to clear cytoplasm in an inflammatory background (hematoxylin and eosin, × 46).

plasma cells, and eosinophils is evident. The endothelial cells of the capillaries may appear normal, but often have a rounded contour, protruding into the lumen giving a "tombstone" or epithelioid appearance. The cytoplasm contains increased numbers of organelles and thin filaments, and occasional cytoplasmic vacuoles suggesting attempts at lumen formation. Nuclei are round to multilobated but lack significant hyperchromasia.

Although the cause of angiolymphoid hyperplasia with eosinophilia is unknown, the prevailing opinion is that it is a reactive proliferation. In a significant number of cases studied histologically, evidence of a large blood vessel rupture or mural damage was associated with the capillary proliferation. Most pathologists consider this entity to be distinct from Kimura disease (3), a condition of lymphadenopathy associated with peripheral blood eosinophilia and a polymorphic inflammatory soft tissue mass occurring almost exclusively in Asian men. Although the histopathological findings are similar, the vascular component of Kimura disease is minor and the endothelial cells lack the epithelioid features seen in angiolymphoid hyperplasia with eosinophilia.

Neoplastic Vascular Proliferations

Benign

Infantile Hemangioma

Infantile hemangioma (capillary hemangioma) is one of the most common neoplasms of the eyelid and orbit, and can present significant problems for the affected child, the parents, and the ophthalmologist. It typically manifests within days to weeks after birth, but only 10% to 15% of cases are present at birth. Rapid enlargement and the cosmetic appearance are causes for parental concern, generally requiring reassurance on the part of the neonatologist or pediatrician as to the disease process and its natural course. Maximum tumor volume is usually reached by 6 to 12 months of age, at which point the mass begins to involute. Speed of regression fails to match that of growth, however, and complete resolution typically is not finished until school age. A slightly depressed, ill-defined dermal scar may be the only residuum of the once prominent vascular tumor. However, infantile hemangioma causing ptosis or proptosis may need treatment to prevent serious sequelae (14). The most common of these is deprivation amblyopia (see Chapter 71) due to blockage of the light into the eye by the ptotic eyelid overlying the pupillary axis; less commonly amblyopia is related to astigmatism induced by the mass effect on the eye. Rarely, facial hemangiomas may be associated with systemic anomalies of the CNS, cardiovascular system, and the eye (PHACE association) (MIM 606519) (6).

Histopathological features of infantile hemangioma are dependent on the stage of tumor development or regression at the time that it is sampled. Excised tissue during the active growth phase shows significant vascular endothelial cell proliferation, which in its early stages may be predominantly a plump spindle cell process with little or no capillary

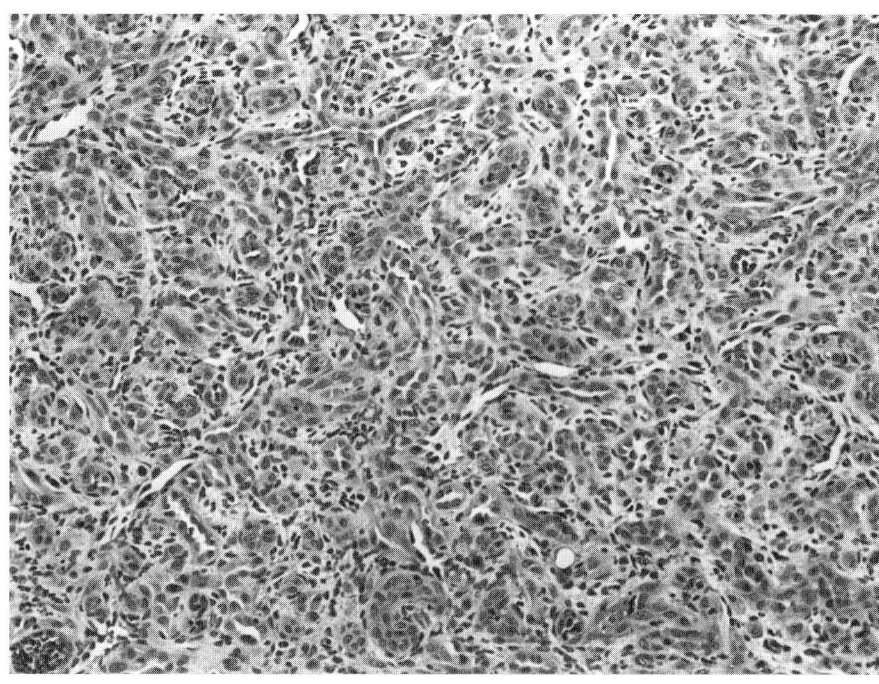

Figure 5 Histological section of infantile hemangioma showing numerous clustered small capillaries with plump endothelial cells either forming solid cores or surrounding round to slit-like lumina (hematoxylin and eosin, ×160).

lumen formation (Fig. 5). Mitotic figures, as might be expected, are easily identified, but do not exhibit atypical patterns. Later in the active phase, the classical appearance of a closely apposed, well-developed capillary proliferation with little intervening stroma is evident. Clusters of capillaries may assume lobular configurations, interspersed among normal tissue elements, or separated by thin fibrous strands. Small arteries may be identified within the lobules. Capillary proliferation within small nerves ("pseudoinvasion") is common, as are mast cells within the capillary proliferation. Fibrin thrombi and/or hemosiderin deposition, however, is unusual. With regression, capillaries gradually diminish in numbers and become, replaced by loose fibrous tissue, until finally only a subtle and easily overlooked focus of loose connective tissue marks the site of the once exuberant capillary proliferation.

Infantile hemangioma has been shown to be immunophenotypically distinct from other proliferations of capillaries in the skin and subcutaneous tissue. Infantile hemangiomas exhibit immunoreactivity not only for vascular endothelial markers (CD31, CD34, Factor VIII, and *Ulex europus*) and pericyte (smooth muscle actin) markers, but also for antigens not normally expressed by cutaneous vasculature (glucose transporter 1 [(GLUT1), Lewis Y antigen (LeY), and others] (27). This distinctive pattern is similar to that seen in placental tissue, and when combined with the usual perinatal appearance of these proliferations, suggests some association between the two, such as embolization of placental tissue during parturition or abnormal receptivity of innate fetal/neonatal tissue to molecular or hormonal events controlling placental vasculogenesis (28). These immunophenotypic markers remain positive even through involution of infantile hemangiomas, and are therefore valuable diagnostic tools in identifying such lesions.

Congenital Nonprogressive Hemangioma

While a small proportion of infantile hemangiomas are present at birth, they behave in the same fashion as those occurring shortly after birth, and should not be combined with another clinically and immunophenotypically distinct group of congenital vascular proliferations now termed congenital nonprogressive hemangioma (29). As the name implies, lesions of this group are present at birth but do not exhibit significant enlargement in the neonatal period or infancy. These proliferations can be subdivided based on their clinical course: those that rapidly involute in a more accelerated fashion than infantile hemangioma (rapidly involuting congenital hemangioma), or those that remain stationary (noninvoluting congenital hemangioma). While histopathologically somewhat similar to infantile hemangioma, congenital nonprogressive hemangioma exhibits a more pronounced lobular architecture of capillary proliferation and separation of lobules by dense connective tissue. In contrast to infantile hemangioma, congenital nonprogressive hemangioma does not react with antibodies to GLUT1 or LeY antigens by immunohistochemistry.

Cavernous Hemangioma

Cavernous hemangioma is a collection of dilated vascular channels lined by flattened endothelium and thin fibrous vessel walls containing variable numbers of smooth muscle elements (Figs. 6 to 8). Thrombosis is common, and organization of thrombi may result in a capillary network simulating a lobular capillary hemangioma or intravascular papillary endothelial hyperplasia (Fig. 9). They may occur in the eyelid, orbit, or intraocularly in the retina or choroid. Eyelid lesions appear as blue-purple papules or nodules either singly or in groups. Orbital involvement is typically intraconal, manifesting in middle age with proptosis but sparing vision or motility disruption. Radiographic studies demonstrate a circumscribed mass with little enhancement using contrast media. Calcification in association with thrombosis may be detected. Pathological examination of the excised tissue demonstrates a slightly bosselated, deep red-purple mass with a thin fibrous covering and a spongy appearance on cut surface (Fig. 10). Those occurring in the choroid are either a localized, disciform to dome-shaped mass (1,36) or a diffuse involvement in cases of Sturge–Weber syndrome (MIM 185300) (see Chapter 55) (7,38). An exudative retinal detachment may supervene due to leakage from the abnormal vessels (45) (Figs. 11 to 13).

While the term cavernous hemangioma remains entrenched in the literature, and connotes distinct clinical, radiographic, and histopathological findings depending on its location, it does not fulfill the currently accepted definition of a "hemangioma" in that it has no proliferative capability. Some authors use the term hamartoma to describe them while others view them as a venous malformation (33). Malformations are present at birth, grow in proportion to the child, and fail to involute over time. Enlargement may result from trauma or hemodynamic changes such as thrombosis and organization (27).

Hemangioblastoma

Capillary proliferations occurring in the retina, particularly when multiple, may represent one component of von Hippel–Lindau disease (VHLD) (see Chapter 55) (37). While present at birth, they routinely do not become evident ophthalmoscopically until adulthood, when they appear as pink-red to yellow vascular tufts fed and drained by a large, variably tortuous artery and vein, respectively (Fig. 14). Significant leakage of proteinaceous fluid may cause localized or even complete exudative retinal detachment. The capillary proliferations in the hemangioblastoma are accompanied by vacuolated stromal cells, which distinguish this entity from the hemangiomas described above (Fig. 15). The vacuolated cells are favored to be of glial origin, but they also contain the same genetic alteration as their endothelial counterparts, namely mutations in the *VHL* gene on chromosome 3 (3p25–26). Germline mutations of this tumor suppressor gene have been detected in 81% of patients with retinal hemangioblastomas (9). Screening of family members of affected individuals by molecular testing is available (40).

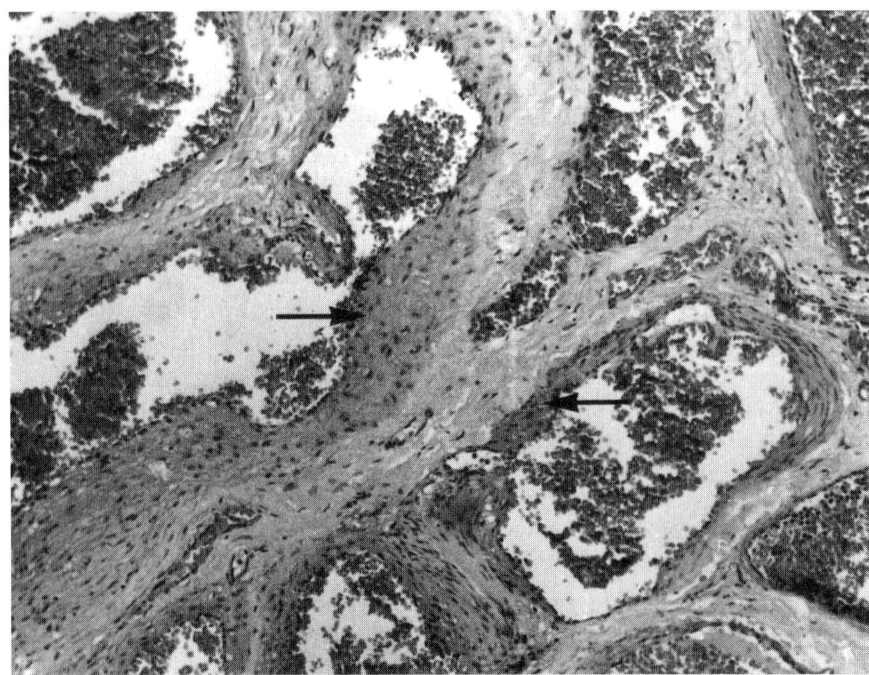

Figure 6 Histological section of venous malformation demonstrating large, somewhat irregular lumina lined by flattened endothelium and containing numerous erythrocytes, with variable degrees of smooth muscle and fibrous tissue in the surrounding walls (hematoxylin and eosin, ×100).

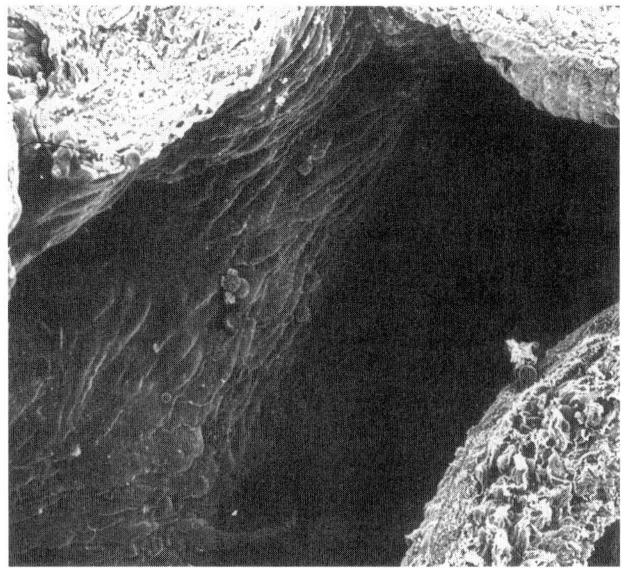

Figure 7 Scanning electron micrograph of the endothelial-lined lumen within a cavernous hemangioma (× 290).

Presumed Acquired Retinal Hemangioma

Solitary red-yellow or peach colored, solid, vascular masses in the peripheral retina, often associated with hemorrhage and exudates, have been described either as isolated findings or in association with other intraocular diseases such as retinitis pigmentosa, retinopathy of prematurity, or Coats disease. Initially termed "presumed acquired retinal hemangioma" (20), the consensus of opinion now is that these are reactive vascular proliferations, either idiopathic or secondary to congenital, inflammatory, traumatic, and degenerative ocular conditions (20,34). Such lesions are characterized by a reactive gliovascular proliferation, which may arise as such or be due to vascularization of a pigment epithelial proliferation (16). In contrast to hemangioblastoma, they are found in older subjects without a personal or family history of VHLD, typically occur in the inferotemporal peripheral retina, and lack dilated, tortuous feeding and draining blood vessels (20).

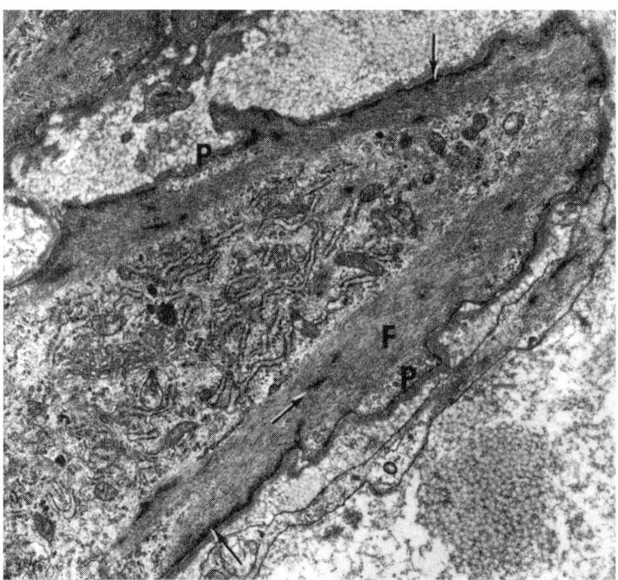

Figure 8 Transmission electron micrograph of a smooth muscle cell, showing subplasmalemmal thin filaments (F) with focal electron-dense areas (*arrows*), flask-like cell membrane pits (P) akin to pinocytotic vesicles, and a prominent basal lamina (×14,000).

Other

Other rare forms of cutaneous or subcutaneous benign vascular proliferations presenting in children include tufted angioma and infantile kaposiform hemangioendothelioma, and neither eyelid nor orbital manifestations of these entities was found in a review of the literature.

Angiogenesis, defined as new capillary formation, occurs in a number of settings in the eye (including corneal neovascularization, iris neovascularization, and neovascularization affecting the retina) are all complications with deleterious consequences for vision, and are further discussed elsewhere (see Chapter 68).

Intermediate Malignant Potential

Hemangioendothelioma

Hemangioendothelioma, a neoplasm derived from the vascular endothelium, is considered to be of intermediate malignant potential. It is capable of local recurrence, metastasis and death, but at a reduced rate as compared to angiosarcoma (42). Although the term hemangioendothelioma is now utilized for those vascular neoplasms with a low but real significant risk of aggressive behavior, historically it has been employed for a range of processes including benign conditions, and thus caution must be exercised in interpreting such reports. Its occurrence in the eye and ocular adnexal is vanishingly rare; only a single choroidal malignant hemangioendothelioma has been reported (8). Histopathologically, hemangioendothelioma is characterized by solid cords or nests of relatively bland polygonal endothelial cells, centered within the occluded lumen of a blood vessel, and infiltrating centrifugally into the surrounding soft tissue. Distinct vascular channels are rare, and when present are located at the periphery of the tumor. Mitotic activity typically is minimal to nonexistent. The principal clue to the endothelial nature of the cells is the presence of intracytoplasmic lumens or vacuoles (so-called "blisters"). Immunohistochemical markers for vascular endothelial cells, such as

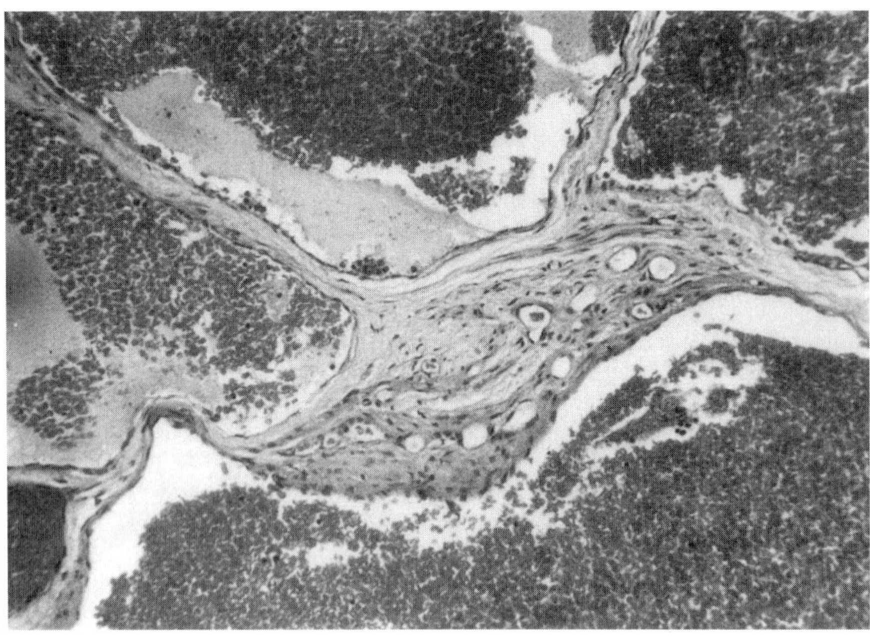

Figure 9 A cluster of capillaries adjacent to a cavernous space suggesting organization of a luminal thrombus and incorporation into the vessel wall (hematoxylin and eosin, ×170).

CD31, CD34, *Ulex europeus*, von Willebrand factor are usually positive and helpful in diagnosis. The intervening stroma may vary from myxoid to hyalinized in appearance. Features portending a more aggressive clinical behavior include the presence of necrosis, spindle cell morphology, nuclear atypia, and mitotic figures >1 per 10 high power fields.

Kaposi Sarcoma

Kaposi sarcoma, although now debated as to its biologic risk, if considered malignant is the most common malignant vascular neoplasm of the ocular adnexae, assuming prominence as one of the constellation of findings associated with AIDS (35). Its rapid increase in incidence in the 1980s in association with infection by the human immunodeficiency virus (HIV) (see Chapter 8) suggested the possibility of a viral etiologic agent, and subsequent immunological and genotypic studies have demonstrated a strong link between human herpes virus 8 and Kaposi sarcoma (4). HIV may promote development of Kaposi sarcoma by production of cytokines, and the tumor itself may produce autocrine cytokines such as VEGF in a positive feedback mechanism. While most common in AIDS, it may

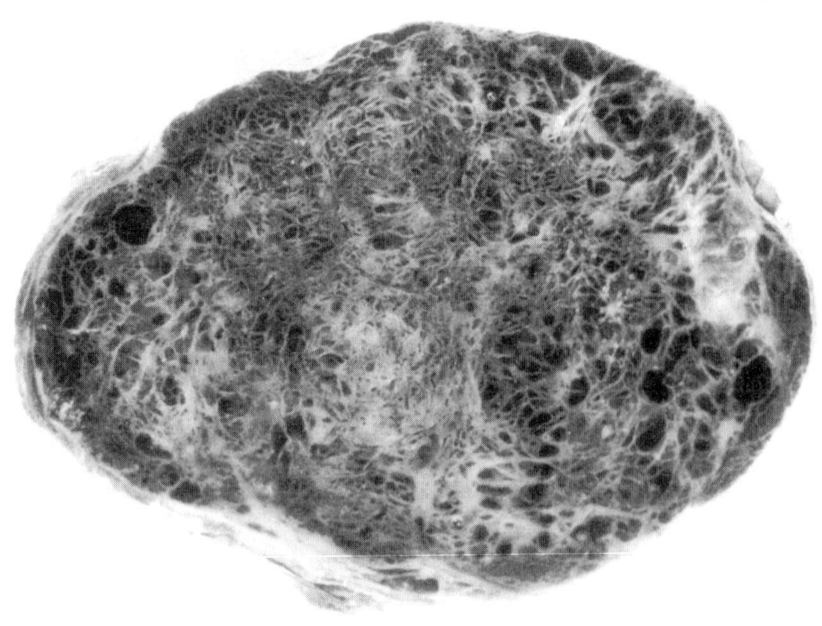

Figure 10 Excision specimen of orbital cavernous hemangioma (venous malformation). Note the overall circumscription of the mass and its honeycomb pattern of vascular spaces (×7).

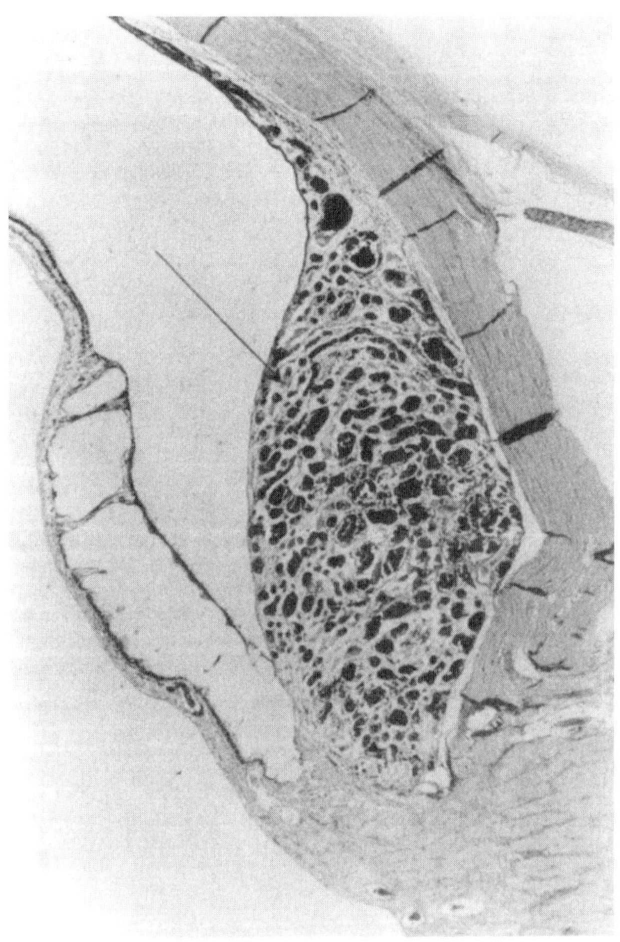

Figure 11 Histological section of a circumscribed peripapillary choroidal venous malformation, with overlying cystoid edema of the retina (hematoxylin and eosin, ×68). *Source*: Courtesy of Dr. D.M. Albert.

also arise in other immunologically altered or deficient states. It may involve the eyelid and/or conjunctiva, and may be solitary or multicentric. Mortality is often due to coexistent opportunistic infections or development of another malignancy.

Histopathologically, Kaposi sarcoma is classically characterized by a relatively circumscribed plaque-like to nodular proliferation of bland spindle cells in arcing fascicles, containing slit-like intercellular spaces and extravasated erythrocytes (Fig. 16). Periodic acid Schiff positive hyaline globules, possibly representing degenerated erythrocytes, may be present either intra- or extracellularly. Well-formed vascular channels may be present in the early stages of the tumor. Mitotic activity is usually low, as is nuclear pleomorphism. An inflammatory component may be present at the periphery of the tumor, comprised principally of lymphocytes and plasma cells.

Immunohistochemical studies of the spindle cells favor a lymphatic endothelial cell phenotype as opposed to vascular endothelium, showing positive reactivity with lymphatic markers D2-40, LYVE-1, and VEGFR3 (31). By transmission electron microscopy (TEM), tumor cells line slit-like spaces, exhibiting few intercellular junctions and incomplete basal lamina, which appears fragmented. Intracytoplasmic Weibel–Palade bodies are not present.

Malignant

Angiosarcoma

Angiosarcoma has only rarely been reported to involve the eyelid, much less the conjunctiva or orbit, and never intraocularly as a primary malignancy (19). Cutaneous angiosarcoma, however, is most common in the head and neck area, particularly the scalp.

Histopathologically, angiosarcoma may exhibit variability in differentiation from well-formed but irregular interconnecting vascular channels with relatively bland nuclear features to the more common pattern of infiltrating cords of cells with nuclear pleomorphism, hyperchromasia, and abnormal mitotic figures (Fig. 17). Endothelial papillary tufting into irregularly shaped lumina is a characteristic finding, and must be distinguished from intravascular papillary endothelial hyperplasia as previously described. Immunohistochemical markers of vascular endothelium, such as CD31 and CD34, are usually positive, even in poorly differentiated tumors (43). No definitive genetic abnormality thus far has been recognized as a precipitating factor in the development of angiosarcoma, although mutations of the *TP53* gene that encodes for p53 may play a role (5).

NONPROLIFERATIVE VASCULAR MALFORMATIONS

Overview

Nonproliferative vascular malformations are relatively common in the orbit, but are far less common intraocularly. Because they are developmental anomalies, they are present at birth, and grow in proportion to the host. They do not undergo cellular hyperplasia, characteristic of the proliferative conditions described above. Due to their slow growth, they may not produce signs or symptoms until some precipitating event occurs, such as hemorrhage. Malformations may exhibit histopathological uniformity in their alterations from normal, such as venous malformation (cavernous hemangioma), and are termed simple malformations, or may display intermediate characteristics making categorization less clear-cut, as in mixed venous–lymphatic malformation, and are classified as combined malformations. It is perhaps best to view vascular malformations in the context of a continuum of anomalies, with the classically

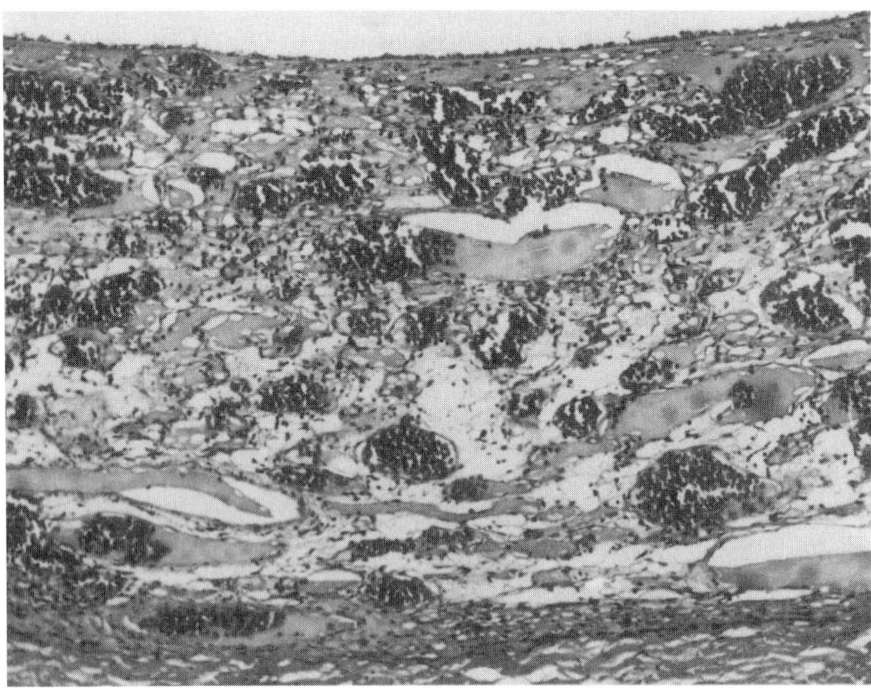

Figure 12 Histological section of venous malformation of the choroid in a 28-year-old male with Sturge–Weber syndrome. Note the plaque-like thickening of the choroid by closely packed, thin-walled vessels (hematoxylin and eosin, ×70).

described arteriovenous, venous, and lymphatic forms as discrete points along that continuum.

Vascular malformations may become apparent as early as the first trimester of gestation. Recent evidence suggests that they may result from abnormalities in vascular remodeling in utero. Alterations in various signaling pathways and their activating sequences, such as platelet-derived growth factor (PDGF) and transforming growth factor β (TGFβ) have been implicated in the development of vascular malformations in genetically engineered mice (5).

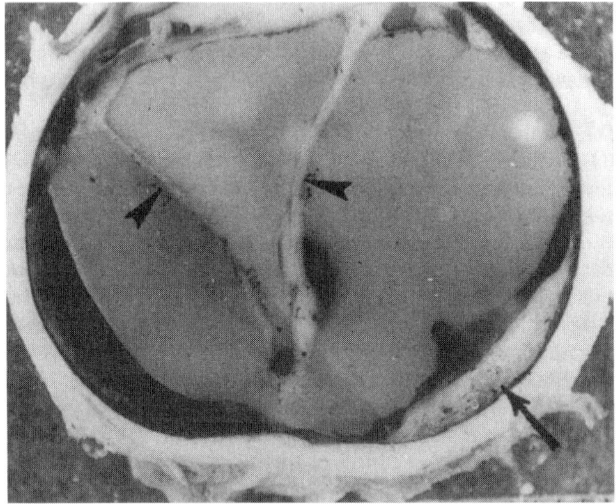

Figure 13 Enucleation specimen of a 27-year-old female with Sturge–Weber syndrome, showing a diffuse venous malformation of the choroid, partially ossified temporally (*arrow*), with an exudative retinal detachment (*arrowheads*). (×3)

Although the pathogenetic mechanism(s) causing vascular malformations are only beginning to be determined experimentally, there appears to be some correlation at the human level. At least in an autosomal-dominant disorder with multiple cutaneous and mucosal venous malformations (MIM #600195), molecular genetic studies have identified missense mutations in the *TEK* gene on chromosome 9 (9p21) that encodes for an endothelial cell-specific tyrosine kinase receptor (2).

Abnormal neural development may secondarily affect the vascular system; such a scenario has been proposed for port-wine stains of the skin as in Sturge–Weber syndrome (see Chapter 55) where nerves around the ectatic blood vessels are reduced in number.

Clinical categorization of vascular malformations is based primarily on their radiographic and ultrasound imaging characteristics. Rheologically, they can be divided into high flow (arterial or arteriovenous malformations), low flow (venous or mixed venous–lymphatic malformations), or no flow, that is, not associated with the arteriovenous circulation (lymphatic malformations) (33).

Arteriovenous Malformations

Arteriovenous malformations as primary developmental anomalies are uncommon; secondary arteriovenous shunts as sequelae of trauma are more likely. Developmental arteriovenous malformations of the

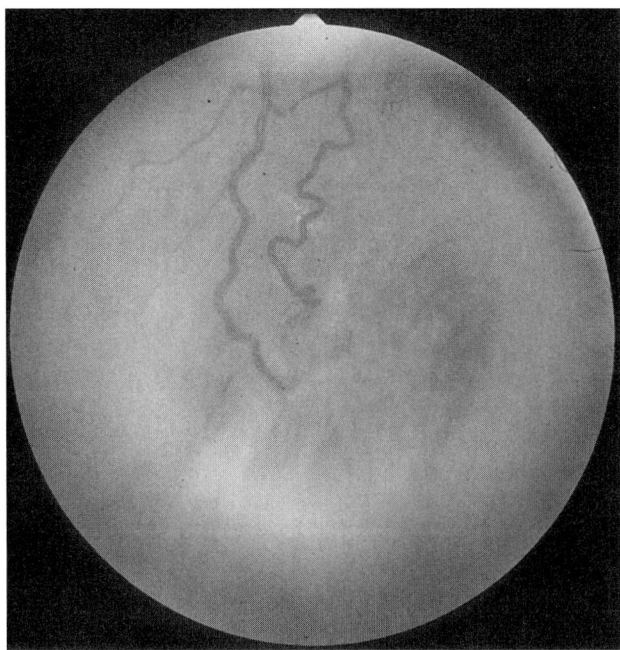

Figure 14 Fundus photograph of retinal hemangioblastoma in von Hippel–Lindau disease (×6). Note the small size of the tumor and increased caliber of the feeding vessels.

orbit may be associated with similar processes in the brain and retina (Wyburn–Mason syndrome) (see Chapter 55) (30). Involvement of the eyelids may also occur. Patients typically present with pulsatile proptosis, epibulbar venous congestion, and/or glaucoma. By definition, arteriovenous malformations are high flow states causing venous congestion and antegrade venous flow. Pulsation and a bruit may be detected on physical examination. Retinal arteriovenous malformations may be visualized on fundoscopy as engorged, tortuous blood vessels entering and exiting the retina from the optic nerve head, forming a tangled mass of arteriovenous connections on the retinal surface. Those in the orbit are highlighted by angiography or Doppler studies.

Histopathological examination of arteriovenous malformations reveals a plethora and variety of blood vessels, ranging from large caliber arteries and veins to small arterioles and venules to capillary beds (Fig. 18). Large blood vessels usually have a dysmorphic architecture, with irregular smooth muscle bundles in the media, intimal and adventitial fibrosis of veins, and an incomplete internal elastic lamina in arteries. The intervening connective tissue varies from being densely fibrotic to myxoid in appearance. Intraluminal foreign material is common as evidence of iatrogenic embolization prior to surgical resection.

Venous Malformations

Venous malformations most commonly involve the orbit, but can occur in the eyelid, and rarely the choroid and retina (17,25). Those in the orbit may be subdivided into two clinical syndromes: distensible malformations with enlargement on Valsalva maneuver and demonstration of ecstatic channels on contrast injection, and nondistensible, without these characteristics (33). Venous malformations are characterized by

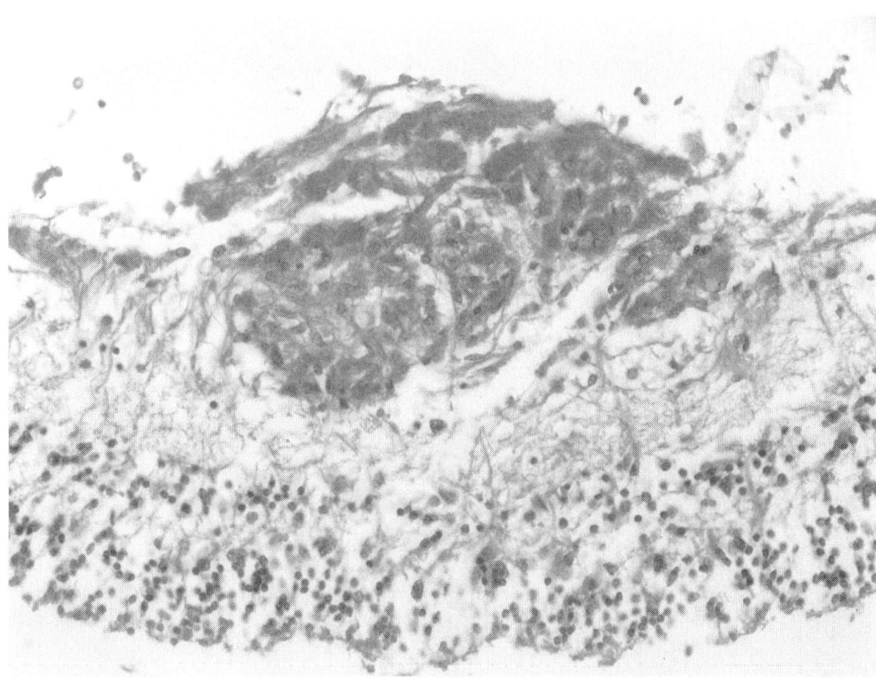

Figure 15 Histological section of hemangioblastoma of the retina in von Hippel–Lindau disease (hematoxylin and eosin, ×115).

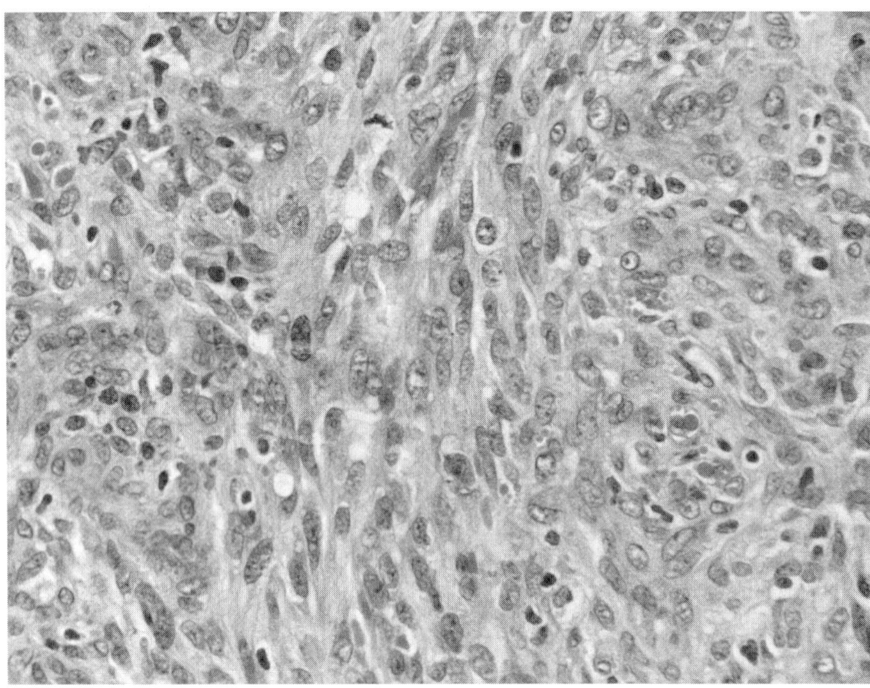

Figure 16 Kaposi sarcoma of the conjunctiva, showing spindle cells, slit-like extracellular spaces, and extravasated erythrocytes (hematoxylin and eosin, ×46).

a conglomeration of dilated venous channels lined by flattened endothelium. Histopathologically, the blood vessel walls are relatively thin, lined by flattened endothelium and contain smooth muscle bundles, although often attenuated or incompletely circumferential. The blood vessels are separated by variably thick fibrous bands, which at the periphery may give the appearance of a fibrous capsule to the malformation. As might be expected with the slow velocity of blood flow through the malformation, luminal thrombosis is relatively common. Organization of thrombosed lumina and recanalization by capillaries sometimes creates the appearance of lobular capillary proliferation or intravascular papillary endothelial

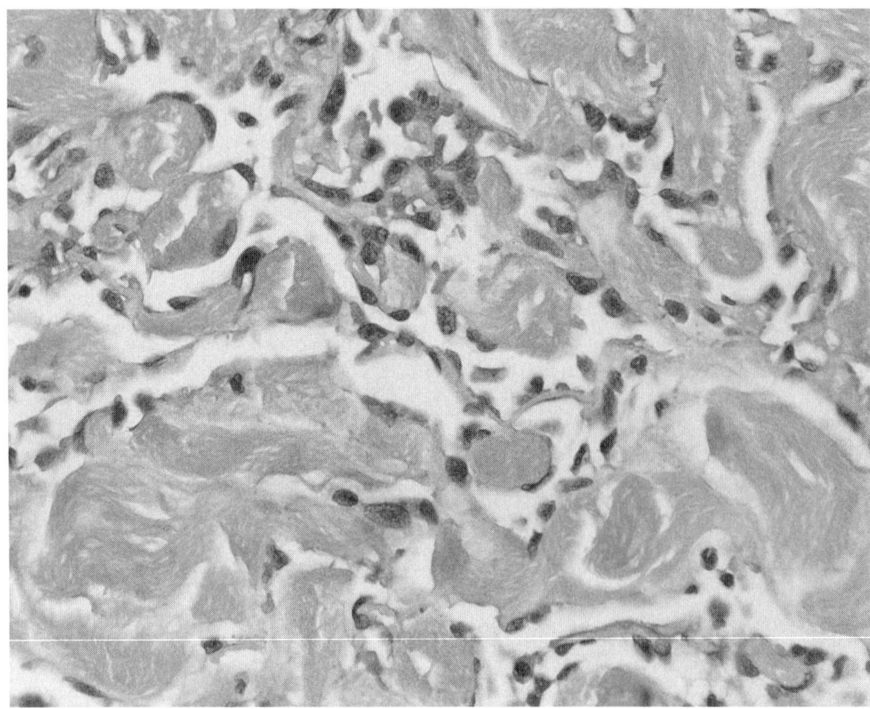

Figure 17 Angiosarcoma involving the skin. Note the interconnecting, irregularly shaped channels infiltrating the dermis, lined by enlarged endothelial cells with nuclear hyperchromasia (hematoxylin and eosin, ×46).

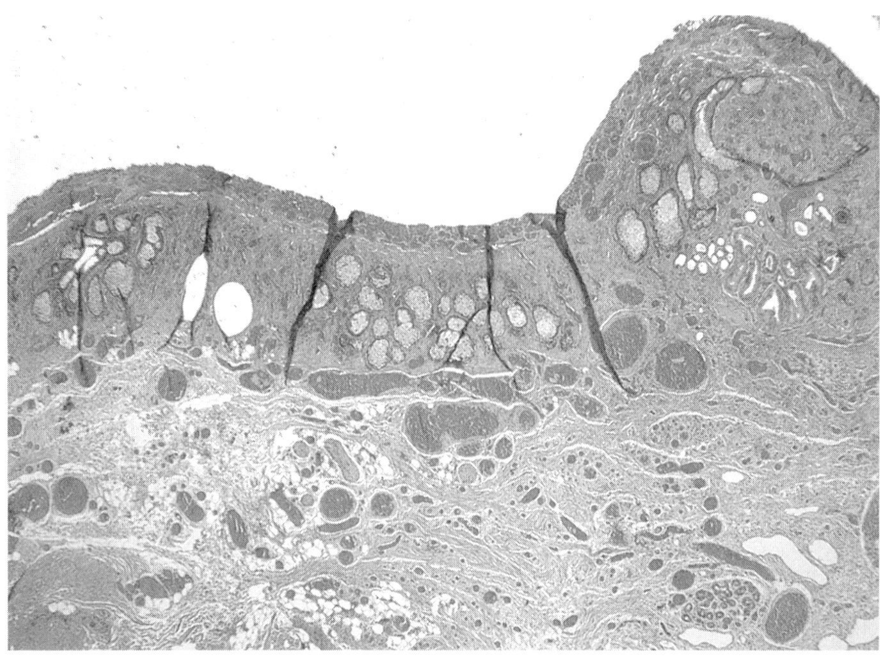

Figure 18 Arteriovenous malformation involving the eyelid, showing variably sized congested vessels predominantly in the pretarsal space (hematoxylin and eosin, ×2.3).

hyperplasia. Hemosiderin deposition and/or calcification are also common sequelae.

Orbital Varix

Orbital varix, if congenital, would fit in the rubric of a venous malformation; however, more commonly it is secondary to orbital or intracranial trauma, or arteriovenous shunting. It may vary in size with changes in pressure or position. Orbital varix may present as an orbital mass, but varies from venous malformation with regard to clinical manifestations, although histological differentiation from a lymphatic or venous malformation may be problematic (24).

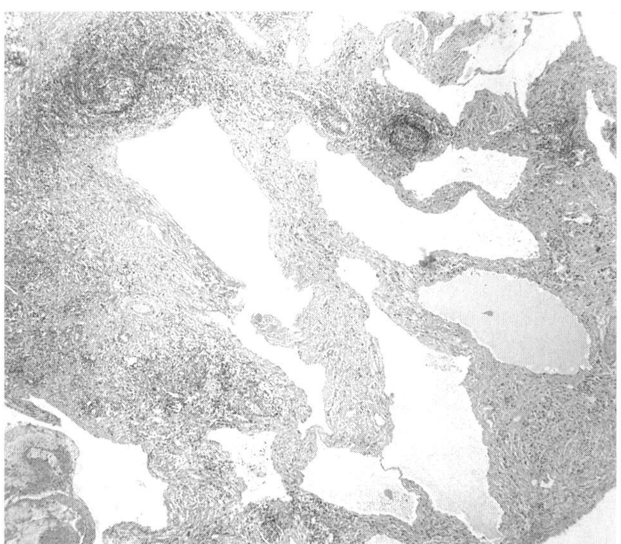

Figure 19 Lymphatic malformation of the orbit at low power demonstrating cavernous spaces, some containing acellular eosinophilic fluid, and intervening stroma with lymphoid tissue (hematoxylin and eosin, ×4.6).

Lymphatic Malformations

Lymphatic malformations (lymphangiomas) are uncommon in the orbit and ocular adnexae, and typically manifest in childhood as proptosis. A sudden onset of proptosis may result from hemorrhage into the malformation (so-called "chocolate cyst"). Initial presentation and/or intermittent exacerbation of the proptosis have also been attributed to reactive lymphoid hyperplasia associated with upper respiratory infections (44).

Lymphatic malformations in their prototypic form are an ill-defined congery of lymphatic channels with intervening admixed lymphoid tissue often containing follicles with germinal centers (Fig. 19). Lymphatic lumina are lined by a flattened endothelium and contain faintly eosinophilic material sometimes with occasional lymphocytes or erythrocytes (Fig. 20). The blood vessel walls may contain scant smooth muscle bundles, usually incompletely circumferential, but if present in significant amounts and combined with paucicellular stroma, may overlap considerably with the histopathological features of venous malformations (32). In fact, some authors consider such lesions to be a separate category, so-called mixed venous–lymphatic malformations. The close developmental relationship between venous and

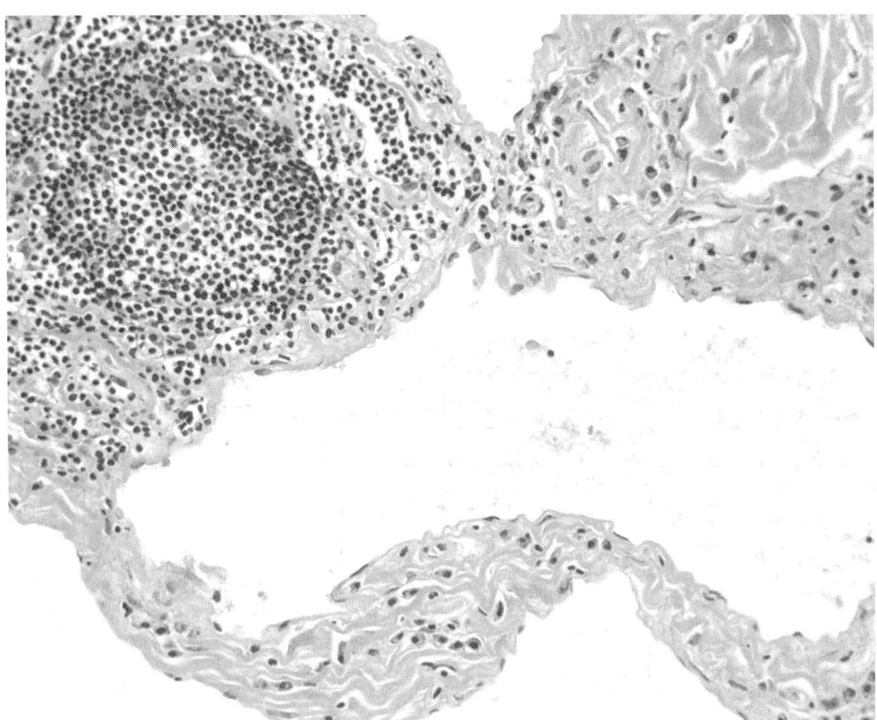

Figure 20 Higher-power view of lymphatic malformation. Endothelial cells are flattened and appear discontinuous. Note the lymphoid germinal center (*top left*) (hematoxylin and eosin, ×23).

lymphatic systems embryologically may explain this overlap and the variability in the histopathological appearances between and within individual malformations. Lymphatic malformations may arise from pluripotential precursor cells that may differentiate along both vascular and lymphatic endothelial pathways. Thus far, no native lymphatic channels have been found within the orbital adipose tissue or extraocular muscles, although lymphatics are present within the lacrimal gland and the optic nerve as demonstrated by enzyme histochemistry (5′ nucleotidase activity) (13). Immunohistochemical reactivity to lymphatic endothelial marker D2-40 has demonstrated positive staining in areas of orbital inflammation, suggesting that lymphatic differentiation may be induced by cytokines as yet undetermined (10).

REFERENCES

1. Anand R, Augsburger JJ, Shields JA. Circumscribed choroidal hemangiomas. Arch Ophthalmol 1989; 107: 1338–42.
2. Boon LM, Mulliken JB, Vikkula M, et al. Assignment of a locus for dominantly inherited venous malformations to chromosome 9p. Hum Mol Genet 1994; 3:1583–7.
3. Buggage RR, Spraul CW, Wojno TH, et al. Kimura disease of the orbit and ocular adnexa. Surv Ophthalmol 1999; 44: 79–91.
4. Cesarman E, Knowles DM. Kaposi's sarcoma-associated herpes virus. Semin Diagn Pathol 1997; 14:54–66.
5. Chiller KG, Frieden IJ, Arbiser JL. Molecular pathogenesis of vascular anomalies: classification into three categories based upon clinical and biochemical characteristics. Lymphat Res Biol 2003; 1:267–81.
6. Coats DK, Paysse EA, Levy ML. PHACE: a neurocutaneous syndrome with important ophthalmologic implications. Ophthalmology 1999; 106:1739–41.
7. Comi AM. Pathophysiology of Sturge–Weber syndrome. J Child Neurol 2003; 18:509–16.
8. Dhermy P, Capron F, Deschatres F. Malignant hemangioendothelioma of the choroid. J Fr Ophtalmol 1984; 7: 363–9.
9. Dollfus H, Massin P, Taupin P, et al. Retinal hemangioblastoma in von Hippel–Lindau disease: a clinical and molecular study. Invest Ophthalmol Vis Sci 2002; 43:3067–74.
10. Fogt F, Zimmerman RL, Daly T, Gausas RE. Observation of lymphatic vessels in orbital fat of patients with inflammatory conditions: a form fruste of lymphangiogenesis? Int J Mol Med 2004; 13:681–3.
11. Font RL. Eyelids and lacrimal drainage system. In: Spencer WH, ed. Ophthalmic Pathology: An Atlas and Textbook, vol. 4. 4th ed. Philadelphia, PA: W.B. Saunders, 1996: 2218–437.
12. Font RL, Wheeler TM, Boniuk M. Intravascular papillary endothelial hyperplasia of the orbit and ocular adnexa: a report of five cases. Arch Ophthalmol 1983; 101:1731–6.
13. Gausas RE, Gonnering RS, Lemke BN, et al. Identification of human orbital lymphatics. Ophthal Plast Reconstr Surg 1999; 15:252–9.
14. Haik BG, Karcioglu ZA, Gordon RA, et al. Capillary hemangioma (infantile periocular hemangioma). Surv Ophthalmol 1994; 38:399–426.
15. Hardwig P, Robertson DM. von Hippel–Lindau disease. A familial, often lethal, multi-system phakomatosis. Ophthalmology 1984; 91:263–70.
16. Heimann H, Bornfeld N, Vij O, et al. Vasoproliferative tumours of the retina. Br J Ophthalmol 2000; 84:1162–9.

17. Hewick S, Lois N, Olson JA. Circumferential peripheral retinal cavernous hemangioma. Arch Ophthalmol 2004; 122:1557–60.
18. Hidayat AA, Cameron JD, Font RL, Zimmerman LE. Angiolymphoid hyperplasia with eosinophilia (Kimura's disease) of the orbit and ocular adnexa. Am J Ophthalmol 1983; 96:176–89.
19. Hufnagel T, Ma L, Kuo TT. Orbital angiosarcoma with subconjunctival presentation: report of a case and literature review. Ophthalmology 1987; 94:72–7.
20. Irvine F, O'Donnell N, Kemp E, Lee WR. Retinal vasoproliferative tumors. Arch Ophthalmol 2000; 118: 563–9.
21. Kanda N, Watanabe S. Regulatory roles of sex hormones in cutaneous biology and immunology. J Dermatol Sci 2005; 38:1–7.
22. Lee WR, Chawla JC, Reid R. Bacillary angiomatosis of the conjunctiva. Am J Ophthalmol 1994; 118:152–7.
23. McEachren TM, Brownstein S, Jordan DR, et al. Epithelioid hemangioma of the orbit. Ophthalmology 2000; 107: 806–10.
24. Menon SV, Shome D, Mahesh L, et al. Thrombosed orbital varix: a correlation between imaging studies and histopathology. Orbit 2004; 23:13–8.
25. Messmer E, Font RL, Laqua H, et al. Cavernous hemangioma of the retina. Immunohistochemical and ultrastructural observations. Arch Ophthalmol 1984; 102:413–8.
26. North PE, Mihm MC Jr. Histopathological diagnosis of infantile hemangiomas and vascular malformations. Facial Plast Surg Clin N Am 2001; 9:505–24.
27. North PE, Waner M, Mizeracki A, et al. A unique microvascular phenotype shared by juvenile hemangiomas and human placenta. Arch Dermatol 2001; 137: 559–70.
28. North PE, Waner M, James CA, et al. Congenital nonprogressive hemangioma: a distinct clinicopathologic entity unlike infantile hemangioma. Arch Dermatol 2001; 137:1607–20.
29. Patel U, Gupta SC. Wyburn–Mason syndrome. A case report and review of the literature. Neuroradiology 1990; 31:544–6.
30. Pyakurel P, Pak F, Mwakigonja AR, et al. Lymphatic and vascular origin of Kaposi's sarcoma spindle cells during tumor development. Int J Cancer 2006; 119:1262–7.
31. Rootman J, Hay E, Graebo D, et al. Orbital-adnexal lymphangiomas: a spectrum of hemodynamically isolated vascular hamartomas. Ophthalmology 1986; 93: 1558–70.
32. Rootman J. Vascular malformations of the orbit: hemodynamic concepts. Orbit 2003; 22:103–19.
33. Shields JA, Decker WL, Sanborn GE, et al. Presumed acquired retinal hemangiomas. Ophthalmology 1983; 113: 1292–300.
34. Shuler JD, Holland GN, Miles SA, et al. Kaposi sarcoma of the conjunctiva and eyelids associated with the acquired immunodeficiency syndrome. Arch Ophthalmol 1989; 107: 858–62.
35. Singh AD, Kaiser PK, Sears JE. Choroidal hemangioma. Ophthalmol Clin North Am 2005; 18:151–61.
36. Singh AD, Shields CL, Shields JA. von Hippel–Lindau disease. Surv Ophthalmol 2001; 46:117–42.
37. Sullivan TJ, Clarke MP, Morin JD. The ocular manifestations of Sturge–Weber syndrome. J Pediatr Ophthalmol Strabismus 1992; 29:349–56.
38. Tsai PS, DeAngelis DD, Spencer WH, et al. Bacillary angiomatosis of the anterior orbit, eyelid, and conjunctiva. Am J Ophthalmol 2002; 134:433–5.
39. Webster AR, Maher ER, Moore AT. Clinical characteristics of ocular angiomatosis in von Hippel–Lindau disease and correlation with germline mutation. Arch Ophthalmol 1999; 117:371–8.
40. Werner MS, Hornblass A, Reifler DM, et al. Intravascular papillary endothelial hyperplasia: collection of four cases and a review of the literature. Ophthal Plast Reconstr Surg 1997; 13:48–56.
41. Weiss SW, Goldblum JR. Hemangioendothelioma: vascular tumors of intermediate malignancy. Enzinger and Weiss' soft tissue tumors. 4th ed. St. Louis: Mosby, 2001: 891–915.
42. Weiss SW, Goldblum JR. Malignant Vascular Tumors. Enzinger and Weiss' Soft Tissue Tumors. 4th ed. St. Louis, MO: Mosby, 2001:917–54.
43. Weiss SW, Goldblum JR. Tumors of Lymph Vessels. Enzinger and Weiss' Soft Tissue Tumors. 4th ed. St. Louis, MO: Mosby, 2001:955–83.
44. Witschel H, Font RL. Hemangioma of the choroid. A clinicopathologic study of 71 cases and a review of the literature. Surv Ophthalmol 1976; 20:415–31.
45. Yuan K, Jin YT, Lin MT. The detection and comparison of angiogenesis-associated factors in pyogenic granuloma by immunohistochemistry. J Periodontol 2000; 71: 701–19.

63

Tumors of the Optic Nerve, Peripheral Nerves, and Autonomic Nervous System

Thomas J. Cummings and Gordon K. Klintworth
Departments of Pathology and Ophthalmology, Duke University, Durham, North Carolina, U.S.A.

INTRODUCTION

This chapter reviews neoplasms of the central, peripheral, and autonomic nervous systems as they relate to the eye, optic nerve, and orbit. Ocular tissues are potential sites of origin for tumors derived from the peripheral and autonomic nervous systems. The tissues of the eye and ocular adnexa are innervated by nerves from the ophthalmic division of the trigeminal nerve and motor fibers from the facial nerve. Within the orbit reside neurogenic derivatives including the ciliary ganglion and Schwann cells, which are also the potential sources of neoplasms and reactive proliferations. The reactive traumatic neuroma is included since it is a hypertrophic peripheral nerve process. The optic nerve is a central rather than a peripheral nerve. It is composed of axons derived from the ganglion cells in the retina, and glial tissue from which gliomas derive. Meningiomas are included because of their origin from the leptomeninges and therefore close alliance with the optic nerve.

GLIOMAS OF THE OPTIC NERVE

Overview

Histogenetically, primary gliomas of the optic nerve derive from the nerve's indigenous population of astrocytes. Although the term "optic nerve glioma" is traditionally regarded as representative of the pilocytic astrocytoma, this terminology is imprecise (58). "Glioma" is a nonspecific term that could describe a tumor of either astrocytic, oligodendroglial, or ependymal lineage. To reduce ambiguity between pathologists and clinicians, it is recommended that astrocytic tumors be subtyped and graded accurately when possible. We prefer the classification scheme of the World Health Organization (WHO) (14).

Gliomas of the optic nerve present within the spectrum of astrocytic neoplasia including pilocytic astrocytoma and the diffusely infiltrative fibrillary astrocytomas (25,30,42). The WHO classifies the pilocytic astrocytoma (WHO Grade I) as well-differentiated fibrillary astrocytomas (WHO Grade II), anaplastic astrocytoma (WHO Grade III), and glioblastoma (WHO Grade IV), all of which can involve the optic nerve (14).

Clinical Features

Low-grade pilocytic (juvenile) astrocytomas are slow-growing tumors that typically are diagnosed within the first two decades of life. They are rare in adults (114). Females appear to be at a slightly higher risk for optic nerve tumors, while both genders are equally affected when the optic chiasm is involved. Clinically, patients may present with ophthalmic abnormalities including visual impairment, optic atrophy, and proptosis (30). Hormonal dysfunction (50) including gigantism (28) and precocious puberty (39) related to hypothalamic or pituitary involvement can also occur. The long-term prognosis of optic nerve pilocytic astrocytomas is favorable. Many tumors remain quiescent for long periods of time and fail to grow or recur even if surgical resection is incomplete, and some have been documented by neuroimaging to regress spontaneously (115). Hypotheses to explain the regression include the resorption of the mucoid material secreted by the tumor, diminished vascular distension, and apoptosis outpacing cellular proliferation (60,80).

Contrarily, some neoplasms grow and infiltrate neighboring structures such as the optic chiasm and hypothalamus, despite years of quiescence resulting in much morbidity and a lethal outcome in contrast to tumors restricted to one optic nerve (5). Pilocytic astrocytomas of the optic nerve rarely undergo malignant transformation and evolve into an anaplastic astrocytoma or glioblastoma (112).

High-grade astrocytomas of the optic nerve are distinct from their low-grade pilocytic counterparts and typically present in adulthood often with visual loss that eventually progresses to blindness. The optic nerve head may disclose papilledema or optic atrophy (42). Histologically these biologically aggressive tumors resemble anaplastic astrocytomas and glioblastomas elsewhere in the central nervous system (CNS) and spread via the leptomeninges or cerebrospinal fluid (CSF) both intracranially and to the spinal neuraxis (78). Although rare in childhood, glioblastomas of the optic nerve have been reported either arising de novo (17), from malignant transformation of a pilocytic astrocytoma (109), or secondary to radiation therapy (95).

Enlargement of the optic foramen and erosion of the anterior and posterior clinoid processes and sphenoidal ridge are features of optic nerve gliomas that can be identified with conventional radiographs (29,32). While computed tomography (CT) may disclose enlargement of the optic nerve or irregular solid thickening along the nerve, magnetic resonance imaging (MRI) is the preferred neuroimaging diagnostic procedure for the evaluation of the optic pathway (41). Although most tumors exhibit contrast-enhancement, this can be variable. Advantages of MRI include superior evaluation of the intracanalicular, chiasmal, and postchiasmal extension of tumor, increased sensitivity in delineating subtle differences in fat content and hydration of neural tissues, and lack of artifact produced by surrounding bone (41). An optic nerve glioblastoma with invasion of the optic chiasm, optic tract, and left medial temporal lobe has been documented by MRI (111).

Histopathology

Optic nerve pilocytic astrocytomas are typically white to tan in color, and often contain abundant mucosubstance within small cystoid spaces, which imparts a glistening or gelatinous appearance. Hemorrhage is sometimes evident in focal regions and if extensive it can rarely cause proptosis (15). As the glioma diffusely expands though the optic foramen during its spread, the optic nerve may acquire an hourglass shape. Tumor may also infiltrate the subarachnoid space causing a rim of tumor around a mildly involved nerve. When the tumor extends to the optic nerve head, the adjacent retina may also be involved (87).

Sometimes it may be difficult, if not impossible, to determine the exact site of origin when large tumors involve the optic nerve, optic chiasm, hypothalamus, thalamus or floor of the third ventricle, despite radiographic, intraoperative, and postmortem examination (27,70).

Optic nerve astrocytomas react with antibodies to glial fibrillary acidic protein (GFAP), vimentin, and S100 protein. GFAP is the most specific and highlights the cytoplasmic filaments and fibrillar processes of the neoplastic cells. An origin from type-1 astrocytes is suggested by their immunoreactivity to HNK-1 (a type-1 astrocyte precursor marker), and immunonegativity to A2B5 (a type-2 astrocyte precursor marker) (26).

Pilocytic Astrocytomas of the Optic Nerve

Pilocytic astrocytomas of the optic nerve are microscopically identical to those elsewhere in the CNS. Three histological patterns (coarsely reticulated, finely reticulated, and coarsely fibrillated) are recognizable and one usually predominates (107), but pattern heterogeneity is often found in any given tumor.

In tumors with the coarsely reticulated pattern, bipolar astrocytes manifest a biphasic pattern whereby the neoplastic cells closely surround blood vessels or loosely arranged around small mucin-containing cystoid spaces. When viewed in cross-section, the optic nerve bundles appear enlarged and hypercellular compared to the normal optic nerve (Fig. 1). Eosinophilic granular bodies, Rosenthal fibers, and protein droplets can be reassuring findings in challenging diagnostic cases; however, they are not always present. Blood vessels may appear hyalinized in long-standing cases, while other blood vessels are hyperplastic with glomeruloid tufting and are thought to be responsible for the contrast-enhancement detected with neuroimaging. Some tumors also display necrosis and cells in mitosis, lending mimicry to higher grade astrocytomas. As with spinal cord and posterior fossa pilocytic astrocytomas, those of the optic nerve possess the ability to invade the subarachnoid space and disseminate within the subarachnoid space (10,58).

In the finely reticulated pattern, small round or ovoid nuclei are embedded within a frail-reticulated syncytium of neuroglial fibers similar to an extension of the indigenous neuroglia of the optic nerve. This pattern may be mistaken with the histological appearance of a well-differentiated infiltrative fibrillary astrocytoma. Fibrillary astrocytomas may exhibit a mild hypercellularity and nuclear pleomorphism, but they usually lack Rosenthal fibers, hyalinized blood vessels, mitoses, microvascular proliferation, and necrosis. Some pilocytic astrocytomas infiltrate among the optic nerve axons (a neurofilament immunohistochemical stain can demonstrate this), and can add additional uncertainty to the precise categorization of some of these tumors. The coarsely fibrillar pattern is seen least commonly and is characterized by spindled neuroglial cells arranged in fairly well-defined bundles similar to schwannoma.

Arachnoid gliomatosis is an uncommon astrocytic proliferation that circumferentially expands the leptomeninges, but typically does not penetrate the dural sheath (100). It may be seen in patients with and without neurofibromatosis type 1 (NF1) (MIM +162200) (see Chapter 55) (64,90). In diffuse hyperplastic gliosis of the optic nerve and chiasm a dense cellular gliosis widely separates the individual nerve fibers. In these cases, the distinction from neoplasia can be difficult. Arachnoidal hyperplasia is not to be confused with meningioma of the optic nerve sheath (20). Iris neovascularization (23), glaucoma (55), and extensive calcification (45) are other rare findings seen in optic nerve pilocytic astrocytomas.

Ultrastructurally, optic nerve pilocytic astrocytomas are found to have cytoplasmic filaments measuring 5 to 10 nm in diameter (Fig. 2). Astrocytes with fewer cytoplasmic filaments but more prominent nucleoli, ribosomes, endoplasmic reticulum (ER), and

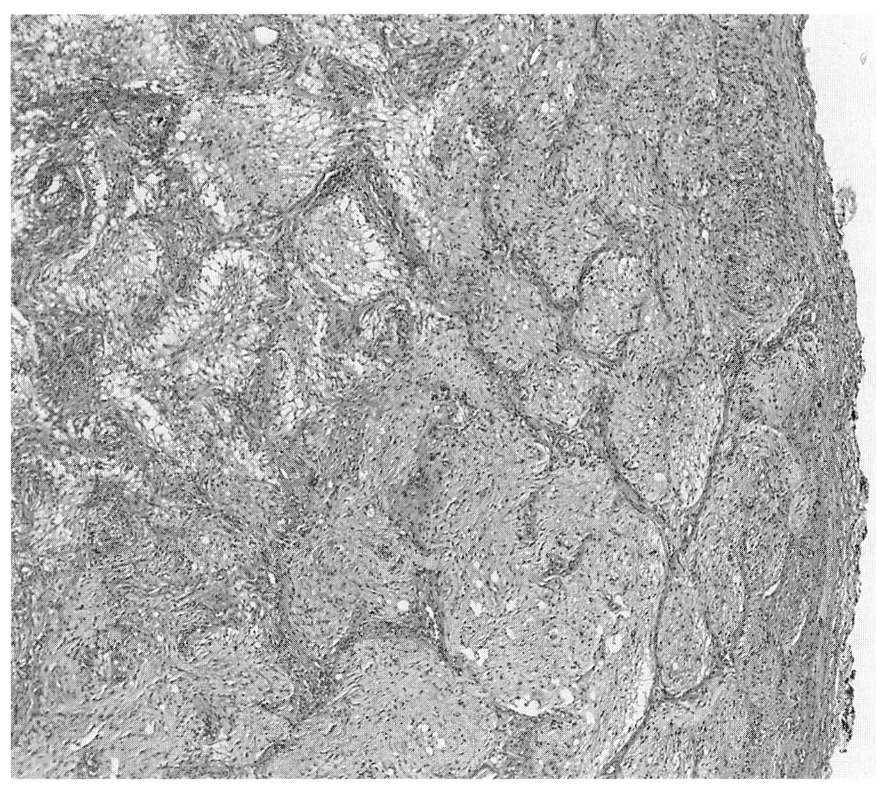

Figure 1 Pilocytic astrocytoma of the optic nerve characterized by an astrocytic proliferation that expands the compartmentalized nerve bundles (hematoxylin and eosin, ×4.5).

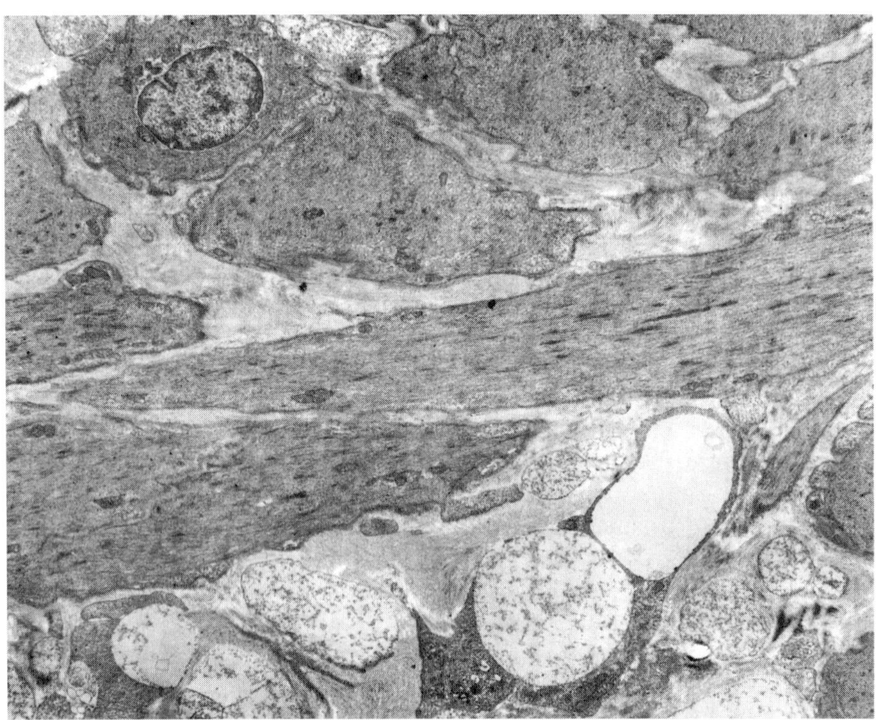

Figure 2 Pilocytic astrocytoma of the optic nerve. The tumor cell processes are composed of many intermediate filaments and occasional mitochondria (×4,400).

Golgi apparati are thought to be metabolically active with the production of mucoid material (3,32).

The Ki-67 (Mib-1) proliferation-related labeling index of many optic nerve pilocytic astrocytomas has been reported as <1% (11,66), but it may also be as high as 19.5% (104). These tumors can increase in size and then stabilize, especially in individuals younger than 20-years-old.

Well-Differentiated Fibrillary Astrocytomas of the Optic Nerve

Similarly histologically to diffuse astrocytomas elsewhere in the CNS, diffuse fibrillary astrocytomas are characterized by hypercellularity and tumor cells, which exhibit cytological pleomorphism. Mitoses, microvascular proliferation, and necrosis are absent. On a small biopsy, the difference between pilocytic astrocytoma and well-differentiated fibrillary astrocytoma can be challenging, especially when the finely reticulated pattern is present. In some tumors, it may be impossible to distinguish between the two. The distinction, however, is of practical importance as clinical decisions related to therapy and prognosis may be based on the grade of the tumor.

Malignant Fibrillary Astrocytomas of the Optic Nerve

Malignant fibrillary astrocytomas of the optic nerve are histologically indistinguishable from those in other parts of the CNS. When there is increased cellularity, cytological pleomorphism, and mitotic activity are present the diagnosis is anaplastic astrocytoma (WHO Grade III), but when glomeruloid microvascular proliferation or necrosis is present the tumor is designated a glioblastoma (Fig. 3). Caution is necessary as some of these seemingly ominous features can also be found occasionally in pilocytic astrocytomas. Attention to the degree of cytological pleomorphism and the presence or absence of Rosenthal fibers, protein droplets, and eosinophilic granular bodies is necessary for correct interpretation.

Oligodendrogliomas of the Optic Nerve

Neoplasms rarely arise from oligodendroglia in the optic nerve, despite the fact that oligodendrocytes are a prominent cellular component of the normal optic nerve. The literature contains rare reports of optic nerve oligodendrogliomas (32,87,89).

Gliomatosis Cerebri Involving the Optic Nerve

In gliomatosis cerebri, glial cells extensively infiltrate CNS but do not form a defined mass lesion (24). The nosological definition and histogenesis of gliomatosis cerebri remain uncertain, and in the WHO classification this tumor is in the category of neuroepithelial neoplasms of unknown origin. The tumor cells migrate along myelinated fiber tracts including the optic pathway, and can result in ophthalmic manifestations such as visual loss, nystagmus, diplopia, homonymous hemianopia, and visual loss (22). Few reports of gliomatosis cerebri have documented involvement of the optic nerves and chiasm, one of which was reported as having the histological features of an anaplastic gemistocytic astrocytoma (35).

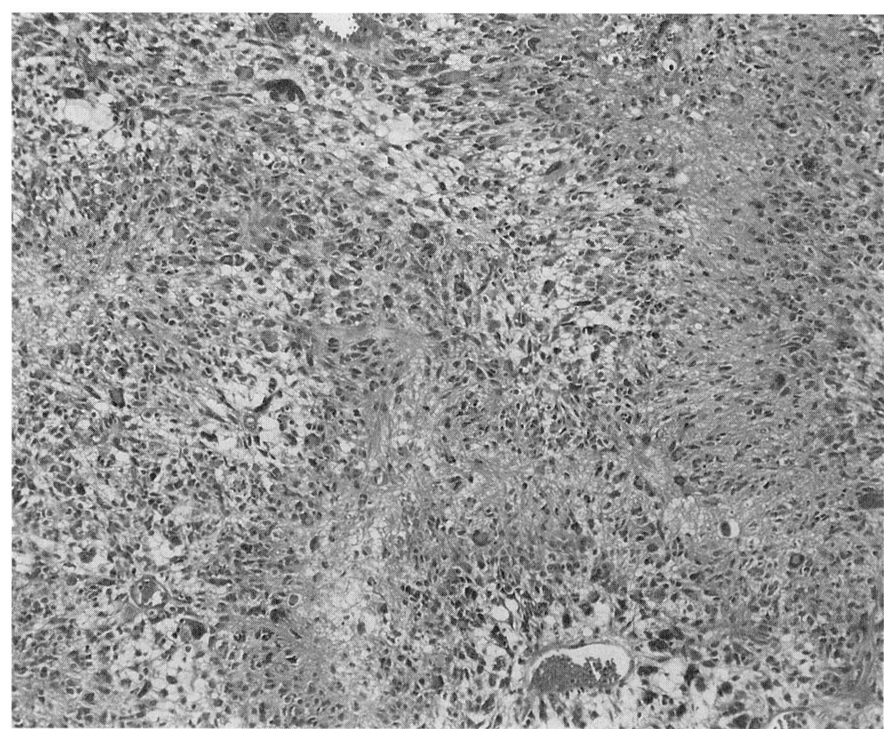

Figure 3 Glioblastoma of the optic nerve exhibiting cytological pleomorphism and serpiginous foci of necrosis (hematoxylin and eosin, ×11).

Multicentric Gliomas Involving the Optic Nerve

Multicentric gliomas are defined as those that form multifocal mass lesions, but without obvious connecting routes. They are rarely associated with the optic nerve. One such case included an anaplastic astrocytoma of the optic chiasm with an occipital lobe glioblastoma (103).

Gangliogliomas of the Optic Nerve

Gangliogliomas are well-differentiated neoplasms of both neuronal and origin usually involving the temporal lobe in young adults. Histologically, gangliogliomas are characterized by the features of a pilocytic astrocytoma admixed with neoplastic ganglion cells. Neurofilament protein and synaptophysin immunostains can be utilized to highlight the neoplastic ganglion cells in gangliogliomas. Rare examples of this tumor have affected the optic nerve and chiasm (59,92), which are normally white matter fiber tracts lacking ganglion cells. To explain the presence of ganglion cells in tumors in this visual pathways an origin from ectopic neurons is suspected (16). Alternatively, a derivation from the undifferentiated neuroepithelium of the optic stalk with concurrent differentiation into glial and ganglionic derivatives with neoplastic potential is possible (63). The prospect of nonneoplastic hypothalamic neurons being entrapped in a pilocytic astrocytoma needs to be excluded when the tumor involves the hypothalamus.

Etiology and Pathogenesis

Pilocytic astrocytomas of the optic pathways are associated with NF1 and generally have a more favorable outcome than non-NF1 associated tumors (38,39,56,57). Both optic nerves are involved in approximately 20% of patients with NF1 (33,41), but extensive bilateral involvement of the visual tracts is rare (96). Loss of expression of the NF1 tumor suppressor gene has been implicated in the development of optic gliomas in patients with NF1, but not in sporadic pilocytic astrocytomas (38,110).

Although most tumors grow slowly or not at all, tumor enlargement and progressive visual impairment occurs occasionally in children with NF1 (44). Individuals with NF1 manifest perineural arachnoidal gliomatosis and sphenoid wing dysplasia, but malignant transformation is rare.

Other rare associations with pilocytic astrocytomas include von Hippel–Lindau disease (MIM #193300) (see Chapter 55) (79) and postradiation vasculopathy of the moyamoya type (bilateral stenosis or occlusion of the internal carotid arteries and their branches) following radiotherapy (69,95).

MENINGIOMAS

Overview

Meningiomas arise from the arachnoid mater of the leptomeninges and are typically slow-growing tumors. They may arise anywhere along the optic nerve sheath (Fig. 4), but the vast majority found within the orbit are direct extensions of intracranial meningiomas from along the wing of the sphenoid bone (sphenoidal ridge meningioma) (36,86), the tuberculum sellae (suprasellar meningioma), or above and adjacent to the cribriform plate (olfactory groove meningioma) (101).

Clinical Features

Patients with these tumors usually come under the initial care of neurosurgeons rather than ophthalmologists because of the associated neurologic symptoms, although proptosis and chorioretinal folds are a rare presentation. Sphenoidal ridge meningiomas are frequently accompanied by an exuberant reactive hyperostosis of the adjacent sphenoid bone, and this is often sufficiently pronounced to produce proptosis by itself (106). A sphenoidal ridge meningioma occasionally spreads anteriorly as far as the globe and may invade the choroid (75).

Ectopic orbital meningiomas may reside outside the muscle cone without an attachment to the optic nerve (48,68), or rarely external to the periosteal coverings of the orbital walls. Orbital meningiomas are seldom bilateral (99), but are sometimes associated with meningiomas in extraorbital sites and even in the thorax. Other meningiomas of ophthalmological importance sometimes arise beneath the conjunctiva or caruncle (67), within the optic canal (49), paranasal sinuses, and the skin around the eye (61).

As with meningiomas elsewhere in the CNS those arising in the orbit occur more often in females than in males, and the majority of those present in younger individuals tend to predominate in males (83). Conceivably, the overall preponderance of females is linked with the demonstration of receptors for progesterone and estrogen in a majority of intracranial tumors (108). In the experience of some investigators (48) about one-fourth of the cases of primary orbital meningiomas become symptomatic before 10 years of age, in sharp contrast to intracranial meningiomas, which are rarely apparent before the age of 20 years (72). However, this early age of onset has not confirmed in other studies (113).

Similar to intracranial and intraspinal meningiomas, the majority of primary orbital meningiomas present in the fifth decade of life. The tumor typically spreads within the optic nerve sheath causing compression and visual loss is the principal complaint. Nerve compression may also be revealed by the emergence of prominent optociliary shunt vessels at the optic disc (93).

Histopathology

Because of variable morphologic patterns, meningiomas are subdivided into numerous histological types. Some meningiomas, the vast majority in the context of the optic nerve, appear as sheets or lobules of polygonal cells with indistinct cytoplasmic membranes and oval vesicular nuclei (syncytial meningioma) (Fig. 5), whereas other meningiomas are composed of densely packed interwoven bundles of spindle-shaped cells with some degree of whorl formation in a collagenous matrix that imparts toughness to the tumor (fibroblastic meningioma). Transitional meningiomas encompass features of both the syncytial and fibroblastic patterns. The diagnosis can be made by fine needle aspiration cytology (71).

Within meningiomas intranuclear invaginations of cytoplasm sometimes confer a light-microscopic appearance of an intranuclear inclusion body, but the

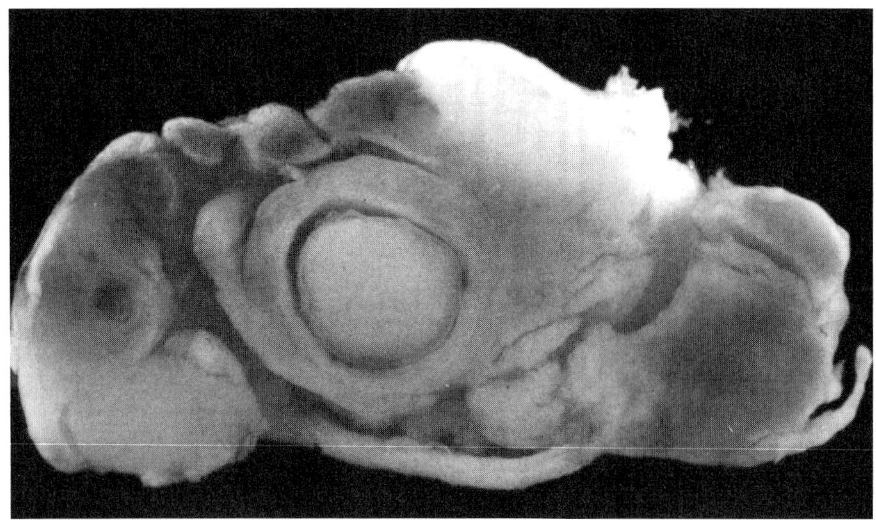

Figure 4 Meningioma of the optic nerve showing thickening of the nerve sheath and extension through the dura mater into the connective tissue of the orbit (resected specimen, ×7.5).

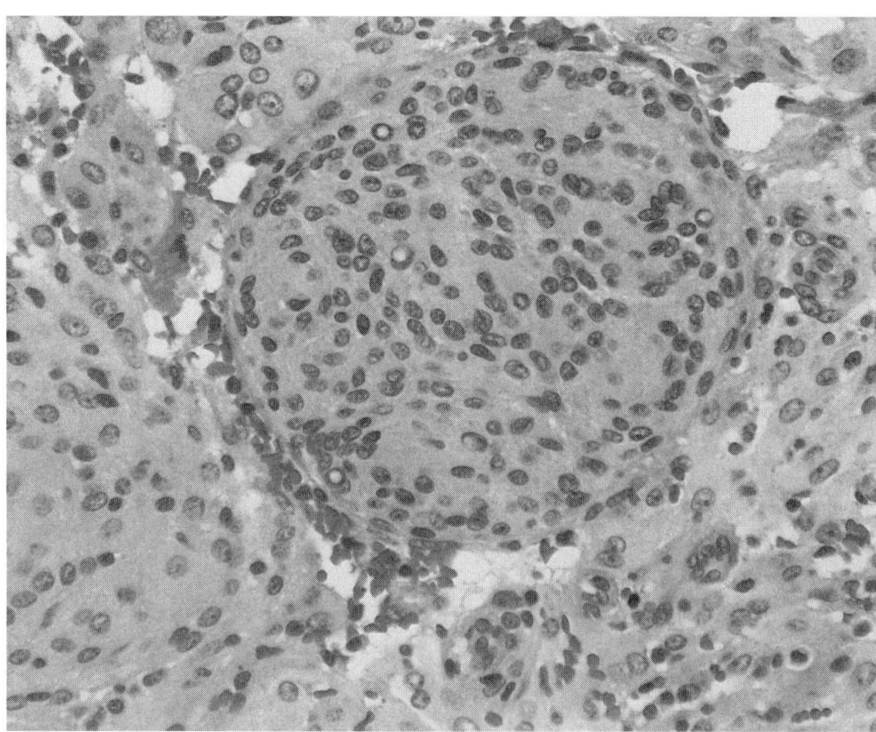

Figure 5 Meningioma of the optic nerve. This well-differentiated meningioma exhibits whorl-like clusters of monomorphic tumor cells, some of which display nuclear pseudoinclusions (hematoxylin and eosin, ×56).

cytoplasmic nature of these pseudoinclusions is readily discernible by transmission electron microscopy (TEM). Spherical bodies with concentric lamellae that are calcified and sometimes also impregnated with iron (psammoma bodies) are common in meningiomas and occasionally obscure most of the cellular component. Provided the degree of calcification is sufficient, many orbital meningiomas are evident radiologically (12.5%). Psammoma bodies occur in areas of high cellularity and may be of diagnostic significance since fibroblastic and Schwann cell tumors do not form them. By TEM the bodies possess a substructure of radially arranged spicules of apatite crystals oriented around an amorphous mass. Ultrastructurally, a striking feature of meningiomas is the complex interdigitating of the cell processes between contiguous tumor cells as well as the presence of desmosomes and hemidesmosomes (Fig. 6) (21). Individual tumor cells often possess vast amounts of intracytoplasmic filaments and unlike some other neoplasms, basement membrane material and microfibrils are not deposited between the tumor cells (21).

Metastasis is an exceedingly rare phenomenon, but meningiomas can be locally infiltrative and subject to recurrence (62).

Meningiomas are one of the most heterogeneous neoplasms encountered by the ophthalmic pathologist and neuropathologist. Although 15 histological subtypes and three histological grades are recognized by the WHOs classification of tumors of the nervous system, many of these are unlikely to present within the orbit (62). Most meningiomas are benign and are associated with a low risk of recurrence and a low risk of aggressive growth. These WHO Grade I subtypes include meningothelial, fibroblastic, transitional, secretory, psammomatous, angiomatous, microcystic, lymphoplasmacyte-rich, and metaplastic.

WHO Grade II meningiomas are associated with a greater likelihood of recurrence and/or aggressive behavior and include the atypical, clear cell, and chordoid histological subtypes. They are defined by the WHO as a meningioma with increased mitotic activity or three or more of the following features: increased cellularity, small cells with high nucleus: cytoplasm ratio, prominent nucleoli, uninterrupted patternless or sheet-like growth, and foci of "spontaneous" or "geographic" necrosis. Increased mitotic activity here has been defined as four or more mitoses per 10 high-power fields in addition to moderately high MIB-1 labeling indices.

Anaplastic (malignant) meningiomas (WHO Grade III) are defined by the WHO as meningiomas exhibiting histological features of frank malignancy far in excess of the abnormalities present in atypical meningioma (62). Such features include malignant cytology with an appearance similar to carcinoma, sarcoma, or malignant melanoma, or a high mitotic index (20 or more mitoses per 10 high-power fields). In these cases the differential

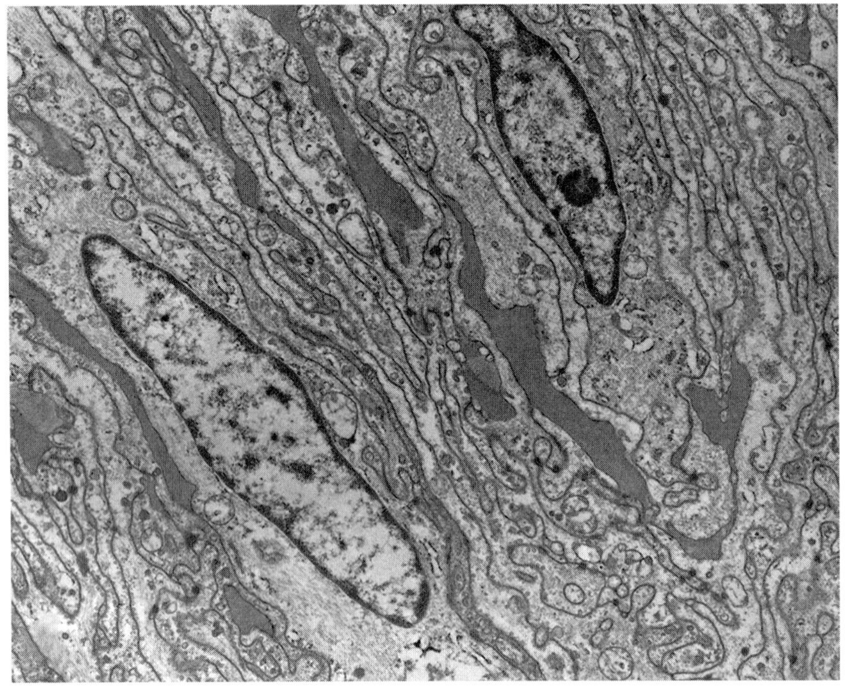

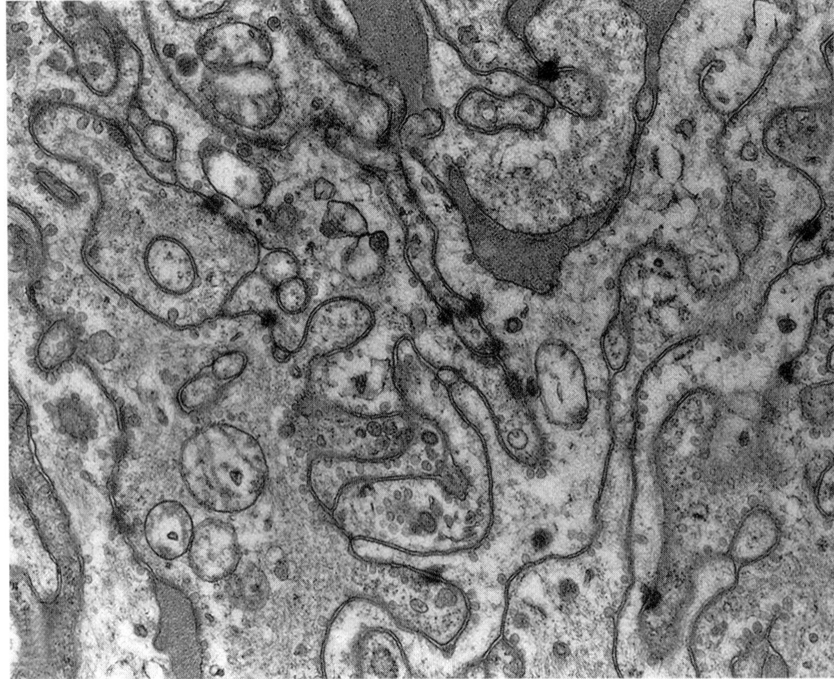

Figure 6 Transmission electron micrographs of a meningioma showing complex interdigitating cytoplasmic processes containing occasional desmosomes that connect adjacent cells (top, ×5,000; bottom, ×13,700).

diagnosis includes the possibility of a systemic malignancy metastatic to a meningioma, a well-documented occurrence.

Etiology and Pathogenesis

Individuals may inherit a predisposition to meningioma. Multiple meningiomas are a hallmark of neurofibromatosis type 2 (MIM #101000) (see Chapter 55), and in these individuals they tend to occur earlier in life than sporadic meningiomas (9,48,72). A tumor suppressor gene for meningioma has been identified on the long arm of chromosome 22 (22q12.3–qter) and this is at a locus different from the gene responsible for NF2 (19,84). Losses of chromosomes 1p, 6q, and 14q have been associated with atypical and anaplastic meningiomas (40,84).

The meningothelial cells of the optic nerve sheath are the source of most primary orbital meningiomas, while other primary orbital meningiomas not connected to the optic nerve probably arise from meningothelial cells in an ectopic location. Clinically and radiographically, meningiomas are often described as "dural-based" tumors. While tumor often invades the dura and appears to be plastered to it, meningiomas are tumors derived from the arachnoid. Distinction is to be made of tumor from meningeal hyperplasia (85). At least some of the latter cells presumably become entrapped in the perineurium of the nerves as they pass beyond the meningeal coverings of the CNS.

TUMORS OF PERIPHERAL NERVES AND THE AUTONOMIC NERVOUS SYSTEM

Neurofibroma

A neurofibroma is composed of a variable mixture of Schwann cells, collagen fibers, and scattered nerve axons that produce fusiform enlargement of the nerve. Perineurial cells may also be involved although there is good evidence that the Schwann cells are themselves able to produce collagen. Frequently the tumor has an appreciable mucin content making it soft and slimy. From a clinicopathological standpoint it is usual to recognize three categories of neurofibroma: localized, plexiform, and diffuse (94).

Most localized neurofibromas in the orbit present as solitary lesions, only some 12% being associated with neurofibromatosis. They are discrete with an indeterminate capsule and are composed of elongated spindle cells with a characteristic wavy nucleus in a stroma with variable mucin content (51). The upper part of the orbit is a preferred location and mild discomfort as well as proptosis is common (52,88).

Plexiform neurofibroma is commonly seen in individuals with NF1 and comprises a convoluted tangle of nerves thickened by Schwann cell proliferation. In contradistinction to the solitary lesions, which occur mainly in adult life, the plexiform tumor usually presents in childhood and may be associated with bony defects of the orbit (7,77). Diffuse neurofibroma is the least common form and is associated with generalized neurofibromatosis in about 10% of cases. The component cells are usually less elongated than those in other neurofibromas and may include clusters of Meissner bodies, but their chief significance lies in an absence of a capsule such that they are intimately bound to the surrounding structures and difficult to excise (13).

Schwannoma

A schwannoma is a benign, slow-growing encapsulated tumor of Schwann cells that gradually enlarges the nerve and has a tendency to arise eccentrically located on the nerve trunk of origin (18,94). This neoplasm is still often inappropriately designated a neurilemoma, which indicates a tumor of the neurilema (sheath of a nerve), but all tumors arise from cells. They tend to occur more commonly in the superior orbit (46), where they may present as a mass lesion and result in slowly progressive unilateral proptosis (98).

Schwannomas uncommonly involve the uvea, including the ciliary body, choroid, and iris (91), where they are often misdiagnosed as malignant melanoma. The two may share similar ophthalmoscopic, angiographic, and ultrasonographic findings, which prevents them from being distinguished clinically (34,91). Rare cases of ocular melanotic (97) and pigmented (91) schwannomas have been reported, and they may share histological and immunohistochemical findings, which overlap, including immunoreactivity to HMB45. TEM can be useful, depending on either the presence or absence of a continuous basal lamina (its presence should indicate schwannoma), and whether or not there is ultrastructural evidence of melanogenesis indicative of in situ melanin synthesis. Melanotic schwannoma has a known association with the Carney complex (MIM #160980) (see Chapter 55), and its occurrence should prompt a clinical investigation for other features of the complex including myxomas, endocrine tumors, and spotty skin pigmentation. An association with the Carney complex does not yet appear to have been demonstrated with the ocular cases of melanotic schwannomas (91).

Although sometimes occurring sporadically, orbital schwannomas may be a manifestation of NF1. *Café-au-lait* spots of the skin may be associated (76) and the only other stigma of this phakomatosis. In contrast to neurofibromas, which tend to be painless, schwannomas compress the nerve of origin so that pain is often a prominent clinical feature.

The schwannoma tends to be firm and rubbery in consistency and after sectioning cystic spaces containing mucoid material are frequently disclosed. Light microscopy presents two different patterns (Fig. 7). One is composed of closely compacted, spindle-shaped cells with eosinophilic cytoplasm, oval nuclei, and indistinct cell membranes (Antoni type-A). The nuclei of the tumor cells are often palisaded, sometimes around hyalinized structures resembling tactile corpuscles known as Verocay bodies. In other schwannomas, stellate cells are haphazardly arranged in a myxomatous matrix (Antoni type-B), which does not stain with alcian blue, in contrast to the mucoid material of neurofibromas (94).

Other histological features frequently encountered in schwannomas are thickened and hyalinized

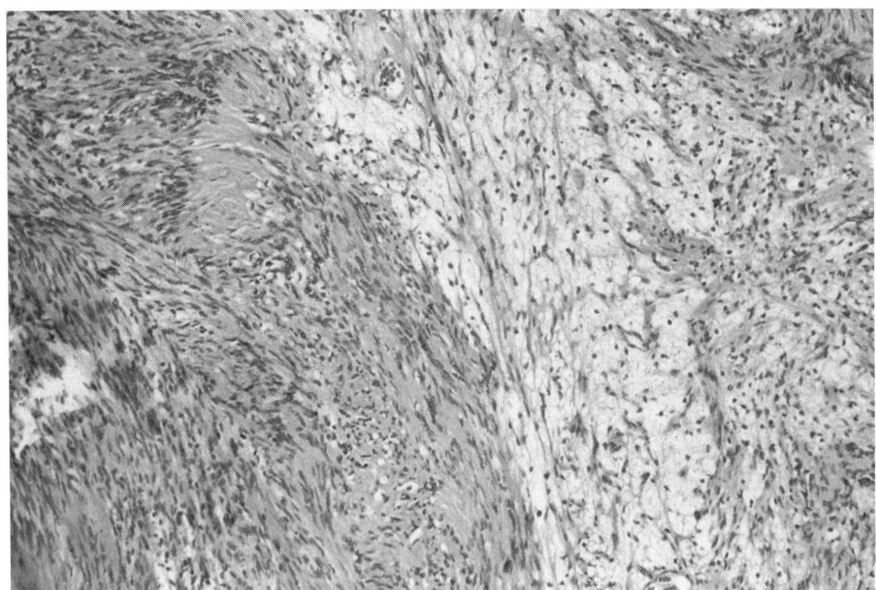

Figure 7 Schwannoma of the orbit. The hypercellular Antoni A component containing a Verocay body is demarcated from the macrophage-rich Antoni B component (hematoxylin and eosin, ×11).

blood vessels, a lymphocytic infiltration, and hemosiderin- or lipid-laden macrophages. The lipidized Antoni B component is often responsible for a macroscopic bright yellow appearance. Vascular thromboses can result in foci of necrosis, which is not to be misinterpreted as an atypical or malignant feature.

Schwannomas can exhibit degenerative features including hyalinization, calcification, and cystic degeneration (102). In some, the nuclear and cytological atypia can be increased but without conspicuous mitoses (74), and are particularly prone to occur in schwannomas of long duration so-called "ancient change." Schwannomas can vary in their ratio of Antoni A and B architecture. Those which are dominant in Antoni A exhibit increased cellularity and are referred to as a cellular schwannoma.

Sometimes there is histological overlap between schwannoma and neurofibroma. Schwannomas are typically more strongly and diffusely immunoreactive for S100 protein than neurofibromas. In addition, a stain for neurofilament protein can be useful because in schwannomas the axons are displaced to the periphery of the tumor where it originates from the parent nerve, whereas these fibers are typically preserved within the fusiform enlargement of the nerve in neurofibromas.

By TEM, schwannomas are characterized by cells with slender cellular processes and minimal rough ER, a basal lamina, and long-spacing collagen with cross-striations of 100 nm periodicity (Fig. 8). Although tumors derived from Schwann cells frequently produce conspicuous quantities of long-spacing collagen, this also forms in some normal tissues and in their pathologic conditions, including nonschwannian tumors. Endoneurial fibroblasts without a surrounding basal lamina are scattered throughout the tumor. Unlike neurofibromas, schwannomas rarely undergo malignant transformation into malignant nerve sheath tumors, but they may recur many years after excision (94).

Malignant Peripheral Nerve Sheath Tumors

Malignant peripheral nerve sheath tumors (MPNST) rarely involve the orbit (65) and about half of such tumors arise in patients with NF1. They either originate from neurofibromas or arise de novo from normal peripheral nerve, and they arise in schwannomas only rarely (94). One orbital MPNST developed in a patient with NF1 after empirical radiotherapy for presumed bilateral optic nerve and chiasm gliomas (31). A predilection for involvement of the supraorbital nerve has been noted (43) and the prognosis is poor, with the majority of patients dying within 5 years.

Traumatic Neuroma

Following the transection of peripheral nerves, the severed axons sprout from the promimal end of the cut nerve and grow in haphazard directions (94). These regenerating small clusters of axons, together with hyperplastic fibroblasts and Schwann cells, may form a swelling of the nerve (traumatic or amputation neuroma). Despite the fact that orbital nerves are severed during enucleations and other surgical procedures around the eye, traumatic neuromas are extremely rare in the orbit (37,73). Perhaps this reflects the small size of the orbital nerves or alternatively a lesser capacity of cranial nerves to regenerate than nerves of the peripheral nervous system. They may be associated with slowly enlarging conjunctival inclusion cysts. Patients may experience persistent pain

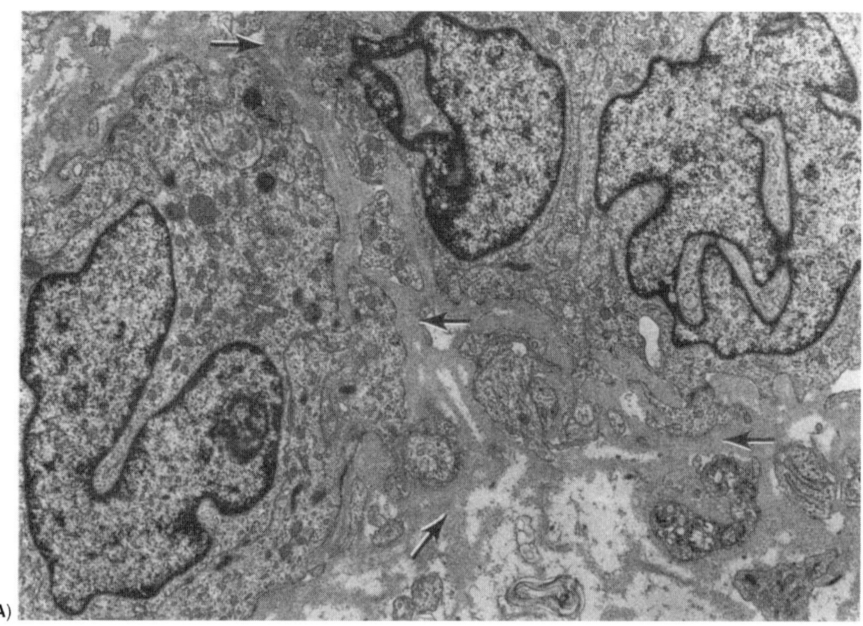

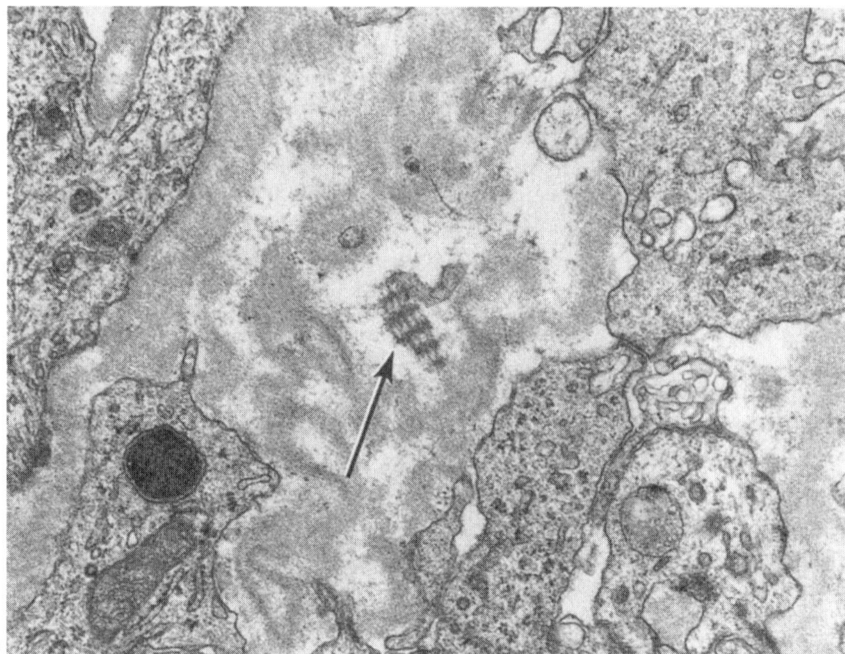

Figure 8 Transmission electron micrographs of a schwannoma. (**A**) The neoplastic Schwann cells are characteristically surrounded by a prominent basal lamina (*arrows*). The cells may encase axons (×10,050). (**B**) Extracellular broad-banded collagen (*arrow*) is frequently adjacent to the basal laminar material of Schwann cell (× 24,400). *Source*: Courtesy of Dr. J. Shelburne.

that is probably caused by mechanical irritation of the amputation neuroma, by retracting scar tissue, or compression from an adjacent cyst (1,73).

Granular Cell Tumor

Originally called granular cell myoblastoma, because of a belief that it stems from striated muscle, granular cell tumor is an extremely rare orbital neoplasm (2,47). This generally benign encapsulated tumor is composed of large, round, or polygonal cells with small, vesicular, or hyperchromatic nuclei (Fig. 9). The eosinophilic cytoplasm contains coarse granules, which are often strongly positive with the periodic acid Schiff stain. The tumor cells are reactive to S100 protein antibodies, evidence that supports the claim that they are of neural or Schwann cell derivation.

By TEM most of the granules appear as amorphous, eosinophilic, lysosomal-like structures, but sheaths of intracytoplasmic filaments (angulated bodies) also occur (Fig. 10) (4). Orbital involvement is associated with a generally good prognosis following local excision. A rare malignant granular cell tumor metastatic from the neck to the orbit has been described (12).

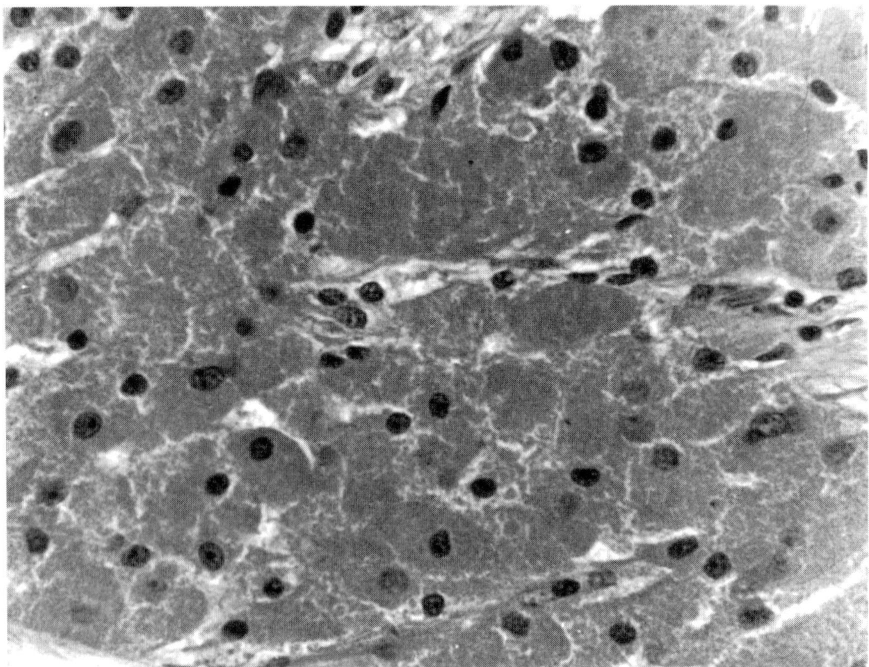

Figure 9 Granular cell tumor of the orbit. The neoplastic cells are characterized by voluminous fine granular eosinophilic cytoplasm and small regular nuclei (hematoxylin and eosin, ×400).

Paraganglioma

The term "chromaffin cells" is used to describe small clusters of epithelioid cells derived from neuroectoderm that are innervated by preganglionic sympathetic fibers and which synthesize and release catecholamines (epinephrine and norepinephrine). These cells develop a brown discoloration when exposed to aqueous solutions of potassium dichromate (chromaffin reaction). Clusters of morphologically similar cells but without a positive chromaffin reaction occur as chemoreceptor cells in the carotid body at the bifurcation of the carotid artery, in the aortic arches, in the glomus jugulare, and at numerous other sites. According to ultrastructural studies, the traditional nonchromaffin paraganglia differ only in number of neuron-secretory granules from the chromaffin cells of the sympathetic nervous system. These various specialized cells on occasion give rise to tumors known as chemodectomas or paragangliomas (53,82).

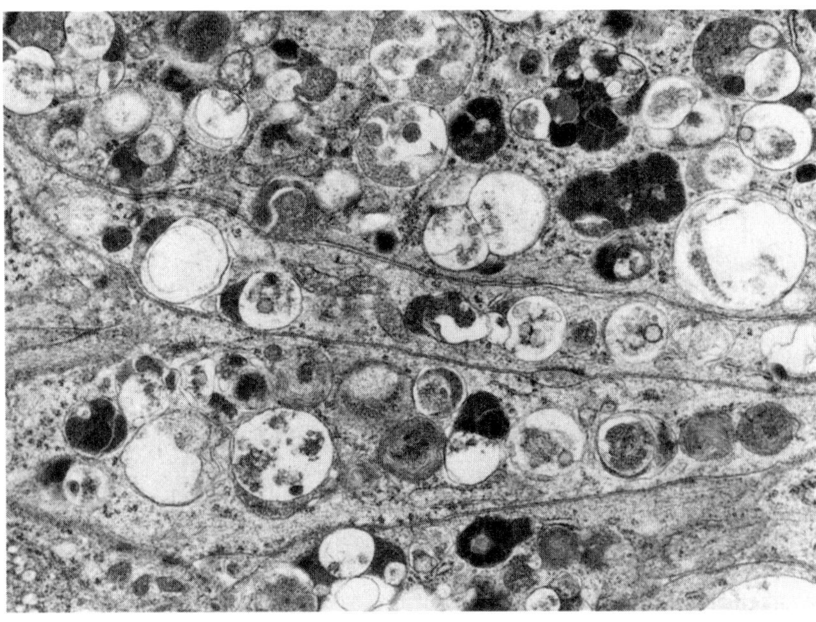

Figure 10 Ultrastructure of granular cell tumor. The cytoplasm contains numerous membrane-bound inclusions of variable size and shape (×14,100). *Source*: Courtesy of Dr. J. Shelburne.

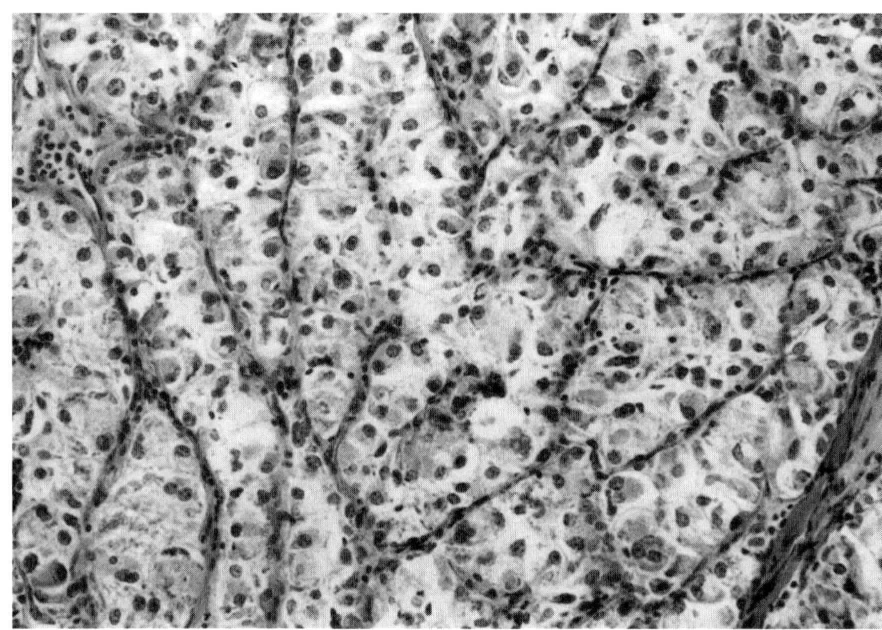

Figure 11 Paraganglioma (chemodectoma) of the orbit. The cells vary in size and have fine granular eosinophilic cytoplasm. The cells tend to form clusters separated by fibrous septa (hematoxylin and eosin, ×180).

Paragangliomas are rare in the orbit, where they are thought to originate in the ciliary ganglion (6,105). There is an exceptional report of an orbital paraganglioma with an admix of melanin (81). Orbital paragangliomas tend to involve the extraocular muscles and if incompletely excised may recur and even undergo malignant change. Extension to the middle cranial fossa has been reported (105), and conversely, intracranial paragangliomas may extend to the orbit (54).

Paragangliomas consist of variable-sized cells with round to oval nuclei and fine-granular eosinophilic cytoplasm arranged in nests, balls ("zellballen"), or cords separated by septa consisting of connective tissue or sinusoids (Fig. 11). Mitotic figures are rarely seen and the vascular component is often marked and suggestive of an angioma. Characteristic dense-core granules (50–200 nm in diameter) are disclosed in the tumor cells by TEM (Fig. 12).

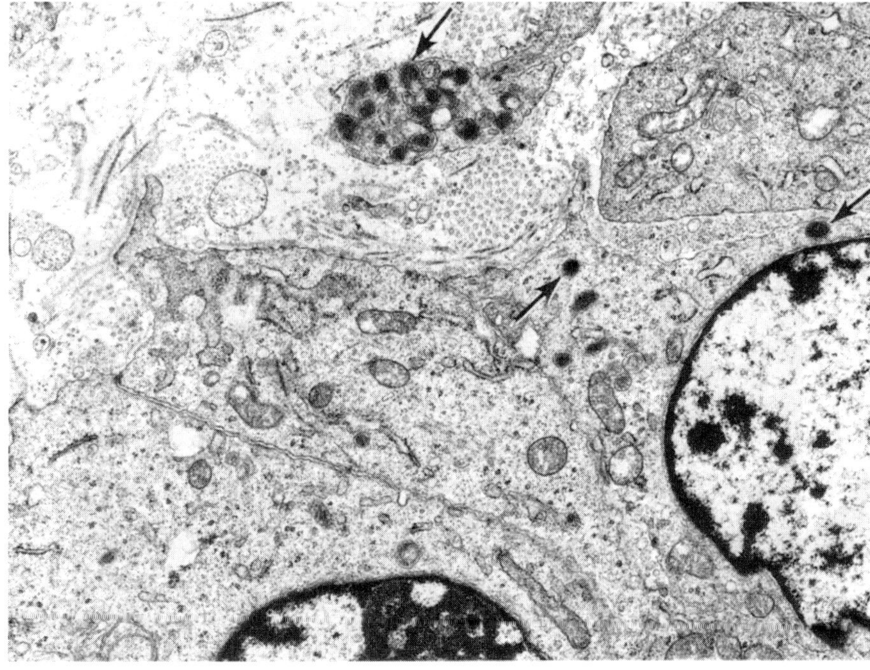

Figure 12 Electron micrograph of paraganglioma, showing characteristic dense-core granules (*arrows*) within the cytoplasm of tumor cells (×33,200) *Source*: Courtesy of Dr. J. Shelburne.

REFERENCES

1. Abramoff MD, Ramos LP, Jansen GH, et al. Patients with persistent pain after enucleation studied by MRI dynamic color mapping and histopathology. Invest Ophthalmol Vis Sci 2001; 42:2188–92.
2. Allaire GS, Laflamme P, and Bourgouin P. Granular cell tumour of the orbit. Can J Ophthalmol 1995; 30:151–3.
3. Anderson DR, Spencer WH. Ultrastructural and histochemical observations of optic nerve gliomas. Arch Ophthalmol 1970; 83:324–35.
4. Aparicio SR, Lumsden CE. Light- and electron-microscope studies on the granular cell myoblastoma of the tongue. J Pathol 1969; 97:339–55.
5. Balcer LJ, Liu GT, Heller G, et al. Visual loss in children with neurofibromatosis type 1 and optic pathway gliomas: relation to tumor location by magnetic resonance imaging. Am J Ophthalmol 2001; 131:442–5.
6. Bednar MM, Trainer TD, Aitken PA, et al. Orbital paraganglioma: case report and review of the literature. Br J Ophthalmol 1992; 76:183–5.
7. Binet EF, Kieffer SA, Martin SH, et al. Orbital dysplasia in neurofibromatosis. Radiology 1969; 93:829–33.
8. Borit A, Richardson EP Jr. The biological and clinical behaviour of pilocytic astrocytomas of the optic pathways. Brain 1982; 105:161–87.
9. Bosch MM, Boltshauser E, Harpes P, et al. Ophthalmologic findings and long-term course in patients with neurofibromatosis type 2. Am J Ophthalmol 2006; 141:1068–77.
10. Bruggers CS, Friedman HS, Phillips PC, et al. Leptomeningeal dissemination of optic pathway gliomas in three children. Am J Ophthalmol 1991; 111:719–23.
11. Burger PC, Shibata T, Kleihues P. The use of the monoclonal antibody Ki-67 in the identification of proliferating cells: application to surgical neuropathology. Am J Surg Pathol 1986; 10:611–7.
12. Callejo SA, Kronish JW, Decker SJ, et al. Malignant granular cell tumor metastatic to the orbit. Ophthalmology 2000; 107:550–4.
13. Carroll GS, Haik BG, Fleming JC, et al. Peripheral nerve tumors of the orbit. Radiol Clin North Am 1999; 37: 195–202.
14. Cavenee WK, Furnari FB, Nagane M, et al. Diffusely infiltrating astrocytomas. In: Kleihues P, Cavenee WK, eds. World Health Organization Classification of Tumours. Pathology and Genetics. Tumours of the Nervous System. Lyon: IARC Press, 2000:10–21.
15. Charles NC, Nelson L, Brookner AR, et al. Pilocytic astrocytoma of the optic nerve with hemorrhage and extreme cystic degeneration. Am J Ophthalmol 1981; 92: 691–5.
16. Chilton J, Caughron MR, Kepes JJ. Ganglioglioma of the optic chiasm: case report and review of the literature. Neurosurgery 1990; 26:1042–5.
17. Cirak B, Unal O, Arslan H, et al. Chiasmatic glioblastoma of childhood. A case report. Acta Radiol 2000; 41: 375–6.
18. Cockerham KP, Cockerham GC, Stutzman R, et al. The clinical spectrum of schwannomas presenting with visual dysfunction: a clinicopathologic study of three cases. Surv Ophthalmol 1999; 44:226–34.
19. Collins VP, Nordenskjold M, Dumanski JP. The molecular genetics of meningiomas. Brain Pathol 1990; 1:19–24.
20. Cooling RJ, Wright JE. Arachnoid hyperplasia in optic nerve glioma: confusion with orbital meningioma. Br J Ophthalmol 1979; 63:596–9.
21. Copeland DD, Bell SW, Shelburne JD. Hemidesmosome-like intercellular specializations in human meningiomas. Cancer 1978; 41:2242–9.
22. Couch JR, Weiss SA. Gliomatosis cerebri. Report of four cases and review of the literature. Neurology 1974; 24: 504–11.
23. Cummings TJ, Chu CT, Pollock SC, et al. Optic nerve astrocytoma with angiogenesis and neovascular glaucoma. Ophthal Pract 2000; 18:227–30.
24. Cummings TJ, Hulette CM, Longee DC, et al. Gliomatosis cerebri: cytologic and autopsy findings in a case involving the entire neuraxis. Clin Neuropathol 1999; 18:190–7.
25. Cummings TJ, Provenzale JM, Hunter SB, et al. Gliomas of the optic nerve: histological, immunohistochemical (MIB-1 and p53), and MRI analysis. Acta Neuropathol 2000; 99:563–70.
26. Cutarelli PE, Roessmann UR, Miller RH, et al. Immunohistochemical properties of human optic nerve glioma. Evidence of type 1 astrocyte origin. Invest Ophthalmol Vis Sci 1991; 32:2521–4.
27. Davis PC, Hoffman JC Jr, Weidenheim KM. Large hypothalamic and optic chiasm gliomas in infants: difficulties in distinction. Am J Neuroradiol 1984; 5: 579–85.
28. Drimmie FM, MacLennan AC, Nicoll JA, et al. Gigantism due to growth hormone excess in a boy with optic glioma. Clin Endocrinol 2000; 53:535–8.
29. Duke-Elder S. Tumours of the optic nerve and its sheaths. In: Duke-Elder S, ed. System of Ophthalmology. St. Louis, MO: C.V. Mosby, 1976:229–68.
30. Dutton JJ. Gliomas of the anterior visual pathway. Surv Ophthalmol 1994; 38:427–52.
31. Dutton JJ, Tawfik HA, DeBacker CM, et al. Multiple recurrences in malignant peripheral nerve sheath tumor of the orbit: a case report and a review of the literature. Ophthal Plast Reconstr Surg 2001; 17:293–9.
32. Eggers H, Jakobiec FA, Jones IS. Tumors of the optic nerve. Doc Ophthalmol 1976; 41:43–128.
33. Ersahin Y, Yunten N. Bilateral optic nerve glioma. Ped Neurosurg 1999; 31:168–8.
34. Fan JT, Campbell RJ, Robertson DM. A survey of intraocular schwannoma with a case report. Can J Ophthalmol 1995; 30:37–41.
35. Felsberg GJ, Glass JP, Tien RD, et al. Gliomatosis cerebri presenting with optic nerve involvement: MRI. Neuroradiology 1996; 38:774–7.
36. Finn JE, Mount LA. Meningiomas of the tuberculum sellae and planum sphenoidale. A review of 83 cases. Arch Ophthalmol 1974; 92:23–7.
37. Folberg R, Bernardino VB, Jr., Aguilar GL, et al. Amputation neuroma mistaken for recurrent melanoma in the orbit. Ophthalmic Surg 1981; 12:275–8.
38. Gutmann DH, Hedrick NM, Li J, et al. Comparative gene expression profile analysis of neurofibromatosis 1-associated and sporadic pilocytic astrocytomas. Cancer Res 2002; 62:2085–91.
39. Habiby R, Silverman B, Listernick R, et al. Precocious puberty in children with neurofibromatosis type 1. J Pediatr 1995; 126:364–7.
40. Heimberger AB, Wiltshire RN, Bronec R, et al. Biphasic malignant meningioma: a comparative genomic hybridization study. Clin Neuropathol 2002; 21:258–64.
41. Hollander MD, FitzPatrick M, O'Connor SG, et al. Optic gliomas. Radiol Clin N Am 1999; 37:59–71.
42. Hoyt WF, Meshel LG, Lessell S, et al. Malignant optic glioma of adulthood. Brain 1973, 96:121–32.

43. Jakobiec FA, Font RL, and Zimmerman LE. Malignant peripheral nerve sheath tumors of the orbit: a clinicopathologic study of eight cases. Trans Am Ophthalmol Soc 1985; 83:332–66.
44. Janss AJ, Grundy R, Cnaan A, et al. Optic pathway and hypothalamic/chiasmatic gliomas in children younger than age 5 years with a 6-year follow-up. Cancer 1995; 75: 1051–9.
45. Jordan DR, Anderson RL, White GL Jr, et al. Acute visual loss due to a calcified optic nerve glioma. Can J Ophthalmol 1989; 24:335–9.
46. Kapur R, Mafee MF, Lamba R, et al. Orbital schwannoma and neurofibroma: role of imaging. Neuroimaging Clin N Am 2005; 15:159–74.
47. Karcioglu ZA, Hemphill GL, and Wool BM. Granular cell tumor of the orbit: case report and review of the literature. Ophthalm Surg 1983; 14:125–9.
48. Karp LA, Zimmerman LE, Borit A, et al. Primary intraorbital meningiomas. Arch Ophthalmol 1974; 91: 24–8.
49. Kennerdell JS, Maroon JC. Intracanalicular meningioma with chronic optic disc edema. Ann Ophthalmol 1975; 7: 507–12.
50. Korsgaard O, Lindholm J, Rasmussen P. Endocrine function in patients with suprasellar and hypothalamic tumours. Acta Endocrinol 1976; 83:1–8.
51. Kottler UB, Conway RM, Schlotzer-Schrehardt U, et al. Isolated neurofibroma of the orbit with extensive myxoid changes: a clinicopathologic study including MRI and electron microscopic findings. Orbit 2004; 23:59–64.
52. Krohel GB, Rosenberg PN, Wright JE, et al. Localized orbital neurofibromas. Am J Ophthalmol 1985; 100: 458–64.
53. Lack EE. Tumors of the Adrenal Gland and Extra-Adrenal Paraganglia. Lack. Washington, D.C.: Armed Forces Institute of Pathology, 1997; 223–59.
54. Laquis SJ, Vick V, Haik BG, et al. Intracranial paraganglioma (glomus tumor) with orbital extension. Ophthal Plast Reconstr Surg 2001; 17:458–61.
55. Listernick R, Charrow J, Greenwald MJ, et al. Optic gliomas in children with neurofibromatosis type 1. J Pediatr 1989; 114:788–92.
56. Listernick R, Charrow J, Gutmann DH. Intracranial gliomas in neurofibromatosis type 1. Am J Med Gen 1999; 89:38–44.
57. Listernick R, Charrow J, Gutmann DH. Comments on neurofibromatosis 1 and optic pathway tumors. Am J Med Gen 2001; 102:105.
58. Listernick R, Louis DN, Packer RJ, et al. Optic pathway gliomas in children with neurofibromatosis 1: consensus statement from the NF1 optic pathway glioma task force. Ann Neurol 1997; 41:143–9.
59. Liu GT, Galetta SL, Rorke LB, et al. Gangliogliomas involving the optic chiasm. Neurology 1996; 46:1669–73.
60. Liu GT, Lessell S. Spontaneous visual improvement in chiasmal gliomas. Am J Ophthalmol 1992; 114:193–201.
61. Lopez DA, Silvers DN, Helwig EB. Cutaneous meningiomas–a clinicopathologic study. Cancer 1974; 34: 728–44.
62. Louis DN, Scheithauer BW, Budka H, et al. Meningiomas. In: Kleihues P, Cavenee WK, eds. Pathology and Genetics. Tumours of the Nervous System. Lyon: IARC Press, 2000: 176–84.
63. Lu WY, Goldman M, Young B, et al. Optic nerve ganglioglioma. Case report. J Neurosurg 1993; 78: 979–82.
64. Lynch TM, Gutmann DH. Neurofibromatosis 1. Neurol Clin 2002; 20:841–65.
65. Lyons CJ, McNab AA, Garner A, et al. Orbital malignant peripheral nerve sheath tumours. Br J Ophthalmol 1989; 73:731–8.
66. Machen SK, Prayson RA. Cyclin D1 and MIB-1 immunohistochemistry in pilocytic astrocytomas: a study of 48 cases. Hum Path 1998; 29:1511–6.
67. Macmichael IM, Cullen JF. Primary intraorbital meningioma. Br J Ophthalmol 1969; 53:169–73.
68. Mandelcorn MS, Shea M. Primary orbital perioptic meningioma: a case report. Can J Ophthalmol 1971; 6: 293–7.
69. Maruyama K, Mishima K, Saito N, et al. Radiation-induced aneurysm and moyamoya vessels presenting with subarachnoid haemorrhage. Acta Neurochir 2000; 142:139–43.
70. McDonnell P, Miller NR. Chiasmatic and hypothalamic extension of optic nerve glioma. Arch Ophthalmol 1983; 101:1412–5.
71. Mehrotra R, Kumar S, Singh K, et al. Fine-needle aspiration biopsy of orbital meningioma. Diagn Cytopathol 1999; 21:402–4.
72. Merten DF, Gooding CA, Newton TH, et al. Meningiomas of childhood and adolescence. J Pediatr 1974; 84:696–700.
73. Messmer EP, Camara J, Boniuk M, et al. Amputation neuroma of the orbit. Report of two cases and review of the literature. Ophthalmology 1984; 91:1420–3.
74. Moloney G, Brewer J, and O'Donnell BA. 'Ancient' schwannoma of the orbit. Clin Experiment Ophthalmol 2004; 32:637–8.
75. Moore CE. Sphenoidal ridge meningioma with optic nerve metastasis. Br J Ophthalmol 1968; 52:636–9.
76. Mortada A. Orbital neurilemmoma with cafe-au-lait pigmentation of the skin. Br J Ophthalmol 1968; 52:262–4.
77. Mortada A. Neurofibromatosis of lid and orbit in early childhood. J Pediatr Ophthalmol 1977; 14:148–50.
78. Murphy M, Timms C, McKelvie P, et al. Malignant optic nerve glioma:metastases to the spinal neuraxis. Case illustration. J Neurosurg 2003; 98:110.
79. Nau JA, Shields CL, Shields JA, et al. Optic nerve glioma in a patient with von Hippel-Lindau syndrome. J Ped Ophthalmol Strabismus 2003; 40:57–8.
80. Parsa CF, Hoyt CS, Lesser RL, et al. Spontaneous regression of optic gliomas: thirteen cases documented by serial neuroimaging. Arch Ophthalmol 2001; 119: 516–29.
81. Paulus W, Jellinger K, Brenner H. Melanotic paraganglioma of the orbit: a case report. Acta Neuropathol 1989; 79: 340–6.
82. Pellitteri PK, Rinaldo A, Myssiorek D, et al. Paragangliomas of the head and neck. Oral Oncol 2004, 40:563–75.
83. Perry A, Dehner LP. Meningeal tumors of childhood and infancy. An update and literature review. Brain Pathol 2003; 13:386–408.
84. Perry A, Gutmann DH, Reifenberger G. Molecular pathogenesis of meningiomas. J Neurooncol 2004; 70: 183–202.
85. Perry A, Lusis EA, Gutmann DH. Meningothelial hyperplasia: a detailed clinicopathologic, immunohistochemical and genetic study of 11 cases. Brain Pathol 2005; 15:109–15.
86. Radhakrishnan S, Lee MS. Optic Nerve Sheath Meningiomas. Curr Treat Options Neurol 2005; 7:51–5.
87. Rao NA, Spencer WH. Optic Nerve. In: Spencer WH, ed. Ophthalmic Pathology. An Atlas and Textbook. Philadelphia, PA: W.B. Saunders, 1996:513–622.

88. Rose GE, Wright JE. Isolated peripheral nerve sheath tumours of the orbit. Eye 1991; 5:668–73.
89. Rubinstein LJ. Pathological features of optic nerve and chiasmatic gliomas. Neurofibromatosis 1988; 1:152–8.
90. Rush JA, Younge BR, Campbell RJ, et al. Optic glioma. Long-term follow-up of 85 histopathologically verified cases. Ophthalmology 1982; 89:1213–9.
91. Saavedra E, Singh AD, Sears JE, et al. Plexiform pigmented schwannoma of the uvea. Surv Ophthalmol 2006; 51:162–8.
92. Sadun F, Hinton DR, Sadun AA. Rapid growth of an optic nerve ganglioglioma in a patient with neurofibromatosis 1. Ophthalmology 1996; 103:794–9.
93. Saeed P, Rootman J, Nugent RA, et al. Optic nerve sheath meningiomas. Ophthalmology 2003; 110:2019–30.
94. Scheithauer BW, Woodruff JM, Erlandson RA. Tumors of the Peripheral Nervous System. Washington, D.C.: Armed Forces Institute of Pathology, 1999.
95. Serdaroglu A, Simsek F, Gucuyener K, et al. Moyamoya syndrome after radiation therapy for optic pathway glioma: case report. J Child Neurol 2000; 15:765–7.
96. Shah JR, Patkar DP, Pungavkar SA, et al. Extensive gliomas of visual tract in a patient of neurofibromatosis-I. Indian J Pediatr 2000; 67:939–40.
97. Shields JA, Font RL, Eagle RC Jr, et al. Melanotic schwannoma of the choroid. Immunohistochemistry and electron microscopic observations. Ophthalmology 1994; 101:843–9.
98. Shields JA, Kapustiak J, Arbizo V, et al. Orbital neurilemoma with extension through the superior orbital fissure. Arch Ophthalmol 1986; 104:871–3.
99. Sood GC, Malik SK, Gupta DK, et al. Bilateral meningiomas of the orbit. Am J Ophthalmol 1966; 61:1533–5.
100. Stern J, Jakobiec FA, Housepian EM. The architecture of optic nerve gliomas with and without neurofibromatosis. Arch Ophthalmol 1980; 98:505–11.
101. Stern WE. Meningiomas in the cranio-orbital junction. J Neurosurg 1973; 38:428–37.
102. Subramanian N, Rambhatia S, Mahesh L, et al. Cystic schwannoma of the orbit-a case series. Orbit 2005; 24: 125–9.
103. Synowitz M, von Eckardstein K, Brauer C, et al. Case history: multicentric glioma with involvement of the optic chiasm. Clin Neurol Neurosurg 2002; 105:66–8.
104. Takeuchi H, Kabuto M, Sato K, et al. Chiasmal gliomas with spontaneous regression: proliferation and apoptosis. Childs Nerv Syst 1997; 13:229–33.
105. Venkataramana NK, Kolluri VR, Kumar DV, et al. Paraganglioma of the orbit with extension to the middle cranial fossa: case report. Neurosurgery 1989; 24:762–4.
106. Verheggen R, Markakis E, Muhlendyck H, et al. Symptomatology, surgical therapy and postoperative results of sphenoorbital, intraorbital-intracanalicular and optic sheath meningiomas. Acta Neurochir Suppl. 1996; 65:95–8.
107. Verhoeff FH. Tumors of the optic Nerve. In: Cytology and Cellular Pathology of the Nervous System. New York: Hafner Publishing Company, 1965:1029–39.
108. Wan WL, Geller JL, Feldon SE, et al. Visual loss caused by rapidly progressive intracranial meningiomas during pregnancy. Ophthalmology 1990; 97:18–21.
109. Wilson WB, Feinsod M, Hoyt WF, et al. Malignant evolution of childhood chiasmal pilocytic astrocytoma. Neurology 1976; 26:322–5.
110. Wimmer K, Eckart M, Meyer-Puttlitz B, et al. Mutational and expression analysis of the NF1 gene argues against a role as tumor suppressor in sporadic pilocytic astrocytomas. J Neuropathol Exp Neurol 2002; 61:896–902.
111. Woiciechowsky C, Vogel S, Meyer R, et al. Magnetic resonance imaging of a glioblastoma of the optic chiasm. J Neurosurg 1995; 83:923–5.
112. Wong JY, Uhl V, Wara WM, et al. Optic gliomas. A reanalysis of the University of California, San Francisco experience. Cancer 1987; 60:1847–55.
113. Wright JE. Primary optic nerve meningiomas: clinical presentation and management. Trans Sect Ophthalmol Am Acad Ophthalmol Otolaryngol 1977; 83:617–25.
114. Wulc AE, Bergin DJ, Barnes D, et al. Orbital optic nerve glioma in adult life. Arch Ophthalmol 1989; 107:1013–6.
115. Yoshikawa G, Nagata K, Kawamoto S, et al. Remarkable regression of optic glioma in an infant. Case illustration. J Neurosurg 2003; 98:1134.

Tumors of Soft Tissue

Hakan Demirci and Victor M. Elner
Kellogg Eye Institute, University of Michigan, Ann Arbor, Michigan, U.S.A.

INTRODUCTION

Soft tissue tumors are an uncommon, heterogeneous group of neoplasms with respect to clinical manifestations, histogenesis, cytogenetics, molecular biology, and prognosis. Overall, their incidence varies from <1% to 16% depending on whether the data is derived from an ophthalmic pathology department or clinical ophthalmology service (60,107,214,221).

FIBROBLASTIC TUMORS

Nodular Fasciitis

Nodular fasciitis is a benign, reactive proliferation of fibroblasts and myofibroblasts in superficial soft tissue that is often confused with a spindle cell sarcoma clinically and histopathologically (253). It may affect any age group but usually occurs in individuals 10 to 60 years of age, with no gender predilection. Head and neck involvement is common (Fig. 1) (2,249). About 25 cases are reported to affect the periorbital region, of which 15 were younger than age 20 years (219). It affects the orbit and anterior ocular structures, including the eyelid, epibulbar surface, and corneoscleral limbus. Nodular fasciitis presents with a short history of onset, usually 1 month or less, and is characterized by the rapid growth of a soft, well-circumscribed mass (73,219).

The pathogenesis of nodular fasciitis is not clear. Bernstein (16) postulated that it is an unusual form of granulation tissue occuring as a reaction to minor trauma (16). A history of trauma is found in up to 15% of cases, favoring the reactive nature of this lesion (16,190). However, the high incidence of trauma compared to the very low incidence of nodular fasciitis suggests that trauma alone is not sufficient for the development of this lesion. Cytogenetic analyses have shown several clonal chromosomal abnormalities (17,63,68,208,249), while flow cytometric studies display an absence of aneuploidy, all consistent with benignity (65,160,179). Other investigations have disclosed that a high proportion of the proliferating cells in nodular fasciitis are in the S and G_2 growth phases of the cell cycle and exhibit polyclonal cellular expansion

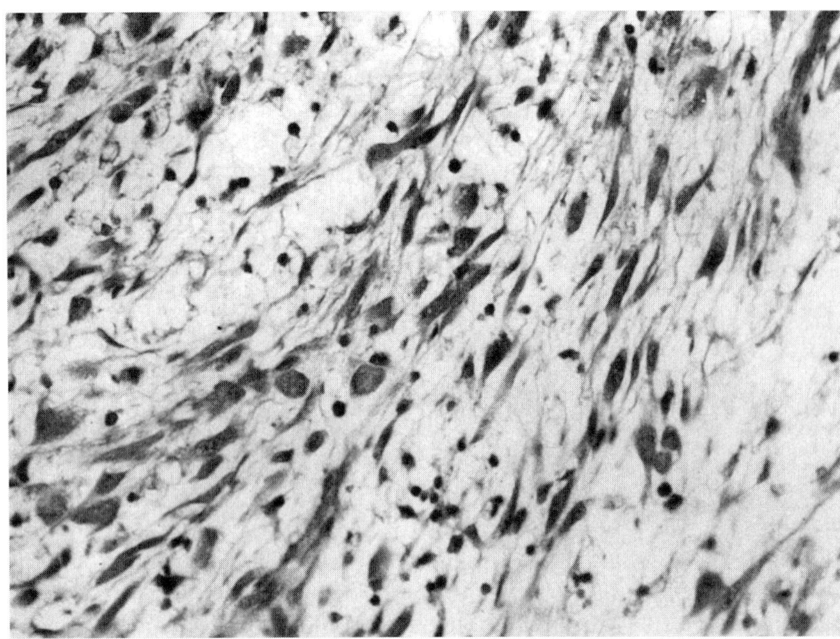

Figure 1 Nodular fasciitis. An exuberant proliferation of fibroblasts presents a superficial resembrance of fibrosarcoma. However, the cell nuclei are small and irregular and there is more collagen synthesis than is seen in most fibrosarcomas. Scattered lymphocytes suggest an inflammatory basis for the lesion (hematoxylin and eosin, × 250). *Source*: Courtesy of Professor A. Garner.

using human androgen-receptor gene (*HUMARA*) methylation-specific polymerase chain reaction (PCR) (136). The latter supports a reactive rather than a neoplastic process, the clonality found by cytogenetic tests being attributed to favored growth of particular cell clones by the culture conditions (136).

Histopathologically, nodular fasciitis is composed of plump, mitotically active stellate, or spindle-shaped fibroblastic cells in an edematous stroma. The cells lack nuclear hyperchromasia and pleomorphism and contain abundant cytoplasm. Variable amounts of myxoid ground substance are intermixed with the cells. Immunohistochemical stains reveal strong positive reactivity with antibodies to smooth muscle-specific actin and vimentin, but no immunoreactivity for S100, desmin, p53, CD34, or epithelial membrane antigens (EMAs) (203,253). These results are consistent with myofibroblastic differentiation and are corroborated by transmission electron microscopy (TEM) findings of elongated cells containing abundant dilated rough endoplasmic reticulum (ER) and parallel bundles of actin-like filaments with fusiform densities (203).

Treatment of periocular nodular fasciitis involves complete excision of the well-circumscribed mass. Local recurrences have not occurred in ocular cases, but have been noted at other sites (<2%) (219). Neither malignant transformation nor metastases have been documented.

Solitary Fibrous Tumor

Solitary fibrous tumor is a rare mesenchymal spindle cell tumor usually occurring in the pleura, but also affecting many other sites including the mediastinum, peritoneum, orbit, and deep soft tissues of the extremities (98,261). About 70 orbital cases have been reported, sometimes with lacrimal sac and lacrimal gland involvement (14,137). It presents as a well-circumscribed mass, which causes insidious, painless proptosis developing during an average of 3 years in middle-aged adults whose mean age is 34 years (9–44 years) (14,137). Only three cases have been reported in children (1,137,149). The tumor enhances intensely with contrast in imaging studies and may result in bony remodeling of orbital walls (14,85,137).

Immunohistochemical and TEM studies have been used to describe the histogenesis of solitary fibrous tumor. The tumor cells are CD34-positive, a property they share with normal and neoplastic endothelial cells, but they lack factor VIII antigen expression (42). Ultrastructural findings of actin filaments, focal intercellular junctions, and cytoplasmic-dense bodies suggest myofibroblastic/fibroblastic differentiation. A recent study, analyzing the ultrastructural spectrum of solitary fibrous tumors concluded that they are heterogeneous in their cellular composition (113). The tumors appear to originate from a perivascular stem cell that gives rise to tumor cells exhibiting endothelial, pericytic, or fibroblastic differentiation, all three cell types being present in normal angiogenesis (113). This interpretation of the histogenesis suggests that the tumor cells have an ability, possibly through stromal cell/matrix interaction, to produce the characteristic hemangiopericytoma-like branching, dilated blood vessels that are present in a patchy distribution in most of these tumors.

Histopathologically, solitary fibrous tumor exhibits variable patterns of cellular architecture, without any tendency to form bundles. It consists of bland spindle cells haphazardly arranged in hypo- and hypercellular areas with intervening thick collagen fibers. Criteria for benignity include low mitotic activity (<4 per 10 high-power microscopic fields) and no abnormal mitotic figures, pleomorphism, or tumor giant cells (95). There is characteristic perivascular fibrosis as well as the dilated, branching hemangiopericytoma-like vessels. Vimentin, CD34, and CD99 immunoreactivity is present in 100%, 90%, and 70% of cases, respectively (172,194,239). Positivity for vimentin and CD34 supports a diagnosis of solitary fibrous tumor, but since they are nonspecific markers, morphologic correlation with routine histopathology is necessary for the pathologic diagnosis. Immunopositivity for EMA and Bcl-2 (both, 20–35%) is less common (161,172,194,239,240), and the cells are negative for desmin, cytokeratin, factor VIII-related antigen, S100 protein, and smooth muscle-specific actin (106).

The treatment for solitary fibrous tumor is excision of the circumscribed growth since most are benign. In about 10% of the cases, however, invasive local growth and/or a frankly malignant phenotype with metastases may occur (59,105). In the orbit, most recurrences are due to incomplete excision (1,14,137). Only one case of malignant solitary fibrous tumor has been reported in the orbit (34). Cytogenetic analysis of solitary fibrous tumor often discloses chromosomal losses at 9p, 13q, and 20p, with losses at 13q being the most frequently observed abnormality (95,138,139, 154,165). Although morphologically similar, recurrent tumors often exhibit increased mitotic activity and show newly acquired abnormalities in clones of tumor cells not present in the primary tumors, correlating with more aggressive behavior (171). A recent study showed that basic fibroblast growth factor (FGF), Ki-67 protein, and p53 antigen can be useful markers for both prognosis and diagnosis of solitary fibrous tumor since they are detected in high levels in tumors with a more aggressive clinical course (237,273).

Hemangiopericytoma

Hemangiopericytoma has classically been used to designate neoplasms of putative pericytic origin (260). Ocular involvement is almost exclusively orbital, affecting middle-aged adults who average 42 to 47 years (46,122,225). A rare exception is the ciliary body hemangiopericytoma (26). There is male predominance in ocular cases, while females are affected more often by tumors at other sites (225). When visible, the neoplasms are violet, highly vascular, and spongy, often with feeder blood vessels (225). The tumors appear well-circumscribed and cause progressive, unilateral proptosis with an average onset of 3 years (46,122,244).

Originally proposed to comprise cells of pericytic origin, ultrastructural studies disclosed five types differentiation among the tumor cells: undifferentiated (48%), pericytic (32%), myoid (8%), histiocytic (8%), and fibroblastic (4%), challenging this concept (53). The tumor cells show basal lamina, cytoplasmic processes, pinocytotic vescicles, cytoplasmic microfilaments with dense bodies, and poorly formed intercellular junctions, features that are not specific for pericytic differentiation, but are also found in cells of fibroblastic origin (Figs. 2–4) (209). These ultrastructural features have been used in conjunction with immunohistochemistry to argue that hemangipericytomas should be reclassified as fibroblastic. Schurch et al. (209) argue that positivity for fibroblast-associated antigens CD34 and CD99 is additional evidence for the need to reclassify these tumors of which only 10% to 20% react with the pericytic markers, muscle-specific actin, and smooth muscle-specific actin (48,53,209). These findings have supported redesignation of most of these tumors as solitary fibrous tumors, which themselves show variable microscopic morphology, including cellular, fat-forming, and giant cell-rich variants (87,95). Tumors remaining as hemangiopericytomas are only those CD34-negative tumors, which react for muscle and/or smooth muscle-specific actins or exhibit clear cut myoid–pericytic ultrastructural features.

Hemangiopericytomas usually exhibit infiltrating margins when examined histopathologically. They have monotonous appearances at low-power microscopic power, with moderate to high cellularity, and the presence of numerous, variably thick-walled, branching dilated vessels with a characteristic staghorn appearance. At high power, closely packed, uniformly sized, spindle-shaped to round cells containing small amounts of pale, eosinophilic cytoplasm and bland, often vesicular nuclei are surrounded by a rich network of the sinusoidal vessels. Reticulin may be stained to reveal its presence around individual or groups of tumor cells and between tumor cells and the sinusoidal vessels (95). Benign hemangiopericytomas are distinguished from frankly malignant tumors by high cellularity, necrosis, mitotic rate of greater than 4 per 10 high-power microscopic fields, and nuclear and cellular pleomorphism (225). The tumor cells react uniformly for vimentin and fairly consistently for CD34 and CD99, both of which may stain only focally (84,95,189). Muscle-specific actin and smooth muscle-specific actin reactivity is seen in 10% to 20% of tumors (84,164,189). The tumor cells are negative for factor VIII-related antigen and CD31 vascular markers (84,164,189). Cytogenetically, disparate chromosomal aberrations have been reported, but break points in

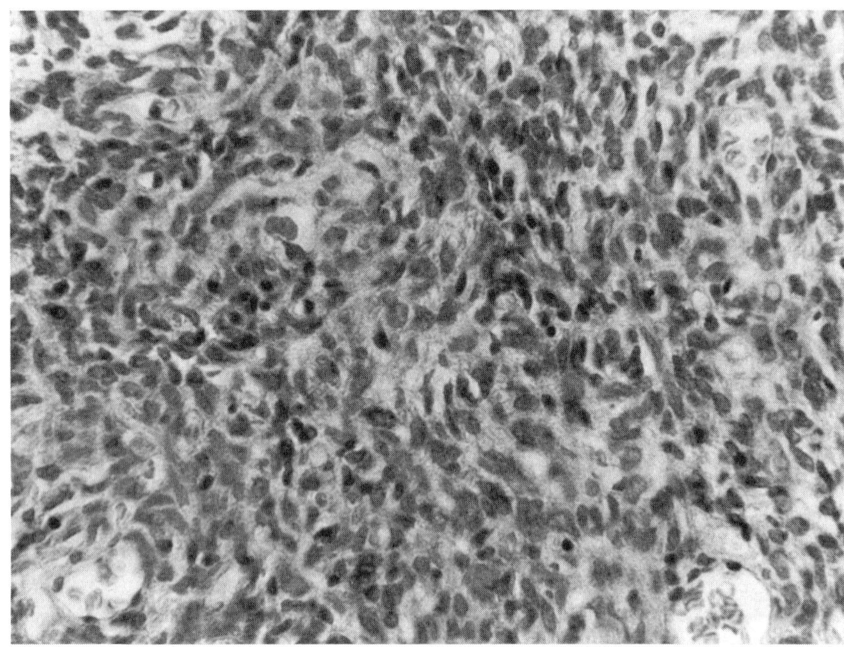

Figure 2 Benign hemangiopericytoma of the orbit. Several small endothelium-lined vascular channels are separated by densely packed spindle cells (hematoxylin and eosin, ×390). *Source*: Courtesy of Professor A. Garner.

12q13–15 and 19q13 have been identified in almost half and one-fourth of cases, respectively (167).

About two-thirds of hemangiopericytomas pursue a benign clinical course, but the clinical course cannot be predicted with assurance based on the histopathologic findings (46,122). Thus, even microscopically benign-appearing tumors may recur. With each recurrence, these and borderline and frankly malignant tumors may become progressively more aggressive with greater tendencies to recur locally and result in distant metastases (140,247). Local recurrence seen in 30% of cases and metastases complicating 15% of cases, have occurred after decades of apparent disease-free survival (46,122). These tumors are relatively radioresistant and radiotherapy may increase their aggressiveness (44). However, some may respond to high dose radiation (11).

Fibrous Histiocytoma

Fibrous histiocytoma is a spindle cell mesenchymal tumor that may involve any soft tissue site (255). Ocular involvement by fibrous histiocytoma includes

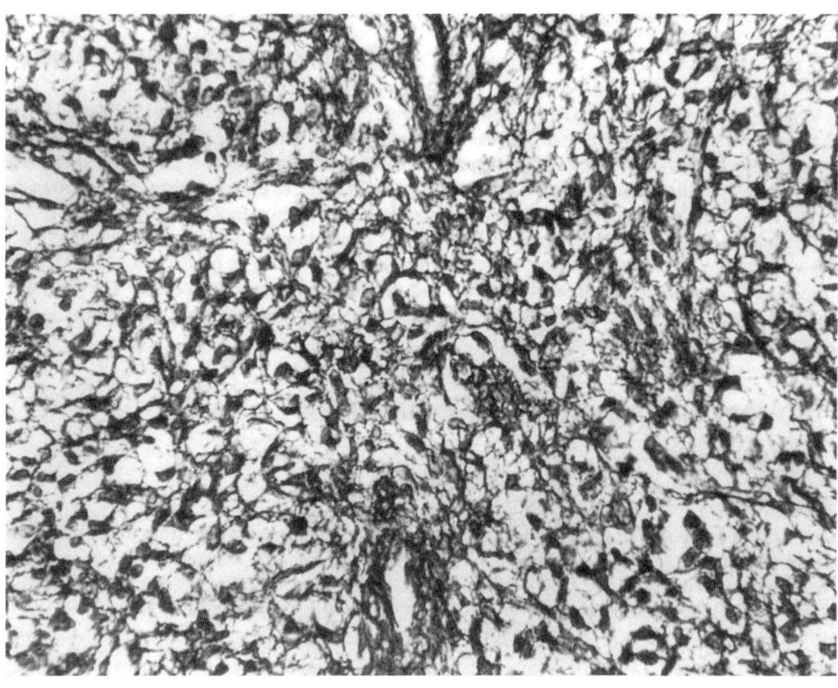

Figure 3 Benign hemangiopericytoma of the orbit, showing a dense network of "reticulin" fibers that enclose individual tumor cells, in contrast to the retuculin distribution in hemangioendotheliomas, here clusters of cells around a central blood vessel are delineated (Gomori reticulin stain, ×390). *Source*: Courtesy of Professor A. Garner.

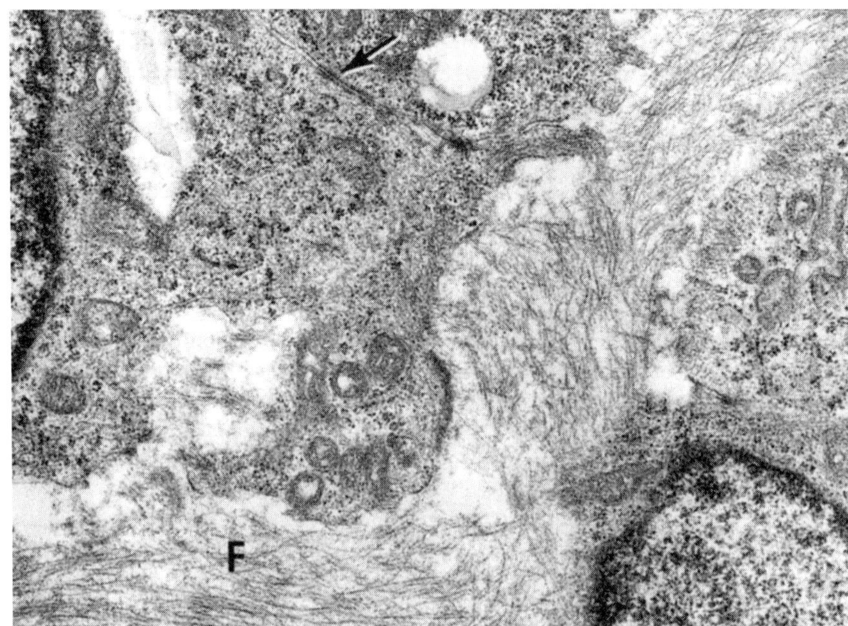

Figure 4 Transmission electron micrograph of hemangiopericytoma. It shows an accumulation of extracellular collagenous fibrils (F), which correspond to the "reticulin" seen by light micrscopy. Adjacent tumor cells are connected by macula adherens cell junctions (*arrow*) (× 20,490). *Source*: Courtesy of Dr. J. Shelburne.

anterior or deep orbit, eyelid, conjunctiva, episclera, and corneoscleral limbus (52,78). Patients are generally middle-aged, averaging 43 years, with a female predominance in tumors affecting nonorbital ocular structures (78). Tumors of the conjunctiva, episclera, and corneoscleral limbus have a history of onset that is generally less than 6 months and appear yellow and circumscribed with prominent superficial vessels (43). Orbital tumors cause proptosis and appear circumscribed on imaging (78).

Most knowledge about fibrous histiocytoma is based on the analysis of skin tumors. The marked variability in the histopathologic features of fibrous histiocytoma has created controversy concerning its cell of origin (Fig. 5). The concept of a primitive mesenchymal cell exhibiting variable expression of histiocytic and fibroblastic phenotypes is supported by tumor cell immunoreactivity for CD68 and vimentin, respectively (43). However, immunoreactivity of dermal tumors for factor XIIIa, an antigen present on dermal dendritic cells, suggests that these tumors may arise from other histiocytic precursor cells (36,227). Some authors have considered fibrous histiocytoma

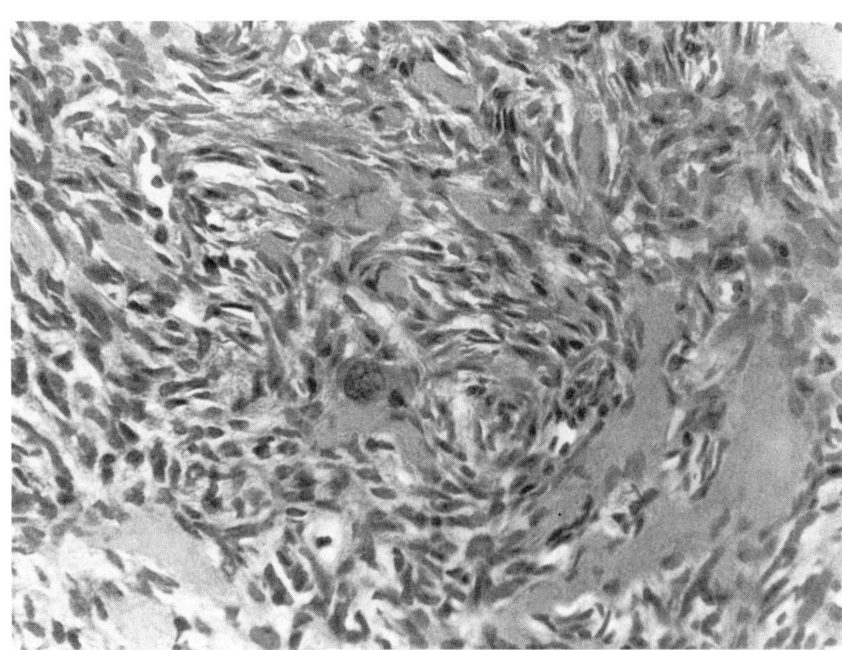

Figure 5 Fibrous histiocytoma in orbit. Spindle-shaped cells intermingled with wisps of collagenous tissue are arranged in a matted and slightly whorled pattern. A multinucleated cell is also present but has no sinister implication, and the overall cytology is regular (hematoxylin and eosin, × 385). *Source*: Courtesy of Professor A. Garner.

to be a reactive fibrosing inflammatory process because of the almost invariable presence of inflammatory cells, frequent spontaneous regression, and tendency to be associated with a history of insect bites or vaccinations (37,51). This interpretation has been challenged by proponents for neoplasia who argue that many neoplasms have an inflammatory component, that local recurrence is frequent, and that the history of trauma is nonspecific (31). Clonal chromosome aberrations found in some of these tumors argues for their claim of a neoplastic process (31).

Microscopically, the tumor has poorly defined margins and extensively infiltrates surrounding tissues making complete surgical excision difficult (30). The tumor cells grow in a prominent cartwheel or storiform pattern, sometimes combined with areas containing spindle-shaped to round cells and sinusoidal or staghorn-shaped blood vessels as observed in hemangiopericytoma. An admixture of fibroblastic and histiocytic cells is present, the latter with characteristically lipid laden with foamy cytoplasm, and intermediate types. Both nuclear pleomorphism and hyperchromasia are absent, and mitoses are usually <5 per 10 high-power microscopic fields. Usually present are scattered inflammatory cells, mostly lymphocytes, plasma cells, and Touton giant cells. Immunohistochemical positivity for C68 and vimentin in almost all tumors, and factor XIIIa, supports the diagnosis (255). Fibrous histiocytomas are negative for cytokeratin, desmin, S100 protein, and CD34 antigens (255).

Clonality may be demonstrated by cytogenetic tests, which show mostly trisomy 7 or a clonal loss or gain of a sex chromosome (31). The local invasiveness of this tumor has been attributed to the production of matrix metalloproteinases 2 and 14, which may facilitate cell migration through the extracellular matrix (ECM) matrix by cleaving collagen I, laminin, and the extracellular domain of the hyaluronan receptor (CD44) (251). The metalloproteinases also activate transforming growth factor β (TGFβ), a molecule that upregulates fibroblast motility and collagen production (251).

Reported recurrence is higher for orbital tumors (about 30%) than those affecting other anterior ocular sites (7%) (43,78).

Malignant Fibrous Histiocytoma

Malignant fibrous histiocytoma has classically been used to designate a group of pleomorphic soft tissue sarcomas thought to be derived from cells exhibiting hybrid histiocytic and fibroblastic differentiation (173,180,256). It is the most common soft tissue sarcoma of adulthood (199,256). The orbit is the most frequent site of ocular involvement. The eyelid, conjunctiva, episclera, and corneoscleral limbus are rarely affected (78). Its demographic and clinical features are very similar to fibrous histiocytoma, but the average history of onset is 4 months (78).

The concept of malignant fibrous histiocytoma, based on histogenetic studies, has evolved in recent years (67,199). Early ultrastructural studies indicated that these tumors comprised four common types of tumor cells: (*i*) fibroblastic spindle cells with a prominent rough ER (*ii*) histiocytic plump cells containing lysosomes, lipid droplets, occasional hyaline globules, and surface pseudopodia; (*iii*) myofibroblasts with a prominent rough ER cisternae, and arrays of actin myofilaments; and (*iv*) undifferentiated cells containing scant cytoplasm and few organelles (256). These tumors frequently expressed putative histiocytic markers, α-1-anti-trypsin, α-1-anti-chymotrypsin, lysozyme, as well as the fibroblastic markers, vimentin, and actin (199). Later studies challenged the concept of histiocytic tumor cell derivation or differentiation. Accordingly, the plump cells have been reinterpreteted as fibroblasts with abundant cytoplasm, prominent Golgi apparatus, and variable numbers of primary and secondary lysosomes while the lysosomal enzyme immunoreactivity is deemed to be nonspecific due to its detection in other tumors, including carcinomas and melanoma (199). This interpretation is supported by the observations that malignant fibrous histiocytoma does not express antigens (e.g., leukocyte common antigen (CD45)) and enzymatic profiles more consistent with those of fibroblasts than histiocytes (115,269). Monoclonal antibodies raised against malignant fibrous histiocytoma cell lines manifest strong reactivity for perivascular mesenchymal cells and fibroblasts, but not for cells of macrophage/monocytes lineage (115,269). Taken together these findings have been used to advance the hypothesis that malignant fibrous histiocytomas are composed of admixtures of neoplastic cells of fibroblastic/myofibroblastic differentiation and reactive, CD68-positive, histiocytic cells of monocyte/macrophage lineage (5,102,236). Based on this notion, these tumors have been reclassified as pleomorphic sarcomas, which, due to their variable microscopic morphology, include: (*i*) storiform–pleomorphic fibrosarcoma, (*ii*) myxofibrosarcoma, (*iii*) pleomorphic fibrosarcoma with giant cells, and (*iv*) inflammatory fibrosarcoma (199).

Histologically, these pleomorphic sarcomas have ill-defined, infiltrative margins. The storiform–-pleomorphic fibrosarcomas usually exhibit a storiform growth pattern in which the spindle cell component appears fibroblastic, myofibroblastic, or smooth muscle-like (Fig. 6). Often admixed with spindle cells are rounded histiocyte-like fibroblastic cells and bizarre tumor giant cells. Marked nuclear and cytologic

(A) 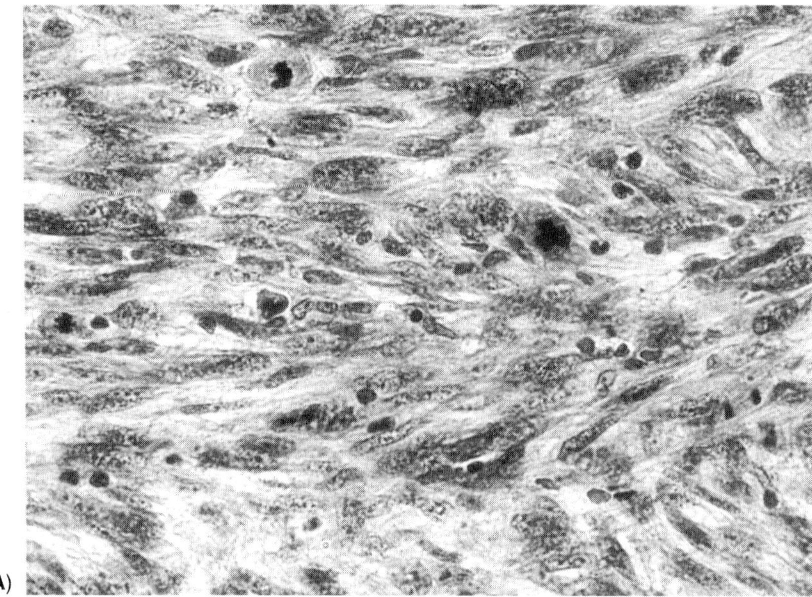

(B) 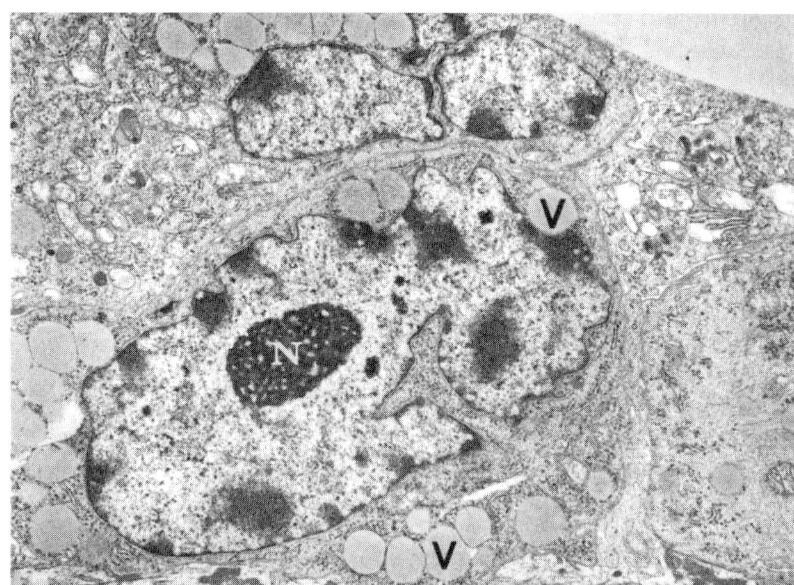

Figure 6 Malignant fibrous histiocytoma. (**A**) The cells remain predominantly spindle shaped but have increased nuclear–cytoplasmic ratios and conspicuous nucleoli and show prominent abnormal mitotic activity (hematoxylin and eosin, ×365). *Source*: Courtesy of Professor A. Garner. (**B**) Ultrastructure of tumor cell in malignant fibrous histiocytoma. Note the prominent nucleolus (N) and numerous cytoplasmic vacuoles (V) (×6,300). *Source*: Courtesy of Dr. J. Shelburne.

pleomorphism and high mitotic activity are common. A chronic inflammatory cell infiltration is a regular feature. Pleomorphic fibrosarcoma with giant cells exhibit a prominent-reactive osteoclast giant cell reaction. Inflammatory fibrosarcoma contains sheets of benign xanthoma cells and numerous reactive inflammatory cells including neutrophils, eosinophils, and fewer lymphocytes and plasma cells. Myxofibrosarcoma adds diffuse or focal areas of myxoid stroma to an otherwise typical storiform-pleomorphic pattern. Consistent immunoreactivity is seen for vimentin, actin, lysozyme, alpha-1-anti-trypsin and alpha-1-anti-chymotrypsin, and CD68 antigens (199). Variably present is reactivity for smooth muscle-specific actin, desmin, cytokeratin, EMA, S100 protein, and neurofilament (199). The presence of myofibroblasts explains why these tumors express actin, smooth muscle-specific actin, and desmin. Typical ultrastructural features of the fibroblastic cells include prominent dilated rough ER reticulum, intermediate filaments, and Golgi apparatus; the myofibroblastic cells also show nuclear contractions, pinocytic vesicles, and thin filaments with associated dense bodies (5,131,236). Cytogenetic studies show no specific abnormalities characteristic for these sarcomas, but teloremic associations, ring chromosomes, and dicentric chromosomes are frequent. Several proto-oncogenes mapping to a region of the long arm of chromosome 12 (12q13–15) appear to participate in the development of pleomorphic sarcomas (9,15,193,202).

The reported recurrence for malignant fibrous histiocytomas, now reclassified as pleomorphic sarcomas following wide excision is two-thirds for orbital tumors and 10-year survival rate is 23% (78).

Fibrosarcoma

Fibrosarcomas are malignant neoplasms composed of mesenchymal cells showing fibroblastic differentiation and variable collagen production. Primary fibrosarcoma rarely involves the ocular region (250). It arises in the orbit and eyelid, primarily in children at a mean age of 4 years (4,28,114,272), and is therefore usually classified as infantile or juvenile fibrosarcoma (250). Primary fibrosarcoma usually presents with rapid onset of proptosis, eyelid swelling, palpable mass, and restriction of ocular motility (250). Computed tomography (CT) demonstrates an irregular, but well-circumscribed mass frequently with adjacent bone destruction. Fibrosarcoma can occur as a secondary orbital malignancy after radiation therapy for hereditary retinoblastoma or due to extension from a primary origin in a paranasal sinus or nasal cavity in which case it is always associated with bone destruction (4).

The histogenesis of fibrosarcoma has been established by ultrastructural and immunohistochemical studies, which indicate an origin from mesenchymal cells that may show fibroblastic or myofibroblastic differentiation. Ultrastructural features include a prominent rough ER and indented nuclear membranes, which may be accompanied by the presence of microfilament bundles with dense bodies in tumor cells with myofibroblastic differentiation (235). The presence of myofibroblastic differentiation is responsible for immunopositivity for muscle-specific actin, smooth muscle-specific actin, and desmin (254).

Histopathologically, juvenile fibrosarcoma is very similar to the classic fibrosarcoma of adults. The typical histologic appearance is of a densely cellular proliferation of uniform spindle cells arranged in interlacing bundles and sharply intersecting fascicles, which sometimes exhibit the classical herringbone pattern. Variants include tumors with small round cells, myxoid matrix, and whorled growth patterns. Immunoreactivity for the nonspecific markers vimentin (100%) and neuron-specific enolase (35%) is common (41). Some tumors are positive for markers signifying myofibroblastic differentiation: alpha-smooth muscle actin (33%), muscle-specific actin (30%), smooth muscle-specific actin (29%), and desmin (20%) (40,134,213). Cytogenetic analysis of most tumors reveals a chromosomal translocation [t(12;15)(p13;q26)] in which the *ETV6* gene on chromosome 12 (12p) become transferred to the NTRK3 locus on chromosome 15 (15q) resulting in fusion of *ETV6* and *NTRK3* genes at the NTRK3 locus, which is activated (22,132,200). The resulting oncoprotein contains the N-terminal aspect of ETV6 fused to the NTRK3 domain, which encodes a tyrosine kinase receptor (132,200) and promotes cell proliferation. Trisomies of chromosomes 8,11,17, and 20 may also occur and are thought to induce mitotic activity (41).

Juvenile fibrosarcoma is regarded as a tumor of borderline or low malignant potential by some authors (75), but carrying a significantly better prognosis than fibrosarcoma in adults. The juvenile type often exhibits diploid DNA consistent with its less aggressive clinical course that results in a 5 year survival of 94% (40). A small series of 5 cases with orbital and eyelid juvenile fibrosarcoma showed recurrence in 2 cases following excision with no metastases (250,272).

ADIPOCYTIC TUMORS

Lipoma

Lipoma is the most common benign mesenchymal neoplasm in adults. About 20 recorded cases with ocular involvement, affecting the orbit, conjunctiva, and lacrimal sac have been reported (51,185). It is a tumor of adults more than 50-years-old and is more common in men. Lipomas usually appear as soft, well-circumscribed, lobulated, yellow-gray tumors.

Histogenetically, lipomas consist of mature lipocytes. Ultrastructural studies show adipocytes, each containing a single centrally positioned large lipid vacuole and peripherally placed cytoplasm and nucleus (129). Also present are small spindle cells, preadipocytes, with occasional lipid vacuoles; these cells are often situated along the interstitial capillaries and are thought to be adipocyte precursors. These spindle cells are more often present in lipomas than in normal fat tissue (228).

Histopathologically, lipoma is composed of lobules of mature adipocytes. These cells are identical to the surrounding tissue except for slight variation in size and shape of the cells. A variant reported to occur in the orbit is spindle cell/pleomorphic lipoma in which there is a variable admixture of spindle cells and rounded pleomorphic cells containing hyperchromatic nuclei, sometimes multiple and arranged in a floret-like pattern. Adipocytes stain immunochemically for vimentin and variably for S100 protein, leptin, and leptin receptor (175,176).

Cytogenetic abnormalities have been found in 55% to 75% of lipomas (205). The 12q13–q15 region of chromosome 12 is the most often affected. A chromosomal translocation [t(3;12)(q27–q28; q13–q15)] accounts for 25% of all these aberrations (205). The 12q13–q15 cytogenetic aberrations may result in a fusion gene containing material from the *HMGA2* and *LPP* genes (187). Transcript of this fusion gene contains domains that regulate transcription and are capable of initiating tumorigenesis. Chromosome 13 abnormalities are the next most common, found in up to 20% of all lipomas, followed by rearrangements of chromosomes 6 and 7 (205).

Liposarcoma

Liposarcoma, a common soft tissue sarcoma of adults, arise from mesenchymal cells demonstrating lipoblastic differentiation. Only 40 cases of liposarcoma have been reported in the orbit (29). Metastatic liposarcoma to the orbit is exceedingly rare (29). Affected patients range in age from 5 to 79 years with females predominating (29). Orbital liposarcomas cause insidious proptosis and globe displacement due to a palpable mass over durations ranging from several months to 7 years, but they may cause pain (230). CT may reveal a mass of variably increased density compared with surrounding fat, but this finding may be extremely subtle and appreciated only by sequential imaging, if at all. Magnetic resonance imaging (MRI) improves the detection of these lesions by discriminating them from surrounding orbital fat using gadolinium enhancement on T1-weighted images (182). These tumors are yellow to yellow-white, gelatinous to firm, lobular, sometimes vascular, and poorly circumscribed to frankly invasive.

Histogenetically, tumor cells appear to derive from lipoblast precursor adventitial cells that arise around capillary-sized blood vessels (188). Degrees of differentiation range from primitive mesenchymal spindle- or stellate-shaped fibroblast-like cells containing little or no lipid to lipoblasts that contain hyperchromatic, indented, or sharply scalloped nuclei and cytoplasmic lipid droplets (13).

The histologic appearance of liposarcomas range from well-differentiated lipoma-like lesions, through intermediate-grade myxoid or round cell subtypes, to poorly differentiated pleomorphic tumors. Well-differentiated liposarcoma is an intermediate, locally aggressive subtype containing a component of mature adipocytes that show significant nuclear atypia and variation in size (69,70,262). These tumors exhibit varying numbers of vacuolated lipoblasts and hyperchromatic, multinucleated stromal cells (Fig. 7) (58,206). Myxoid and round-cell liposarcomas are subtypes composed of uniform round- to oval-shaped, primitive, mesenchymal cells and variable numbers of small lipoblasts containing nuclei displaced by large lipid droplets resulting in a signet-ring appearance (Fig. 8). The tumor cells are imbedded in a prominent myxoid stroma containing an intricate, arborizing vascular pattern (58,206). Pleomorphic liposarcomas contain variable numbers of pleomorphic multivacuolated lipoblasts that vary in cell diameter in a background of high-grade pleomorphic sarcoma (malignant fibrous histiocytoma-like sarcoma). The pleomorphic cells may be small and round or spindle-shaped, the latter often arranged in fascicles. Scattered multinucleated tumor giant cells may be present in this pleomorphic variant. Dedifferentiated liposarcoma is composed of mild to markedly atypical cells often in abrupt histological transition from low- to high-grade patterns. Immunoreactivity for S100 protein may be present in the lipoblasts (55).

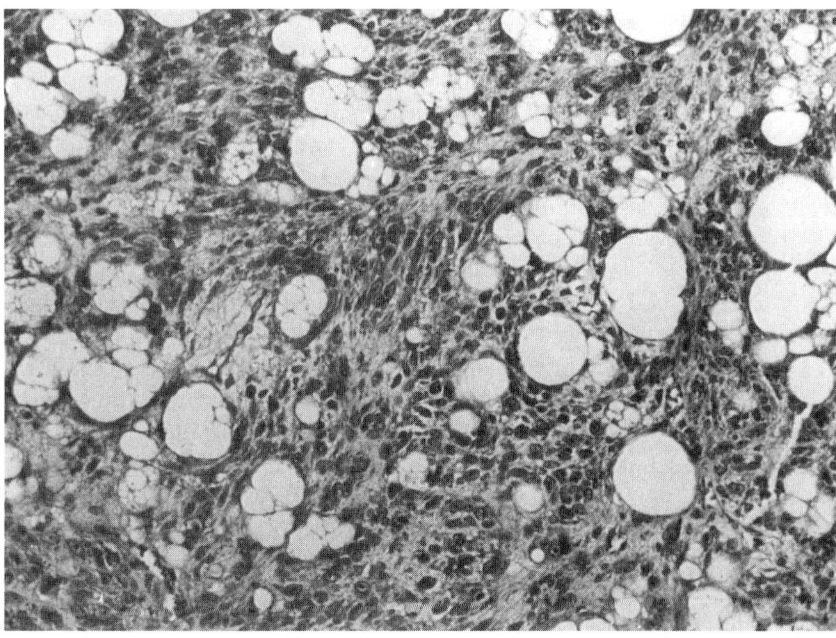

Figure 7 Liposarcoma of the orbit. Pleomorphic and frequently undifferentiated cells are shown. Some cells contain multiple vacuoles within the cytoplasm. However, in places the lipid content has been liberated to create larger vacuolar spaces. Oil red O-staining of frozen sections serves to confirm the lipid nature of the material within the vacuoles (hematoxylin and eosin, ×155). *Source*: Courtesy of Professor A. Garner.

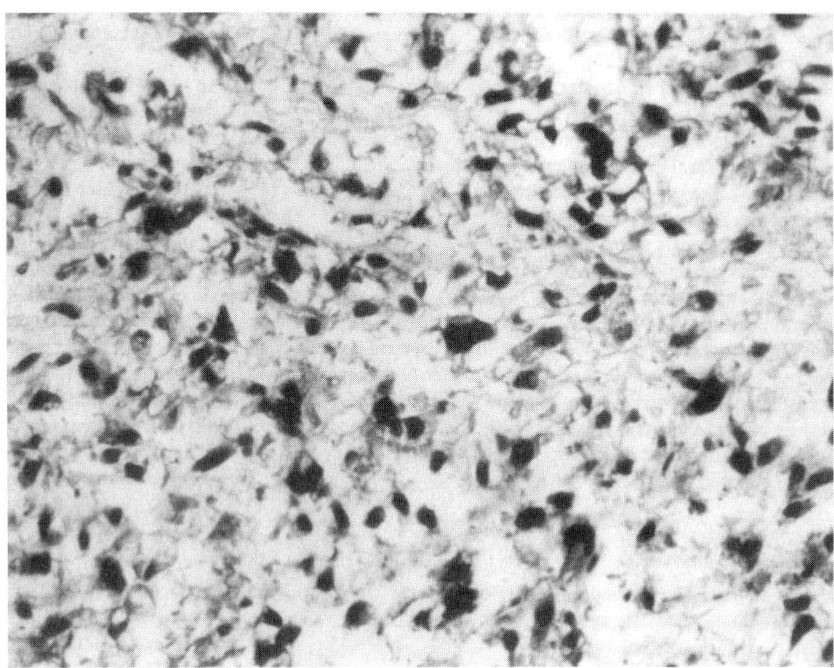

Figure 8 Myxoid liposarcoma. Scatttered signet ring and otherwise vacuolated cell forms are seen within a loose stroma, and the cell nuclei show moderate pleomorphism (hematoxylin and eosin, ×455). *Source*: Courtesy of Professor A. Garner.

Cytogenetically, well-differentiated liposarcomas show supernumerary ring and/or giant marker chromosomes, which contain amplified sequences derived from different chromosomes, particularly from a region of chromosome12 (2q13–15) where several proto-oncogenes such as *MDM2*, *CDK4*, *HMGI-C*, are encoded (49,197,198). *HMGI-C* assists in adipocyte differentiation, *CDK4* plays a role in cell cycle regulation, and *MDM2* regulates cell proliferation. Ring and/or giant marker chromosomes are found in dedifferentiated liposarcoma (76). In high-grade areas, overexpression of *MDM2* and a mutation of *TP53*, a gene that reduces cell proliferation, may be responsible for tumor aggressiveness (57). Myxoid and round cell liposarcoma show unique chromosomal reciprocal translocation [t(12;16) (q13;p11)], resulting in the formation of a chimeric *CHOP-TLS* gene (121,158). An alternative translocation [t(12;22) (q13;q12)] involving *CHOP* and the 5′ end of the *EWS* gene mapping to a region on chromosome 22 (22q12) can be detected in 10% of these tumors (50,186). *CHOP*, on chromosome 12, encodes a DNA transcription factor while *TLS*, on chromosome 16, encodes an RNA-binding protein. The *CHOP-TLS* and *CHOP-EWS* chimeric proteins function as potent transcription factors that promote oncogenic proliferation (47). Pleomorphic liposarcomas lack distinct cytogenetic alterations and exhibit complex chromosomal abnormalities with pronounced aneuploidy (47).

Low immunohistochemical expression of p27, a cell cycle regulator, in myxoid and round cell liposarcoma correlates with decreased survival (29). Metastasis has not been reported in patients with orbital liposarcoma (29,118).

SMOOTH MUSCLE TUMORS

Leiomyoma

Leiomyoma is a benign tumor of smooth muscle origin that can develop in any part of the body. Ocular involvement is most common in adult women, occurring at an average age of 34 years (195). The ciliary body and peripheral choroid are the eye tissues in which this tumor most often arises, but may rarely present in the conjunctiva and orbit (18,24,215, 216,243) or iris (Fig. 9). When the tumor involves the ciliary body or peripheral choroid, diagnosis is often delayed until secondary complications of lens subluxation, glaucoma, or retinal detachment occur (18,24,195,215,216,243). Examination reveals an amelanotic, dome-shaped tumor that transmits light and is often associated with overlying dilated episcleral vessels. It may be difficult to distinguish clinically from an amelanotic malignant melanoma.

Leiomyomas arise wherever smooth muscle cells are present. When they develop from ciliary body smooth muscle, a neural crest derivative, they are described as mesectodermal. At other sites the tumors are of mesodermal origin, arising from smooth muscle precursors within blood vessel walls, adnexal structures, and deep soft tissues (116,117,195,257). The histogenesis of leiomyomas is based on light microscopic, ultrastructural, and immunohistochemical features. The tumor cells resemble normal smooth muscle cells with cigar-shaped, round, or ovoid nuclei

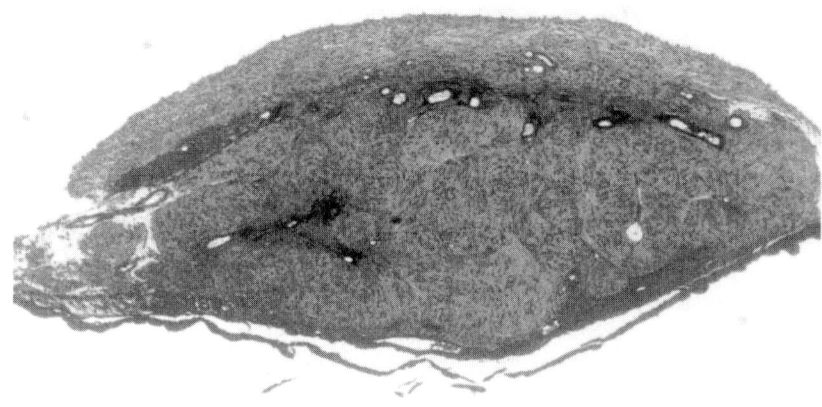

(A)

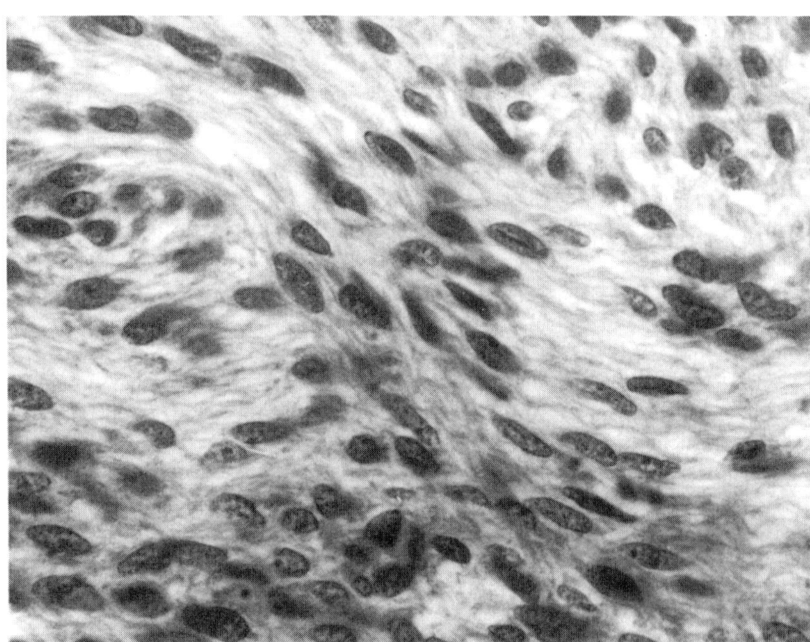

(B)

Figure 9 Leiomyoma. (**A**) Small iris leiomyoma in a surgically enucleated eye of a 16-year-old girl who was thought to have a malignant ocular melanoma (hematoxylin and eosin, ×56). (**B**) The tumor cells have spindle-shaped nuclei with blunted ends and small nucleoli. The cells are separated by an abundant fibrillary material and contain no melanin pigment (hematoxylin and eosin, ×740). *Source*: Courtesy of Drs. H.E. Grossniklaus and W.R. Green.

and red, eosinophilic, or fuchsinophilic cytoplasm when stained with the hematoxylin and eosin and Masson trichrome methods, respectively (257). Ultrastructurally, leiomyomas contain 12 nm thick myosin filaments associated with 6 to 8 nm thin actin filaments, 10 nm intermediate filaments, and dense bodies and plaques (Fig. 10) (97). Immunohistochemically, the filaments in these tumors are regularly positive for smooth muscle-specific actin, muscle-specific actin, desmin, and h-caldesmon, an actin-binding protein (101).

Histopathologically, leiomyomas have interlacing and tightly packed bundles of spindle cells arranged in palisades, with minimal or no collagenous stroma. The tumor cells contain blunt-ended or oval nuclei and moderate amounts of fibrillar eosinophilic cytoplasm whose fibrils stain with the Masson trichrome stain (163). Immunohistochemically, the tumor cells are always positive for vimentin and the aforementioned filamentary antigens. They do not stain for S100 protein even though they are thought to be of neural crest origin (101). Ultrastructural studies show abundant mitochondria, rough ER, and free ribosomes (97). Intracytoplasmic myofilaments oriented along the long axis of cells, intermediate filaments around dense bodies, and micropinocytotic vesicles are also visible (97). Common cytogenetic abnormalities of deep soft tissue leiomyomas include translocation between chromosomes 12 and 14 (20%), deletions in chromosome 7 (17%), trisomy of chromosome 12 (12%), and aberrations of chromosome 6 (5%) (6). Potentially involved are high mobility group genes on chromosomes 6 and 12 that encode for DNA-binding proteins, which regulate transcription by influencing the access of other DNA-binding proteins. Microarray gene chip analyses demonstrate that genes regulating retinoid synthesis, insulin growth factor metabolism, TGF signaling, and ECM

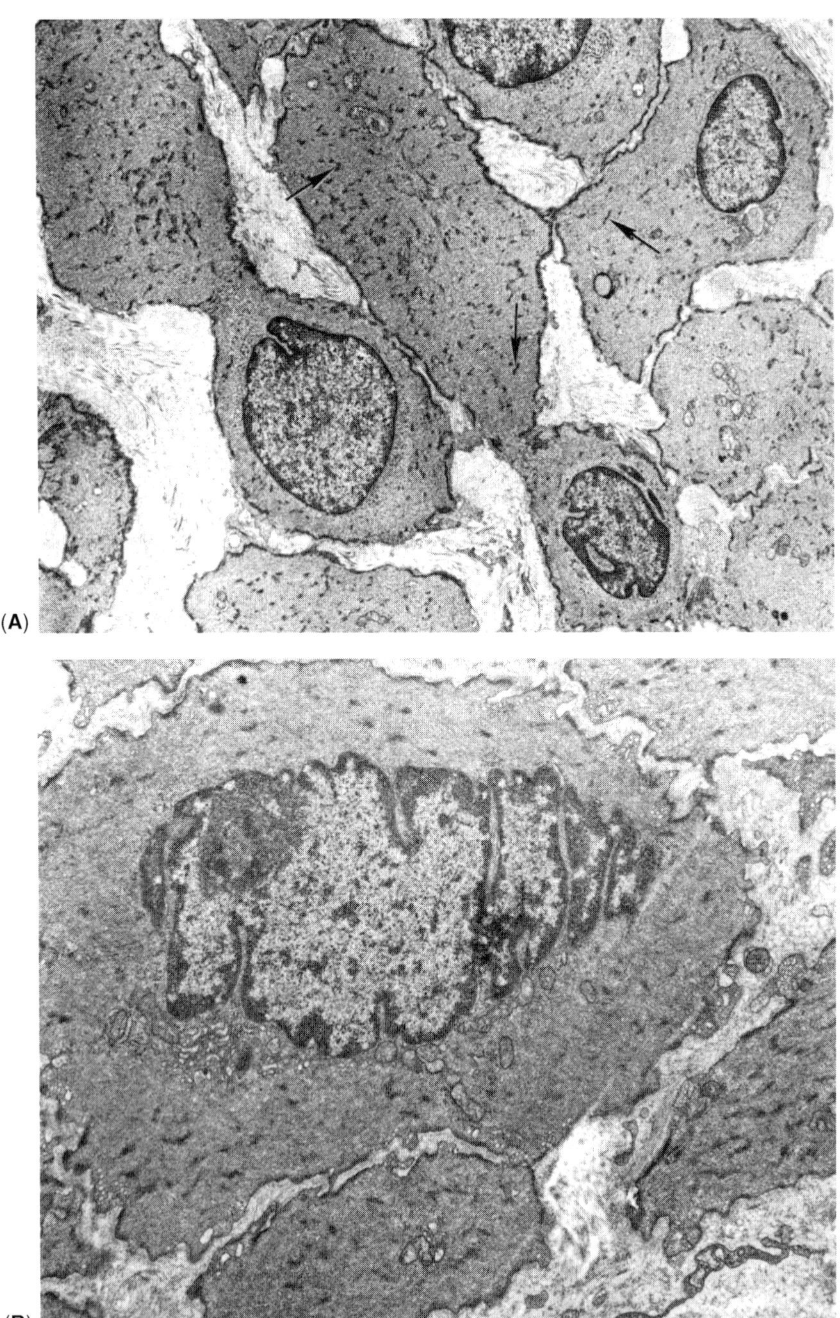

Figure 10 Leiomyoma. (**A**) Note the relatively uniform appearance of the cytoplasm of the smooth muscle cells caused by abundant, closely packed cytoplasmic filaments of myosin. Scatttered throughout the cytoplasm are ill defined densities (*arrows*), and these are particularly prominent on the inner surface of the cell membrane (× 4,000). (**B**) Higher magnification of smooth muscle cell (× 10,400). *Source*: Courtesy of Dr. G.K. Klintworth.

formation may be important to the development of leiomyoma (6). Leiomyomas also express receptors for FGF, which enhances collagen and glycosaminoglycan (GAG) synthesis, facilitating tumor–ECM interactions that may enhance tumor growth (268).

Leiomyosarcoma

Leiomyosarcoma is a malignant mesenchymal tumor with features of smooth muscle differentiation. It is rare in the periocular region, where it primarily involves the orbit, but it may also arise in the conjunctiva (265), iris, and ciliary body (183) and is a tumor of adults, with a peak incidence in the sixth decade of life, affecting women more than men. The main clinical presentations are proptosis, visual disturbance, diplopia, and mass effect developing over the course of weeks to months. Leiomyosarcoma can occur in younger patients with previous hereditary retinoblastoma, especially in those treated with external beam radiotherapy during the first year of life. The latency period between radiotherapy and the diagnosis of leiomyosarcoma varies from 12 to 50 years (77,80,166).

Leiomyosarcomas are generally classified in three main categories: deep soft tissue, cutaneous, and vascular. In the ocular region, the tumors are best categorized as deep soft tissue leiomyosarcomas and are thought to arise from smooth muscle precursors around vascular structures, mostly small veins (71). The histogenesis of leiomyosarcomas is based on light microscopic, ultrastructural, and immunohistochemical features. The tumor cells have features of smooth muscle cells with elongated profiles, abundant, deeply eosinophilic cytoplasm with fuchsinophilic myofibrils, and centrally located, blunt-ended nuclei. Ultrastructurally, leiomyosarcomas contain numerous 6 to 8 nm thin myofilaments, dense bodies, pinocytic vesicles, conspicuous intercellular junctions, and basal lamina (72). Immunohistochemical staining of filamentary proteins, smooth muscle-specific actin, muscle-specific actin, and desmin as well as the actin-binding protein, h-caldesmon, regularly occurs in these tumors and supports a smooth muscle progenitor cell of origin (8,99,248).

Histopathologically, the tumors are nonencapsulated. Well-differentiated leiomyosarcomas exhibit intersecting fascicles or bundles of spindle cells in palisades, eosinophilic fibrillar cytoplasm containing vacuoles, and elongated, cigar-shaped nuclei (47). Nuclei are hyperchromatic and pleomorphic and tumor giant cells may be present. The mitotic index is generally greater than 5 mitoses per 10 high-power microscopic fields, but orbital leiomyosarcomas with small numbers of mitoses have been reported (157,258). The tumors are highly cellular, but fibrosis or myxoid change may be present and hyalinized, hypocellular zones or areas of necrosis are frequent in larger leiomyosarcomas (66). Glycogen can be demonstrated by periodic acid Schiff stain in the cytoplasm. Differentiated cells have numerous myofibrils oriented along the long axis of the cell and react with these myofibrils are positive with the Masson trichrome or phosphotungstic acid–hematoxylin stains. In poorly differentiated cells, the longitudinal striations are less numerous and are disorganized with clumping of the myofilamentous material to give a clotted appearance. Immunoreactivity for filamentary proteins as noted earlier is present in the great majority of tumors. Ultrastructurally, the tumors have deeply clefted nuclei and the aforementioned features of smooth muscle cells, including cytoplasmic filaments with densities, cell junctions, pinocytic vesicles, and investing basement membrane. Poorly differentiated tumors show fewer myofilaments and more rough ER and free ribosomes (72). Cytogenetic analysis shows structural aberrations in less than 20% of tumors, affecting several chromosomes (207). Aberrations in the *RB1* retinoblastoma gene, consistent with loss of chromosome 13 material, and abnormalities in the genes and proteins in the Rb-cyclin D pathway have been reported (56,232). Correlations between the cytogenetic changes and age, sex, grade, depth, or size have not been made (153). Molecular studies of most tumors show overexpression and point mutations in *p53* and *MDM2* genes, which regulate cell proliferation and survival (21,56). Immunosuppression and infection with the human immunodeficiency virus (HIV) or with Epstein–Barr virus may predispose to tumor development (207). Accordingly, leiomyosarcoma has become the second leading malignancy in immunodeficient children.

A review of literature showed tumor recurrence in 4 of 7 cases (57%) between 5 and 36 months after resection and 3 of 7 cases (43%) died of metastasis after between 12 and 47 months (159).

SKELETAL MUSCLE TUMORS

Rhabdomyosarcoma

Rhabdomyosarcoma is the most common malignant orbital tumor of childhood and the most common soft tissue sarcoma of children (150). The most often involved sites are the genitourinary system (29%), parameninges (24%), limb extremities (15%), retroperitonum (13%), orbit (8%), and other parts of the head and neck (7%) (25). It may also involve the iris (170,270). The mean age of onset of primary and secondary orbital rhabdomyosarcomas is 7 and 12 years, respectively, with predilection for boys (107). Most tumors are sporadic, but a few arise in children with neurofibromatosis type I (MIM +162200), Li–Fraumeni syndrome (MIM #151653), Costello syndrome (MIM #218040), Noonan syndrome (MIM #163950), and miscellaneous congenital anomalies (33,92,120,145,201,226,238,271). Typical clinical manifestations for orbital rhabdomyosarcoma include progressive proptosis, ptosis, and a palpable mass with a history of onset of days to weeks (217,218). The tumor tends to arise superiorly and medially in the orbit. It may arise from the paranasal sinuses to invade the orbit secondarily and bone destruction is often evident on CT, and may arise from the paranasal sinuses to invade the orbit secondarily (12). Intracranial extension with bone destruction worsens the prognosis.

The histogenesis of rhabdomyosarcoma was initially established on the basis of histochemical stains and TEM studies. The Masson trichrome and phosphotungstic acid–hematoxylin stains were used to visualize cross striations due to arrays of actin and myosin filaments (myofibrils) in well-differentiated tumor cells, leading to the contention that these tumors originate from mesenchymal cells with skeletal muscle differentiation. Strongly supporting this proposed origin were ultrastructural studies that confirmed, with increasing differentiation, the presence of 6 to 8 nm actin myofilaments arranged in parallel bundles, 12 to 15 nm myosin filaments with attached ribosomes, and partially formed Z-bands (Figs. 11–15) (66). The advent of immunohistochemical staining provided further support for this histogenesis and supplanted TEM as the diagnostic method of choice. The tumors were found to exhibit positive immunoreactivity for the skeletal muscle-specific intermediate filament proteins, desmin and muscle-specific actin, as well as myoglobin, the oxygen transport protein of muscle. Later, positive immunostaining for nuclear MyoD and myogenin, two nuclear regulatory proteins, was found to be highly specific and sensitive for rhabdomyosarcoma, including those with poorly differentiated cells (37). Transfection of MyoD into multipotential mesodermal cells was found to stimulate myogeneic differentiation and skeletal muscle formation (252).

Rhabdomyosarcomas are highly cellular neoplasms exhibiting considerable pleomorphism and high mitotic activity and often have a high nucleocytoplasmic ratio. However, these tumors may be divided into four histopathologic subtypes, each associated with distinctive clinical, genetic, and prognostic features. Children are overwhelmingly affected by three subtypes of rhabdomyosarcoma: all of which may involve the ocular region (embryonal, alveolar, and spindle cell). Embryonal rhabdomyosarcoma is the most common type (123). It is composed of spindle or ovoid rhabdomyoblasts showing variable degrees of myogenic differentiation. The tumors vary in cellularity from scattered tumor cells in a loose, myxoid or collagenous stroma, to highly cellular tumors of densely arrayed cells with little stromal support (259). The botryoid variant of embryonal rhabdomyosarcoma generally involves the mucosa of the genitourinary tract and derives its name from the grossly visible grapelike protrusions that it forms (259). In the ocular region, botryoidal rhabdomyosarcoma affects the anterior orbit, eyelid, and conjunctiva (123,217,218,220). Microscopically, it contains a dense band of rhabdomyoblasts separated from the epithelium by a layer of loose, myxoid stroma as well as deeper stromal involvement in larger tumors. The alveolar subtype of rhabdomyosarcoma occurs in older children and tends to involve the inferior portion of the orbit (220). It is composed of large primitive round cells with hyperchromatic nuclei, coarse chromatin, and prominent nucleoli. These highly cellular tumors exhibit poorly cohesive cells in large collections that are separated by thin fibrous septae. The central cells frequently degenerates and becomes necrotic, leaving a single layer of well-preserved tumor cells adherent to the fibrovascular septae, the so-called alveolar pattern (20,81). The solid variant of the alveolar subtype is deemed to be present if central degeneration does not occur. Often present are tumor giant cells with multiple

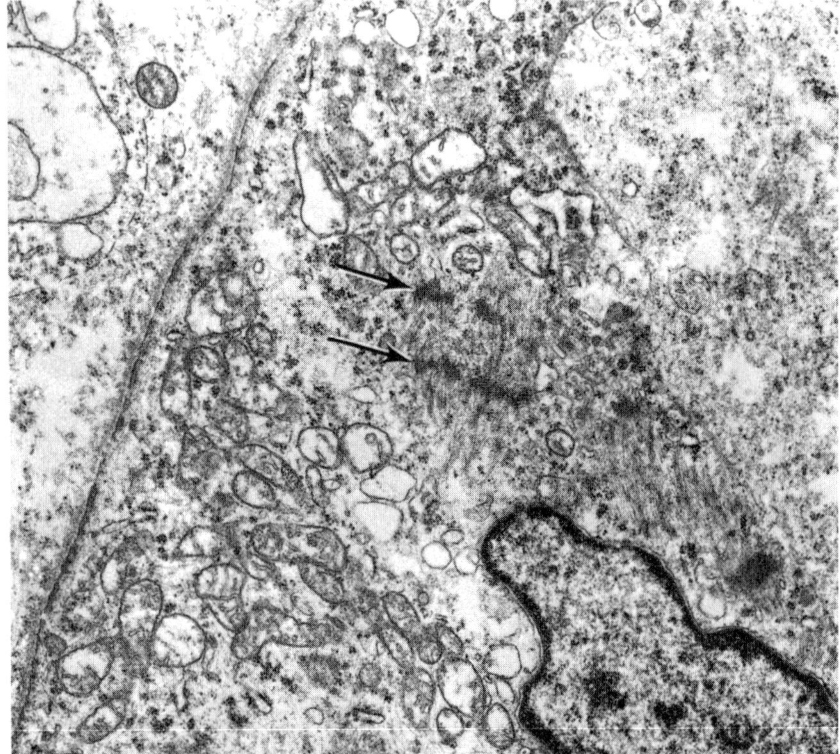

Figure 11 Rhabdomyosarcoma. The diagnosis of rhabdomyosarcoma can be established by transmission electron microscopy when the 15 nm thick cytoplasmic filaments of myosin have a parallel arrangement and are organized into sarcomere-like units with *Z* lines (*arrows*). The cells contain both thick (myosin) and thin (actin) filaments (× 12,900). *Source*: Courtesy of Dr. G.K. Klintworth.

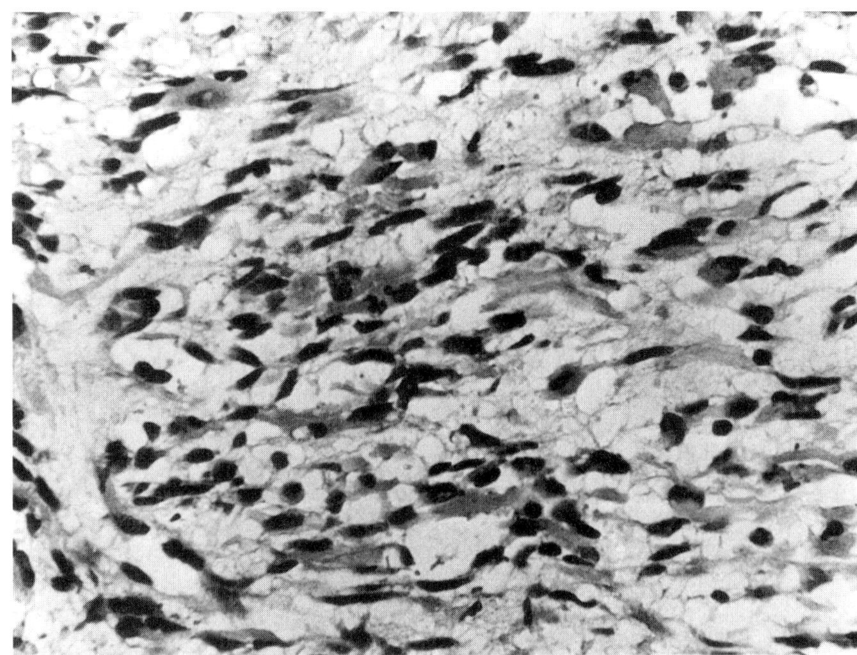

Figure 12 Rhabdomyosarcoma. Well-differentiated embryonal rhabdomyosarcoma of the orbit, showing numerous strap-shaped cells, the cytoplasm of which is deeply eosinophilic (hematoxylin and eosin, $\times$ 390). *Source*: Courtesy of Professor A. Garner.

peripheral nuclei and weakly eosinophilic cytoplasm that lacks cross striations, but contains rhabdomyoblastic elements. These giants cell are thought to develop by fusion of rhabdomyoblasts (20,81).

The spindle subtype of rhabdomyosarcoma is composed almost exclusively of elongated cells with eosinophilic, fibrillar cytoplasm, and tapered or blunt-ended nuclei containing prominent nucleoli (259). One variant of the spindle type contains prominent collagen fiber separating tumor cells; the other variant is more cellular with tumor cells arranged in fascicles or bundles. These cells may possess cross striations. The pleomorphic type of rhabdomyosarcoma almost exclusively affects adults whose average age is 56 years (83). A rarity in the ocular region, these tumors are composed of loosely

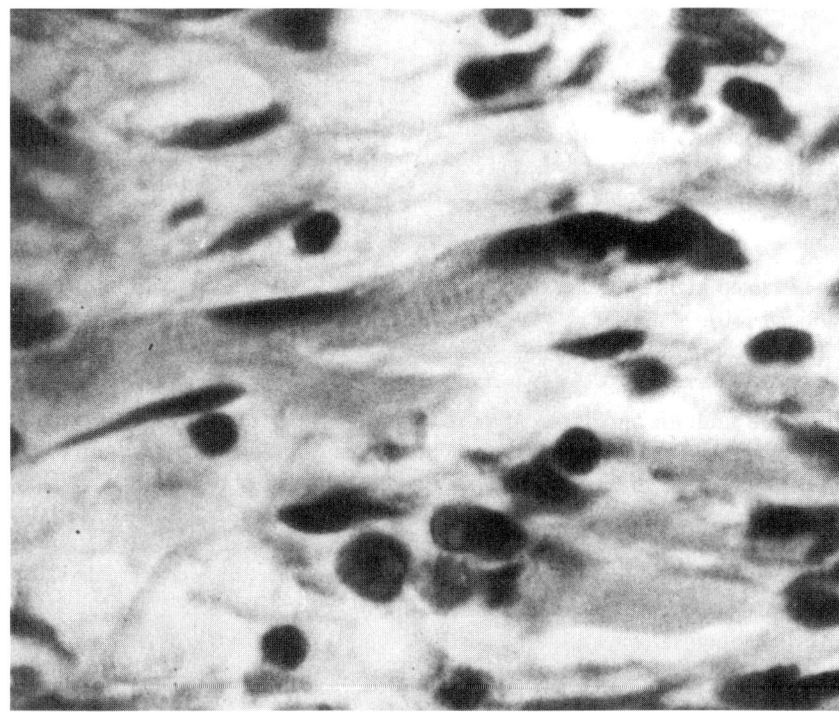

Figure 13 Embryonal rhabdomyosarcoma of the orbit. At higher magnification occasional strap-shaped cells exhibit readily recognized cross-striations (hematoxylin and eosin, $\times$ 1,050). *Source*: Courtesy of Professor A. Garner.

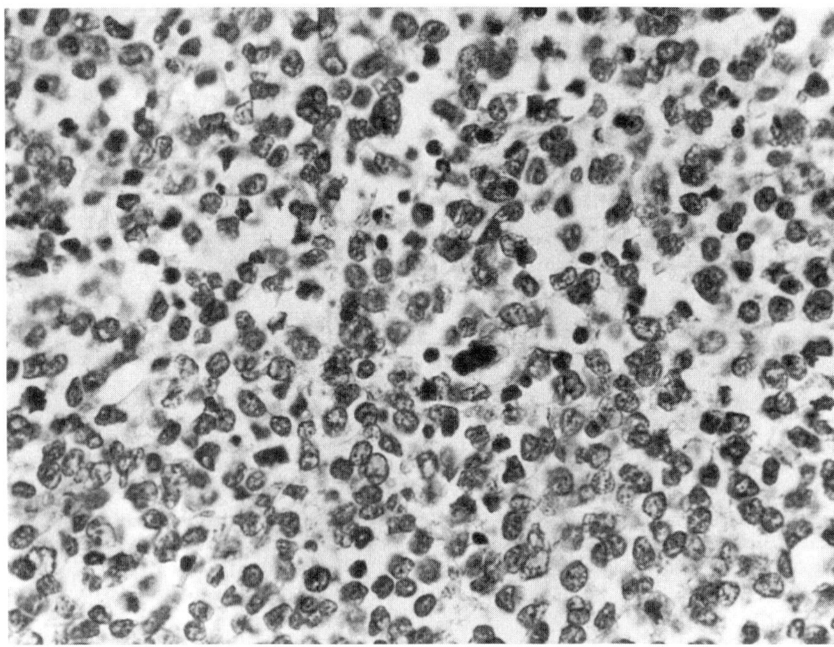

Figure 14 Undifferentiated rhabdomyosarcoma of the orbit. The cells have only scanty cytoplasm, and the nuclei are irregular and hyperchromatic (hematoxylin and eosin, ×390). *Source*: Courtesy of Professor A. Garner.

and haphazardly arranged undifferentiated and pleomorphic cells. The pleomorphic cells comprise variable proportions of rhabdomyoblasts with polygonal, spindle, tadpole, and racquet-like contours, all with eosinophilic cytoplasm and hyperchromatic nuclei (82). Special stains disclose that cross striations are present in more than one-half of embryonal variant, common in the spindle type, and rare in the alveolar and pleomorphic subtypes of rhabdomyosarcoma. Glycogen, stainable with the periodic acid Schiff stain is present in most tumors, regardless of subtype. In general, the presence of immunohistochemical markers correlates with the degree of myogenic differentiation. Only nonspecific vimentin immunoreactivity may be detected in poorly differentiated tumor cells. Reactivity for desmin and

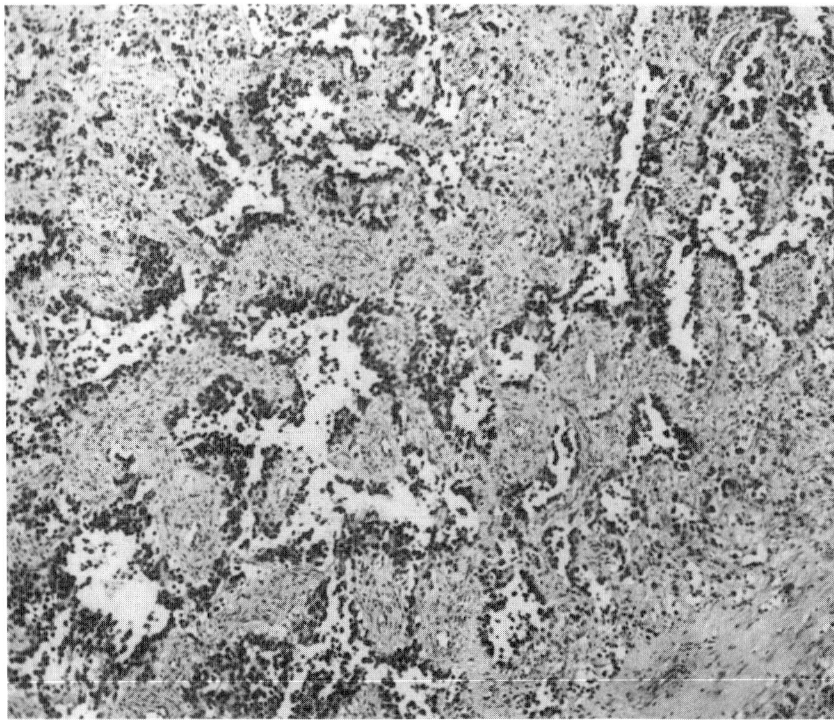

Figure 15 Alveolar rhabdomyosarcoma of the orbit. Interlacing bands of fibrous tissue are associated with irregular spaces lined by hyperchromatic tumor cells. Similar neoplasmic rhabdomyoblasts are shed into the "alveoli" (hematoxylin and eosin, ×70). *Source*: Courtesy of Professor A. Garner.

muscle-specific actin is found in developing rhabdomyoblasts and staining for myoglobin, myosin, and creatine kinase M are evident in well-differentiated cells (212). Immunostaining for desmin and muscle-specific actin are present in 95% to 100% of the rhabdomyosarcomas and a positive immunoreactivity is less often present for myogenin (91%), MyoD (91%), and myoglobin (28%) (267).

Recent studies suggest that rhabdomyoblasts forming tumors of the embryonal subtype demonstrate features of early myogenesis, whereas tumor cells of the alveolar subtype show more advanced myogenic differentiation (62). Molecular genetic studies of embryonal rhabdomyosarcoma characteristically show loss of heterozygosity at a region of chromosome 11 (11p15) harboring the insulin-like growth factor 2 (ILGF2), H19, p57 oncogenes, with loss of maternal chromosomal material (162). More than 80% of alveolar rhabdomyosarcomas have unique chromosomal translocations, [(2;13)(q35;q14) or (1;13)(p36;q14)], resulting in the formation of two chimeric *PAX3-FKHR* and *PAX7-FHKR* genes, respectively. These aberrant fusion products are very rare in embryonal rhabdomyosarcoma (10,178). Each fusion product is a hybrid that contains one *PAX* DNA-binding domain and one *FKHR* transcription domain that render them more potent than the separate wild-type proteins, partly because they are also insensitive to inhibitory effects (109). Moreover, they are expressed at high levels because they are transcript at a high rate due to the presence of fusion products in a positive feedback loop. These molecular aberrations contribute to the malignant behavior of the alveolar subtype by promoting cellular growth, apoptosis, and differentiation (10,234). Expression of the PAX-FKHR product stimulates genes associated with myogenic differentiation, including the induction of MyoD and myogenin that may be stained immunohistochemically (127,128). MyoD binds to DNA and controls transcription of genes involved in rhabdomyoblast differentiation and proliferation (212). In rhabdomyosarcoma, MyoD loses its ability to cause cell cycle arrest even though it retains its ability to bind DNA and promote muscle differentiation (191,241). In addition, MyoD expression may be down regulated by a number of factors, including stimulation of growth factor receptors and oncogene products associated with other malignancies, such as retinoblastoma (111,152,162,191).

Based on results of the Intergroup Rhabdomyosarcoma Study (45,135), primary orbital rhabdomyosarcomas demonstrate almost 100% survival with current therapy involving surgical bulking and combination of chemotherapy and external beam radiotherapy compared to all rhabdomyosarcomas where survival was 84% at 5 years. Embryonal subtype also compares favorably with the alveolar subtype, with 87% and 71% 5-year survivals, respectively.

TUMORS OF UNCERTAIN HISTOGENESIS

Myxoma

Myxoma is a benign soft tissue tumor that usually affects subcutaneous tissue and deep skeletal muscles (3). Involvement of the ocular region by myxoma is uncommon, but this neoplasm has been reported in the conjunctiva, eyelid, orbit, or cornea have been reported, principally in middle-aged adults without gender predilection (125,126,148,184). In the conjunctiva, it appears as a well-circumscribed, yellow–pink, translucent, cystic and/or solid mass (61). Rare in the orbit, the presenting symptom is proptosis (146). It shows an infiltrative, well-circumscribed, enhancing soft tissue mass on CT (146). It can be a solitary lesion or a component of Carney complex (MIM #160980), Mazabraud syndrome (intramuscular myxoma with fibrous dysplasia), and McCune–Albright syndrome (MIM #174800) (125,126).

Histogenetically, Stout (233) regarded myxoma as a tumor of primitive mesenchyme. Since then, proposed cells of origin include vascular endothelium, neural crest cells of the nerve sheath, dendritic cells, and fibroblasts, or their precursors (74,143). Whatever their origin, the tumor cells appear to be modified mesenchymal cells that produce excessive amounts of GAGs rich in hyaluronic acid, but little collagen (3). Most ultrastructural studies show predominantly fibroblast or myofibroblast-like tumor cells with dilated rough ER, Golgi complexes, pinocytic vesicles and intracytoplasmic microfilaments with focal densities (100,233).

Myxomas of soft tissue are generally classified in 5 major categories: intramuscular, cutaneous (superficial angiomyxoma), juxta-articular, nerve sheath (neurothekeoma), and aggressive angiomyxoma (263). However, these categories have not been applied to myxomas involving the ocular region. Myxomas are non-encapsulated, hypocellular, and hypovascular with a mucoid ECM that is intensely basophilic upon hematoxylin and eosin staining. The main histologic components are sparse spindle- and stellate-shaped stromal cells, fine fibrillary reticulin fibers, and interstitial mucin and variable numbers of fibrous strands or trabeculae. Scattered mast cells and occasional macrophages are present. The abundant mucoid material stains positive with alcian blue, mucicarmine, and the Hale colloidal iron method that is reduced by hyaluronidase treatment of tissue sections prior to staining (130). The ultrastuctural features mentioned above and immunohistochemical positivity for vimentin, but not S100 protein, is consistent with the diagnosis (100). Rare cells may stain for smooth muscle-specific actin. Genetic studies of myxomas are extremely limited (159,174).

Alveolar Soft Part Sarcoma

Alveolar soft part sarcoma is a rare tumor of uncertain differentiation (147). It affects young adults and adolescents between 15 to 35 years of age with a 4:1 female-to-male ratio (79,124,144). The usual presenting findings are proptosis, edema, and conjunctival hyperemia due a slowly growing, painless mass that is soft and friable at surgery (79,124). CT or MRI shows a poorly circumscribed intraconal or extraconal mass with diffuse contrast enhancement and curvilinear flow voids similar to benign hemangioma (39).

The histogenesis of alveolar soft part sarcoma is uncertain. Several immunohistochemical studies have suggested a myogenic origin, based on the expression of MyoD1 protein and filamentary proteins, namely desmin and muscle-specific actin (211). However, other immunohistochemical studies failed to confirm these findings (197). A neural crest cell origin has been suggested based on S100 protein and neuron-specific enolase immunoreactivity in 25% of cases as well as ultrastructural findings of Schwann cell differentiation including well defined myelin sheaths, myelinated axons, and aggregated fine filamentous structures, termed angulated bodies (88,177).

Histopathologically, the tumor is poorly circumscribed, highly vascular neoplasm. It receives its name from its pseudoalveolar histological appearance, characterized by nests of noncohesive, polygonal cells arranged in clusters separated by delicate septae containing sinusoidal vascular channels lined by flattened endothelium (264). Especially in children, the tumor sometimes grows as diffuse sheets of cells without an apparent nesting pattern. The tumor cells are large, round or polygonal, with little pleomorphism, and contain abundant eosinophilic, finely granular cytoplasm with sharply defined borders conferring a distinctly epithelioid appearance. They contain one or two vesicular nuclei with prominent nucleoli. Mitotic figures are scarce, there is little pleomorphism, and nuclear atypia is uncommon. Intracytoplasmic rhomboid- or rod-shaped crystalline inclusions, sometimes faintly visible on hematoxylin and eosin staining, are well demonstrated with the periodic acid Schiff staining that is resistant to diastase digestion. Immunoreactivity for MyoD1 is common, with fewer cases staining positively for desmin and a minority for S100 and neuron-specific enolase (178,246). Ultrastructurally, cell membranes of adjacent cells are joined by a few poorly developed junctions; and the cytoplasm contains numerous mitochondria, abundant rough ER, and a prominent Golgi complex. Characteristic is the presence of membrane-bound or free electron-dense polygonal crystals with a periodicity of 10 nm (147,177,223). A recent study showed these crystals contain monocarboxylate transporter 1 and its chaperone CD147, which regulate lactate and metalloproteinases (142). Cytogenetic studies often reveal a nonreciprocal chromosomal translocation [der(17)t(X;17)(p11;q25)] that results in the formation of the *ASPL-TFE3* fusion gene (109). Occurring during the G2 phase of the cell cycle the translocation results in a fusion protein product. The later localizes to the nucleus and function as an aberrant transcription factor causing transcription deregulation in tumorigenesis (141). The availability in females of two X-chromosomes capable of providing material for translocation to chromosome 17 where it is not subject to X inactivation, appears to impart gender proclivity to this tumor (27).

Metastatic disease and death may occur many years after resection with 20-year survival of only 15% (147).

Extraskeletal Mesenchymal Chondrosarcoma

Extraskeletal mesenchymal chondrosarcoma is a tumor of cartilaginous differentiation (93,112,169). Orbital involvement, responsible for about 10% of cases, is most common in women averaging 25 years of age with an age range of 10 to 38 years (242). The main presenting clinical manifestations are proptosis, decreased vision, pain, swelling, tearing, and a palpable mass. CT shows a well-defined mass, multiple areas of fine and coarse calcification, and moderate contrast enhancement of this highly vascular tumor (222). The history of onset of reported cases is highly variable, ranging from days to over one year.

The histogenesis of extraskeletal mesenchymal chondrosarcoma has been established by the invariable histopathologic presence of islands of well-differentiated cartilaginous tissue in the tumors (204). Because of the presence of this cartilaginous tissue, this tumor has been considered a variant of chondrosarcoma. However, immunoreactivity for the *MIC2* gene product (CD99) and a chromosomal translocation [t(11;22)(q24;q12)] in the primitive cells of this tumor, both typical of extraskeletal Ewing sarcomas and primitive neuroectodermal tumors, have raised the possibility of a common progenitor cell for these tumors (91).

Histopathologically, extraskeletal mesenchymal chondrosarcomas have a bimorphic pattern composed of sheets of undifferentiated, primitive round, oval, or spindle-shaped mesenchymal cells and small, discrete islands of well differentiated, benign-appearing cartilaginous tissue, which may show calcification or ossification (204). The undifferentiated cells are arranged in small aggregates around sinusoidal vascular channels lined by a single layer of endothelium, imparting a hemangiopericytoma-like pattern. These cells contain ovoid or elongated, hyperchromatic nuclei and scanty, poorly outlined cytoplasm. Immunohistochemically, the cartilaginous areas are strongly S100-positive and show weak positivity for desmin. Undifferentiated regions are positive for CD99, neuron-specific enolase, and CD57, a molecule involved in cell–cell and cell–ECM adhesion (108). Ultrastructurally, well-differentiated cells are irregularly round, stellate, or scalloped with large ovoid nuclei, short cytoplasmic processes, abundant rough ER with focal sac-like dilatations, well-developed Golgi apparatus, and variable amounts of glycogen (156). Undifferentiated tumor cells have large nuclei, prominent nucleoli, and inconspicuous cytoplasm with few organelles.

Overall, the 10-year survival is poor at 25% to 30%, but orbital cases may have a better prognosis, presumably due to their relatively smaller size at the time of diagnosis (158,242).

EXCEPTIONAL SOFT CONNECTIVE TISSUE TUMORS

Ocular presentations of some soft connective tissue neoplasms are exceedingly rare and subjects of individual case reports and small case series. Benign tumors of this nature include: glomus tumor (38,119), infantile myofibromatosis (64,229), giant cell angiofibroma (54,94,104), desmoid fibromatosis (86,151,210), juvenile fibromatosis (32), elastofibroma (7,110), giant cell fibroblastoma (35), and rhabdomyoma (103, 133,168). Malignant entities include: synovial sarcoma (192,224), epithelioid sarcoma (266), desmoplastic small round cell tumor (274), malignant extrarenal rhabdoid tumor (90,96,196,231), malignant mesenchymoma and ectomesenchymoma (19,23,155,181,245), and congenital undifferentiated sarcoma (89).

REFERENCES

1. Alexandrakis G, Johnson TE. Recurrent orbital solitary fibrous tumor in a 14-year-old girl. Am J Ophthalmol 2000; 130:373–6.
2. Allen PW. Nodular fasciitis. Pathology 1972; 4:9–26.
3. Allen PW. Myxoma is not a single entity: a review of the concept of myxoma. Ann Diagn Pathol 2000; 4:99–123.
4. Alvord EC Jr., Lofton S. Gliomas of the optic nerve or chiasm: outcome by patient's age, tumor site, and treatment. J Neurosurg 1988; 68:85–98.
5. Antonescu CR, Erlandson RA, Huvos AG. Primary fibrosarcoma and malignant fibrous histiocytoma of bone-a comparative ultrastructural study: evidence of a spectrum of fibroblastic differentiation. Ultrastruct Pathol 2000; 24:83–91.
6. Arslan AA, Gold LI, Mittal K, et al. Gene expression studies provide clues to the pathogenesis of uterine leiomyoma: new evidence and a systematic review. Hum Reprod 2005; 20:852–63.
7. Austin P, Jakobiec FA, Iwamoto T, et al. Elastofibroma oculi. Arch Ophthalmol 1983; 101:1575–9.
8. Azumi N, Ben-Ezra J, Battifora H. Immunophenotypic diagnosis of leiomyosarcomas and rhabdomyosarcomas with monoclonal antibodies to muscle-specific actin and desmin in formalin-fixed tissue. Mod Pathol 1988; 1:469–74.
9. Baird K, Davis S, Antonescu CR, et al. Gene expression profiling of human sarcomas: insights into sarcoma biology. Cancer Res 2005; 65:9226–35.
10. Barr FG. Gene fusions involving PAX and FOX family members in alveolar rhabdomyosarcoma. Oncogene 2001; 20:5736–46.
11. Bastin KT, Mehta MP. Meningeal hemangiopericytoma: defining role for radiation therapy. J Neurooncol 1992; 14: 277–87.
12. Benedict WF, Fung YK, Murphree AL. The gene responsible for the development of retinoblastoma and osteosarcoma. Cancer 1988; 8:1691–4.
13. Bennett JH, Shousha S, Puddle B, et al. Immunohistochemical identification of tumours of adipocytic differentiation using an antibody to a P2 protein. J Clin Pathol 1995; 48:950–4.
14. Bernardini FP, de Conciliis C, Schneider S, et al. Solitary fibrous tumor of the orbit: is it rare? Report of a case series and review of the literature. Ophthalmology 2003; 110:1442–8.
15. Berner JM, Meza-Zepeda LA, Kools PF, et al. HMGIC, the gene for an architectural transcription factor, is amplified and rearranged in a subset of human sarcomas. Oncogene 1997; 14:2935–41.
16. Bernstein KE, Lattes R. Nodular (pseudosarcomatous) fasciitis, a non recurrent lesion: clinicopathologic study of 134 cases. Cancer 1982; 49:1668–78.
17. Birdsall SH, Shipley JM, Summersgill BM, et al. Cytogenetic findings in a case of nodular fasciitis of the breast. Cancer Genet Cytogenet 1995; 81:166–8.
18. Biswas J, Kumar SK, Gopal L, et al. Leiomyoma of the ciliary body extending to the anterior chamber: clinicopathologic and ultrasound biomicroscopic correlation. Surv Ophthalmol 2000; 44:336–42.
19. Bittinger A, Rossberg C, Rodehuser M. Primary malignant ectomesenchymoma of the orbit. Gen Diagn Pathol 1997; 142:221–5.
20. Blodi FC. Pathology of orbital bones. Am J Ophthalmol 1976; 81:1–26.
21. Blom R, Guerrieri C, Stal O, et al. Leiomyosarcoma of the uterus: a clinicopathologic, DNA flow cytometric, p53 and mdm-2 analysis of 49 cases. Gynecol Oncol 1998; 68: 54–61.
22. Bourgeois JM, Knezevich SR, Mathers JA, et al. Molecular detection of the ETV6–NTRK3 gene fusion differentiates congenital fibrosarcoma from other childhood spindle cell tumors. Am J Surg Pathol 2000; 24:937–46.
23. Brannan PA, Schneider S, Grossniklaus HE, et al. Malignant mesenchymoma of the orbit: case report and review of the literature. Ophthalmology 2003; 110:314–7.
24. Brannan SO, Cheung D, Trotter S, et al. A conjunctival leiomyoma. Am J Ophthalmol 2003; 136:749–50.
25. Breitfeld PP, Meyer WH. Rhabdomyosarcoma: New windows of opportunity. Oncologist 2005; 10:518–27.
26. Brown HH, Brodsky MC, Hembree K, Mrak RE. Supraciliary hemangiopericytoma. Ophthalmology 1991; 98:378–9.
27. Bu X, Bernstein L. A proposed explanation for female predominance in alveolar soft part sarcoma. Nonincativation of X; Autosome translocation fusion gene. Cancer 2005; 103:1245–53.

28. Buchanan TA, Hoyt WF. Optic nerve glioma and neovascular glaucoma: report of a case. Br J Ophthalmol 1982; 66:96–8.
29. Cai YC, McMenamin ME, Rose G, et al. Primary liposarcoma of the orbit: a clinicopathologic study of seven cases. Ann Diagn Pathol 2001; 5:255–66.
30. Calonje E, Fletcher CDM. Cutaneous fibrohistiocytic tumors: an update. Adv Anat Pathol 1994; 1:2–15.
31. Calonje E. Is cutaneous benign fibrous histiocytoma (dermatofibroma) a reactive inflammatory process or a neoplasm? Histopathol 2000; 37:278–80.
32. Campbell RJ, Garrity JA. Juvenile fibromatosis of the orbit: a case report with review of the literature. Br J Ophthalmol 1991; 75:313–6.
33. Carnevale A, Lieberman E, Cardenas R. Li-Fraumeni syndrome in pediatric patients with soft tissue sarcoma or osteosarcoma. Arch Med Res 1997; 28:383–6.
34. Carrera M, Prat J, Quintana M. Malignant solitary fibrous tumour of the orbit: report of a case with 8 years follow-up. Eye 2001; 15:102–4.
35. Carroll G, Haik BG, Karcioglu ZA. Orbital giant cell fibroblastoma. Orbit 1999; 18:25–32.
36. Cerio R, Griffiths CE, Cooper KD, et al. Characterization of factor XIIIa positive dermal dendritic cells in normal and inflamed skin. Br J Dermatol 1989; 121: 421–31.
37. Cessna MH, Zhou H, Perkins SL, et al. Are myogenin and myoD1 expression specific for rhabdomyosarcoma? A study of 150 cases, with emphasis on spindle cell mimics. Am J Surg Pathol 2001; 25:1150–7.
38. Charles NC. Multiple glomus tumors of the face and eyelid. Arch Ophthalmol 1976; 94:1283–5.
39. Chu WC, Howard RG, Roebuck DJ, et al. Periorbital alveolar soft part sarcoma with radiologic features mimicking haemangioma. Med Pediatr Oncol 2003; 41: 145–6.
40. Coffin CM, Fletcher JA. Infantile fibrosarcoma. In: Fletcher CDM, Unni KK, Mertens F, eds. Tumors of Soft Tissue and Bone. Pathology and Genetics. Lyon, France: IARC Press, 2002:98–100.
41. Coffin CM, Jaszcz W, O'Shea PA, et al. So-called congenital-infantile fibrosarcoma: does it exist and what is it? Pediatr Pathol 1994; 14:133–50.
42. Cohen PR, Rapini RP, Farhood AI. Expression of the human hematopoietic progenitor cell antigen CD34 in vascular and spindle cell tumors. J Cutan Pathol 1993; 20: 15–20.
43. Conway RM, Holbach LM, Naumann GO, et al. Benign fibrous histiocytoma of the corneoscleral limbus: unique clinicopathologic features. Arch Ophthalmol 2003; 121: 1776–9.
44. Craven JP, Quigley TM, Bolen JW, et al. Current management and clinical outcome of hemangiopericytoma. Am J Surg 1992; 162:490–3.
45. Crist WM, Anderson JR, Meza JL, et al. Intergroup rhabdomyosarcoma study-IV: results for patients with nonmetastatic disease. J Clin Oncol 2001; 19: 3091–102.
46. Croxatto JO, Font RL. Hemangiopericytoma of the orbit: a clinicopathologic study of 30 cases. Hum Pathol 1982; 13: 210–8.
47. Czerniak B. Pathologic and molecular aspects of soft tissue sarcomas. Surg Oncol Clin N Am 2003; 12:263–303.
48. d'Amore ESG, Manivel JC, Sung JH. Soft tissue and meningeal hemangiopericytomas: an immunohistochemical and ultrastructural study. Hum Pathol 1990; 21: 414–23.
49. Dal Cin P, Kools P, Sciot R, et al. Cytogenetic and fluorescence in situ hybridization investigation of ring chromosomes characterizing a specific pathologic subgroup of adipose tissue tumors. Cancer Genet Cytogenet 1993; 68:85–90.
50. Dal Cin P, Sciot R, Panagopoulos I, et al. Additional evidence of a variant translocation t(12;22) with EWS/CHOP fusion in myxoid liposarcoma: clinicopathological features. J Pathol 1997; 182:437–41.
51. Daniel CS, Beaconsfield M, Rose GE, et al. Pleomorphic lipoma of the orbit: a case series and review of literature. Ophthalmology 2003; 110:101–5.
52. Daniels CS, Clark BJ, Tuft SJ. Corneoscleral fibrous histiocytoma. Br J Ophthalmol 2002; 86:477–8.
53. Dardick I, Hammar SP, Scheithauer BW. Ultrastructural spectrum of hemangiopericytoma: a comparative study of fetal, adult, and neoplastic pericytes. Ultrastruct Pathol 1989; 13:111–54.
54. Dei Tos AP, Seregard S, Calonje E, et al. Giant cell angiofibroma. A distinctive orbital tumor in adults. Am J Surg Pathol 1995; 19:1286–93.
55. Dei Tos AP, Wadden C, Fletcher CD. S-100 protein staining in liposarcoma. Its diagnostic utility in the high grade myxoid (round cell) variant. Appl Immunohistochem 1996; 4:95–101.
56. Dei Tos AP, Doglioni C, Piccinin S, et al. Molecular abnormalities of the p53 pathway in dedifferentiated liposarcoma. J Pathol 1997; 181:8–13.
57. Dei Tos AP. Liposarcoma: New entities and evolving concepts. Ann Diag Pathol 2000; 4:252–66.
58. Dei Tos AP, Maestro R, Doglioni C, et al. Tumor suppressor genes and related molecules in leiomyosarcoma. J Pathol 2006; 148:1037–45.
59. de Leval L, Defraigne JO, Hermans G, et al. Malignant solitary fibrous tumor of the pleura: report of a case with cytogenetic analysis. Virchows Arch 2003; 442:388–92.
60. Demirci H, Shields CL, Shields JA, et al. Orbital tumors in the older adult population. Ophthalmology 2002; 109: 243–8.
61. Demirci H, Shields CL, Eagle RC Jr, et al. Report of a conjunctival myxoma case and review of the literature. Arch Ophthalmol 2006; 124:735–8.
62. Dias P, Chen B, Dilday B, et al. Strong immunostaining for myogenin in rhabdomyosarcoma is significantly associated with tumors of the alveolar subclass. Am J Pathol 2000; 156:399–408.
63. Donner LR, Silva T, Dobin SM. Clonal rearrangement of 15p11.2, 16p11.2, and 16p13.3 in a case of nodular fasciitis additional evidence favoring nodular fasciitis as a benign neoplasm and not a reactive tumefaction. Cancer Genet Cytogenet 2002; 139:138–40.
64. Duffy MT, Harris M, Hornblass A. Infantile myofibromatosis of orbital bone. A case report with computed tomography, magnetic resonance imaging, and histologic findings. Ophthalmology 1997; 104:1471–4.
65. el-Jabbour JN, Wilson GD, Bennett MH, et al. Flow cytometric study of nodular fasciitis, proliferative fasciitis, and proliferative myositis. Hum Pathol 1991; 22: 1146–9.
66. Erlandson RA. The ultrastructural distinction between rhabdomyosarcoma and other undifferentiated "sarcomas". Ultastruct Pathol 1987; 11:83–101.
67. Erlandson RA, Antonescu CR. The rise and fall of malignant fibrous histiocytoma. Ultrastructural Pathol 2004; 28:283–9.
68. Evans H, Bridge JA. Nodular fasciitis. In: Fletcher CDM, Unni KK, Mertens F, eds. Tumors of Soft Tissue and Bone.

Pathology and Genetics. Lyon, France: IARC Press, 2002: 48–9.
69. Evans HL. Liposarcoma: a study of 55 cases with a reassessment of its classification. Am J Surg Pathol 1979; 3:507–23.
70. Evans HL. Liposarcomas and atypical lipomatous tumors: a study of 66 cases followed for a minimum of 10 years. Surg Pathol 1988; 1:41.
71. Farshid G, Pradhan M, Goldblum J, et al. Leiomyosarcoma of somatic soft tissues: a tumor of vascular origin with multivariate analysis of outcome in 42 cases. Am J Surg Pathol 2002; 26:14–24.
72. Ferenczy A, Richart RM, Okagaki TA. A comparative ultrastructural study of leiomyosarcoma, cellular leiomyoma, and leiomyoma of the uterus. Cancer 1971; 28: 1004–18.
73. Ferry AP, Sherman SE. Nodular fasciitis of the conjunctiva apparently originating in the fascia bulbi (Tenon's capsule). Am. J. Ophthalmol 1974; 78:516–7.
74. Fetsch JF, Laskin WB, Miettinen M. Nerve sheath myxoma: a clinicopathologic and immunohistochemical analysis of 57 morphologically distinctive, S-100 protein- and GFAP-positive, myxoid peripheral nerve sheath tumors with a predilection for the extremities and a high local recurrence rate. Am J Surg Pathol 2005; 29: 1615–24.
75. Fisher C. Fibromatosis and fibrosarcoma in infancy and childhood. Eur J Cancer 1996; 32A:2094–100.
76. Fletcher CD, Akerman M, Dal Cin P, et al. Correlation between clinicopathological features and karyotype in lipomatous tumors. A report of 178 cases from the Chromosomes and Morphology (CHAMP) Collaborative Study Group. Am J Pathol 1996; 148:623–30.
77. Folberg R, Cleasby G, Flanagan JA, et al. Orbital leiomyosarcoma after radiation therapy for bilateral retinoblastoma. Arch Ophthalmol 1983; 101:1562–5.
78. Font RL, Hidayat AA. Fibrous histiocytoma of the orbit. Hum Pathol 1982; 13:199–209.
79. Font RL, Jurco S III, Zimmerman LE. Alveolar soft-part sarcoma of the orbit: a clinicopathologic analysis of seventeen cases and a review of the literature. Hum Pathol 1982; 13:569–79.
80. Font RL, Jurco S 3rd, Brechner RJ. Postradiation leiomyosarcoma of the orbit complicating bilateral retinoblastoma. Arch Ophthalmol 1983; 101:1557–61.
81. Fu YS, Perzin KH. Non-epithelial tumors of the nasal cavity, paranasal sinuses, and nasopharynx. A clinicopathologic study. II. Osseous and fibro-osseous lesions, including osteoma, fibrous dysplasia, ossifying fibroma, osteoblastoma, giant cell tumors, and osteosarcoma. Cancer 1974; 3:1289–305.
82. Furlong MA, Mentzel T, Fanburg-Smith JC. Pleomorphic rhabdomyosarcoma in adults: a clinicopathologic study of 38 cases with emphasis on morphologic variants and recent skeletal muscle-specific markers. Mod Pathol 2001; 14:595–603.
83. Gaffney EF, Dervan PA, Fletcher CDM. Pleomorphic rhabdomyosarcoma in adulthood: analysis of 11 cases with definition of diagnostic criteria. Am J Surg Pathol 1993; 17:601–9.
84. Gengle, C, Guillou L. Solitary fibrous tumor and haemangiopericytoma: evolution of a concept. Histopathol 2006; 48:63–74.
85. Gigantelli JW, Kincaid MC, Soparkar CN, et al. Orbital solitary fibrous tumor: radiographic and histopathologic correlations. Ophthal Plast Reconstr Surg 2001; 17:207–14.
86. Gnepp DR, Henley J, Weiss S, et al. Desmoid fibromatosis of the sinonasal tract and nasopharynx. A clinicopathologic study of 25 cases. Cancer 1996; 78:2572–9.
87. Goldsmith JD, van de Rijn M, Syed N. Orbital hemangiopericytoma and solitary fibrous tumor: a morphologic continuum. Int J Surg Pathol 2001; 9:295–302.
88. Gomez JA, Amin MB, Ro JY, et al. Immunohistochemical profile of myogenin and MyoD1 does not support skeletal muscle lineage in alveolar soft part sarcoma. A study of 19 tumors. Arch Pathol Lab Med 1999; 123:503–7.
89. Gormley PD, Thompson J, Aylward GW, et al. Congenital undifferentiated sarcoma of the orbit. J Pediatr Ophthalmol Strabismus 1994; 31:59–61.
90. Gottlieb C, Nijhawan N, Chorneyko K, et al. Congenital orbital and disseminated extrarenal malignant rhabdoid tumor. Ophthal Plast Reconstr Surg 2005; 21:76–9.
91. Granter SR, Renshaw AA, Fletcher CD, et al. CD99 reactivity in mesenchymal chonrosarcoma. Hum Pathol 1996; 27:1273–6.
92. Gripp KW, Scott CI Jr, Nicholson L, et al. Five additional Costello syndrome patients with rhabdomyosarcoma: proposal for a tumor screening protocol. Am J Med Genet 2002; 108:80–7.
93. Guccion JG, Font RL, Enzinger FM, et al. Extraskeletal mesenchymal chondrosarcoma. Arch Pathol 1973; 95: 336–40.
94. Guillou L, Gebhard S, Coindre JM. Orbital and extraorbital giant cell angiofibroma: a giant cell-rich variant of solitary fibrous tumor? Clinicopathologic and immunohistochemical analysis of a series in favor of a unifying concept. Am J Surg Pathol 2000; 24:971–9.
95. Guillou L, Fletcher JA, Fletcher CDM, et al. Extrapleural solitary fibrous tumor and hemangiopericytoma. In: Fletcher CDM, Unni KK, Mertens F, eds. Tumors of Soft Tissue and Bone. Pathology and Genetics. Lyon, France: IARC Press, 2002:86–90.
96. Gunduz K, Shields JA, Eagle RC Jr, et al. Malignant rhabdoid tumor of the orbit. Arch Ophthalmol 1998; 116: 243–6.
97. Harman JW, O'Hegarty MT, Byrnes CK. The ultrastructure of human smooth muscle. I. Studies of cell surface and connections in normal and achalasia esophageal smooth muscle. Exp Mod Pathol 1962; 1:204–8.
98. Hasegawa T, Matsuno Y, Shimoda T, et al. Extrathoracic solitary fibrous solitary tumors: their histological variability and potentially aggressive behavior. Hum Pathol 1999; 130:1464–73.
99. Hasegawa T, Hasegawa F, Hirose T, et al. Expression of smooth muscle markers in so called malignant fibrous histiocytomas. J Clin Pathol 2003; 56:666–71.
100. Hashimoto H, Tsuneyoshi M, Daimaru Y, et al. Intramuscular myxoma. A clinicopathologic, immunohistochemical, and electron microscopic study. Cancer 1986; 58:740–7.
101. Hashimoto H, Quade B. Leiomyoma of deep soft tissue In: Fletcher CDM, Unni KK, Mertens F, eds. Tumors of Soft Tissue and Bone. Pathology and Genetics. Lyon, France: IARC Press 2002:130.
102. Hatano H, Tokunaga K, Ogose A, et al. Origin of histiocyte-like cells and multinucleated giant cells in malignant fibrous histiocytoma: neoplastic or reactive? Pathol Int 1999; 49:14–22.
103. Hatsukawa Y, Furukawa A, Kawamura H, et al. Rhabdomyoma of the orbit in a child. Am J Ophthalmol 123:142–4, 1997.
104. Hayashi N, Borodic G, Karesh JW, et al. Giant cell angiofibroma of the orbit and eyelid. Ophthalmology 1999; 106:1223–9.

105. Hayashi S, Kurihara H, Hirato J, et al. Solitary fibrous tumor of the orbit with extraorbital extension: case report. Neurosurg 2001; 49:1241–5.
106. Heathcote JG. Pathology update: solitary fibrous tumour of the orbit. Can J Ophthalmol 1997; 32:432–5.
107. Henderson JW, Campbell RJ, Farrow GM, et al. Orbital Tumors. 3rd ed. New York, NY: Raven Press, 1993:165.
108. Hoang MP, Suarez PA, Donner LR, et al. Mesenchymal chondrosarcoma: a small cell neoplasm with polyphenotypic differentiation. Int J Surg Patho 2000; 8:291–301.
109. Hollenbach AD, Sublett JE, McPherson CJ, et al. The Pax3-FKHR oncoprotein is unresponsive to the Pax3-associated repressor hDaxx. EMBO J 1999; 18:3702–11.
110. Hsu JK, Cavanagh HD, Green WR. An unusual case of elastofibroma oculi. Cornea 1997; 16:112–9.
111. Husmann I, Soulet L, Gautron J, et al. Growth factors in skeletal muscle regeneration. Cytokine Growth Factor Rev 1996; 7:249–58.
112. Huvos AG, Rosen G, Dabska M, et al. Mesenchymal chondrosarcoma. A clinicopathologic analysis of 35 patients with emphasis on treatment. Cancer 1983; 51: 1230–7.
113. Ide F, Obara K, Mishima K, et al. Ultrastructural spectrum of solitary fibrous tumor: a unique perivascular tumor with alternative lines of differentiation. Virchows Arch 2005; 446:646–52.
114. Imes RK, Hoyt WF. Childhood chiasmal gliomas: update on the fate of patients in the 1969 San Francisco Study. Br J Ophthalmol 1986; 70:179–82.
115. Iwasaki H, Isayama T, Johzaki H, et al. Malignant fibrous histiocytoma. Evidence of perivascular mesenchymal cell origin immunocytochemical studies with monoclonal anti-MFH antibodies. Am J Pathol 1987; 128:528–37.
116. Jakobiec FA, Font RL, Tso MO, et al. Mesectodermal leiomyoma of the ciliary body: a tumor of presumed neural crest origin. Cancer 1977; 39:2102–13.
117. Jakobiec FA, Iwamoto T. Mesectodermal leiomyoma of the ciliary body associated with a nevus. Arch Ophthalmol 1978; 96:692–5.
118. Jakobiec FA, Rini F, Char D, et al. Primary liposarcoma of the orbit. Problems in the diagnosis and management of five cases. Ophthalmology 1989; 96:180–91.
119. Jensen OA. Glomus tumor (Glomangioma) of eyelid. Arch Ophthalmol 1965; 73:511–3.
120. Jung A, Bechthold S, Pfluger T, et al. Orbital rhabdomyosarcoma in Noonan syndrome. J Pediatr Hematol Oncol 2003; 25:330–2.
121. Kanoe H, Nakayama T, Hosaka T, et al. Characteristics of genomic breakpoints in TLS-CHOP translocations in liposarcomas suggest the involvement of translin and topoisomerase II in the process of translocation. Oncogene 1999; 18:721–9.
122. Karcioglu Z, Nasr AM, Haik BG. Orbital hemangiopericytoma: Clinical and morphologic features. Am J Ophthalmol 1997; 124:661–72.
123. Karcioglu ZA, Hadjistilianou D, Rozans M, et al. Orbital rhabdomyosarcoma. Cancer Control 2004; 11: 328–33.
124. Kashyap S, Sen S, Sharma MC, et al. Alveolar soft-part sarcoma of the orbit: report of three cases. Can J Ophthalmol 2004; 39:552–6.
125. Kennedy RH, Flanagan JC, Eagle RC Jr, et al. The Carney complex with ocular signs suggestive of cardiac myxoma. Am J Ophthalmol 1991; 111:699–702.
126. Kennedy RH, Waller RR, Carney JA. Ocular pigmented spots and eyelid myxomas. Am J Ophthalmol 1987; 104: 533–8.
127. Khan J, Bittner ML, Saal LH, et al. cDNA microarrays detect activation of a myogenic transcription program by the PAX3-FKHR fusion oncogene. Proc Natl Acad Sci USA 1999; 96:3264–9.
128. Khan J, Bittner ML, Saal LH, et al. cDNA microarrays detect activation of a myogenic transcription program by the PAX3-FLHR fusion oncogene. PNAS 1999; 96:13264–9.
129. Kim YH, Riener L. Ultrastructure of lipoma. Cancer 1982; 50:102–6.
130. Kindblom LG, Stener B, Angervall L. Intramuscular myxoma. Cancer 197; 34:1737–44.
131. Kindblom LG, Widehn S, Meis-Kindblom JM. The role of electron microscopy in the diagnosis of pleomorphic sarcomas of soft tissue. Semin Diagn Pathol 2003; 20:72–81.
132. Knezevich SR, McFadden DE, Tao W, et al. A novel ETV6–NTRK3 gene fusion in congenital fibrosarcoma. Nat Genet 1998; 18:184–7.
133. Knowles DM II, Jakobiec FA. Rhabdomyoma of the orbit. Am J Ophthalmol 1975; 80:1011–8.
134. Kodet R, Stejskal J, Pilat D, et al. Congenital-infantile fibrosarcoma: a clinicopathological study of five patients entered on the Prague children's tumor registry. Pathol Res Pract 1996; 192:845–53.
135. Kodet R, Newton WA Jr, Hamoudi AB, et al. Orbital rhabdomyosarcomas and related tumors in childhood: relationship of morphology to prognosis-an Intergroup Rhabdomyosarcoma study. Med Pediatr Oncol 1997; 29: 51–60.
136. Koizumi H, Mikami M, Doi M, et al. Clonality analysis of nodular fasciitis by HUMARA-methylation-specific PCR. Histopathology 2005; 47:320–34.
137. Krishnakumar S, Subramanian N, Mohan ER, et al. Solitary fibrous tumor of the orbit: a clinicopathologic study of six cases with review of the literature. Surv Ophthalmol 2003; 48:544–54.
138. Krisman M, Adams H, Jaworska M, et al. Patterns of chromosomal imbalances in benign solitary fibrous tumours of the pleura. Virchows Arch 2000; 437: 248–55.
139. Krisman M, Adams H, Jaworska M, et al. Benign solitary fibrous tumour of the thigh: morphological, chromosomal and differential diagnostic aspects. Langenbecks Arch Surg 2000; 385:521–5.
140. Kupersmith MJ, Warren FA, Newa J, et al. Irradiation of meningiomas of the intracranial anterior visual pathway. Ann Neurol 1987; 21:313–7.
141. Ladanyi M, Lui MY, Antonescu CR, et al. The der(17)t (X;17)(p11;q25) of human alveolar soft part sarcoma fuses the transcription factor gene to ASPL, a novel gene at 17q25. Oncogene 2001; 20:48–57.
142. Ladanyi M, Antonescu CR, Drobnjak M, et al. The precrystalline cytoplasmic granules of alveolar soft part sarcoma contain monocarboxylate transporter 1 and CD147. Am J Pathol 2002; 160:1215–21.
143. Landon G, Ordonez NG, Guarda LA. Cardiac myxoma: an immunohistochemical study using endothelial, histiocytic and smooth muscle cell markers. Arch Pathol Lab Med 1986; 110:116–20.
144. Lee DA, Campbell RJ, Waller RR, et al. A clinicopathologic study of primary adenoid cystic carcinoma of the lacrimal gland. Ophthalmology 1985; 92:128–34.
145. Li FP, Fraumeni JF Jr. Prospective study of a family cancer syndrome. JAMA 1982; 247:2692–4.

146. Lieb WE, Goebel HH, Wallenfang T. Myxoma of the orbit: a clinicopathologic report. Graefes Arch Clin Exp Ophthalmol 1990; 228:28–32.
147. Lieberman PH, Brennan MF, Kimmel M, Erlandson RA, Garin-Chesa P, Flehinger BY. Alveolar soft-part sarcoma. A clinico-pathologic study of half a century. Cancer 1989; 63:1–13.
148. Lo GG, Biswas J, Rao NA, et al. Corneal myxoma. Case report and review of the literature. Cornea 1990; 9: 174–8.
149. Lucci LM, Anderson RL, Harrie RP, et al. Solitary fibrous tumor of the orbit in a child. Ophthal Plast Reconstr Surg 2001; 17:369–73.
150. Mack TM. Sarcomas and other malignancies of soft tissue, retroperitoneum, peritoneum, pleura, heart, mediastinum and spleen. Cancer 1995; 275:211–44.
151. Maillard AA, Kountakis SE. Pediatric sino-orbital desmoid fibromatosis. Ann Otol Rhinol Laryngol 1996; 105: 463–6.
152. Maione R, Amati P. Interdependence between muscle differentiation and cell-cycle control. Biochim Biophys Acta 1997; 1332:M19–30.
153. Mandahl N, Fletcher CDM, Dal Cin P, et al. Comparative cytogenetic study of spindle cell and pleomorphic leiomyosarcomas of soft tissues. A report from CHAMP study group. Cancer Genet Cytogenet 2000; 116:66–73.
154. Martin AJ, Summersgill BM, Fisher C, et al. Chromosomal imbalances in meningeal solitary fibrous tumors. Cancer Genet Cytogenet 2002; 135:160–4.
155. Matsko TH, Schmidt RA, Milam AH, et al. Primary malignant ectomesenchymoma of the orbit. Br J Ophthalmol 1992; 76:438–41.
156. Mawad JK, Mackay B, Raymond AK, et al. Electron microscopy in the diagnosis of small round cell tumors of bone. Ultrastruct Pathol 1994; 18:263–8.
157. Meis-Kindblom JM, Bergh P, Gunterberg B, et al. Extraskeletal myxoid chondrosarcoma: a reappraisal of its morphologic spectrum and prognostic factors based on 117 cases. Am J Surg Pathol 1999; 23:636–50.
158. Meis-Kindblom JM, Sjogren H, Kindblom LG, et al. Cytogenetic and molecular analyses of liposarcoma and its soft tissue simulators: recognition of new variants and differential diagnosis. Virchows Arch 2001; 439: 141–51.
159. Meekins BB, Dutton JJ, Proia AD. Primary orbital leiomyosarcoma. A case report and review of the literature. Arch Ophthalmol 1988; 106:82–6.
160. Mellin W, Niezabitowski A, Brockmann M, et al. DNA ploidy in soft tissue tumors: An evaluation of the prognostic implications in different tumor types. Curr Topics Pathol 89:95–122.
161. Mentzel T, Bainbridge TC, Katenkamp D. Solitary fibrous tumor: clinicopathological, immunohistochemical, and ultrastructural analysis of 12 cases arising in soft tissues, nasal cavity and nasopharynx, urinary bladder and prostate. Virchows Arch 1997; 430: 445–53.
162. Merlino G, Helman LJ. Rhabdomyosarcoma-working out the pathways. Oncogene 1999; 18:5340–8.
163. Meyer SL, Fine BS, Font RL, et al. Leiomyoma of the ciliary body: electron microscopic verification. Am J Ophthalmol 1968; 66:1061–8.
164. Middleton LP, Duray PH, Merino MJ. The histological spectrum of hemangiopericytoma: application of immunohistochemical analysis including proliferative markers to facilitate diagnosis and predict prognosis. Hum Pathol 1998; 29:636–40.
165. Miettinen MM, el-Rifai W, Sarlomo-Rikala M, et al. Tumor size-related DNA copy number changes occur in solitary fibrous tumors but not in hemangiopericytomas. Mod Pathol 1997; 10:1194–200.
166. Mihara F, Gupta KL, Kartchner ZA, et al. Leiomyosarcoma after retinoblastoma radiotherapy. Radiat Med 1991; 9: 183–4.
167. Mitelman Database of Chromosome Aberrations in Cancer. 2002 http://cgap.nci.nih.gov/Chromosomes/Mitelman
168. Myung J, Kim IO, Chun JE, et al. Rhabdomyoma of the orbit: a case report. Pediatr Radiol 2002; 32:589–92.
169. Nakashima Y, Unni KK, Shives TC, et al. Mesenchymal chondrosarcoma of bone and soft tissue. A review of 111 cases. Cancer 1986; 57:2444–53.
170. Naumann G, Font RL, Zimmeman LE. Electron microscopic verification of primary rhabdomyosarcoma of the iris. Am J Ophthalmol 1972; 74:110–7.
171. Ness GO, Lybaek H, Arnes J, et al. Chromosomal imbalances in a recurrent solitary fibrous tumor of the orbit. Cancer Genet Cytogenet 2005; 162:38–44.
172. Nielsen GP, O'Connell JX, Dickersin GR, et al. Solitary fibrous tumor of soft tissue: a report of 15 cases, including 5 malignant examples with light microscopic, immunohistochemical and ultrastructural data. Mod Pathol 1997; 10:1028–37.
173. O'Brian JE, Stout AP. Malignant fibrous xanthomas. Cancer 1964; 17:1446–55.
174. Okamoto S, Hisaoka M, Ushijima M, et al. Activating G_s(alpha)mutation in intramuscular myxomas with or without fibrous dysplasia of bone. Virchows Arch 2000; 437:133–7.
175. Oliveira AM, Nascimento AG, Okuno SH, et al. P27 (kip1) protein expression correlates with survival in myxoid and round cell liposarcoma. J Clin Oncol 2000; 18:2888–93.
176. Oliveira AM, Nascimento AG, Lloyd RV. Leptin and leptin receptor mRNA are widely expressed in tumors of adipocytic differentiation. Mod Pathol 2001; 14:549–55.
177. Ordonez NG, Ro JY, Mackay B. Alveolar soft part sarcoma. An ultrastructural and immunocytochemical investigation of its histogenesis. Cancer 1989; 63: 1721–36.
178. Ordonez NG, Mackay B. Alveolar soft-part sarcoma: a review of the pathology and histogenesis. Ultrstryct Pathol 1998; 22:275–92.
179. Oshiro Y, Fukada T, Tsuneyoshi M. Fibrosarcoma versus fibromatoses and cellular nodular fasciitis. A comparative study of their proliferative activity using proliferating cell nuclear antigen, DNA flow cytometry, and p53. Am J Surg Pathol 1994; 18:712–9.
180. Ozzello L, Stout AP, Murray MR. Cultured characteristics of malignant histiocytomas and fibrous xanthomas. Cancer 1963; 16:331–44.
181. Paikos P, Papathanassiou M, STafanaki K, et al Malignant ectomesenchymoma of the orbit in a child: Case report and review of the literature. Surv Ophthalmol 2002; 4: 368–74.
182. Panzarella MJ, Naqvi AH, Cohen HE, et al. Predictive value of gadolinium enhancement in differentiating ALT/WD liposarcomas from benign fatty tumors. Skeletal Radiol 2005; 34:272–8.
183. Park SW, Kim HJ, Chin HS, et al. Mesectodermal leiomyosarcoma of the ciliary body. AJNR Am J Neuroradiol 2003; 24:1765–8.

184. Pe'er J, Hydayat AA. Myxomas of the conjunctiva. Am J Ophthalmol 1986; 2:80–6.
185. Pe'er JJ, Stefanyszyn M, Hidayat AA. Nonepithelial tumors of the lacrimal sac. Am J Ophthalmol 1994; 118: 650–8.
186. Pellin A, Boix J, Blesa JR, et al. EWS/FLI-1 rearrangement in small round cell sarcomas of bone and soft tissue detected by reverse transcriptase polymerase chain reaction amplification. Eur J Cancer 1994; 30A:827–31.
187. Petit MM, Mols R, Schoenmakers EF, et al. LPP, the preferred fusion partner gene of HMGIC in lipomas, is a novel member of the LIM protein gene family. Genomics 1996; 36:118–29.
188. Poissonet CM, La Velle M, Burds AR. Growth and development of adipose tissue. J Pediatr 1988; 113:1–9.
189. Porter PL, Bigler SA, McNutt M, et al. The immunophenotype of hemangiopericytomas and glomus tumors, with special reference to muscle protein expression: an immunohistochemical study and review of the literature. Mod Pathol 1991; 4:46–52.
190. Price EB, Silliphant WM, Shuman R. Nodular fasciitis: a clinicopathologic analysis of 65 cases. Am J Clin Path 1961; 35:122–36.
191. Puri PL, Sartorelli V. Regulation of muscle regulatory factors by DNA-binding, interacting proteins and post-transcriptional modifications. J Cell Physiol 2000; 185: 155–73.
192. Ratnatunga N, Goodlad JR, Sankarakumaran N, et al. Primary biphasic synovial sarcoma of the orbit. J Clin Pathol 1992; 45:265–7.
193. Reid AH, Tsai MM, Venzon DJ, et al. MDM2 amplification, P53 mutation, and accumulation of the P53 gene product in malignant fibrous histiocytoma. Diagn Mol Pathol 1996; 5:65–73.
194. Renshaw AA. O13 (CD99) in spindle cell tumors. Reactivity with hemangiopericytoma, solitary fibrous tumor, synovial sarcoma, and meningioma but rarely with sarcomatoid mesotheioma. Appl Immunohistochem 1995; 3:250–6.
195. Richter MN, Bechrakis NE, Stoltenburg-Didinger G, et al. Transscleral resection of a ciliary body leiomyoma in a child: case report and review of the literature. Graefes Arch Clin Exp Ophthalmol 2003; 241:953–7.
196. Rootman J, Damji KF, Dimmick JE. Malignant rhabdoid tumor of the orbit. Ophthalmology 1989; 96:1650–4.
197. Rosai J, Dias P, Parham DM, et al. MyoD1 protein expression in alveolar soft part sarcoma as confirmatory evidence of its skeletal muscle nature. Am J Surg Pathol 1991; 15:974–81.
198. Rosai J, Akerman M, Dal Cin P, et al. Combined morphologic and karyotypic study of 59 atypical lipomatous tumors. Evaluation of their relationship and differential diagnosis with other adipose tissue tumors (a report of the CHAMP Study Group). Am J Surg Pathol 1996; 20:1182–9.
199. Rosenberg AE. Malignant fibrous histiocytoma: past, present, and future. Skeletal Radiol 2003; 32:613–8.
200. Rubin BP, Chen CJ, Morgan TW, et al. Congenital mesoblastic nephroma t(12;15) is associated with ETV6–NTRK3 gene fusion: cytogenetic and molecular relationship to congenital (infantile) fibrosarcoma. Am J Pathol 1998; 153:1451–8.
201. Ruymann FB, Maddux HR, Ragab A, et al. Congenital anomalies associated with rhabdomyosarcoma: an autopsy study of 115 cases. A report from the Intergroup Rhabdomyosarcoma Study Committee (representing the Children's Cancer Study Group, the Pediatric Oncology Group, the United Kingdom Children's Cancer Study Group, and the Pediatric Intergroup Statistical Center). Med Pediatr Oncol 1988; 16:33–9.
202. Sakabe T, Shinomiya T, Mori T, et al. Identification of a novel gene, MASL1, within an amplicon at 8p23.1 detected in malignant fibrous histiocytomas by comparative genomic hybridization. Cancer Re 1999; 59:511–5.
203. Sakamot T, Ishibashi T, Ohnishi Y, et al. Immunohistological and electron microscopical study of nodular fasciitis of the orbit. Br J Ophthalmol 1991; 75: 636–8.
204. Salvador AH, Beabout JW, Dahlin DC. Mesenchymal chrondrosarcoma: observations on 30 new cases. Cancer 1971; 28:605–15.
205. Sandberg AA. Updates on the cytogenetics and molecular genetics of bone and soft tissue tumors: lipoma. Cancer Genet Cytogenet 2004; 150:93–115.
206. Sandberg AA. Updates on the cytogenetics and molecular genetics of bone and soft tissue tumors: liposarcoma. Cancer Genet Cytogenet 2004; 155:1–24.
207. Sandberg AA. Updates on the cytogenetics and molecular genetics of bone and soft tissue tumors: leiomyosarcoma. Cancer Genet Cytogenet 2005; 161:1–19.
208. Sawyer JR, Sammartino G, Baker GF, Bell JM. Clonal chromosome aberrations in a case of nodular fasciitis. Cancer Genet Cytogenet 1994; 76:154–6.
209. Schurch W, Skalli O, Lagace R, et al. Intermediate filament proteins and actin isoforms as markers for soft-tissue tumor differentiation and origin. III. Hemangiopericytomas and glomus tumors. Am J Pathol 1990; 136:771–86.
210. Schutz JS, Rabkin MD, Schutz S. Fibromatous tumor (desmoid type) of the orbit. Arch Ophthalmol 1979; 97:703–4.
211. Sciot R, Dal Cin P, de Vos R, et al. Alveolar soft part sarcoma: evidence for its myogenic origin and for the involvement 17q25. Histopathology 1993; 23:439–44.
212. Sebire NJ, Malone M. Myogenin and MyoD1 expression in paediatric rhabdomyosarcomas. J Clin Pathol 2003; 56:412–6.
213. Sheng WQ, Hisaoka M, Okamoto S, et al. Congenital-infantil fibrosarcoma. A clinicopathologic study of 10 cases and molecular detection of the ETV6–NTRK3 fusion transcripts using paraffin-embedded tissues. Am J Clin Pathol 2001; 115:348–55.
214. Shields JA, Bakewell B, Augsburger JJ, et al. Classification and incidence of space-occupying lesions of the orbit. A survey of 645 biopsies. Arch Ophthalmol 1984; 102: 1606–11.
215. Shields CL, Shields JA, Varenhorst MP. Transcleral leiomyoma. Ophthalmology 1991; 98:84–7.
216. Shields JA, Shields CL, Eagle RC, et al. Observations on seven cases of intraocular leiomyoma. Arch Ophthalmol 1994; 112:521–8.
217. Shields CL, Shields JA, Honavar SG, et al. Primary ophthalmic rhabdomyosarcoma in 33 patients. Trans Am Ophthalmol Soc 2001; 99:133–42.
218. Shields CL, Shields JA, Honavar SG, et al. Clinical spectrum of primary ophthalmic rhabdomyosarcoma. Ophthalmology 2001; 108:2284–92.
219. Shields JA, Shields CL, Christian C, et al. Orbital nodular fasciitis simulating a dermoid cyst in an 8-month-old child. Case report and review of the literature. Ophthal Plast Reconstr Surg 2001; 17:144–8.
220. Shields JA, Shields CL. Rhabdomyosarcoma: review for the ophthalmologist. Surv Ophthalmol 2003; 48:39–57.

221. Shields JA, Shields CL, Scartozzi R. Survey of 1264 patients with orbital tumors and simulating lesions: The 2002 Montgomery Lecture, part 1. Ophthalmology 2004; 111:997–1008.
222. Shinaver CN, Mafee MF, Choi KH. MRI of mesenchymal chondrosarcoma of the orbit: case report and review of the literature. Neuroradiology 1997; 39:296–301.
223. Shipkey FH, Lieberman PH, Foote FW Jr, et al. Ultrastructure of alveolar soft part sarcoma. Cancer 1964; 17:821–30.
224. Shukla PN, Pathy S, Sen S, et al. Primary orbital calcified synovial sarcoma: a case report. Orbit 2003; 22:299–303.
225. Sibony PAA, Krauss HR, Kennerdell JS, et al. Optic nerve sheath meningiomas: clinical manifestations. Ophthalmology 1984; 91:1313–26.
226. Smith AC, Squire JA, Thorner P, et al. Association of alveolar rhabdomyosarcoma with the Beckwith-Wiedemann syndrome. Pediatr Dev Pathol 2001; 4: 550–8.
227. Solis E, Moreno A, Rodriguez-Enriquez B, Sanchez-Vizcaino JS, et al. Benign fibrous histiocytoma with indeterminate cells and eosinophils: collision, differentiation, or involution? Am J Dermatopathol 2004; 26: 237–41.
228. Solvonuk PF, Taylor GP, Hancock R, et al. Correlation of morphologic and biochemical observations in human lipomas. Lab Invest 1984; 51:469–74.
229. Stautz CC. CT of infantile myofibromatosis of the orbit with intracranial involvement: a case report. AJNR Am J Neuroradiol 1991; 12:184–5.
230. Stewart WB, Krohel GB, Wright JE. Lacrimal gland and fossa lesions: an approach to diagnosis and management. Ophthalmology 1979; 86:886–95.
231. Stidham DB, Burgett RA, Davis MM, et al. Congenital malignant rhabdoid tumor of the orbit. JAAPOS 1999; 3: 318–20.
232. Stratton MR, Moss S, Warren W, et al. Mutation in p53 gene in human soft tissue sarcomas: association with abnormalities of the RB1 gene. Oncogene 1990; 5: 1297–301.
233. Stout AP. Myxoma, the tumor of primitive mesenchyme. Ann Surg 1948; 127:706–19.
234. Sublett JE, Jeon IS, Shapiro DN. The alveolar rhabdomyosarcoma PAX3/FKHR fusion protein is a transcriptional activator. Oncogene 1995; 11:545–52.
235. Suh CH, Ordonez NG, Mackay B. Fibrosarcoma: observations on the ultrastructure. Ultrastruct Pathol 1993; 17: 221–9.
236. Suh CH, Ordonez NG, Mackay B. Malignant fibrous histiocytoma: an ultrastructural perspective. Ultrastruct Pathol 2000; 24:243–50.
237. Sun Y, Naito Z, Ishiwata T, et al. Basic FGF and Ki-67 proteins useful for immunohistological diagnostic evaluations in malignant solitary fibrous tumor. Path Int 2003; 53:284–90.
238. Sung L, Anderson JR, Arndt C, et al. Neurofibromatosis in children with Rhabdomyosarcoma: a report from the Intergroup Rhabdomyosarcoma study IV. J Pediatr 2004; 144:666–8.
239. Suster S, Nascimento AG, Miettinen M, et al. Solitary fibrous tumors of soft tissue. A clinicopathologic and immunohistochemical study of 12 cases. Am J Surg Pathol 1995; 19:1257–66.
240. Suster S, Fisher C, Moran CA. Expression of bcl-2 oncoprotein in benign and malignant spindle cell tumors of soft tissue, skin, serosal surfaces and gastrointestinal tract. Am J Surg Pathol 1998; 22:863 72.
241. Tintignac LA, Leibovitch MP, Leibovitch SA. New insight into MyoD regulation: involvement in rhabdomyosarcoma pathway? Bul Cancer 2001; 88:545–8.
242. Tuncer S, Kebudi R, Peksayar G, et al. Congenital mesenchymal chondrosarcoma of the orbit. Case report and review of the literature. Ophthalmology 2004; 111: 1016–22.
243. van den Broek PP, de Faber JT, Kliffen M, et al. Anterior orbital leiomyoma: possible pulley smooth muscle tissue tumor. Arch Ophthalmol 2005; 123:1614.
244. Verheggen R, Markakis E, Muhlendyck H, et al. Symptomatology, surgical therapy and postoperative results of sphenoorbital, intraorbital-inttracanalicular and optic nerve sheaths. Acta Neurochir Suppl 1996; 65: 95–8.
245. Vlvo A. Malignant mesodermal mixed tumor (mesenchymoma) of the orbit. Am J Ophthalmol 1968; 66:919–23.
246. Wang NP, Bacchi CE, Jiang JJ, et al. Does alveolar soft part sarcoma exhibit skeletal muscle differentiation? An immunocytochemical and biochemical study of myogenic regulatory protein expression. Am J Pathol 1995; 147:1799–810.
247. Wara WM, Sheline GE, Newman H, et al. Radiation therapy of meningiomas. AJR Radium Ther Nucl Med 1975; 123:453–8.
248. Watanabe K, Kusakabe T, Hoshi N, et al. h-Caldesmon in leiomyosarcoma and tumors with smooth muscle cell-like differentiation: its specific expression in the smooth muscle cell tumor. Hum Pathol 1999; 30:392–6.
249. Weibolt VM, Buresh CJ, Roberts CA, et al. Involvement of 3q21 in nodular fasciitis. Cancer Genet Cytogenet 1998; 106:177–9.
250. Weiner JM, Hidayat AA. Juvenile fibrosarcoma of the orbit and eyelid: a study of five cases. Arch Ophthalmol 1983; 101:253–9.
251. Weinrach DM, Wang KL, Wiley EL, et al. Immunohistochemical expression of matrix metalloproteinase 1,2,9, and 14 in dermatofibrosarcoma protuberans and common fibrous histiocytoma (dermatofibroma). Arch Pathol Lab Med 2004; 128:1136–41.
252. Weintraub H, Davis R, Tapscott S, et al. The myoD gene family: nodal point during specification of the muscle cell lineage. Science 1991; 251:761–6.
253. Weiss SW, Goldblum JR. Nodular fasciitis. In: Weiss SW, Goldblum JR, eds. Soft Tissue Tumors. 4th ed. St. Louis, MO: Mosby, 2001:250–66.
254. Weiss SW, Goldblum JR. Fibrosarcoma. In: Weiss SW, Goldblum JR, eds. Soft Tissue Tumors. 4th ed. St. Louis, MO: Mosby, 2001:409–39.
255. Weiss SW, Goldblum JR. Benign fibrohisticytic tumors. In: Weiss SW, Goldblum JR, eds. Soft Tissue Tumors. 4th ed. St. Louis, MO1: Mosby, 2001:441–90.
256. Weiss SW, Goldblum JR. Malignant fibrous histiocytoma. In: Weiss SW, Goldblum JR, eds. Soft Tissue Tumors. 4th ed. St. Louis, MO: Mosby, 2001:539–67.
257. Weiss SW, Goldblum JR. Benign tumors of smooth muscle. In: Weiss SW, Goldblum JR, eds. Soft Tissue Tumors. 4th ed. St. Louis, MO: Mosby, 2001:695–726.
258. Weiss SW, Goldblum JR. Leiomyosarcoma. In: Weiss SW, Goldblum JR, eds. Soft Tissue tumors. 4th ed. St. Louis, MO: Mosby, 2001:727–48.
259. Weiss SW, Goldblum, JR. Rhabdomyosarcoma. In: Weiss SW, Goldblum JR, eds. Soft Tissue Tumors. 4th ed. St. Louis, MO: Mosby, 2001:785–835.
260. Weiss SW, Goldblum JR. Hemangiopericytoma and solitary fibrous tumor family. In: Weiss SW, Goldblum JR, eds. Soft Tissue Tumors. 4th ed. St. Louis, MO: Mosby, 2001:1001–21.

261. Weiss SW, Goldblum JR. Solitary fibrous tumor. In: Weiss SW, Goldblum JR, eds. Soft Tissue Tumors. 4th ed. St. Louis, MO: Mosby, 2001:1021–31.
262. Weiss SW, Rao VK. Well differentiated liposarcoma (atypical lipoma) of deep soft tissue of the extremities, retroperitoneum and miscellaneous sites: a follow-up study of 92 cases with analysis of the incidence of dedifferentiation. Am J Surg Pathol 1992; 16:1051–8.
263. Weiss SW, Goldblum JR. Benign soft tissue tumors and pseudotumors of miscellaneous type. In: Weiss SW, Goldblum JR, eds. Soft Tissue Tumors. 4th ed. St. Louis, MO: Mosby, 2001:1419–81.
264. Weiss SW, Goldblum JR. Malignant soft tissue tumors of uncertain type. In: Weiss SW, Goldblum JR, eds. Soft Tissue Tumors. 4th ed. St. Louis, MO: Mosby, 2001: 1483–571.
265. White VA, Damji KF, Richards JSF, Rootman J. Leiomyosarcoma of the conjunctiva. Ophthalmol ogy 1991; 98:1560–4.
266. White VA, Heathcote JG, Hurwitz, et al. Epithelioid sarcoma of the orbit. Ophthalmology 1994; 101: 1680–7.
267. Wijnaendts LC, van der Linden JC, van Unnik, et al. The expression pattern of contractile and intermediate filament proteins in developing skeletal muscle and rhabdomyosarcoma of childhood: diagnostic and prognostic utility. J Pathol 1994; 174:283–92.
268. Wolanska M, Bankowski E. Fibroblast growth factors (FGF) in human myometrium and uterine leiomyomas in various stages of tumour growth. Biochimie 2006; 88: 141–6.
269. Wood GS, Beckstead JH, Turner RR, et al. Malignant fibrous histiocytoma tumor cells resemble fibroblasts. Am J Surg Pathol 1986; 10:323–35.
270. Woyke S, Chwirot R. Rhabdomyosarcoma of the iris: report of the first recorded case. Br J Ophthalmol 1972; 56: 60–4.
271. Yang P, Grufferman S, Khoury MJ, et al. Association of childhood rhabdomyosarcoma with neurofibromatosis type I and birth defects. Genet Epidemiol 1995; 12:467–74.
272. Yanoff M, Scheie HG. Fibrosarcoma of the orbit. Report of two patients. Cancer 1966; 19:1711–6.
273. Yokoi T, Tsuzuki T, Yatabe Y, et al. Solitary fibrous tumour: significance of p53 and CD34 immunoreactivity in its malignant transformation. Histopathology 1998; 32: 423–32.
274. Yoon M, Desai K, Fulton R, et al. Desmoplastic small round cell tumor: a potentially lethal neoplasm manifesting in the orbit with associated visual symptoms. Arch Ophthalmol 2005; 123:565–7.

65

Tumors of Bone and Cartilage

Bret M. Wehrli
Department of Pathology, University of Western Ontario, London, Ontario, Canada

J. Godfrey Heathcote
Departments of Pathology and Ophthalmology and Visual Sciences, Dalhousie University, Halifax, Nova Scotia, Canada

INTRODUCTION

Many pathological processes may involve the bony walls of the orbit. Inflammatory processes, such as sinusitis, and structural lesions, such as mucocele, may destroy the bone, as may deposits of metastatic carcinoma. Secondary involvement of the bone may occur with benign neoplasms, (e.g., meningioma of the sphenoid wing), and with infiltrative carcinomas of adnexal origin, (e.g., basal cell carcinoma). In this chapter, we shall concentrate on lesions that arise within the orbital bone and manifest as space-occupying tumors. Such lesions are relatively rare, comprising <2% of all orbital tumors (128).

A variety of reactive and neoplastic processes give rise to space-occupying lesions in orbital bones and their nature exerts some influence on the clinical presentation. Thus, benign fibro-osseous lesions generally produce a slowly progressive displacement of the globe whereas malignant neoplasms grow rapidly within the orbit and may cause pain. Reactive lesions sometimes show a sudden increase in size as a result of intralesional hemorrhage. In the orbit, as with bony tumors elsewhere, the final diagnosis must be derived from correlation of the clinical findings with the imaging studies and the histopathology.

REACTIVE BONE LESIONS

Cholesterol Granuloma

Cholesterol granuloma, a reactive inflammatory lesion most often seen in the middle ear and petrous temporal bone, can infrequently involve the orbit (3,39,46,51,68, 79,85,96,127,134). In a review of 3100 orbital lesions, Selva et al. identified only six cases of cholesterol granuloma (127). Males in their fourth to fifth decades are primarily affected. The lesion almost exclusively arises within the diploe of the frontal bone above the lacrimal fossa and then enlarges, with eventual breach of the outer table and extension into the periorbital tissues (3,79,85,127).

Presenting complaints typically include fullness of the upper orbit and downward and medial displacement of the globe with proptosis. Other symptoms and clinical findings may include dull aches, blurred or double vision, ptosis, and a palpable mass or defect in the orbital rim (85). Plain radiographs reveal a well-defined, superotemporal, osteolytic lesion with rounded edges and without associated sclerosis or bony spicules but computed tomography (CT) and magnetic resonance imaging (MRI) allow better appreciation of the locally destructive nature of this lesion and its extent (39,53).

Grossly, the lesion appears cystic and is filled with brown fluid and yellow granular material. The histological features of cholesterol granuloma are distinctive, consisting of cholesterol clefts surrounded by inflamed granulation tissue, foreign body-type multinucleated giant cells, lipid- and hemosiderin-laden macrophages, fibrosis, and recent hemorrhage. Epithelial cells and keratin flakes are not present, distinguishing this lesion from epidermoid/dermoid cysts.

While the cause of cholesterol granuloma is unknown, several mechanisms have been proposed (79,85,96,127). Trauma with associated hemorrhage has been suggested as the primary event in cholesterol granuloma of the orbit and the predilection for the frontal bone and the preponderance of males, many of them manual laborers, have been taken as evidence in favor of this. However, a history of trauma has been documented in only a minority of cases. Abnormal pneumatization of orbital bone has also been postulated. Cholesterol granuloma in normally aerated bones, such as the petrous temporal bone and paranasal sinuses, has been attributed to ventilatory obstruction secondary to chronic inflammation or mechanical blockage. According to this theory, negative pressure develops within the obstructed space as the entrapped air is resorbed, leading to mucosal engorgement and eventual hemorrhage. Several animal studies that have reproduced lesions histologically identical to cholesterol granuloma following deliberate obstruction of normally aerated bones lend support to this idea. Alternatively, the presence of an unrecognized anomaly within the diploe could result in hemorrhage and consequent cholesterol granuloma formation. Reports of cholesterol granuloma within Pagetic bone (96) and bone involved by fibrous dysplasia (127) also lend credence to this theory. It is likely that cholesterol granuloma represents an unusual reaction to hemorrhage and, regardless of the inciting cause, subsequent degradation of blood leads to the formation of cholesterol crystals and a foreign body reaction. The release of prostaglandins from entrapped platelets may result in bone resorption and in the exposure of new blood vessels, further extending the process (85,127). Curettage is usually curative, although rare recurrences have been attributed to incomplete removal, particularly from the bony base of the lesion (46,79). Clinically, the differential diagnosis includes: lacrimal gland carcinoma, epidermoid/dermoid cysts, aneurysmal bone cyst, ossifying fibroma, eosinophilic granuloma, and metastasis. Histopathological examination should readily distinguish cholesterol granuloma from these entities.

Giant Cell Granuloma

Giant cell (reparative) granuloma, first described by Jaffe (63), is thought to be a reaction to intraosseous hemorrhage. The mandible and maxilla are most commonly affected (33) but a few cases involving the orbit have been reported (43,44,57,94,128,137). Patients with orbital giant cell granuloma have ranged in age from 5 to 54 years (average 18.6 years) with a 3:2 male preponderance. Presenting complaints have included proptosis, eyelid retraction, and displacement of the globe. Giant cell granuloma appears on plain radiographs as a round or oval area of lucency with distinct borders, but minimal reactive sclerosis (33). The cortex is often markedly thinned but usually intact and without a periosteal reaction.

The lesional tissue is friable, gritty, and tan-gray or brown. Cystic change and hemorrhage are often present. Histologically, giant cell granuloma consists of multinucleated osteoclast-type giant cells in a background of reactive spindle cells, collagen and areas of hemorrhage. The giant cells have a tendency to cluster around the areas of hemorrhage. Irregular trabeculae of woven bone lined by reactive osteoblasts may be present, as may secondary aneurysmal bone cyst-like changes. Ultrastructurally, the spindle cells resemble myofibroblasts and the giant cells have the properties of macrophages (33).

Curettage is the treatment of choice and recurrence is rare. Although metastasis and malignant transformation have not been documented, giant cell granuloma may be locally aggressive and one exceptional case required radiotherapy following two recurrences (137). The main differential diagnostic considerations are: giant cell tumor of bone, brown tumor of hyperparathyroidism, aneurysmal bone cyst, and nonossifying fibroma. The etiopathogenesis of giant cell granuloma is uncertain. The lesion may represent an exuberant reparative reaction to intraosseous hemorrhage secondary to trauma. However, a history of trauma is infrequently elicited. Other proposed causes include infections, developmental anomalies, and hormonal influences (100). Because of clinical and histological similarities between giant cell granuloma and cherubism, de Lange et al. analyzed four cases of giant cell granuloma for mutations in the *SH3BP2* gene that encodes for the Sh3 domain-binding protein 2 and which is mutated in cherubism. No mutations were identified suggesting that giant cell granuloma and cherubism are distinct entities (28).

Brown Tumor of Hyperparathyroidism

The brown tumor of hyperparathyroidism derives its name from the red-brown color resulting from the accumulation of hemosiderin. Another osteoclast-type giant cell-rich lesion of bone, the brown tumor is most commonly identified in the setting of hyperparathyroidism secondary to chronic renal failure of any cause (77). Brown tumors arise in association with primary hyperparathyroidism and in several instances have led to the discovery of the underlying condition (92). Individuals of all ages may be affected and brown tumors may arise in all parts of the axial and appendicular skeleton. They may be single or multiple. On plain radiographs, brown tumors typically appear as well-circumscribed osteolytic lesions without marginal sclerosis (149). Multiple radiolucent foci, salt-and-pepper osteopenia of the skull, and subperiosteal bone resorption of the terminal phalanges may suggest a diagnosis of brown tumor prior to histological confirmation (149).

A review of brown tumors of the orbit revealed that affected patients ranged in age from 10 to 70 years (average 33 years) with a female predominance (115). In these patients orbital maxillary, frontal, and ethmoid bones were involved and the underlying hyperparathyroidism was either primary or secondary (55,77,92,102,115,135). Patients presented with proptosis, displacement of the globe, decreased visual acuity, headaches, and facial numbness.

Regardless of the cause of hyperparathyroidism, the excess circulating parathyroid hormone stimulates osteoclastic activity and causes significant bone resorption. This leads to the formation of macroscopic cysts, which are initially filled with fibrovascular tissue. It is felt that subsequent microfractures and hemorrhage into these cysts provokes a reparative response characterized by the presence of reactive fibroblasts, blood vessels, blood and its breakdown products (mostly hemosiderin), and multinucleated osteoclast-type giant cells. Hence, the histological features of brown tumor are virtually indistinguishable from those of giant cell reparative granuloma. Subtle features that may aid in this distinction include intracortical and intratrabecular osteoclast tunneling resorption cones. The distinction is more readily made from a clinical history of renal failure or abnormal blood chemistry (elevated serum calcium, alkaline phosphatase, and parathyroid hormone). It is essential that, whenever a diagnosis of "giant cell lesion of bone" is made, biochemical analysis be performed to rule out the possibility of a brown tumor. Most brown tumors regress upon correction of the underlying cause of hyperparathyroidism, but curettage is the treatment of choice for symptomatic tumors.

Aneurysmal Bone Cyst

Aneurysmal bone cysts are blood-filled, multiloculated, cystic lesions that, although benign, are often locally destructive. They primarily occur in individuals younger than 20 years of age and, although most arise in the metaphyses of long tubular bones, vertebrae, and small tubular bones of the hands and feet, any bone may be affected (36,88). Craniofacial aneurysmal bone cysts account for approximately 18% of all cases (36). The roof of the orbit is the most common orbital site but cases primarily involving the ethmoid, sphenoid, and zygomatic bones have been documented (17,20,26,48,54,58,66,82,93,117). No significant sex predilection exists. Like other orbital masses, aneurysmal bone cyst most often produces proptosis with painless swelling. Optic nerve and oculomotor nerve deficits, diplopia, partial loss of vision, and papilledema may arise secondary to the space-occupying lesion. Imaging features of orbital aneurysmal bone cyst are similar to those of long tubular bones and are distinctive (20,26,54,82). On plain radiographs, lesions are typically well-circumscribed and radiolucent, with distention of the bone and extensive disruption of the cortex, leaving only a paper-thin shell of bone produced by an intact residual periosteum. A soap bubble appearance reflects multiloculation caused by fibrous septa. The multilocular, cystic nature of the lesion with internal fluid levels is better demonstrated by CT and MRI.

Grossly, the lesion has a dark spongy appearance and exudes thick red-brown material consistent with partially coagulated blood. Since aneurysmal bone cysts are typically treated by curettage, numerous collapsed ribbons of moderately cellular fibrovascular tissue are observed microscopically, rather than complete cysts. The tissue within these ribbons resembles granulation tissue but may be mitotically active. Irregular trabeculae of variably mineralized woven bone are frequently found within the fibrous septa and are covered by plump reactive osteoblasts and osteoclast-type giant cells. Rare endothelial cells may be identified, although the great majority of fibrous septa lack an endothelial lining. Large amounts of blood, clotted and unclotted, are present between the fibrous septa, with hemosiderin within both macrophages and the fibrous septa. Solid areas may appear identical to giant cell reparative granuloma. Rare lesions that almost entirely resemble giant cell reparative granuloma but are found in locations more typical of aneurysmal bone cysts have been called solid variants of aneurysmal bone cyst. The adjacent cancellous and cortical bone show active resorption and a shell of fibrous tissue with reactive bone and residual periosteum may be seen at the periphery of the lesion.

Aneurysmal bone cysts are benign but locally destructive and may cause severe deformity and functional impairment. Most lesions increase in size, often rapidly, and require attention. The most effective treatment is complete surgical resection (36,88), although this may cause major functional impairment and often is not possible for orbital lesions. For these reasons, curettage with bone grafting is most often performed although it is associated with a significant rate of recurrence, usually within 2 years (58). Various agents, such as liquid nitrogen or phenol, have been used to reduce the recurrence rate but not in controlled studies (36,88). Despite these instances of recurrence, most aneurysmal bone cysts are eventually brought under control by repeated curettage alone. Radiotherapy is reserved for exceptional cases and is generally to be avoided owing to the risk of radiation-induced sarcoma (36,88).

Different theories of pathogenesis of aneurysmal bone cyst have been proposed and include the development of local circulatory disturbances such as thrombosis or the formation of an intraosseous arteriovenous malformation, secondary to either trauma or a preexisting bone lesion (17,36,66). Aneurysmal bone cyst-like areas may be found in a number of different bone lesions, e.g., fibrous dysplasia, osteoblastoma, giant cell tumor of bone, non-ossifying fibroma, and osteosarcoma, and are referred to as secondary aneurysmal bone cysts. Regardless of whether an aneurysmal bone cyst is primary or secondary, all of the proposed mechanisms suggest a reactive process resulting from expansile blood flow causing erosion and resorption of the adjacent bone and resulting in a labyrinth of blood-filled channels bounded by a shell of periosteal bone. Recent molecular studies, however, have demonstrated the consistent presence of chromosome 17p13 rearrangements that upregulate transcription of the ubiquitin-specific protease 6 (*USP6*) oncogene, indicating that primary aneurysmal bone cyst may be a neoplasm (27,109,110). The common theme in each of these translocations is fusion of noncoding promoter regions of highly expressed genes to the USP6 coding sequence. Each of the identified five fusion partner genes (*ZNF9*, *CDH11*, *COL1A1*, *TRAP150*, and *OMD*) is highly expressed in cells of mesenchymal lineage and three have known roles in osteogenesis. Given that aneurysmal bone cysts contain little mature bone, and only minor components of immature bone, it has been proposed that transformation of the progenitor cell might occur prior to the point of osteoblastic commitment (111). Similar gene rearrangements have not been identified in secondary aneurysmal bone cysts, suggesting that secondary aneurysmal bone cyst may be a common endpoint of differentiation in several bone tumors (111).

BENIGN FIBRO-OSSEOUS LESIONS

Ossifying Fibroma and Fibrous Dysplasia

It has been proposed that ossifying fibroma is a variant of fibrous dysplasia (78). Both are benign fibro-osseous tumors that frequently arise within the craniofacial bones and demonstrate such striking histological overlap that, solely on this basis, distinction between the two may be impossible. To confidently distinguish between these two entities, attention must also be given to clinical and radiographic features. Ossifying fibromas generally occur in individuals in their third and fourth decades, whereas fibrous dysplasia most often presents in the second decade of life, although both may occur at any age (8,9,64,78,103,112,128,152). Radiographically, ossifying fibroma is often better circumscribed or sharply demarcated, with smooth contours and surrounded by a radiodense rim. In contrast, the limits of fibrous dysplasia are often less well-defined and a radiodense rim is lacking. Both lesions, by virtue of their mixture of varying amounts of fibrous and osseous tissue, have a heterogeneous appearance with a mixed pattern of osteoblastic and osteolytic areas, although fibrous dysplasia classically has a ground glass appearance on plain radiographs. MRI images are similar for both with a low- to intermediate-signal intensity on T1-weighted images and low-signal intensity on T2-weighted images. While certain features are more characteristic of one lesion over the other, there is considerable overlap and imaging studies alone cannot be considered diagnostic.

Microscopically, both lesions consist of varying amounts of fibrous and osseous stroma, but some subtle features may help to distinguish between them. The bony trabeculae within ossifying fibroma are composed of lamellar bone, lined by plump, reactive osteoblasts, and demonstrate greater continuity. However, the trabeculae within fibrous dysplasia consist almost entirely of woven bone, lack osteoblastic rimming, and are more irregular and discontinuous (Fig. 1). The trabeculae are classically described as having the appearance of Chinese characters at a low magnification. The presence of myxomatous matrix is also typical of ossifying fibroma. A variant of ossifying fibroma, aggressive psammomatoid ossifying fibroma, is characterized by large numbers of cementum-like structures, both within the fibrous stroma and within the bony trabeculae (Fig. 2) (50,90,91,153). As the name suggests, this variant is more aggressive locally, with frequent breach of the cortex and extension into

(A) 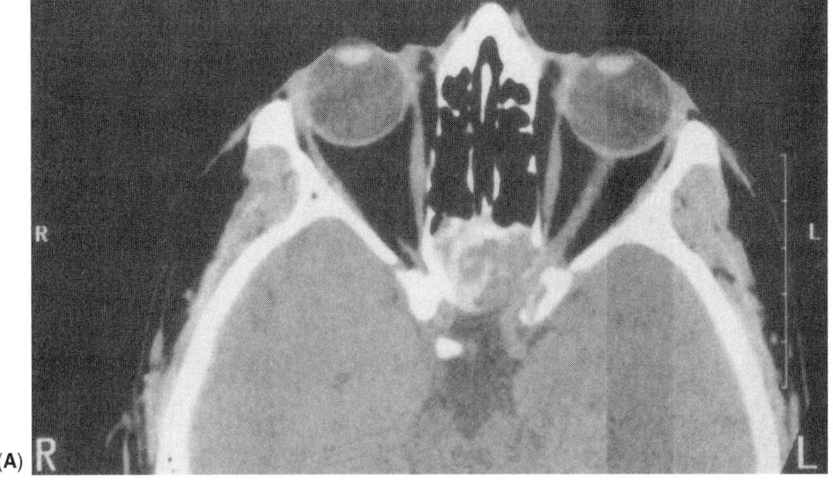

(B) 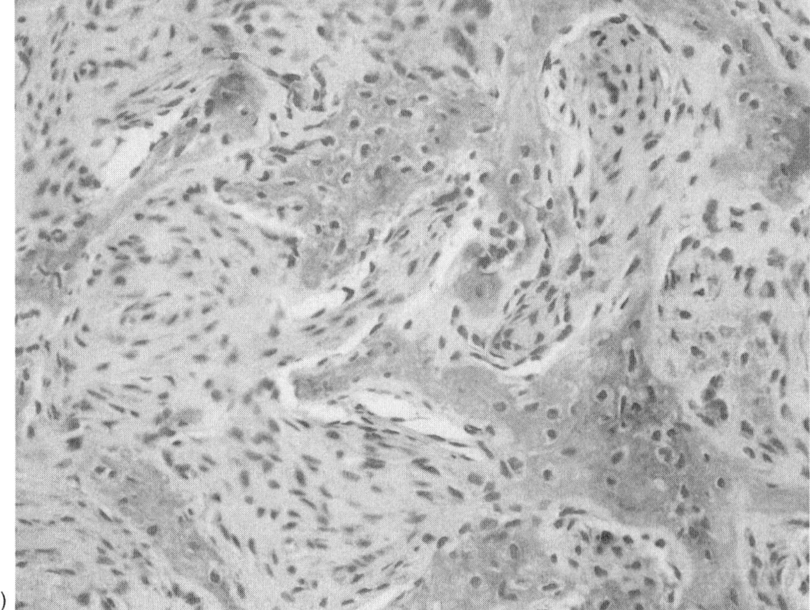

Figure 1 Fibrous dysplasia. A young woman presented with a 6-month history of severe headaches followed by diminished vision in the left eye. A computed tomography scan (**A**) revealed a mass in the sphenoid sinus displacing the left optic nerve with a differential diagnosis of chordoma versus chondrosarcoma. A transnasal biopsy (**B**) revealed irregular trabeculae of woven bone in a fibrocellular matrix, consistent with fibrous dysplasia.

adjacent tissues. Lesions of similar appearance occurring within the gnathic bones are called either "cementifying fibroma" or "cemento-osseous fibroma," depending on the absence or presence of osseous trabeculae.

The importance of trying to distinguish ossifying fibroma from fibrous dysplasia stems from differences in management. The treatment of choice for ossifying fibroma is en bloc resection, which limits local recurrence (118,152). Curettage or conservative excision has historically been utilized for foci of fibrous dysplasia that compromise functions or cause deformity, pain, or fracture. When involving the orbit, ossifying fibroma generally manifests as a slow-growing, painless mass with associated globe displacement and proptosis (8,64,78,103,128,152). The frontal bone is most commonly involved, followed by the ethmoidal and maxillary bones. Most tumors attain a significant size (up to 5 cm in diameter) for which orbitocranial or orbitorhinological approaches are necessary for complete excision.

Fibrous dysplasia may affect one (monostotic) or multiple (polyostotic) bones. Furthermore, the polyostotic form may be associated with cutaneous pigmentation and endocrine disorders, of which sexual precocity is most common (McCune–Albright syndrome) (MIM #174800). Most cases involving the orbit are of the monostotic form (9,112,128,152). The frontal bone is most frequently involved, followed by the sphenoid and ethmoid bones. Proptosis, globe displacement, and facial asymmetry are the most frequent presentations. However, diplopia, cranial nerve palsies, raised intracranial pressure, and nasal

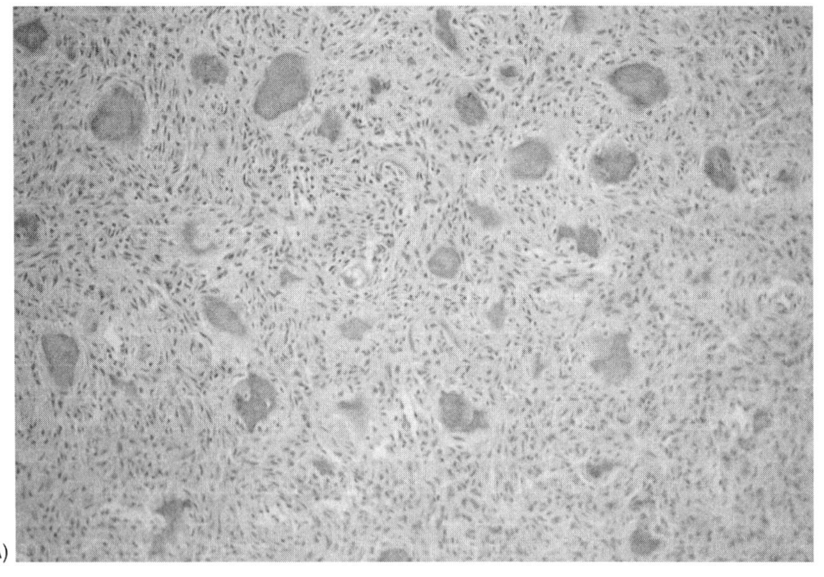

(A)

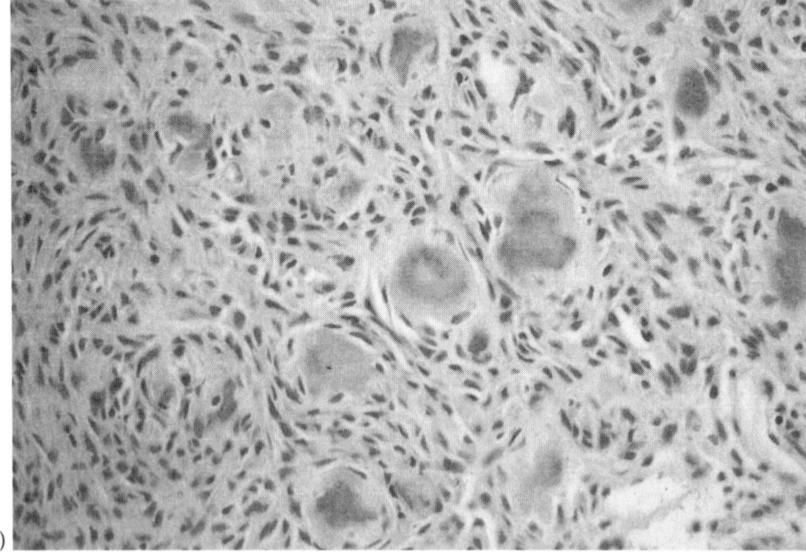

(B)

Figure 2 Psammomatoid ossifying fibroma. (**A**) A tumor removed from the orbit of a 28-year-old woman shows structures resembling psammoma bodies and cementum within a cellular stroma. (**B**) The spindle-shaped cells are moderately pleomorphic and arranged in whorls.

obstruction have all been reported secondary to orbital fibrous dysplasia. These lesions demonstrate slow growth and may spontaneously involute. Malignant transformation to osteosarcoma, chondrosarcoma, fibrosarcoma, and giant cell-rich sarcoma has been documented and the risk increases from 0.5% to 15% following radiotherapy.

Although characterized by the arrest of bone maturation in the woven bone stage, hence the use of the term dysplasia, recent molecular findings suggest that fibrous dysplasia may be a neoplasm (22). Activating *GNAS1* mutations have been identified in both polyostotic and monostotic forms. These mutations lead to increased cyclic adenosine monophosphate (cAMP) levels that may in turn result in high levels of c-*fos*, which have also been detected in fibrous dysplasia. In studies of transgenic mice, overexpression of c-*fos* has resulted in bony lesions that closely resemble fibrous dysplasia. Most mutations occur sporadically and in postzygotic somatic cells. Whether an individual develops monostotic or polyostotic disease is dependent on the size of the cell mass during embryogenesis when the mutation occurs and the location of the mutation within the cell mass (22).

The pathogenesis of ossifying fibroma is less clear. Sawyer et al. identified identical chromosomal breakpoints occurring in three separate cases of (cemento-) ossifying fibromas of the orbit involving bands on the X-chromosome and chromosome 2 (Xq26 and 2q33) suggesting a role in the pathogenesis of this tumor (124). Another unexplored and interesting possibility is the role of *HRPT2* in the pathogenesis of ossifying fibromas. *HRPT2* has been identified as the tumor-suppressor gene responsible for the hyperparathyroidism-jaw tumor syndrome (hyperparathyroidism type 2) (MIM #145001). In this autosomal-dominant syndrome, patients develop parathyroid tumors and "jaw tumors" that have been variably called cementifying fibroma, ossifying fibroma, cemento-ossifying fibroma, and ossifying jaw fibroma. Linkage analysis has assigned the *HRPT2* gene to chromosome 1 at the q21–q31 region. The *HRPT2* gene encodes a 531 amino acid tumor suppressor called parafibromin. Although *HRPT2* mutations have been identified in the parathyroid carcinomas, to date the presence of *HRPT2* mutations in the ossifying fibromas has not been investigated (1,97).

Cherubism

A reactive, fibro-osseous disorder that primarily affects the jaws, cherubism (MIM #118400) derives its name from the characteristic facial appearance of affected patients whose marked fullness of cheeks and upward gaze bear a striking resemblance to the cherubs depicted in Baroque art (24). This disease is most often inherited in an autosomal-dominant fashion, although sporadic cases and autosomal recessive inheritance patterns have also been documented (72,89). Regardless of the inheritance pattern, affected individuals appear normal at birth and do not typically develop signs of the disease until the second or third year of life (69,126). Males appear to be affected twice as often as females possibly due to variable penetrance (100% in males, 50–70% in females) and expressivity, the latter ranging from subclinical disease to classic cherubism. Besides the characteristic findings of bilateral expansion of the mandible and maxilla and upward gaze, other abnormalities include: irregular deciduous teeth that are misplaced, malformed, become loose and are lost early; bilateral chronic enlargement of the submandibular lymph nodes; and a narrow high arched palate. Ocular manifestations of cherubism include increased visibility of the sclera and proptosis and are attributable either to lower eyelid retraction from diffuse enlargement of the lower half of the face or to upward displacement of the eyes from a mass involving the orbital floor (24,69,72,89,126,143). Decreased visual acuity secondary to optic nerve compression has been documented. Imaging studies alone are virtually diagnostic and may allow early recognition of disease. Plain radiographs reveal irregular, multilocular, bilateral, well demarcated, lucent, cystic lesions causing bony expansion. A thinned but intact cortex remains and there is no periosteal reaction. Teeth are often displaced or unerupted and may appear to float within cyst-like spaces. Clinical laboratory measurements, in particular serum calcium and parathyroid hormone levels, are usually normal, although alkaline phosphatase may be elevated secondary to osteolysis.

Although initially thought to be a severe form of fibrous dysplasia, biopsy of the lesions of cherubism reveals histologic features that are similar to those of giant cell reparative granuloma. The distinction between cherubism, giant cell reparative granuloma, and giant cell tumor of bone is based mainly on the extent of the lesion (72). The lesions of cherubism gradually progress until puberty at which point growth stops and involution begins, such that most patients eventually have relatively normal faces (138). Because of the tendency to spontaneous involution, conservative therapy has been recommended. However, removal of teeth and curettage may stimulate this process. Compared to other giant cell-rich lesions of the gnathic bones, recurrence is rare. At the molecular level, Ueki et al. (147) have identified different point mutations in the SH3-binding protein SH3BP2 encoded by a gene on chromosome 4 (4p16.3), which provides compelling evidence for the role of this protein in the pathogenesis of at least a subset of cases of cherubism. They postulated that mutations in the protein may lead to a gain of function or act in a dominant-negative manner and that the onset of cherubism and its organ-restricted characteristics may be related to the process of dental development in children. In the presence of altered SH3BP2, signaling pathways involved in coordinating osteoclast and osteoblast activity in the mandible and maxilla that are essential for normal eruption of secondary teeth could be disrupted, resulting in cherubism.

Myxoma

Myxomas are benign neoplasms with a gross gelatinous appearance owing to their high content of myxoid ground substance. They occur most frequently in soft tissues but may also arise within bones, most commonly the mandible and maxilla with very rare cases occurring in extragnathic bones (15,74,83,86,100,113,120,136). Two cases of intraosseous myxomas arising in the posterolateral orbital wall with extension into both the orbit and cranial cavity have been documented (15,86). Both patients presented with swelling, proptosis, and discomfort of the affected eye without diplopia or loss of visual acuity. Additionally, Landa et al. reported a recurrent myxoma of the zygoma with associated mild proptosis (74). Radiographically, the lesions were well-circumscribed and osteolytic. CT imaging revealed lesions of soft tissue density without evidence of bone matrix production. There was focal destruction of bone but no periosteal reaction.

Grossly, the tumors have a gray-white appearance and a slimy, mucoid consistency. Histologically, the characteristic features of myxomas include the presence of scattered spindled to stellate cells with bland nuclear features set in a prominent background of extracellular acid mucin, a loose network of reticulin fibers with sparse mature collagen fibers, and a poorly developed vasculature. Ultrastructural examination of myxomas discloses cells with features of fibroblasts and myofibroblasts (100). Myxoma is a diagnosis of exclusion as myxoid change can be seen in virtually all bone or soft tissue tumors and the immunophenotype (with expression of vimentin and occasionally actin) is nonspecific. Much of the evidence suggests that myxomas arise from modified fibroblasts, which produce excessive quantities of extracellular acid mucin. The occasional association with fibrous dysplasia (Mazabraud syndrome) suggests an underlying error in tissue metabolism but whether intraosseous myxomas arise from dental (odontogenic) or nondental (osteogenic) tissue is still a matter of controversy (100,136).

While myxomas appear grossly circumscribed, local infiltration into adjacent cortical bone or soft tissues is often present. This may account for the significant local recurrence rate associated with intraosseous myxomas and adequate surgical margins and long-term follow-up are recommended (15,74,86). Little is known of the pathogenesis of intraosseous myxoma although activating mutations in the Arg 201 codon of the *GNAS* gene encoding the alpha subunit of stimulatory guanine nucleotide G proteins that stimulate cAMP formation, have been recognized in McCune–Albright syndrome (MIM #174800), and isolated fibrous dysplasia (108). These mutations have also been identified in intramuscular myxomas but interestingly not in juxta-articular myxomas suggesting that different types of myxoma may be distinct despite their histological similarities (107).

Myofibroma/Myofibromatosis

Presenting as painless nodules, most frequently at birth or within the first 2 years of life, these myofibroblastic proliferations are one of the most common "fibrous" tumors of childhood (18,41). Clinically, two distinct forms are recognized, with presentation as either a solitary nodule (myofibroma) or multiple nodules (myofibromatosis), the latter ranging in number from a few to greater than 50 (41). Most solitary myofibromas arise within the dermis and subcutaneous tissue of the head and neck (18,41), but rare cases of isolated bone lesions have been reported (37). In myofibromatosis, dermal and subcutaneous lesions again predominate, although skeletal muscle and bone lesions are also frequent. Although newborns, infants, and children are predominantly affected, both solitary and multifocal myofibromas have been reported in adults (18,41,150).

Several cases involving orbital bone, soft tissue, or both, have been documented (14,25,41,52,105, 131,139,141,144,150,154). Most reported lesions have been solitary but the orbit has also been involved as a part of multifocal disease (105). Frontal, sphenoid, and zygomatic bones have been involved (25,37,52,131) and affected individuals have variably presented with proptosis and a firm, painless mass. CT imaging typically reveals a heterogeneous, well-circumscribed mass with moderate vascularity (73,81).

Macroscopically, most lesions are small (at most several centimeters in diameter), unencapsulated but circumscribed, firm with a rubbery consistency, and have a cut-surface with a whorled, fascicular appearance. Microscopically, all lesions have a similar biphasic appearance. Spindle cells with abundant eosinophilic cytoplasm are arranged in fascicles and resemble smooth muscle. In addition there is a population of more primitive, small, round cells, or spindle cells with limited cytoplasm that is associated with a prominent hemangiopericytoma-like vascular pattern. This primitive component is typically central and surrounded by the better differentiated fascicles of myofibroblasts. Intravascular growth is a well-documented feature and should not be mistaken for a sign of malignancy. The better differentiated areas express vimentin, smooth muscle actin and occasionally desmin, consistent with their myofibroblastic nature. Actin is also expressed within the primitive areas but is typically more focal and weaker.

Local recurrence following simple excision is uncommon and the prognosis for individuals with multifocal disease with visceral involvement is poor and, for this reason, once a diagnosis of myofibroma is rendered, imaging studies should be immediately performed to determine whether visceral involvement is present. Although most cases of myofibromatosis are sporadic, rare incidents of affected cousins, half-siblings, and parent–offspring pairs suggests in some cases an autosomal-dominant inheritance pattern. As the majority of lesions are small, asymptomatic, and tend to disappear spontaneously, it is difficult to determine the significance of this.

BENIGN BONE NEOPLASMS

Intraosseous Hemangioma

Hemangiomas account for less than 1% of all detected primary bone tumors (35). While the majority arise within the vertebral bodies, the temporal and parietal bones of the skull are the next most common sites (35). Hemangiomas involving the orbital bones account for less than 5% of cranial intraosseous hemangiomas (4,13,23,56,59,98,122,142,143). Affected individuals are usually in their third to fifth decades and typically present with a slow-growing, nontender, bony mass that may, depending on its size and location, cause proptosis, globe displacement, diplopia, loss of vision, optic atrophy, papilledema, and ptosis. Plain film images characteristically reveal a lucent, well-demarcated, intraosseous defect that expands the bone and has a bubbly or trabeculated appearance described as a honeycomb or sunburst pattern. While the cortex is often expanded and thinned, it remains intact and soft tissue extension is not present. CT imaging demonstrates similar features but is better for assessing the cortex and periosteum (4,98,122,142). Although the above features are diagnostic, they are not present in all lesions. The differential diagnosis of a well-circumscribed, intraosseous lesion in this region includes: fibrous dysplasia, dermoid cyst, meningioma, eosinophilic granuloma, metastatic carcinoma, and multiple myeloma and biopsy or complete excision will often be required for definitive diagnosis, particularly for isolated lesions. Preoperative angiography may be useful to confirm the vascular nature of the lesion (4,98).

The gross appearance of intraosseous hemangioma is that of a dark, loose, friable, spongy lesion (4,23,35). As in other parts of the body hemangiomas have been divided microscopically into capillary and cavernous types based on the size of the constituent blood vessels (see Chapter 62). However, a mixture of blood vessels of various sizes is usually present and classification is somewhat arbitrary and, more importantly, bears no significance on treatment and outcome. Regardless of histological subtype, all the blood vessels within hemangiomas have flat to plump endothelial cells without atypia and mitotic activity. A lobular growth pattern is present, indicative of a benign vascular tumor. A complex, anastomosing, invasive growth pattern, solid sheets of epithelioid or spindle cells with nuclear atypia and mitotic activity should suggest a more aggressive lesion such as a hemangioendothelioma or angiosarcoma. Papillary endothelial hyperplasia (Masson-type change) can also be present and should not be mistaken for malignancy (35). Thromboses and calcifications may be identified, particularly in cavernous hemangiomas. The intervascular connective tissue may show myxoid change and residual cancellous bone is usually thickened.

Osteoma

Osteomas are largely confined to the craniofacial skeleton, with a prevalence approaching 1% in imaging studies. They are more common in men and below the age of 50 years. Most arise from the frontal and ethmoid sinuses and may secondarily extend into the orbit pushing before them a covering of sinus mucosa, although isolated osteomas of the orbital bones also occur. Overall, osteomas comprise approximately 1% of orbital tumors. Multiple osteomas of the facial bones are usually associated with Gardner syndrome (MIM +175100) (84).

The presenting symptoms of sinonasal osteomas depend on their location and size. Frontal sinus osteomas generally cause headaches and ethmoidal osteomas nasal discharge. Tumors that involve the orbit may produce ocular symptoms and signs, such as proptosis, pain on ocular movement, and diminution of visual acuity. Transient amaurosis has occasionally been described (155).

Osteomas are generally classified according to their histological appearance into ivory osteomas, composed of compact bone with small Haversian systems and a scanty, hypocellular stroma and mature osteomas composed of cancellous bone with a more cellular stroma, bony trabeculae rimmed by osteoblasts and osteoclasts and often dilated, thin-walled blood vessels. It is well known that osseous lesions of the sinonasal region are difficult to differentiate and that individual tumors may show several histological patterns (45). Mature osteomas may be difficult to distinguish from ossifying fibroma or fibrous dysplasia. Ivory osteomas are easily recognized and are particularly found in the calvarium, with less dense lesions more common in the facial bones. The compact bone is often of woven as well as lamellar type.

In general, osteomas range in size from 1 to 5 cm in diameter and small tumors are often asymptomatic. Tumors may be round with a smooth surface or be bosselated. Their color varies from white (ivory) to pink-tan, depending on the proportion of compact bone within the lesion (Fig. 3). They are benign, with a limited potential for extension or recurrence after incomplete removal. Small, asymptomatic tumors may be observed but larger symptomatic tumors should be removed by open surgery or endonasal endoscopic resection (104).

There is still debate over the true nature of osteomas. Although those in the mature category may resemble an osteoblastoma and appear neoplastic, the hypocellular ivory type may represent osseous hamartomas. The increased incidence after puberty and the common location at the junction of frontal and ethmoid sinuses suggests a developmental origin. There is evidence that trauma may trigger the growth of the lesions and inflammation may also play a role (87). Similar mechanisms may underlie the occasional occurrence of osteomas within the orbital and periocular soft tissue (61).

Osteoblastoma

Osteoid osteoma, osteoblastoma, and aggressive osteoblastoma represent a continuum of benign bone-forming lesions with increasing growth potential (30). Of the three, osteoid osteoma is the most common, has the most limited growth potential, usually measures less than 1 cm in diameter, and occurs predominantly in the long tubular bones of the

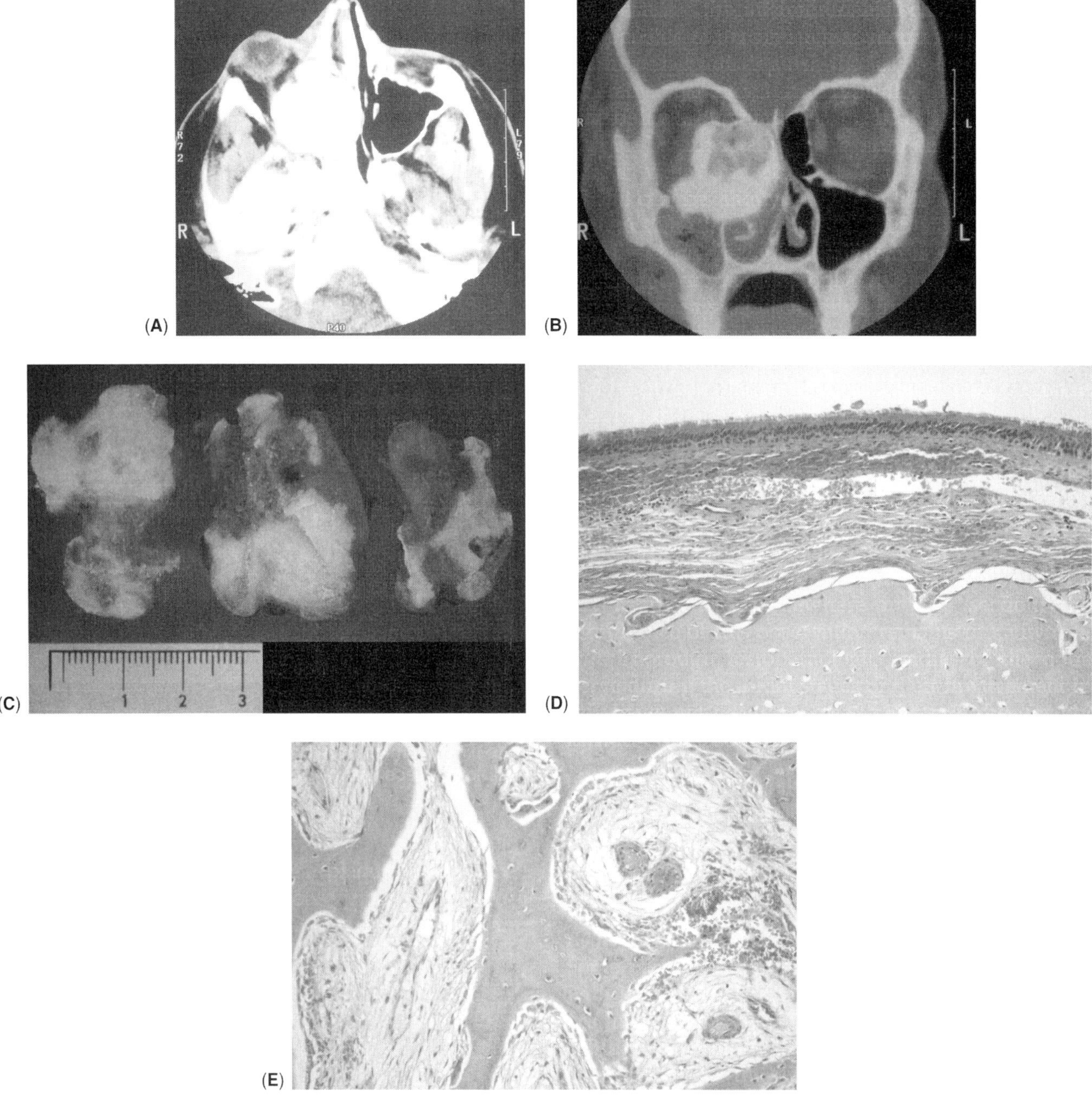

Figure 3 Sino-orbital osteoma. A 14-year-old boy presented with proptosis and a transient loss of vision on looking to the right. A CT scan confirmed the presence of a calcified mass of variable density in the right ethmoid sinus extending into the medial orbit, maxillary antrum, and nasal passage (**A, B**). Sections through the excised bony mass show dense (ivory) and mature areas (**C**), corresponding to compact bone beneath the sinus epithelium (**D**), and cancellous bone (**E**), respectively.

extremities, followed by the small bones of the hands and feet. Osteoid osteoma arising within the craniofacial bones is distinctly uncommon (30). Aggressive osteoblastoma, usually measuring more than 4 cm in diameter and consisting of epithelioid osteoblasts, has not been documented within the orbital bones. In contrast, nearly 20% of osteoblastomas arise within the craniofacial bones (30).

Osteoblastomas of the orbit most often arise in the orbital roof but may secondarily involve the ethmoidal cells, sphenoid bone, and maxillary or frontal sinuses (2,7,19,21,60,76,81,148). Although the age range of affected individuals is broad (3–76 years), most patients are young (mean age of 24 years). A sex predilection is not evident. Growth of osteoblastomas is usually slow but continuous, resulting in painless proptosis and globe displacement. Other symptoms resulting include: periorbital swelling, frontal headaches, visual loss, and, rarely, epileptic seizures and manifestations of increased intracranial pressure. Imaging studies usually reveal a well-demarcated, round/oval, lytic defect surrounded by a rim of reactive sclerosis. On CT images, the lesion has a high bone density but is less dense and more heterogeneous than an ivory osteoma. Intraoperatively, a central nidus is evident which has a red, granular, friable appearance, and is well-circumscribed by sclerotic bone.

The histopathological features of osteoid osteoma and osteoblastoma are virtually identical, consisting of an interlacing network of evenly distributed trabeculae of woven bone in a loose fibroblastic stroma with a prominent vasculature (Fig. 4). The bony trabeculae are lined by plump osteoblasts with reactive nuclear changes that should not be mistaken for evidence of malignancy. Scattered osteoclastic activity is also typical. Mitotic activity is usually low, occasionally brisk, but morphologically normal. Since osteoblastoma and osteoid osteoma have identical histology, distinction between them relies heavily on tumor location and size, the presence of pain relieved by aspirin (typical of osteoid osteoma) and the amount of perilesional sclerosis visible on imaging studies (30). Given a local recurrence rate of nearly 25%, en bloc resection of osteoblastoma is the treatment of choice (30). However, in the orbital milieu this is often not achievable particularly if there is cranial base extension (2,21,60). In a review of 13 cases of orbital osteoblastoma, only 2 cases recurred locally and no postoperative deaths or serious deficits were reported (2). Parodi et al. reported an orbital osteoblastoma that was only partially ablated but had not recurred 4 years later (114). Radiotherapy is reserved for cases in which only subtotal resection has been achieved or for unresectable lesions in symptomatic patients. Malignant transformation of osteoblastoma, while extremely rare, is possible and long-term follow-up is recommended (30,42).

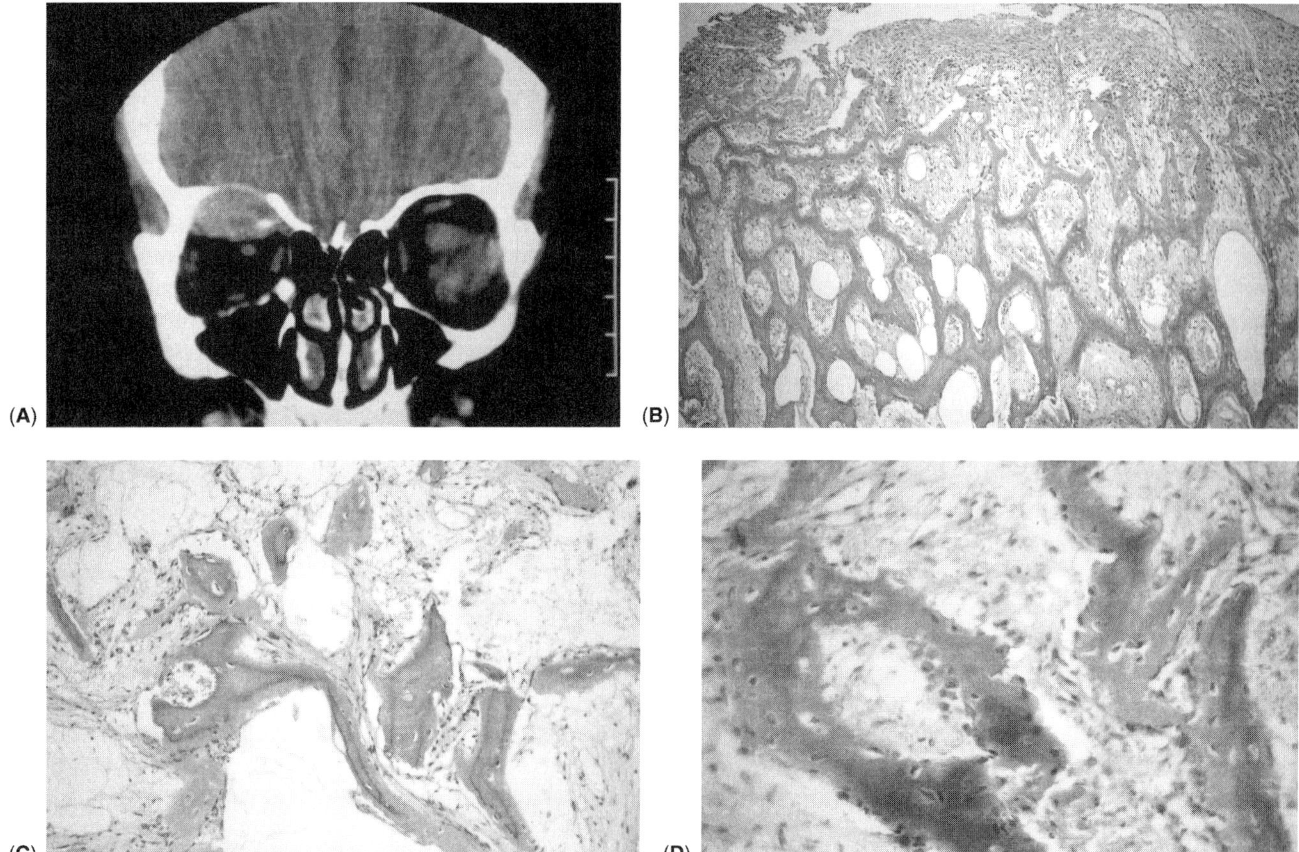

Figure 4 Osteoblastoma. A 60-year-old woman presented with proptosis and a bony defect in the orbital roof (**A**). Histological sections show a network of trabeculae of woven bone with prominent thin-walled blood vessels in the stroma (**B, C**). The trabeculae were lined by plump osteoblasts (**D**).

MALIGNANT BONE NEOPLASMS

Osteosarcoma

Osteosarcoma is the most common primary malignant bone tumor and comprises a large group of malignant neoplasms, which demonstrate diverse biological behavior and histomorphology (70). They are defined by the direct production, at least focally, of osteoid or mineralized bone by tumor cells, without a cartilaginous precursor. The vast majority of osteosarcomas affect young individuals in their second and third decades of life, with a male predominance (31). Most osteosarcomas are primary tumors arising de novo. However, it is well recognized that osteosarcoma can arise secondarily from a number of preexisting bone lesions including fibrous dysplasia, Paget disease of bone (MIM #602080) and chronic osteomyelitis, as well as following radiotherapy or a metallic implant (31). Osteosarcoma may also arise in several clinical settings, including hereditary retinoblastoma (see Chapter 60) (31).

Osteosarcomas can be divided into intramedullary forms, by far the most common, and surface and intracortical forms, both of which are rare. The most frequent sites are the metaphyses of the appendicular skeleton, where the highest rates of bone growth occur, and less than 10% of osteosarcomas affect the craniofacial bones, with mandibular and maxillary involvement accounting for 50% and 25% of cases, respectively (31). A significant number of osteosarcomas of the orbit arise in the setting of long-standing Paget disease of bone (MIM #602080) or following radiotherapy for the treatment of retinoblastoma some 10 to 30 years previously (49,145). Long et al. reported a rare case of osteosarcoma arising within a phthisical eye (80). Imaging features of osteosarcoma are similar regardless of location and typically demonstrate a mixed lytic and sclerotic lesion with evidence of aggressive growth, including frequent breaches of the bony cortex, extension into adjacent soft tissues and structures, and a periosteal reaction (31).

There are several histological variants of osteosarcoma (70). The conventional form often demonstrates areas of osteogenic, chondroblastic, and fibroblastic differentiation within the same lesion. As the diagnosis of osteosarcoma relies on identifying direct osteoid/bone production by tumor cells, which can be focal, generous sampling of lesions is necessary so as to not render an erroneous diagnosis of chondrosarcoma, the treatment of which is significantly different. Less common histological variants of osteosarcoma include small cell osteosarcoma, which mimics other "small blue round cell" tumors and is distinguishable only by the presence of osteoid; telangiectatic osteosarcoma, which resembles aneurysmal bone cyst at low-magnification but is readily distinguished at high magnification by marked cellular atypia; and even rarer osteoblastoma-like, giant cell-rich, and well-differentiated variants that may mimic osteoblastoma, giant cell granuloma, and fibrous dysplasia or ossifying fibroma, respectively.

Osteosarcomas, save for the well-differentiated variant, generally are aggressive neoplasms that are treated by preoperative chemotherapy, wide resection, and postoperative chemotherapy adjusted to the percentage of residual viable tumor identified in the resection specimen (31). While the 5-year survival rate is in the order of 70% for peripheral osteosarcoma, the prognosis for craniofacial osteosarcoma is only 35%, with a negligible 5-year survival rate for osteosarcomas arising in Paget disease of bone (39,49,145).

Almost all osteosarcomas contain complex clonal chromosomal aberrations comprising numerous numerical and structural alterations. Frequently affected chromosomal regions include 1p11–13, 1q11–12, 1q21–22, 11p14–15, 14p11–13, 15p11–13, 17p, and 19q13. However, the karyotypic changes vary from case to case and no specific translocation or any other diagnostically consequential structural alteration has been assigned to conventional osteosarcoma (121).

Ewing Sarcoma

Ewing sarcoma belongs to a large group of tumors that morphologically resemble one another and are collectively referred to as the "small blue round cell" tumors. Although morphological features may aid in their distinction, they are often subtle and ancillary techniques are required to accurately subtype these primitive tumors. Since the biological behavior and treatment of the different tumors vary significantly, exact subtyping is critical. There has been much debate as to the cell of origin or line of differentiation of Ewing sarcoma but currently it is considered a neuroectodermal neoplasm (34). Ewing sarcoma comprises approximately 10% of all primary malignant bone tumors and the great majority of cases occur in children, with a peak incidence between 5 and 13 years of age (34). Only 2% to 3% involve the craniofacial bones (34). Orbital involvement occurs most frequently in the form of a metastasis from distant sites, although several cases of primary orbital Ewing sarcoma, both intraosseous and extraosseous, have been reported (38,128,130,156). The presenting signs and symptoms of these orbital tumors included proptosis, a mass, pain, visual loss, and motility restriction. Imaging studies have shown diffuse, unevenly enhancing lesions with mottled bony destruction, with or without an associated periosteal reaction.

Ewing sarcoma is characterized histologically by sheets and nests of monomorphic cells with scant cytoplasm. The nuclei are small to intermediate in size, with open, fine chromatin, and small nucleoli. Nuclear atypia is mild but mitoses and apopotic cells are numerous. Rosettes, cross-striations, adipocytic differentiation, and bone matrix are not identified. Areas of hemorrhage and necrosis are frequently seen. Histochemical stains reveal significant amounts of intracellular glycogen and a paucity of supportive reticulin fibers. Immunohistochemically, the tumor cells typically demonstrate strong, membranous staining with antibodies against CD99, which reacts with an epitope in the cell surface antigen $p30/32^{MIC2}$, a glycoprotein of unknown function. While this antibody is very sensitive, it is not very specific and a number of other tumors included in the group of "small blue round cell" tumors demonstrate positivity. Therefore, positive staining for CD99 in the absence of staining for epithelial, lymphoma, skeletal muscle, and neuroblastoma markers is necessary to render a diagnosis of Ewing sarcoma. Occasionally the primitive cells express antigens associated with intercellular tight junctions, indicating some degree of epithelial differentiation (125). Transmission electron microscopic (TEM) studies of Ewing sarcoma cells demonstrate few cytoplasmic organelles, large amounts of intracellular glycogen, and sparse and poorly developed cell junctions (34). Neurosecretory granules, prominent cell junctions, and myofilaments are absent. Most cases of Ewing sarcoma are also characterized by the presence of a specific t(11;22) or t (21;22) translocation, which can be detected in paraffin-embedded tissues (34).

Ewing sarcoma is aggressive and frequently metastasizes (34). Once an almost invariably fatal disease, with advances in surgery, radiation therapy, and chemotherapy, the 5-year survival for Ewing sarcoma is currently in the order of 74% (128).

CARTILAGINOUS NEOPLASMS

Enchondroma/Chondroma

Benign, purely cartilaginous tumors of the orbit are exceedingly rare. They may either arise within bone (enchondroma) or within the orbital soft tissues (chondroma), the latter being more common. Orbital chondromas are believed to arise from either the trochlea (65), the only cartilaginous structure in the normal orbit, or from pluripotential orbital mesenchyme (12). Regardless of origin, the clinical, radiographic, and histological features of these cartilaginous lesions are similar (128,152). A slowly growing, painless lump is often noted by patients. Other symptoms depend on the location of the lesion but may include proptosis, headaches, and sinus obstruction. On plain radiographs, enchondromas are usually well-circumscribed, lytic lesions which may expand the bone and cause cortical thinning. However, breach of the cortex, periosteal reaction, and extension into adjacent soft tissue do not occur (116). Similarly, chondromas often appear as circumscribed radiolucencies. CT imaging often discloses intralesional calcifications, which appear as signal voids on MRI.

On gross examination, enchondromas and chondromas are composed of well-demarcated lobules of soft, opalescent-blue to hard and gritty, ivory-white tissue. Microscopically, lobules of hyaline cartilage separated by fibrovascular septa show slightly increased cellularity and more disorderly architecture compared with normal articular cartilage. A lacunar pattern is maintained in that the chondrocytes are round or polyhedral and reside in spaces (lacunae) surrounded by hyaline cartilage. Myxoid areas should not be prominent and, if present, should raise the possibility of chondrosarcoma. Clustering of the chondrocytes is common but spindling of the cells is very limited and, when present, is usually at the periphery of lobules. The chondrocyte nuclei are small with dense chromatin. Mild nuclear atypia and binucleated forms may be seen and should not be interpreted as unequivocal features of malignancy. Mitoses are not identifiable. Unlike chondrosarcomas, enchondromas do not demonstrate infiltrative growth between the bony trabeculae of the medullary cavity but rather have expanding borders with encasement by a rim of lamellar bone.

Because of the rarity of craniofacial chondromas, purely cartilaginous lesions in this region should be viewed with suspicion, since many subsequently prove to be chondrosarcomas (152). Distinguishing enchondroma or chondroma from low-grade chondrosarcoma by histology alone may be impossible and for this reason, complete but conservative surgical excision of all craniofacial cartilaginous tumors is recommended (128,152).

Chondrosarcoma

The second most frequent primary malignant tumor of bone, accounting for a quarter of all primary bone sarcomas, chondrosarcoma comprises a group of heterogeneous lesions. They may be divided into primary and secondary forms, the former arising de novo and the latter arising via malignant transformation of a preexisting benign cartilaginous lesion, most often an enchondroma or osteochondroma, or in relation to underlying Paget disease of bone or previous radiotherapy (32). Chondrosarcomas may be further subdivided based on their location into intramedullary, which comprise the great majority of chondrosarcomas, or as rare surface chondrosarcomas. Further subtyping into conventional, dedifferentiated, clear cell, or mesenchymal forms reflects differences in clinical behavior and morphologic features. More than 90% of chondrosarcomas are of the conventional subtype, consisting of lobules of hyaline cartilage which, depending on their cellularity and degree of nuclear atypia, are classified as grade 1, 2, or 3 (32).

The grade 1 and 2 lesions generally behave indolently, with a propensity for local recurrence when inadequately excised. Metastases usually occur late in the course of the disease. These low- to intermediate-grade neoplasms are most often treated by surgery alone and show little response to radiotherapy or chemotherapy. The grade 3 lesions, on the other hand, have a high metastatic potential and are often treated with combinations of systemic chemotherapy and radiotherapy, in addition to surgical resection (32).

Most chondrosarcomas affect the pelvic and thoracic bones, femur, scapula, and humerus, with only 2% arising in the craniofacial bones, the majority in the skull base (32). The orbit is usually secondarily affected and chondrosarcomas arising within the orbital bone are extremely rare (32,47,123, 128,140,156). Given the predilection for the skull base, patients often present with orbital, paranasal sinus, or pharyngeal symptoms. Patients are usually in their fifth to sixth decade and men are affected twice as often as women (47,123,140). Imaging studies reveal a destructive lesion with an admixture of radiolucent and radiodense areas. A popcorn or ring-like calcification pattern is typical. Expansion of the involved bone and thinning of the cortex is common and periosteal reactions may also occur (32,47,123, 128,140,152).

Grossly, the cartilaginous nature of the lesion is often evident by the presence of multiple translucent, gray-blue lobules, which resemble normal cartilage. Mineralization is grossly appreciable in the form of opaque, chalk-like, or granular and yellow hard areas. Microscopically, although low-grade tumors may resemble enchondromas, there is usually greater cellularity, greater nuclear enlargement and atypia, greater spindling of the tumor cells, myxoid stroma, mitotic activity, and infiltrative growth between medullary trabeculae. However, because of significant overlap of histological features, clinical and radiographic correlation is necessary to accurately diagnose cartilaginous lesions of bone.

Complete resection is necessary to eradicate the disease, although this is often impossible in the case of craniofacial tumors, resulting in frequent local recurrences (47,123,140). The outcome for patients with chondrosarcoma of the craniofacial bones has improved and Ruark et al. reported 43% of their patients to be alive and free of disease 5 years following surgery (123). The most common cause of death was uncontrolled local disease. Poorer prognosis was associated with incomplete excision and high-grade lesions. A poor prognosis is also associated with overexpression of cyclooxygenase (cox)-2, which correlates with the histological grade (40). Surgery, with the intent of obtaining histologically clear margins at the first attempt, remains the most effective treatment for chondrosarcoma.

Occasionally, areas within low-grade conventional chondrosarcomas may undergo malignant progression to high-grade sarcoma, resulting in the juxtaposition of both components within the same lesion (32). This phenomenon is known as dedifferentiation and may occur in chondrosarcoma at any site, including the orbit (118). Acceleration of tumor growth or a new onset of pain often herald dedifferentiation, which may be appreciated by the presence of purely lytic areas with a complete loss of bony architecture or a permeative growth pattern within a lesion which otherwise demonstrates the characteristic imaging features of chondrosarcoma (32). The dedifferentiated component is much more biologically aggressive and can take the form of malignant fibrous histiocytoma, osteosarcoma, fibrosarcoma, rhabdomyosarcoma or, rarely, angiosarcoma. Dedifferentiated chondrosarcoma metastasizes with alacrity and long-term survival rates are dismal (32).

Because of its frequent occurrence in the craniofacial bones, mesenchymal chondrosarcoma warrants particular consideration (16,62,129,132,133). This variant has a biphasic appearance and is characterized by the presence of nodules of low-grade conventional chondrosarcoma surrounded by large number of primitive small blue round cells. Evidence suggests that the latter component has phenotypic features corresponding to the early condensational phase of cartilaginous differentiation (75,151). Mesenchymal chondrosarcoma affects younger patients and is more aggressive (32). The tumors may arise within bone or soft tissues at most sites in the body. Tuncer et al. identified 17 cases of orbital mesenchymal chondrosarcoma in a literature review and found the mean age of presentation was 25 years (range 10–84 years), with a female preponderance (72%) (146). To this series they added a case presenting in a newborn. Although imaging studies may suggest the cartilaginous nature of the lesion (71), biopsy is needed to confirm the diagnosis, which in most cases is straightforward. With limited tissue sampling, the diagnosis may be more difficult, particularly if only the small blue round cell component has been sampled, in which case the differential diagnosis includes the spectrum of small blue round cell tumors. Immunohistochemical studies will help to rule out several tumors in the differential diagnosis and expression of collagen type II in the tumor matrix has been postulated as a specific marker of mesenchymal chondrosarcoma (101). Mesenchymal chondrosarcomas are frequently CD99 positive and caution must be taken not to interpret CD99 immunopositivity as unequivocal evidence for a Ewing sarcoma. Antibodies against SOX9, a transcription factor and master regulator of chondrogenesis, have also been shown to be potentially useful in diagnosis (151). Mesenchymal chondrosarcoma is considered a high-grade tumor and is treated primarily with a combination of surgery and chemotherapy (32). In contrast to conventional chondrosarcoma, it is moderately responsive to systemic chemotherapy. The prognosis for this form of chondrosarcoma is poor, with reported survival rates at 5 and 10 years of 54.6% and 27.3%, respectively (146). Long-term follow-up is recommended as metastases can occur more than 20 years after initial surgery (32).

MISCELLANEOUS NEOPLASMS

Oral Melanotic Neuroectodermal Tumor of Infancy

The oral melanotic neuroectodermal tumor of infancy (OMNTI) is a rare unusual tumor of infancy, with only two cases identified over a 20-year period at the Children's Hospital of Philadelphia (119). Over 90% of cases occur in the head and neck region and of these approximately 80% arise in the maxilla. At least four cases with orbital involvement have been reported (73). Of particular interest to ophthalmic pathologists, the histological appearance of the tumor bears a startling resemblance to the primitive optic vesicle and has been given names such as retinal anlage tumor and pigmented retinal choristoma.

Over 90% of cases of OMNTI occur in infants less than 1-year-old and there is no definite sex predilection. In the maxilla the tumor presents as a purple, soft tissue swelling beneath intact mucosa. It may be noted at birth but, if not clinically pigmented, it may only be detected when there are feeding problems. Imaging studies reveal an intraosseous radiolucency with poorly demarcated margins. There may be calcification within the tumor and, because of its locally aggressive growth, there is often displacement of primary teeth. CT imaging provides the best delineation of the extent of the tumor. Despite the characteristic clinical presentation, an incisional biopsy is usually performed before resection is undertaken. Definitive treatment involves either local excision with curettage or en bloc resection. Reconstructive surgery may be required around 6 years of age when the permanent teeth begin to erupt. Chemotherapy and radiotherapy are generally regarded as ineffective.

Histologically, the tumor is composed of two types of cells in a dense fibrous stroma (Fig. 5). Small "neuroblastic" cells with hyperchromatic nuclei and scanty cytoplasm are partially surrounded by larger epithelioid cells with vesicular nuclei and abundant cytoplasm. The epithelioid cells contain melanin granules of elliptical shape, similar to those in the retinal pigment epithelium (RPE). Further similarity with RPE is indicated by their propensity to form tubular and alveolar structures and by their expression of both vimentin and cytokeratin 8/18. The aggregates of "neuroblastic" cells may contain delicate neurofibrillary material but do not form rosettes. In general, despite its rapid growth, the tumor does not display necrosis, nuclear atypia, or mitotic activity.

Although the two cell types are different, there is considerable overlap in immunophenotype and evidence from cell culture studies suggests that they may not be distinct in origin (6,29,67,95). Both express neural markers such as PGP 9.5, synaptophysin and neuron-specific enolase but only the epithelioid cells express cytokeratins, vimentin, and HMB45. Occasional tumors may express S100 protein, but the neuroblastoma marker NB84 is not expressed (6). In a study of eight examples of OMNTI, Barrett et al. identified one that expressed CD99, the marker of primitive neuroectodermal tumors, on the membranes of the epithelial cells and, to a lesser extent, the "neuroblastic" cells (6). This particular tumor had a less-differentiated epithelial component, a high mitotic count (7 per 10 high power fields) and a high proliferative fraction (25% of both small and large cells were Ki67-positive). This tumor's natural history was also aggressive: following initial excision, the tumor recurred within 1 month and expanded quickly to involve the entire upper jaw, necessitating a bilateral maxillectomy.

The behavior of OMNTI is generally unpredictable. Although occasional tumors can be large enough to cause severe disfigurement (11), they usually do not exceed 4 cm in diameter, and size does not appear to influence prognosis (67). No histological features have been clearly linked to outcome although aneuploidy may be an indicator of likely recurrence (67). The overall recurrence rate is 10% to 15% and recurrences are thought to grow more aggressively. Metastases may occur in about 7% of cases and are composed of the "neuroblastic" element; they may be widespread and cause death within a few months.

Since the tumor was first described, there has been controversy over its histogenesis. There is little support for either an odontogenic or melanocytic origin and OMNTI is now regarded as a congenital dysembryogenetic neoplasm arising from neural crest cells that recapitulates the early stages of retinal

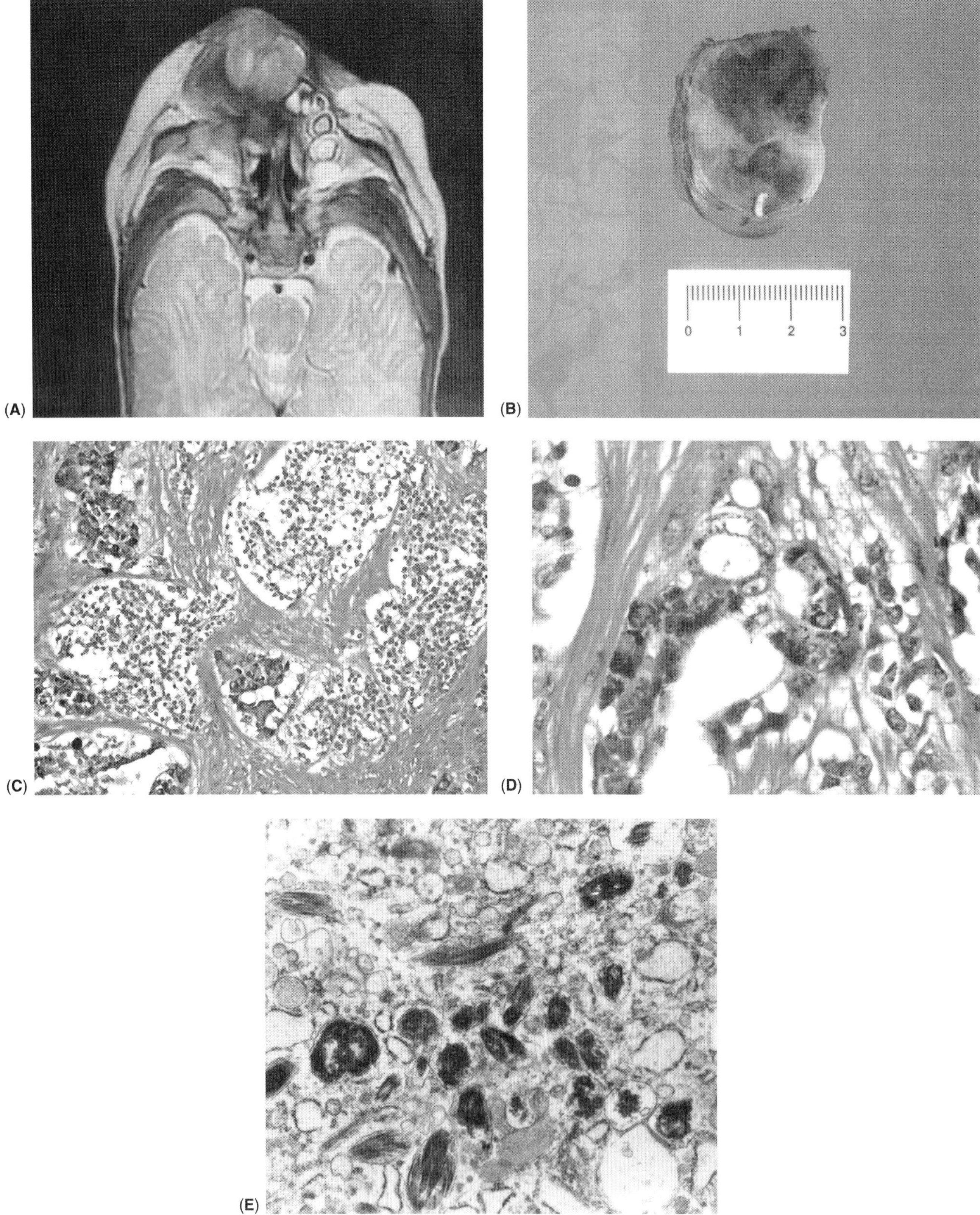

Figure 5 Oral melanotic neuroectodermal tumor of infancy. A 2-month-old boy presented with a mass in the maxilla (**A**) that infiltrated the floor of the orbit. The maxillary alveolus was expanded by a tumor with a blue-black cut surface, which surrounded a primary tooth (**B**). Histological sections revealed a biphasic tumor composed of small "neuroblastic" cells and large pigmented epithelioid cells (**C, D**). By transmission electron microscopy, the melanin granules within the epithelioid cells had an elliptical shape resembling those of retinal pigment epithelium cells (**E**).

development (29). The name retinal anlage tumor has fallen out of favor because the eyes in these patients are normal and it is unlikely that sequestration of developing retina within the maxilla would occur when this develops after retinal morphogenesis is complete. Zimmerman proposed the name pigmented retinal choristoma but the neoplastic behavior of the lesion makes this unsuitable (158). It is difficult to explain the origin of a neoplasm that resembles a collection of microscopic optic vesicles but transformation of a displaced anterior neuroepithelial anlage remains a possibility.

Chordoma

This low-grade malignant bone tumor, although rare (annual incidence of only 1 per million), has excited considerable interest because of its unusual anatomical distribution and histopathology. It originates within the axial skeleton and is thought to arise from remnants of the notochord. The average age of diagnosis is in the fifth decade, although patients with tumors arising in the base of skull, approximately 35% of the total, are generally about 10 years younger (5). When located in the clivus the tumor may extend to the sella turcica and produce disturbances of ocular function, such as an abducent nerve palsy, and visual field defects. Invasion of orbital bone is secondary, although an ectopic chordoma arising in the sphenozygomatic portion of the orbital wall has been described (99).

Although the large lobular tumors in the sacrococcygeal region may be resectable, those at the base of the skull are generally removed piecemeal. Microscopically, the conventional type of chordoma consists of epithelioid cells arranged in sheets and cords in an abundant mucinous stroma. Large epithelioid cells (physaliferous cells) contain large cytoplasmic mucin vacuoles and uniform nuclei, whereas smaller cells have eosinophilic cytoplasm and pleomorphic nuclei. The cells express a variety of keratins and other epithelial antigens, which may help in distinguishing the tumor from a chondrosarcoma (106). The chondroid variant contains areas of hyaline cartilage as well as more conventional chordoma cells and is more frequently found at the skull base. The cartilage may appear histologically benign or malignant. The distinction of chondroid from conventional chordoma is of no clinical significance but the true nature of the lesion remains intriguing. Some probably represent unrecognized chondrosarcomas and others may be examples of divergent differentiation. The dedifferentiated variant, in which the conventional chordoma is accompanied by a malignant mesenchymal component, may arise spontaneously or following radiotherapy. This variant has a poorer prognosis with frequent local recurrences and ultimately death from metastases (5).

The recognition of the existence of benign notochordal cell tumors has provided fresh insight into the histogenesis of chordoma. Yamaguchi et al. have described intraosseous collections of epithelioid cells with vacuolated or eosinophilic cytoplasm without associated myxoid matrix (157). The cells express epithelial markers, vimentin and S100 protein, as do the cells of the conventional chordoma. In addition to these microscopic tumors, there were small extraosseous tumors with an infiltrative growth pattern, in which the cells were more atypical cytologically and were associated with a myxoid intercellular matrix. These extraosseous tumors were designated incipient chordomas, to indicate their miniature size and their intermediate position in the transformation of a benign notochordal cell tumor into a classic chordoma (56).

REFERENCES

1. Aldred MJ, Talacko AA, Savarirayan R, et al. Dental findings in a family with hyperparathyroidism—jaw tumor syndrome and a novel HRPT2 gene mutation. Oral Surg Oral Med Oral Pathol Oral Radiol Endod 2006; 101:212–8.
2. Akhaddar A, Gazzaz M, Rimani M, et al. Benign fronto-orbital osteoblastoma arising from the orbital roof: case report and literature review. Surg Neurol 2004; 61: 391–7.
3. Arat YO, Chaudhry IA, Boniuk M. Orbitofrontal cholesterol granuloma: distinct diagnostic features and management. Ophthal Plast Reconstr Surg 2003; 19:382–7.
4. Banerji D, Inao S, Sugita K, et al. Primary intraosseous orbital hemangioma: a case report and review of the literature. Neurosurgery 1994; 35:1131–4.
5. Barnes LM. Chordoma. In: Barnes L, ed. Surgical Pathology of the Head and Neck. New York: Marcel Dekker, 2001:1151–6.
6. Barrett AW, Morgan M, Ramsay AD, et al. A clinicopathologic and immunohistochemical analysis of melanotic neuroectodermal tumor of infancy. Oral Surg Oral Med Oral Pathol Oral Radiol Endod 2002; 93:688–98.
7. Batay F, Savas A, Ugur HC, et al. Benign osteoblastoma of the orbital part of the frontal bone: case report. Acta Neurochir 1998; 140:729–30.
8. Baumann I, Zimmermann R, Dammann F, et al. Ossifying fibroma of the ethmoid involving the orbit and the skull base. Otolaryngol Head Neck Surg 2005; 133:158–9.
9. Bibby K, McFadzean R. Fibrous dysplasia of the orbit. Br J Ophthamol 1994; 78:266–70.
10. Boedeker CC, Kayser G, Jurgen G, et al. Giant-cell reparative granuloma of the temporal bone: a case report and review of the literature. Ear Nose Throat J 2003; 82: 926–9.
11. Bouckaert MMR, Raubenheimer EJ. Gigantiform melanotic neuroectodermal tumor of infancy. Oral Surg Oral Med Oral Pathol Oral Radiol Endod 1998; 86: 569–72.

12. Bowen JH, Christensen FH, Klintworth GK, et al. A clinicopathologic study of a cartilaginous hamartoma of the orbit: a rare cause of proptosis. Ophthalmology 1981; 88:1356–60.
13. Brackup AH, Haller ML, Danber MM. Hemangioma of the bony orbit. Am J Ophthalmol 1980; 90:258–61.
14. Campbell RJ, Garrity JA. Juvenile fibromatosis of the orbit: a case report with review of the literature. Br J Ophthalmol 1991; 75:313–6.
15. Candy EJ, Miller NR, Carson BS. Myxoma of bone involving the orbit. Arch Ophthalmol 1991; 109: 919–20.
16. Cardenas-Ramirez L, Albores-Saavedra J, de Buen S. Mesenchymal chondrosarcoma of the orbit: report of the first case in orbital location. Arch Ophthal 1971; 86: 410–3.
17. Carmichael F, Malcolm AJ, Ord RA. Aneurysmal bone cyst of the zygomatic bone. Oral Surg Oral Med Oral Pathol 1989; 68:558–62.
18. Chung EB, Enzinger FM. Infantile myofibromatosis. Cancer 1981; 48:1807–18.
19. Chynn EW, Rubin PA. Metastatic Ewing cell sarcoma of the sinus and osteoid osteoma of the orbit. Am J Ophthalmol 1997; 123:565–7.
20. Citardi MJ, Janjua T, Abrahams JJ, et al. Orbitoethmoid aneurysmal bone cyst. Otolaryngol Head Neck Surg 1996; 114:466–70.
21. Clutter DJ, Leopold DA, Gould LV. Benign osteoblastoma: report of a case and review of the literature. Arch Otolaryngol 1984; 110:334–6.
22. Cohen MM Jr. Fibrous dysplasia is a neoplasm. Am J Med Genet 2001; 98:290–3.
23. Colombo F, Cursiefen C, Hofmann-Rummelt C, et al. Primary intraosseous cavernous hemangioma of the orbit. Am J Ophthalmol 2001; 131:151–2.
24. Colombo F, Cursiefen C, Neukam FW, et al. Orbital involvement in cherubism. Ophthalmology 2001; 108: 1884–8.
25. Cruz AA, Maia, EM, Burmamm TG, et al. Involvement of the bony orbit in infantile myofibromatosis. Ophthal Plast Reconstr Surg 2004; 20:252–4.
26. Dailey R, Gilliland G, McCoy GB. Orbital aneurysmal bone cyst in a patient with renal cell carcinoma. Am J Ophthalmol 1994; 117:643–6.
27. Dal Cin P, Kozakewich HP, Goumnerova L, et al. Variant translocations involving 16q22 and 17p13 in solid variant and extraosseous forms of aneurysmal bone cyst. Genes Chromosomes Cancer 2000; 28:233–4.
28. de Lange J, van Maarle MC, van den Akker HP, et al. DNA analysis of the SH3BP2 gene in patients with aggressive central giant cell granuloma. Br J Oral Maxillofac Surg 2007; 45:499–500.
29. De Oliveira MG, Thompson LDR, Chaves ACM, et al. Management of melanotic neuroectodermal tumor of infancy. Ann Diag Path 2004; 8:207–12.
30. Dorfman HD, Czerniak B. Benign osteoblastic tumors. In: Dorfman HD, Czerniak B, eds. Bone Tumors. St. Louis, MO: Mosby, 1998:85–127.
31. Dorfman HD, Czerniak B. Osteosarcoma. In: Dorfman HD, Czerniak B, eds. Bone Tumors. St. Louis, MO: Mosby, 1998:128–252.
32. Dorfman HD, Czerniak B. Malignant cartilage tumors. In: Dorfman HD, Czerniak B, eds. Bone Tumors. St. Louis, MO: Mosby, 1998:353–440.
33. Dorfman HD, Czerniak B. Giant-cell lesions. In: Dorfman HD, Czerniak B, eds. Bone Tumors. St. Louis, MO: Mosby, 1998:598–604.
34. Dorfman HD, Czerniak B. Ewing's sarcoma and related entities. In: Dorfman HD, Czerniak B, eds. Bone Tumors. St. Louis, MO: Mosby, 1998:607–63.
35. Dorfman HD, Czerniak B. Vascular lesions. In: Dorfman HD, Czerniak B, eds. Bone Tumors. St. Louis, MO: Mosby, 1998:729–46.
36. Dorfman HD, Czerniak B. Cystic lesions. In: Dorfman HD, Czerniak B, eds. Bone Tumors. St. Louis, MO: Mosby, 1998:855–79.
37. Duffy MT, Harris M, Hornblass A. Infantile myofibromatosis of orbital bone. A case report with computed tomography, magnetic resonance imaging, and histologic findings. Ophthalmology 1997; 104:1471–4.
38. Dutton JJ, Rose JG, DeBacker CM, et al. Orbital Ewing's sarcoma of the orbit. Ophthal Plast Reconstr Surg 2000; 16:292–300.
39. Eijpe AA, Koornneef L, Verbeeten B Jr, et al. Cholesterol granuloma of the frontal bone: CT diagnosis. J Comput Assist Tomogr 1990; 14:914–7.
40. Endo M, Matsumura T, Yamaguchi T, et al. Cyclooxygenase-2 overexpression associated with a poor prognosis in chondrosarcomas. Hum Pathol 2006; 37:471–6.
41. Enzinger FM, Weiss SW. Fibrous tumors of infancy and childhood. In: Weiss SW, Goldblum JR, eds. Enzinger and Weiss's Soft Tissue Tumors. 4th ed. St Louis, MO: Mosby; 2001:357–63.
42. Figarella-Branger D, Perez-Castillo M, Garbe L, et al. Malignant transformation of an osteoblastoma of the skull: an exceptional occurrence. J Neurosurg 1991; 75: 138–42.
43. Font RL, Blanco G, Soparkar CN, et al. Giant cell reparative granuloma of the orbit associated with cherubism. Ophthalmology 2003; 110:1846–9.
44. Friedberg SA, Eisenstein R, Wallner LJ. Giant cell lesions involving the nasal accessory sinuses. Laryngoscope 1969; 79:763–76.
45. Fu YS, Perzin KH. Non-epithelial tumors of the nasal cavity, paranasal sinuses and nasopharynx: a clinicopathologic study. II. Osseous and fibro-osseous lesions, including osteoma, fibrous dysplasia, ossifying fibroma, osteoblastoma, giant cell tumor and osteosarcoma. Cancer 1974; 33:1289–305.
46. Fukuta K, Jackson IT. Epidermoid cyst and cholesterol granuloma of the orbit. Br J Plast Surg 1990; 43:521–7.
47. Gadwal SR, Fanburg-Smith JC, Gannon FH, et al. Primary chondrosarcoma of the head and neck in pediatric patients: a clinicopathologic study of 14 cases with a review of the literature. Cancer 2000; 88:2181–8.
48. Gan YC, Mathew B, Salvage D, et al. Aneurysmal bone cyst of the sphenoid sinus. Br J Neurosurg 2001; 15:51–4.
49. Goldberg S, Slamovits TL, Dorfman HD, et al. Sarcomatous transformation of the orbit in a patient with Paget's disease. Ophthalmology 2000; 107:1464–7.
50. Hartstein ME, Grove AS, Woog JJ, et al. The multidisciplinary management of psammomatoid ossifying fibroma of the orbit. Ophthalmology 1998; 105:591–5.
51. Heaton RB, Ross JJ, Jochum JM, et al. Cytologic diagnosis of cholesterol granuloma. A case report. Acta Cytol 1993; 37:713–6.
52. Hidayat AA, Font RL. Juvenile fibromatosis of the periorbital region and eyelid. Arch Ophthalmol 1980; 98:280–5.
53. Hill CA, Moseley IF. Imaging of orbitofrontal cholesterol granuloma. Clin Radiol 1992; 46:237–42.
54. Hino N, Ohtsuka K, Hashimoto M, et al. Radiographic features of an aneurysmal bone cyst of the orbit. Ophthalmologica 1998; 212:198–201.

55. Holzer NJ, Croft CB, Walsh JB, et al. Brown tumor of the orbit. JAMA 1977; 238:1758–9.
56. Hook SR, Font RL, McCrary JA, et al. Intraosseous capillary hemangioma of the frontal bone. Am J Ophthalmol 1987; 103:824–7.
57. Hoopes PC, Anderson RL, Blodi FC. Giant cell (reparative) granuloma of the orbit. Ophthalmology 1981; 88: 1361–6.
58. Hunter JV, Yokoyama C, Moseley IF, et al. Aneurysmal bone cyst of the sphenoid with orbital involvement. Br J Ophthalmol 1990; 74:505–8.
59. Hwang K. Intraosseous hemangioma of the orbit. J Craniofac Surg 2000; 11:386–7.
60. Imai K, Tsujiguchi K, Toda C, et al. Osteoblastoma of the nasal cavity invading the anterior skull base in a young child: case report. J Neurosurg 1997; 87:625–8.
61. Ing EB, Heathcote JG. Congenital isolated osteoma cutis of the lateral canthus. Can J Ophthalmol 2001; 36: 408–10.
62. Jacobs JL, Merriam JC, Chadburn A. Mesenchymal chondrosarcoma of the orbit: report of three new cases and review of the literature. Cancer 1994; 73:399–405.
63. Jaffe HL. Giant cell reparative granuloma, traumatic bone cyst and fibrous (fibro-osseous) dysplasia of the jaw bones. Oral Surg Oral Med Oral Pathol 1953; 6: 159–75.
64. Janecka IP, Housepian E. Cranio-facial approach to ossifying fibromas. Laryngoscope 1985; 95:305–6.
65. Jepson CN, Wetzig PC. Pure chondroma of the trochlea: a case report. Surv Ophthalmol 1966; 11:656–9.
66. Johnson TE, Bergin DJ, McCord CD. Aneurysmal bone cyst of the orbit. Ophthalmology 1988; 95:86–9.
67. Kapadia SB, Frisman DM, Hitchcock CL, et al. Melanotic neuroectodermal tumor of infancy. Clinicopathological, immunohistochemical and flow cytometric study. Am J Surg Pathol 1993; 17:566–73.
68. Karim MM, Inoue M, Hayashi Y, et al. Orbital cholesterol granuloma with destruction of the lateral orbital roof. Jpn J Ophthalmol 2000; 44:179–82.
69. Kaugars GE, Niamtu J III, Svirsky JA. Cherubism: diagnosis, treatment, and comparison with central giant cell granulomas and giant cell tumors. Oral Surg Oral Med Oral Pathol 1992; 73:369–74.
70. Klein MJ, Siegal GP. Osteosarcoma: anatomic and histologic variants. Am J Clin Pathol 2006; 125:555–81.
71. Koeller KK. Mesenchymal chondrosarcoma and simulating lesions of the orbit. Radiol Clin North Am 1999; 37: 203–17.
72. Kozakiewicz M, Perczynska-Partyka W, Kobos J. Cherubism—clinical picture and treatment. Oral Dis 2001; 7:123–30.
73. Lamping KA, Albert DM, Lack E, et al. Melanotic neuroectodermal tumor of infancy. Ophthalmology 1985; 92:143–9.
74. Landa LE, Hedrick MH, Nepomuceno-Perez MC, et al. Recurrent myxoma of the zygoma: a case report. J Oral Maxillofac Surg 2002; 60:704–8.
75. Lefebvre V, de Crombrugghe B. Toward understanding Sox9 function in chondrocyte differentiation. Matrix Biol 1998; 16:529–40.
76. Leone CR Jr, Lawton AW, Leone RT. Benign osteoblastoma of the orbit. Ophthalmology 1988; 95:1554–8.
77. Levine MR, Chu A, Abdul-Karim FW. Brown tumor and secondary hyperparathyroidism. Arch Ophthalmol 1991; 109:847–9.
78. Levine PA, Wiggins R, Archibald RWR, et al. Ossifying fibroma of the head and neck: involvement of the temporal bone—an unusual and challenging site. Laryngoscope 1981; 91:720–5.
79. Loeffler KU, Kommerell G. Cholesterol granuloma of the orbit—pathogenesis and surgical management. Int Ophthalmol 1997; 21:93–8.
80. Long JA, Lolley VR, Kelly AG. Osteogenic sarcoma and phthisis bulbi: a case report. Ophthal Plast Reconstr Surg 2000; 16:75–8.
81. Lowder CY, Berlin AJ, Cox WA, et al. Benign osteoblastoma of the orbit. Ophthalmology 1986; 93:1351–4.
82. Lucarelli MJ, Bilyk JR, Shore JW, et al. Aneurysmal bone cyst of the orbit associated with fibrous dysplasia. Plast Reconstr Surg 1995; 96:440–2.
83. McClure DK, Dahlin DC. Myxoma of bone: report of three cases. Mayo Clin Proc 1977; 52:249–53.
84. McNab AA. Orbital osteoma in Gardner's syndrome. Aust N Z J Ophthalmol 1998; 26:169–70.
85. McNab AA, Wright JE. Orbitobfrontal cholesterol granuloma. Ophthalmology 1990; 97:28–32.
86. Maiuri F, Corriero G, Galicchio B, et al. Myxoma of the skull and orbit. Neurochirurgia 1988; 31:136–8.
87. Ma'luf RN, Ghazi NG, Zein, WM, et al. Orbital osteoma arising adjacent to a foreign body. Ophthal Plast Reconstr Surg 2003; 19:327–30.
88. Mankin HJ, Hornicek FJ, Oriz-Cruz E, et al. Aneurysmal bone cyst: a review of 150 patients. J Clin Oncol 2005; 23: 6756–62.
89. Marck PA, Kudryk WH. Cherubism. J Otolaryngol 1992; 21:84–7.
90. Margo CE, Ragsdale BD, Perman KI, et al. Psammomatoid (juvenile) ossifying fibroma of the orbit. Ophthalmology 1985; 92:150–9.
91. Margo CE, Weiss A, Habal MB. Psammomatoid ossifying fibroma. Arch Ophthalmol 1986; 104:1347–51.
92. Martinez-Gavidia EM, Bagan JV, Milian-Masanet MA, et al. Highly aggressive brown tumour of the maxilla as first manifestation of primary hyperparathyroidism. Int J Oral Maxillofac Surg 2000; 29:447–9.
93. Menon J, Brosnahan DM, Jellinek DA. Aneurysmal bone cyst of the orbit: a case report and review of the literature. Eye 1999; 13:764–8.
94. Mercado GV, Shields CL, Gunduz K, et al. Giant cell reparative granuloma of the orbit. Am J Ophthalmol 1999; 127:485–7.
95. Metwaly H, Chung J, Maruyama S, et al. Establishment and characterization of new cell lines derived from melanotic neuroectodermal tumor of infancy arising in the mandible. Pathol Int 2005; 55:331–42.
96. Miller NR, McCarthy EF, Carter N, et al. Lytic Paget disease as a cause of orbital cholesterol granuloma. Arch Ophthalmol 1999; 117:1084–6.
97. Moon S-D, Park J-H, Kim E-M, et al. A novel IVS2-1G>A mutation causes aberrant splicing of the HRPT2 gene in a family with hyperparathyroidism—jaw tumor syndrome. J Clin Endocrinol Metab 2005; 90: 878–83.
98. Moore SL, Chun JK, Mitre SA, et al. Intraosseous hemangioma of the zygoma: CT and MR findings. AJNR Am J Neuroradiol 2001; 22:1383–5.
99. Moshari A, Bloom EE, McLean IW, Buckwalter NR. Ectopic chordoma with orbital invasion. Am J Ophthalmol 2001; 131:400–1.
100. Moshiri S, Oda D, Worthington P, et al. Odontogenic myxoma: histochemical and ultrastructural study. J Oral Pathol Med 1992; 21:401–3.
101. Mueller S, Soeder S, Olineira AM, et al. Type II collagen as a specific marker for mesenchymal chondrosarcomas

compared to other small cell sarcomas of the skeleton. Modern Pathol 2005; 18:1088–94.
102. Naiman J, Green WR, D'Heurle D, et al. Brown tumor of the orbit associated with primary hyperparathyroidism. Am J Ophthalmol 1980; 90:565–71.
103. Nakagawa K, Takasato Y, Ito Y, et al. Ossifying fibroma involving the paranasal sinuses, orbit, and anterior cranial fossa: case report. Neurosurgery 1995; 36:1192–5.
104. Naraghi M, Kashfi A. Endonasal endoscopic resection of ethmoido-orbital osteoma compressing the optic nerve. Am J Otolaryngol 2003; 24:408–12.
105. Nasr AM, Blodi FC, Lindahl S, et al. Congenital generalized multicentric myofibromatosis with orbital involvement. Am J Ophthalmol 1986; 102:779–87.
106. O'Hara BJ, Paetau A, Miettinen M. Keratin subsets and monoclonal antibody HBME-1 in chordoma: immunohistochemical differential diagnosis between tumors simulating chordoma. Hum Pathol 1998; 29:119–26.
107. Okamato S, Hisaoka M, Meis-Kindblom JM, et al. Juxta-articular myxoma and intramuscular myxoma are two distinct entities. Activating Gsα mutation at Arg 201 codon does not occur in juxta-articular myxoma. Virchows Arch 2002; 440:12–5.
108. Okamato S, Hisaoka M, Ushijima M, et al. Activating Gsα mutation in intramuscular myxomas with and without fibrous dysplasia of bone. Virchows Arch 2000; 437:133–7.
109. Oliveira AM, His BL, Weremowicz S, et al. USP6 (Tre2) fusion oncogenes in aneurysmal bone cyst. Cancer Res 2004; 64:1920–3.
110. Oliveira AM, Perez-Atayde AR, Dal Cin P, et al. Aneurysmal bone cyst variant translocations upregulate USP6 transcription by promoter swapping with the ZNF9, COL1A1, TRAP150, and OMD genes. Oncogene 2005; 24:3419–26.
111. Oliveira AM, Perez-Atayde AR, Inwards CY, et al. USP6 and CDH11 oncogenes identify the neoplastic cell in primary aneurysmal bone cysts and are absent in so-called secondary aneurysmal bone cysts. Am J Pathol 2004; 165:1773–80.
112. Osguthorpe JD, Gudeman SK. Orbital complications of fibrous dysplasia. Otolaryngol Head Neck Surg 1987; 97: 403–5.
113. Osterdock RJ, Greene S, Mascott CR, et al. Primary myxoma of the temporal bone in a 17-year-old boy: case report. Neurosurgery 2001; 48:945–8.
114. Parodi MB, Iustulin D, Isola V. Partial ablation of benign osteoblastoma: a case report. 1993; 16:43–5.
115. Parrish CM, O'Day DM. Brown tumor of the orbit: case report and review of the literature. Arch Ophthalmol 1986; 104:1199–202.
116. Pasternak S, O'Connell JX, Verchere C, et al. Enchondroma of the orbit. Am J Ophthalmol 1996; 122:444–5.
117. Patel BC, Sabir DI, Flaharty PM, et al. Aneurysmal bone cyst of the orbit and ethmoid sinus. Arch Ophthalmol 1993; 111:586–7.
118. Potts MJ, Rose GE, Milroy C, et al. Dedifferentiated chondrosarcoma arising in the orbit. Br J Ophthalmol 1992; 76:49–51.
119. Puchalski R, Shah UK, Carpentieri D, et al. Melanotic neuroectodermal tumor of infancy (MNTI) of the hard palate: presentation and management. Int J Pediatr Otorhinolaryngol 2000; 53:163–8.
120. Rambhatla S, Subramanian N, Gangadhara Sundar JK, et al. Myxoma of the orbit. Indian J Ophthalmol 2003; 51:85–7.
121. Raymond AK, Ayala AG, Knuutila S. Conventional osteosarcoma. In: Fletcher CDM, Unni KK, Mertens F, eds. World Health Organization Classification of Tumours. Pathology & Genetics. Tumours of Soft Tissue and Bone. Lyon: IARC Press, 2002: 264–70.
122. Relf SJ, Bartley GB, Unni KK. Primary orbital intraosseous hemangioma. Ophthalmology 1991; 98:541–7.
123. Ruark DS, Schlehaider UK, Shah JP. Chondrosarcomas of the head and neck. World J Surg 1992; 16:1010–6.
124. Sawyer JR, Tryka AF, Bell JM, et al. Nonrandom chromosome breakpoints at Xq26 and 2q33 characterize cemento-ossifying fibromas of the orbit. Cancer 1995; 76: 1853–9.
125. Schuetz AN, Rubin BP, Goldblum JR, et al. Intercellular junctions in Ewing sarcoma/primitive neuroectodermal tumor: additional evidence of epithelial differentiation. Modern Pathology 2005; 18:1403–10.
126. Schultze-Mosgau S, Holbach LM, Wiltfang J. Cherubism: clinical evidence and therapy. J Craniofac Surg 2003; 110: 1846–9.
127. Selva D, Phipps SE, O'Connell JX, et al. Pathogenesis of orbital cholesterol granuloma. Clin Experiment Ophthalmol 2003; 31:78–82.
128. Selva D, White VA, O'Connell JX, et al. Primary bone tumors of the orbit. Surv Ophthalmol 2004; 49:328–42.
129. Sevel D. Mesenchymal chondrosarcoma of the orbit. Brit J Ophthal 1974; 58:882–7.
130. Sharma A, Garg A, Mishra N, et al. Primary Ewing's sarcoma of the sphenoid bone with unusual imaging features: a case report. Clin Neurol Neurosurg 2005; 107: 528–31.
131. Shields CL, Husson M, Shields JA, et al. Solitary intraosseous infantile myofibroma of the orbital roof. Arch Ophthalmol 1998; 116:1528–30.
132. Shimo-Oku M, Okamoto N, Ogita Y, et al. A case of mesenchymal chondrosarcoma of the orbit. Acta Ophthalmol 1980; 58:831–40.
133. Shinaver CN, Mafee MF, Choi KH. MRI of mesenchymal chondrosarcoma of the orbit: case report and review of the literature. Neuroradiology 1997; 39: 296–301.
134. Shykhon ME, Trotter MI, Morgan DW, et al. Cholesterol granuloma of the frontal sinus. J Laryngol Otol 2002; 116: 1041–3.
135. Slem G, Varinli S, Koker F. Brown tumor of the orbit. Ann Ophthalmol 1983; 15:811–2.
136. Slootweg PJ, Wittkampf ARM. Myxoma of the jaws. An analysis of 15 cases. J Maxillofac Surg 1986; 14:46–52.
137. Sood GC, Malik SRK, Gupta DK, et al. Reparative granuloma of the orbit causing unilateral proptosis. Am J Ophthalmol 1967; 63:524–7.
138. Southgate J, Sarma U, Townend JV, et al. Study of the cell biology and biochemistry of cherubism. J Clin Pathol 1998; 51:831–7.
139. Soylemezoglu F, Tezel GG, Koybasoglu F, et al. Cranial infantile myofibromatosis: report of three cases. Childs Nerv Syst 2001; 17:524–7.
140. Stapleton SR, Wilkins PR, Archer DJ, et al. Chondrosarcoma of the skull base: a series of eight cases. Neurosurgery 1993; 32:348–55.
141. Stautz CC. CT of infantile myofibromatosis of the orbit with intracranial involvement: a case report. AJNR Am J Neuroradiol 1991; 12:184–5.
142. Sweet C, Silbergleit R, Mehta B. Primary intraosseous hemangioma of the orbit: CT and MR appearance. AJNR Am J Neuroradiol 1997; 18:379–81.

143. Tang Chen YB, Wornom IL III, Whitaker LA. Intraosseous vascular malformations of the orbit. Plast Reconstr Surg 1991; 87:946–9.
144. Tokano H, Ishikawa N, Kitamura K, et al. Solitary infantile myofibromatosis in the lateral orbit floor showing spontaneous regression. J Laryngol Otol 2001; 115:419–21.
145. Trevisani MG, Fry CL, Hesse RJ, et al. A rare case of orbital osteogenic sarcoma. Arch Ophthalmol 1996; 114: 494–5.
146. Tuncer S, Kebudi R, Peksayar G, et al. Congenital mesenchymal chondrosarcoma of the orbit: case report and review of the literature. Ophthalmology 2004; 111: 1016–22.
147. Ueki Y, Tiziani V, Santanna C, et al. Mutations in the gene encoding c-Abl-binding protein SH3BP2 cause cherubism. Nat Genet 2001; 28:125–6.
148. Ungkanont K, Chanyavanich V, Benjarasamerote S, et al. Osteoblastoma of the ethmoid sinus in a nine-year-old child—an unusual occurrence. Int J Pediatr Otorhinolaryngol 1996; 38:89–95.
149. Vigorita VJ. Metabolic bone disease: part II. In: Vigorita VJ, Ghelman B, eds. Orthopaedic pathology. Philadelphia, PA: Lippincott Williams & Wilkins, 1999: 143–57, 178–9.
150. Waeltermann JM, Huntrakoon M, Beatty EC, et al. Congenital fibromatosis (myofibromatosis) of the orbit: a rare cause of proptosis at birth. Ann Ophthalmol 1988; 20:394–9.
151. Wehrli BM, Huang W, de Crombrugghe B, et al. Sox9, a master regulator of chondrogenesis, distinguishes mesenchymal chondrosarcoma from other small blue cell blue round cell tumors. Hum Pathol 2003; 34:263–9.
152. Wenig BM, Mafee MF, Ghosh L. Fibro-osseous, osseous, and cartilaginous lesions of the orbit and paraorbital region: correlative clinicopathologic and radiographic features, including the diagnostic role of CT and MRI imaging. Radiol Clin North Am 1998; 36:1241–59.
153. Wenig BM, Vinh TN, Smirniotopoulos JG, et al. Aggressive psammomatoid ossifying fibromas of the sinonasal region. A clinicopathologic study of a distinct group of fibro-osseous lesions. Cancer 1995; 76:1155–65.
154. Westfall AC, Mansoor A, Sullivan SA, et al. Orbital and periorbital myofibromas in childhood. Ophthalmology 2003; 110:2000–5.
155. Wilkes SR, Trautmann JC, DeSanto LW, et al. Osteoma. An unusual cause of amaurosis fugax. Mayo Clin Proc 1979; 54:258–60.
156. Woodruff G, Thorner P, Skarf B. Primary Ewing's sarcoma of the orbit presenting with visual loss. Br J Ophthalmol 1988; 72:786–92.
157. Yamaguchi T, Watanabe-Ishiiwa H, Suzuki S, et al. Incipient chordoma: a report of two cases of early-stage chordoma arising from benign notochordal cell tumors. Modern Pathol 2005; 18:1005–10.
158. Zimmerman LE. Discussion paper. Ophthalmology 1985; 92:148–9.

66

Tumors of Lymphoid Tissue

Anand Shreeram Lagoo
Department of Pathology, Duke University, Durham, North Carolina, U.S.A.

INTRODUCTION

Lymphoid infiltrates of the conjunctiva and orbit are common and it has been long recognized that the differentiation of benign infiltrates from malignant lymphomas can be challenging not only for the clinician but also for the pathologist (63). The introduction of immunohistochemistry, flow cytometry, and molecular methods has progressively improved our ability to differentiate between benign lymphoid infiltrates and lymphomas in the past two decades. It is also widely recognized that the outcome of different types of lymphomas in the same location can be diverse and therefore an accurate subclassification of the lymphoma is equally crucial. The current classification of lymphomas is based to a large extent on our understanding of the development of the immune system and the molecular and cellular biology of processes controlling cell cycle progression, cell division, and cell death. The demonstration of specific cytogenetic abnormalities associated with specific lymphomas and leukemia spurred further this study. More recently the molecules involved in these chromosomal events have been defined in detail, revealing a fascinating picture of complex molecular interactions, often converging on a few key molecules that control cell division and cell death, leading ultimately to an uncontrolled proliferation and accumulation of a clone of lymphoid cells. In an important departure from a purely morphologically based classification systems, the current World Health Organization (WHO) classification (52) and its forerunner the Revised European American Lymphoma (REAL) classification (43), define the various types of lymphomas as different diseases with unique clinical behavior (122). This behavior is predicated on the putative cell of origin and the aberration of cellular processes brought about by specific cytogenetic abnormalities. The use of gene chips, which allow the simultaneous examination of the expression of hundreds of genes, has led to further subclassification of certain common categories of lymphomas based on reproducible patterns of expression of gene cohorts. Rather unexpectedly, these studies have also emphasized the importance of the host immune system in determining the ultimate outcome of the lymphoma in a particular patient. A related development of major significance in our understanding of the biology of lymphomas is the role of viruses and bacteria in their causation.

This chapter summarizes the current classification of lymphomas and details the incidence of the various types of lymphomas in the eye, orbit, and other ocular adnexa. The molecular mechanisms considered important in controlling the biology of the various lymphomas is explained in some detail. Other factors that determine the outcome of various lymphomas in general and of orbital and ocular lymphomas in particular, are also considered. Finally, some special techniques crucial for accurate diagnosis are described.

When considering lymphomas in and around the eye, the fundamental distinction between intraocular lymphomas and lymphomas involving ocular adnexal structures must be borne in mind. The former represent a subcategory of primary central nervous system (CNS) lymphomas while the latter are extranodal lymphomas involving soft tissues, including lining and glandular epithelia. The biology of the lymphomas in these two locations is different and the treatment and outcome for the patient are also often distinct. For this reason, throughout this chapter lymphomas in these two locations are treated separately, with greater emphasis on the ocular adnexal lymphomas.

INCIDENCE OF LYMPHOMAS

Worldwide, the incidence of lymphoma has increased dramatically in the past three decades. The annual rate of increase has been nearly 4% starting in the 1970s, tapering to under a 2% annual increase since the 1990s (90). Overall, this translates to an incidence that has nearly doubled in the last 30 years. In a study involving over 60,000 cases of lymphoma diagnosed in the United States over a 17-year period (42), the incidence of non-Hodgkin lymphoma (NHL) was estimated to be 17.1 and 11.5 per 100,000 person-years among white males and females, respectively, and about 40% lower in blacks. More recently it has been estimated that in 2004 there were over 54,000 cases of lymphoma leading to over 19,000 deaths (36). Incidence rises with age, especially after 65 years, and lymphomas occur about 50% more often in males than in females. The proportion of primary extranodal lymphomas is between 20% and 34% of all lymphomas, depending on the criteria used to define primary extranodal lymphoma (65).

Orbital or ocular adnexal lymphomas are much more common than intraocular lymphomas. A large French series (86) found only 7 intraocular tumors compared to 135 orbital tumors in the same period. Indeed orbital lymphomas are the third commonest site of extranodal involvement by lymphoma after the gastrointestinal tract and skin (42) and most studies show that lymphomas are the single most common type of malignant tumor of the orbit. The proportion of all orbital malignant tumors that are lymphomas varies from a low of about 10% (108) to a high of over 50% (79). The latter study, conducted in Florida over a 12-year period (1981 through 1993), recorded an alarming increase in the reported cases of lymphoma in the second half of the study period compared to the first half, this exceeding the overall increase in incidence. The combined incidence of all lymphomas during the entire study period was 149 per million population and that of orbital lymphoma was 1 per million. However, at the beginning of the study period, the incidence of orbital lymphoma was only 0.5 per million and increased to 2.1 per million in 1991. In other studies in the United States (32) and Japan (95), lymphomas constituted about a quarter of all orbital tumors and were the most frequent type of malignant orbital tumor. In East Africa, Burkitt lymphoma was the second commonest orbital tumor (60) but occurred less frequently elsewhere (1). Most studies in the United States have found that Caucasians are affected much more commonly than African Americans and females outnumber males slightly. Although lymphomas were noted over a wide age range (15–96 years), most patients were older (median 71 years) (79). Some studies have examined only conjunctival lymphomas alone (107) finding that the age, sex, and ethnic mix of the patients are similar to other orbital lymphomas.

Intraocular lymphoma is rare. After the first case was published in 1951 only 14 additional cases were described over the next 25 years (7,25). Intraocular lymphoma is often, although not exclusively, a component of multifocal brain lymphoma and the rapid increase in the incidence of primary CNS lymphomas in the past two decades has translated into an increased detection of intraocular lymphomas. Ocular involvement is seen in 15% to 25% of patients presenting with brain lymphoma and between 60% and 80% of patients with intraocular lymphoma have or will develop brain lymphomas (19,61) Intraocular lymphoma may present before, concurrently, or upon relapse of a primary brain lesion, although most patients (70–80%) it precedes brain tumor formation by months to years (15,37,45,81).

CLINICAL PRESENTATIONS

The presentation varies according to the location of the lymphoma.

Orbital Lymphomas

In one series (32), the most common clinical features at presentation were a mass (26%), proptosis (18%), and pain (15%). The mean duration of symptoms was 11 months before referral but has been much longer (23 months) in other studies (39). In another large series of patients (86) the presenting symptoms were ophthalmologic in over 90% patients: pink conjunctival mass or redness in 32% of patients, exophthalmia in 27%, orbital and/or palpebral mass in 19% cases, decreased visual acuity and ptosis in about 6%, and diplopia in less than 2% of patients. The median interval between onset of the first symptoms and the date of diagnosis was 4 months (range: 1 month to 10 years). In general 80% to 90% of cases were unilateral, but bilateral involvement has been reported in some patients in most studies.

Intraocular Lymphomas

The presenting symptoms of intraocular lymphoma are most often blurred vision and floaters (19,46). Less commonly, red eye, photophobia, and ocular pain may be observed. Intraocular lymphoma is bilateral in the majority of cases, although it is often asymmetric (15). Because the lesion of primary intraocular lymphoma is usually a tumor cell infiltrate of the retina, the associated retinochoroiditis leads to marked vitreous clouding and eventual retinal detachment, and glaucoma may occur. In contrast, choroidal involvement is the norm in secondary intraocular lymphoma accompanying generalized systemic lymphoma (37). In one series, all patients with a prior history of systemic lymphoma showed anterior uveitis upon examination, in contrast to those associated with primary CNS lymphoma, where involvement was almost always in the form of vitritis (46). Rarely, primary ocular lymphoma may present as a hypopyon or with involvement of the iris (73,123).

MODERN CLASSIFICATION OF LYMPHOMAS

The Basis for Current Lymphoma Classification

The modern classification of lymphoma is best understood in the context of the normal composition of the acquired immune system. A simplified scheme of B-cell and T-cell development and the various NHL thought to arise from each developmental stage are shown in Figure 1. It is worth emphasizing that lymphocytic leukemias and lymphomas are generally considered to be expressions of the same disease, whereas the various types of lymphomas are distinct disease entities. All modern classifications of lymphoma recognize the basic difference in the biology of lymphomas arising from B cells and T/NK-cells. Another fundamental difference in the organization of both the T/natural killer (NK) cell and B-cell arms of the immune system reflects the concept of precursor cells and terminally differentiated lymphocytes. Lymphomas arising from either precursor B cells or T cells are more similar to each other than they are to those arising from the terminally differentiated cells of the same lineage. Both B cells and T cells show characteristic cytological and molecular changes following activation with antigen, which are described in detail elsewhere in Chapter 3. Here only the morphological and molecular features directly relevant to the classification of lymphomas are summarized briefly. The naïve B-cells, which originate in the bone marrow and undergo rearrangements of the immunoglobulin heavy and light chain genes to produce immunoglobulin unique molecules are localized in the dark-staining mantle zones of lymphoid follicles. After encounter with antigen(s) the B cells downregulate their *BCL2* genes, enter the dark zone of the follicle center, and proliferate. The immunoglobulin heavy chain gene (such as *IGHM*, *IGHE*, or *IGHD*) undergoes somatic hypermutations in the follicle center. Memory cells produced after the antigenic challenge wanes exit through the marginal zones (the lighter staining zone outside the mantle zone). In other circumstances antibody secreting plasma cells are produced. These stages of activation and differentiation can be defined based on the expression of certain molecules on the cell surface, and more recently, through the identification of characteristic gene expression profiles using microarrays (41) or proteomic experiments (59). When the nucleotide sequence of the variable heavy chain region of lymphoma cells is identical to that of the germ line, the lymphoma cells can be assumed to be in the pregerminal center (GC) stage [e.g., mantle cell lymphoma:). If the mutations vary among lymphoma cells but are clonally related (ongoing mutation), the cells can be assumed to be in the GC stage (e.g., follicular lymphoma). If the mutation is fixed among the lymphoma cells, they can be assumed to be in the post-GC stage [e.g., diffuse large B-cell lymphoma and extranodal marginal zone B-cell lymphoma of mucosa-associated lymphoid tissue (MALT)]. In T cells the anatomical sites and sequence of events after antigen activation and memory cell generation are less well defined.

WHO Classification of Lymphomas

The monograph published by WHO (52) provides the definitions of the various types of lymphomas and gives a comprehensive description of clinical, morphological, and molecular genetic characteristics

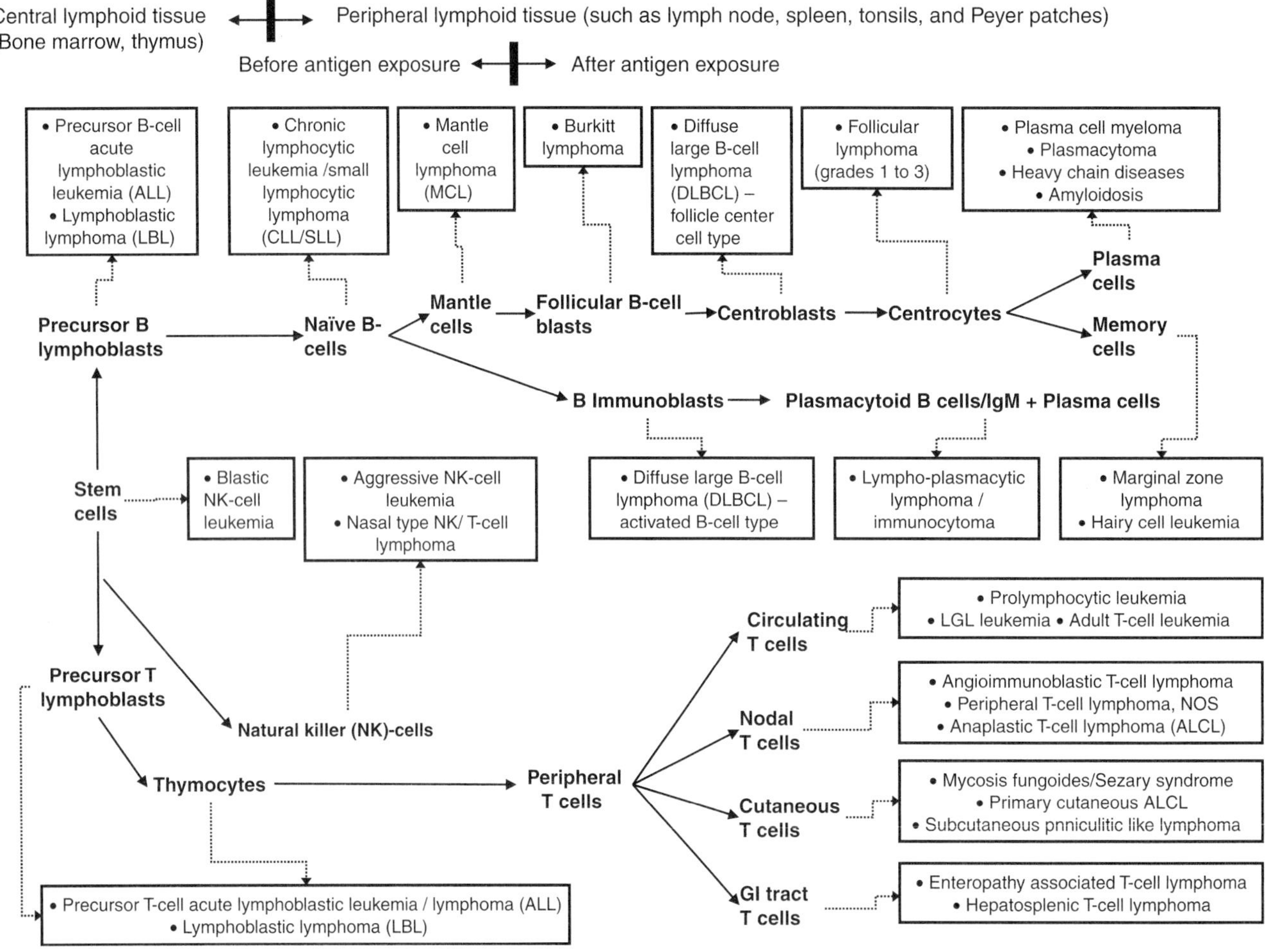

Figure 1 A simplified scheme of B-cell and T-cell development and the lymphomas thought to arise from each stage. The developmental stages are shown in boldface, with solid arrows showing the direction of development. The lymphomas are shown in textboxes connected to the corresponding developmental stage by broken arrows.

useful in their identification. Like all earlier classifications, the WHO classification (52) also recognizes the fundamental distinction between Hodgkin lymphomas and NHL. Hodgkin lymphomas are classified into classical and nodular lymphocyte predominant types. The immunophenotype of the Reed Sternberg cell in classical Hodgkin lymphoma (CD15+, CD30+, CD20–, CD45–) differs from the lymphocytic (L) and histiocytic (H) or "popcorn" cell in nodular lymphocyte-predominant Hodgkin lymphoma (CD15–, CD30–, CD20+, CD45+). However, the malignant cells (Reed Sternberg cells or L and H cells) in both types of Hodgkin lymphoma are in the minority, the majority of cells in the involved organ being reactive lymphocytes and histiocytes (98).

The B-cell lymphomas are divided into precursor B-cell neoplasms, which primarily include acute lymphoblastic leukemia and the related lymphoblastic lymphoma. These tumors are characterized by a blast morphology, rapid growth and an aggressive, but potentially curable, course. The mature B-cell lymphomas comprise about a dozen different entities. From a diagnostic perspective they can be divided on the basis of their cytological features into small cell, mixed small and large cell, and large cell neoplasms, on architectural features into diffuse, follicular, and nodular tumors, or on immunophenotypic characteristics into those expressing CD5 or CD10 or neither. In practice all of these features, often with key cytogenetic features, are used to make the definitive diagnosis. Among CD5+ lymphomas, chronic lymphocytic leukemia/small lymphocytic lymphoma and Mantle cell lymphoma are composed of small cells and usually show a diffuse infiltration of the lymph nodes, except in some mantle cell lymphoma, which can show a nodular pattern. A third type, B-cell prolymphocytic leukemia has intermediate size cells and a diffuse pattern. Among CD10+ lymphomas, acute lymphoblastic leukemia/lymphoblastic lymphoma and Burkitt lymphoma have small to medium-sized cells with a diffuse pattern of infiltration, while follicular lymphomas have a mixture of small and large cells in a follicular pattern. Some diffuse large B-cell lymphomas can be CD10+ and some follicular lymphomas can be composed of mainly large cells. Diffuse large B-cell lymphomas may be negative for both CD5 and CD10 and related conditions like mediastinal (thymic) B-cell lymphoma, primary effusion lymphoma, and intravascular lymphoma may lack other B-cell antigens such as CD20 and surface immunoglobulin. Many B-cell lymphomas lacking both CD5 and CD10 are composed of small- to medium-sized cells and have a diffuse pattern. Included in this broad category are marginal zone lymphoma of MALT type, nodal marginal zone lymphoma, splenic marginal zone lymphoma, lymphoplasmacytic lymphoma, hairy cell leukemia, and plasma cell dyscrasias. Characteristic and often pathognomonic cytogenetic abnormalities are reciprocal translocations between two chromosomes. Chromosome 14, bearing the immunoglobulin heavy chain locus is involved in translocations such as t(14;18) in follicular lymphoma, t(11;14) in mantle cell lymphoma, and t(8;14) in Burkitt lymphoma. The latter involves the cMYC locus on chromosome 8 and alternative translocations with kappa chain locus on chromosome 2 or lambda chain locus on chromosome 22 producing t(2;8) or t(8;22) are also encountered in Burkitt lymphoma. The translocations occurring in MALT lymphomas are discussed more fully later (see the section entitled Molecular Mechanisms in MALT Lymphoma). The cytogenetic abnormalities provide a molecular explanation for the malignant nature of the lymphoma cells, which are discussed more fully later. In B-cell lymphomas, large cell morphology is associated with a more proliferative and aggressive behavior. A notable exception is mantle cell lymphoma, which is clinically aggressive even though the lymphoma cells are small. Small blast cells in acute lymphoblastic leukemia, lymphoblastic lymphoma, and Burkitt lymphoma are highly aggressive.

T-cell lymphomas and NK-cell lymphomas are closely related. They often demonstrate characteristic morphological findings and manifest a predilection for involvement of certain extranodal locations. They are much less frequently encountered in the Western hemisphere for reasons that are not completely clear. They often do not respond predictably to the multidrug chemotherapy regimens that are so effective in B-cell lymphomas (42,76) and the prognosis in most cases remains guarded. Besides the highly aggressive precursor T-cell lymphoblastic lymphoma/leukemia, T-cell prolymphocytic leukemia, human T-cell leukemia virus 1 (HTLV 1) associated adult T-cell leukemia/lymphoma, aggressive NK/T-cell leukemia, hepatosplenic gamma/delta T-cell lymphoma and enteropathy-associated T-cell lymphoma also show aggressive behavior. Peripheral T-cell lymphoma not otherwise specified, angioimmunoblastic T-cell lymphoma and nodal anaplastic large cell lymphoma are less aggressive and primarily involve lymph nodes. Primary skin involvement is seen in the form of either mycosis fungoides, primary cutaneous anaplastic large cell lymphoma, or subcutaneous panniculitis-like T-cell lymphoma, while a nasal-type NK/T-cell lymphoma shows locally destructive behavior. Large granular lymphocyte leukemia represents an unusually indolent T-cell process.

The cell surface markers used in the diagnosis of lymphomas as well as the immunophenotype, cytogenetic abnormalities, and biological properties of the more common lymphomas are summarized in Table 1 and Table 2.

Extranodal lymphomas, such as those occurring in the eye, orbit, or other ocular adnexa raise some additional considerations. The frequency of the different types of lymphomas seen in the lymph node and the orbit and eye differ. The distinction between a primary extranodal lymphoma and secondary involvement of an extranodal site by a lymphoma originating in a lymphoid organ is not always easy. Due to their superficial location many primary ocular adnexal lymphomas, they are likely to be diagnosed in an early stage. However, imaging and additional staging studies, such as bone marrow biopsy, are necessary to establish the true extent of the disease. The differential diagnosis of lymphomas of the orbit and eye differ from those in lymph nodes. Furthermore, extranodal lymphomas that morphologically resemble nodal lymphomas may also differ in behavior. Cutaneous lymphomas provide several good examples of this principle (127). Lastly, the close association of chronic inflammation and marginal zone lymphomas of MALT type raises questions about the etiopathogenesis of orbital lymphomas.

MOLECULAR MECHANISMS OF LYMPHOMAGENESIS

Specific chromosomal translocations have been identified in different lymphomas and the genes present in the translocation junction region are considered to play a crucial role in the pathogenesis of the corresponding lymphoma. The translocations lead to either overexpression of certain genes (such as BCL2, BCL6, BCL10, c-MYC) or the production of chimeric proteins (such as API2-MALT1). Functionally the translocations can be classified into three categories—those causing enhanced proliferation, those causing inhibition of differentiation, and those inhibiting apoptosis. A review of the role of these proteins in normal lymphocyte biology is helpful in understanding their involvement in lymphomagenesis.

Table 1 Significance of Markers Commonly Used in Lymphoma Diagnosis

Antigen	Primary cellular distribution	Significance in lymphoma diagnosis
CD1a	Thymocytes, immature T cells	Expressed in precursor T-cell neoplasms
CD2	All T cells, NK cells	May be lost in T-cell lymphoma
CD4	Helper T cells, monocytes (lower expression)	Coexpression with CD8 or absence of both CD4 and CD8 in precursor T-cell neoplasms
CD3	All T cells	Most specific for T-cell lineage Only cytoplasmic expression may be seen
CD5	All T cells, some naïve B cells	When expressed in B cells, indicates either CLL or MCL May be lost in T-cell lymphoma
CD7	All T cells	Most commonly lost in T-cell lymphomas Most commonly expressed in acute myeloid leukemia
CD10 (CALLA)	Follicular B cells, hematogones	Expressed in precursor B-lymphoblastic lymphoma, Burkitt lymphoma, and follicular lymphoma Expressed in AILD type T-cell lymphoma
CD15	Monocytes, granulocytes	Reed–Sternberg (R–S) cells in classical Hodgkin lymphoma
CD20	B cells	Loss on B cells indicates precursor B cells or plasma cells
CD23	Follicular dendritic cells	Used to differentiate CD5+ B-cell lymphomas: CLL, CD23+ and MCL, CD23−
CD30	Immunoblasts (B and T)	R–S cells in classical Hodgkin lymphoma
CD34	Hematopoietic stem cells	Acute leukemia
CD38	Plasma cells, many other lymphoid cells	Expression on CLL/SLL cells is a poor prognostic indicator
CD45 (LCA)	Leukocytes	Absent in erythroid precursors, plasma cells, and R–S cells
CD56		
CD57	NK cells, T-cell subset	Increased in lymphocyte-predominant Hodgkin lymphoma
CD68	Histiocytes, monocytes	
CD79a	B cells (expressed before CD20), plasma cells	Precursor B-cell, mature B-cell, and plasma cell neoplasms
CD99	*MIC2* gene product	25% to 80% lymphomas, especially precursor cell and T-cell lymphomas, Ewing sarcoma/PNET
CD117	Promyelocytes, mast cells	
Alk1		Anaplastic large cell lymphoma with t(2;5)
BCL2	Many lymphocytes, but not in reactive follicle centers	Expressed in follicle in follicular lymphoma
BCL6	Follicle center cells	Indicates origin from follicle center cells in DLBCL
Cyclin D1		Nuclear expression characteristic for MCL
EBNA-2	EBV infected cells	Endemic Burkitt, some Hodgkin lymphomas, nasal type NK/T-cell lymphoma
EBV-LMP	EBV infected cells	Same as EBNA2
EMA	Epithelial tissue	"Popcorn" cells in lymphocyte-predominance Hodgkin lymphoma, ALCL
Ki-67 (MIB 1)	Proliferating cells	Burkitt-like lymphoma and Burkitt lymphoma have >99% nuclear staining
MPO	Promyelocytes and more mature myeloid cells	Distinction between monocytic and myeloid type of granulocytic sarcoma
TdT	Thymocytes, immature T-, B-, and myeloid blasts	Distinction between Burkitt lymphoma and precursor Bcell lymphoblastic lymphoma Distinction between peripheral T-cell and lymphoblastic lymphomas
TIA-1	Cytotoxic T cells and NK cells	Lymphomas arising from these cells

Molecular Mechanisms of Lymphocyte Development and Activation

B-cell development before antigen stimulation is tightly controlled and the nuclear factor PAX5, the cytokine interleukin 7 (IL7), and histone deacylation have key roles in this process (55). In antigen-induced activation of T-cell and B-cell nuclear factor kappa B (NFκB) is a key nuclear factor that regulates many crucial events leading to cellular proliferation (77). NFκB proteins are normally sequestered in the cytoplasm in an inactive form bound to inhibitory κB (IκB) proteins (119). The primary effect of the signaling cascade that starts with the binding of the antigen to the specific antigen receptors is to free NFκB from the inhibitory protein, which can then translocate to the nucleus. This complex signaling cascade involves many proteins located in the translocation junction region of various lymphomas.

Table 2 Salient Diagnostic and Clinical Features of the Common Non-Hodgkin Lymphomas

Lymphoma	Immunophenotype	Cytogenetic abnormality	Clinical behavior
B-cell lymphomas			
Precursor B-cell lymphoblastic lymphoma/acute lymphoblastic leukemia	CD45+/−, CD19+, CD22+, CD20−/+, CD10+, TdT+/−, sIg−	Hyperdiploidy or other numeric, t(9;22)	Aggressive, curable (80%) Bad prognostic indicator
Burkitt lymphoma/ leukemia	CD45+/−, CD19+, CD22+, CD20+, CD10+, TdT−, sIg+	t(8;14) or less commonly t(2;14) or t(14;22)	Aggressive, curable (90%)
Follicular lymphoma (FCL)	CD45+/−, CD19+, CD22+, CD20+, CD10+, TdT−, sIg+, BCL2+, BCL6+	t(14;18)	Indolent (grade 1 and 2), incurable Moderately aggressive (grade 3), incurable
Diffuse large B-cell lymphoma (DLBCL)	CD45+/−, CD19+, CD22+, CD20+, CD10−/+, TdT−, sIg+, BCL2−/+, BCL6+/−		Aggressive, curable (50%)
Small lymphocytic lymphoma (SLL)	Pan B antigens+, CD5+, CD23+, cyclin D1−	Abnormalities of chromosomes 11, 12, 13, or 17	Indolent, incurable
Mantle cell lymphoma (MCL)	Pan B antigens+, CD5+, CD23−/+, cyclin D1+	t(11;14)	Moderately aggressive, bulky disease, incurable
Marginal zone lymphoma (MZL)	Pan B antigens+, CD5, CD10−	t(11;18)	Localized; curable Bad prognostic indicator
T-cell lymphomas			
Precursor T-cell lymphoblastic lymphoma/acute lymphoblastic leukemia	CD3−/+, CD5+, CD7+, CD1a+, TdT+		Aggressive, curable (50%)
Peripheral T-cell lymphoma, NOS	CD3+, CD5+/−, CD7−/+, CD1a−, TdT−		Variable, incurable
Anaplastic large cell lymphoma	CD3+, CD5+/−, CD7−/+, CD1a−, TdT−, CD30+, ALK1+/	t(2;5)	Good if t(2;5) present

Engagement of the antigen receptor by the cognate antigen leads to the formation of a highly ordered, membrane-associated complex termed the immunological synapse, in which a central signaling zone surrounds clustered antigen receptors. This is known as the supramolecular activation cluster with central and peripheral regions. Different sets of signaling proteins appear to be distributed in these regions, where they can generate unique signals (see Table 3 for names and abbreviations of principle signaling molecules). The first step in antigen receptor-mediated signaling is activation of membrane-associated tyrosine kinases including the *SRC* kinases (LCK and FYN), a Syk-family kinase (zeta-associated protein 70, ZAP70) and Tec-family kinases. These enzymes phosphorylate and activate several downstream adaptor molecules, including SLP76, Lat, and Grb2, which play a major role in organizing the supramolecular signaling complex in the membrane microdomain. They also recruit downstream signaling intermediates to this cluster, such as kinases like phospholipase C $\gamma 2$, phosphoinositide 3-kinase and Akt, as well as the Rho-family guanine nucleotide exchange factor Vav1. Diacyl glycerol generated from the plasma membrane by the action of phospholipase C activates the specific protein kinase C subtype (either β type in B cells or θ type in T cells) recruited to the complex.

At least three intermediate molecules are known to be involved in the downstream cascade leading to the activation of a multisubunit complex termed the inhibitory κB kinase (IKK) complex, which is composed primarily of two catalytic subunits (IKKa and IKKb) and a regulatory subunit (NEMO/IKKg). The first is a member of the membrane-associated guanylate kinase (MAGUK) superfamily, called is an N-terminal protein–protein interaction domain present within several signaling intermediates involved in the apoptosis machinery (see Chapter 2). Typically, the caspase-recruitment domain (CARD) domains of two proteins can juxtapose and allow those proteins to interact physically in specific signaling pathways. CARD of CARD-containing MAGUK (CARMA1) interacts with CARD of the second molecule in the cascade (BCL10) and allows these molecules to dimerize. BCL10 binds tightly to the third molecule in this cascade, MALT1, leading to the oligomerization of

Table 3 Names and Abbreviations of Some Molecules Involved in Activation Signaling Cascade in Lymphocytes

Name	Abbreviation
B-cell lymphoma-associated oncogenes	BCL1, BCL2, BCL6, BCL10
Caspase-recruitment domain	CARD
Membrane-associated guanylate kinase	MAGUK
CARD-containing MAGUK	CARMA1
BCL10 interacting MAGUK protein-1	BIMP1
Nuclear factor kappa B	NFκB
Inhibitor of NFκb	IκB
Inhibitory κ B kinase	IKK
X box-binding protein-1	XBP1
Zeta associated protein-70	ZAP70

the latter. This step is necessary for activation of the caspase-like proteolytic site in the C-terminus of MALT1. Activated MALT1 may cleave a yet to be identified substrate, which probably activates the IKK complex. Upon activation of the IKK complex, the catalytic subunits phosphorylate IkB proteins, thereby marking them for ubiquitylation and subsequent degradation. This process frees NFκB dimers, which then translocate into the nucleus and regulate expression of a wide variety of genes.

Antigen-mediated lymphocyte activation can also lead to apoptosis if the antigen receptor interaction is weak or appropriate costimulatory signals are not present. BCL2 is a key protein involved in preventing apoptosis. API2 may have a similar role. The cells that escape apoptosis mature to plasma cells or memory cells. B lymphocyte-induced maturation protein (Blimp-1) appears to be the key factor responsible for maturation to plasma cells, acting partially through a direct suppression of PAX5. Blimp-1 blocks a proliferative program, in part through direct repression of c-MYC causes upregulation of genes involved in immunoglobulin secretion including heavy and light chain genes and the transcription factor. It also represses numerous genes required in mature B cells, including those involved in GC functions (such as BCL6, AIDS, DNA–protein kinases, Ku70, Ku80, Ku86), intracellular signaling (such as SYK, BTK, BLNK, LYN, FYN), receipt of extracellular information (such as surface immunoglobulin, MHCII, CD19, CD21, CD69, CD86), and follicular homing (such as CXCR5). BCL6 may be involved in preventing terminal differentiation of GC cells, thus permitting continued proliferation under appropriate circumstances. XBP1 also appears to be important, mainly to facilitate the handling of the large amounts of antibody produced in plasma cells.

Mucosa-Associated Lymphoid Tissue (MALT) and Marginal Zone Lymphomas of MALT Type

A major theoretical advance in the understanding of extranodal lymphomas has been the concept of MALT and the B-cell lymphomas arising from such sites, known as marginal zone lymphoma of MALT type (17,50,88). The marginal zone is a rim of pale-staining B cells that lie outside the dark-staining mantle zone of the lymphoid follicles. It is most prominent in mesenteric lymph nodes and the spleen. The B cells in this zone have abundant weakly eosinophilic or clear cytoplasm and a small, slightly cleaved nucleus. These cells are known as "marginal zone cells" or monocytoid B cells. Immunological studies indicate that they are predominantly post-GC, memory B cells (75). The lymphomas arising from the marginal zones of lymph nodes and spleen are known as nodal and splenic marginal zone lymphomas, respectively (9,52) and are distinct from the MALT type marginal zone lymphomas. MALT is normally most prominent as intraepithelial lymphocytes and Peyer patches in the intestine. Other epithelial-lined organs, such as the stomach, salivary glands, and skin, may have only a few intraepithelial lymphocytes as components of MALT (12,14). However, chronic inflammation due to infection or autoimmunity causes a significant increase in this lymphoid tissue. This "induced" MALT may further evolve into indolent B-cell lymphoma known as "marginal zone lymphoma of MALT type" (49,51). Some postulate that the chronic antigenic stimulation by the infectious agent or autoantigen selects a few B cells reactive to that antigen. At this stage, oligoclonal B-cell populations can be detected by molecular methods of immunoglobulin heavy chain analysis (102). Eventually, a clone becomes dominant and subsequently becomes independent of the antigenic stimulation through an accumulation of genetic changes that appear to culminate in activation of NFκB (40). However, even after the detection of a monoclonal population, eradication of the inciting inflammatory stimulus can lead to complete regression of the "lymphoma" in a large proportion of cases (71,72). Even if regression does not occur, the MALT lymphomas typically remain localized to the site of origin and surgical removal of the tumor often leads to long-lasting cure. It is noteworthy that, the same clonal B cells can be found in the regional lymph nodes but, without the antigenic stimulation and/or without help from antigenically stimulated T cells, these clonal B cells do not grow into recognizable lymphomas. These findings suggest the existence of a continuum from chronic inflammation to a completely autonomous B-cell lymphoma.

MALT lymphomas were first described as a consequence of chronic gastritis, most notably due to *Helicobacter pylori* infection (49–51). *H. pylori* infection is common and up to 20% of infected individuals have symptoms of gastritis. A small fraction, probably less than 0.1%, develops gastric carcinoma or lymphoma (30). Subsequently lymphomas associated with chronic thyroiditis and chronic sialadenitis were found to be MALT lymphomas and so were some periorbital and cutaneous lymphomas. Many of these conditions were previously referred to as "pseudolymphomas" or "lymphoid pseudotumors" due to the polymorphous nature of the infiltrate and the indolent nature of the process. More recently, specific cytogenetic abnormalities have been documented in MALT lymphomas (97,128,132). Gastric MALT lymphomas harboring certain specific abnormalities, such as t(11;18), were found to be unresponsive to antibiotic therapy aimed at eradicating the *H. pylori* infection (71,72). This observation has now been extended to MALT lymphomas of other tissues (132,133) and other cytogenetic abnormalities (113,128,131).

Molecular Mechanisms in MALT Lymphoma

Four recurring cytogenetic abnormalities have been identified in MALT lymphomas t(1;14), t(11;18), t(14;18), and t(3;14) (4,113,114,128). The first leads to an overexpression of the *BCL10* gene located on chromosome 1 under the influence of the immunoglobulin heavy chain promoter on chromosome 14. The overexpressed BCL10 can dimerize spontaneously (without the need for the normal activation cascade described above), activate the IKK complex and cause nuclear translocation of NFκB. On the other hand, t(11;18) leads to the formation of a chimeric protein, API2–MALT1, which can dimerize and activate IKK complex without the help of BCL10. The third translocation t(14;18), which rarely occurs as a sole abnormality (113), results in an overexpression of MALT1, leading to excessive activation of the IKK complex. The most recently described t(3;14) involves the *FOXP1* gene, which codes for a transcription factor that is known to be overexpressed in about 10% of diffuse large B-cell lymphomas and confers a poor prognosis in these cases (8). Only in a small minority of these cases, the overexpression is due to t(3;14) (129). The molecular mechanisms connecting *FOXP1* overexpression to MALT lymphomas are not clear (10).

Possible Cause of Orbital MALT Lymphomas

Because normal orbital tissue lacks lymphoid cells and lymphatics it is difficult to explain why lymphomas develop in this site. As mentioned earlier, chronic inflammation can induce abnormal MALT. The nature of the stimulus that induces inflammation in cases of orbital lymphoma remains unknown, but recent evidence implicates *Chlamydia psittaci* as eliciting the chronic inflammation that leads to lymphoma. A recent study (35) has shown that *C. psittaci* DNA is present in many orbital MALT lymphomas and that the lesions regress following effective antibiotic therapy to eradicate the organism. However, other studies (100) have failed to corroborate these findings and have only found *C. psittaci* DNA in rare examples of orbital MALT lymphoma. *H. pylori,* so convincingly implicated in the causation of gastric MALT lymphoma, is an unlikely candidate as the causative agent of orbital MALT lymphoma for several reasons. In gastric MALT lymphomas, infection by *H. pylori* can be demonstrated by direct microscopy and the presence of gastritis is likewise clearly demonstrable. This has never been done in orbital MALT lymphomas. *H. pylori* grows in the acid environment of the stomach and is unlikely to survive in the orbital tissue at normal body pH. In the search for a possible bacterial cause of orbital MALT lymphomas relying solely on polymerase chain reaction (PCR) amplification techniques to identify an organism, ignoring the known biology of the microorganism and in the complete absence of any other evidence of infection by that microbe, may be a risky strategy given that DNA amplification techniques can produce false-positive results through contamination at various steps of tissue processing. A continued search for an infectious or autoimmune cause for chronic inflammation in the orbit that may lead to a MALT lymphoma is required.

Molecular Mechanisms in Other Lymphomas

An excessive proliferation of lymphocytes occurs in Burkitt lymphoma due to an overexpression of c-MYC, while in mantle cell lymphoma overexpression of cyclin-D1 leads to the same effect. In follicular lymphoma, on the other hand, overexpression of BCL2 suppresses apoptosis leading to an accumulation of lymphoma cells. In some diffuse large B-cell lymphomas, t(3;14) causes an overexpression of BCL6 (117), which prevents terminal differentiation (93).

Other Factors Involved in Lymphomagenesis

Chromosomal translocations alone do not lead to lymphomas. For example, translocations-like t(14;18) have been demonstrated in the blood of 15% to 45% of normal individuals but follicular lymphomas occur at a far lower frequency in the same population. In most cases the other putative factors culminating in the lymphoma remain unknown. In MALT lymphomas a multistep process initiated by chronic inflammation appears to culminate in autonomous lymphoid growth through the acquisition of certain chromosomal translocations that confer a survival advantage to the cells by overexpressing genes involved in cell cycle control as described above. In follicular lymphoma the follicular dendritic cells may provide crucial signals required for the survival of lymphoma cells, even in the presence of t(14;18).

Role of Viruses in Lymphoma Development

A wide variety of B-lymphotropic and T-lymphotropic viruses have been described in association with primary CNS lymphoma and, by implication, in intraocular lymphoma. These include Epstein–Barr virus (EBV), human herpes virus 6 (HHV6), human herpes virus 8 (HHV8), simian virus 40 (SV40), human T-cell lymphotropic virus 1 (HTLV1), and hepatitis C virus (89). Epidemiological data suggest an association of hepatitis C virus with gastric MALT lymphomas as well (104). However, association does not imply causality because the viruses may either be involved in inducing proliferation of lymphocytes or merely infect lymphocytes after proliferation. If the viral nucleic acid sequences are found to be clonal, the infection can be assumed to have occurred before lymphoid proliferation. It is also important to demonstrate a neoplastic transforming ability in culture systems and animal models and to consider the epidemiology of human infection and lymphoma formation. It is well established that EBV is present in more than 90% of CNS lymphomas documented in AIDS patients and transplant recipients but only in a minority (10–20%) of those arising in immunocompetent populations (62). The strains of virus found in primary CNS lymphoma are similar to those found in nontumor-bearing populations, suggesting that there is no specific oncogenic variant. A high EBV viral burden and the presence of this virus in nonneoplastic lymph nodes is a risk factor for development of lymphoma. The presence of EBV in a systemic lymphoma is a risk factor for the synchronous or metachronous development of CNS lymphoma. Immunocompromised patients at risk for developing primary CNS lymphoma have very high numbers of circulating EBV-infected cells and their peripheral blood lymphocytes display increased activation antigens and an ability to spontaneously proliferate or transform in vitro.

Intraocular Lymphoma

As a type of primary CNS lymphoma, intraocular lymphoma probably shares many of the pathogenetic mechanisms for brain lymphoma. When bilateral, it is a clonal lesion, as demonstrated in a molecular study of bilateral ocular lymphoma without apparent CNS involvement. Higashide et al. (44) reported the identical B-cell clone in both eyes, possibly from spread through the optic chiasm, in the absence of detectable brain disease. Dysregulation of the immune axis doubtless has a role in tumorigenesis. Intraocular lymphomas have been reported in the setting of AIDS and, similar to brain lesions, appear to be related to EBV in these patients (47,82,87,96,103,110). Posttransplantation lymphoproliferative disorders inclusive of vitreal lymphomas have also been described (23,58,134). It has been recently shown that a majority (55%) of primary intraocular lymphomas have the t(14;18) translocation, usually associated with follicular lymphomas (124). However, this does not appear to alter the overall prognosis in these patients. There may be some pathogenetic mechanisms unique to the intraocular environment. It has long been established that there is an altered immunological environment in the anterior chamber of the eye, responsible for a phenomenon called "anterior chamber-associated immune deviation" (111,112) (see Chapter 3). Multiple soluble factors in the aqueous humor, including transforming growth factor β2 (TGFβ2), contribute to an immunosuppressive microenvironment that prevents activation of primed T cells and suppresses NK-cell activity. Tumor growth is unabetted in this environment and experimentally NK-sensitive tumors that fail to grow in systemic locations are able to grow in the eye (3). Intraocular lymphoma may benefit from this microenvironment and in addition promote secretion of other immunosuppressive factors. Although not definitively diagnostic of lymphoma an elevated IL10 is relatively constant in intraocular B-cell (but not T-cell) lymphomas and may be responsible for some of the immunosuppressive properties of the ocular contents (2,85). Levels of IL10 in the vitreous are elevated relative to that of IL6, and IL10 mRNA can be detected in lymphoma cells when assayed (18). Thus, intraocular lymphoma may secrete additional immunosuppressive factors into the already quiescent ocular microenvironment.

PATHOLOGY OF ORBITAL AND OCULAR LYMPHOMAS

Orbital and Other Ocular Adnexal Lymphomas

Since the landmark paper by Knowles and Jakobiec (63) describing 400 ocular adnexal lymphoid neoplasms, many small and large series detailing the clinical and pathological findings in these tumors have been published (16,29,54,56,64,78,83,86, 91,101,125,126) and reviews have also been published (6,24,67). Other studies are notable because they are limited to bilateral lesions (84), T/NK cell tumors (26), MALT lymphomas (20,69), mantle cell lymphoma (74), early stage disease (120), disease in Africa (1,60) or Asia (22) or emphasize the molecular (21,109,130), cytogenetic (92,116), or flow cytometry (106) findings. Primarily clinical findings related to outcome (5,38,53,80,94,115) or treatment (33,118) are also described in the literature. Lymphoid proliferations confined to specific sites such as the lacrimal gland (34) or conjunctiva (121) have also been described. All studies found that the vast majority (98–100%) of orbital lymphomas are of B-cell origin, even in Asia (22), where T-cell lymphomas occur at a higher incidence. Figure 2 shows the microscopic features of some of the common orbital lymphomas. Marginal zone lymphoma of the MALT type is the commonest type of lymphoma in almost all series, constituting about 45% to 60% of tumors. One series of 47 patients published by radiation oncologists (11) contains only 17% marginal zone lymphoma, possibly reflecting a bias for surgical treatment for this condition at that center (University of Iowa College of Medicine). On the other hand, in a study of 68 cases (22) marginal zone lymphoma constituted 98% of all primary lymphomas in the orbit. Diffuse large B-cell lymphomas and follicular lymphomas each constitute about 10% to 20% of all lymphomas in the orbit. Mantle cell lymphomas are about 3% to 5% in most series and lymphoplasmacytic lymphomas and plasmacytomas have been occasionally reported. Many reports have included all lymphoid proliferations in the orbit and most use a combination of histological features and demonstration of monoclonality in B cells to differentiate lymphomas from other lymphoid proliferations. In the older literature such proliferations are often referred to as "pseudolymphoma." A typical MALT type marginal zone lymphoma has a polymorphous infiltrate, including small and large lymphoid cells and plasma cells, which in its early stage can mimic an inflammatory process. In fact, with our current understanding of the continuum of chronic inflammation and MALT lymphomas, the biological distinction between the two processes may be impossible.

Intraocular Lymphomas

Primary intraocular lymphoma can be histologically diverse but, as in the brain, large B-cell lesions predominate (46). Figure 3 shows the microscopic features of a typical large B-cell lymphoma in the eye. Other forms are described, which span both high- and low-grade lesions, including T-cell lymphomas, mantle-cell lymphomas, and null-cell lymphomas (27,46). Additionally, intraocular involvement by Burkitt lymphoma, mycosis fungoides, HTLV1-associated lymphoma, Hodgkin lymphoma, and plasma cell myeloma have been documented (13,57,66,70,99,105). A special and unusual intraocular presentation is that of primary uveal extranodal marginal zone B-cell lymphomas (MALT-lymphomas) (27), which are unusual both in terms of their anatomic location (uvea, rather than the more common retinal presentation of primary lesions) and their typically indolent clinical course (rather than the aggressive course of the more common diffuse large B-cell lymphomas in the eye). The low-grade nature of these lymphomas is reflected in their past identification as "uveal pseudotumors." The high-grade nature of the lymphoma may not be apparent if the large lymphoma cells are in a minority and reactive small lymphocytes predominate as in the case of a T-cell-rich large B-cell lymphoma (31).

PROGNOSTIC FACTORS IN LYMPHOMAS OF THE ORBIT AND EYE

Orbital and Other Ocular Adnexal Lymphomas

Earlier studies recognized the presence of extraorbital disease in patients with orbital lymphoma as the primary indicator of poor outcome. Knowles et al. (64) found that lymphomas of the conjunctiva were less often associated with systemic involvement than were lymphomas involving the orbit or eyelid. More recent studies have emphasized that accurate classification according to the REAL/WHO classification is important in predicting behavior (16,94) and the stage of disease at presentation is still a significant factor in determining prognosis (5,80). Another recent study (53) found that the presence of bilateral disease, or involvement of the eyelid or lacrimal gland, was more often associated with subsequent systemic involvement and therefore with poorer overall outcome. A high-proliferation fraction or expression of CD43 is also noted to be associated with a poorer outcome (28,94). Chromosomal imbalances detected by comparative genomic hybridization were more commonly present in higher stage disease and were present in all patients who developed recurrent disease (92). A relatively small study of 23 patients (20) found that the presence or absence of chromosomal translocations and clinical stage were less important than the mode of therapy in determining outcome: combined chemotherapy and radiation therapy producing better results than either modality alone. However, the follow-up in this series of Charlotte et al. was relatively short (median 39 months) for indolent lymphomas-like MALT lymphomas (20). Others have found radiation therapy alone to be effective (33,68,80), at least for the MALT lymphomas. In a larger series with a median follow up of 7.5 years (86), age greater than 59 years, elevated lactate dehydrogenase level, disseminated (stage IV) disease, high-grade histology, and the presence of B-cell lymphoma symptoms had a negative impact on overall survival.

Intraocular Lymphoma

Excluding uveal MALT lymphomas, patients with intraocular lymphoma have a poor prognosis.

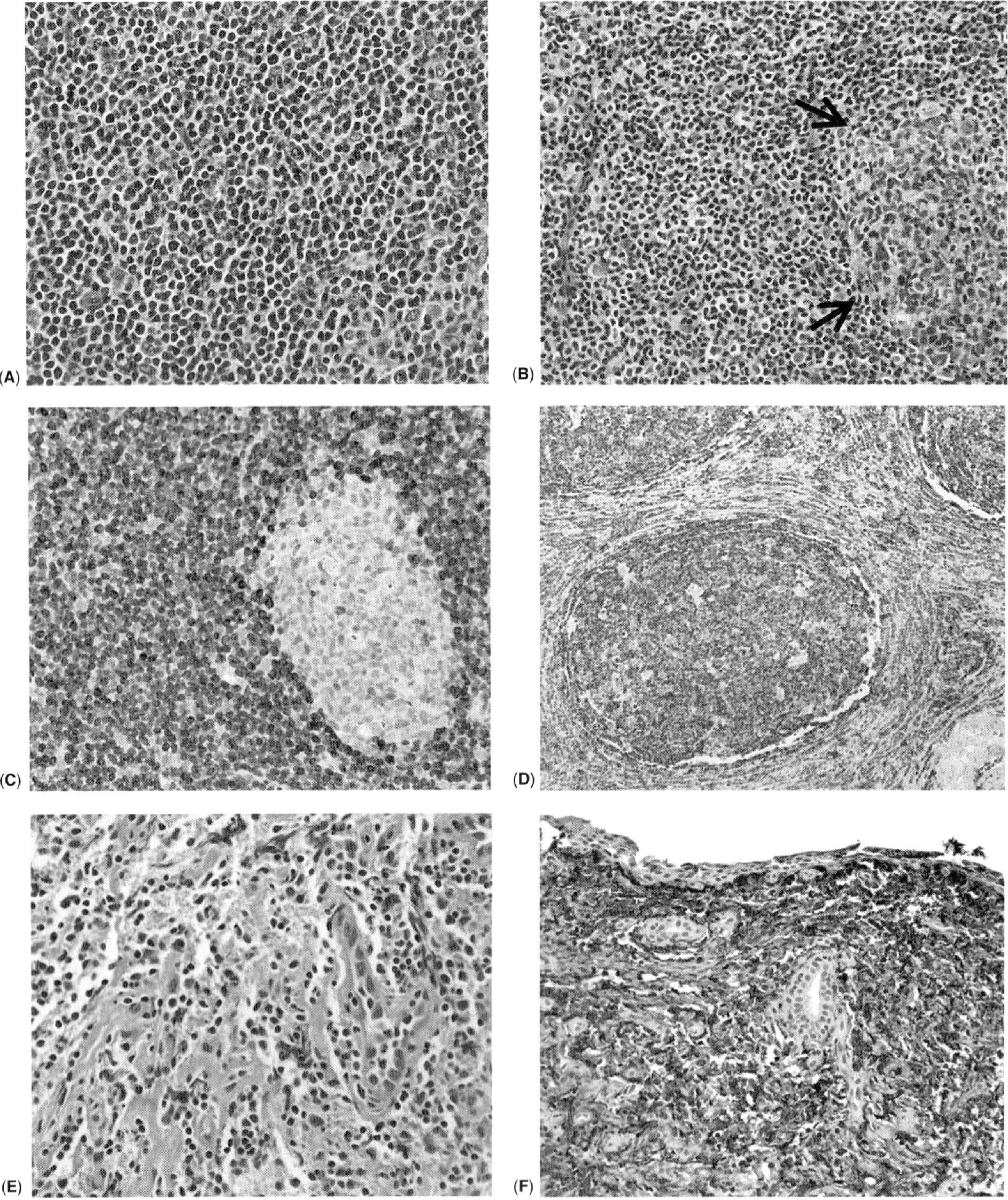

Figure 2 Microscopic features of representative orbital lymphomas. (**A**) MALT-type lymphomas characteristically show the so-called "monocytoid B-cells," which are medium-sized lymphoid cells with moderate, clear cytoplasm (hematoxylin and eosin, × 460). (**B**) Reactive lymphoid follicles (*arrows*) are not unusual in MALT lymphomas (hematoxylin and eosin, × 230). (**C**) The reactive (benign) nature of these follicles is apparent by their negative staining reaction with BCL2 (× 460). (**D**) In contrast, the follicles in follicular lymphoma stain positive for immunohistochemical staining for BCL2 (× 115). (**E**) MALT lymphomas may show an infiltrative pattern in the orbital soft tissues (hematoxylin and eosin, × 460). (**F**) MALT lymphoma in a subconjunctival location can be differentiated from reactive infiltrates by demonstrating that nearly all cells are B cells (CD20, × 230). (*Caption continues on next page.*)

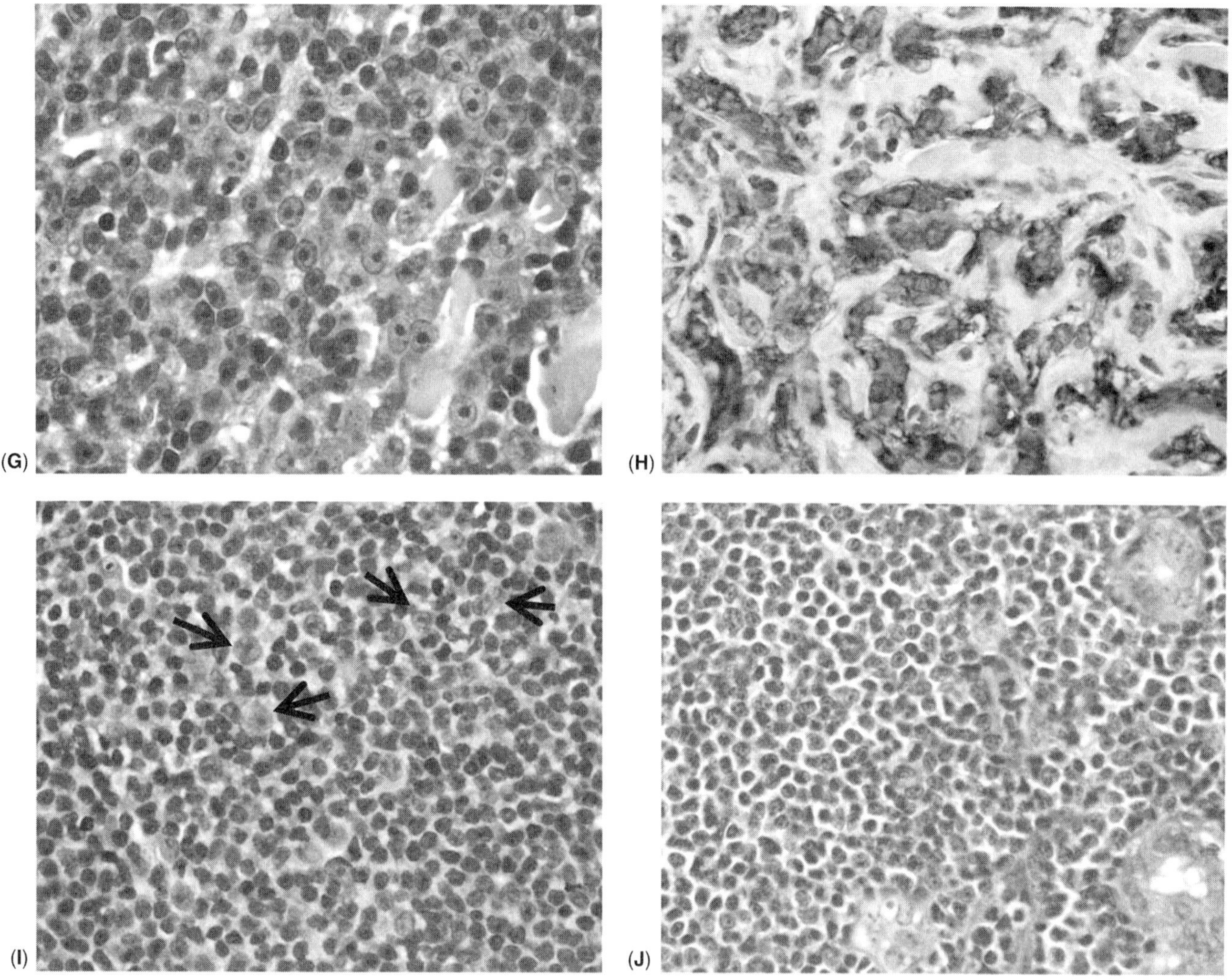

Figure 2 (*Continued*) (**G**) A diffuse large B-cell lymphoma with sheet-like arrangement of immunoblastic cells with prominent central nuclei usually poses no diagnostic problem (hematoxylin and eosin, × 690). (**H**) When present as an infiltrative growth in the soft tissue, immunohistochemical stains are useful to identify the B-cell origin of the tumor (CD20, × 690). (**I**) Chronic lymphocytic leukemia/small lymphocytic lymphoma produces sheet-like infiltrates of small lymphoid cells. Invariably, some centroblast-like large cells are present in small groups called proliferation centers (*arrows*) (hematoxylin and eosin, × 460). (**J**) Mantle cell lymphoma closely mimics CLL/SLL except that proliferation centers are usually absent. Unlike MALT lymphomas, these lymphomas do not show a propensity to attack epithelial structures. The demonstration of immunohistochemial staining for cyclin D1 in the nuclei of the lymphoma cells, or presence of the translocation between chromosomes 11 and 14 is required for diagnosis (hematoxylin and eosin, × 460).

Current therapeutic modalities are controversial and include chemotherapy with or without radiation (19). The blood–ocular barrier is a hindrance to standard chemotherapies, as is the blood–brain barrier and intravitreal delivery of chemotherapeutic agents has been employed. In general, median survivals after diagnosis are in the range of 2 to 3 years, and are significantly shorter when the brain is involved (46,48). Hormigo et al. demonstrated median survivals of up to 60 months in patients with isolated intraocular tumors, compared to 35 months in those with brain involvement at the time of therapy (48).

SPECIAL DIAGNOSTIC CONSIDERATIONS IN INTRAOCULAR, ORBITAL, AND OCULAR ADNEXAL LYMPHOMAS

Lymphoid neoplasms are clonal proliferations of B cells, T cells, or NK cells. When morphological features are not diagnostic of lymphoma, demonstration of clonality is an important confirmatory test. Flow cytometry and DNA-based molecular techniques may be used for this purpose. Additionally, the modern WHO classification of lymphomas is dependent on the immunophenotypic and cytogenetic/molecular properties of malignant cells. Flow

(A)

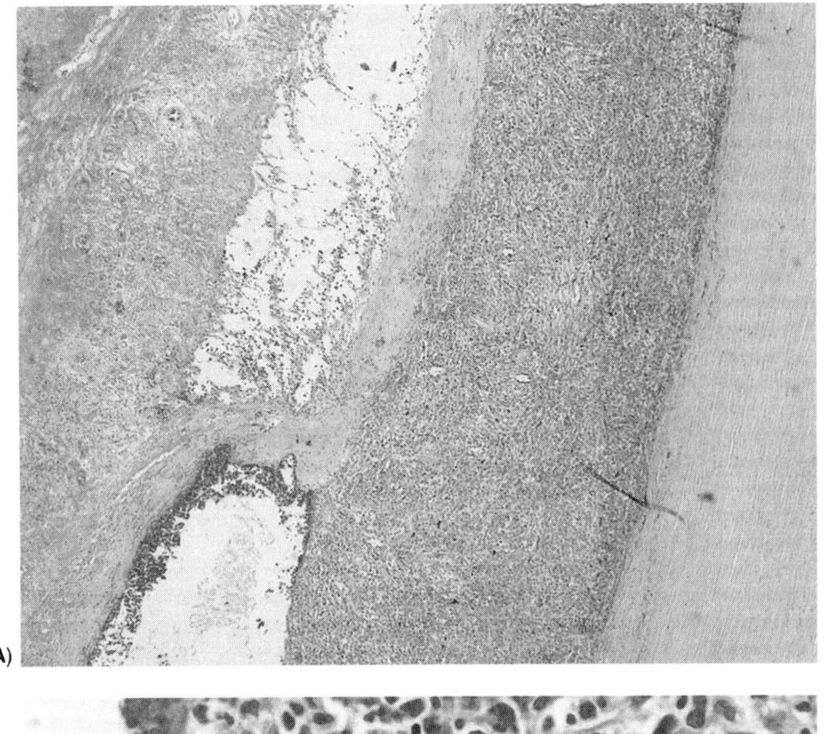

(B)

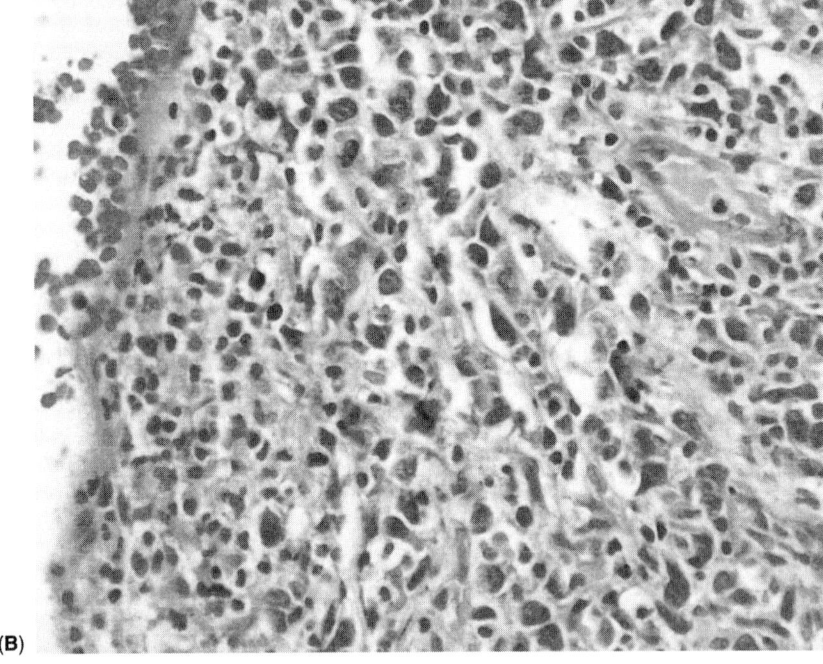

Figure 3 Intraocular large B-cell lymphoma. (**A**) The lymphoma cells grow in sheets under the retina (hematoxylin and eosin, × 115). (**B**) The anaplastic morphology, with large, irregular nuclei, and variably prominent nucleoli are common features of large cell lymphomas in any site (hematoxylin and eosin, × 690).

cytometry is particularly useful in defining the immunophenotype of malignant cells while fluorescence in situ hybridization (FISH) can supplement conventional cytogenetic studies in identifying specific chromosomal abnormalities. Flow cytometry requires living cells in suspension. The cells may be naturally in single cell suspension as in the cerebrospinal fluid (CSF), a fine needle aspirate of a brain lesion, or a vitrectomy specimen. A biopsy may be processed to yield a suspension of single cells but there can be substantial cell loss in processing, especially in cases of large cell lymphoma, plasma cell myeloma, as well as of Reed Sternberg cells in Hodgkin lymphoma. Additionally, the architectural detail available in a biopsy is irretrievably lost. Therefore, the decision to submit any part of a small biopsy specimen for flow cytometry should not be made automatically, but only when appropriate to the case. Availability of cells for analysis is often limited in CSF, fine needle aspirations or vitrectomy specimens and a careful decision has to be made as to which antigens should be tested. The experience of the pathologist and previous history of the patient are critical in making this choice.

Molecular Diagnostic Tests

Molecular diagnosis of CNS lymphoma may include polymerase chain reaction (PCR) based tests, which can be used to detect extremely small amounts of target DNA or RNA. FISH, defined earlier in this chapter, is an extension of cytogenetics using the molecular method of DNA hybridization. It can detect specific cytogenetic abnormalities in cells and tissues after fixation and with higher sensitivity than conventional cytogenetics. More recently, expression of several hundred genes can be tested using gene-chip technology and reverse transcription PCR. The first two are routinely used for diagnosis and the last is an investigational tool at this time.

Tissue Biopsy

Biopsy is the mainstay of diagnosis in orbital lymphomas. Due to the small size of the lesions or their location, only limited tissue may be available for examination. Many of the architectural features associated with particular types of lymphoma may not be readily apparent. Histological features such as follicle formation and lymphoepithelial lesions, may not be well developed or absent. Often, crush artifact introduced in the performance of the biopsy further reduces the quality of the histological material. A great deal of reliance has to be placed on immunohistochemical-staining patterns and an intimate knowledge of the expected staining patterns in the different types of lymphoma, particularly the unusual variations, is necessary to obtain the maximum information from the limited tissue available. As discussed above, many molecular diagnostic techniques can now be applied on paraffin-embedded tissue and are often necessary to make an accurate diagnosis. When a definitive diagnosis of lymphoma cannot be established with all available techniques, the lesion should be designated as an "atypical lymphoid infiltrate." This should prompt a search for systemic involvement and follow up to watch for persistent or worsening disease.

REFERENCES

1. Abiose A, Adido J, Agarwal SC. Childhood malignancies of the eye and orbit in northern Nigeria. Cancer 1985; 55: 2889–93.
2. Akpek EK, Maca SM, Christen WG, et al. Elevated vitreous interleukin-10 level is not diagnostic of intraocular–central nervous system lymphoma. Ophthalmology 1999; 106:2291–5.
3. Apte RS, Mayhew E, Niederkorn JY. Local inhibition of natural killer cell activity promotes the progressive growth of intraocular tumors. Invest Ophthalmol Vis Sci 1997; 38:1277–82.
4. Auer IA, Gascoyne RD, Connors JM, et al. T(11;18)(q21; q21) is the most common translocation in MALT lymphomas. Ann Oncol 1997; 8:979–85.
5. Auw-Haedrich C, Coupland SE, Kapp A, et al. Long-term outcome of ocular adnexal lymphoma subtyped according to the REAL classification. Revised European and American Lymphoma. Br J Ophthalmol 2001; 85: 63–9.
6. Bardenstein DS. Ocular adnexal lymphoma: classification, clinical disease, and molecular biology. Ophthalmol Clin North Am 2005; 18:187–97.
7. Barr CC, Green WR, Payne JW, et al. Intraocular reticulum-cell sarcoma: clinico-pathologic study of four cases and review of the literature. Surv Ophthalmol 1975; 19:224–39.
8. Barrans SL, Fenton JA, Banham A, et al. Strong expression of FOXP1 identifies a distinct subset of diffuse large B-cell lymphoma (DLBCL) patients with poor outcome. Blood 2004; 104:2933–5.
9. Berger F, Felman P, Thieblemont C, et al. Non-MALT marginal zone B-cell lymphomas: a description of clinical presentation and outcome in 124 patients. Blood 2000; 95: 1950–6.
10. Bertoni F, Zucca E. Delving deeper into MALT lymphoma biology. J Clin Invest 2006; 116:22–6.
11. Bhatia S, Paulino AC, Buatti JM, et al. Curative radiotherapy for primary orbital lymphoma. Int J Radiat Oncol Biol Phys 2002; 54:818–23.
12. Bienenstock J, Befus D. Gut- and bronchus-associated lymphoid tissue. Am J Anat 1984; 170:437–45.
13. Bishop JE, Salmonsen PC. Presumed intraocular Hodgkin's disease. Ann Ophthalmol 1985; 17:589–92.
14. Brandtzaeg P, Farstad IN, Johansen FE, et al. The B-cell system of human mucosae and exocrine glands. Immunol Rev 1999; 171:45–87.
15. Buettner H, Bolling JP. Intravitreal large-cell lymphoma. Mayo Clin Proc 1993; 68:1011–5.
16. Cahill M, Barnes C, Moriarty P, et al. Ocular adnexal lymphoma-comparison of MALT lymphoma with other histological types. Br J Ophthalmol 1999; 83:742–7.
17. Cavalli F, Isaacson PG, Gascoyne RD, et al. MALT lymphomas. Hematology (Am Soc Hematol Educ Program) 2001: 241–58.
18. Chan CC. Molecular pathology of primary intraocular lymphoma. Trans Am Ophthalmol Soc 2003; 101:275–92.
19. Chan CC, Wallace DJ. Intraocular lymphoma: update on diagnosis and management. Cancer Control 2004; 11: 285–95.
20. Charlotte F, Doghmi K, Cassoux N, et al. Ocular adnexal marginal zone B cell lymphoma: a clinical and pathologic study of 23 cases. Virchows Arch 2005; 1–11.
21. Chen PM, Chiou TJ, Yu IT, et al. Molecular analysis of mucosa-associated lymphoid tissue (MALT) lymphoma of ocular adnexa. Leuk Lymphoma 2001; 42:207–14.
22. Cho EY, Han JJ, Ree HJ, et al. Clinicopathologic analysis of ocular adnexal lymphomas: extranodal marginal zone B-cell lymphoma constitutes the vast majority of ocular lymphomas among Koreans and affects younger patients. Am J Hematol 2003; 73:87–96.
23. Clark WL, Scott IU, Murray TG, et al. Primary intraocular posttransplantation lymphoproliferative disorder. Arch Ophthalmol 1998; 116:1667–9.
24. Cockerham GC, Jakobiec FA. Lymphoproliferative disorders of the ocular adnexa. Int Ophthalmol Clin 1997; 37: 39–59.

25. Cooper EL, Riker JL. Malignant lymphoma of the uveal tract. Am J Ophthalmol 1951; 34:1153–8.
26. Coupland SE, Foss HD, Assaf C, et al. T-cell and T/natural killer-cell lymphomas involving ocular and ocular adnexal tissues: a clinicopathologic, immunohistochemical, and molecular study of seven cases. Ophthalmology 1999; 106:2109–20.
27. Coupland SE, Heimann H, Bechrakis NE. Primary intraocular lymphoma: a review of the clinical, histopathological and molecular biological features. Graefes Arch Clin Exp Ophthalmol 2004; 242:901–13.
28. Coupland SE, Hellmich M, Auw-Haedrich C, et al. Prognostic value of cell-cycle markers in ocular adnexal lymphoma: an assessment of 230 cases. Graefes Arch Clin Exp Ophthalmol 2004; 242:130–45.
29. Coupland SE, Krause L, Delecluse HJ, et al. Lymphoproliferative lesions of the ocular adnexa. Analysis of 112 cases. Ophthalmology 1998; 105:1430–41.
30. Crowe SE. Helicobacter infection, chronic inflammation, and the development of malignancy. Curr Opin Gastroenterol 2005; 21:32–8.
31. Cummings TJ, Stenzel TT, Klintworth G, et al. Primary intraocular T-cell-rich large B-cell lymphoma. Arch Pathol Lab Med 2005; 129:1050–3.
32. Demirci H, Shields CL, Shields JA, et al. Orbital tumors in the older adult population. Ophthalmology 2002; 109: 243–8.
33. Esik O, Ikeda H, Mukai K, et al. A retrospective analysis of different modalities for treatment of primary orbital non-Hodgkin's lymphomas. Radiother Oncol 1996; 38: 13–8.
34. Farmer JP, Lamba M, Lamba WR, et al. Lymphoproliferative lesions of the lacrimal gland: clinicopathological, immunohistochemical and molecular genetic analysis. Can J Ophthalmol 2005; 40:151–60.
35. Ferreri AJ, Ponzoni M, Guidoboni M, et al. Regression of ocular adnexal lymphoma after *Chlamydia psittaci*-eradicating antibiotic therapy. J Clin Oncol 2005; 23:5067–73.
36. Fisher SG, Fisher RI. The epidemiology of non-Hodgkin's lymphoma. Oncogene 2004; 23:6524–34.
37. Freeman LN, Schachat AP, Knox DL, et al. Clinical features, laboratory investigations, and survival in ocular reticulum cell sarcoma. Ophthalmology 1987; 94:1631–9.
38. Fung CY, Tarbell NJ, Lucarelli MJ, et al. Ocular adnexal lymphoma: clinical behavior of distinct World Health Organization classification subtypes. Int J Radiat Oncol Biol Phys 2003; 57:1382–91.
39. Galieni P, Polito E, Leccisotti A, et al. Localized orbital lymphoma. Haematologica 1997; 82:436–9.
40. Gascoyne RD. Molecular pathogenesis of mucosal-associated lymphoid tissue (MALT) lymphoma. Leuk Lymphoma 2003; 44:S13–20.
41. Gascoyne RD. Emerging prognostic factors in diffuse large B-cell lymphoma. Curr Opin Oncol 2004; 16: 436–41.
42. Groves FD, Linet MS, Travis LB, et al. Cancer surveillance series: non-Hodgkin's lymphoma incidence by histologic subtype in the United States from 1978 through 1995. J Natl Cancer Inst 2000; 92:240–51.
43. Harris NL, Jaffe ES, Stein H, et al. A revised European–American classification of lymphoid neoplasms: a proposal from the International Lymphoma Study Group. Blood 1994; 84:1361–92.
44. Higashide T, Takahira M, Okumura H, et al. Bilaterally identical monoclonality in a case of primary intraocular lymphoma. Am J Ophthalmol 2004; 138:306–8.
45. Hochberg FH, Miller DC. Primary central nervous system lymphoma. J Neurosurg 1988; 68:835–53.
46. Hoffman PM, McKelvie P, Hall AJ, et al. Intraocular lymphoma: a series of 14 patients with clinicopathological features and treatment outcomes. Eye 2003; 17: 513–21.
47. Hofman P, Le Tourneau A, Negre F, et al. Primary uveal B immunoblastic lymphoma in a patient with AIDS. Br J Ophthalmol 1992; 76:700–2.
48. Hormigo A, Abrey L, Heinemann MH, et al. Ocular presentation of primary central nervous system lymphoma: diagnosis and treatment. Br J Haematol 2004; 126: 202–8.
49. Isaacson P, Wright DH. Malignant lymphoma of mucosa-associated lymphoid tissue. A distinctive type of B-cell lymphoma. Cancer 1983; 52:1410–6.
50. Isaacson PG. Gastric MALT lymphoma: from concept to cure. Ann Oncol 1999; 10:637–45.
51. Isaacson PG, Spencer J. Malignant lymphoma of mucosa-associated lymphoid tissue. Histopathology 1987; 11: 445–62.
52. Jaffe ES, Harris NL, Stein H, et al. Pathology and genetics of tumours of haematopoietic and lymphoid tissues. In: Kleihues P, Sobin LH, eds. World Health Organization Classification of Tumours. Lyon, France: IARC Press, 2001.
53. Jenkins C, Rose GE, Bunce C, et al. Clinical features associated with survival of patients with lymphoma of the ocular adnexa. Eye 2003; 17:809–20.
54. Jenkins C, Rose GE, Bunce C, et al. Histological features of ocular adnexal lymphoma (REAL classification) and their association with patient morbidity and survival. Br J Ophthalmol 2000; 84:907–13.
55. Johnson K, Shapiro-Shelef M, Tunyaplin C, et al. Regulatory events in early and late B-cell differentiation. Mol Immunol 2005; 42:749–61.
56. Johnson TE, Tse DT, Byrne GE Jr, et al. Ocular-adnexal lymphoid tumors: a clinicopathologic and molecular genetic study of 77 patients. Ophthal Plast Reconstr Surg 1999; 15:171–9.
57. Keltner JL, Fritsch E, Cykiert RC, et al. Mycosis fungoides. Intraocular and central nervous system involvement. Arch Ophthalmol 1977; 95:645–50.
58. Kheterpal S, Kirkby GR, Neuberger JM, et al. Intraocular lymphoma after liver transplantation. Am J Ophthalmol 1993; 116:507–8.
59. Kim DR. Proteomic changes during the B cell development. J Chromatogr B Analyt Technol Biomed Life Sci 2005; 815:295–303.
60. Klauss V, Chana HS. Ocular tumors in Africa. Soc Sci Med 1983; 17:1743–50.
61. Klingele TG, Hogan MJ. Ocular reticulum cell sarcoma. Am J Ophthalmol 1975; 79:39–47.
62. Knowles DM. Etiology and pathogenesis of AIDS-related non-Hodgkin's lymphoma. Hematol Oncol Clin North Am 2003; 17:785–820.
63. Knowles DM II, Jakobiec FA. Ocular adnexal lymphoid neoplasms: clinical, histopathologic, electron microscopic, and immunologic characteristics. Hum Pathol 1982; 13:148–62.
64. Knowles DM, Jakobiec FA, McNally L, et al. Lymphoid hyperplasia and malignant lymphoma occurring in the ocular adnexa (orbit, conjunctiva, and eyelids): a prospective multiparametric analysis of 108 cases during 1977 to 1987. Hum Pathol 1990; 21:959–73.
65. Krol AD, le Cessie S, Snijder S, et al. Primary extranodal non-Hodgkin's lymphoma (NHL): the impact of alternative definitions tested in the Comprehensive Cancer

Centre West population-based NHL registry. Ann Oncol 2003; 14:131–9.
66. Kumar SR, Gill PS, Wagner DG, et al. Human T-cell lymphotropic virus type I-associated retinal lymphoma. A clinicopathologic report. Arch Ophthalmol 1994; 112: 954–9.
67. Lauer SA. Ocular adnexal lymphoid tumors. Curr Opin Ophthalmol 2000; 11:361–6.
68. Le QT, Eulau SM, George TI, et al. Primary radiotherapy for localized orbital MALT lymphoma. Int J Radiat Oncol Biol Phys 2002; 52:657–63.
69. Lee JL, Kim MK, Lee KH, et al. Extranodal marginal zone B-cell lymphomas of mucosa-associated lymphoid tissue-type of the orbit and ocular adnexa. Ann Hematol 2005; 84:13–8.
70. Leitch RJ, Rennie IG, Parsons MA. Ocular involvement in mycosis fungoides. Br J Ophthalmol 1993; 77:126–7.
71. Liu H, Ruskon-Fourmestraux A, Lavergne-Slove A, et al. Resistance of t(11;18) positive gastric mucosa-associated lymphoid tissue lymphoma to *Helicobacter pylori* eradication therapy. Lancet 2001; 357:39–40.
72. Liu H, Ye H, Ruskone-Fourmestraux A, et al. T(11;18) is a marker for all stage gastric MALT lymphomas that will not respond to *Helicobacter pylori* eradication. Gastroenterology 2002; 122:1286–94.
73. Lobo A, Larkin G, Clark BJ, et al. Pseudo-hypopyon as the presenting feature in B-cell and T-cell intraocular lymphoma. Clin Experiment Ophthalmol 2003; 31:155–8.
74. Looi A, Gascoyne RD, Chhanabhai M, et al. Mantle cell lymphoma in the ocular adnexal region. Ophthalmology 2005; 112:114–9.
75. Lopes-Carvalho T, Kearney JF. Marginal zone B cell physiology and disease. Curr Dir Autoimmun 2005; 8: 91–123.
76. Lopez-Guillermo A, Cid J, Salar A, et al. Peripheral T-cell lymphomas: initial features, natural history, and prognostic factors in a series of 174 patients diagnosed according to the REAL classification. Ann Oncol 1998; 9:849–55.
77. Lucas PC, McAllister-Lucas LM, Nunez G. NF-kappaB signaling in lymphocytes: a new cast of characters. J Cell Sci 2004; 117:31–9.
78. Mannami T, Yoshino T, Oshima K, et al. Clinical, histopathological, and immunogenetic analysis of ocular adnexal lymphoproliferative disorders: characterization of malt lymphoma and reactive lymphoid hyperplasia. Mod Pathol 2001; 14:641–9.
79. Margo CE, Mulla ZD. Malignant tumors of the orbit. Analysis of the Florida Cancer Registry. Ophthalmology 1998; 105:185–90.
80. Martinet S, Ozsahin M, Belkacemi Y, et al. Outcome and prognostic factors in orbital lymphoma: a Rare Cancer Network study on 90 consecutive patients treated with radiotherapy. Int J Radiat Oncol Biol Phys 2003; 55:892–8.
81. Matsuo T, Yamaoka A, Shiraga F, et al. Two types of initial ocular manifestations in intraocular–central nervous system lymphoma. Retina 1998; 18:301–7.
82. Matzkin DC, Slamovits TL, Rosenbaum PS. Simultaneous intraocular and orbital non-Hodgkin lymphoma in the acquired immune deficiency syndrome. Ophthalmology 1994; 101:850–5.
83. McKelvie PA, McNab A, Francis IC, et al. Ocular adnexal lymphoproliferative disease: a series of 73 cases. Clin Experiment Ophthalmol 2001; 29:387–93.
84. McNally L, Jakobiec FA, Knowles DM II. Clinical, morphologic, immunophenotypic, and molecular genetic analysis of bilateral ocular adnexal lymphoid neoplasms in 17 patients. Am J Ophthalmol 1987; 103:555–68.
85. Merle-Beral H, Davi F, Cassoux N, et al. Biological diagnosis of primary intraocular lymphoma. Br J Haematol 2004; 124:469–73.
86. Meunier J, Lumbroso-Le Rouic L, Vincent-Salomon A, et al. Ophthalmologic and intraocular non-Hodgkin's lymphoma: a large single centre study of initial characteristics, natural history, and prognostic factors. Hematol Oncol 2004; 22:143–58.
87. Mittra RA, Pulido JS, Hanson GA, et al. Primary ocular Epstein–Barr virus-associated non-Hodgkin's lymphoma in a patient with AIDS: a clinicopathologic report. Retina 1999; 19:45–50.
88. Miyamoto M, Haruma K, Hiyama T, et al. High incidence of B-cell monoclonality in follicular gastritis: a possible association between follicular gastritis and MALT lymphoma. Virchows Arch 2002; 440:376–80.
89. Morgello S, Lagoo AS. Nervous system involvement by lymphoma, leukemia, and other hematopoietic cell proliferations. In: McLendon RE, Bigner D, Bigner S, et al., eds. Pathology of Tumors of the Central Nervous System: A Guide to Histologic Diagnosis. Oxford: Oxford University Press, 2006.
90. Muller AM, Ihorst G, Mertelsmann R, et al. Epidemiology of non-Hodgkin's lymphoma (NHL): trends, geographic distribution, and etiology. Ann Hematol 2005; 84:1–12.
91. Nakata M, Matsuno Y, Katsumata N, et al. Histology according to the Revised European–American Lymphoma Classification significantly predicts the prognosis of ocular adnexal lymphoma. Leuk Lymphoma 1999; 32:533–43.
92. Ness GO, Lybaek H, Arnes J, et al. Chromosomal imbalances in lymphoid tumors of the orbit. Invest Ophthalmol Vis Sci 2002; 43:9–14.
93. Niu H. The proto-oncogene BCL-6 in normal and malignant B cell development. Hematol Oncol 2002; 20:155–66.
94. Nola M, Lukenda A, Bollmann M, et al. Outcome and prognostic factors in ocular adnexal lymphoma. Croat Med J 2004; 45:328–32.
95. Ohtsuka K, Hashimoto M, Suzuki Y. High incidence of orbital malignant lymphoma in Japanese patients. Am J Ophthalmol 2004; 138:881–2.
96. Ormerod LD, Puklin JE. AIDS-associated intraocular lymphoma causing primary retinal vasculitis. Ocul Immunol Inflamm 1997; 5:271–8.
97. Ott G, Katzenberger T, Greiner A, et al. The t(11;18)(q21; q21) chromosome translocation is a frequent and specific aberration in low-grade but not high-grade malignant non-Hodgkin's lymphomas of the mucosa-associated lymphoid tissue (MALT-) type. Cancer Res 1997; 57: 3944–8.
98. Papadaki T, Stamatopoulos K. Hodgkin disease immunopathogenesis: long-standing questions, recent answers, further directions. Trend Immunol 2003; 24:508–11.
99. Payne T, Karp LA, Zimmerman LE. Intraocular involvement in Burkitt's lymphoma. Arch Ophthalmol 1971; 85: 295–8.
100. Rosado MF, Byrne GE Jr, Ding F, et al. Ocular adnexal lymphoma: a clinicopathological study of a large cohort of patients with no evidence for an association with *Chlamydia psittaci*. Blood 2005; 15:15.
101. Sasai K, Yamabe H, Dodo Y, et al. Non-Hodgkin's lymphoma of the ocular adnexa. Acta Oncol 2001; 40: 485–90.
102. Saxena A, Moshynska O, Kanthan R, et al. Distinct B-cell clonal bands in *Helicobacter pylori* gastritis with lymphoid hyperplasia. J Pathol 2000; 190:47–54.

103. Seerp Baarsma G, Roland Smit LM. Presumed intraocular lymphoma in a 60-year-old man with AIDS. Eur J Ophthalmol 1992; 2:203–4.
104. Seve P, Renaudier P, Sasco AJ, et al. Hepatitis C virus infection and B-cell non-Hodgkin's lymphoma: a cross-sectional study in Lyon, France. Eur J Gastroenterol Hepatol 2004; 16:1361–5.
105. Shakin EP, Augsburger JJ, Eagle RC Jr, et al. Multiple myeloma involving the iris. Arch Ophthalmol 1988; 106: 524–6.
106. Sharara N, Holden JT, Wojno TH, et al. Ocular adnexal lymphoid proliferations: clinical, histologic, flow cytometric, and molecular analysis of forty-three cases. Ophthalmology 2003; 110:1245–54.
107. Shields CL, Shields JA, Carvalho C, et al. Conjunctival lymphoid tumors: clinical analysis of 117 cases and relationship to systemic lymphoma. Ophthalmology 2001; 108:979–84.
108. Shields JA, Shields CL, Scartozzi R. Survey of 1264 patients with orbital tumors and simulating lesions: the 2002 Montgomery Lecture, part 1. Ophthalmology 2004; 111:997–1008.
109. Sigurdardottir M, Sigurdsson H, Barkardottir RB, et al. Lymphoid tumours of the ocular adnexa: a morphologic and genotypic study of 15 cases. Acta Ophthalmol Scand 2003; 81:299–303.
110. Stanton CA, Sloan B III, Slusher MM, et al. Acquired immunodeficiency syndrome-related primary intraocular lymphoma. Arch Ophthalmol 1992; 110:1614–7.
111. Streilein JW, Ohta K, Mo JS, et al. Ocular immune privilege and the impact of intraocular inflammation. DNA Cell Biol 2002; 21:453–9.
112. Streilein JW, Okamoto S, Sano Y, et al. Neural control of ocular immune privilege. Ann N Y Acad Sci 2000; 917: 297–306.
113. Streubel B, Lamprecht A, Dierlamm J, et al. T(14;18)(q32; q21) involving IGH and MALT1 is a frequent chromosomal aberration in MALT lymphoma. Blood 2002; 24:24.
114. Streubel B, Vinatzer U, Lamprecht A, et al. T(3;14)(p14.1; q32) involving IGH and FOXP1 is a novel recurrent chromosomal aberration in MALT lymphoma. Leukemia 2005; 19:652–8.
115. Sullivan TJ, Whitehead K, Williamson R, et al. Lymphoproliferative disease of the ocular adnexa: a clinical and pathologic study with statistical analysis of 69 patients. Ophthal Plast Reconstr Surg 2005; 21: 177–88.
116. Takada S, Yoshino T, Taniwaki M, et al. Involvement of the chromosomal translocation t(11;18) in some Mucosa-associated lymphoid tissue lymphomas and diffuse large B-Cell lymphomas of the ocular adnexa evidence from multiplex reverse transcriptase-polymerase chain reaction and fluorescence in situ hybridization on using formalin-fixed, paraffin-embedded specimens. Mod Pathol 2003; 16:445–52.
117. Takahashi N, Miura I, Ohshima A, et al. Translocation (3;14)(q27;q11): a new variant translocation in a patient with non-Hodgkin's lymphoma of B-cell type with BCL6 rearrangement. Cancer Genet Cytogenet 1996; 90:49–53.
118. Takamura H, Terashima K, Yamashita H. Diagnosis and treatment of orbital malignant lymphoma: a 14-year review at Yamagata University. Jpn J Ophthalmol 2001; 45:305–12.
119. Thome M. CARMA1, BCL-10 and MALT1 in lymphocyte development and activation. Nat Rev Immunol 2004; 4:348–59.
120. Tranfa F, Di Matteo G, Strianese D, et al. Primary orbital lymphoma. Orbit 2001; 20:119–24.
121. Turner RR, Egbert P, Warnke RA. Lymphocytic infiltrates of the conjunctiva and orbit: immunohistochemical staining of 16 cases. Am J Clin Pathol 1984; 81: 447–52.
122. Unassigned: a clinical evaluation of the International Lymphoma Study Group classification of non-Hodgkin's lymphoma. The non-Hodgkin's Lymphoma Classification Project. Blood 1997; 89:3909–18.
123. Velez G, de Smet MD, Whitcup SM, et al. Iris involvement in primary intraocular lymphoma: report of two cases and review of the literature. Surv Ophthalmol 2000; 44: 518–26.
124. Wallace DJ, Shen D, Reed GF, et al. Detection of the bcl-2 t (14;18) translocation and proto-oncogene expression in primary intraocular lymphoma. Invest Ophthalmol Vis Sci 2006; 47:2750–6.
125. White VA, Gascoyne RD, McNeil BK, et al. Histopathologic findings and frequency of clonality detected by the polymerase chain reaction in ocular adnexal lymphoproliferative lesions. Mod Pathol 1996; 9:1052–61.
126. White WL, Ferry JA, Harris NL, et al. Ocular adnexal lymphoma. A clinicopathologic study with identification of lymphomas of mucosa-associated lymphoid tissue type. Ophthalmology 1995; 102:1994–2006.
127. Willemze R, Jaffe ES, Burg G, et al. WHO-EORTC classification for cutaneous lymphomas. Blood 2005; 105:3768–85.
128. Willis TG, Jadayel DM, Du MQ, et al. Bcl10 is involved in t(1;14)(p22;q32) of MALT B cell lymphoma and mutated in multiple tumor types. Cell 1999; 96: 35–45.
129. Wlodarska I, Veyt E, de Paepe P, et al. FOXP1, a gene highly expressed in a subset of diffuse large B-cell lymphoma, is recurrently targeted by genomic aberrations. Leukemia 2005; 19:1299–305.
130. Yan J, Wu Z, Huang S, et al. The clinical value of rearrangement of IgH gene and bcl-2/J(H) fuse gene in the diagnosis of orbital lymphoproliferative disorders. Chung Hua Yen Ko Tsa Chih 2002; 38:388–91.
131. Ye H, Gong L, Liu H, et al. MALT lymphoma with t(14;18) (q32;q21)/IGH-MALT1 is characterized by strong cytoplasmic MALT1 and BCL10 expression. J Pathol 2005; 205: 293–301.
132. Ye H, Liu H, Attygalle A, et al. Variable frequencies of t(11;18)(q21;q21) in MALT lymphomas of different sites: significant association with CagA strains of *H. pylori* in gastric MALT lymphoma. Blood 2003; 3:3.
133. Ye H, Liu H, Raderer M, et al. High incidence of t(11;18) (q21;q21) in *Helicobacter pylori*-negative gastric MALT lymphoma. Blood 2003; 101:2547–50.
134. Ziemianski MC, Godfrey WA, Lee KY, et al. Lymphoma of the vitreous associated with renal transplantation and immunosuppressive therapy. Ophthalmology 1980; 87: 596–601.

67

Vascular Diseases

Geoffrey G. Emerson, Peter J. Francis, and David J. Wilson
Casey Eye Institute, Oregon Health and Science University, Portland, Oregon, U.S.A.

Alec Garner
Institute of Ophthalmology, Moorfields Eye Hospital, London, U.K.

INTRODUCTION

As in other parts of the body the ocular tissues are dependent on the vascular system for nutrients and many diseases of the vascular system affect the eye and adnexa. This chapter summarizes the structure of the normal blood vessels. It also reviews general aspects of vascular disease in the eye and specific vascular disorders and their ocular effects.

NORMAL BLOOD VESSELS

Development

In contrast to angiogenesis (see Chapter 68) the vascular system develops by vasculogenesis from mesenchymal tissue in the mesoderm as endothelial and fibrous supportive tissue primordia (angioblastic mesoderm) (1). Endothelial cells proliferate to form of chords of cells. The chords of angioblasts produce an early laminin basement membrane, generate a partial lumen (37) and migrate over a transient matrix of fibronectin to contact neighboring chords. Arcades of vessels are produced, the earliest sign of a capillary network (Fig. 1). With the establishment of blood flow to meet local metabolic demand of developing tissues the characteristics of arteries and veins will appear (78). Solid cords of endothelium are created and link with other cords to form a network of lumenized capillaries. Subsequent growth is increasingly dependent on sprouting from these early vessels.

A major factor influencing the proliferation and maturation of the vasculature in the later stages of embryogenesis and fetal development is local metabolic demand, and this control persists throughout life. The smaller blood vessels especially are dependent on an active circulation for their maturation.

Initial activity is concerned with cell proliferation and migration, functions facilitated by fibronectin secretion. There then follows a switch to laminin production, which induces further differentiation so

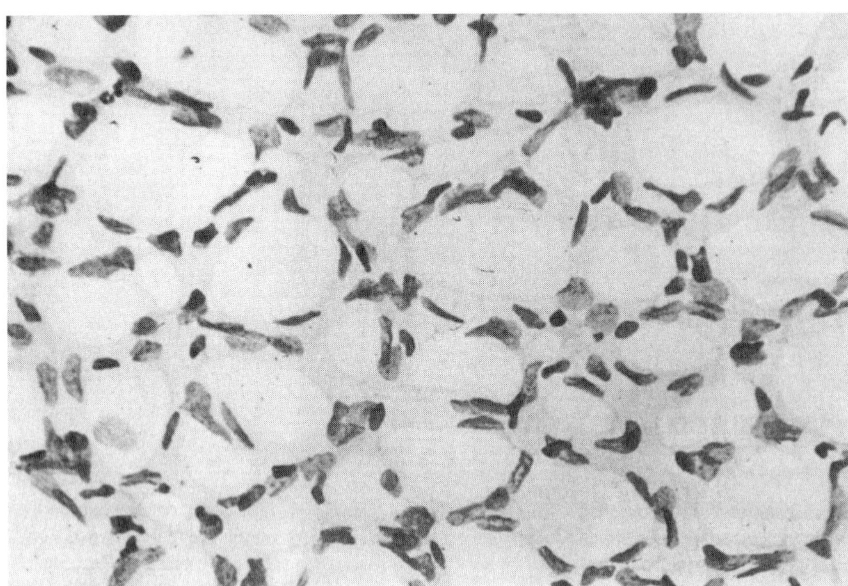

Figure 1 Embryonic development of peripheral vascular bed. Enzyme digest preparation of the developing vasculature in the retina of a 20-week-old fetus shows a network of endothelium-lined capillaries. Subsequent development involves the selective atrophy of some capillaries and the hypertrophy of others before the definitive circulation is established (hematoxylin and eosin, × 175). *Source*: From Ref. 57.

that a lumen is formed (37) and cell-to-cell attachments develop. Anchorage of the developing vascular endothelium to the extracellular matrix (ECM) is necessary, and is accomplished by the production of heparan sulfate proteoglycan and the cell adhesion-promoting nidogen/entactin molecule encourages stability, collagen type IV serving to bind the various components and form a basement membrane on the abluminal side of the capillary. The addition of pericytes, smooth muscle cells, and fibroblasts to the outer aspect of the blood vessel continue the maturation process.

These general principles are similarly observed in the embryogenesis of the ocular circulation, the latter having been studied most thoroughly in the retina, where a close meshwork of capillaries is laid down by in situ mesenchyme (32), possibly emanating from the adventitia of established blood vessels at the optic nerve head. Subsequently, some capillaries become acellular by a process of retraction or degeneration of the endothelial lining and are reduced to mere strands of basement membrane, whereas others hypertrophy and become recognizable arterioles and venules, depending on their relationship to the parent artery and vein. The importance of tissue oxygenation in determining the density of the vascular bed in the retina is demonstrated by the wide capillary-free zone formed around the arterioles (67); that surrounding the veins is considerably narrower (Fig. 2)

Structure

The active tissue of the vascular system is the endothelial cell layer that modulates both intralumina viscosity and selective vascular permeability. Architectural support of the endothelium varies throughout the system. The most support is necessary for the large conductive channels (such as the aorta) that must accommodate high and variable intraluminal pressure. Architectural support is least at the capillary level where the intraluminal pressure is low and there is a premium established for selective transport of substances into and out of the vascular lumen. The venous system has intermediate degrees of architectural support.

Arteries

The arterial wall is composed of three zones external to the endothelium bounded by elastic lamina. The innermost is composed of smooth muscle and fibroblasts. The centered zone is composed mainly of smooth muscle cells, and the external layer is primarily loose fibrovascular tissue. Arteries have three coats; an inner intima provided by a single layer of endothelium resting on a collagenous zone in which smooth muscle cells and fibroblasts can be recognized, a media formed by smooth muscle, collagen, and elastic fibers, and an outer adventitia consisting of loose connective tissue. Between the coats of the larger blood vessels are elastic laminae, formed by condensation and cross-linkage of multiple elastic fibers, which completely encircle the wall.

The largest arteries (aorta, carotid, femoral) contain elastic tissue in the medial coat to withstand the wide fluctuation in intraluminal tension that takes place between cardiac systole and diastole. The elastic tissue acts as an energy reservoir and serves to propagate the onward movement of a pulse wave.

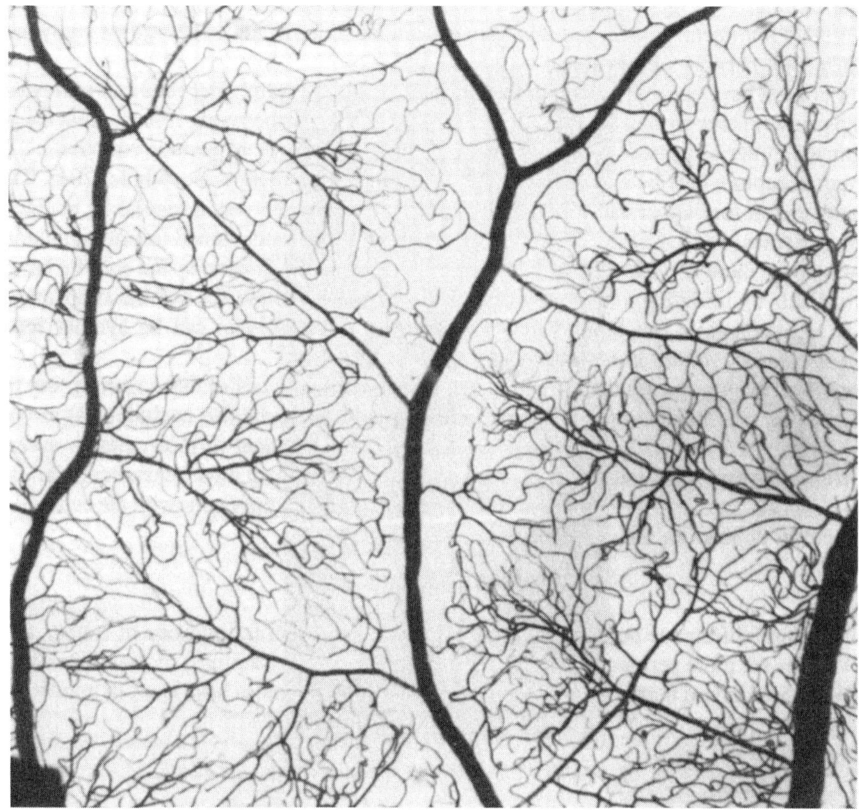

Figure 2 Flat preparation of a human retina injected with colloidal carbon to demonstrate the patent blood vessels. Next to the arteriole there is a zone free of perfused capillaries and considered a measure of the relatively high oxygen tension on the arterial side of the circulation since no such zone is adjacent to the venule (× 25).

The tensile properties of the collagen fibers, on the other hand, prevent overdistension during systole.

Arteries of smaller caliber, such as the ophthalmic artery and its branches, have rather less elastic tissue since they are required to withstand smaller distending forces. Conversely, they have a greater proportion of muscular tissue, individual smooth muscle cells being wrapped around the intimal lining in a predominantly helical fashion, to facilitate the regulation of blood flow through the lumen.

Arterioles

As their name implies, arterioles are minute arteries and the distinction between a small artery and a large arteriole is arbitrary the number of smooth muscle cells in cross sections of the wall. Definitions have been based, variously, on internal diameter, absence of a continuous internal elastic lamina, and the number of smooth muscle cells in cross sections of the wall. Rhodin (82) makes a distinction between arterioles measuring 50 to 100 μm with more than one layer of smooth muscle and a well-developed internal elastic lamina and terminal arterioles, with a caliber of 30 to 50 μm, a single layer of smooth muscle, and scanty or absent elastic tissue. As the capillary bed is approached, the elastic component diminishes and the muscle coat becomes discontinuous. The terminal or precapillary arterioles are the final arbiters of blood supply to the capillaries. It is within the small arteries and arterioles that the drop from an arterial pressure of around 100/70 mmHg to nonpulsatile flow at approximately 25 mmHg takes place.

Capillaries

Capillaries consist of a lumen lined by a single layer of endothelium attached to a basement membrane. In most capillaries, a second type of contractile cell, the pericyte, that is located external to the endothelial cell but within basement membrane produced by the endothelial cell and the pericyte.

Myofilaments have been described in the cytoplasm of both endothelial cells and pericytes, and both smooth muscle actin and myosin are present in pericytes (51). Pericytes in the ocular vascular system possess receptors for the potent vasoconstrictor peptide endothelin-1 (76). Endothelin-1 is secreted in a paracrine fashion by the endothelial cells (103). Similarly, the endothelium produces vasodilatory paracrine factors, including prostaglandin E_2, thromboxane, and nitric oxide. Endothelial cells and smooth muscle cells communicate directly via gap junctional coupling.

The cells of the systemic vascular endothelium are generally linked to each other by desmosomes (similar to those found in epithelial cells), but those in the retinal circulation are linked to each other by tight encircling junctions (zonulae occludentes) making up the retinal vascular portion of the blood–retinal barrier. The blood–retinal barrier restricts movement of molecules in excess of a few hundred daltons between the lumen of retinal vessels and the extravascular retinal environment.

Venules
The only structural difference between the smallest venules and capillaries is one of caliber. Venules are more permeable, more susceptible to vasoactive amines, such as histamine, and more apt to become thrombosed than are capillary vessels. The larger venules have smooth muscle cells in their walls.

Veins
Veins have a narrow layer of smooth muscle in their walls and a little elastic tissue. Both are less conspicuous than in arteries of the same size, and in consequence, veins are relatively more distensible and are able to function as capacitance vessels.

Cellular and Other Vascular Components

Endothelium
Endothelial cells vary in morphology and function throughout the circulatory system depending on vessel size and the nature of the organ or tissue. All vascular endothelial cells share certain general properties (53): (*i*) preservation of vascular integrity by triggering the clotting cascade, (*ii*) inhibition of inappropriate intravascular thrombosis and lysis of established clots, (*iii*) regulation of vascular permeability, (*iv*) control of blood flow distribution (via arterial and arteriolar tone), (*v*) source of growth factors involved in angiogenesis and wound repair, (*vi*) recruitment of inflammatory cells and mediators, and (*vii*) production of extracellular proteins, such as components of basement membrane.

Contractile filaments have been demonstrated in the cytoplasm of the vascular endothelium, including that of the retina (Fig. 3) (75). Filaments containing actin and myosin are particularly prominent in newly formed endothelium and may be related to the capacity of new blood vessels to infiltrate surrounding tissue.

The vascular endothelial cell is a manifestly complex cell with diverse functions (84), and it has a seminal role in the pathogenesis of most vasculopathies, including those affecting the eye.

Smooth Muscle
Vascular smooth muscle cells are spindle shaped and measure 20 to 50 μm in length. Their distinctive feature is a uniformly high density of contractile protein filaments, mostly in the form of a cell-specific actin, in the cytoplasm aligned parallel to the long axis of the cells. Contraction can be stimulated by mechanical stretching, metabolic factors, and, in all but intraretinal blood vessels, by adrenergic nerves.

Pericytes
Contractile cells lying external to the endothelial lining are a feature of capillaries in all ocular tissues. Each pericyte has multiple pseudopodial processes that envelop the capillary and are sandwiched between layers of basement membrane; in the retina about 85% of the lining endothelium is covered in this way (34).

The location of the pericytes is similar to the location of smooth muscle of larger vessels (51). When transmural pressure be increased, as occurs in shunt vessels, pericytes will transform into muscle cells (5) and, as previously noted, have receptors for endothelin-1. Nevertheless, there is no good evidence that they exercise an appreciable contractile function under normal conditions.

Basement Membrane
The basic component of vascular basement membranes, as with basement membranes elsewhere, is collagen type IV, which acts as a structural backbone and binds to the other membrane components. Laminin and fibronectin function in cell attachment to ECMs such as basement membrane. The role of the entactin and nidogen molecules is less well defined but again may have to do with cell attachment and general binding activities. Proteoglycans, especially heparan sulfate proteoglycan, are crucial to the selective barrier function of vascular basement membranes (5).

The membranes covering the outer surfaces of the smaller blood vessels have a second layer in which fibrils of up to 10 nm diameter are observed. Such fibrils are probably contributed by adjacent connective tissue cells, including, possibly, pericytes. This second layer is likely to correspond to the argyrophilic network of fibers seen to surround the vessels of the retina in digest preparations (Fig. 4).

Age-Related Changes
As with vessels in other parts of the cardiovascular system, those of the eye and its contents are subject to degeneration with age.

Arteries
From middle age onward, the smooth muscle cells of the media are slowly replaced by collagen, and the elastic tissue becomes progressively calcified and frayed. As a result there is loss of recoil capacity in

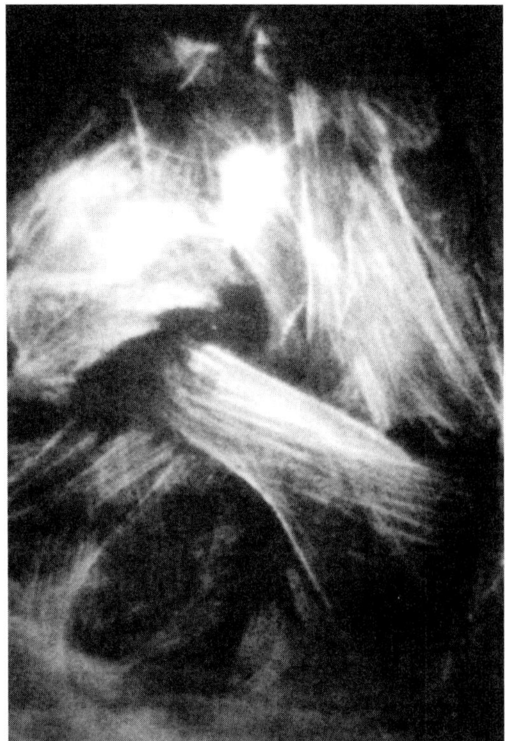

(A)

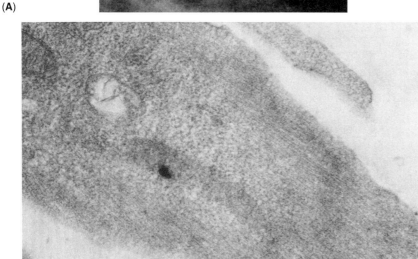

(B)

Figure 3 Contractile protein filaments in the cytoplasm of newly formed vascular endothelium in tissue culture. (**A**) Indirect immunofluorescence using antibody to actin shows bundles of myofilaments in the cytoplasm (× 750). (**B**) Transmission electron microscopy shows numerous 4 to 7 nm diameter filaments aligned parallel to the long axis of the cell (× 39,900).

response to the pulse wave, and the wall of the artery becomes fixed in a relatively dilated state to constitute senile arteriosclerosis. Some increase in intimal collagen also occurs, and commonly there is associated atherosclerosis. A progressive increase in interfibrillar cross-linkage of collagen fibers adds to the lack of distensibility and, morphologically, can be equated with increasing hyalinization of the media.

Arterioles

Arteriolar smooth muscle is likewise gradually replaced by collagen (Fig. 4), especially in the presence of hypertension. The mural thickening that results has the effect of reducing the caliber of the arteriole, whereas the reduced muscle content is paralleled in the retina by a reduced ability to autoregulate in response to changes in oxygen tension (77). A further complication of mural thickening in retinal arterioles is compression of branch veins as they pass beneath the arteriole.

The various degrees of mural thickening cause vascular dilation and progressive opacification of the vessel wall. Where venous channels pass under the arteriole the loss of vessel wall transparency produces a variety of defects when the arterioles cross over the

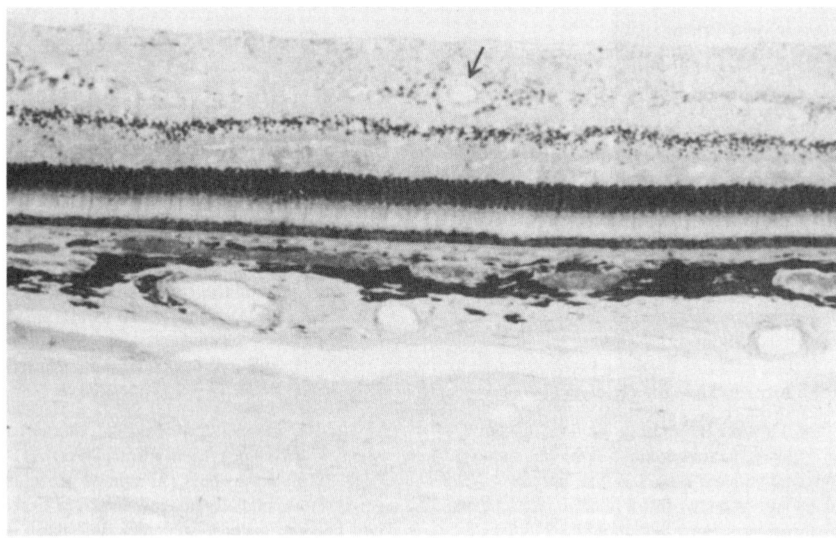

Figure 4 The wall of an arteriole in the retina of an individual with diabetes mellitus is thickened by the accumulation of a homogeneous eosinophilic (hyaline) material beneath the endothelium (*arrow*) (hematoxylin and eosin, × 165).

veins that may or may not be associated with interruption of intraluminal flow.

Capillaries

Involution of retinal endothelial cells and pericytes occurs in the retinal periphery attributed to a progressive decrease in blood flow through aging vessels (21) and is probably attributable to a impaired perfusion through sclerosed arterioles. Capillary aneurysms may also develop in the periphery of the retina and in some instances may be preceded by perivascular reticulin deposition with loop formation (Fig. 5) (see section entitled Aneurysms). An analysis by Ashton (7), however, suggests that microaneurysms are more commonly a feature of concomitant vascular disease and are unusual as a function of aging alone.

Veins

Collagen accumulates in the walls of veins and may lead to loss of tone with dilatation and increased tortuosity.

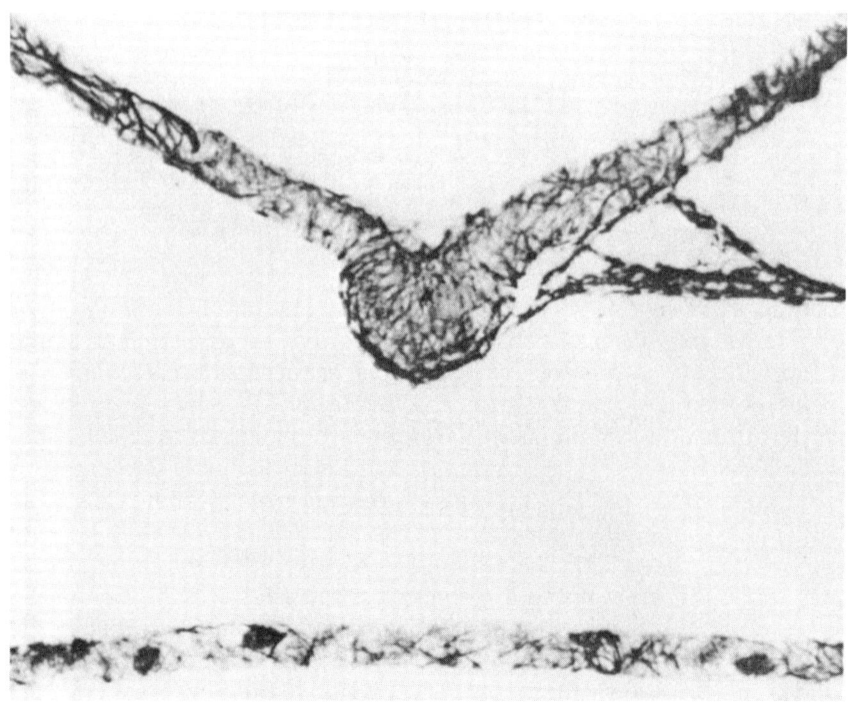

Figure 5 Retinal digest preparation stained to show a network of argyrophilic reticulin fibers surrounding the capillary blood vessels (vascular basement membrane). They are especially prominent in diabetic microangiopathy (× 480).

COMMON MANIFESTATIONS OF VASCULAR DISEASE IN THE EYE

Increased Permeability

Edema

Edema is the accumulation of fluid in the extravascular compartment. Both intracellular and extracellular edema are recognized, but in the context of the eye discussion is confined to extracellular fluid accumulation. The interstitial fluid may be in the form of an ultrafiltrate of the circulating blood and contain very little protein (transudative edema), or it may include large amounts of protein (exudative edema). In general there are three important physiological mechanisms in regulating fluid balance between the vascular and tissue compartments, exchange occurring predominantly through the vascular endothelium of the capillaries: (*i*) hydrostatic pressure: between the arterial and the venous sides of the capillary bed there is a steady fall in intravascular tension of about 20 mmHg (from about 32 to 12 mmHg in most extraocular tissues and from about 45 to 18 mmHg within the globe); (*ii*) oncotic pressure: plasma proteins, especially albumin, exert an osmotic pressure of about 25 mmHg and serve to keep the circulating fluid within the blood vessels; and (*iii*) permeability: of the endothelium determines how quickly and to what extent equilibrium occurs between intravascular and extravascular fluid compartments.

Fluid exchange between the vascular and extravascular compartments depends on the interplay of oncotic and hydrostatic pressures modulated by vascular endothelium, and is such that fluid tends to leave the capillaries on the arterial side and return at the venous end. Edema results if this delicate balance is upset.

Transudates

Transudative edema usually reflects an increase in hydrostatic pressure within blood vessels. Reduced oncotic pressure secondary to hypoproteinemia is not clinically significant for the eye.

Intraretinal transudation is frequently a feature of systemic hypertension and retinal vein occlusion. Increased hydrostatic pressure related to vascular dilatation may be a factor in edema associated with acute inflammation (including allergic reactions) in ocular and orbital tissue. A net balance in favor of increased transudation into the tissues is also a feature of hypotony, particularly in the uvea. A primary defect in the vascular endothelium resulting in increased permeability to small molecules is an early feature of diabetic retinopathy. Transudation from superficial capillaries in the retina causes retinal nebular opacification and diminished light reflexes and, in the neighborhood of the optic nerve head, is associated with separation of individual nerve fibers so that they are rendered unduly distinct.

Exudates

Exudative edema may occur in the general circulation because of physiologic separation between adjacent vascular endothelial cells. Such separation is mediated by vasoactive amine released in acute inflammation and hypersensitivity. The retinal vascular components of the blood–retinal barrier prevent significant plasma leakage in both hypertensive and inflammatory states (26). As a rule, the appearance of retinal exudates is due to structural damage to the endothelial lining, although observation of experimental and spontaneous hypertension in rats indicates that minor amounts of plasma protein might cross intact endothelium by means of increased pinocytosis (65). Malformed blood vessels allow transudation, as in the aneurysmal or telangiectatic capillary bed of Coats disease, to such an extent that the exudate causes a total serous retinal detachment.

Once beyond the vessel wall, the exuded plasma spreads between the cellular components of the tissues along paths of least resistance, but because of fibrinogen content, the exudates soon coagulate. The aqueous component is gradually reabsorbed, leaving progressively inspissated residues, which because they contain exuded lipid as well as protein may appear waxy. In the retina such exudates also tend to have discrete edges and have a hard appearance (Fig. 6). Eventually, through fibrinolytic activity, the exudates begin to resolve, macrophages accumulating to take up and degrade residual material. Since lipid, especially cholesterol (73), is more difficult to degrade than protein, thus lipid residues tend to resolve more slowly.

Parafoveal exudates are likely to be arranged in a ring or circinate manner around the macula. Retinal exudates are inclined to pool in the outer plexiform layer, where the tissue is less supported and the resorption capacity is limited because of the absence of blood vessels in the outer retina. The natural movement of intraocular fluid toward the choriocapillaris may also be a factor in outer retinal accumulation, large molecular complexes being held back by the intercellular junctional complexes of the outer limiting membrane. Exudates from vessels in the macula are distributed between the radially disposed fibers of Henle layer and assume a characteristic stellate pattern. Henle layer consists of the axons of the foveal cones, which connect with the internal retina along an oblique course. A circinate distribution is also common around microaneurysms in diabetic retinopathy and around foci of capillary

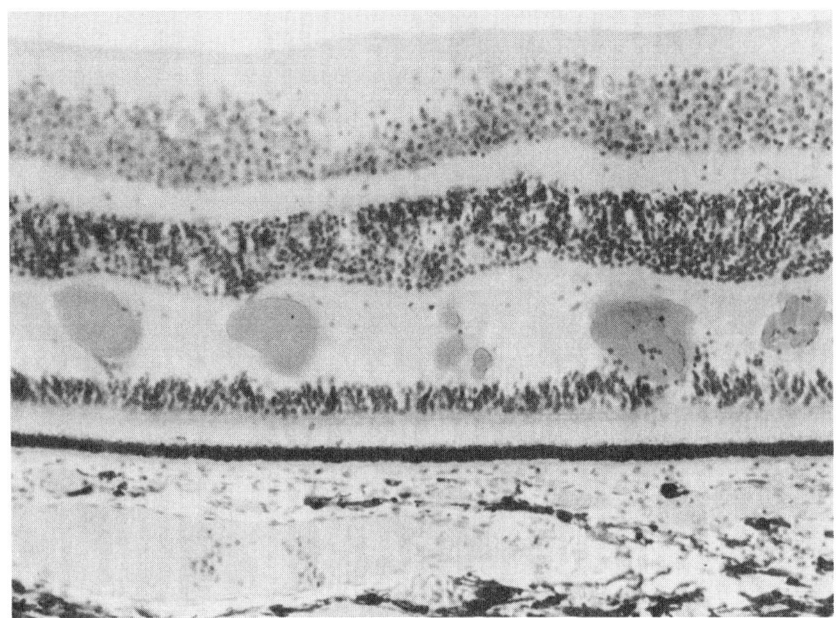

Figure 6 Retinal exudates collect in the outer plexiform layer, where they become inspissated to form eosinophilic masses with characteristically well defined or "hard" borders (hematoxylin and eosin, × 135).

closure in retinal vascular occlusion. The annular distribution of the exudates is likely to reflect centrifugal drainage from a focal origin, the initial fluid becoming progressively inspissated as the aqueous component drains unimpeded toward the choriocapillaris. Ultimately the solubility product of the residual protein and lipid is exceeded, and deposition forms a ring of opaque hard exudates at some distance from the source.

Papilledema

The term "papilledema" was defined in the classic paper of Paton (71) as passive edema due to raised intracranial pressure. However, a number of conditions give rise to passive or inflammatory optic nerve head swelling in which there is no concomitant rise in cerebrospinal fluid (CSF) pressure, including vascular hypertension. Edema of the optic disc can develop in a variety of situations with one or more of the following features: (*i*) a shift in the pressure differential across the lamina (e.g., ocular hypotony); (*ii*) mechanical distortion of the lamina cribrosa: posterior bowing in acute pressure elevating glaucoma and anterior bowing in ocular hypotony; and (*iii*) impaired vascular perfusion of the optic nerve head (e.g., nonarteritic ischemic optic neuropathy).

The pathophysiologic basis for optic disc swelling was assumed to be tissue distortion of the optic disc because of transudation from impaired venous return. However, histopathological studies provide little evidence of increased interstitial volume, implying that other factors are involved. The current mechanism is thought to be an alteration of axoplasmic flow leading to optic disc tissue distortion (i.e., not true "edema"). The movement of cytoplasmic contents along the axon composed of solutes and organelles is essential to the viability of the neuron and, of necessity, is bidirectional. Movement of axoplasm from cell nucleus to synapse, i.e., from retina to lateral geniculate body is known as orthograde flow. The return (or retrograde) flow is distinctly slower. Ischemia initially interferes with rapid transport, both orthograde and retrograde, with slow axoplasmic flow being particularly vulnerable to moderate degrees of mechanical compression (2). Prolonged ischemia results in axonal necrosis and cessation of all flow of whatever rate, as does compression if it is sufficient to mechanically crush the axon.

The nerve head swelling in both acute (rapid pressure elevation) glaucoma and ocular hypotony may be attributable in part to posterior and anterior bowing, respectively, of the lamina cribrosa. Such distortion constricts the available space for the nerve axons and thus interferes primarily with the slow orthograde phase of axoplasmic transport (both orthograde and retrograde in hypotony) (69). Inadequate capillary perfusion due to primary vascular disease within the nerve head may be important in the papilledema of hypertension (56) and giant cell arteritis. The papilledema associated with raised intracranial pressure is mediated by increased CSF pressure within the optic nerve sheath. This too causes impaired slow orthograde axoplasmic transport (92).

Interference with axoplasmic transport is almost certainly partial rather than complete, as tracer studies and the fairly minor impairment of visual acuity testify. Even so, some nerve fibers eventually succumb to unrelieved obstruction, causing necrosis and the disrupted ends undergo further distension due to the inflow of more axoplasm. Such swollen and disrupted axons are seen as cytoid bodies by light microscopy and are identical to those seen in retinal nerve fiber layer infarcts (RNFLI) (cotton-wool spots[a]) (102). Swelling of the optic nerve head occurs in both anterior and lateral directions, the latter causing blurring of the optic disc margins and sometimes producing tenting and limited detachment of the immediate peripapillary retina.

Hemorrhage

Hemorrhage is the result of loss of structural integrity of the blood vessel wall. There may be several mechanisms acting singly or simultaneously: (*i*) mechanical rupture, whether accidental or surgical, (*ii*) intraluminal pressure elevation, (*iii*) inflammation of the vessel wall, (*iv*) weakening of the vessel wall to form aneurysmal or telangiectatic dilation, (*v*) developmental malformations, especially of the conjunctiva and orbit, (*vi*) new vessel formation with thin adventitial support, and (*vii*) blood-clotting abnormalities (e.g., platelet deficiency in leukemia).

Hemorrhages from blood vessels in the inner retina tend to infiltrate among the axons in the nerve fiber layer and, consequently, assume a linear- or flame-shaped distribution. With deeper retinal hemorrhage the blood is confined by vertical organization of the middle and outer retina that leads to a spherical or "blot" configuration. Bleeding from capillaries in the outer retina tends to remain localized around the defective vessels.

Intraluminal blood when in contact with extravascular tissues activates the blood-clotting process. Ultimately the clot is removed by macrophages as the tissue recovers. Removal of the spent clot is facilitated by proteolytic enzymes derived from both injured tissue and participating polymorphonuclear neutrophils (PMNs). Subsequently the hematoma is organized by fibroblasts (or glia in the retinal tissue) and proliferating blood vessels to leave a fibrous (or glial) scar. Hemoglobin (Hb) pigment from degenerating red blood cells is converted to hemosiderin and may persist for months or even years in the tissues usually in macrophages. The lipid content of the extravasated red blood cells, especially free cholesterol, is similarly liable to persist as cholesterol clefts in tissue sections and occasionally become the focus of a multinucleated giant cell reaction (Fig. 7).

The pattern of hemorrhage resolution varies according to the tissue involved. Hemorrhage in the subhyaloid space internal to the retina may remain fluid with only a limited tendency toward organization and a correspondingly greater potential for proteolysis and complete resolution. The lack of clot formation may be related to the absence of a fibrous response in this location (24).

Ischemia

Reduced ocular blood flow damages tissues with high metabolic requirements, such as the retina. Initially damage is reversible, but becomes irreversible if ischemia is prolonged. In general, the complications are a direct outcome of the metabolic deprivation, but there is also a risk of tissue damage during reprofusion. Reperfusion damage is directed at the blood vessels themselves, by free oxygen radicals formed by activation of PMNs or formation of xanthine oxidase by compromised vascular endothelium (88).

Causes of Ischemia

Thrombosis

There are three basic elements leading to the formation of a thrombus: modulation of the luminal surface of vascular endothelial cells, activation in the circulating platelets, and launching the coagulation cascade. Normally the vascular endothelium is antithrombogenic partially because it is able to secrete a number of antithrombotic factors, such as prostacyclin. Platelets will adhere to a damaged endothelial luminal surface and will release thromboxane A, and other agents that promote further platelet aggregation and initiate the clotting process. The clotting process is conversion of fibrinogen to fibrin and the formation of a definitive thrombus containing enmeshed blood cells.

Intravascular thrombosis as a pathological event is prone to occur under the following conditions: (*i*) extensive or sustained endothelial damage (e.g., atheromatous plaque, vasculitis, or diabetes mellitus) (64), (*ii*) disturbance of laminar flow, which may develop over an atheromatous plaque or because of a localized narrowing of the blood vessel, brings platelets into contact with the vascular endothelium, and (*iii*) increased coagulability. This is a feature of several diverse conditions, such as disseminated cancer, the aftermath of severe trauma, during and immediately after pregnancy, and a genetic predisposition.

[a] Focal areas of the retina that were extensively studied by British ophthalmologists were called "cotton-wool spots" because of the resemblance of their color to cotton-wool (known as cotton by Americans). They are a feature of many retinal diseases in which ischemia is a feature. By light microscopy the lesions are located in the retinal nerve fiber layer and resemble cells and were once designated "cytoid bodies." It is now known that the cotton-wool spots result from swollen axons within the nerve fiber layer caused by impaired axoplasmic flow. Some designate the abnormality as retinal nerve fiber layer infarct, despite the fact that unlike true infarcts they are reversible. Despite shortcomings in the designation retinal nerve fiber layer infarct (RNFLI) is used throughout this text for want of a brief precise better term.

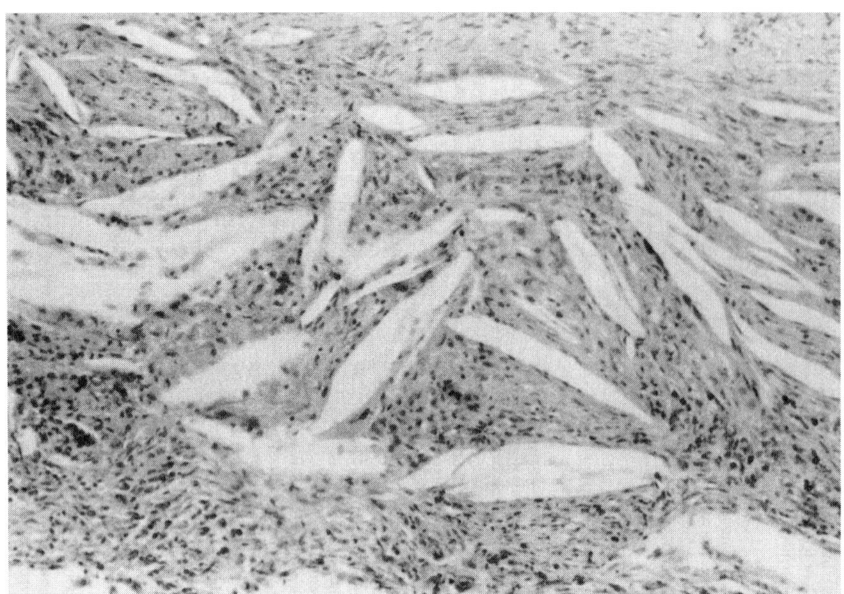

Figure 7 Part of an organizing hematoma in the orbit. Clefts that contained cholesterol crystals before tissue embedding are surrounded by multinucleated giant cells. Numerous macrophages with engulfed hemosiderin are also present (hematoxylin and eosin, × 135).

Once formed the thrombus may propagate and totally occlude the affected blood vessel. Fragments of the clot may break away and cause embolic ischemia downstream. Ultimately intraluminal clots will organize and may recanalize through action of the fibrinolytic system of plasminogen activators and other proteolytic enzyme systems.

Embolism

Ocular ischemia can result from arterial emboli, the principal source of which is ulcerated atheromatous plaques. Amaurosis fugax is a complication in up to 40% of patients with occlusive carotid atherosclerosis (29). The embolus consists largely of cholesterol and aggregated platelets. The embolus is often present in the ocular circulation for periods varying between a few minutes and several hours before breaking. Other sources of intraocular emboli include the mural thrombus from a fibrillating left atrium, infected vegetations from diseased cardiac valves, fat from fractured bones, and nitrogen bubbles in decompression sickness. Fragments of endocardial myxoma, amniotic fluid, radio-opaque dyes used in arteriography, and periocular injections have also been reported as causing retinal embolism.

Spasm

Along with other muscular arteries, the central retinal artery and its principal branches are susceptible to intense focal constriction. Spasm sufficient to obstruct flow can occasionally be responsible for visual loss in migraine (13) or may result from medication with ergot and its derivatives. The spasm is usually short-lived, and irreversible damage to the dependent tissues is avoided, although rarely permanent visual disturbance has been reported.

Inadequacy of Perfusion

Intraluminal narrowing or occlusion of the carotid arteries and their ophthalmic and orbital branches can impair ocular nutrition. Causes include atherosclerosis, Takayasu arteritis, giant cell arteritis, and other forms of vasculitis (see Chapter 69).

Ocular Complications of Ischemia

Globe: Chronic Ocular Ischemia

Ischemia of the whole eye follows occlusion of the ophthalmic artery and is usually a complication of carotid artery disease. Anterior segment findings include protein-rich exudation into the aqueous humor as a result of a blood–ocular barrier breakdown, atrophy of the iris, and ciliary body, anterior subcapsular cataract, and corneal edema as a sequel to the failure of energy-dependent corneal endothelial cell function. Iris neovascularization and peripheral anterior synechiae leading to secondary glaucoma may also develop from associated retinal hypoxia or a direct response to the anterior segment ischemia. Posterior segment damage involves panretinal atrophy with peripheral hemorrhages and microaneurysms, optic disc neovascularization, and vitreous exudates. Trypsin digest preparations reveal widespread acellularity of the retinal capillaries (29).

Uvea

The uvea is less vulnerable to ischemia than the retina because of extensive anastamoses among choroidal vessels. Major ciliary arteries, both anterior and posterior, can also be occluded without apparent harm because of anastomotic compensation. Nevertheless, uveal ischemia sometimes occurs, as a result of trauma, hypertensive fibrinous necrosis, sickle cell disease, and various types of vasculitis.

Acute iris ischemia produces an initial separation of iris stromal fibers as well as disruption of iris pigment epithelium and loss of neurosensory melanin pigment. The pigment will disperse throughout the anterior and posterior chambers. More gradual ischemia results in thinning by atrophy, with marked loss of cellular components.

Choroidal ischemia, as observed in malignant or accelerated systemic hypertension, causes degeneration of retinal pigment epithelium (RPE). The depigmentation may be expressed as focal area of RPE atrophy. Pigment released from damaged RPE may aggregate centrally in the area of damage to form an Elschnig spot or may be dispersed along damaged choroidal vessels to form Siegrist streaks. More widespread ischemia is likely to cause the degeneration of the outer layers of the neuroretina as well.

Retina

Central Retinal Artery Occlusion. Central retinal artery occlusion is usually caused by atherosclerosis, possibly as a result of the plaque (27), and is often associated with systemic hypertension. Embolism and occasionally arteritis may be also cause occlusion. The obstruction usually occurs where the central retinal artery is narrowest, i.e., at or immediately behind the lamina cribosa.

With occlusion, complete loss of vision is usually immediate. Studies suggest irreversible neuronal changes are present after 2 h (42). Initially, the retina becomes opaque, due to intracellular edema and necrosis of the inner layers. The outer layers of the retina (deep to the outer plexiform layer) are preserved, because nutrition is supplied by the choriocapillaris. Mitochondrial damage is due to breakdown of Na^+-K^+-ATPase-dependent electrolyte balance across mitochondrial cell membranes. Eventually, the necrotic tissue is phagocytosed to leave an atrophic inner retina. There is no glial reaction because astrocytes are also located in the internal retina and are destroyed by ischemia. The presence of a cilioretinal circulation in about 25% of individuals means that the immediate peripapillary retina may be preserved. Preretinal and iris neovascularization are unusual complications.

Branch Retinal Artery Occlusion. This is usually the result of embolism from atheromatous plaques and occurs mainly at blood vessel bifurcations. Direct thrombosis is unusual since the atherosclerotic process rarely extends beyond the optic disc. The effects on the dependent retina are identical to those described for central artery occlusion, although the risk of secondary iris neovascularization is slight less.

Retinal Nerve Fiber Layer Infarcts. Cotton-wool spots are discrete ischemic lesions in the nerve fiber layer of the retina characterized by an elevation of the inner retinal surface and poorly demarcated fluffy whitish opacification. RNFLIs are most commonly located in the posterior retina, where the nerve fiber layer is thickest and are a feature of several vascular retinopathies as well as a frequent retinal finding in patients with acquired immunodeficiency syndrome (AIDS) (97) with human immunodeficiency virus (HIV) retinopathy (97).

Focal aggregates of globular structures within the nerve fiber layer are apparent by light microscopy, which have been called cytoid bodies (Fig. 8), particularly because they commonly have a central weakly basophilic "nucleus." However, the absence of DNA, as evidenced by histochemical staining reactions, indicates that the central component is not a true nucleus; teased preparations and transmission electron microscopy (TEM) show that cytoid bodies are the swollen ends of disrupted nerve axons (4). Furthermore, the nucleus-like structure consists of amorphous electron-dense material derived from the lipid-protein residues of degenerate cytoplasmic organelles. Not all axons in the region of a RNFLI are disrupted; those lying immediately beneath the inner limiting membrane (ILM) in particular often being preserved. Ganglion cells and parts of the inner nuclear layer in the involved region are also necrotic, but cells in the deeper retinal layers are not affected.

Understanding of the RNFLIs has come from experimental embolization of the retinal circulation combined with TEM and tracer studies of axoplasmic transport. If artificial emboli are introduced into the carotid circulation of a laboratory animal, some lodge in the smaller arterioles of the retina and are likely to be followed by the development of a RNFLI (4). Focal swelling related to fusiform expansion of nerve fibers in the territory supplied by the obstructed arteriole is present within 1h and at this stage the swelling appears to be largely due to imbibition of water, since the distended region is unduly electron lucent, with few organelles and sparse neurofilaments (Fig. 9). Such intracellular edema is most readily explained by hypoxia and failure of the sodium pump mechanism, with additional damage caused by failure to remove the products of glycolysis and the development of

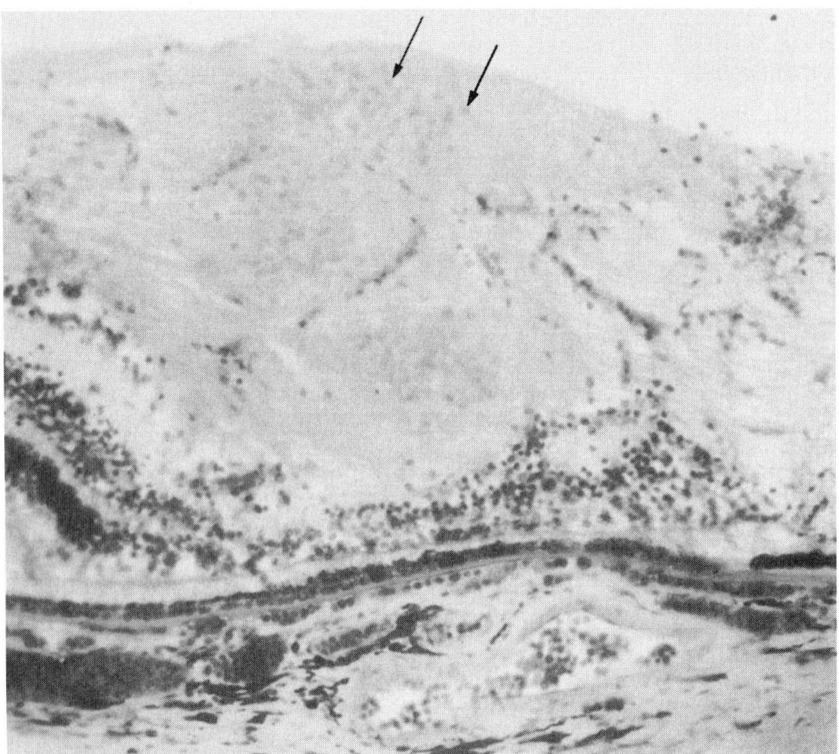

Figure 8 Retinal nerve fiber layer infarcts (RNFLIs) are made up of numerous cytoid bodies and, in the upper lesions, a central zone of necrosis. The cytoid bodies lie in the nerve fiber layer and represent the distended stumps of disrupted axons; the pseudonuclei (*arrows*) are formed by coalescence of the lipoprotein membranes of degenerate cytoplasmic organelles (hematoxylin and eosin, × 175).

intracellular acidosis. Thereafter, many of the distended axons become increasingly rich in mitochondria and other organelles (Fig. 10). This change is best seen toward the edges of the lesion, since the central part becomes necrotic with loss of axonal continuity. Much of this later nerve fiber swelling and mitochondrial increase is due to interference with axoplasmic transport (66). Axoplasmic flow is normally bidirectional and requires local supply of energy from the surrounding tissue fluids along the entire length of the axon. Consequently, focal vascular insufficiency results in axonal distension, because while axoplasm continues to be fed into the damaged region, there is no local source of energy necessary to pump it away (Fig. 11).

In the healing phase of RNFI, the necrotic debris is removed through autolysis and phagocytosis. Eventually a glial scar is formed, from surviving astrocytes withstanding ischemia more successfully than nerve tissue. Although the nonperfused capillaries may reopen, there is no improvement in the focal scotoma or in the partial nerve fiber bundle defect caused by loss of axons passing through the ischemic zone.

Central Retinal Vein Occlusion. Central retinal vein occlusion presents acutely with tortuous congested veins, hemorrhages, and angiographic evidence of vascular stasis caused by thrombotic occlusion of the vein at or behind the lamina cribrosa. Such occlusion can complicate any number of diseases, complete loss of vision is usually immediate. Nonhuman primate studies suggest irreversible neuronal changes are the retina becomes opaque and pale, due mainly to intracellular edema but also in part to necrosis of the inner layers. The outer layers of the retina (deep to the outer plexiform layer) are preserved, because nutrition is supplied by the choriocapillaris. Experimental occlusion of the central retinal artery in monkeys (61) causes early swelling of mitochondria with subsequent degeneration and accumulation of water in the neuronal cytoplasm.

Reduced arterial perfusion in retinal vein occlusion is reduced because of a combination of obstructed venous outflow and reduced arterial inflow (48). Impaired perfusion with a consequently reduced shear rate could be expected to cause thrombosis in the veins, where the circulation is in any case most sluggish, especially if there is an associated increase in intrinsic viscosity.

Central retinal vein occlusion presents acutely with tortuous congested veins, hemorrhages, and angiographic evidence of vascular stasis caused by thrombotic occlusion of the vein at or behind the lamina cribrosa. Such occlusion can complicate any of a number of diseases, some of which have been substantiated but others merely postulated.

Hyperviscosity States

Hyperviscosity is often associated with retinal vein occlusion. It may be due to an increased concentration of circulating red blood cells (polycythemia),

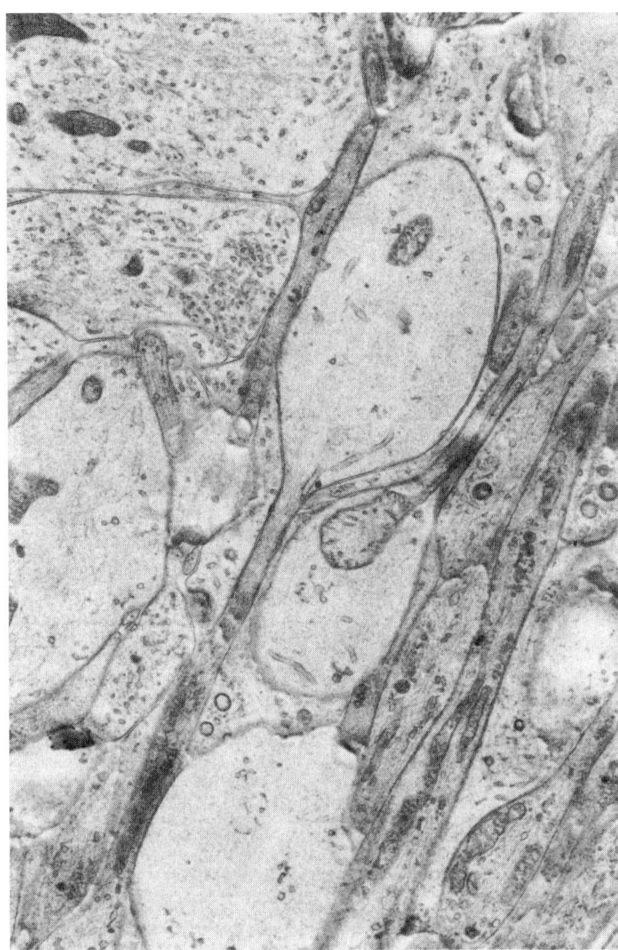

Figure 9 Transmission electron micrograph of a retinal nerve fiber layer infarct at an early stage in its evolution. Individual axons in an area of retinal ischemia have become focally distended by the accumulation of relatively electron-lucent material containing few organelles. From experimentally induced lesions in a pig retina 1 hour after embolic occlusion of a terminal arteriole. (× 10,400).

increased concentration of plasma proteins, or metabolic disorders (e.g., homocystinuria) (12,91).

Vasculitis. Vasculitis, particularly phlebitis, is sometimes present in younger persons with retinal vein occlusion. The cause of the phlebitis is usually obscure, but possible causes include sarcoidosis, Behcet disease, systemic lupus erythematosus, or Eales disease.

Reduced Arterial Perfusion. Retinal arterial perfusion is reduced in retinal vein occlusion because of a combination of obstructed venous outflow and reduced arterial inflow (48). Impaired perfusion with a consequently reduced shear rate could be expected to cause thrombosis in the veins, where the circulation is in any case most sluggish, especially if there is an associated increase in intrinsic viscosity.

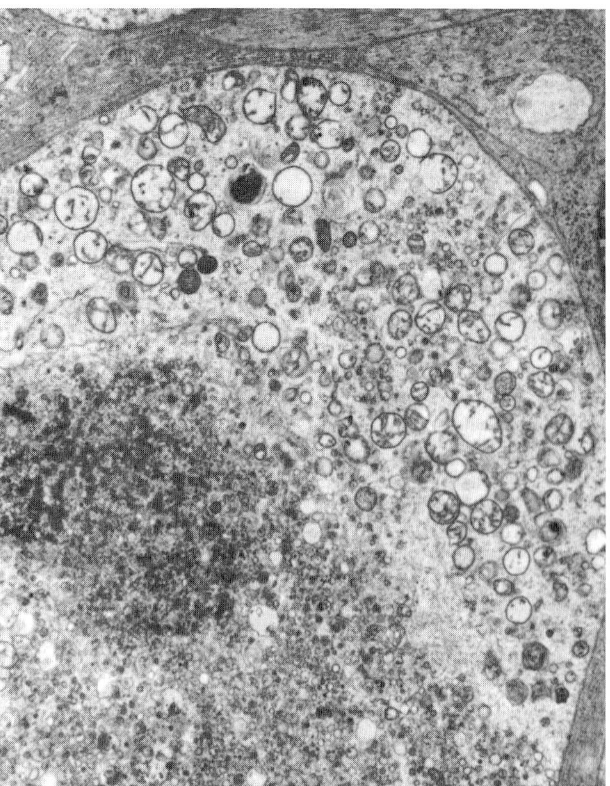

Figure 10 Transmission electron micrograph of cytoid body showing accumulated cytoplasmic organelles, mainly mitochondria, with a central electron-dense pseudonucleus formed by the residues of degenerate organelles (× 10,600).

Turbulence. Turbulence of blood flow is present in the region of the lamina cribrosa where the artery and the vein share a common adventitial sheath. Also any thickening and dilatation of the artery wall tends to impinge on and compress the vein within the rigid tunnel imposed by the lamina. Swelling of the venous endothelium has also been reported in association with atheromatous disease of the central retinal artery (57). Compression by massive drusen of the optic

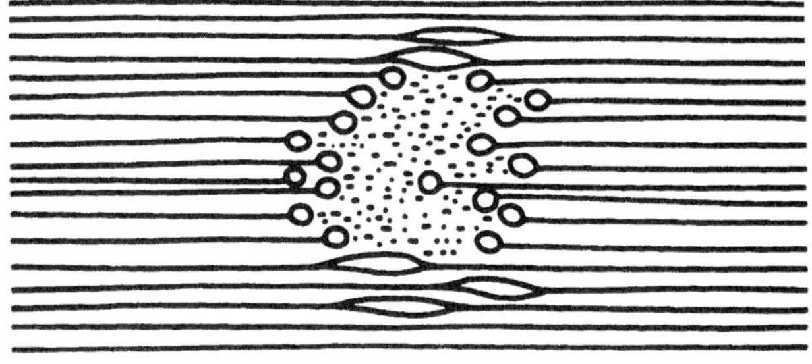

Figure 11 A large retinal nerve fiber layer infarct. In the center, where the energy deprivation is most severe, axonal necrosis is liable to occur, and nerve fiber swelling because of the disrupted flow of axoplasm develops at the edges of the infarcted zone. Clinically, the central necrotic zone may be relatively gray compared with the fluffy white edges.

nerve head has also been described in central retinal vein thrombosis (39). Developments of this kind are expected to disturb the normal laminar flow and favor a thrombotic event.

Obstructed Outflow. Interference with retinal vein drainage predisposing to retinal vein occlusion may be secondary to raised intraocular pressure (IOP), raised intracranial pressure, or an adjacent neoplasm.

There are two main forms of central retinal vein occlusion: ischemic and nonischemic. The ischemic form is much the more serious type but also the less common, accounting for between 20% (49) and 36% (74) of all central retinal vein occlusions. Then it is characterized by numerous hemorrhages, RNFLIs, and loss of visual function. Fluorescein angiography frequently reveals areas of capillary closure. Systemic arterial disease, such as atherosclerosis or, migraine may precipitate a thrombotic event. Nonhuman primate studies suggest that reduced perfusion may not be permanent in the context of experimental vein occlusion (46).

The nonischemic form is a more benign condition thought to represent a central retinal vein occlusion in the absence of detectable inflow deficiency. Hemorrhages are fewer than in the ischemic form, RNFLIs are rare, and, although there is circulatory stasis, there is no progression to permanent capillary closure.

Up to half of patients with the nonischemic form of central retinal vein occlusion recover spontaneously, however there is a risk of developing cystoid macular edema and degeneration. The ischemic form of retinal vein occlusion is more likely to lead to severe macular degeneration; a third is at risk of iris neovascularization and angle-closure glaucoma. Less commonly neovascularization of the optic disc or retinal surface may be stimulated by angiogenic factors, such as vascular endothelial growth factor (VEGF).

Branch Retinal Vein Occlusion. The events that follow acute occlusion have been studied experimentally in the nonhuman primate (83). Photocoagulation of a branch vein gives an immediate reduction in arterial caliber and inflow, which may well represent an autoregulatory response to increased venous backpressure. Within the next few hours the capillaries and postcapillary venules in the drainage area become progressively distended so that transudative edema and plasma leakage develops. Eventually some of the distended blood vessels rupture and bleed, but in many of those remaining intact, stagnation, and thrombosis supervene. In consequence there is complete cessation of blood flow through the affected capillaries and venules, resulting, in some instances, in ischemia sufficient to provoke RNFLIs. The blood vessels themselves are liable to become acellular. In addition to interstitial edema, there is also intracellular swelling, which probably reflects tissue hypoxia. A collateral circulation is often established in monkeys with artificially induced branch vein obstruction within 2 to 3 days, and this may mitigate some of the tissue changes. In older humans, with varying degrees of arteriolosclerosis, this capacity is likely to be impaired, and collateral channels providing an alternative drainage route usually take weeks or months to develop. With the emergence of a collateral circulation the nonperfused vessels may regain their endothelial lining, but in some instances the capillaries remain closed with lumina invaded by glial processes (Fig. 12). Chronic cystoid macular edema can persist after a vein occlusion as growth factors such as VEGF may play a role in patients with persistent edema.

Occlusion produces visual defects in its drainage area and can be either acute or chronic. Acute occlusion presents with distension and tortuosity of the affected vein, with both superficial and deep retinal edema. Deep hemorrhages from capillaries or small venules are common, although superficial flame-shaped hemorrhages may be present if the obstruction takes place close to the optic nerve head. RNFLIs may also develop in relation to peripapillary venous occlusions, and microaneurysms are common in the later stages.

Occlusion of the retinal vein occurs almost always at the site of arteriovenous crossing, particularly where the artery crosses in front of the vein (100); here the artery and vein have a shared adventitial sheath, which is commonly thickened and responsible for some localized vascular narrowing. Systemic hypertension was reported in 93% of patients in a study reported by Kohner and Shilling (59). Endothelial cell proliferation or swelling has been described at these sites (101) and hyperviscosity may be a contributory factor in some patients (70).

The events that follow acute occlusion have been studied experimentally in the nonhuman primate (83). Photocoagulation of a branch vein gives an immediate reduction in arterial caliber and inflow, which may well represent an autoregulatory response to increased venous backpressure. Within the next few hours the capillaries and postcapillary venules in the drainage area become progressively distended so that transudative edema and plasma leakage develops. Eventually some of the distended blood vessels rupture and bleed, but in many of those remaining intact, stagnation, and thrombosis supervene. In consequence there is complete cessation of blood flow through the affected capillaries and venules, resulting, in some instances, in ischemia sufficient to provoke RNFLIs. The blood vessels themselves are liable to become acellular. In addition to interstitial edema, there is also intracellular swelling, which probably reflects tissue hypoxia. A collateral circulation is often established in monkeys with artificially induced branch vein obstruction within 2 to 3 days, and this may mitigate some of the tissue changes. In older humans, with varying degrees of arteriolosclerosis, this capacity is likely to be impaired, and collateral channels providing an alternative drainage route usually take weeks or months to develop. With the emergence of a collateral circulation the nonperfused vessels may regain their endothelial lining, but in some instances the capillaries remain closed with lumina invaded by glial processes (Fig. 12). Chronic cystoid macular edema can persist after a vein occlusion as growth factors may play a role in patients with persistent edema as is evidenced by its resolution after inhibition of VEGF with the drugs pegaptanib or bevacizumab.

Persistence of capillary closure is associated with a poor prognosis for visual recovery. Iris neovascularization and neovascular glaucoma are infrequent, possibly because there is an inadequate stimulus (51).

Anterior Ischemic Optic Neuropathy

Anterior ischemic optic neuropathy (AION) presents with a sudden onset of monocular blindness, usually in the absence of pain, associated with optic disc edema. Eventually the other eye commonly becomes involved. Arteritic and nonarteritic forms are recognized.

In nonarteritic AION, vascular insufficiency caused by atherosclerosis is likely to be a principal factor, with an enhanced predisposition in diabetic and hypertensive individuals (15). However, a convincing association with an absent or reduced physiological optic cup has been established (15), and it has been reasoned that because this implies a small scleral canal, through which the nerve fibers pass through the correspondingly restricted gap in Bruch membrane. Blood vessels at the optic disc are more vulnerable to minor degrees of compression. Thus, an otherwise inconsequential level of impaired arterial perfusion could provoke defective axoplasmic flow, with swelling that compresses the optic nerve capillaries and leads to further ischemic damage. Nonarteritic AION can also complicate severe hemorrhage, and although hypotension may be an adequate explanation in some cases, autoregulatory vasoconstriction has been suggested in others (47).

Arteritic AION is less common than the nonarteritic form and is almost always attributable to occlusion of the posterior ciliary arteries by giant cell arteritis, although it may be secondary to pulseless disease (Takayasu arteritis).

Aneurysms

Aneurysmal dilatation of the ocular and orbital vasculature can be congenital or acquired and, although sometimes seen in the orbit and conjunctiva, is most frequent and of greatest consequence in the retina.

Congenital Aneurysms

Leber miliary aneurysms occur as telangiectasis or varicosity of circumscribed areas of the retinal capillary bed. By virtue of their excessive permeability, they are a cause of intra- and subretinal exudation, leading eventually to retinal detachment.

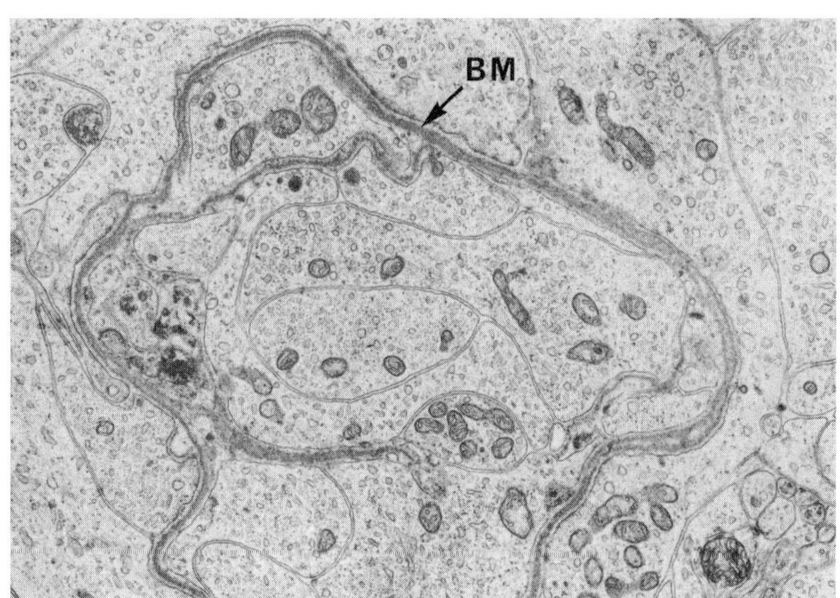

Figure 12 Transmission electron micrograph of a capillary in the retina of a monkey subjected to experimental branch vein occlusion. Deprived of effective circulation, the endothelium and pericytes have sloughed off, leaving a basement membrane outline. The lumen of the defunct capillary is invaded by glial processes (× 12,600). *Abbreviation*: BM, basement membrane. *Source*: From Ref. 60.

The affected blood vessels have thin walls at first, but gradually they become increasingly thickened by inspissated plasma, perhaps representing a primary focal defect in the blood-retina barrier.

Racemose retinal aneurysms are arteriovenous malformations presenting either as an isolated phenomenon or in conjunction with similar anomalies in the midbrain (Wyburn–Mason syndrome) (see Chapter 55). Similar aneurysms also occur in the orbit, where they are liable to cause proptosis.

Acquired Aneurysms

Microaneurysms

Although capillary aneurysms are described in the conjunctiva, especially in diabetic subjects, they are most common and of greatest significance in vascular disorders of the retina, being encountered in macroglobulinemia, sickle cell disease, retinal vein occlusion, and diabetes mellitus. They occur chiefly, but not exclusively, on the venous side of the capillary bed. Microaneurysms on the arterial side are associated particularly with systemic hypertension. Sometimes developing in clusters, they are not uncommonly found encircling areas of capillary closure (Fig. 13).

The walls of microaneurysms are particularly permeable making them a ready source of local serous exudation and hemorrhage. The wall of the aneurysms becomes thickened by accumulated plasma residues, which can be observed in flat mounts as a periodic acid Schiff-positive cap covering the distended segment, and eventually many of them become coated on the internal aspect by a thrombus. Thrombotic occlusion of the aneurysm can manifest itself clinically as disappearance or apparent resolution (Fig. 14). The life of a microaneurysm can vary from months in hypertensive retinopathy to a year or more in diabetes mellitus.

Microaneurysms appear to originate in two different ways (Fig. 15); by focal dilatation of the wall or by the fusion of the two arms of a capillary loop (7). Ballantyne and Loewenstein (11) considered that they may be related to venous stasis, a view that finds support in the occurrence of microaneurysms in retinal vein occlusion and hyperviscous states, as in macroglobulinemia and diabetes mellitus. Others have sought an intrinsic defect in the capillary wall to explain aneurysm formation since changes in the basement membrane are an integral part of diabetic microangiopathy. Another explanation, focal pericyte degeneration (20), was originally based on the assumption that this cell has a contractile function, it is still conceivable that loss of passive support from a cell wrapped around the endothelial lining could weaken the wall sufficiently for focal distension to occur. A subsequent hypothesis linking pericyte loss with microaneurysms takes their putative inhibitory affect on endothelial cell proliferation as an explanation for the frequently observed hypercellular aneurysms. Should microaneurysms be formed in this way, they can be regarded as limited attempts at new vessel formation (43).

Microaneurysms preceded by capillary loops may perhaps more readily be attributed to attempted revascularization of ischemic foci in the retina, the loops being associated with localized endothelial cell hyperplasia and capillary elongation. Nevertheless, loop aneurysms and neovascularization can each occur in the absence of the other, and the relationship is speculative. Commonly, reticulin fibers that enmesh the outer surfaces of the capillaries straddle the base of a loop (Fig. 16) and may be an additional or alternative factor in the approximation of the arms of the loop. Increased amounts of perivascular reticulin are especially prominent in diabetic retinopathy (9).

Macroaneurysms

Arteriolar aneurysms are much less common than their capillary counterparts and are found mainly on the second- or third-order branches. Structurally the aneurysms have been compared to those found on small intracerebral arteries, which show a subendothelial accumulation of hyaline material and focal deficiency of the internal elastic lamina. Moreover, like those in the brain, retinal macroaneurysms are usually a feature of aging and poorly controlled systemic hypertension, especially in women. The frequent occurrence of macroaneurysms at points of branching is suggestive of mechanical injury related to turbulence. Some macroaneurysms have a tendency to leak and, should they be present on blood vessels near the posterior pole, be a cause of macular edema and circinate exudates. Others are asymptomatic.

SPECIFIC VASCULAR DISORDERS AND THEIR OCULAR EFFECTS

Atherosclerosis

Atherosclerosis is primarily a disease of large and medium-sized arteries and is characterized by focal intimal thickening, which, commencing with lipid accumulation is ultimately associated with fibrous and smooth muscle cell proliferation. In the context of the orbit and its contents, atherosclerosis is seen chiefly in the ophthalmic artery, although potentiating factors, such as systemic hypertension and diabetes mellitus, can be associated with extension of the process into smaller arteries of central retinal and ciliary artery size. An autopsy study of diabetic subjects showed that although 34 of 60 eyes had

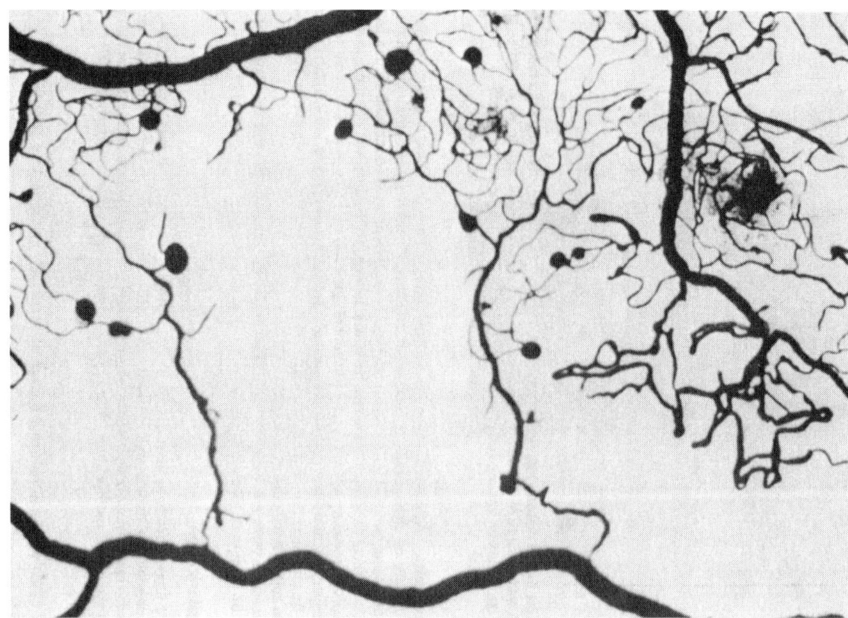

Figure 13 Flat preparation of retina from a diabetic subject, showing crops of capillary aneurysms around a focal area of ischemia. The patent vessels are perfused with colloidal carbon (× 40).

atherosclerosis of the ophthalmic artery, 13 with reduction of the orifice to less than half its normal caliber, only 3 eyes showed central retinal artery involvement, and this of a trivial degree (36). The incidence of central retinal artery atheroma in the general population is probably even less. Nevertheless, the same study indicated that ophthalmic artery stenosis may contribute to the development of diabetic retinopathy. Moreover, the few subjects with central retinal artery involvement occasionally succumb to thrombotic occlusion. Retinal vein obstruction has also been attributed to atherosclerotic thickening of the adjacent artery.

Indirect involvement of the eye can be a feature of carotid artery atherosclerosis in a number of ways. Occlusion or severe stenosis of the internal carotid

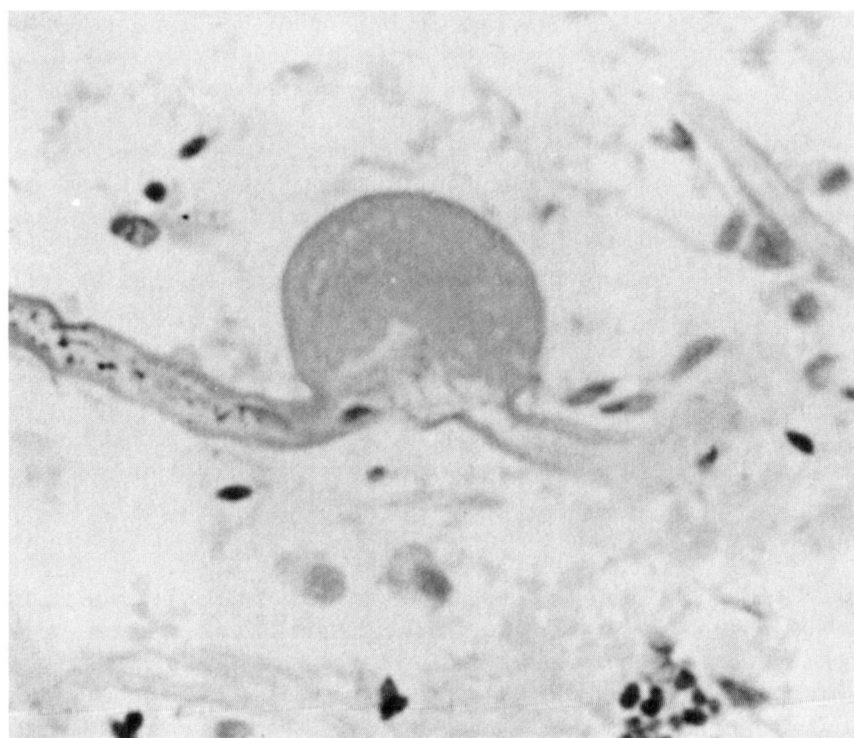

Figure 14 Retina from a diabetic individual sectioned parallel to the surface, showing a thrombosed microaneurysm. Such vessels appear normal in fluorescein angiograms and could lead to an erroneous clinical impression that the aneurysm has regressed (periodic acid Schiff and hematoxylin, × 375).

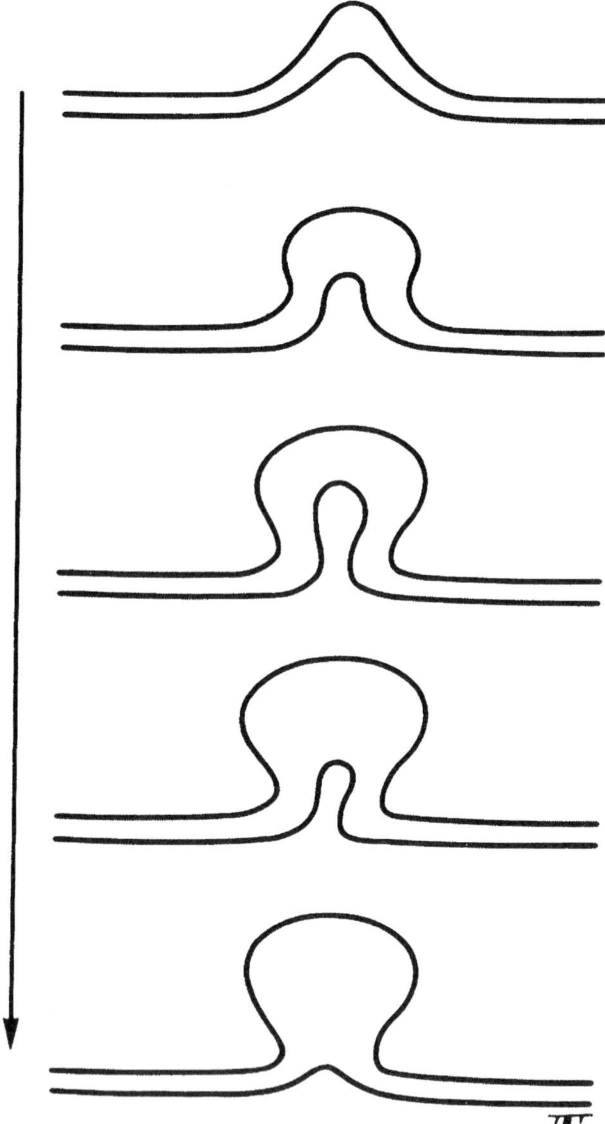

Figure 15 Sequence of events that appear to precede the formation of a "loop" capillary aneurysm. An initial focal proliferation of endothelial cells in the capillary wall produces dilatation and kinking of the vessel, which is tethered to the surrounding tissues by its surrounding network of reticulin fibers and glial attachments. Progressive proliferation leads to further dilatation and the development of a loop.

artery can affect vision by reducing flow through the middle cerebral artery and interfering with occipital lobe function.

Reduction in ocular blood flow is conditioned by the capacity of the external carotid artery to provide a collateral condition, and should persistent loss of vision occur it is more commonly due to shedding of emboli and their lodgement in the central retinal artery. Other less severely compromised patients may show compensatory dilatation of the retinal arteries and scattered areas of RNFLIs associated with ophthalmodynamometric evidence of reduced arterial perfusion pressure.

Transient amaurosis may be a feature of shock or heart failure should the arterial supply to the eye be compromised by atherosclerotic narrowing, but a more frequent cause is embolism from a plaque close to the origin of the internal carotid artery. Both cholesterol and platelet emboli have been described. Emboli to the retina usually break up after a few minutes and permanent visual loss is rare, but repeated attacks are not uncommon and may presage more serious embolization of the cerebral vessels. Presumably emboli also lodge in the uveal circulation, but because of the rich potential for anastomotic compensation, are not expected to cause significant functional disturbance.

Hypertension

Over 90% of clinical hypertension is idiopathic (essential), renal disease accounting for most of the remainder. Other rare causes include certain endocrine disorders, such as pheochromocytoma, toxemia of pregnancy, and coarctation of the aorta. Ocular signs of hypertension can be an early indication of the extent of disease and need for systemic therapy.

Hypertensive Retinopathy

Benign Phase

Retinopathy in the benign phase of systemic hypertension is unusual but, should it occur, is generally limited to tiny glistening whitish foci presumed to be serous exudates and exceptionally, small RNFLIs, and isolated linear hemorrhages.

The larger arterioles surrounding the optic disc may exhibit opacification of the vessel from sclerosis due to collagenous replacement of the muscle elements. The consequent loss of elasticity probably accounts for both the distension of these blood vessels seen in the later stages of benign hypertension (52) and the infrequency of malignant retinopathy in patients with long-standing mild hypertension and in those with age-related arteriolosclerosis. The presence of increased collagen appears to protect against the distortion of the vessel wall from an excessive elevation of blood pressure (62).

Generalized narrowing of the smaller arterioles has been confirmed by measurement of fundus photographs, although casual ophthalmoscopy can give a misleading impression. The narrowing is due to vasoconstriction, probably autoregulatory, and is most common in the early stages before vessel opacification has developed.

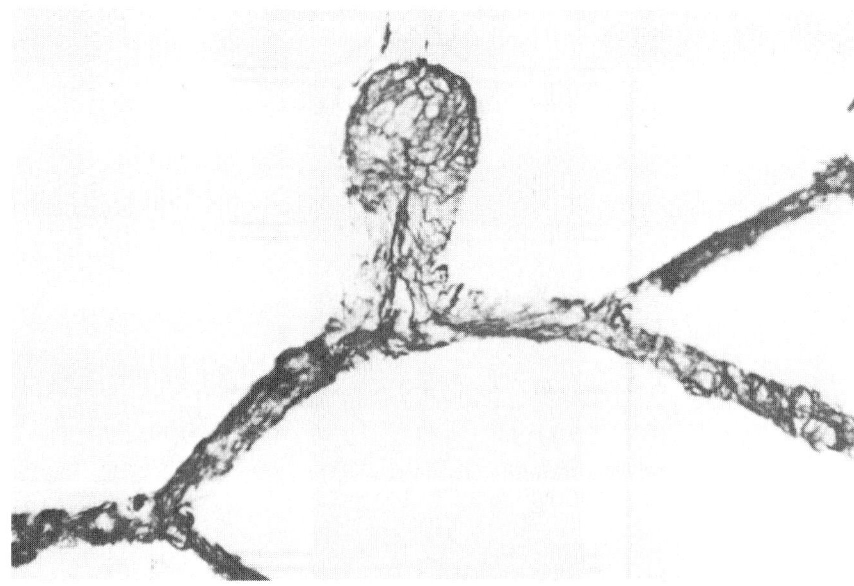

Figure 16 Retina in diabetic microangiopathy studied by trypsin digestion and reticulin staining. Perivascular reticulin fibers are prominent in many places and can be seen surrounding and straddling the base of a microaneurysm (× 420).

Malignant (Accelerated) Phase

The malignant phase is uncommon, affecting less than 5% of hypertensive patients, with a predilection for younger, male subjects, and blacks. As a rule, elevation of the diastolic blood pressure to levels commensurate with vascular necrosis and the development of retinopathy occur as a complicating event in patients with a previous history of benign hypertension. Situations in which the hypertension increases rapidly to diastolic levels in excess of 130 mmHg de novo include ischemic renal disorders, toxemia of pregnancy, and pheochromocytoma.

Retinopathy is a measure of arteriolar damage and is heralded by the emergence of linear hemorrhages and RNFLIs in the posterior fundus. Retinal edema quickly develops, and eventually serous exudates are observed; papilledema becomes apparent as the condition persists.

The retinal arteries may be narrowed (77), although overlying edema and congestion of the retinal veins can make subjective assessment deceptive. In the smaller, ophthalmoscopically unrecognizable terminal arterioles fibrinous necrosis occurs, and represents the replacement of damaged smooth muscle fibers by fibrin and other plasma proteins leaking through defects in the endothelial lining of the affected vessels (Fig. 17).

Pathogenesis

Vasoconstriction can be regarded as an autoregulatory attempt to prevent overperfusion of the capillary bed, retinal, and other ocular lesions developing should this attempt prove inadequate. In the benign phase of hypertension there is compensatory hypertrophy and hyperplasia of arteriolar smooth muscle to accommodate the process, but the malignant phase appears to be associated with a blood pressure rise sufficient to overcome the capacity for autoregulation.

The regulatory arteriolar constriction can be marked before failure occurs, even to the point of virtual closure (Fig. 18) (35). However, the extensive and detailed analyses with fluorescein angiography (FA) by Hayreh of a similar experimental model point to focal leakage (focal intraretinal periarteriolar transudates) as constituting the initial manifestation of a retinopathy (50). This suggests that the constriction, marked though it is, does not result in significant capillary closure and is not a likely cause of the subsequent RNFLIs. The leakage probably corresponds to the endothelial cell damage described in a TEM study of hypertensive primate retinas, the damage being in the form of holes or tears attributable to loss of support by a necrotic muscle wall (Fig. 19) (35).

RNFLI is linked with foci of capillary nonperfusion and is perhaps a sequel to structural, as opposed to functional, obliteration of the lumen of a damaged terminal arteriole. The cessation of blood flow may be a result of secondary thrombosis or the accumulation of fibrin and other plasma components in the blood vessel wall beneath the defective endothelium (35).

A possible sequence of events is as follows: (*i*) autoregulatory vasoconstriction of arterioles, (*ii*) failure of autoregulatory capacity manifested by muscle necrosis and focal leakage, (*iii*) secondary closure of the necrotic arteriolar segment, and (*iv*) capillary nonperfusion and RNFLIs (Fig. 20).

Capillary microaneurysms may develop and are more prominent on the arterial side of the retinal

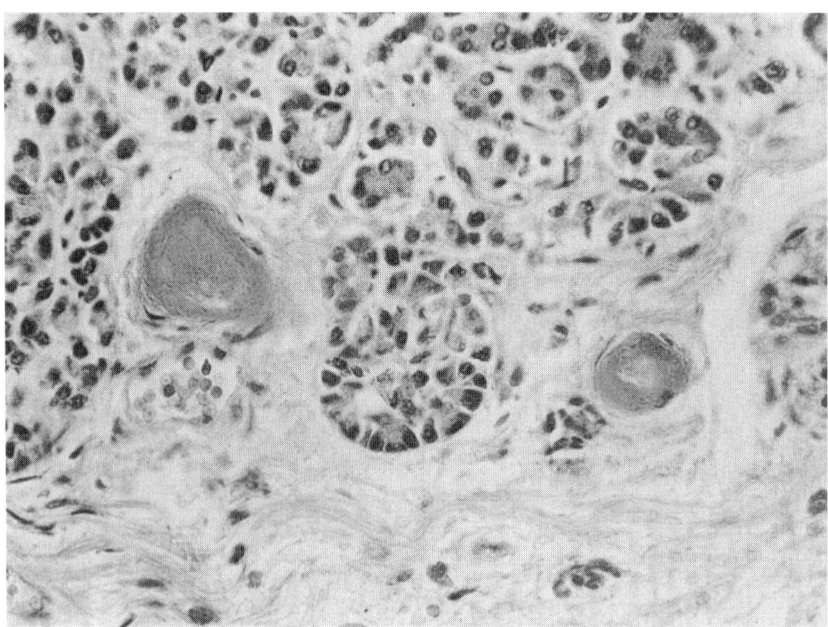

Figure 17 Arteriolar lesion in malignant hypertension. The "smudgy" appearance is caused by seepage of plasma into the vessel wall allied to necrosis of the smooth muscle cells. Such fibrinous necrosis increases the thickness of the wall of the arteriole, with consequent reduction in the lumen and blood flow (hematoxylin and eosin, $\times$ 320).

circulation, in contradistinction to the predominantly venous distribution in most other retinopathies. Possibly they reflect inadequate autoregulation and elevated perfusion pressure. Retinal hemorrhages may have a similar explanation: they originate predominantly from the radial peripapillary capillaries located in the nerve fiber layer, which gives them their characteristic linear or flame-shaped configuration.

Hypertensive Optic Neuropathy

The papilledema of hypertensive vascular disease involves both anterior and lateral swelling associated with plasma leakage and disruption of the nerve fibers as they pass through the region of the optic nerve head. As with RNFLI, this represents the effect of ischemia and consequent interference with axoplasmic transport. Axolemmal swelling, both anterior and posterior to the lamina cribrosa, has been described in animal studies (56), and there is subsequent loss of axons with replacement gliosis. Both the exudation and the ischemia are the outcome of fibrinous necrosis of the smaller arterioles supplying the optic disc, although other factors, such as impeded venous outflow (as a result of raised intracranial pressure transmitted into the optic nerve sheath), may also be involved.

Hypertensive Choroidopathy

Choroidal involvement in malignant hypertension is a common histological finding and clinically usually takes the form of Elschnig spots. These are discrete serous exudates beneath the RPE with secondary epithelial degeneration and, as with the retinal leakages, probably represent failed autoregulation culminating in fibrinous arteriolar necrosis (56). Animal studies also indicate that extensive choroidal ischemia may supervene (45).

Diabetes Mellitus

Vascular lesions are an important manifestation of diabetes mellitus. Diabetes type I (insulin dependent) is a consequence of autoimmune pancreatic islet β cell loss. The genetic susceptibility is associated with an aberrant expression of class II major histocompatibility products on the β cells (63). Diabetes type II (noninsulin dependent) accounts for 80% of primary diabetes in North America and Europe, with a generally much later onset than the type I disease. Patients with diabetes type II have a wide range of resistance to insulin at the level of the insulin receptor (22).

Diabetic Vascular Disease

Few parts of the body are spared the vascular complications of the diabetic process, the incidence generally correlating with the duration of the metabolic defect. Circulatory disturbances are at the root of the renal complications, the neuropathy, and the tendency to gangrene, as well as the retinal complications. Microangiopathy develops after the onset of diabetes mellitus and may be delayed if the carbohydrate disturbance is kept under rigid control (3, 22).

One way in which hyperglycemia can affect the vasculature is by inducing nonenzymatic glycosylation of protein. At first the changes are reversible, but ultimately stable complexes are formed, especially where collagen and other protein components of the

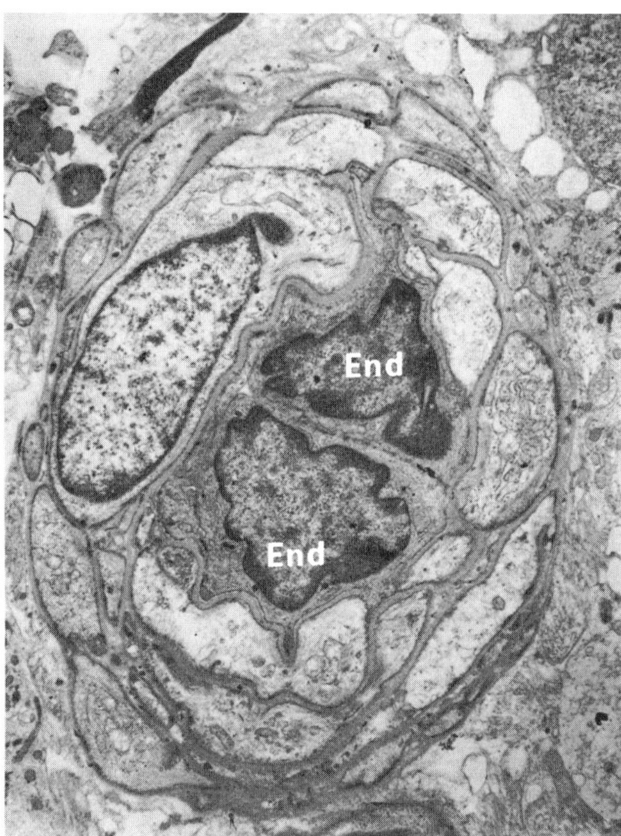

Figure 18 Experimentally induced hypertensive retinopathy in a monkey. Marked vasoconstriction resulted in obliteration of the arteriolar lumen. The endothelial lining (End) is compressed but otherwise normal, and although there is some increase in electron lucency in some cells, the smooth muscle coat shows no sign of necrosis (× 7,500).

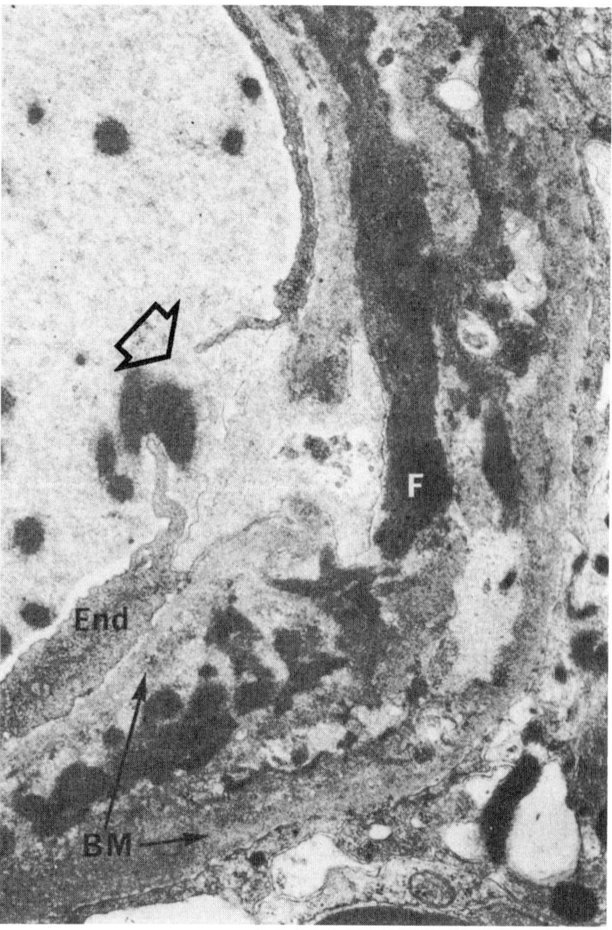

Figure 19 Transmission electron micrograph of part of the wall of a precapillary retinal arteriole in an acutely hypertensive monkey. The endothelium (End) is attenuated and at one point is ruptured (*arrow*). The smooth muscle coat is degenerate and infiltrated with fibrin (F), BM, basement membrane (× 20,500).

vascular wall are concerned. There are then a number of ways in which the blood vessels and circulating blood can be adversely affected (17): (*i*) the collagen-attached end products of glycosylation have an affinity for plasma protein, and this can interfere with transmural transport and contribute to basement membrane thickening; (*ii*) cross-linkage of insoluble basement membrane components through their glycosylated units leads to abnormal permeability; (*iii*) the glycosylated elements may react with PMNLs and macrophages with subsequent inflammation; and (*iv*) glycosylation of hemoglobin (HbA_{1c}) decreases oxygenation of target tissues.

A second way for hyperglycemia to damage the microvasculature is by causing increased utilization of the polyol route of glucose metabolism, resulting in its conversion to sorbitol under the influence of aldose reductase. The accumulation of sorbitol reduces the capacity for cellular uptake of myoinositol from the plasma. This in turn reduces the level of Na^+-K^+-ATPase activity, with consequent impairment of the ability of smooth muscle cells and pericytes to control vascular tone (99).

Capillary Changes

The hallmark of diabetic capillaropathy is a thickening of the basement membrane of up to five times the normal 80 to 120 nm width, a development that accompanies the metabolic disturbance and occurs in many tissues. As with most developments in diabetes mellitus, it would be wrong to look to a single causative factor, but there is good evidence that hyperglycemia may have a direct effect. Thus it has been shown that the capillary basement membranes of eels with physiological hyperglycemia induced by keeping them in water at 4°C are several times thicker than those of eels swimming in warmer water (14). Moreover, incorporation of proline and lysine by rat lens capsule can be enhanced in vitro by adding glucose to the incubation substrate.

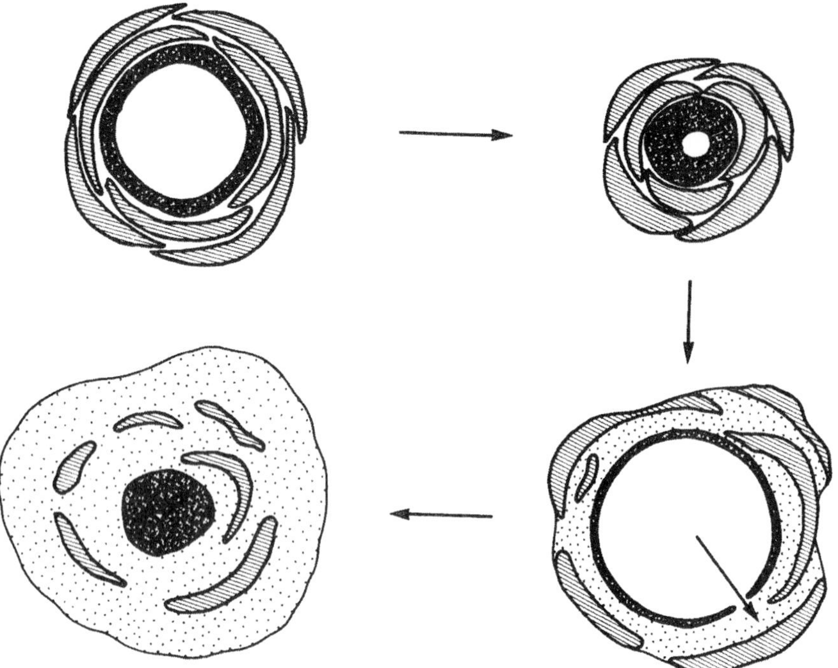

Figure 20 Postulated sequence of events in the pathogenesis of arteriolar fibrinous necrosis in hypertensive retinopathy. Initially, precapillary arterioles undergo extreme constriction, possibly as a result of an autoregulatory process. Subsequently, smooth muscle cell necrosis occurs in the face of persistently raised blood pressure, with resultant arteriolar dilatation and leakage of plasma into the degenerate wall through focal breaks in the unsupported lining endothelium. Ultimately, continued plasma insudation may produce a secondary reduction in the arteriolar lumen.

Reduced turnover as well as increased synthesis may also play a part in the thickening and account for the lamination that is sometimes seen. Increased permeability develops at an early stage in the diabetic process. Cytokines and growth factors, in particular VEGF, are believed to play a role in this process (44).

Arteriolar Changes

It has long been recognized that hyaline arteriosclerosis of the type commonly identified with the benign phase of hypertension is particularly prominent in diabetes mellitus. The hyaline contains fibrin and lipid from the circulating plasma, leakage possibly being facilitated by alterations in the permeability of the endothelial lining and basement membrane integrity.

Arterial Disease

Apart from microangiopathy, the larger arteries are prone to develop excessively severe atherosclerosis such that all patients with diabetes mellitus of more than 10 years duration tend to have clinically significant plaque formation. Several factors are likely to be responsible for this accelerated atherogenesis, including associated hyperlipidemia, platelet abnormalities, and glycosylation of subendothelial and lipoprotein molecules. There is evidence that plaque formation at the origin of the ophthalmic artery sufficient to cause stenosis aggravates an established diabetic retinopathy (Fig. 21) (35).

Diabetic Retinopathy

Not all diabetics develop retinal disease, but the incidence rises with the duration of the metabolic defect, so that patients with juvenile-onset diabetes (type I) are at greatest risk. From an incidence of 12% after 0 to 5 years of diabetes, the figure in one series rose to 91% after 21 years (54). Moreover, the risk of developing a significant retinopathy is influenced by the quality of metabolic control. Visual impairment attributable to retinopathy sufficient to rate admission to the blind register affects just under 2% of the diabetic population in the United Kingdom, but this is likely to rise with the increasing prevalence of both diabetes type I and type II (67).

From a clinical standpoint it is convenient to recognize four grades of diabetic retinopathy: background retinopathy (which rarely leads to blindness), macular edema, a severe nonproliferative diabetic retinopathy, and proliferative diabetic retinopathy. Inevitably, however, the biochemical complications of the diabetic state precede the clinical manifestations, and it is expected that functional disturbances constitute a preretinopathy phase.

Preretinopathy: Blood–Retina Barrier Changes

Vitreous fluorophotometry points to limited breakdown of the blood–retina barriers at an early stage (25) that is reversible with good glycemic control. The permeability appears to be confined to small molecules initially, and leakage of protein, as judged by immunohistochemical examination of human retinas (94), does not occur until retinopathy is clinically evident.

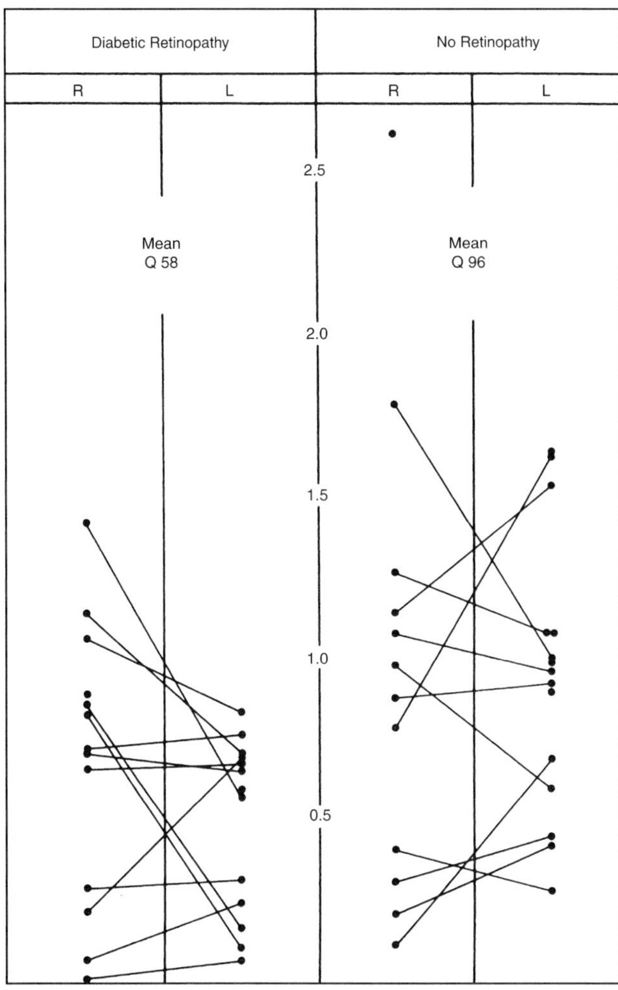

Figure 21 Comparison of the area (mm^2) of the ophthalmic artery ostium at autopsy in diabetic subjects with and without retinopathy. Although the means of the areas were significantly different, the considerable overlap between the two groups and the variation in caliber between the right and left sides suggest that ophthalmic artery narrowing as a result of atherosclerosis is unlikely to be a major factor in diabetic retinopathy, although it may contribute.

Retinal Blood Flow

Increased blood flow occurs in the early and preretinopathy phases of diabetes, implying a degree of vasodilatation within the retinal vasculature. This contention is supported by the observation that in vitro cultures of vascular endothelium secrete reduced amounts of the vasoconstrictor substance endothelin when subjected to a hyperglycemic milieu, and pericytes are less responsive under such conditions. Perhaps the increased flow is a response to tissue hypoxia, a view supported by the demonstration that the increase can be partially negated if the patient is subjected to 100% oxygen breathing (40).

Background Retinopathy: Clinical Features

The initial clinical manifestations of diabetic retinopathy are microaneurysms, exudates, punctate hemorrhages, and foci of capillary closure.

Microaneurysms. Aneurysmal dilatation of the retinal capillaries is a constant finding in background retinopathy and may be its presenting sign. They predominate on the venous side of the circulation in the posterior retina and are usually most frequent around foci of closed capillaries (Fig. 22). Their importance lies in their excessive permeability and liability to rupture, resulting in focal serous exudation and hemorrhage. Accumulated thrombus within the aneurysmal sac causes many aneurysms to be obliterated, the life of individual lesions being of the order of several months (58). When the thrombosis obliterates the sac but does not obstruct flow, fluorescein angiography may give a misleading impression of regression (Fig. 14).

Exudates. Serous exudation implies breakdown of the blood–retina barrier, and although endothelial cell degeneration and loss may be involved in leakage from microaneurysms and the later stages of the retinopathy, its occurrence in the earlier stages is probably a functional event. Animal experiments suggest that reversible dysfunction of the intercellular junctions may be involved (96). Intravascular hypoxia occurring on the venous side of the circulation, by exaggerating any tendency to hyperviscosity and in this way raising the intraluminal pressure, may add to the risk of leakage. Increased permeability of the thickened basement membranes may further promote exudation.

Hemorrhages. The extravasation of blood cells is contingent on a substantial endothelial cell deficit and is most often encountered in the vicinity of microaneurysms.

Capillary Closure. Small foci in the posterior fundus in which the capillaries are not perfused are an early feature of background retinopathy. The capillaries in these areas are devoid of both pericytes and endothelium and are represented merely by tubes of basement membrane. Thrombotic occlusion of the feeding arteriole is one possible explanation for these areas. The capillaries are also subject to external compression by surrounding tissue made edematous by ischemic hypoxia. The clinical significance of capillary closure is considerable because scotomata are caused by degeneration of nerve fibers and ganglion cells and microaneurysms and neovascularization are prone to develop in these areas (Fig. 23). There is some evidence that limited attempts at revascularization

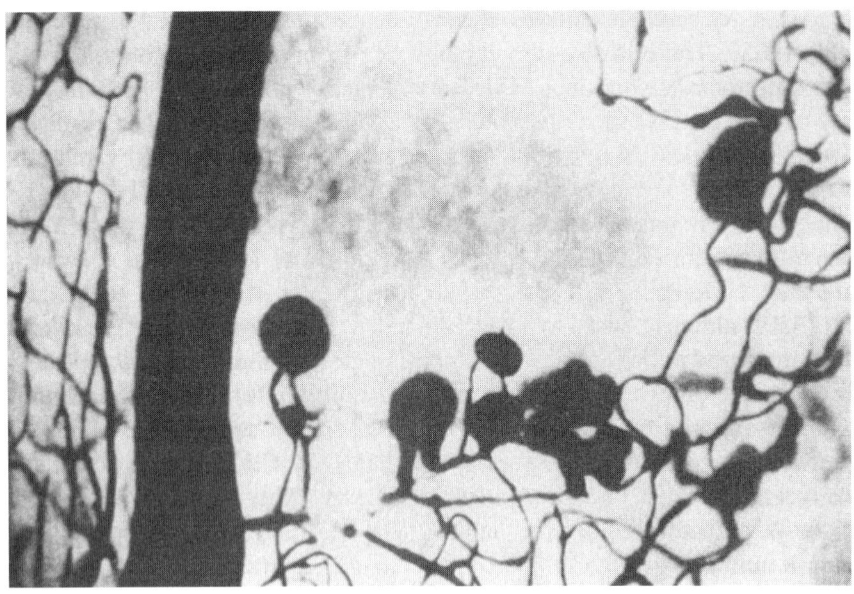

Figure 22 Diabetic retinopathy flat mount of retina perfused with colloidal carbon, showing a cluster of capillary aneurysms surrounding a zone of nonperfusion in which a cotton-wool spot developed ($\times$110).

may occur, possibly due to reendothelialization of residual basement membrane tubes where these have not been invaded by glia.

Background Retinopathy: Underlying Vascular Pathology

Endothelial Cells. The retinal endothelium is associated with an enhanced risk of thrombotic vascular occlusion caused not only by hypercoagulability of the circulating blood but also by intrinsic abnormalities.

Pericytes. An invariable feature of diabetic retinopathy is selective degeneration of capillary pericytes. In retinal digest preparations stained with periodic acid Schiff and hematoxylin, the nuclei of these cells fail to stain and have been termed ghost cells, but staining with hematoxylin and eosin produces an intense pink color (8). Eventually there is total degeneration of the pericyte nucleus and, presumably, of its cytoplasmic processes. Loss of pericytes is sometimes accompanied by loss of endothelium. A study of bovine capillaries suggests that both the endothelium and pericytes degenerate but that

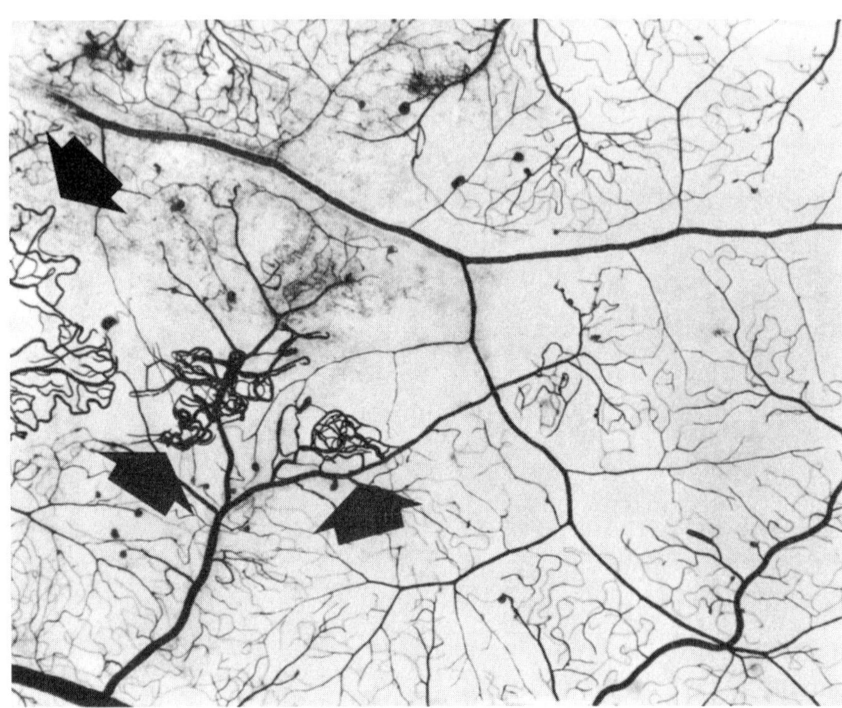

Figure 23 Flat mount of retina in proliferative diabetic retinopathy. The patent blood vessels have been perfused with colloidal carbon. Leashes of new capillaries on the surface of the retina (*arrows*) originated from venules at the edges of inadequately perfused foci in the underlying tissue ($\times$ 21).

the former has a greater capacity for regeneration than the latter.

The cause of the degeneration is not clear, but hyperglycemia seems to be directly involved. Cultured pericytes multiply at a much reduced rate in the presence of supplemental glucose, and glucose inhibits ascorbate transport within these cells. The metabolism of excessive blood glucose through the polyol pathway may be involved in the toxicity, aldose reductase inhibitors having a protective effect on the retinal pericytes of galactosemic dogs (55). Apart from a putative role in microaneurysm formation, as described earlier, the absence of pericytes may have a permissive effect on endothelial cell multiplication in the context of ensuing proliferative disease.

Basement Membrane. The retinal capillaries share the basement membrane changes seen in other tissues (Fig. 24), the thickening possibly representing incorporation of plasma residues as well as increased synthesis.

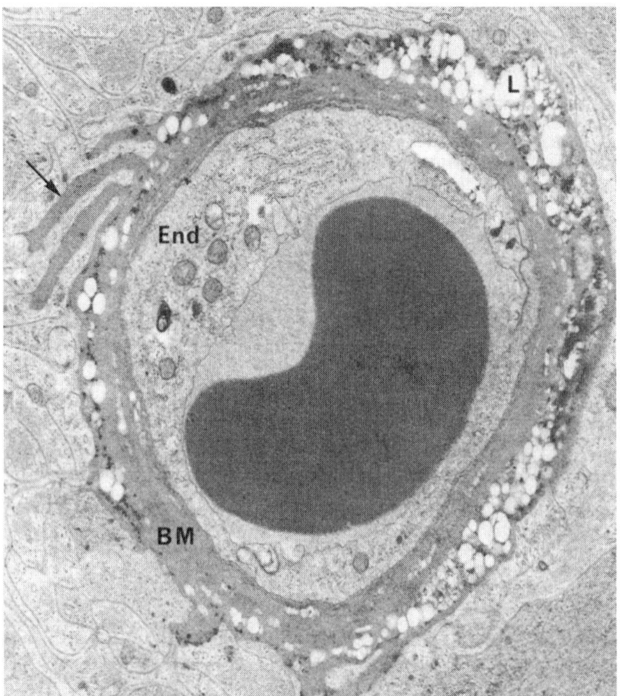

Figure 24 Retinal capillary in diabetic retinopathy showing marked thickening of the basement membrane (BM). Globular spaces in the membrane probably represent lipid insudation, with much of the lipid (L) filling the site of a necrotic pericyte. Extension of the basement membrane material between adjacent neural tissue (*arrow*) is the likely counterpart of the argyrophilic membrane, which invests retinal capillaries and is particularly prominent in diabetes. *Abbreviation*: End, endothelium ($\times$ 13,400). *Source*: Courtesy of the late Professor N. Ashton.

Arterioles. Hyalinization of the retinal arterioles with gradual reduction in the arteriolar lumen is one result of background diabetic retinopathy. Eventual occlusion of these terminal arterioles due to presumed thrombus formation is the likely cause of the increasing number of foci of capillary closure. It seems that the occlusion in these circumstances is a relatively gradual process since it does not give rise to detectable tissue necrosis. On the other hand, occlusion of precapillary arterioles developing as a fairly rapid event would account for the RNFLIs seen in approximately a third of diabetic retinas.

Veins. Retinal vein caliber increases in about 10% of patients with diabetic retinopathy (85). Initially the dilation may be reversed with improved control of the metabolic state and may be a consequence of increased arterial flow in hypoxic conditions. Eventually the abnormality is likely to become fixed as the vessel wall thickens and becomes sclerotic and opaque.

Maculopathy

Some diabetic patients have minimal background retinopathy but present with incapacitating visual loss attributable to macular edema (16). Histological examination reveals cystoid spaces presumed to represent edema fluid located mainly in the outer plexiform (Henle) layer but also extending into the inner retinal layers. Transudation and even exudation from perifoveal vessels may be a factor, although this is probably a minor consideration, and an ultrastructural analysis pointed to a primary swelling of Müller cells that only later rupture to spill their contents into the extracellular space and form cysts. In view of the reduced circulation demonstrable in the maculae of affected patients, it may be more reasonable to look to ischemia for an explanation of the maculopathy, a conclusion supported by experimental models (93).

Severe Nonproliferative Retinopathy

Retinal Nerve Fiber Layer Infarction

The emergence of RNFLI is indicative of accelerating focal ischemia and as such is a harbinger of subsequent neovascularization. Their presence suggests that the causative arteriolar occlusions not only involve larger areas of the capillary bed but occur more rapidly.

Intraretinal Microvascular Anomalies

Dilated and elongated capillary loops, frequently forming bizarre hairpin or corkscrew patterns, are sometimes seen invading focal avascular zones of the retina. Such blood vessels are likely to be new endothelial cell proliferations in the form of either completely new capillaries or reendothelializations of previously defunct vessels.

Proliferative Diabetic Retinopathy

Proliferation of new blood vessels on the inner surface of the retina and within the vitreous cavity is usually a late manifestation of diabetic retinopathy, with an incidence of around 60% after 15 to 20 years of diabetes (60), although this incidence is diminished when glycemic control is improved. As a rule it is preceded by a worsening of the background retinopathy and is associated with increasing areas of capillary closure. There is good reason, as with proliferative retinopathy in other disease states, to impute tissue hypoxia as the key pathogenetic factor. A number of angiogenic factors have been implicated in the formation of proliferative diabetic retinopathy, including VEGF (86), angiopoietin (41), basic fibroblast growth factor (FGF) (10), insulin-like growth factor 1 (ILGF1) (38), and erythropoietin (98).

The new blood vessels usually stem from larger veins near areas of capillary closure or near the optic disc. Initially they proliferate in the potential space between the ILM and the posterior face of the vitreous, where they appear flat (Fig. 25), but eventually they can invade the vitreous, using condensations of the vitreal collagen as a support. Alternatively they may be dragged forward as a consequence of becoming bound to the posterior face of a retreating vitreous. At first the proliferating capillaries are leaky, but this is largely corrected as the vessels mature and permanent intercellular junctions are formed. Fenestrations of the endothelium of new vessels are rare. Pericyte development and the formation of a fibrous adventitia also ensues, the responsible myofibroblasts exerting traction in a way that incurs the risk of retinal detachment. It is at this stage that new blood vessels are prone to bleed, since they are incompletely formed, poorly supported, and subject to traction by a retracting vitreous.

Sickle Cell Disease

Deformation of erythrocytes into a sickle shape under hypoxic conditions is a feature of a group of familial disorders characterized by the presence of an abnormal Hb variant (see Chapter 36).

Sickle cell disease (SS disease, MIM #603903) results from a specific homozygous mutation in the betaglobin gene (*HBB*), which causes HbS and virtually all the Hb is abnormal. As the partial pressure of the blood oxygen drops during its passage through the tissues, there is a risk that sickling will occur, and this interferes with the pliability of the affected erythrocytes so that they do not easily pass through narrow capillaries. In consequence vasoocclusion readily occurs with untoward effects on the dependent tissues. Moreover, such cells are unduly fragile and give rise to hemolytic anemia.

The sickle cell trait represents the heterozygous carrier state and is usually asymptomatic. Nevertheless, the red cells contain 25% to 43% HbS and can be made to sickle in vitro and under exceptional circumstances, such as flying at high altitude in vivo. Factors governing the degree of sickling include the following: (*i*) the proportion of HbS within the erythrocyte, (*ii*) the level of hypoxia, (*iii*) circulation time, and (*iv*) cellular Hb concentration.

HbC, in which the glutamic acid at the 6 position of the chain is replaced by lysine, can occur in combination with HbS in geographically defined

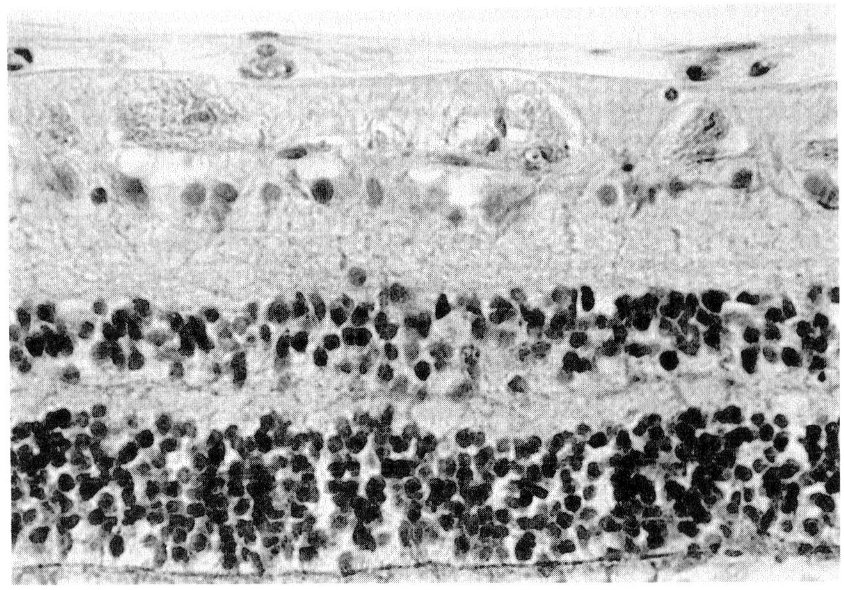

Figure 25 Section showing newly formed capillary blood vessels spreading between the inner limiting membrane of the retina and the posterior face of the vitreous (hematoxylin and eosin, $\times$ 385).

communities where the genes for both abnormalities are rife. Patients with combined sickle cell and HbC disease (SC disease) usually have fewer occlusive and hemolytic complications but, perversely, the incidence of retinopathy is higher. Thus, proliferative retinopathy has been reported as involving 32.8% of patients with HbS–HbC disease compared with 2.6% of patients with pure HbS–HbS disease (23).

Sickle cell-β-thalassemia is another double heterozygous state that can be associated with retinal lesions. As much as 60% to 80% of the Hb may be of the HbS type, and the symptoms of the disease resemble those of sickle cell disease more closely than those of beta thalassemia (MIM +141900).

Sickle Cell Retinopathy

Although sludging of conjunctival capillaries and occlusion of uveal vessels occur, the ocular complications of serious proportions are confined to the retina. This is probably because there are fewer alternative anastomotic sources of blood supply in the retina compared with other tissues.

The retinal manifestations of sickle cell disease and its variants resemble those of diabetes mellitus to a considerable degree, the principal difference relating to their distribution. Whereas the retinopathy of diabetes is essentially central (posterior), that due to sickling is mainly peripheral, although the macula may be involved in sickle cell retinopathy. Typical features of sickle cell retinopathy are retinal and vitreal hemorrhages, neovascularization, and, in some instances, retinal detachment (31).

Pathogenesis

Arteriolar Occlusion

The primary event is vaso-occlusion. Clinical experience supported by FA and a study of retinal digest preparations shows that arterioles, particularly the precapillary branches, are the most common sites. The reason for this is not clear, although a number of observations may be relevant: (*i*) the drop in pO_2 at precapillary level is sufficient to initiate sickling, (*ii*) the precapillary arteriole has a very narrow lumen and is a potential bottleneck, (*iii*) the arterial blood is unusually viscous, because of the presence of erythrocytes that have undergone irreversible sickling, (*iv*) irreversibly sickled cells can act as microemboli. Given these findings it is conceivable that irreversibly sickled cells arriving at the narrow precapillary arteriole become lodged and impede the passage of other erythrocytes so that they, too, begin to sickle. Furthermore, once started, a vicious cycle is established because stagnation and sickling are mutually stimulatory.

Occasionally the occluded arteriole reopens. Reopening within a few hours of the occlusion is probably due to break up of the red cell aggregate, whereas reopening after a delay of weeks or months is a result of recanalization. Delayed reopening is associated with endothelial cell and pericyte loss in the dependent capillary bed, and although some limited revascularization from the recanalized arteriole may take place, the number of new closures outweighs the reopenings. As a result, the zone of ischemia enlarges and gradually spreads from the periphery of the retina toward the posterior pole. A similar pattern of closure develops around the terminal blood vessels at the macula, beginning at the horizontal raphe on the temporal side of the fovea.

The predilection of the peripheral and perimacular regions of the retina for occlusive lesions is unexplained but may be connected with the minimal capacity of the functional end vessels in these sites to establish collateral compensation.

Retinal Hemorrhage

Vascular necrosis at or adjacent to the site of occlusion predisposes to bleeding into the retina, and within a matter of days or weeks the hematoma assumes an orange-red color recognizable clinically as a "salmon patch." The hemorrhage at this stage is intraretinal, but eventually it may spill into the subhyaloid space and vitreous or dissect between the photoreceptor outer segments and RPE. Subretinal hemorrhage of the latter kind is usually associated with dispersion and hyperplasia of the RPE to produce a black sunburst spot. Alternatively, the hematoma may remain localized and ultimately be organized to leave a cavity or focal retinoschisis. Macrophages containing hemosiderin may appear as iridescent granules on ophthalmic examination.

Neovascularization

When a precapillary arteriole is occluded, blood flow is diverted through proximal capillaries to the venous drainage channels. Such centripetal recession of the vascular arcades renders the preequatorial retina ischemic, and some 8 to 36 months later new capillary formations may arise from the sites of arteriolar-venular anastomosis. Initially, the new vessels lie on the surface of the retina, but gradually further proliferation results in delicate tufts of capillaries, each with a feeding arteriole and draining venule, projecting into the vitreous cavity. At first the tufts have little surrounding fibrous tissue and have been likened to sea fans.

The new capillaries are unduly permeable, and leakage of plasma into the vitreous, by virtue of its disruptive effect on gel stability, may be a factor in the commonly observed collapse of the vitreous body.

Collapse and retraction of the vitreous stresses sea fans adherent to its posterior foci and predisposes to tearing and bleeding into the vitreal cavity. Traction on the subjacent retina may also develop and produce retinal tears or holes, and possibly rhegmatogenous retinal detachment. Ultimately, a minority of the new vessels are themselves subject to occlusion and may regress. This pattern of events, first defined on the basis of direct observation and FA has since been demonstrated histologically.

Proliferative retinopathy is rare in childhood and should it develop in later life predominates in males and, as previously noted, is more common in SC than SS disease. The reason for this is not immediately apparent, but the suggestion has been made that the moderate level of vascular occlusion seen in patients with SC disease would in time lead to a commensurate degree of proliferative retinopathy, whereas the higher risk of occlusion expected of SS disease might relate to nascent as well as to established blood vessels and so abort most of the emergent neovascular tufts.

Retinopathy of Prematurity

Retinopathy of prematurity (ROP) occurs in a retina that is still undergoing active vascularization as part of normal fetal development and is characterized by the proliferation of fibrovascular tissue at the border between vascularized and as yet unvascularized retina. Abnormal fibrovascular tissue extends from the inner retina onto the surface of the retina, and creates a risk for retinal detachment.

Terry (89) was the first to define the clinical aspects of ROP (then called retrolental fibroplasia), but it took a decade for its true nature to be recognized. One of the more intriguing pieces of evidence was the discovery that premature infants born in a private hospital in Melbourne, Australia had a lower incidence of ROP than those born in a state-aided hospital; the essential difference in the nursing care was more sparing use of oxygen where the cost of supplemental oxygen was a factor (18). The relationship was confirmed in a controlled clinical trial by Patz and colleagues (72) and subsequently verified with experimental studies on laboratory animals. Accordingly, the administration of oxygen in neonatal units came to be much more rigorously monitored, and the incidence of ROP decreased dramatically.

Even so, despite these measures, recent years have witnessed a minor resurgence of ROP, and although several factors may be operative, the primary factor appears to be the survival of increasingly premature (and lower birth weight) newborns.

Clinicopathological Development

The primary clinical sign is irregular branching of the most recently formed retinal vessels with increased tortuosity of the more posteriorly located parent vessels. This may occur as a premonitory sign, however it is not specific. The pathognonomic changes of ROP begin at the margin of the developing vasculature and can be divided into five clinical stages that correlate with tissue changes. The disease process may arrest spontaneously, however, especially in the early stages, and progression to the final cicatricial state is not inevitable.

Stage 1. Demarcation Lines

Anterior to the fringes of the developing retinal blood vessels there is normally a narrow rim of tissue made up of a "vanguard" of spindle-shaped cells associated with posterior differentiating endothelium. The early clinical phase of ROP is characterized by hyperplasia of both spindle cells and endothelial cells creating an opaque (white) line separating the avascular and vascularized retina.

Stage 2. Ridge

Continued proliferation of the cells responsible for the demarcation line, particularly the endothelial cells thicken and elevate the retinal surface to form a ridge. Initially white, the ridge becomes increasingly pink as capillaries begin to form in the abnormal tissue.

Stage 3. Ridge with Extraretinal Fibrovascular Proliferation

The angiogenic tissue within the ridge is able to breach the ILM and extend onto the inner retinal surface (Fig. 26). Glial cells from the retina are also present supporting the neovascular tissue.

Stage 4. Subtotal Retinal Detachment

Proliferation of fibroglial neovascular tissue creates an extension into the vitreal cavity. Contraction of the fibrous component of the neovascular tissue causes tractional detachment of the underlying retina.

Stage 5. Total Retinal Detachment

Depending on the degree and circumferential extent of the vitreoretinal proliferation, the retina is at risk of being completely detached and deformed by fixed retinal folds. The combined retinal and extraretinal fibrovascular tissue may then be drawn forward and come to lie against the back of the lens (retrolental fibroplasia) (Fig. 27) significantly limiting or extinguishing visual function potential (81).

Because the obliterative effect of oxygen is in large measure a function of vascular maturity in the retina, infants of lower birth weight are at most risk for developing the advanced cicatricial stages of ROP.

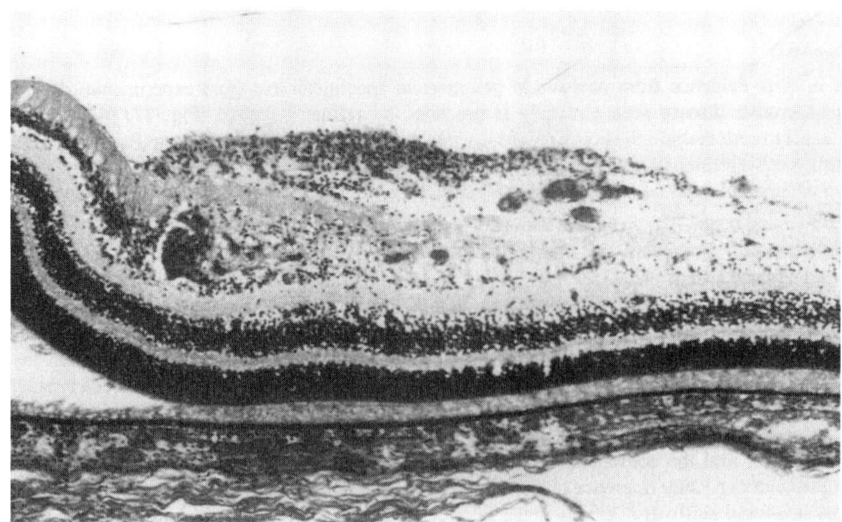

Figure 26 Retinopathy of prematurity, stage 3. The inner retina is thickened by a proliferation of vanguard (spindle) cells and endothelial cell precursors to constitute an elevated ridge. The cells lying on the surface of the retina represent a leash of developing new vessels that have broken through the inner limiting lamina in the region of the ridge (hematoxylin and eosin, ×95). *Source*: Reproduced with permission from Garner A. The pathology of retinopathy of prematurity. In: Silverman WA, Flynn JT, eds. Contemporary Issues in Fetal and Neonatal Medicine, 2. Retinopathy of Prematurity. Boston: Blackwell Scientific, 1986: 19–52.

In older infants nearing a full 40-week gestation, blood vessels at the retinal periphery alone are affected. Because the circulation on the temporal side of the eye is the last to be established, being farthest from the optic disc, the effects of oxygen toxicity at this stage neovascularization is more likely to occur in this region alone (Fig. 28). Subsequent cicatrization of such peripheral fibrovascular proliferation can cause temporal traction on the retina and temporal displacement of the macula.

Pathogenesis

There is clear evidence from analyses of postmortem specimens and from experimental data that the vasoproliferative disease seen clinically is preceded by retinal ischemia (Fig. 29). This is attributable to incomplete vascularization of the retina as well as endothelial cell necrosis and consequent obliteration of parts of the capillary bed; and as with the proliferative retinopathies as a whole, there is reason to interpret the relationship as causal, in which case an understanding of the pathogenesis of ROP requires knowledge of the factors giving rise to the initial ischemia (63).

Hyperoxia

Following the identification of hyperoxia on clinical grounds, experiments involving animal neonates have

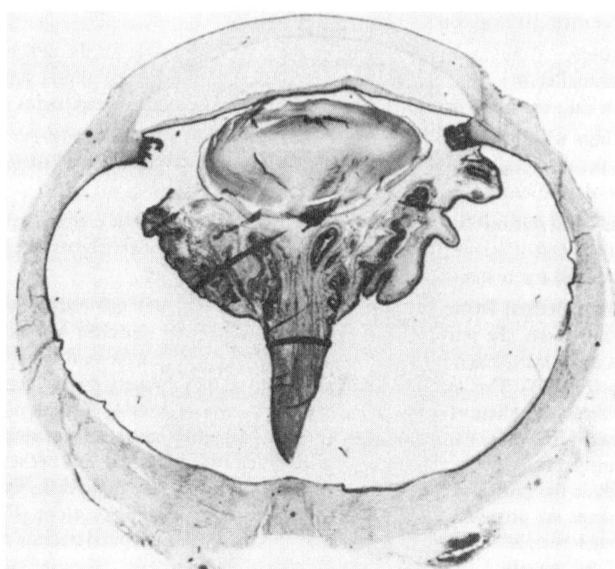

Figure 27 Retrolental fibroplasia. The retina is completely detached in conjunction with marked fibrovascular tissue proliferation on the anterior surface (hematoxylin and eosin, ×3.5). *Source*: Courtesy of the late Professor N. Ashton.

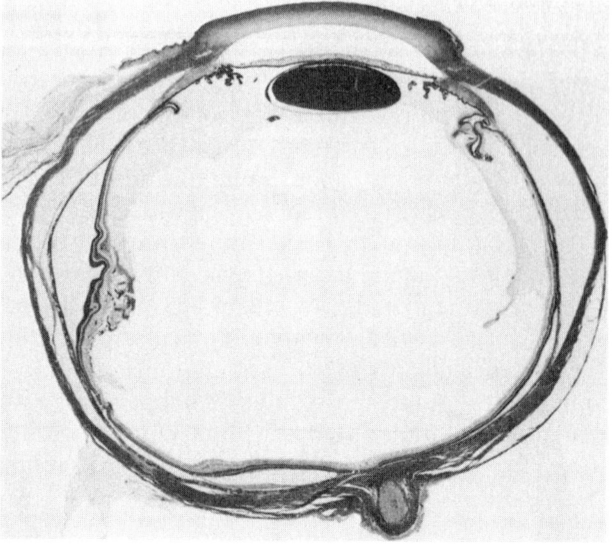

Figure 28 Retrolental fibroplasia of mild degree. Since the least mature retinal vessels are most vulnerable to oxygen excess and since the temporal periphery is the last part of the retina to be vascularized, in mild cases subsequent vasoproliferation may be confined to this zone (Masson trichrome, ×3.4).

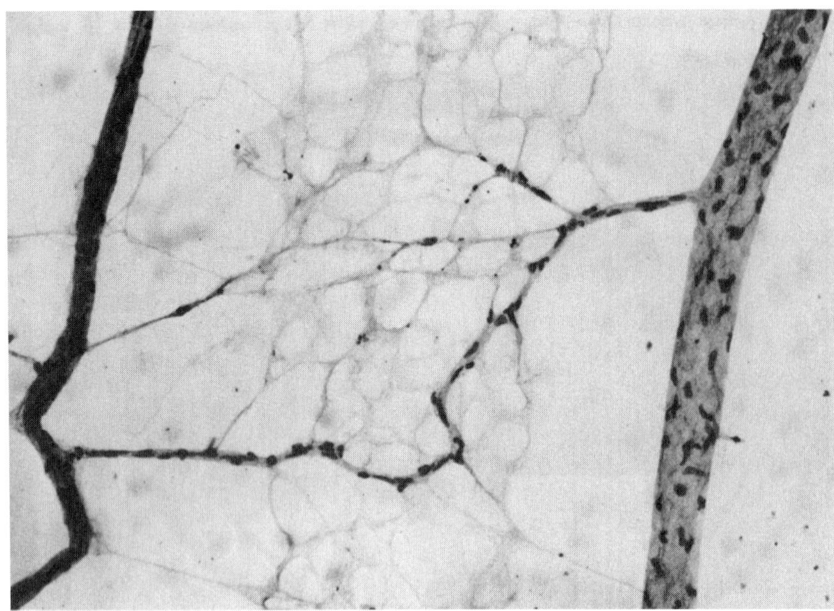

Figure 29 Retina of a premature infant subjected to excessive oxygen. There is marked obliteration of the capillary bed, leaving acellular basement membrane remnants. The main arterial and venous channels are also attenuated (periodic acid Schiff and hematoxylin, × 145).

provided further evidence that oxygen can be toxic to developing retinal capillary endothelium. Animal studies indicate an initial autoregulatory vasoconstriction in response to high levels of inspired oxygen (6). Endothelial cell degeneration ensues, however, beginning with the most recently differentiated cells.

Retinal Maturity

The possibility that retinal immaturity is important is emphasized by the preponderance of infants with birth weights under 1000 g in the most recently encountered cases.

Coats Disease

As Coats himself recognized, the condition that bears his name may well have more than one cause (19), and correspondingly some prefer the term "Coats lesion" or "Coats syndrome" to Coats disease. Coats lesion is characterized by extensive creamy or yellowish exudates within and beneath the retina, as well as hemorrhage and reflective material. The affected retina is often detached with subretinal serous fluid. The vascular abnormality is usually unilateral, most commonly of the temporal retina. Although cases are recognized in adulthood children are more commonly affected, with a peak incidence at age of 9 or 10 years. The majority of those affected are males.

Histopathology

The basic defect in Coats lesion is abnormal capillary blood vessels with loss of integrity of the vascular endothelium causing gradual leakage of plasma into the retina. Minor hemorrhage may occur. Phagocytic cells, from circulating monocytes and the RPE, remove the lipid and protein residues. Free cholesterol crystallizes appearing as iridescent particles surrounded by a multinucleated giant cells. New blood vessels may develop on the outer surface of the retina due to relative hypoxia of a detached retina. Fibrous organization follows; the retina becomes progressively more degenerate and disorganized, from outer to inner retina.

Etiology and Pathogenesis

The nature of the underlying vascular defect is not always clear, and it is important to recognize that primary inflammatory states, e.g., toxocariasis, can produce a vascular response similar to Coats disease. A proportion of the cases described in the original report by Coats were hemangioblastomas as reported by von Hippel (95). The two entities are now considered to be distinct. Coats divided the remaining cases into those with and those without discernible vascular anomalies, i.e., focal dilatation of capillaries to form congenital aneurysms or areas of more generalized telangiectasis (Fig. 30) (79). Tripathi and Ashton (90) showed, by TEM that the dilated capillaries were thickened. They postulated that the primary cause was a breakdown in the blood-retina barrier, with secondary damage to the capillary wall leading to irregular dilatation and aneurysm formation.

Eales Disease

Idiopathic retinal vasculitis (Eales disease) is recurrent hemorrhages and perivascular sheathing by leukocytes in the periphery of the retinas of young adult

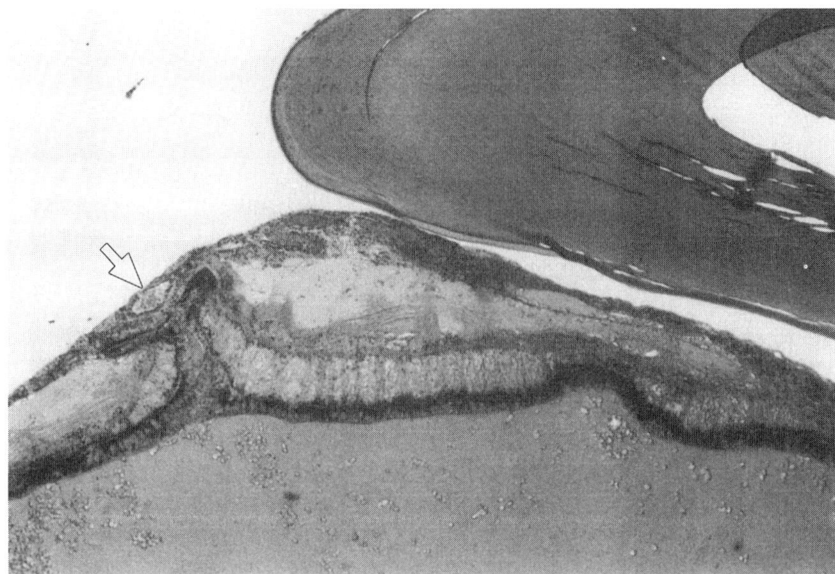

Figure 30 Coats disease. Section of an enucleated eye showing detachment of the retina associated with a serous subretinal exudate. A zone of telangiectasia is seen in the retina (*arrow*) and appears to be the source of the exudation (hematoxylin and eosin, × 26).

males (30). However, similar lesions can occur in the central retina, in older individuals, and in women. Thus "idiopathic retinal vasculitis" is probably a more appropriate term for what was known as Eales disease.

Pathology

The most common histologic feature is an accumulation of lymphocytes around and within the walls ("perivascular cuffing") of retinal veins (28) Plasma cells may also be present, and occasionally there is a granulomatous reaction with multinucleated giant cells. Retinal vasculitis (Fig. 31) can spread from the retinal periphery to the posterior retina. Occasionally the vasculitis progresses from posterior to periphery.

Retinal vasculitis may be an isolated lesion or be associated with uveitis, and in some instances there is little or no vasculitis, the vascular sheathing apparently being due to retinal vessel wall thickening.

Abnormalities caused by vascular thrombosis and necrosis are common. Thrombotic branch vein occlusion with capillary closure and tissue hypoxia is probably responsible for preretinal neovascularization that occurs. Aneurysmal dilatation and more extensive varicosities giving a beaded appearance to the venules and veins is also caused by inflammation and necrosis. Weakened blood vessels, together with the intravitreal neovascular proliferation, produce recurrent hemorrhage. Intravitreal hemorrhage can develop even in the absence of preretinal vessels as an extension of intraretinal bleeding, a phenomenon that

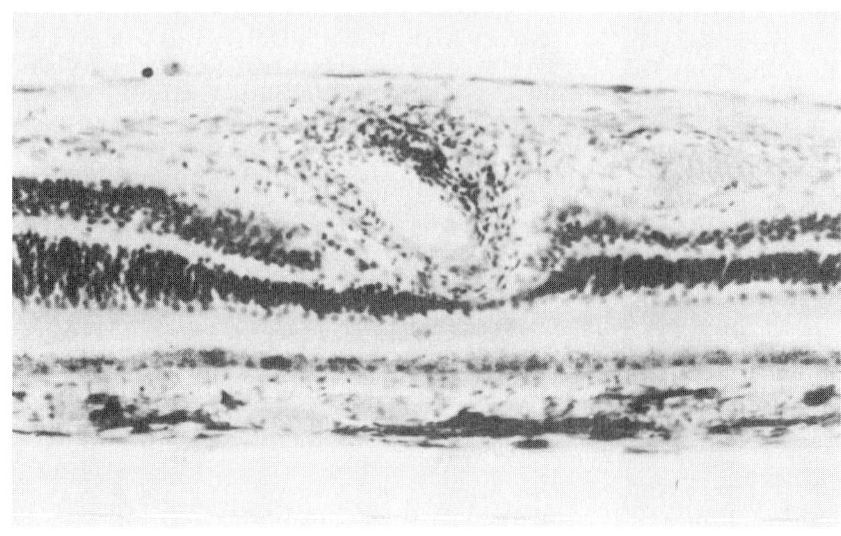

Figure 31 Eales disease. Section of retina showing a venule sheathed with lymphocytes and scanty plasma cells (hematoxylin and eosin, × 165).

may be linked with damage to the ILM in the vicinity of inflamed venous channels. Frequently the ILM is thickened, possibly due to inspissation of proteinaceous exudates.

The fibrosis that accompanies the preretinal vasoproliferation can predispose eventually to retinal detachment and iris neovascularization with secondary angle closure glaucoma.

Etiology and Pathogenesis

The cause of Eales disease is believed to be an autoimmune process possibly triggered by an exogenous agent. The histological finding of a lymphocytic and occasionally granulomatous vasculitis is supportive of an immunological process without providing any etiological clues. Hematological abnormalities, particularly of the clotting the clotting mechanism and blood viscosity, are described, as are plasma protein irregularities. Many patients with Eales disease are tuberculin hypersensitive (80).

Ocular Ischemic Syndrome

The ocular ischemic syndrome is caused by gradual narrowing and ultimate occlusion of arteries arising from the aortic arch. The occlusion affects cerebral, cardiac, and ocular vascular systems.

In the western hemisphere, atherosclerosis is the most common cause of ocular ischemic syndrome. Occasionally giant cell arteritis has been implicated. In Eastern Asia Takayasu arteritis (pulseless disease) is a significant cause, particularly in young women.

Presenting symptoms of transient blindness (amaurosis fugax) may be precipitated by a sudden movement of the head, by postural hypotension, or by exertion. There are no objective ocular signs at this stage although there may be a progressive reduction in the central retinal artery pressure. As ischemia progresses, the retina becomes translucent (a result of ischemic atrophy), the circulation time becomes prolonged, and dilated peripheral vessels may occlude. Arteriolovenular shunts at vascular crossings have been described in patients with Takayasu arteritis. Petechiae and occasional nerve fiber layer hemorrhages may also develop. Preretinal neovascularization in the region of the optic disc occasionally develop. Optic disc atrophy occurs in association with absent posterior ciliary artery perfusion. Anterior segment ischemia is also frequent, particularly in patients with severe bilateral carotid artery disease. Mild enophthalmos may be caused by ischemic atrophy of the orbital tissues surrounding the eye. Cataracts may also appear.

Arteriovenous Fistulas

The internal carotid artery is immobile as it passes through the cavernous sinus. Indirect contusion or direct skull fracture of the sphenoid may cause focal arterial wall weakening and dilation or a frank rupture to form a fistula between the internal carotid and the cavernous sinus.

Once the fistula is established there is a sudden increase in venous pressure in the cavernous sinus causing reversal of blood flow into the venous system including the ophthalmic vein. The orbital veins become markedly congested and incompetent leading to pre- and postseptal soft tissue swelling and pulsatile proptosis. Swelling of the eyelid is also common, and eventually periorbital and facial venous dilatation may be marked as alternative anastomotic drainage channels become established. The rapid progression of swelling is associated with severe pain.

Simultaneous with the rise in venous pressure is a drop in ophthalmic artery pressure to the degree that ocular ischemia may develop. The cornea may become edematous, and the retina may show superficial hemorrhages and microaneurysms. There is a risk of secondary neovascular glaucoma occuring.

Cavernous sinus dural arteriovenous fistulas are typically less severe than cavernous sinus-carotid fistulas. They too can present with proptosis, orbital congestion, increased IOP, or retinal hemorrhages and edema, however, the presentation is far more gradual (87).

REFERENCES

1. Aeby C. Der Bau Des Menschlichen Korpers. Leipzig: 1868.
2. Anderson DR. Axonal Transport in the Retina and Optic Nerve. St. Louis, MO: Mosby, 1977.
3. Anonymous. Retinopathy and nephropathy in patients with type 1 diabetes four years after a trial of intensive therapy. The diabetes control and complications trial/epidemiology of diabetes interventions and complications research group. N Engl J Med 2000; 342:381–9.
4. Ashton N, Harry J. The pathology of cotton wool spots and cytoid bodies in hypertensive retinopathy and other diseases. Trans Ophthalmol Soc UK 1963; 83:91–114.
5. Ashton N, Henkind P. Experimental occlusion of retinal arterioles: using graded glass ballotini. Br J Ophthalmol 1965; 49:225–34.
6. Ashton N, Ward B, Serpell G. Role of oxygen in the genesis of retrolental fibroplasias: a preliminary report. Br J Ophthalmol 1953; 37:513–20.
7. Ashton N. Retinal micro-aneurysms in the non-diabetic subject. Br J Ophthalmol 1951; 35:189–212.
8. Ashton N. Studies of the retinal capillaries in relation to diabetic and other retinopathies. Br J Ophthalmol 1963; 47:521–38.
9. Ashton N. Vascular basement membrane changes in diabetic retinopathy. Montgomery lecture, 1973. Br J Ophthalmol 1974; 58:344–66.
10. Baird A, Esch F, Gospodarowicz D, Guillemin R. Retina- and eye-derived endothelial cell growth factors: partial

molecular characterization and identity with acidic and basic fibroblast growth factors. Biochemistry 1985; 24: 7855–60.
11. Ballantyne AJ, Loewenstein A. Retinal microaneurysms and punctate haemorrhages. Br J Ophthalmol 1944; 28: 593–8.
12. Bearelly S, Fekrat S. Controversy in the management of retinal venous occlusive disease. Int Ophthalmol Clin 2004; 44:85–102.
13. Behrman S. Amaurosis fugax et amaurosis fulminas. Arch Ophthalmol 1951; 45:458–67.
14. Bendayan M, Rasio EA. Hyperglycemia and microangiopathy in the eel. Diabetes 1981; 30:317–25.
15. Beri M, Klugman MR, Kohler JA, Hayreh SS. Anterior ischemic optic neuropathy. VII. Incidence of bilaterality and various influencing factors. Ophthalmology 1987; 94: 1020–8.
16. Bodansky HJ, Cudworth AG, Whitelocke RA, Dobree JH. Diabetic retinopathy and its relation to type of diabetes: review of a retinal clinic population. Br J Ophthalmol 1982; 66:496–9.
17. Brownlee M, Cerami A, Vlassara H. Advanced glycosylation end products in tissue and the biochemical basis of diabetic complications. N Engl J Med 1988; 318: 1315–21.
18. Campbell K. Intensive oxygen therapy as a possible cause of retrolental fibroplasia: a clinical approach. Med J Aust 1951; 2:48–50.
19. Coats G. Forms of retinal disease with massive exudation. R Land Ophthalmol Hasp Rep 1908; 17:440–525.
20. Cogan DG, Toussaint D, Kuwabara T. Retinal vascular patterns. IV. Diabetic retinopathy. Arch Ophthalmol 1961; 66:366–78.
21. Cogan DG. Development and senescence of the human retinal vasculature. Trans Ophthalmol Soc UK 1963; 83: 465–89.
22. Colwell JA. Effect of diabetic control on retinopathy. Diabetes 1966; 15:497–9.
23. Condon PI, Serjeant GR. Ocular findings in hemoglobin SC disease in Jamaica. Am J Ophthalmol 1972; 74:921–31.
24. Constable IJ. Pathology of vitreous membranes and the effect of haemorrhage and new vessels on the vitreous. Trans Ophthalmol Soc UK 1975; 95:382–6.
25. Cunha-Vaz J, Faria de Abreu JR, Campos AJ. Early breakdown of the blood–retinal barrier in diabetes. Br J Ophthalmol 1975; 59:649–56.
26. Cunha-Vaz JG. The blood-retinal barriers. Doc Ophthalmol 1976; 41:287–327.
27. Dahrling BEII. The Histopathology of Early Central Retinal Artery Occlusion. Arch Ophthalmol 1965; 73: 506–10.
28. Donders PC. Eales' disease. Doc Ophthalmol Proc Ser 1958; 12:1–105.
29. Dugan JD Jr, Green WR. Ophthalmologic manifestations of carotid occlusive disease. Eye 1991; 5(Pt 2):226–38.
30. Eales H. Cases of retinal haemorrhage associated with epistaxis and constipation. Birmingham Meet Rev 1880; 9:262–72.
31. Emerson GG, Harlan JB, Fekrat S, Lutty GA. Goldberg MF. Hemoglobinopathies In: Ryan SJ, ed. Retina, 4th ed.. Elsevier Mosby, 2006; 1428–45.
32. Flower RW, McLeod DS, Lutty GA, et al. Postnatal retinal vascular development of the puppy. Invest Ophthalmol Vis Sci 1985; 26:957–68.
33. Foulis AK. C.L. Oakley lecture (1987). The pathogenesis of beta cell destruction in type I (insulin-dependent) diabetes mellitus. J Pathol 1987; 152:141–8.
34. Frank RN, Turczyn TJ, Das A. Pericyte coverage of retinal and cerebral capillaries. Invest Ophthalmol Vis Sci 1990; 31:999–1007.
35. Garner A, Ashton N, Tripathi R, et al. Pathogenesis of hypertensive retinopathy. An experimental study in the monkey. Br J Ophthalmol 1975; 59:3–44.
36. Garner A, Ashton N. Ophthalmic artery stenosis and diabetic retinopathy. Trans Ophthalmol Soc UK 1972; 92: 101–10.
37. Grant DS, Tashiro K, Segui-Real B, et al. Two different laminin domains mediate the differentiation of human endothelial cells into capillary-like structures in vitro. Cell 1989; 58:933–43.
38. Grant M, Russell B, Fitzgerald C, Merimee TJ. Insulin-like growth factors in vitreous. Studies in control and diabetic subjects with neovascularization. Diabetes 1986; 35: 416–20.
39. Green WR, Chan CC, Hutchins GM, Terry JM. Central retinal vein occlusion: a prospective histopathologic study of 29 eyes in 28 cases. Retina 1981; 1:27–55.
40. Grunwald JE, Riva CE, Baine J, Brucker AJ. Total retinal volumetric blood flow rate in diabetic patients with poor glycemic control. Invest Ophthalmol Vis Sci 1992; 33: 356–63.
41. Hackett SF, Wiegand S, Yancopoulos G, Campochiaro PA. Angiopoietin-2 plays an important role in retinal angiogenesis. J Cell Physiol 2002; 192:182–7.
42. Hamasaki DI, Kroll AJ. Experimental central retinal artery occlusion. An electrophysiological study. Arch Ophthalmol 1968; 80:243–8.
43. Hammes HP. Pericytes and the pathogenesis of diabetic retinopathy. Horm Metab Res 2005; 37(Suppl. 1):39–43.
44. Harhajn NS, Antonetti DA. Regulation of tight junctions and loss of barrier function in pathophysiology. Int J Biochem Cell Biol 2004; 36:1206–37.
45. Hayreh SS, Servais GE, Virdi PS. Fundus lesions in malignant hypertension. VI. Hypertensive choroidopathy. Ophthalmology 1986; 93:1383–400.
46. Hayreh SS, van Heuven WA, Hayreh MS. Experimental retinal vascular occlusion. I. Pathogenesis of central retinal vein occlusion. Arch Ophthalmol 1978; 96:311–23.
47. Hayreh SS. Anterior ischemic optic neuropathy. VIII. Clinical features and pathogenesis of post-hemorrhagic amaurosis. Ophthalmology 1987; 94:1488–502.
48. Hayreh SS. Central Retinal Vein Occlusion. St. Louis, MO: Mosby, 1980.
49. Hayreh SS. Classification of central retinal vein occlusion. Ophthalmology 1983; 90:458–74.
50. Hayreh SS. Classification of hypertensive fundus changes and their order of appearance. Ophthalmologica 1989; 198:247–60.
51. Herman IM, D'Amore PA. Microvascular pericytes contain muscle and nonmuscle actins. J Cell Biol 1985; 101:43–52.
52. Hill DW, Dollery CT. Calibre changes in retinal arterioles. Trans Ophthalmol Soc UK 1963; 83:61–70.
53. Jaffe EA. Cell biology of endothelial cells. Hum Pathol 1987; 18:234–9.
54. Jerneld B, Algvere P. Relationship of duration and onset of diabetes to prevalence of diabetic retinopathy. Am J Ophthalmol 1986; 102:431–7.
55. Kador PF, Akagi Y, Terubayashi H, et al. Prevention of pericyte ghost formation in retinal capillaries of galactose-fed dogs by aldose reductase inhibitors. Arch Ophthalmol 1988; 106:1099–102.
56. Kishi S, Tso MO, Hayreh SS. Fundus lesions in malignant hypertension. I. A pathologic study of experimental

hypertensive choroidopathy. Arch Ophthalmol 1985; 103: 1189–97.
57. Klien BA. Occlusion of the central retinal vein: clinical importance of certain histopathologic observations. Am J Ophthalmol 1953; 36:316–24.
58. Kohner EM, Dollery CT. The rate of formation and disappearance of microaneurysms in diabetic retinopathy. Trans Ophthalmol Soc UK 1970; 90:369–74.
59. Kohner EM, Shilling JS. Retinal vein occlusion. In: Medical Ophthalmology. London: Chapman & Hall, 1976.
60. Kohner EM. The natural history of proliferative diabetic retinopathy. Eye 1991; 5(Pt 2):222–5.
61. Kroll AJ. Experimental central retinal artery occlusion. Arch Ophthalmol 1968; 79:453–69.
62. Leishman R. The eye in general vascular disease: hypertension and arteriosclerosis. Br J Ophthalmol 1957; 41:641–701.
63. Lutty GA, Chan-Ling T, Phelps DL, et al. Proceedings of the Third International Symposium on Retinopathy of Prematurity: An Update on ROP From the Lab to the Nursery (November 2003, Anaheim, California). Mol Vis 2006; 12:532–80.
64. Lutty GA, Ikeda K, Chandler C, McLeod DS. Immunolocalization of tissue plasminogen activator in the diabetic and nondiabetic retina and choroid. Invest Ophthalmol Vis Sci 1991; 32:237–5.
65. Martinez-Hernandez A, Amenta PS. The basement membrane in pathology. Lab Invest 1983; 48:656–77.
66. McLeod D. Ophthalmoscopic signs of obstructed axoplasmic transport after ocular vascular occlusions. Br J Ophthalmol 1976; 60:551–6.
67. Metcalfe MA, Baum JD. Incidence of insulin dependent diabetes in children aged under 15 years in the British Isles during 1988. BMJ 1991; 302:443–7.
68. Michaelson IC. Retinal Circulation in Man and Animals. Springfield, 1954.
69. Minckler DS, Bunt AH. Axoplasmic transport in ocular hypotony and papilledema in the monkey. Arch Ophthalmol 1977; 95:1430–6.
70. Miyashita K, Tanahashi N, Akiya S. Red blood cell aggregability in diabetic retinopathy. Nippon Ganka Gakkai Zasshi 1988; 92:1166–70 [in Japanese].
71. Paton L. The pathology of papilloedema: a histological study of sixty eyes. Brain 1911; 33:389–432.
72. Patz A, Hoeck LE, De La Cruz E. Studies on the effect of high oxygen administration in retrolental fibroplasia. I. Nursery observations. Am J Ophthalmol 1952; 35: 1248–53.
73. Peters TJ, De Duve C. Lysosomes of the arterial wall. II. Subcellular fractionation of aortic cells from rabbits with experimental atheroma. Exp Mol Pathol 1974; 20:228–56.
74. Quinlan PM, Elman MJ, Bhatt AK, et al. The natural course of central retinal vein occlusion. Am J Ophthalmol 1990; 110:118–23.
75. Rahi A, Ashton N. Contractile proteins in retinal endothelium and other non-muscle tissues of the eye. Br J Ophthalmol 1978; 62:627–43.
76. Ramachandran E, Frank RN, Kennedy A. Effects of endothelin on cultured bovine retinal microvascular pericytes. Invest Ophthalmol Vis Sci 1993; 34:586–95.
77. Ramalho PS, Dollery CT. Hypertensive retinopathy. Caliber changes in retinal blood vessels following blood-pressure reduction and inhalation of oxygen. Circulation 1968; 37:580–8.
78. Reagan FR. Vascularisation phenomena on fragments of embryonic bodies completely isolated from yolk sac entoderm. Am J Anat 1915; 9:329–41.
79. Reese AB. Telangiectasis of the retina and Coats' disease. Am J Ophthalmol 1956; 42:1–8.
80. Renie WA, Murphy RP, Anderson KC, et al. The evaluation of patients with Eales' disease. Retina 1983; 3:243–8.
81. Repka MX, Tung B, Good WV, et al. Outcome of eyes developing retinal detachment during the early treatment for retinopathy of prematurity study (ETROP). Arch Ophthalmol 2006; 124:24–30.
82. Rhodin JÁ. The ultrastructure of mammalian arterioles and precapillary sphincters. J Ultrastruct Res 1967; 18:181–223.
83. Rosen DA, Marshall J, Kohner EM, et al. Experimental retinal vein occlusion in the rhesus monkey. Radioactive microsphere and radioautographic studies [proceedings]. Trans Ophthalmol Soc UK 1976; 96:198.
84. Silverman MD, Babra B, Pan Y, et al. Differential E-selectin expression by iris versus retina microvascular endothelial cells cultured from the same individuals. Microvasc Res 2005; 70:32–42.
85. Skovborg F, Nielsen AV, Lauritzen E, Hartkopp O. Diameters of the retinal vessels in diabetic and normal subjects. Diabetes 1969; 18:292–8.
86. Spaide RF, Fisher YL. Intravitreal bevacizumab (Avastin) treatment of proliferative diabetic retinopathy complicated by vitreous hemorrhage. Retina 2006; 26:275–8.
87. Stiebel-Kalish H, Setton A, Nimii Y, et al. Cavernous sinus dural arteriovenous malformations: patterns of venous drainage are related to clinical signs and symptoms. Ophthalmology 2002; 109:1685–91.
88. Szabo ME, Droy-Lefaix MT, Doly M, et al. Ischemia and reperfusion-induced histologic changes in the rat retina. Demonstration of a free radical-mediated mechanism. Invest Ophthalmol Vis Sci 1991; 32:1471–8.
89. Terry TL. Extreme prematurity and fibroblastic overgrowth of persistent vascular sheath behind each crystal line lens. I. Preliminary report. Am J Ophthalmol 1942; 25: 203–4.
90. Tripathi R, Ashton N. Electron microscopical study of Coat's disease. Br J Ophthalmol 1971; 55:289–301.
91. Trope GE, Lowe GD, McArdle BM, et al. Abnormal blood viscosity and haemostasis in long-standing retinal vein occlusion. Br J Ophthalmol 1983; 67:137–42.
92. Tso MO, Hayreh SS. Optic disc edema in raised intracranial pressure. IV. Axoplasmic transport in experimental papilledema. Arch Ophthalmol 1977; 95: 1458–62.
93. Tso MO. Pathological study of cystoid macular oedema. Trans Ophthalmol Soc UK 1980; 100:408–13.
94. Vinores SA, Gadegbeku C, Campochiaro PA, Green WR. Immunohistochemical localization of blood-retinal barrier breakdown in human diabetics. Am J Pathol 1989; 134:231–5.
95. von Hippel E. Über eine sehr seltene erkrankung der netzhaut: klinische beobaehtungen. Graefes Arch Ophthalmol 1904; 59:83–106.
96. Wallow IH, Engerman RL. Permeability and patency of retinal blood vessels in experimental diabetes. Invest Ophthalmol Vis Sci 1977; 16:447–61.
97. Ward RC, Weiner MJ, Albert DM. The eye. In: Pathology and Pathophysiology of AIDS and HIV-Related Diseases. London: Chapman & Hall, 1989.
98. Watanabe D, Suzuma K, Matsui S, et al. Erythropoietin as a retinal angiogenic factor in proliferative diabetic retinopathy. N Engl J Med 2005; 353:782–92.
99. Webb RC, Loekette WF, Vanhoutte PM, Bohr DH. Sodium Potassium Adenosine Triphosphate and Vasodilatation. New York: Raven Press, 1981.

100. Weinberg D, Dodwell DG, Fern SA. Anatomy of arteriovenous crossings in branch retinal vein occlusion. Am J Ophthalmol 1990; 109:298–302.
101. Wetzig PC, Thatcher DB. The treatment of acute and chronic central venous occlusion by light coagulation. Mod Prob Ophthalmol 1974; 12:247–53.
102. Whiter JR. Pathology of a cotton-wool spot. Am J Ophthalmol 1959; 48:473–85.
103. Yanagisawa M, Masaki T. Endothelin, a novel endothelium-derived peptide. Pharmacological activities, regulation and possible roles in cardiovascular control. Biochem Pharmacol 1989; 38:1877–83.

68

Angiogenesis

Ming Lu
Vantage Eye Center, Monterey, California, U.S.A.

Anthony P. Adamis
Eyetech Pharmaceuticals, New York, New York, U.S.A.

INTRODUCTION

Angiogenesis is the development of new capillaries from a pre-existing vascular network. The term "neovascularization" has been used to describe the development of new vessels in pathologic states and is considered synonymous with angiogenesis in this chapter. In adults, the vasculature is quiescent except during wound healing (108), hair growth (149), and the menstrual cycle (38). Otherwise, endothelial cells are almost dormant within the cell cycle, but they respond to angiogenic factors released by hypoxic issues by undergoing migration, proliferation and differentiation to form new capillaries, as in tumor growth and myocardial infarction (39).

Angiogenesis may occur in a variety of ocular disorders such as corneal alkali burn, retinopathy of prematurity (ROP), retinal artery or vein occlusion, diabetic retinopathy (see Chapter 67) and age-related macular degeneration (AMD) (see Chapter 18) (1,22,144). Angiogenic and angiostatic factors are pivotal in the pathogenesis of these diseases and the identification of these factors as well as their mechanisms of action has led to the development of drugs specifically targeting the molecules or their signal transduction pathways. An important angiogenic factor is vascular endothelial growth factor (VEGF) and it appears to be one of the major regulators in ocular neovascularization (38,98).

ANGIOGENESIS

Basic Process

Angiogenesis begins with the stimulation of the quiescent vascular endothelial cells and a focal increased vascular permeability (Fig. 1). The degradation of the surrounding matrix allows the activated and proliferating endothelial cells from the existing vasculature to migrate and form tubes (52). A phase of maturation and re-modeling of these new vessels ensues to form a vascular network. Endothelial cell

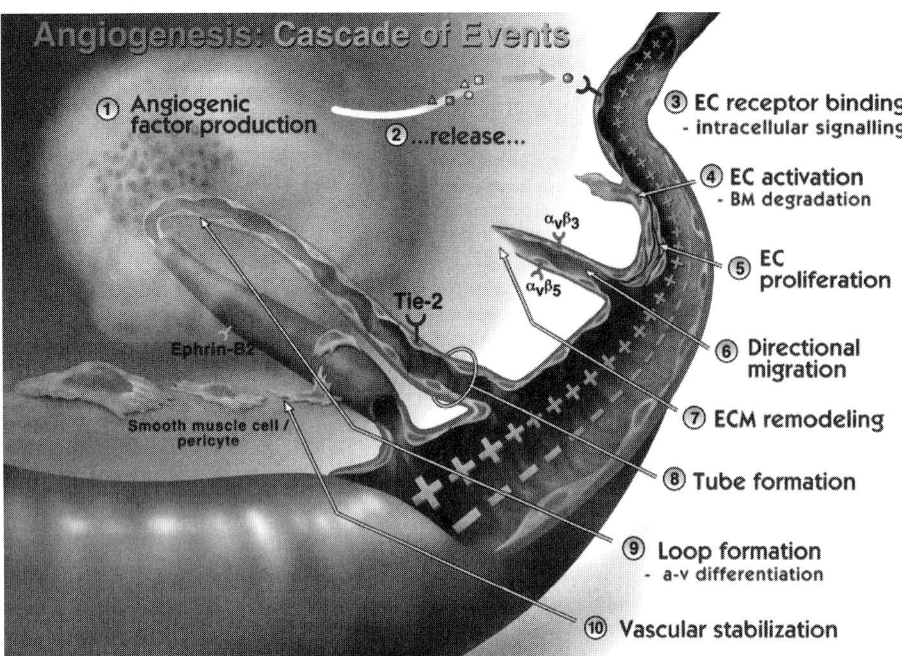

Figure 1 The process of angiogenesis occurs as an orderly series of events. *Abbreviations*: EC, endothelial cell; ECM, extracellular matrix. *Source*: Information provided by the Angiogenesis Foundation, Inc.

invasion and migration require co-operative activity of the urokinase-type plasminogen activator, matrix metalloproteinases (MMPs), and the cysteine proteinase systems (88). These enzymes are upregulated by cytokines and the angiogenic factors such as basic fibroblast growth factor (FGF) and VEGF. Endogenous inhibitors of proteolytic enzymes, such as plasminogen activator inhibitors and tissue inhibitors of metalloproteinases (TIMPs) are simultaneously down-regulated. Activated endothelial cells express integrins such as αvβ3 and αvβ5, assist their migration through the degraded matrix. Subsequently, endothelial cells proliferate, form new capillaries, and synthesize a new basal lamina. The recruitment of pericytes and smooth muscle cells, a process regulated by platelet-derived growth factor (PDGF) (56), helps stabilize the newly formed blood vessels (29).

The angiogenic cascade is coordinated by multiple angiogenic and angiostatic factors. When the new blood vessel formation is sufficient to cope with local demands for oxygen and nutrients, the levels of angiogenic factors decrease and/or the expression of factors that inhibit new vessel formation (angiogenic inhibitors/angiostatic factors) become prominent. Neovascularization is a response, not only to a rise in the local concentration of angiogenic molecules, but likely also to a concomitant fall in the levels of endogenous angiogenic inhibitors (18).

Angiogenic Factors

Angiogenic factors include VEGF, FGF2, angiopoietins, transforming growth factor alpha and beta (TGFα, TGFβ), hepatocyte growth factor (HGF), connective tissue growth factor (CTGF), and interleukin 8 (IL8). VEGF is a prime regulator of angiogenesis (38), stimulating endothelial cells to degrade their basement membrane and to migrate with concomitant release of MMPs and plasminogen activators. This stimulates endothelial cell expression of αvβ3 and αvβ5 integrins, endothelial cell proliferation, and vascular tube formation.

The VEGF family includes VEGF-A, VEGF-B, VEGF-C, VEGF-D, VEGF-E (85), and placenta growth factor (PGF) (38,144). VEGF-A plays a pivotal role in the development of angiogenesis in ischemic and inflammatory diseases. PGF acts synergistically with VEGF-A in angiogenesis and plasma extravasation in pathological conditions (27). VEGF-E is encoded by the parapoxvirus Orf virus. It is a potent angiogenic factor expressed in mammalian cells (85). The abbreviation VEGF in this chapter represents VEGF-A since it is widely accepted in the research field of angiogenesis.

VEGF is a 35–45 kDa homodimeric protein which was originally isolated as a vasopermeability factor (123) and later cloned and identified as an angiogenesis factor (37). The structure and function of VEGF and its gene regulation have been extensively reviewed (38,144). Six different isoforms of VEGF are derived through alternative splicing of mRNA (21,38). The smaller isoforms ($VEGF_{110}$, $VEGF_{121}$, $VEGF_{144}$, and $VEGF_{165}$) are secreted and freely diffusible, whereas the larger isoforms ($VEGF_{189}$ and $VEGF_{208}$) are bound to heparin-containing proteoglycans on the cell surface or basement membrane (59). $VEGF_{165}$ appears to be the main one responsible for pathological ocular neovascularization (61,81,150). In terms of permeability, VEGF is 50,000 times more potent at increasing dermal micro-vascular permeability than histamine (122). VEGF induces the expression of urokinase-type and tissue-type plasminogen activators, as well as metalloproteinase interstitial collagenase. This co-induction promotes degradation of the local extracellular matrix and facilitates vascular endothelial cell migration (11). VEGF is an endothelial cell-specific mitogen (112,128) and it is involved in normal vascular development, ovulation, and tumor angiogenesis (38). Hypoxia is a major regulator of VEGF expression (38), which distinguishes VEGF from other growth factors postulated to have a role in ocular neovascular diseases, including insulin-like growth factor 1 (IGF1), FGF, epidermal growth factor (EGF), PGF, and VEGF-B (24). VEGF expression is also up-regulated by EGF, TGFα and TGFβ, IGF1, FGF, and PGF (38). Many ocular cells produce VEGF, including retinal pigment epithelial cells (RPE), pericytes, vascular endothelial cells, glial cells, Müller cells, and ganglion cells (92). Among the identified angiogenic factors VEGF-A plays a central role in the development of ocular neovascularization.

VEGF preferentially binds to high affinity receptors on vascular endothelial cells (135) and three members of the VEGF receptor (VEGFR) family have been identified: VEGFR1, VEGFR2, and VEGFR3. VEGFR1 (fms-like tyrosine kinase-1, Flt-1) is predominantly expressed in inflammatory cells and is implicated in blood vessel survival (144). VEGFR2 (kinase insert domain-containing receptor or KDR) is considered to be the receptor that mediates functional VEGF signaling in vascular endothelial cells (32,89). VEGFR3 is implicated in the genesis of lymphatic vessels (66).

VEGF receptors appear to be tyrosine kinases capable of phosphorylating other proteins involved in cellular signal transduction (145). One mechanism through which VEGF increases vascular permeability is via fenestrae induction (117,118). An intravitreal injection of VEGF promotes capillary non-perfusion and vascular permeability through the adhesion of leukocytes to endothelium, which is mediated by up-regulation of intercellular adhesion molecule-1 (ICAM-1) (72,94). Murine $VEGF_{164}$ ($VEGF_{165}$ in humans) has been identified as a pathological isoform due to its preferential up-regulation in pathological conditions (141). It was found that $VEGF_{164}$ induces retinal vascular leukostasis through increased expression of ICAM-1 (61,72,141). VEGF is a chemoattractant for endothelial cell precursors, inducing their mobilization and promoting their differentiation (14). Nitric oxide is a mediator of VEGF-induced endothelial cell proliferation (109). VEGF acts as an endothelial survival factor by inhibiting apoptosis (7).

The attractiveness of VEGF as a therapeutic target derives from its roles in two of the most basic processes within the typical lesions of advanced diabetic retinopathy, ROP, retinal vascular occlusions and AMD, namely neovascularization and vascular leakage. The role of VEGF as a critical factor in the control of the growth of abnormal blood vessels from the retina and choroid directly addresses a central problem in these ocular diseases.

Angiostatic Factors

Known angiostatic factors include thrombospondin, angiostatin, endostatin, pigment epithelium-derived factor (PEDF), and soluble VEGFR1 (9,26,39). Numerous inhibitors of angiogenesis counteract the effects of VEGF. PEDF is one such putative inhibitor found in the normal eye and suspected of being responsible for the avascularity of cornea and vitreous (31). PEDF is increased by hyperoxia and decreased by hypoxia (31), unlike other angiostatic factors, such as angiostatin (105) and endostatin (104). PEDF expression causes ocular neovascularization to regress by promoting apoptosis of cells within neovascular lesions (33,95). PEDF expression is decreased within choroidal neovascular tissues, whereas the VEGF level is increased (100,102). PEDF expression is inversely correlated with the formation of choroidal neovascularization (CNV) in an experimental animal model (116). An intraocular injection of adenoviral vectors expressing PEDF decreases CNV in a mouse model (96) and a phase 1 study of gene therapy with an adenovirus vector containing the PEDF gene has been completed for advanced CNV in patients with AMD (23). However, the role of PEDF in CNV remains controversial since PEDF levels are elevated in CNV-derived RPE (80) and proliferative diabetic retinopathy (33).

Recently, soluble VEGFR1 has been shown to be essential for the maintenance of corneal avascularity, despite the presence of VEGF in this tissue. Experimental suppression of soluble VEGFR1, whether by neutralizing antibodies, RNA interference, or conditional gene ablation, can abolish corneal avascularity in mice (9). Moreover, immunohistochemical and Western blot measurements in human corneas have demonstrated the presence of high levels of soluble VEGFR1, together with its sequestration of VEGF; neovascularized corneas, by contrast, show significantly reduced levels of soluble VEGFR1, as well as reduced binding of VEGF (10).

Additional angiogenesis modulators have been discovered during the past decade. Regulators of vascular integrity known as angiopoietins, regulators of vascular integrity, are involved in pathologic neovascularization (147). Angiopoietin-1 (ANG1) protects established vasculature against plasma leakage (136). Angiopoietin-2 (ANG2) enhances the VEGF effect in ischemia-induced angiogenesis. Both hypoxia and VEGF up-regulate the expression of ANG2 but not ANG1 in vascular endothelial cells (101). The angiopoietins owe their opposite effect to respective agonist and antagonist signaling actions through the endothelial Tie2 receptor. Vessels in ANG1-overexpressing mice are resistant to leaks caused by inflammatory agents. Co-expression of ANG1 and VEGF has an additive effect on angiogenesis but results in leakage-resistant vessels typical of ANG1 (136). Therefore, ANG1 may be useful for reducing micro-vascular leakage and, in combination with VEGF, for promoting growth of non-leaky vessels. Angiopoietins also play a role in CNV formation. Immunohistochemical examination of CNV in AMD and other diseases disclosed that ANG1 and ANG2 were present (106). The Tie2 receptor is expressed in vascular structures, RPE and in fibroblast-like cells. VEGF up-regulates ANG1 synthesis and secretion by RPE (53). Systemically expressed soluble Tie2 receptor via adenoviral-mediated gene delivery markedly inhibits the development of laser-induced CNV in mice (54). ANG1 may have a potential therapeutic use as it suppresses VEGF-induced leukostasis and inflammation by inhibiting expression of ICAM-1, vascular cell adhesion molecule-1, and E-selectin (63).

The extracellular matrix (ECM) is a repository for a variety of angiogenic factors and vascular endothelial cells interact with the ECM for migration through integrin receptors (51). The ECM degrading enzymes, such as matrix metalloproteinases and their inhibitors, TIMPs, play a role in the penetration of blood vessels into the ECM. Promising strategies have been developed to inhibit CNV by suppressing integrin function (51,62,73) or by overexpression of TIMP3 (134).

Physiological Angiogenesis

The critical role of VEGF in developmental angiogenesis and vasculogenesis is demonstrated by the fact that deletion of the VEGF gene, or its receptor, results in abnormal blood vessel development and death in utero (25,34,40,124,144). Experimental manipulation of VEGF levels in transgenic mice have demonstrated that VEGF levels need to be closely regulated. Not only does knockout of a single VEGF allele lead to embryonic lethality (25,35), but modest over-expression is also lethal (93).

VEGF expression can be detected in giant cells of the trophoblast within a few days following implantation (19). In the human fetus at 16–22 wks after gestation, VEGF mRNA is detectable in virtually all tissues (126). Gene-targeting studies have demonstrated that all three VEGFRs are essential for the normal development of embryonic vasculature as well (38). In the human adult, VEGF is involved in physiological angiogenesis, such as the female reproductive system (36).

The retinal vasculature develops by both vasculogenesis and angiogenesis (114). A primordial vasculature originates at the optic nerve head and spreads over the inner surface of the retina (vasculogenesis). Subsequently, blood vessels sprout by means of angiogenesis from these primordial vessels into the retina, forming the deep vasculature of the inner retina (60). VEGF and its receptors are expressed in the normal retina (64,143). VEGF regulates endothelial cell survival via anti-apoptotic signaling, suggesting a function to maintain endothelial cell integrity (45,46).

Angiogenesis in Ocular Diseases

Aside from VEGF, FGF2 has been implicated in the pathogenesis of ocular neovascularization. This growth factor is present within the RPE in surgically removed CNV membranes (12,41) and FGF2 mRNA is up-regulated in RPE, choroidal vascular endothelial cells, and fibroblasts in laser-induced CNV in rats (99,150). Sustained release of *Fgf2* by subretinal pellets induces CNV in pigs (131) and rabbits (65). However, a targeted disruption of the FGF2 gene does not inhibit the development of laser-induced CNV in mice, suggesting that it is not essential for the development of CNV (138). A retinal over-expression of FGF2 may be angiogenic only in the setting of cellular injury that unmasks intracellular FGF2 (146). Adenovirus expressed $VEGF_{165}$ can cause CNV in mouse models (30). Furthermore, *in vitro* inhibition experiments have identified VEGF as the sole endothelial cell mitogen synthesized and secreted by hypoxic retinal cells (6,127). Moreover VEGF can promote CNV by stimulating endothelial cell expression of metalloproteinases, which degrade the ECM and facilitate tissue invasion by new blood vessels. This is co-ordinated by a down-regulation of endothelial expression of TIMPs (69).

Retina and Iris Neovascularization

VEGF levels correlate both spatially and temporally with iris neovascularization in a monkey model (90). This study demonstrated that VEGF expression was increased in the retina prior to the development of neovascularization. In addition, the VEGF levels declined as the neovascularization regressed. An injection of VEGF alone into normal primate eyes is sufficient to produce retinal edema, hemorrhage, venous beading, capillary occlusion with ischemia, microaneurysms and retinal, and iris neovascularization and neovascular glaucoma, characteristic findings of all stages of diabetic retinopathy (139,140). Moreover, the inhibition of intraocular VEGF suppresses retinal ischemia-associated iris (3) and retinal neovascularization (6). Blockade of VEGF receptor signaling is sufficient to completely prevent retinal neovascularization (107). Therefore, VEGF appears to be the mediator of ischemia-induced ocular angiogenesis in iris and retina (98).

In the human eye, elevated vitreous and aqueous humor VEGF levels strongly correlate with retinal ischemia-associated neovascularization in diabetic retinopathy, retinal vein occlusion, and ROP (2,4,77,110). The vitreous concentrations of VEGF are higher than aqueous humor levels, suggesting the existence of an intraocular VEGF concentration gradient between the vitreous and aqueous humor. After successful laser panretinal photo-coagulation for retinal neovascularization, the intraocular concentration of VEGF is reduced after therapy by an average of 75% (4). Furthermore, the VEGF present in the vitreous of individuals with active intraocular neovascularization is capable of binding VEGF receptors, as well as stimulating retinal endothelial cell growth in vitro (4). VEGF is consistently expressed in neovascular membranes obtained from diabetic patients (77). High VEGF mRNA levels are detected in the retina of enucleated eyes from patients with retinal neovascularization secondary to diabetes mellitus, central retinal vein occlusion, retinal detachment, and intraocular tumors (110). These data demonstrate a close correlation of elevated intraocular VEGF concentration with active intraocular neovascularization in humans.

Diabetic Retinopathy

Diabetic retinopathy can be classified into non-proliferative and proliferative stages (5) both characterized by multiple progressive micro-vascular changes. Diabetic retinopathy is discussed in detail in Chapter 67. The hallmark of the proliferative stage is neovascularization. Increased VEGF expression has also been demonstrated in the retinal and choroidal blood vessels of subjects with diabetes using immunohistochemical studies of post-mortem tissue (74). Theories to explain the pathological findings of the three stages of diabetic retinopathy, include non-enzymatic glycosylation (20), sorbitol accumulation (42), and activation of protein kinase C (78,125). There are also a number of hemodynamic theories for the pathogenesis of diabetic retinopathy, including retinal leukostasis (82), blood viscosity (83) and erythrocyte deformability (91). The retinal leukostasis theory states that endothelial cell death and retinal vessel leakage are secondary to adherence of activated leukocytes. It has also been postulated that platelet abnormalities in diabetics may contribute to diabetic retinopathy by causing focal capillary occlusion and focal areas of ischemia in the retina (83). The hemodynamic theories can potentially explain the leakage and ischemia seen at the non-proliferative stage of diabetic retinopathy. The endocrine theory states that growth hormone and IGF1 are involved in the pathogenesis of diabetic retinopathy (84). IGF1 is also called somatomedin because it mediates the effect of growth hormone. At least three pieces of evidence suggest that IGF1 is involved in the pathogenesis of diabetic retinopathy. The first is that ablation of the pituitary gland has been associated with regression of retinal neovascularization (113). Secondly, the incidence and severity of diabetic retinopathy in growth hormone-deficient dwarfs are much lower than in other diabetic patients (8). Moreover, the concentration of IGF1 in the vitreous correlates positively with serum concentrations in patients with diabetes but not in normal subjects (47,86). Thus, leakage is probably the primary source of this factor, although local production cannot be ruled out. Since IGF1 is mitogenic to endothelial cells, the endocrine theory seems the best to explain the final neovascular stage of diabetic retinopathy.

It is evident that none of the above theories alone is adequate to explain the development and progression of diabetic retinopathy. Conceivably, the pathogenesis of diabetic retinopathy is best understood by integrating these categories, with particular emphasis on their temporal sequence. A hypothesis involving VEGF as a fundamental element in combination with the above theories is preferable to any of the theories in isolation (70). At the mild non-proliferative stage of diabetic retinopathy, the increase in VEGF by hyperglycemia (13,130,137) and advanced glycation end-products (AGEs) may cause the leakage of the retinal vasculature (97). At the severe non-proliferative stage, VEGF induces retinal ischemia by enhancing endothelial cell ICAM-1 expression and neutrophil adhesion (72,94). Ischemia further increases VEGF gene expression (38). Thus there is a positive feedback loop that increases VEGF production in an accelerated manner. The positive feedback loop of VEGF and ischemia contributes to the accelerated accumulation of VEGF seen at the advanced stages of diabetic retinopathy. The marked increase of VEGF by hyperglycemia, AGEs and ischemia, makes the retina–blood barrier leaky enough to allow a sufficient amount of IGF1 to enter the vitreous from the systemic circulation, further stimulating VEGF gene expression (115). Once the VEGF concentration in the retina and vitreous exceeds the threshold of angiogenesis, new vessels grow, and the proliferative stage ensues.

Proliferative diabetic retinopathy is primarily an ischemic disease, since neovascularization of the retina, optic nerve and iris is preceded temporally and associated spatially by retinal capillary nonperfusion (15,87). Ablation of ischemic retinas by laser photo-coagulation, which has been the mainstay of treatment for diabetic retinopathy in the past 30 yrs, leads to stabilization and regression of neovascularization (4). These observations support the hypothesis that an angiogenic factor released from the ischemic retina stimulates angiogenesis both locally and at a distance (92). The responsible factor must meet at least three criteria: mitogenic for endothelial cells, secreted and freely diffusible, and induced by ischemia (15,87). To date only VEGF fits all three criteria.

Age-Related Macular Degeneration

As mentioned in Chapter 18 where AMD is considered in detail, AMD patients with larger and more extensive drusen and pigmentary abnormalities have a relatively higher chance of developing neovascular AMD, with the development of choroidal new vessels that break through the Bruch membrane into the subretinal pigment epithelial space and/or into the sub-retinal space, frequently affecting the fovea and producing substantial visual loss. CNV is a major cause of visual loss in AMD. One of the earliest signs of CNV often is sub-retinal or sub-RPE hemorrhage. Appearing as a greenish gray sub-retinal lesion, CNV leaks fluorescein on angiography. However, sub-retinal blood or lipid exudates, also signs of CNV, may block the angiographic hyperfluorescence. CNV may not exhibit fluorescein leakage if it has undergone involution or is enveloped by RPE proliferation. Repeated leakage of blood, serum, and lipid can stimulate fibroglial organization leading to a cicatricial (disciform) scar. The histopathologic features of surgically excised CNV in patients with AMD indicates the presence of RPE, vascular endothelium, fibrocytes, macrophages, photoreceptors and the extracellular components including collagen, fibrin, basal laminar deposit, and fragments of the Bruch membrane (50).

Retinal angiomatous proliferation (RAP) has been recognized as a unique form of neovascular AMD (148). RAP refers to new vessel development extending outward from the neurosensory retina, sometimes anastomosing with the choroidal circulation. Typically, RAP commences as intraretinal capillary proliferation, later extending into the sub-retinal space, and finally terminates with frank CNV.

Choroidal Neovascularization

Any condition that produces a disruption or break in Bruch membrane may predispose the eye to CNV, such as myopic degeneration, ocular histoplasmosis, angioid streaks, punctate inner choroidopathy, and choroidal rupture due to trauma (44). CNV may be initiated by reduction in blood flow, accumulation of metabolic byproducts, oxidative stress, and alterations in Bruch membrane (11,48). In response to a metabolic and/or hypoxic stress, the RPE and the retina produce factors which lead to vascular endothelial cell proliferation and migration.

The prognosis for patients with CNV without intervention is disappointing (75,76). Although the Macular Photocoagulation Study Group found thermal laser photo-coagulation for extra-foveal and juxta-foveal CNV beneficial, as well as a select group of sub-foveal CNV, the majority (87%) of patients with newly diagnosed exudative AMD do not meet Macular Photo-coagulation Study criteria for laser photo-coagulation (43). A two-component model for CNV has been proposed (132). The vascular component of CNV is comprised of vascular endothelial cells, endothelial cell precursors, and pericytes. The extra-vascular component is comprised of inflammatory, glial and RPE cells, and fibroblasts. VEGF plays an important role in the vascular component of CNV (11,22,98,144). VEGF is over-expressed in the RPE of autopsy eyes with AMD and in trans-differentiated RPE cells of surgically excised CNV membranes (41,49). Vitreous VEGF levels are significantly higher in patients with AMD and CNV as compared to healthy controls (57,142). Intravitreous injections of VEGF induce proliferation of choroidal endothelial cells in non-human primates (139). RPE secretion of VEGF is polarized with higher basal secretion towards the Bruch membrane than apical secretion towards photoreceptors (17). VEGF receptors are preferentially localized to the inner choriocapillaris endothelium. The increased thickness and hydrophobicity of Bruch membrane with lipophilic material may decrease the diffusion of oxygen from the choroid to retina (58). Hypoxia is a potent stimulus of VEGF expression. Other factors implicated in AMD, such as advanced glycation endproducts and reactive-oxygen intermediates, are potent stimuli of VEGF expression in RPE cells (67,71). Transgenic mice and other animal models over-expressing VEGF in RPE cells lead to CNV formation (16,121,133). These findings suggest an important role for VEGF in the pathogenesis of AMD-related CNV and make VEGF a suitable target for anti-angiogenic therapy in AMD patients. Macrophages secrete VEGF and in an animal model, macrophage depletion inhibits CNV (120).

Retinopathy of Prematurity

ROP, which is a cause of blindness in children (129), begins with delayed retinal vascular growth after premature birth (see Chapter 67). The avascular retina-associated hypoxia releases VEGF to stimulate new blood vessel growth. Both oxygen-regulated and non-oxygen-regulated factors contribute to normal vascular development and retinal neovascularization (111,119). VEGF is the oxygen-regulated factor as discussed earlier. VEGF level is increased in ROP retina and decreased after laser treatment (151). A critical non-oxygen-regulated growth factor is IGF1. Lack of IGF1 prevents normal retinal vascular growth and impairs vascular endothelial cell survival (55). Premature infants who develop ROP have low levels of serum IGF1 compared to age-matched infants without disease. Low IGF1 predicts ROP in premature infants. See Chapter 67 for further remarks on ROP.

Corneal Neovascularization

Invasion of new blood vessels into the normally avascular cornea, also called corneal neovascularization, is a sight-threatening condition usually associated with inflammatory or infectious disorders of the ocular surface (28). Epithelial trauma and/or hypoxia may stimulate the production of angiogenic factors by local epithelial cells, keratocytes, and infiltrating leukocytes (macrophages, neutrophils). Some of these factors [i.e., acidic and basic FGF, interleukin 1 (IL1), and VEGF] have been identified and isolated from cornea and tears. Angiogenic factors stimulate a localized enzymatic degradation of the basement membrane of perilimbal vessels at the apex of a vascular loop. Activated vascular endothelial cells migrate and proliferate to form new blood vessels. A balance exists between angiogenic factors (such as FGF2 and VEGF) and angiostatic molecules (such as angiostatin, endostatin, or PEDF) in the cornea. Basic FGF is normally sequestered within Descemet membrane and may be mobilized by injury. Inflammatory cells, such as macrophages and monocytes, also contain VEGF and corneal inflammation is a common stimulus for neovascularization. Corneal neovascularization also occurs in infectious (as in viral and bacterial keratitis), immune (such as rejection of corneal transplant), and degenerative corneal diseases. Angiostatic steroids, nonsteroidal inflammatory agents, and VEGF antagonists have been effective in animal models to inhibit corneal neovascularization (68,79,103).

REFERENCES

1. Adamis AP, Aiello LP, D'Amato RA. Angiogenesis and ophthalmic disease. Angiogenesis 1999 3:9–14.
2. Adamis AP, Miller J, Bernal M et al. Increased vascular endothelial growth factor levels in the vitreous of eyes with proliferative diabetic retinopathy. Am J Ophthalmol 1994 118:445–50.
3. Adamis AP, Shima DT, Tolentino M et al. Inhibition of vascular endothelial growth factor prevents retinal ischemia-associated iris neovascularization in a nonhuman primate. Arch Ophthalmol 1996 114:66–71.
4. Aiello LP, Avery RL, Arrigg PG et al. Vascular endothelial growth factor in ocular fluid of patients with diabetic retinopathy and other retinal disorders. N Eng J Med 1994 331:1480–7.
5. Aiello LP, Gardner TW, King GL et al. Diabetic retinopathy. Diabetes Care 1998 21:143–56.
6. Aiello LP, Pierce EA, Foley ED et al. Suppression of retinal neovascularization in vivo by inhibition of vascular endothelial growth factor (VEGF) using soluble VEGF-receptor chimeric proteins. Proc Natl Acad Sci USA 1995 92:10457–61.
7. Alon T, Hemo I, Itin A et al. Vascular endothelial growth factor as a survival factor for newly formed retinal vessels and has implications for retinopathy of prematurity. Nature Med 1995 1:1024–8.
8. Alzaid AA, Dinneen SF, Melton LJ 3rd, Rizza RA. The role of growth hormone in the development of diabetic retinopathy. Diabetes Care 1994 17:531–4.
9. Ambati BK, Nozaki M, Singh N et al. Corneal avascularity is due to soluble VEGF receptor-1. Nature 2006 443: 993–7.
10. Ambati BK, Patterson E, Jani P, et al. Soluble vascular endothelial growth factor receptor-1 contributes to the corneal anti-angiogenic barrier. Br J Ophthalmol 2006; [Epub ahead of print].
11. Ambati J, Ambati BK, Yoo SH et al. Age-related macular degeneration: etiology, pathogenesis, and therapeutic strategies. Surv Ophthalmol 2003 48:257–93.
12. Amin R, Puklin JE, Frank RN. Growth factor localization in choroidal neovascular membranes of age-related macular degeneration. Invest Ophthalmol Vis Sci 1994 35:3178–88.
13. Amin RH, Frank RN, Kennedy A et al. Vascular endothelial growth factor is present in glial cells of the retina and optic nerve of human subjects with nonproliferative diabetic retinopathy. Invest Ophthalmol Vis Sci 1997 38:36–47.
14. Asahara T, Takahashi T, Masuda H et al. VEGF contributes to postnatal neovascularization by mobilizing bone marrow-derived endothelial progenitor cells. EMBO J 1999 18:3964–72.
15. Ashton N. Neovascularization in ocular disease. Trans Ophthalmol Soc (UK) 1961 81:145–61.
16. Baffi J, Byrnes G, Chan CC, Csaky KG. Choroidal neovascularization in the rat induced by adenovirus mediated expression of vascular endothelial growth factor. Invest Ophthalmol Vis Sci 2000 41:3582–9.
17. Blaauwgeers HG, Holtkamp GM, Rutten H et al. Polarized vascular endothelial growth factor secretion by human retinal pigment epithelium and localization of vascular endothelial growth factor receptors on the inner choriocapillaris. Evidence for a trophic paracrine relation. Am J Pathol 1999 155:421–8.
18. Bouck N. PEDF: anti-angiogenic guardian of ocular function. Trends Mol Med 2002 8:330–4.
19. Breier G, Albrecht U, Sterrer S, Risau W. Expression of vascular endothelial growth factor during embryonic angiogenesis and endothelial cell differentiation. Development 1992 114:521–32.
20. Brownlee M. Glycation and diabetic complications. Diabetes 1994 43:836–41.
21. Burchardt M, Burchardt T, Chen MW et al. Expression of messenger ribonucleic acid splice variants for vascular endothelial growth factor in the penis of adult rats and humans. Biol Reprod 1999 60:398–404.
22. Campochiaro PA, Hackett SF. Ocular neovascularization: a valuable model system. Oncogene 2003 22:6537–48.
23. Campochiaro PA, Nguyen QD, Shah SM et al. Adenoviral vector-delivered pigment epithelium-derived factor for neovascular age-related macular degeneration: results of a phase I clinical trial. Hum Gene Ther 2006 17:167–76.

24. Cao Y, Linden P, Shima D et al. in vivo angiogenic activity and hypoxia induction of heterodimers of placenta growth factor/vascular endothelial growth factor. J Clin Invest 1996 98:2507–11.
25. Carmeliet P, Ferreira V, Breir G et al. Abnormal blood vessel development and lethality in embryos lacking a single VEGF allele. Nature 1996 380:435–9.
26. Carmeliet P, Jain RK. Angiogenesis in cancer and other diseases. Nature 2000 407:249–57.
27. Carmeliet P, Moons L, Luttun A et al. Synergism between vascular endothelial growth factor and placental growth factor contributes to angiogenesis and plasma extravasation in pathological conditions. Nat Med 2001 7:575–83.
28. Chang JH, Gabison EE, Kato T, Azar DT. Corneal neovascularization. Curr Opin Ophthalmol 2001 12:242–9.
29. Crocker DJ, Murad TM, Geer JC. Role of the pericyte in wound healing. An ultrastructural study. Exp Mol Pathol 1970 13:51–65.
30. Csaky KG, Baffi JZ, Byrnes GA et al. Recruitment of marrow-derived endothelial cells to experimental choroidal neovascularization by local expression of vascular endothelial growth factor. Exp Eye Res 2004 78:1107–16.
31. Dawson DW, Volpert OV, Gillis P et al. Pigment epithelium-derived factor: a potent inhibitor of angiogenesis. Science 1999 285:245–8.
32. de Vries C, Escobedo JA, Ueno H et al. The fms-like tyrosine kinase, a receptor for vascular endothelial growth factor. Science 1992 255:989–91.
33. Duh EJ, Yang HS, Haller JA et al. Vitreous levels of pigment epithelium-derived factor and vascular endothelial growth factor: implications for ocular angiogenesis. Am J Ophthalmol 2004 137:668–74.
34. Dumont DJ, Jussila L, Taipale J et al. Cardiovascular failure in mouse embryos deficient in VEGF receptor-3. Science 1998 282:946–9.
35. Ferrara N, Carver-Moore K, Chen H, et al. Heterozygous embryonic lethality induced by targeted inactivation of the VEGF gene. Nature 1996 380:439–42.
36. Ferrara N, Chen H, Davis-Smyth T et al. Vascular endothelial growth factor is essential for corpus luteum angiogenesis. Nat Med 1998 4:336–40.
37. Ferrara N, Leung DW, Cachianes G et al. Purification and cloning of vascular endothelial growth factor secreted by pituitary folliculostellate cells. Methods Enzymol 1991 198:391–405.
38. Ferrara N. Vascular endothelial growth factor: basic science and clinical progress. Endocr Rev 2004 25: 581–611.
39. Folkman J. Angiogenesis and angiogenesis inhibition: an overview. EXS 1997 79:1–8.
40. Fong G-H, Rossant J, Gertssenstein M, Breitman ML. Role of the Flt-1 receptor tyrosine kinase in regulating the assembly of vascular endothelium. Nature 1995 376: 66–70.
41. Frank RN, Amin RH, Eliott D et al. Basic fibroblast growth factor and vascular endothelial growth factor are present in epiretinal and choroidal neovascular membranes. Am J Ophthalmol 1996 122:393–403.
42. Frank RN. The aldose reductase controversy. Diabetes 1994 43:169–72.
43. Freund KB, Yannuzzi LA, Sorenson JA. Age-related macular degeneration and choroidal neovascularization. Am J Ophthalmol 1993 115:786–91.
44. Gass JDM. Stereoscopic Atlas of Macular Diseases: diagnosis and Treatment. Vol. 2. St. Louis, MO: C.V. Mosby Company, 1997.
45. Gerber HP, Dixit V, Ferrara N. Vascular endothelial growth factor induces expression of the antiapoptotic proteins Bcl-2 and A1 in vascular endothelial cells. J Biol Chem 1998 273:13313–6.
46. Gerber HP, McMurtrey A, Kowalski J et al. Vascular endothelial growth factor regulates endothelial cell survival through the phosphatidylinositol 3′-kinase/Akt signal transduction pathway. Requirement for Flk-1/KDR activation. J Biol Chem 1998 273:30336–43.
47. Grant M, Russel B, Fitzgerald C, Merimee TJ. Insulin-like growth factors in vitreous:studies in control and diabetic subjects with neovascularization. Diabetes 1986 35: 416–20.
48. Green WR. Histopathology of age-related macular degeneration. Mol Vis 1999 5:27–36.
49. Grossniklaus HE, Ling JX, Wallace TM et al. Macrophage and retinal pigment epithelium expression of angiogenic cytokines in choroidal neovascularization. Mol Vis 2002 8:119–26.
50. Grossniklaus HE, Martinez JA, Brown VB et al. Immunohistochemical and histochemical properties of surgically excised subretinal neovascular membranes in age-related macular degeneration. Am J Ophthalmol 1992 114:464–72.
51. Hammes HP, Brownlee M, Jonczyk A et al. Subcutaneous injection of a cyclic peptide antagonist of vitronectin receptor-type integrins inhibits retinal neovascularization. Nat Med 1996; 2:529–33.
52. Hanahan D, Folkman J. Patterns and emerging mechanisms of the angiogenic switch during tumorigenesis. Cell 1996 86:353–64.
53. Hangai M, Moon YS, Kitaya N et al. Systemically expressed soluble Tie2 inhibits intraocular neovascularization. Hum Gene Ther 2001 12:1311–21.
54. Hangai M, Murata T, Miyawaki N et al. Angiopoietin-1 upregulation by vascular endothelial growth factor in human retinal pigment epithelial cells. Invest Ophthalmol Vis Sci 2001 42:1617–25.
55. Hellstrom A, Perruzzi C, Ju M, et al. Low IGFI suppresses VEGF-survival signaling in retinal endothelial cells: direct correlation with clinical retinopathy of prematurity. Proc Natl Acad Sci USA 2001 98:5804–8.
56. Hellstrom MH, Gerhardt H, Kalen M et al. Lack of pericytes leads to endothelial hyperplasia and abnormal vascular morphogenesis. J Cell Biol 2001 153:543–53.
57. Holekamp NM, Bouck N, Volpert O. Pigment epithelium-derived factor is deficient in the vitreous of patients with choroidal neovascularization due to age-related macular degeneration. Am J Ophthalmol 2002 22134:220–7.
58. Holz FG, Sheraidah G, Pauleikhoff D, Bird AC. Analysis of lipid deposits extracted from human macular and peripheral Bruch's membrane. Arch Ophthalmol 1994 112:402–6.
59. Houck KA, Leung DW, Rowland AM et al. Dual regulation of vascular endothelial growth factor bioavailability by genetic and proteolytic mechanisms. J Biol Chem 1992 267:26031–7.
60. Hughes S, Yang H, Chan-Ling T. Vascularization of the human fetal retina: roles of vasculogenesis and angiogenesis. Invest Ophthalmol Vis Sci 2000 41:1217–28.
61. Ishida S, Usui T, Yamashiro K et al. VEGF164-mediated inflammation is required for pathological, but not physiological, ischemia-induced retinal neovascularization. J Exp Med 2003 198:483–9.
62. Kamizuru H, Kimura H, Yasukawa T et al. Monoclonal antibody-mediated drug targeting to choroidal neovascularization in the rat. Invest Ophthalmol Vis Sci 2001 42: 2664–72.

63. Kim I, Moon SO, Park SK et al. Angiopoietin-1 reduces VEGF-stimulated leukocyte adhesion to endothelial cells by reducing ICAM-1, VCAM-1, and E-selectin expression. Circ Res 2001 89:477–9.
64. Kim I, Ryan AM, Rohan R et al. Constitutive expression of VEGF, VEGFR1, and VEGFR2 in normal eyes. Invest Ophthalmol Vis Sci 1999 40:2115–21. Erratum in: Invest Ophthalmol Vis Sci 2000 41:368.
65. Kimura H, Sakamoto T, Hinton DR et al. A new model of subretinal neovascularization in the rabbit. Invest Ophthalmol Vis Sci 1995 36:2110–9.
66. Kukk E, Lymboussaki AS, Taira S et al. VEGF-C receptor binding and pattern of expression with VEGFR3 suggests a role in lymphatic vascular development. Development 1996 122:3829–37.
67. Kuroki M, Voest EE, Amano S et al. Reactive oxygen intermediates increase vascular endothelial growth factor expression in vitro and in vivo. J Clin Invest 1996 98: 495–504.
68. Kvanta A. Ocular angiogenesis: the role of growth factors. Acta Ophthalmol Scand 2006 84:282–8.
69. Lamoreaux WJ, Fitzgerald ME, Reiner A, et al. Vascular endothelial growth factor increases release of gelatinase A and decreases release of tissue inhibitor of metalloproteinases by microvascular endothelial cells in vitro. Microvasc Res 1988 55:29–42.
70. Lu M, Adamis AP. Vascular endothelial growth factor gene regulation and action in diabetic retinopathy. Ophthalmol Clin North Am 2002 15:69–79.
71. Lu M, Kuroki M, Amano S et al. Advanced glycation end products increase retinal vascular endothelial growth factor expression. J Clin Invest 1998 101:1219–24.
72. Lu M, Perez VL, Ma N et al. VEGF increases retinal vascular ICAM-1 expression in vivo. Invest Ophthalmol Vis Sci 1999 40:1808–12.
73. Luna J, Tobe T, Mousa, SA et al. Antagonists of integrin αvβ3 inhibit retinal neovascularization in a murine model. Lab Invest 1996 75:563–73.
74. Lutty GA, McLeod S, Merges C et al. Localization of VEGF in human retina and choroid. Arch Ophthalmol 1996 114:971–7.
75. Macular Photocoagulation Study Group. Laser photocoagulation for juxtafoveal choroidal neovascularization. Five-year results from randomized clinical trials. Arch Ophthalmol 1994 112:500–9.
76. Macular Photocoagulation Study Group. Visual outcome after laser photocoagulation for subfoveal choroidal neovascularization secondary to age-related macular degeneration. The influence of initial lesion size and initial visual acuity. Arch Ophthalmol 1994 112:480–8.
77. Malecaze, F, Clamens S, Simorre-Pinatel V et al. Detection of vascular endothelial growth factor messenger RNA and vascular endothelial growth factor-like activity in proliferative diabetic retinopathy. Arch. Ophthalmol 1994 112:1476–82.
78. Mandarino LJ. Current hypotheses for the biochemical basis of diabetic retinopathy. Diabetes Care 1992 15: 1892–901.
79. Manzano R, Peyman G, Khan P et al. Inhibition of experimental corneal neovascularization by Bevacizumab (Avastin). Br J Ophthalmol 2006; 91: 804–7.
80. Martin G, Schlunck G, Hansen LL, Agostini HT. Differential expression of angioregulatory factors in normal and CNV-derived human retinal pigment epithelium. Graefes Arch Clin Exp Ophthalmol 2004 242:321–6.
81. McColm JR, Geisen P, Hartnett ME. VEGF isoforms and their expression after a single episode of hypoxia or repeated fluctuations between hyperoxia and hypoxia: relevance to clinical ROP. Mol Vis 2004; 21(10):512–20.
82. McLeod DS, Lefer DJ, Merges C, Lutty GA. Enhanced expression of intracellular adhesion molecule-1 and P-selectin in the diabetic human retina and choroid. Am J Pathol 1995 147:642–53.
83. McMillan DE. The effect of diabetes on blood flow properties. Diabetes 1983; 32(Suppl 2):56–63.
84. Merimee TJ. Diabetic retinopathy. N Eng J Med 1990 322: 978–83.
85. Meyer M, Clauss M, Lepple-Wienhues A et al. A novel vascular endothelial growth factor encoded by Orf virus, VEGF-E, mediates angiogenesis via signaling through VEGFR2 (KDR) but not VEGFR1 (Flt-1) receptor tyrosine kinases. EMBO J 1999 18:363–74.
86. Meyer-Schwickerath R, Pfeiffer A, Blum WF, et al. Vitreous levels of the insulin-like growth factors I and II, and the insulin-like growth factor binding proteins 2 and 3, increase in neovascular eye disease. Studied in nondiabetic and diabetic subjects. J Clin Invest 1993 92: 2620–5.
87. Michaelson IC. The mode of development of retinal vessels. Trans Ophthalmol Soc (UK) 1948 68:137–80.
88. Mignatti P, Rifkin DB. Plasminogen activators and matrix metalloproteinases in angiogenesis. Enzyme Protein 1996 49:117–37.
89. Millauer B, Wizigmann-Voos S, Schnurch H et al. High affinity VEGF binding and developmental expression suggest Flk-1 as a major regulator of vasculogenesis and angiogenesis. Cell 1993 72:835–46.
90. Miller J, Adamis AP, Shima DT et al. Vascular endothelial growth factor/vascular permeability factor is temporally and spatially correlated with ocular angiogenesis in a primate model. Am J Pathol 1994 145:574–84.
91. Miller JA, Gravallese E, Bunn HF et al. Non-enzymatic glycosylation of erythrocyte membrane proteins: relevance to diabetes. J Clin Invest 1980 65:896–901.
92. Miller JW, Adamis AP, Aiello LP. Vascular endothelial growth factor in ocular neovascularization and proliferative diabetic retinopathy. Diabetes/Metabolism Rev 1997 13:37–50.
93. Miquerol L, Langille BL, Nagy A. Embryonic development is disrupted by modest increases in vascular endothelial growth factor gene expression. Development 127:3941–6.
94. Miyamoto K, Khosrof S, Bursell SE et al. Vascular endothelial growth factor (VEGF)-induced retinal vascular permeability is mediated by intercellular adhesion molecule-1 (ICAM-1). Am J Pathol 2000 156:1733–9.
95. Mori K, Gehlbach P, Ando A et al. Regression of ocular neovascularization in response to increased expression of pigment epithelium-derived factor. Invest Ophthalmol Vis Sci 2002 43:2428–34.
96. Mori K, Gehlbach P, Yamamoto S, et al. (AAV-mediated gene transfer of pigment epithelium-derived factor inhibits choroidal neovascularization. Invest Ophthalmol Vis Sci 2000 43:1994–2000.
97. Murata TK, Nakagawa A, Khalil T et al. The relation between expression of vascular endothelial growth factor and breakdown of the blood retinal barrier in diabetic rat retinas. Lab Invest 1996 74:819–25.
98. Ng EW, Adamis AP. Targeting angiogenesis, the underlying disorder in neovascular age-related macular degeneration. Can J Ophthalmol 2005 40:352–68.
99. Ogata N, Matsushima M, Takada Y et al. Expression of basic fibroblast growth factor mRNA in developing choroidal neovascularization. Curr Eye Res 1996 15:1008–18.

100. Ogata N, Nishikawa M, Nishimura T et al. Inverse levels of pigment epithelium-derived factor and vascular endothelial growth factor in the vitreous of eyes with rhegmatogenous retinal detachment and proliferative vitreoretinopathy. Am J Ophthalmol 2002 133:851–2.
101. Oh H, Takagi H, Suzuma K, et al. Hypoxia and vascular endothelial growth factor selectively up-regulate angiopoietin-2 in bovine microvascular endothelial cells. J Biol Chem 1999 274:15732–9.
102. Ohno-Matsui K, Morita I, Tombran-Tink J et al. Novel mechanism for age-related macular degeneration: an equilibrium shift between the angiogenesis factors VEGF and PEDF. J Cell Physiol 2001 189:323–33.
103. Oliver A, Ciulla TA. Corticosteroids as antiangiogenic agents. Ophthalmol Clin North Am 2006 19:345–351.
104. O'Reilly MS, Boehm T, Shing Y et al. Endostatin: an endogenous inhibitor of angiogenesis and tumor growth. Cell 1997 88:277–85.
105. O'Reilly MS, Holmgren L, Shing Y et al. Angiostatin: a circulating endothelial cell inhibitor that suppresses angiogenesis and tumor growth. Cold Spring Harb Symp Quant Biol 1994 59:471–82.
106. Otani A., Takagi H, Oh H et al. Expressions of angiopoietins and Tie2 in human choroidal neovascular membranes. Invest Ophthalmol Vis Sci 1999 40:1912–20.
107. Ozaki H, Seo MS, Ozaki K, et al. Blockade of vascular endothelial growth factor receptor signaling is sufficient to completely prevent retinal neovascularization. Am J Pathol 2000 156:697–707.
108. Paavonen K, Puolakkainen P, Jussila L et al. Vascular endothelial growth factor receptor-3 in lymphangiogenesis in wound healing. Am J Pathol 2000 156:1499–504.
109. Papapetropoulos A, Garcia-Cardena G, Madri JA, Sessa WC. Nitric oxide production contributes to the angiogenic properties of vascular endothelial growth factor in human endothelial cells. J Clin Invest 1997 100: 3131–9.
110. Pe'er J, Shweiki D, Itin A et al. Hypoxia-induced expression of vascular endothelial growth factor by retinal cells is a common factor in neovascularizing ocular diseases. Lab Invest 1995 72:638–45.
111. Penn JS, Rajaratnam VS, Collier RJ, Clark AF. The effect of an angiostatic steroid on neovascularization in a rat model of retinopathy of prematurity. Invest Ophthalmol Vis Sci 2001 42:283–90.
112. Plate KH, Brier G, Weich HA, Risau W. Vascular endothelial growth factor is a potential tumor angiogenesis factor in human gliomas in vivo. Nature 1992 359: 845–8.
113. Poulsen JE. Recovery from retinopathy in a case of diabetes with Simmonds' disease. Diabetes 1953 2:7–12.
114. Provis JM. Development of the primate retinal vasculature. Prog Retina Eye Res 2001 20:799–821.
115. Punglia RS, Lu M, Hsu J, et al. Regulation of vascular endothelial growth factor expression by insulin-like growth factor I. Diabetes 1997 46:1619–26.
116. Renno RZ, Youssri AI, Michaud N et al. Expression of pigment epithelium-derived factor in experimental choroidal neovascularization. Invest Ophthalmol Vis Sci 2002 43:1574–80.
117. Roberts WG, Palade GE. Increased microvascular permeability and endothelial fenestration induced by vascular endothelial growth factor. J Cell Sci 1995 108:2369–79.
118. Roberts WG, Palade GE. Neovasculature induced by vascular endothelial growth factor is fenestrated. Cancer Res 1997 57:765–72.
119. Saishin Y, Saishin Y, Takahashi K et al. VEGF-TRAP (R1R2) suppresses choroidal neovascularization and VEGF-induced breakdown of the blood–retinal barrier. J Cell Physiol 2003 195:241–8.
120. Sakurai E, Anand A, Ambati BK et al. Macrophage depletion inhibits experimental choroidal neovascularization. Invest Ophthalmol Vis Sci 2003 44:3578–85.
121. Schwesinger C, Yee C, Rohan RM et al. Intrachoroidal neovascularization in transgenic mice overexpressing vascular endothelial growth factor in the retinal pigment epithelium. Am J Pathol 2001 158:1161–72.
122. Senger D, Connolly D, Van De Water L et al. Purification and NH2-terminal amino acid sequence of guinea pig tumor secreted vascular permeability factor. Cancer Res 1990 50:1774–8.
123. Senger DR, Galli SJ, Dvorak AM et al. Tumor cells secrete a vascular permeability factor that promotes accumulation of ascites fluid. Science 1983 219:983–85.
124. Shalaby F, Rossand J, Yamaguchi TP et al. Failure of blood-island formation and vasculogenesis in Flk-1 deficient mice. Nature 1995 376:62–6.
125. Sheetz MJ, King GL. Molecular understanding of hyperglycemia's adverse effects for diabetic complications. JAMA 2002 288:2579–88.
126. Shifren JL, Doldi N, Ferrara N et al. In the human fetus, vascular endothelial growth factor is expressed in epithelial cells and myocytes, but not vascular endothelium: implications for mode of action. J Clin Endocrinol Metab 1994 79:316–22.
127. Shima DT, Deutsch U, D'Amore PA. Hypoxic induction of vascular endothelial growth factor (VEGF) in human epithelial cells is mediated by increases in mRNA stability. FEBS Letters 1995 370:203–8.
128. Shweiki D, Itin A, Soffer D, Keshet E. Vascular endothelial growth factor induced by hypoxia may mediate hypoxia-initiated angiogenesis. Nature 1992 359:843–5.
129. Smith LE. IGF1 and retinopathy of prematurity in the preterm infant. Biol Neonate 2005 88:237–344.
130. Sone H, Kawakami Y, Okuda Y, Sekine Y. Ocular vascular endothelial growth factor levels in diabetic rats are elevated before observable retinal proliferative changes. Diabetologia 1997 40:726–30.
131. Soubrane G, Cohen SY, Delayre T et al. Basic fibroblast growth factor experimentally induced choroidal angiogenesis in the minipig. Curr Eye Res 1994 13:183–95.
132. Spaide RF. Rationale for combination therapies for choroidal neovascularization. Am J Ophthalmol 2006 141:149–56.
133. Spilsbury K, Garrett KL, Shen WY et al. Overexpression of vascular endothelial growth factor (VEGF) in the retinal pigment epithelium leads to the development of choroidal neovascularization. Am J Pathol 2000 157:135–44.
134. Takahashi T, Nakamura T, Hayashi A et al., Inhibition of experimental choroidal neovascularization by overexpression of tissue inhibitor of metalloproteinases-3 in retinal pigment epithelium cells. Am J Ophthalmol 2000 130:774–81.
135. Thieme H, Aiello LP, Takagi H, et al. Comparative analysis of vascular endothelial growth factor receptors on retinal and aortic vascular endothelial cells. Diabetes 1995 44:98–103.
136. Thurston G, Rudge JS, Ioffe E et al. Angiopoietin-1 protects the adult vasculature against plasma leakage. Nat Med 2000 6:460–3.
137. Tilton RG, Kawamura T, Chang KC et al. Vascular dysfunction induced by elevated glucose levels in rats

is mediated by vascular endothelial growth factor. J Clin Invest 1997 99:2192–202.

138. Tobe T, Ortega S, Luna JD et al. Targeted disruption of the FGF2 gene does not prevent choroidal neovascularization in a murine model. Am J Pathol 1998 153:1641–6.
139. Tolentino MT, Miller JW, Gragoudas ES et al. Vascular endothelial growth factor is sufficient to produce iris neovascularization and neovascular glaucoma in a non-human primate. Arch Ophthalmol 1996 114: 964–70.
140. Tolentino MT, Miller JW, Gragoudas ES, et al. Intravitreal injections of vascular endothelial growth factor produce retinal ischemia and microangiopathy in an adult primate. Ophthalmology 1996 103:1820–8.
141. Usui T, Ishida S, Yamashiro K et al. VEGF164(165). as the pathological isoform: differential leukocyte and endothelial responses through VEGFR1 and VEGFR2. Invest Ophthalmol Vis Sci 2004 45:368–74.
142. Wells JA, Murthy R, Chibber R et al. Levels of vascular endothelial growth factor are elevated in the vitreous of patients with subretinal neovascularisation. Br J Ophthalmol 1996 80:363–6.
143. Witmer AN, Blaauwgeers HG, Weich HA et al. Altered expression patterns of VEGF receptors in human diabetic retina and in experimental VEGF-induced retinopathy in monkey. Invest Ophthalmol Vis Sci 2002 43:849–57.
144. Witmer AN, Vrensen GF, Van Noorden CJ, Schlingemann RO. Vascular endothelial growth factors and angiogenesis in eye disease. Prog Retin Eye Res 2003 22:1–29.
145. Xia P, Aiello LP, Ishii H et al. Characterization of vascular endothelial growth factor's effect on the activation of protein kinase C, its isoforms, and endothelial cell growth. J Clin Invest 1996 98:2018–26.
146. Yamada H, Yamada E, Kwak N et al. Cell injury unmasks a latent proangiogenic phenotype in mice with increased expression of FGF2 in the retina. J Cell Physiol 2000 185: 135–42.
147. Yancopoulos GD, Davis S, Gale NW et al. Vascular-specific growth factors and blood vessel formation. Nature 2000 407:242–8.
148. Yannuzzi LA, Negrao S, Iida T et al. Retinal angiomatous proliferation in age-related macular degeneration. Retina 2001 21:416–34.
149. Yano K, Brown LF, Detmar M. Control of hair growth and follicle size by VEGF-mediated angiogenesis. J Clin Invest 2001 107:409–17.
150. Yi X, Ogata N, Komada M, et al. Vascular endothelial growth factor expression in choroidal neovascularization in rats. Graefes Arch Clin Exp Ophthalmol 1997 235:313–9.
151. Young TL, Anthony DC, Pierce E et al. Histopathology and vascular endothelial growth factor in untreated and diode laser-treated retinopathy of prematurity. J AAPOS 1997 1:105–10.

69

Vasculitides

Andrew Flint
Department of Pathology, University of Michigan, Ann Arbor, Michigan, U.S.A.

INTRODUCTION

Vasculitis can be defined as inflammation and subsequent injury to a blood vessel wall that may result in vessel wall necrosis and thrombosis with subsequent ischemia of organs. Vasculitis may present as a primary disorder in various organs including the eye (105).

The vasculitides have been the subject of numerous reports since a gross pathologic description by Rokitansky in 1852 (124). Subsequently, descriptions of polyarteritis nodosa (PN), giant cell arteritis (GCA), Takayasu arteritis (TA), Kawasaki disease (KD), Wegener granulomatosis (WG), Churg–Strauss syndrome (CSS), and other primary inflammatory conditions of blood vessels have appeared in the literature (76). The majority of the vasculitides affect small vessels including post-capillary venules, capillaries, arterioles, and small arteries. In contrast, other vasculitides such as GCA exclusively affect large to medium-sized arteries (95), or both small and medium-sized arteries and veins as in the case of WG. The vasculitides are usually classified by the type or size of blood vessel involved. Three main groups of vasculitides have been defined: (*i*) large-vessel vasculitis (GCA, TA); (*ii*) medium-sized vessel vasculitis (classic PN which may also involve small vessels, KD); and (*iii*) small-vessel vasculitis (WG, CSS, microscopic polyangiitis, Henoch–Schonlein purpura, essential cryoglobulinemic vasculitis, and cutaneous leukocytoclastic angiitis) (73).

An alternative approach to classification is based on presumed pathogenic mechanisms. Proposed mechanisms include immune complex-mediated injury, anti-endothelial cell antibody injury, cell-mediated injury, and injury mediated by anti-lysosomal antibody (74,139).

Immune complex formation with subsequent binding to endothelial cells can lead to complement fixation, activation of the complement cascade, and the release of inflammatory mediators. Inflammation and necrosis of vessel walls may be a result and is marked by the presence of karryorhectic debris in arterial walls. Examples of immune complex-mediated disorders include lupus vasculitis, Behçet disease (BD), and sulfonamide-induced vasculitis. Antibodies to endothelial cells and collagen and matrix proteins can damage blood vessel walls via antibody-dependent-cell-mediated cytotoxicity (99,139). Cell-mediated injury can also result in granuloma formation as occurs in GCA and TA. Cell-mediated injury is also thought to be a mechanism that gives rise to the vessel wall necrosis, hemorrhage, and thrombosis that affects both blood vessels and soft tissues in WG (139).

Autoantibodies to leukocyte proteins are incriminated in the causation of WG, microscopic polyangiitis, and CSS (139). Antineutrophil cytoplasmic autoantibody-mediated vasculitis is characterized by the presence of autoantibodies directed to antigens contained in the granules of neutrophils and the lysosomes of monocytes. The antineutrophil cytoplasmic antibodies (cANCA) are thought capable of activating polymorphonuclear leukocytes (PMNs) and monocytes. These activated inflammatory cells release toxic oxygen metabolites, causing vascular inflammation. PMN activation can injure endothelial cells in such cases.

In addition to the primary vasculitides where the vessels themselves are the target of inflammation, other systemic disorders may secondarily produce inflammation of blood vessels. Connective tissue disorders such as systemic lupus erythematosus (SLE) and rheumatoid arthritis (RA) are examples, as are some infections such as syphilis. Both primary and secondary vasculitides can involve the eye and its arteries, veins, and capillaries. GCA, WG (58,123), BD, SLE, PN, syphilis, and herpes infection represent a few of these disorders. Ophthalmic manifestations of vasculitis may be manifested in part by scleritis, keratitis, uveitis, retinal vasculitis, and optic neuropathy (104,105,143). Collagen vascular disorders are responsible for approximately one half of noninfectious cases of peripheral ulcerative keratitis (140). Some of the disorders involve the blood vessels of the eye directly, whereas other disorders affect the eye indirectly by causing inflammation of extraocular blood vessels.

GIANT CELL ARTERITIS

An inflammatory disease primarily occurring in the elderly, GCA (also known as cranial or temporal arteritis) is marked by inflammation of large and medium-sized arteries. GCA occurs most commonly in individuals older than 50 years and is related to polymyalgia rheumatica (118) with which it often coexists. Ocular manifestations include vision loss, diplopia, ptosis, and amaurosis fugax. Other signs and symptoms include headache (the main symptom in more than 60% of patients), jaw and tongue claudication, low-grade fever, and anorexia (118). Upper extremity claudication, carotid artery bruits, and myocardial infarction secondary to coronary arteritis have been reported (118). When inflamed, the temporal arteries become swollen and tender. Fundoscopy performed early in the clinical course reveals slight pallor and edema of the optic disc, scattered cotton-wool spots (see Chapter 67), and small hemorrhages. Infarction of the optic nerve may occur (83) if the arteries supplying the anterior portion of the optic nerve become inflamed. Choroidal infarction has also been reported (117).

As with most of the other vasculitides, the pathogenesis and nature of the initial arterial injury is unknown. Neutrophils infiltrate the injured vessel and secrete toxic reactive oxygen species and matrix metalloproteinases. T lymphocytes are thought to play a role in the injury as CD4+ T cells are found in association with macrophages that form granulomas. Neovascularization of the intima and media of the inflamed vessels is postulated to play a role in the intimal proliferation that may lead to occlusion of the lumen. Vascular endothelial growth factor expression is associated with this process (151) as is the elaboration of platelet-derived growth factor (PDGF) (80,81). Investigations by Weyand and colleagues suggest that cases of GCA with significant intimal hyperplasia are associated with both higher levels of gamma interferon (IFNγ), interleukin 1(IL), and PDGF (152,153). In addition, myofibroblasts account for some of the cellular proliferation of the intima as the inflammation develops. A prominent systemic inflammatory response develops as well and is manifested by elevated erythrocyte sedimentation rate (ESR) and increased levels of C-reactive protein (CRP).

The arteritis most often involves arteries arising from the aorta, though other medium and large arteries may also be involved. The superficial temporal, ophthalmic, posterior ciliary, and vertebral arteries are particularly affected. Inflammation is irregularly distributed along the length of these vessels. The histopathologic hallmark of GCA is granulomatous inflammation that takes the form of multinucleated giant cells. The media of the artery wall is most often affected, and manifests collections of multinucleated giant cells, macrophages, and lymphocytes that are largely centered about a fragmented internal elastic lamina. With severe inflammation, the media undergoes necrosis. The adventitia is infiltrated by similar inflammatory cells, and the intima often becomes hyperplastic, and can result in occlusion of the lumen. Occlusion can also result from thrombosis. Biopsy samples usually show lesser degrees of inflammation and intimal proliferation; multinucleated giant cells are not always observed.

WEGENER GRANULOMATOSIS

Wegener granulomatosis typically occurs in the fourth to fifth decades and men are more commonly involved. Early descriptions of WG emphasized a triad of pathologic features: a systemic necrotizing vasculitis involving both small arteries and veins, necrotizing granulomatous inflammation of the upper or lower respiratory tract, or both, and a necrotizing glomerulonephritis (34,40,148). Chest radiographs manifest infiltrates, nodules, and cavities. Nasal septal perforation and collapse of the nasal arch can eventually develop. A widespread vasculitis involves both small arteries and veins (64). Subsequent reports have described patients with a more limited form of the disease that involves only the lower and upper respiratory tract (19,20).

WG is an example of a pauci-immune small-vessel vasculitis. Pauci-immune vasculitis has a paucity or absence of vessel wall staining for immunoglobulin and is often associated with ANCA (126). ANCA toward proteinase 3 can be detected by cytoplasmic immunofluorescence staining of PMNs (cANCA) (96). The appearance of these antibodies has a specificity of almost 90% in biopsy-documented cases of WG and the sensitivity of cANCA determination is almost 100% in patients with active generalized disease (72,114,144). Experiments have shown that antiproteinase 3 can lyse cultured endothelial cells (108) and exert direct cytotoxic effects on cytokine-activated vascular endothelium (100). In addition, excessive production of tumor necrosis factor (TNF) and IFNγ is postulated to initiate and perpetuate the granulomatous inflammatory lesion characteristic of WG (132). Peripheral blood lymphocytes from patients with active WG produce markedly increased amounts of IFNγ and increased production of TNF (97). In addition, most patients manifest elevated titers of cANCA; however, some patients with limited disease produce elevated titers of pANCA, an antibody to myeloperoxidase (134). ANCA positivity is not regarded as specific for WG, and approximately 10% of patients with WG have negative assays for ANCA (75). Aberrant helper T-cell type 1 cytokine production may play a role in a cell-mediated immune response (31,132).

Orbital and ocular involvement commonly occurs in both the classic and limited forms of WG and does not differ in frequency or severity (17,136). Ocular involvement may be seen in 29% to 58% of patients (18,29,41), and often coexists with other head and neck sites of involvement. Ocular manifestations include peripheral ulcerative keratitis, episcleritis, scleritis, uveitis, dacryoadenitis, nasolacrimal duct obstruction, and retinal vasculitis (14,30,56,57, 63,93,137). Inflammation of the anterior ciliary arteries and perilimbal arteries may lead to peripheral ulcerative keratitis and necrotizing scleritis (8). Proptosis with orbital pseudotumor may develop rapidly, accompanied by pain and eyelid erythema. Rarely, destruction of the globe results (89). Haynes et al. have reported that ocular involvement may also result from contiguous granulomatous sinusitis (58), leading to ocular muscle involvement, nasolacrimal duct obstruction, and optic neuropathy.

Pathologically, an occlusive necrotizing vasculitis is present, involving the anterior and posterior ciliary arteries, optic nerve vessels, and the perilimbal blood vessels (46). The anterior and posterior segments of the eye may be involved, as may the lacrimal system, periocular, and orbital soft tissues (92). The inflammation involves medium-sized arteries, arterioles, capillaries, and venules and may be granulomatous or nongranulomatous. Granulomatous vasculitis is characterized by transmural infiltrates of PMNs, lymphocytes and monocytes, and smaller numbers of plasma cells and eosinophils. Multinucleated giant cells (Langhans type) are found within the vessel wall, often accompanied by fibrinoid necrosis and karryorhectic debris. Extravascular lesions are usually present and consist of loose collections of monocytes and PMNs with scattered multinucleated giant cells. Central zones of fibrinoid necrosis may be present and small, discrete collections of PMNs ("microabscesses") are often observed. Larger lesions may also contain extensive areas of necrosis encompassing nuclear debris. Granulomatous inflammation of the sclera may also occur, though not directly based upon blood vessel involvement.

BEHÇET DISEASE

A chronic, multisystem, small-vessel vasculitis, BD produces a variety of clinical manifestations including oral and genital aphthous ulcers, arthralgias, cutaneous lesions, and meningoencephalitis (50,121). Patients in the second and third decades of life are most often affected by the recurrent cutaneous and mucous membrane ulcerations that appear suddenly and regress spontaneously. Behçet was among the first observers to emphasize the relationship between ocular inflammation and the mucocutaneous lesions (11). Ocular involvement occurs after the other body sites become involved. Nonocular involvement seems to be more prevalent among women, while ocular involvement is more common among men (42). A panuveitis may develop, characterized by bilateral nongranulomatous inflammation of the iris and ciliary body, vitritis, and an occlusive retinal vasculitis.

Fenton and Easom have described a constellation of pathologic features in eyes enucleated from a series of patients with BD (42). Lymphoid infiltrates of the iris blood vessels were observed as were thrombi. These observers also noted marked inflammation of the retinal arteries and veins and their surrounding supporting tissues as well as ischemic necrosis of the retina, ciliary body, and iris. Other lesions included anterior chamber inflammatory exudates, lymphocyte infiltrates of iris, ciliary body, choroid, and secondary scarring of the retina. While the blood vessel wall infiltrates were composed of T lymphocytes, PMNs, and macrophages, a small vessel neutrophilic vasculitis was often observed (98). Other observers have described nongranulomatous uveitis and retinal detachment (51).

Rarely, BD may be complicated by aortitis and phlebitis, likely secondary to inflammation of the much smaller vasa vasorum (76). Large and medium-sized artery involvement may produce myocardial infarction, the Budd–Chiari syndrome, claudication, and obstruction of the vena cavae. Chronically inflamed vessels manifest intramural as well as perivascular infiltrates of lymphocytes and monocytes; the vessel wall itself undergoes scarring. Aneurysm and thrombus formation may complicate the inflammation.

It is postulated that BD results from humoral and cellular immunologic mechanisms (51). Immune complex-mediated damage and disordered T-lymphocyte functions have been reported. Charteris et al. described T-lymphocyte infiltrates of the iris and ciliary body that extended into the choroid. Lymphocytes had also infiltrated retinal blood vessels (23). Nonocular sites of T-lymphocyte infiltration have also been found and lend support to the postulate that T-lymphocyte-mediated immune mechanisms underlie much of the tissue damage (22,24). Immunochemical characterization of the inflammatory infiltrates have demonstrated a preponderance of CD4+ T cells and a relative absence of CD8+ T cells within the intramural and perivascular infiltrates. In addition, the cellular infiltrate in the choroid consisted mainly of CD4+ T cells and macrophages (23). Complement or immunoglobulin deposition was not identified, in contrast to a case report by Mullaney and Collum (111). Subsequently, the vascular endothelium has been shown to extensively express adhesion molecules and major histocompatibility class II antigens (51). Increased adhesion molecule expression has been associated with uveitis and retinal vasculitis (154,155,158). The preponderance of CD4+ T cells and relative lack of CD8+ T cells could lead to B-cell stimulation and antibody production.

CONNECTIVE TISSUE DISORDERS

Systemic disorders not usually regarded in terms of vascular inflammation may on occasion provoke blood vessel inflammation. For example, vasculitis may complicate the clinical course of RA and SLE.

Rheumatoid Arthritis

An autoimmune disorder, RA is characterized by a generalized, chronic polyarthritis that characteristically involves the small joints of the hands and feet in a symmetrical fashion. Other peripheral joints may be involved as well as the heart, lung, skin, and blood vessels (88,127).

Ocular involvement may take the form of keratoconjunctivitis sicca, episcleritis, anterior scleritis, marginal corneal furrows, and retinal vasculitis secondary to posterior scleritis (61,105). Scleritis is likely due to a vasculitis (101). A microangiopathy with fibrinoid necrosis, neutrophil invasion of the vessels, and immune deposits have been observed in scleral and conjunctival biopsy samples obtained from patients with necrotizing scleritis (106). In long-standing RA, the vascular inflammation may result in arteriolar occlusive changes, resulting in a necrotizing anterior scleritis (scleromalacia perforans). A small group of patients develop severe keratoconjunctivitis sicca that results in corneal perforation (62). Rheumatoid nodules are thought to develop around inflamed blood vessels. Jones and Jayson found a significant incidence of rheumatoid subcutaneous nodules and other features of microvasculitis in patients with rheumatoid scleritis (78). A microangiopathy with fibrinoid necrosis, PMN invasion of the vessels and immune deposits have been observed in scleral and conjunctival biopsy samples obtained from patients with necrotizing scleritis (106). Rheumatoid episcleritis and rheumatoid scleritis are also associated with widespread systemic disease, particularly of the cardiovascular and respiratory systems. The presence of scleritis may portend serious systemic disease (147).

Inflammation and tissue destruction is postulated to be caused by cellular interactions involving CD4+ T cells, macrophages, and antigen-presenting cells. Numerous inflammatory cytokines are released, including IL1 and TNF (150). Cytokine release leads to collagen and proteoglycan degeneration and tissue necrosis (36). Rheumatoid factors (RFs), such as IgM antibodies formed against the patient's IgG, can lead to immune complex formation and deposition in joints and blood vessels. Immune complex deposition in vessel walls leads to complement activation and subsequent endothelial swelling, perivascular cellular infiltration, and thrombosis (133,146).

Scleritis occurs not only in association with RA, but also with other connective tissue disorders, including PN, relapsing polychondritis, WG, and SLE.

Systemic Lupus Erythematosus

An autoimmune inflammatory disease, SLE is characterized by the presence of circulating autoantibodies to one or more components of cell nuclei and by the formation of immune complexes (1). Polyclonal

B-lymphocyte activation results in the production of several autoantibodies, including anti-lymphocyte, antinuclear, and anti-thyroid antibodies. Immune complex formation and deposition also characterize SLE and lead to local inflammation and tissue injury. Activation of complement leads to the intravascular release of C3a and C5a with the subsequent activation of inflammatory cells and endothelial cell damage. Damage to blood vessels may also occur at sites remote from immune complex deposition (105).

SLE is characterized by multiple organ system involvement, including the joints, skin, kidneys, lungs, central nervous system (CNS), and eyes. Approximately 90% of patients are women of child-bearing age (96). Collagen vascular diseases are responsible for approximately one half of noninfectious cases of peripheral ulcerative keratitis, and. keratoconjunctivitis sicca is the most frequent corneal complication of SLE (105,140). Deep keratopathy and peripheral ulcerative keratitis may occur infrequently (122). In such cases, deposition of immune complexes in the limbal blood vessels of the peripheral cornea with activation of the complement system has been shown to produce collagenase (37). An inflammatory microangiopathy is typically found in conjunctival biopsy samples (140). Heiligenhaus and colleagues examined tissue samples obtained from patients with SLE-associated peripheral ulcerative keratitis, scleritis, and cicatrizing conjunctivitis and observed subepithelial and perivascular cellular infiltration and granuloma formation (59). These workers also demonstrated the presence of immune deposits along epithelial basement membranes and in vessel walls, compatible with an immune complex-mediated disorder. Immune complex deposition in CNS capillaries has also been documented in patients with coexistent CNS and occlusive retinal disease (69).

Retinopathy is also a well-described complication of SLE and may parallel the activity of the systemic disease (56,87,135). The most common findings are cotton-wool spots (localized accumulations of axoplasmic debris in the retinal nerve fiber layer due to an interruption in axonal organelle transport), retinal hemorrhages, and optic disc edema. This lesion is usually due to focal inner retinal ischemia, and is thought to result from an immune complex-mediated vasculopathy (52). A rarely occurring but severe vaso-occlusive retinopathy can develop in SLE patients (68). This complication has been thought to be based on an immune complex-mediated vasculitis. Pathologically, the retinal vessel walls manifests fibrinoid change and thrombosis though actual inflammation of the vessel is sparse (54). Retinal capillary dilatation and microaneurysms have been documented by fluorescein angiography of the fundus (91). This form of retinopathy results in vision loss in about 80% of affected SLE patients. An association between severe vaso-occlusive retinopathy and the presence of antiphospholipid antibodies has been described (3,21,51,53,109). This pattern of arteriolar vaso-occlusive retinopathy may occur in patients who do not have SLE (3,22). In addition, an association between antiphospholipid antibodies, retinopathy, and CNS lupus has been described (7). Neovascularization or vitreous hemorrhage occurs in about 40% of the reported cases.

POLYARTERITIS NODOSA

Polyarteritis nodosa primarily involves small and medium-sized muscular arteries; PN spares veins and venules. PN typically affects the kidneys (renal involvement accounts for most of the mortality resulting from PN), the musculoskeletal system, CNS, gastrointestinal system, the skin, and the heart. Men are more commonly affected than woman and the onset of disease usually occurs in patients between 20 and 40 years of age. A variety of clinicopathologic manifestations are associated with PN, depending on the organ(s) involved. Localized muscle pain or weakness, peripheral and cranial nerve neuropathies, bowel pain or bleeding, hypertension, tender cutaneous nodules, skin ulceration, and gangrene are manifestations of PN (43). In contrast to WG, the respiratory tract is not involved. Constitutional symptoms and signs include fever, malaise, arthralgias, and myalgias. The diagnosis of PN is based on clinical signs and symptoms and the pathologic examination of biopsy samples obtained from involved tissues, usually kidney, muscle, or sural nerve. PN has been subdivided into classic and microscopic forms. The classic form is defined as a systemic vasculitis involving medium-sized arteries (frequently with aneurysm formation), usually without glomerular involvement (32). Microscopic PN is characterized by a small-vessel vasculitis, usually accompanied by necrotizing glomerulonephritis (3). Classic PN is associated with negative cANCA titers whereas microscopic PN may be accompanied by elevated pANCA titer. Close correlation between myeloperoxidase antibodies and disease activity in patients with microscopic PN has been reported (31).

Ocular involvement is found in 10% to 20% of patients and may represent the initial clinical presentation (13,156). Inflammation of the branches of the ophthalmic artery can result in retinal and optic nerve ischemia (55). Choroidal vessel and anterior ciliary artery involvement have been documented (105). Such vascular inflammation is manifested as papilledema or papillitis, hemorrhages, and cotton-wool spots (4,44). A necrotizing scleritis and peripheral ulcerative keratitis are other manifestations of ocular involvement (29,30,110). CNS involvement may result in extraocular muscle palsies, nystagmus, and homonymous hemianopia (43). Inflammation of the orbital blood vessels can lead to exophthalmos (145).

PN is manifested by vascular mural fibrinoid necrosis with an accompanying infiltrate of PMNs, eosinophils, and mononuclear leukocytes. The choroidal, retinal, and ciliary arteries are typically involved. Fibrinoid necrosis is characterized by the accumulation of plasma proteins, including fibrin, at sites of tissue destruction. The inflammation may vary in its appearance from one vessel to another, and even within different areas of the same vessel. The inflammation is often distributed in an eccentric rather than concentric manner about the vessel's circumference. Thrombosis may result from the alteration of the endothelium by the inflammation, and weakened portions of the vessel wall may dilate, leading to microaneurysm formation (66). Healing of the lesions takes the form of fibrosis with recanalization of thrombi. Granulomatous inflammation is not a feature of PN.

Most cases of PN are idiopathic though infection is thought to be responsible for some cases of immune complex-mediated PN (76). Hepatitis B antigen or HBV antibodies are present in 30% to 55% of patients with PN (49,130). Deposits of hepatitis B antigen, IgM, and complement in vessel walls have been found in patients with PN (49,120). The pathogenesis of PN has been attributed to immune complex deposition involving small arteries as well as vessels smaller than arteries, especially glomerular capillaries. Classic PN, involving medium-sized arteries, does not manifest immune complex deposits.

KAWASAKI DISEASE

Eighty percent of cases of KD occur in children younger than 5 years old (157). Asian children appear to be most susceptible to developing this disorder, especially Japanese children (142). KD is characterized by inflammation of medium-sized blood vessels and the presence of the mucocutaneous lymph node syndrome (84). The principal clinical features include: fever, nonexudative conjunctivitis, oropharyngeal changes including erythema, swelling and fissuring of the lips, diffuse erythema of the oropharynx or strawberry tongue, peripheral extremity changes including erythema of the palms and soles, induration and edema of the hands and feet, desquamation of the skin of the hands and feet, transverse grooves in the nails, a polymorphous rash, and cervical lymphadenopathy (9). The presence of five of these features (fever must be present) are required for an absolute diagnosis (9). Other clinical manifestations include electrocardiogram abnormalities (in almost 90% of cases), myocarditis, diarrhea, arthralgia or arthritis, proteinuria, and sterile pyuria. Laboratory abnormalities include a leukocytosis with left shift, an elevated ESR and an elevated CRP level. A lymphocytosis characterized by a predominance of polyclonal B cells develops during the clinical course. Serum markers associated with collagen vascular disorders, such as ANCA, RF, ANA, and anti-DNA, are absent. Thrombocytosis develops by the third week of illness.

KD is regarded in large part as a systemic vasculitis. Medium and large vessels subsequently become inflamed, with the coronary arteries being at greatest risk, though any artery and vein may also be inflamed, such as the femoral, renal, and iliac arteries. Angiographic abnormalities of the coronary vasculature are demonstrable in 30% to 60% of patients (48,82). In most patients, the angiographic abnormalities improve, however, one-third of patients develop ischemic heart disease (82). The panvasculitis is initially manifested as intimal collections of inflammatory cells. Edema and leukocyte infiltrates extend transmurally to involve the adventitia. The inflammatory cells are predominantly macrophages, CD8– T cells, and smaller numbers of PMNs and plasma cells (16,77). As the inflammation progresses, the media is destroyed and aneurysm formation may result. The inflamed wall eventually becomes fibrotic, leading to stenosis or thrombosis. These pathologic features are similar to those of PN and both conditions occur at points of arterial branching (159). However, unlike PN, fibrinoid necrosis of the blood vessel walls is not prominent in KD. Unlike PN, KD has a strong predilection for the coronary arteries and there is only minimal participation by PMNs.

The ophthalmic manifestations include mild to marked conjunctival congestion and a mild to moderate anterior uveitis that is most commonly bilateral (18). Conjunctival inflammation is found in 88% to 96% of patients (71,85). Small vessel vasculitis is postulated to account for the conjunctivitis. In a series reported by Jacob et al., one of nine patients developed posterior segment inflammation (70). This inflammation took the form of macular edema, disc swelling, and retinal vessel engorgement. The vitreous may become filled with moderate numbers of inflammatory cells.

The pathogenesis of KD is incompletely understood. The presence of numerous macrophages and T lymphocytes and the scarcity of PMNs suggest that activation of T cells and monocytes plays a central role in the pathogenesis. Activated monocytes have been detected in the tissues and peripheral blood of patients with KD (6). The clinical features and epidemiologic data suggest that a bacterial or viral infection is the likely cause. A large variety of infectious agents has been postulated, though a specific agent has not been identified (9,10,28).

CHURG–STRAUSS SYNDROME

Churg and Strauss described 13 patients with a multisystem syndrome characterized by fever, peripheral blood eosinophilia, asthma, and a rapidly progressive clinical course (27). Symptomatology was primarily the result of cardiac failure, renal damage, and peripheral neuropathy. The CSS, or allergic granulomatous angiitis as it is also called, has been subsequently described in additional detail by other observers (26,27,33,61,149). A peripheral eosinophilia >1000/mm^3 is observed in 85% of patients at some point during the clinical course (149). Mononeuritis multiplex may be present, as might purpura and urticaria (27). Cardiac, renal, and gastrointestinal involvement has also been described. Pathologically, a necrotizing arteritis, extravascular granulomas, and tissue eosinophilia have been observed (141). Small arterioles, capillaries, and small venules undergo fibrinoid necrosis, and eosinophils infiltrate vessel walls as well as extravascular tissues (60).

There have been very few reports of ocular involvement in CSS (2). By 1986, only six cases of ocular involvement had been reported. The earliest report may be that of Cury et al. who described a patient with unilateral episcleritis and panuveitis that ultimately required enucleation (33). The pathologic features included necrotizing granulomatous inflammation. Foci of fibrinoid necrosis were observed in the sclera and were accompanied by infiltrates of eosinophils, epithelioid histiocytes, and giant cells. Small blood vessels manifested perivascular infiltrates of inflammatory cells. Weinstein et al. described two patients who developed ischemic optic neuropathy, retinal infarcts, and superior oblique muscle palsy (149). Meisler et al. reported a patient with conjunctival inflammation and amyloidosis in association with CSS (103). The patient had developed bilateral upper eyelid swelling and bloody ocular discharge. The upper tarsal conjunctivae were yellow, waxy, and nodular. A biopsy sample manifested tissue infiltrates of eosinophils and amyloid deposits. Granulomatous inflammation, however, was not observed.

CSS is distinguished from PN by the presence of asthma as asthma is infrequently associated with PN (103). PN affects small and medium-sized arteries, and a PMN infiltrate is characteristic. CSS, in contrast, affects small arteries, capillaries, and veins; eosinophils, plasma cells, and lymphocytes are the early cellular actors, histiocytes appear in the chronic stage. Extravascular foci of fibrinoid necrosis develop and are surrounded by radially arranged histiocytes and epithelioid cells. Necrotic eosinophils are also found within the necrotic centers of the granulomas (103).

A patient reported by Shields et al. developed right upper eyelid swelling (131). Clinically, a vascularized diffuse thickening of the tarsal conjunctiva was observed as was a separate but similar lesion involving the plica semilunaris. Biopsy samples manifested noncaseating granulomas with lymphocytes, plasma cells, histiocytes, giant cells, and numerous eosinophils. Although a vasculitis was not observed, the authors reported that extraocular manifestations of CSS subsequently developed over 6 months. Nissim et al. described a single patient whose initial manifestation of CSS was conjunctivitis (113). A conjunctival biopsy sample revealed necrotizing granulomatous inflammation and tissue eosinophilia. The necrotic material was composed of nuclear debris from eosinophils and fibrinoid necrosis.

Finally, a series of 30 patients with CSS was reported that included a single patient with ocular involvement, a marginal corneal ulcer (27).

TAKAYASU ARTERITIS

Takayasu arteritis involves large blood vessels such as the aorta and its branches, including the coronary arteries. Pulmonary arteries may also become inflamed (115). The inflammation involves the media and results in the destruction of the elastin framework; progressive destruction of the media leads to subsequent atrophy and fibrosis of the smooth muscle of the media. In some cases, aneurysm formation or actual rupture of the weakened walls occurs. Clinically, patients often manifest dizziness, syncope, weak or absent pulses, and differences in blood pressure readings between the arms. Women are more commonly affected, usually between the ages of 15 and 45 years (86).

The inflammation first centers on the vasa vasorum that nourish the media; the adjacent adventitia is also inflamed. Natural killer cells, cytotoxic T lymphocytes, helper T cells, monocytes, granulocytes, and dendritic cells populate the inflammatory infiltrate (129). The infiltrates may also become granulomatous and multinucleated giant cells are often present. The granulomatous inflammation is mediated by sensitized CD4+ T cells and macrophages. Various cytokines and elevated plasma levels of IL1 and IL6 have been measured in affected patients (116). Additionally, release of IL6 by circulating inflammatory cells appears to be closely linked to disease activity (116). An association has been noted between HLA types and TA, and the arteritis has also been linked to rheumatic fever, streptococcal infections, tuberculosis, and collagen vascular disorders (67,125). Antibodies directed against vascular endothelial cells have been detected in TA and it has been postulated that these antibodies could produce vascular damage via complement fixation as well as through antibody-dependent cellular cytotoxicity (33,35,79).

INFECTIOUS VASCULITIDES

Infectious agents can cause vasculitis and are the most common cause of secondary vasculitis. Tissue injury is usually initiated by microbial invasion of the vascular endothelium, which triggers a chemotactic response for neutrophils and generates immune complex formation (74). Inflammation results from the host's immune response to the organisms and also from bacterial products that can attract and activate leukocytes and humoral inflammatory mediators. Immune complex deposits in the walls of blood vessels can produce inflammatory damage to the vessel walls. Rickettsial, bacterial, and fungal infections have all been documented to produce vasculitis (45,46,107,112,128,138).

Viral Vasculitis

Viral infections can predispose a patient to vasculitis that apparently does not involve viral proliferation within vessel walls (94). Infection with the human immunodeficiency virus is such an example. Retinal microangiopathy is the most common ophthalmic manifestation of AIDS. Jabs et al. reported that retinopathy was present in approximately two-thirds of patients with AIDS (69). HIV retinopathy is manifested by cotton-wool spots that occur following periods of retinal ischemia (47,65). Cotton-wool spots that reflect swollen axons in the retinal nerve fiber layer from a disruption of axonal transport occur (102). They are most commonly found in the posterior pole of the eye, cotton-wool spots appear as distinct, well demarcated opacifications of the nerve fiber layer without any accompanying intraocular inflammatory changes. Over 50% of patients with AIDS manifest microaneurysms and intra- and pre-retinal hemorrhages. The pathogenesis of HIV retinopathy remains controversial but seems to be related to immune complex deposition, actual infection of the retinal vascular endothelium, and local release of cytotoxic factors (39). A true vasculitis is not present. Ultrastructural studies demonstrate nonspecific findings of retinal arterioles with narrowed lumens, swollen endothelial cells, thickened basal lamina, loss of pericytes, and immunoglobulin and complement deposits within vessel walls (119). Red cell aggregation, elevated fibrinogen levels, circulating immune complexes, and plasma viscosity have all been reported as being correlated with the occurrence of ocular microangiopathy (37,38).

While ocular complications are commonplace in cases of herpes zoster ophthalmicus, retinal vascular involvement is very uncommon (12). Brown and Mendis described sheathing and narrowing of the branches of the temporal arterioles in a patient with herpes zoster ophthalmicus (15). Herpes zoster vasculitis can pathologically mimic GCA, as described in a report by Al-Abdulla et al. (5). In situ hybridization of an inflamed temporal artery demonstrated herpes zoster DNA within the temporal artery wall (5).

Vascular inflammation resulting from direct vessel wall invasion by viruses is uncommon. In such cases, a cell-mediated immune response is thought to be responsible for the inflammatory reaction. Varicella zoster infection can also account for retinal vasculitis (24). In a case reported by Kuo et al. a patient with varicella zoster infection developed keratitic precipitates, and numerous inflammatory cells in the anterior chamber and vitreous, and perivenous exudates (90).

REFERENCES

1. Aaronson AJ, Ordofiez NG, Diddie KR, Ernest T. Immune complex deposition in the eye in systemic lupus erythematosus. Arch Intern Med 1979; 139:1312–3.
2. Acheson JF, Cockerell OC, Bentley Cr, Sanders MD. Churg–Strauss vasculitis presenting with severe visual loss due to bilateral sequential optic neuropathy. Br J Ophthalmol 1993; 77:118–9.
3. Acheson JF, Gregson MC, Merry P, Schulenberg WE. Vasocclusive retinopathy in the primary antiphospholipid antibody syndrome. Eye 1991; 5:48–55.
4. Akova YA, Jabbur NS, Foster S. Ocular presentation of polyarteritis nodosa. Ophthalmology 1993; 100:1775–81.
5. Al-Abdulla NA, Rismondo V, Minkowski JS, Miller NR. Herpes zoster vasculitis presenting as giant cell arteritis with bilateral internuclear ophthalmoplegia. Am J Ophthalmology 2002; 134:912–4.
6. Ariga S, Koga M, Takahasi M, et al. Maturation of macrophages from peripheral blood monocytes in Kawasaki disease: immunocytochemical and immunoelectron microscopic study. Pathol Int 2000; 51:257–63.
7. Au AK, O'Day J. Review of severe vaso-occlusive retinopathy in systemic lupus erythematosus and the antiphospholipid syndrome: associations, visual outcomes, complications and treatment. Clin Exp Ophthalmol 2004; 32:87–100.
8. Austin P, Green WR, Sallyer DC, et al. Peripheral corneal degeneration and occlusive vasculitis in Wegener's granulomatosis. Am J Ophthalmol 1978; 85:311–7.
9. Barron KS. Kawasaki disease: etiology, pathogenesis, and treatment. Cleveland Clin J Med 2002; 69(Suppl.): SII-69–SII-78.
10. Barron KS, Shulman ST, Rowley A, et al. Report of the National Institutes of Health Workshop on Kawasaki Disease. J Rheumatol 1999; 26:170–90.
11. Behçet H. Uber rezidivierende, aphthose, durch ein Virus verursachte Geschwure am Mund, am Auge und den Genitalien. Dermatol Wochenschr 1937; 105:1152–7.
12. Bodaghi B, Rozenberg F, Cassoux N, et al. Nonnecrotizing herpetic retinopathies masquerading as severe posterior uveitis. Ophthalmology 2003; 110:1737–43.
13. Boeck J. Ocular changes in periarteritis nodosa. Am J Ophthalmol 1956; 42:567–76.
14. Bredvik BK, Trocme SD. Ocular manifestations of immunological and rheumatological inflammatory disorders. Curr Opin Ophthalmol 1995; 6:92–6.
15. Brown RM, Mendis U. Retinal arteritis complicating herpes zoster ophthalmicus. Br J Ophthal 1973; 57:344–6.

16. Brown TJ, Crawford SE, Cornwall ML et al. CD8 T lymphocytes and macrophages infiltrate coronary artery aneurysms in acute Kawasaki disease. J Infect Dis 2001; 184:940–3.
17. Bullen CL, Liesegan TJ, McDonald TJ, DeRemee RA. Ocular complications of Wegener's granulomatosis. Ophthalmology 1983; 90:279–90.
18. Burke MJ, Rennebohm RM. Eye involvement in Kawasaki disease. J Pediatr Ophthalmol Strabismus 1981; 18:7–11.
19. Carrington CB, Liebow AA. Limited forms of angiitis and granulomatosis of Wegener's type. Am J Med 1966; 41: 497–527.
20. Cassan SM, Divertie MB, Hollenhorst RW, Harrison EG Jr. Pseudotumor of the orbit and limited Wegener's granulomatosis. Ann Intern Med 1970; 72:687–93.
21. Castanon C, Amigo MC, Banales JV, et al. Ocular vaso-occlusive disease in primary antiphospholipid syndrome. Ophthalmology 1995; 102:256–62.
22. Charteris DG, Barton K, McCartney AC, Lightman SL. CD4+ lymphocyte involvement in ocular Behçet's disease. Autoimmunity 1992; 12:201–6.
23. Charteris DG, Champ C, Rosenthal AR, Lightman SL. Behçet's disease: activated T-lymphocytes in retinal perivasculitis. Br J Ophthalmol 1992; 76:499–501.
24. Chen S, Weinberg GA. Acute retinal necrosis syndrome in a child. Pediatr Infect Dis J 2002; 21:78–80.
25. Chowdhury T, Jalali S, Majji AB. Successful treatment of fungal retinitis and retinal vasculitis with oral itraconazole. Retina 2002; 22:800–2.
26. Chumbley LC, Harison EG, DeRemee RA. Allergic granulomatosis and angiitis (Churg–Strauss syndrome): report and analysis of 30 cases. Mayo Clin Proc 1977; 52: 477–84.
27. Churg J, Strauss L. Allergic granulomatosis, allergic angiitis, and periarteritis nodosa. Am J Pathol 1951; 27: 277–301.
28. Cimaz R, Falcini F. An update on Kawasaki disease. Autoimmun Rev 2003; 2:258–63.
29. Cogan DG. Corneoscleral lesions in periarterits nodosa and Wegener's granulomatosis. Trans Am Ophthalmol Soc 1955; 53:321–44.
30. Cohen Tervaert JW, Goldschmeding R, Elema JD, et al. Association of autoantibodies to myeloperoxidase with different forms of vasculitis. Arthritis Rheum 1990; 33: 1264–72.
31. Csernok E, Trabandt Am Muller A, et al. Cytokine profiles in Wegener's granulomatosis: predominance of type 1 (Th1) in the granulomatous inflammation. Arthritis Rheum 1999; 42:472–750.
32. Cupps TR, Fauci AS. Systemic necrotizing vasculitis of the polyarteritis nodosa group. In: Smith LH, ed. The Vasculitides: Major Problems in Internal Medicine. Philadelphia: WB Saunders Co., 1981; 21:26–49.
33. Cury D, Breakey AS, Payne BF. Allergic granulomatous angiitis associated with uveoscleritis and papilledema. Arch Ophthalmol 1956; 55:261–6.
34. DeRemee RA, McDonald TJ, Harrison EG, Coles DT. Wegener's granulomatosis: anatomic correlates, a proposed classification. Mayo Clin Proc 1976; 51:777–81.
35. Eichhorn J, Sima D, Thiele B, et al. Anti-endothelial cell antibodies in Takayasu's arteritis. Circulation 1996; 94: 2396–401.
36. Eiferman RA, Carothers DJ, Yankeelov JA. Peripheral rheumatoid ulceration and evidence for conjunctival collagenase production. Am J Ophthalmol 1979; 87:703–9.
37. Engstrom RE, Holland GN, Hardy WD, Meiselman HJ. Hemorrheologic abnormalities in patients with human immunodeficiency virus infection and ophthalmic microvasculopathy. Am J Ophthalmol 1990; 109:153–61.
38. Ewert BH, Jennette JC, Falk RJ. Anti-myeloperoxidase antibodies stimulate neutrophils to damage human endothelial cells. Kidney Int 1992; 41:375–83.
39. Faber DW, Wiley CA, Lynn GB, et al. Role of HIV and CMV in the pathogenesis of retinitis and retinal vasculopathy in AIDS patients. Invest Ophthalmol Vis Sci 1992; 33:2345–53.
40. Fauci AS, Haynes BF, Katz P, Wolff SM. Wegener's granulomatosis: prospective clinical and therapeutic experience with 85 patients for 21 years. Ann Intern Med 1983; 98:76–85.
41. Fauci AS, Wolff SM. Wegener's granulomatosis: studies in eighteen patients and a review of the literature. Medicine 1973; 52:535–61.
42. Fenton R, Easom H. Behçet's syndrome. Arch Ophthalmol 1964; 72:71–81.
43. Ford RG, Siekert RG. Central nervous system manifestations of periarteritis nodosa. Neurology 1965; 15:114–22.
44. Foster CS. Ocular manifestations of the nonrheumatic acquired collagen vascular diseases. In: Smolin G, Thoft RA, eds. The Cornea: Scientific Foundations and Clinical Practice. 2nd ed. Boston: Little, Brown, 1987:352–7.
45. Fountain JA, Werner RB. Tuberculous retinal vasculitis. Retina 1984; 4:48–50.
46. Frayer WC. The histopathology of perilimbal ulceration in Wegener's granulomatosis. Arch Ophthalmol 1960; 64: 58–64.
47. Freeman WR, Lerner CW, Mines JA, et al. A prospective study of the ophthalmologic findings in the acquired immune deficiency syndrome. Am J Ophthalmol 1984; 97:133–42.
48. Fujiwara H, Hamashima Y. Pathology of the heart in Kawasaki disease. Pediatrics 1978; 61:100–7.
49. Fye KH, Becker MJ, Theofilopoulos AN, et al. Immune complexes in hepatitis B antigen-associated periarteritis nodosa: detection by antibody dependent cell-mediated cytotoxicity and the Raji cell assay. Am J Med 1977; 62: 783–91.
50. George RK, Chan C-C, Whitcup SM, Nussenblatt RB. Ocular immunopathology of Behçets disease. Surv Ophthalmol 1997; 42:157–62.
51. Glace-Bernard A, Bayani N, Chretien P, et al. Antiphospholipid antibodies in retinal vascular occlusions. A prospective study of 75 patients. Arch Ophthalmol 1994; 112:790–5.
52. Glueck HI, Kant KS, Weiss MA, et al. Thrombosis in systemic lupus erythematosus: relation to the presence of lupus anticoagulants. Arch Intern Med 1985; 145: 1389–95.
53. Gold DH, Feiner L, Henkind P. Retinal arterial occlusive disease in systemic lupus erythematosus. Arch Ophthalmol 1977; 95:1580–5.
54. Gold DH, Morris A, Henkind P. Ocular findings in systemic lupus erythematosus. Br J Ophthalmol 1972; 56: 800–4.
55. Goldsmith J. Periarteritis nodosa with involvement of the choroidal and retinal arteries. Am J Ophthalmol 1946; 29: 435–46.
56. Harman LE, Margo CE. Wegener's granulomatosis. Surv Ophthalmol 1998; 42:458–80.
57. Harper SL, Letko E, Samson CM, et al. Wegener's granulomatosis: the relationship between ocular and systemic disease. J Rheumatol 2001; 28:1025–32.
58. Haynes BF, Fishman ML, Fauci AS, Wolff SM. The ocular manifestations of Wegener's granulomatosis. Fifteen

years experience and review of the literature. Am J Med 1977; 63:131–41.
59. Heiligenhaus A, Dutt JE, Foster CS. Histology and immunopathology of systemic lupus erythematosus affecting the conjunctiva. Eye 1996; 10:425–32.
60. Hellmich B, Ehlers S, Csernok E, Gross WL. Update on the pathogenesis of Churg–Strauss syndrome. Clin Exp Rheumatol 2003; 21(Suppl. 32):S69–77.
61. Hemady R, Chu W, Foster CS. Keratoconjunctivitis sicca and corneal ulcers. Cornea 1990; 9:170–3.
62. Henkind PK, Gold DH. Ocular manifestations of rheumatic disorders. Natural and iatrogenic. Rheumatology 1973; 4:13–59.
63. Herbort CP, Cimino L, Abu EL, Asrar AM. Ocular vasculitis: a multidisciplinary approach. Curr Opin Rheumatol 2005; 17:25–33.
64. Hoffman GS, Kerr GS, Leavitt RY, et al. Wegener granulomatosis: an analysis of 158 patients. Ann Intern Med 1992; 116:488–98.
65. Holland GN, Pepose JS, Petit TH, et al. Acquired immune deficiency syndrome: ocular manifestations. Ophthalmology 1983; 90:859–73.
66. Hsu CT, Kerrison JB, Miller NR, Goldberg MF. Choroidal infarction, anterior ischemic optic neuropathy, and central retinal artery occlusion from polyarteritis nodosa. Retina 2001; 21:348–51.
67. Ishohisa I, Numano F, Maezawa H, Sasazuki T. HLA-Bw52 in Takayasu's disease. Tissue Antigens 1978; 12: 246–8.
68. Jabs DA, Fine SL, Hochberg MC, et al. Severe retinal vaso-occlusive disease in systemic lupus erythematosus. Arch Ophthalmol 1986; 104:558–63.
69. Jabs DA, Green WR, Fox R, et al. Ocular manifestations of acquired immune deficiency syndrome. Ophthalmology 1989; 96:1092–9.
70. Jacob JL, Polomeno RC, Chad Z, Lapointe N. Ocular manifestations of Kawasaki disease (mucocutaneous lymph node syndrome). Can J Ophthalmol 1982; 17: 199–202.
71. Jennette JC. Implications for pathogenesis of patterns of injury in small- and medium-sized-vessel vasculitis. Cleve Clin J Med 2002; 69(Suppl.):SII-33–SII-38.
72. Jennette JC, Ewert BH, Falk RJ. Do antineutrophil cytoplasmic autoantibodies cause Wegener's granulomatosis and other forms of necrotizing vasculitis? Rheum Dis Clin North Am 1993; 19:1–14.
73. Jennette JC, Falk RJ. Vasculitis affecting the skin. Arch Dermatol 1994; 130:899–906.
74. Jennette JC, Falk RJ. Small-vessel vasculitis. N Engl J Med 1997; 337:1512–23.
75. Jennette JC, Falk RJ, Anddrassy K, et al. Nomenclature of systemic vasculitides. Proposal of an international consensus conference. Arthritis Rheum 1994; 37:187.
76. Jennette JC, Rosen J. Vasculitis. In: Damjanov I, Linden J, eds. Anderson's Pathology. Vol. 1, Chapter 47, 10th ed. St Louis, MO: Mosby, 1996:1421–45.
77. Jennette JC, Sciarrotta J, Takahashi K, Naoe S. Predominance of monocytes and macrophages in the inflammatory infiltrates of acute Kawasaki disease arteritis. Pediatr Res 2003; 53:173.
78. Jones DEP, Jayson MIV. Rheumatoid scleritis: a long-term follow up. Proc R Soc Med 1973; 66:1161–3.
79. Kallenberg CG. Autoantibodies in vasculitis: current perspectives. Clin Exp Rheumatol 1993; 11:355–60.
80. Kallenberg CG, Cohen Tervaeert JW, et al. Autoimmunity to lysosomal enzymes: new clues to vasculitis and glomerulonephritis? Immunol Today 1991; 12:61–4.
81. Kaiser M, Weyand CM, Bjomsson J, Goronzy JJ. Platelet derived growth factor, intimal hyperplasia, and ischaemic complications in giant cell arteritis. Arthritis Rheum 1998; 41:623–33.
82. Kato H, Koike S, Yamamoto M, et al. Coronary aneurysms in infants and young children with acute febrile mucocutaneous lymph node syndrome. J Pediatr 1975; 86:892–8.
83. Kattah JC, Mejico L, Chrousos GA, et al. Pathologic findings in a steroid-responsive optic nerve infarct in giant-cell arteritis. Neurology 1999; 53:177–80.
84. Kawasaki T. Mucocutaneous lymph node syndrome showing particular skin desquamation from the finger and toe in infants. Allergy 1967; 16:178–89.
85. Kawasaki T, Kosaki F, Okawa S, et al. A new infantile acute febrile mucocutaneous lymph node syndrome (MLNS) prevailing in Japan. Pediatrics 1974; 54:271–6.
86. Kerr GS, Hallahan CW, Giordano J, et al. Takayasu's arteritis. Ann Intern Med 1994; 120:919–29.
87. Klinhoff AV, Beatti CW, Chalmers A. Retinopathy in systemic lupus erythematosus: relationship to disease activity. Arthritis Rheum 1986; 29:1152–6.
88. Koffler D. The immunology of rheumatoid arthritis. Clin Symp 1979; 31:21–5.
89. Koyama T, Matsuo N, Watanabe Y, et al. Wegener's granulomatosis with destructive ocular manifestations. Am J Ophthalmol 1984; 98:736–40.
90. Kuo Y-H, Yip Y, Chen S-N. Retinal vasculitis associated with chickenpox. Am J Ophthalmol 2001; 132:584–5.
91. Lanham JG, Barrie T, Kohner EM, Hughes GR. SLE retinopathy: evaluation by fluorescein angiography. Ann Rheum Dis 1982; 41:473–8.
92. Lanza JT, Ku Y, Lucente FE, Har-El G. Wegener's granulomatosis of the orbit: lacrimal gland involvement as a major sign. Am J Otolaryngol 1995; 16:119–22.
93. Leavitt JA, Butrus SI. Wegener's granulomatosis presenting as dacryoadenitis. Cornea 1991; 10:542–5.
94. Levy-Clarke GA, Burrager R, Shen D, et al. Human T-cell lymphotropic virus type-1 associated T-cell leukemia/ lymphoma masquerading as necrotizing retinal vasculitis. Ophthalmology 2002; 109:1717–22.
95. Lie JT. Illustrated histopathologic classification criteria for selected vasculitis syndromes. Arthritis Rheum 1990; 33: 1074–87.
96. Locke IC, Cambridge G. Autoantibodies to neutrophil granule proteins: pathogenic potential in vasculitis? Br J Biomed Sci 1996; 53:302–16.
97. Ludviksson BR, Sneller MC, Chua KS, et al. Active Wegener's granulomatosis is associated with HLA-DR+ CD4+ cells exhibiting an unbalanced Th1-type T cell cytokine pattern: reversal with IL-10. J Immunol 1998; 160:3602–9.
98. Mamo J, Baghdassarian A. Behçet's disease. Arch Ophthalmol 1964; 71:38–48.
99. Mayet WJ, Hermann EM, Csernok E, Gross WL, Meyer zum Buschenfelde KHI. In vitro interactions of c-ANCA (antibodies to proteinase 3) with human endothelial cells. Adv Exp Med Biol 1993; 336:109–13.
100. Mayet WJ, Schwarting A, Meyer zum Buschenfelde K-H. Cytotoxic effects of antibodies to proteinase 3 (C-ANCA) on human endothelial cells. Clin Exp Immunol 1994; 97:458–65.
101. McGavin DD, Williamson J, Forrester JV, et al. Episcleritis and scleritis. A study of their clinical manifestations and association with rheumatoid arthritis. Br J Ophthalmol 1976; 60:192–226.
102. McLeod D, Marshall J, Kohner EM, Bird AC. The role of axoplasmic transport in the pathogenesis of cotton-wool spots. Br J Ophthalmol 1977; 61:177–91.

103. Meisler DM, Stock ES, Wertz RD, et al. Conjunctival inflammation and amyloidosis in allergic granulomatosis and angiitis (Churg–Strauss syndrome). Am J Ophthal 1981; 91:216–9.
104. Menezo V, Lightman S. The eye in systemic vasculitis. Clin Med 2004; 4:250–4.
105. Messmer EM, Foster CS. Vasculitic peripheral ulcerative keratitis. Surv Ophthalmol 1999; 43:379–96.
106. Messmer EM, Foster CS. Destructive corneal and scleral disease associated with rheumatoid arthritis. Cornea 1995; 14:408–17.
107. Mikkila HO, Seppala IJ, Viljanen MK, et al. The expanding clinical spectrum of ocular lyme borreliosis. Ophthalmology 2000; 107:581–7.
108. Monecucco C. Role of ANCA in the pathogenesis of Wegener's granulomatosis: a short review. Monaldi Arch Chest Dis 1994; 49:323–6.
109. Montehermoso A, Cervera R, Font J, et al. Association of antiphospholipid antibodies with retinal vascular disease in systemic lupus erythematosus. Semin Arthritis Rheum 1999; 28:326–32.
110. Moore JG, Sevel D. Corneo-scleral ulceration in periarteritis nodosa. Br J Ophthalmol 1966; 50:651–5.
111. Mullaney J, Collum LMT. Ocular vasculitis in Behçet's disease. Int Ophthalmol 1985; 7:183–91.
112. Nenoff P, Kellermann S, Horn LC, et al. Case report. Mycotic arteritis due to *Aspergillus fumigatus* in a diabetic with retrobulbar aspergillosis and mycotic meningitis. Mycoses 2001; 44:407–14.
113. Nissim F, Von der Valde J, Czernobilsky. A limited form of Churg–Strauss syndrome. Arch Pathol Lab Med 1982; 106:305–7.
114. Nolle B, Specks U, Ludemann J, et al. Anticytoplasmic autoantibodies, their immunodiagnostic value in Wegener's granulomatosis. Ann Intern Med 1989; 111:28–36.
115. Noris M. Pathogenesis of Takayasu's arteritis. J Nephrol 2001; 14:506–13.
116. Noris M, Daina E, Gamba S, et al. Interleukin-6 and RANTES in Takayasu's arteritis. A guide for therapeutic decisions? Circulation 1999; 100:55–60.
117. Novak MA, Green WR, Miller NR. Ophthalmological manifestations: a case of familial giant cell arteritis. Md Med J 1984; 33:817–20.
118. Penn H, Dasgupta B. Giant cell arteritis. Autoimmun Rev 2003; 2:199–203.
119. Pepose JS, Holland GN, Nestor MS, et al. Acquired immune deficiency syndrome: pathogenic mechanisms of ocular disease. Ophthalmology 1985; 92:472–84.
120. Purcell JJ, Birkenkamp R, Tsai CC. Conjunctival lesions in periarteritis nodosa. Arch Ophthalmol 1984; 102: 736–8.
121. Ramsay A, Lightman S. Hypopyon uveitis. Surv Ophthalmol 2001; 46:1–18.
122. Reeves JA. Keratopathy associated with systemic lupus erythematosus. Arch Ophthalmol 1965; 74:159–60.
123. Robinson MR, Lee SS, Sneller MC, et al. Tarsal-conjunctival disease associated with Wegener's granulomatosis Ophthalmology 2003; 110:1770–80.
124. Rokitansky K. Ueber einige der wichtigsten Krankheiten der Arterien. Denkschrift Kais Akad der Wissensch 1852; 4:49.
125. Sagar S, Ganguly NK, Koicha M, Sharma BK. Immunopathogenesis of Takayasu arteritis. Heart Vessels, Supplement, 1992; 7:85–90.
126. Savige J, Davies D, Falk RJ, et al. Antineutrophil cytoplasmic antibodies (ANCA) and associated diseases. Kidney Int 2000; 57:846–62.
127. Schilder DP, Harvey WP, Hufnagel C. Rheumatoid spondylitis and aortic insufficiency. Circulation 1955; 12: 770 [Abstract].
128. Schlaegel TF Jr, Kao SF. A review (1970–1980) of 28 presumptive cases of syphilitic uveitis. Am J Ophthalmol 1982; 93:412–4.
129. Seko Y, Minota S, Kawasaki A, et al. Perforin-secreting killer cell infiltration and expression of a 65-kD heat-shock protein in aortic tissue of patients with Takayasu's arteritis. J Clin Invest 1994; 93:750–8.
130. Sergent JS, Lockshin MD, Christian CL, Gocke DJ. Vasculitis with hepatitis B antigenemia: long-term observations in 9 patients. Medicine 1976; 55:1–18.
131. Shields CL, Shields JA, Rozanski TI. Conjunctival involvement in Churg–Strauss syndrome. Am J Ophthalmol 1986; 102:601–5.
132. Sneller MC. Granuloma formation, implications for the pathogenesis of vasculitis. Cleveland Clin J Med 2002; 69 (Suppl. 2):SII40–3.
133. Sneller MC, Fauci AS. Pathogenesis of vasculitis syndromes. Adv Rheum 1997; 81:221–42.
134. Soukiasian SH, Foster CS, Niles JL, Raizman MB. Diagnostic value of antineutrophil cytoplasmic antibodies in scleritis associated with Wegener's granulomatosis. Ophthalmology 1992; 99:125–32.
135. Stafford-Brady FJ, Urowitz MB, Gladman DD, Easterbrook M. Lupus retinopathy: patterns, associations and prognosis. Arthritis Rheum 1988; 31:1105–10.
136. Stavrou P, Deutsch J, Rene C, et al. Ocular manifestations of classical and limited Wegener's granulomatosis. Q J Med 1993; 86:719–25.
137. Straatsma BR. Ocular manifestations of Wegener's granulomatosis. Am J Ophthalmol 1957; 44:789–99.
138. Sulewski ME, Green WR. Ocular histopathologic features of a presumed case of Rocky Mountain spotted fever. Retina 1986; 6:125–30.
139. Sundy JS, Haynes BF. Pathogenic mechanisms of vessel damage in vasculitis syndromes. Rheum Dis Clin North Am 1995; 21:861–81.
140. Taauber J, Sainz de la Maza M, Hoang-Xuan T, Foster CS. An analysis of therapeutic decision making regarding immunosuppressive chemotherapy for peripheral ulcerative keratitis. Cornea 1990; 9:66–73.
141. Takanashi T, Uchida S, Arita M, et al. Orbital inflammatory pseudotumor and ischemic vasculitis in Churg–Strauss syndrome: report of two cases and review of the literature. Ophthalmology 2001; 108:1129–33.
142. Taubert KA. Epidemiology of Kawasaki disease in the United States and worldwide. Prog Pediatr Cardiol 1997; 6:181–5.
143. Thomas JE, Jabs JA. Ocular manifestations of vasculitis. Rheum Dis Clin North Am 2001; 27:761–79.
144. van der Woude FJ, Rasmussen N, Lobatto S, et al. The TH: autoantibodies against neutrophils and monocytes: tools for diagnosis and marker of disease activity in Wegener's granulomatosis. Lancet 1985; 1:425–9.
145. Van Wien S, Merz EH. Exophthalmos secondary to periarteritis nodosa. Am J Ophthalmol 1963; 56:204–8.
146. Vollertson RS, Conn DL. Vasculitis associated with rheumatoid arthritis. Rheum Dis Clin North Am 1990; 16:445–6.
147. Watson PG, Hayreh SS. Scleritis and episcleritis. Brit J Ophthalmol 1976; 60:163–91.
148. Wegener F. Uber eine eigenartige rhinogene Granulomatose mit besonderer Beteiligung des Arteriensystems und der Nieren. Beitr Pathol Anat 1939; 102:36 68.

149. Weinstein JM, Chui H, Lane S, Corbett J, Towfighi J. Churg–Strauss syndrome (allergic granulomatous angiitis). Neuro-ophthalmologic manifestations. Arch Ophthalmol 1983; 101:1217–20.
150. Weyand CM, Goronzy JJ. The molecular basis of rheumatoid arthritis. J Mol Med 1997; 75:772–85.
151. Weyand CM, Goronzy JJ. The pathogenesis of giant cell arteritis. Bull Rheum Dis 2002; 51:111.
152. Weyand CM, Hicok KC, Hunder GG, Goronzy JJ. Tissue cytokine patterns in patients with polymyalgia rheumatica and giant cell arteritis. Ann Intern Med 1994; 121:484–91.
153. Weyand CM, Tetzlaff N, Bjomsson J, et al. Disease patterns and tissue cytokine profiles in giant cell arteritis. Arthritis Rheum 1997; 40:19–26.
154. Whitcup SM. Involvement of cell adhesion molecules in the pathogenesis of experimental autoimmune uveoretinitis. Ocular Immunol Inflamm 1995; 3:53–6.
155. Whitcup SM, Chan CC, Li Q, Nussenblatt RB. Expression of cell adhesion molecules in posterior uveitis. Arch Ophthalmol 1992; 110:662–6.
156. Wise GN. Ocular periarteritis nodosa. Report of two cases. Arch Ophthalmol 1952; 48:1–11.
157. Yanagawa H, Nakamura Y, Yashiro M, Hirose K. Results of 12 nationwide surveys of Kawasaki disease. In: Kato H, ed. Kawasaki Disease. New York: Elsevier, 1995:14.
158. Zaman AG, Edelsten C, Stanford MR, et al. Soluble intercellular adhesion molecule-1 (sICAM-1) as a marker of disease relapse in idiopathic uveoretinitis. Clin Exp Immunol 1994; 95:60–5.
159. Zeek P, Smith CC, Weeter JC. Studies on periarteritis nodosa. III. The differentiation between the vascular lesions of periarteritis nodosa and of hypersensitivity. Am J Pathol 1948; 24:889–917.

70

Ocular Involvement in Disorders of the Nervous System

Gordon K. Klintworth and Thomas J. Cummings
Departments of Pathology and Ophthalmology, Duke University, Durham, North Carolina, U.S.A.

INTRODUCTION

Vision, one of the most complex of all sensations interpreted by the nervous system, is dependent upon the integrity of pathways within the brain that comprise neurons, neuroglia, as well as blood vessels and other connective tissue elements.

Apart from the usual pathologic processes such as inflammation, developmental anomalies, vascular disorders and neoplasia that affect most tissues the brain is prone to unique disorders that can be arbitrarily divided into diseases primarily of white matter (disorders of myelin) or gray matter (neuronal disorders). The optic nerve is involved in many conditions that affect the white matter of the central nervous system (CNS) and optic nerve demyelination, optic neuritis and optic atrophy are features of numerous neurologic disorders.

DISORDERS OF MYELIN

The myelin sheaths of axons within the optic nerve and other parts of the CNS are synthesized by oligodendrocytes and consist of this cell's external plasma membrane in the form of bimolecular lipid leaflets twisted in a spiral manner around the nerve axons. Oligodendrocytes express several specific antigens and enzymes (galactocerebroside, galactosulphatide, carbonic anhydrase C, 2′,3′-cyclic nucleotide 3′-phosphohydrolase, glycerol-3-phosphate dehydrogenase and lactate dehydrogenase). Myelin is composed of aggregates of lipid (such as monogalactosylceramide, ethanolamine phospholipid, long-chain fatty acids, galactosyl ceramides and cholesterol), proteins [myelin-associated glycoprotein and myelin basic proteins—A_1, P_1, P_2, small basic protein, pre-basic proteins, intermediate protein, proteolipid protein (see section on Pelizaeus–Merzbacher disease), Wolfgram protein, peripheral myelin glycoprotein P0] and glycosaminoglycans (GAGs) (72). The metabolic turnover of most of these components is slow, but some proteins are metabolized more rapidly (193).

Disorders of myelin include conditions in which the myelin sheath becomes destroyed after it has formed (demyelinating diseases) as well as entities in which the myelin sheath does not form normally (leukodystrophies or dysmyelinating diseases). Myelin may be destroyed non-specifically under natural circumstances as a result of viral infections, nutritional deficiencies, anoxic and toxic insults, immunopathologic reactions, as well as experimentally (59,159). The connotation demyelinating diseases designates disorders with early myelin destruction often disproportionate to the injury noted in the axons, neurons, and neuroglia. Demyelinating diseases include multiple sclerosis (MS), neuromyelitis optica, subacute sclerosing panenecephalitis (SSPE) (see Chapter 8), progressive multifocal leukoencephalopathy (PML) (see Chapter 8), and acute disseminated encephalomyelitis. Depending on the cause axonal damage may be conspicuous. Since myelin represents the cell membrane of oligodendrocytes, degenerative changes in this cell type are usually prominent in demyelinating states. Microglia and blood-derived macrophages phagocytose degenerated myelin following its destruction. Loss of phospholipids, an increase of esterified cholesterol, proteolysis, and GAG breakdown accompanies demyelination. Astrocytes later proliferate and impart a sclerotic texture to the lesions, but fibroblasts because of their paucity within the CNS other than in the optic nerve do not contribute significantly to this reaction.

Multiple Sclerosis

Introduction

MS, also called disseminated sclerosis, is the most common disease of the human CNS in which myelin is destroyed without damage to axons. The disease with its characteristic pathological features first became recognized as an entity slightly more than a century ago (36). The phenotype of multiple sclerosis is wide-ranging with fulminating as well as chronic forms.

Clinical Features

This chronic relapsing and remitting disorder is typified by symptoms and signs pointing to multiple episodes of randomly located lesions in the CNS, which are disseminated in both time of onset and place. The term "multiple sclerosis" stresses the multitude of lesions, whereas "disseminated sclerosis" underscores their temporal and spatial dissemination. Poor health, fatigue, acute infections, trauma, allergic conditions, exposure to cold, and emotional upsets appear to provoke the acute episodes of MS, but how these factors operate remains unknown. Classical MS (Charcot type) usually commences in early adulthood during the second to fourth decades of life. It rarely becomes symptomatic in childhood or in persons older than 50 years of age. The onset is generally rather abrupt, often within a period of hours or days, and may be manifest as visual, or other neurological disturbances. As a rule this is followed within a few days or weeks by significant improvement with little functional deficit, probably when edema regresses and axonal conduction is restored. Nystagmus, intention tremor, and scanning speech (Charcot triad) may be present in the early stages. At first the clinical diagnosis is difficult; a requirement being that various lesions appear at different times in different parts of the CNS. Occasionally, the manifestations such as a reduction in visual acuity are accentuated by vigorous exercise (Uhthoff syndrome) or by a hot bath.

The clinical picture of MS is highly variable not only with regard to the symptoms and signs, which depend on the location of the lesions, but also in the severity, time course, and progression of the disease. Ninety percent of patients have spontaneous remissions and relapses in the early stages with intervals of months or years preceding a relapse. MS is usually progressive with increasingly more severe episodes, each of which results in additional, permanent disability due to the accumulated incomplete recovery from each lesion. A slow, continuous deterioration of the neurologic status often becomes apparent late in the course of the disease, with fatality in 5 to 25 years or more. In some individuals, MS is inexorably progressive, giving rise to almost total disability and death within 1 to 2 years of onset. In most patients MS is more indolent; relapses develop at intervals of several years. Some patients experience only one or two attacks or appear to recover completely after each of a series of attacks. Rarely, the disorder is asymptomatic, the only evidence of MS being old plaques found postmortem in brains of individuals with no history of neurological disease. In about one-third of patients, MS progresses so slowly, without serious disability, as not to reduce the life span. In a series of 241 patients studied by McAlpine (125) and followed for a minimum of 10 years, approximately one-third were dead, one-third were disabled, and one-third had no physical restrictions or disabilities. The longer the interval between the initial attack and the first relapse, the better the prognosis. Younger patients occasionally experience a severe fulminating illness from the onset, whereas an onset in middle life is usually associated with a more indolent course.

Presumably, some demyelinated axons transmit impulses, as vision may still be present in an eye that has a completely demyelinated optic nerve. Remission of symptoms can be accounted for on the assumption that demyelinated axons can transmit impulses. Nerve conduction becomes temporarily impaired during acute demyelination, while permanent disability follows the axonal degeneration or interference with nerve conduction by poorly understood mechanisms.

Ocular Manifestations

The visual system and ocular motor apparatus are affected by disorders such as optic neuritis and internuclear ophthalmoplegia (63). The myelinated axons within the CNS which are concerned with visual function are commonly affected in MS. Ophthalmologic findings include nystagmus from involvement of the vestibular system in the brainstem (about 70% of cases). Palsies of nerves that innervate the extraocular muscles, disturbances of conjugate gaze, and visual field defects occur due to plaques in the various parts of the visual pathways. Diplopia in most instances is of the type known as internuclear ophthalmoplegia (from involvement of the medial longitudinal fasciculus), and bilateral internuclear ophthalmoplegia is virtually pathognomonic of MS.

The optic nerve of one or both eyes is frequently affected in MS, particularly in Asia, where it is frequently bilateral and severe from the onset. The initial clinical manifestations of MS may be a sudden visual field loss or a loss of central visual acuity. The maculopapillary fibers of the optic nerve appear to be preferentially involved. As with lesions elsewhere in the CNS, the first incident in the optic nerve frequently causes a transient loss of function (impaired central visual acuity and visual field defects) that persists for only several days or weeks before complete or almost total recovery; less often the lesion is serious and culminates in permanent visual loss. Succeeding incidents may affect the same or the contralateral eye. Acute optic neuritis or retrobulbar neuritis is the first clinical evidence of the disease in 15% of patients, and about 70% of patients hospitalized for MS eventually develop optic neuritis. Traub and Rucker (206) followed 87 patients 10 to 15 years after an initial bout of retrobulbar neuritis and found that 28 (32.2%) developed evidence of MS. Twenty-six of these patients were 20 to 40 years old at the time of the first bout, indicating that an individual in this age group who has an initial episode of retrobulbar neuritis has a 40% to 50% chance of developing other manifestations of MS within 10 to 15 years. When retrobulbar neuritis begins in persons older than 40 years, the chance of acquiring MS is remote (206). Since this study by Traub and Rucker, however, others have found subsequent demyelinating episodes in 11.5% to 85% of cases of retrobulbar neuritis (32,106,126). The risk of a patient with uncomplicated optic neuritis developing MS has been found in a prospective study to be about 35% (40).

During the course of the illness, visual impairment is a feature of 34% of cases in the United States, but in Japan, where MS is rare and differs clinically from that of the so-called Western countries, 70% of patients develop visual symptoms. In Japan, visual impairment is common at the onset, the optic nerves and the spinal cord are predominantly involved and the disease tends to be severe and rapidly progressive (189).

In 1944, Rucker (176) drew attention to the frequent perivenous sheathing of retinal veins in patients with MS, an observation that has been repeatedly confirmed (Fig. 1). Although this fundoscopic abnormality is extremely common in patients with peripheral uveitis due to various causes, the small white clouds and sheaths about retinal veins in MS form without the usual visible accompaniments of uveitis, such as hemorrhage, cells in the vitreous, or a pigment disturbance. Such lesions may remain unchanged for many months or years, and in some instances round dot-like opacities with the diameter of a medium-sized vein are visible in the vitreous close of the retina (Rucker bodies) (179). The incidence of perivenous sheathing in MS ranges from 1.5% to 42% of cases (10,54,79,178,179). The sheathing of retinal veins in MS corresponds to a perivenous infiltrate of lymphocytes sometimes with plasma cells (7,58,62,187,204) (Fig. 2). Some histopathologic studies of the retina in MS have disclosed an apparent rarefaction of the ganglion cells (67,204) and perhaps relevant to this is the finding of tissue-bound IgG on ganglion cells in several cases of MS, but not in controls (123).

Several authors have drawn attention to the higher incidence of peripheral uveitis (pars planitis, chronic cyclitis) in patients with MS compared with the general population (6,10,24,26,68). In a study of 53 patients with MS, Breger and Leopold (24) detected a peripheral uveitis in 14 subjects (27%) and in nine of these patients the disease was active while the other five were quiescent. The uveal disease may antecede the neurologic involvement by several years (68), yet the significance of the association between uveitis and MS remains uncertain, and histologic examinations of eyes in such cases have not been performed. The retinal arterioles appear unaffected (94,105,146, 177,178,207,226), but the venous branches peripheral to the area of sheathing may become engorged and bleed. Yet, unlike the peripheral periphlebitis of Eales disease (see Chapter 67), hemorrhages are not associated with most of these mild perivascular lesions. Sheathing and progressive obliteration of peripheral retinal veins, peripheral and posterior uveitis, retinitis proliferans, retinal neovascularization, and retinal microaneurysms have been documented in patients with MS (6,26,138). Although some of these nonspecific ocular manifestations (perivenous sheathing and peripheral uveitis) seem to be more frequent in

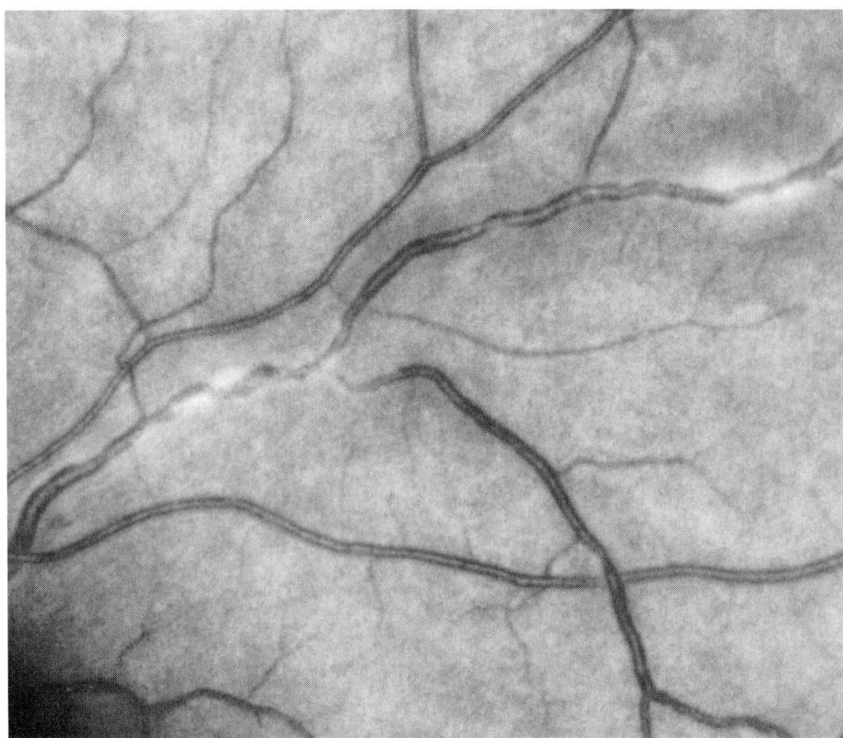

Figure 1 Periphlebitic venous sheathing in a patient with multiple sclerosis. *Source*: Reproduced from Wise GN, Dollery CT, Henkind P. The Retinal Circulation. New York: Harper and Row, 1971; p. 208.

subjects with MS than in the general population, others (microaneurysms, retinal neovascularization) are not significantly more common in MS than one would expect by the chance association of coincidental diseases.

Histopathology

In patients dying with MS, specific lesions are restricted to the CNS with those occurring elsewhere being either unrelated to the disease or secondary to it such as the muscle contractures that eventually develop in many cases. Peripheral nerves are not involved and all other organs are normal in the uncomplicated case.

In classic MS numerous circumscribed areas of focal demyelination of different ages are found throughout the CNS, where any part can be affected. The lesions are usually readily apparent to the naked

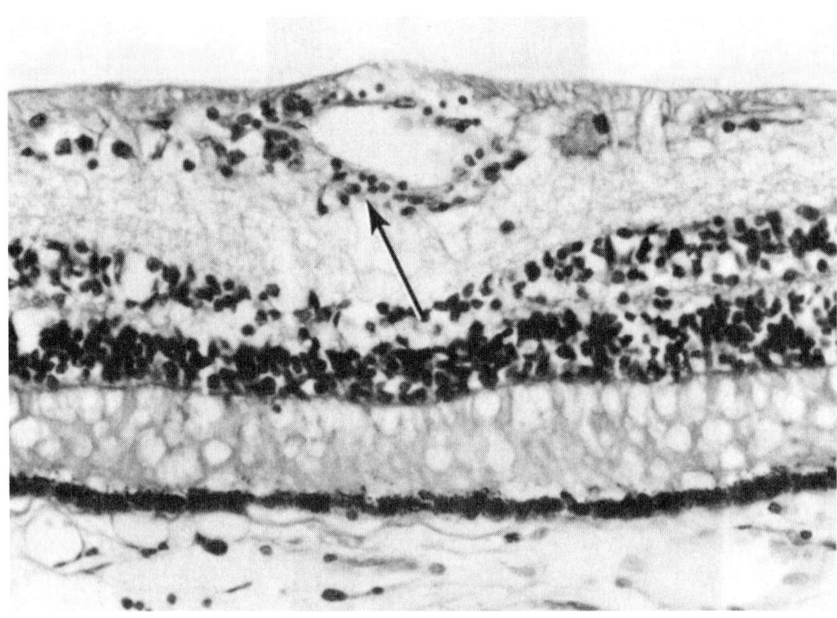

Figure 2 Perivenous lymphocytic infiltrate (*arrow*) in retina of patient with multiple sclerosis (hematoxylin and eosin, ×305).

eye in cross sections of the brain, appearing in the gray and white matter as patches with sharply demarcated edges (Figs. 3 and 4). In the living patient MS plaques are readily visualized with magnetic resonance imaging (MRI) (Fig. 5). The larger areas of demyelination are usually irregular in shape with a lobulated outline. The abnormal regions vary in color; the recent ones tend to be pink while the older ones, which are firm in the unfixed brain, are gray. Although the word sclerosis is descriptive of the firm texture of the numerous gliotic (sclerotic) foci, early lesions are softer in consistency than normal brain. Traditionally, the areas of myelin destruction have been termed plaques; however, they are not flat discs but have spherical, ovoid, or other three-dimensional configurations. The axons or nerve cell bodies are more or less uninvolved, but destruction of axons may be noted in some of the oldest lesions. Although, as mentioned above, the distribution of the "plaques" varies considerably from case to case, they are commonly contiguous with the ventricles, especially the outer angles of the lateral ventricles, the floor of the sylvian aqueduct, and the fourth ventricle (62). Demyelinated foci in the cerebral white matter tend to stop short of the cerebral cortex leaving intact about 1 mm of subcortical myelin. In the spinal cord, a thin rim of subpial white matter is also frequently spared. In contrast to other neurologic diseases, the myelin sheaths and axons distal to the lesions either do not undergo a series of morphologic degenerative changes (Wallerian degeneration) or such alterations are minimal.

In tissue sections MS plaques are optimally visualized in preparations stained for myelin, such as luxol fast blue (LFB) or the Weil stain. Dyes, like the Holzer stain, that accentuate glial tissue may be useful in disclosing older gliotic lesions. The dimensions, distribution, and age of MS plaques vary extensively from case to case. The preserved axons and cell bodies within the plaques of MS differentiate the lesions of MS from infarcts.

While the histologic appearance of the plaques in MS varies considerably with their age, loss of myelin in the presence of preservation of axons and nerve cell bodies is a striking feature. In long-standing plaques, as well as in some recent lesions, a loss of oligodendrocytes is conspicuous. However, in some recent plaques, that are believed to be slightly older than the acute lesions, numerous cells of oligogendrocyte origin are abundant, presumably secondary to a reactive hyperplasia (158). These cells, which appear on the basis of immunocytochemical markers to be phenotypically undifferentiated oligodendrocytes, are thought to account for the extensive remyelination present in some plaques (157). Some plaques do not entirely lack myelin (shadow plaques) and in long-standing plaques there is commonly a partial destruction of axons. Perivascular lymphocytic cuffing, usually modest in degree, commonly occurs within or around the lesions; this feature is often more

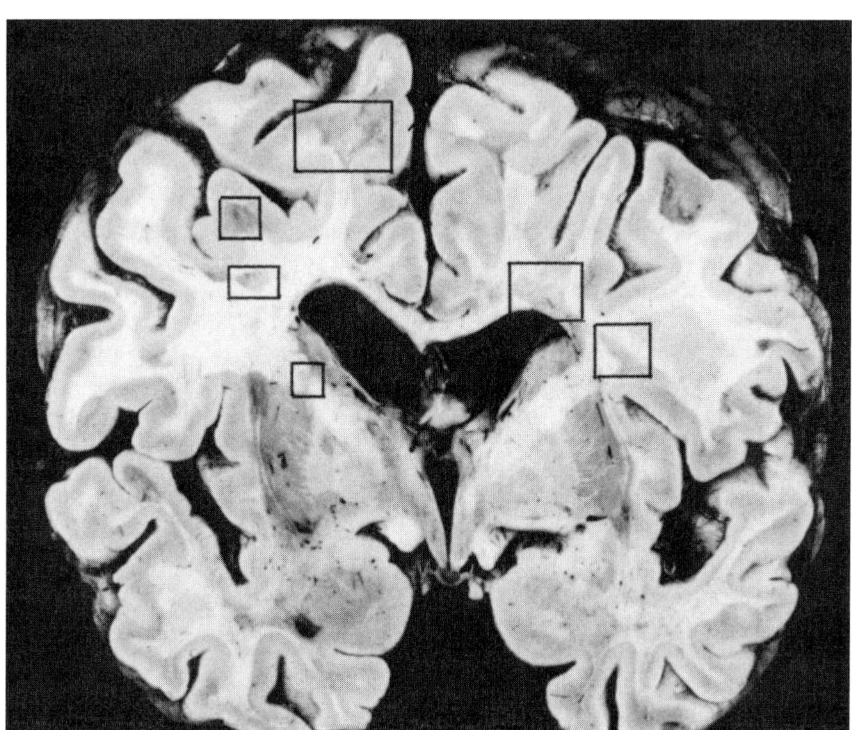

Figure 3 Coronal section through cerebral hemispheres showing plaques (*in boxes*) in a brain with multiple sclerosis.

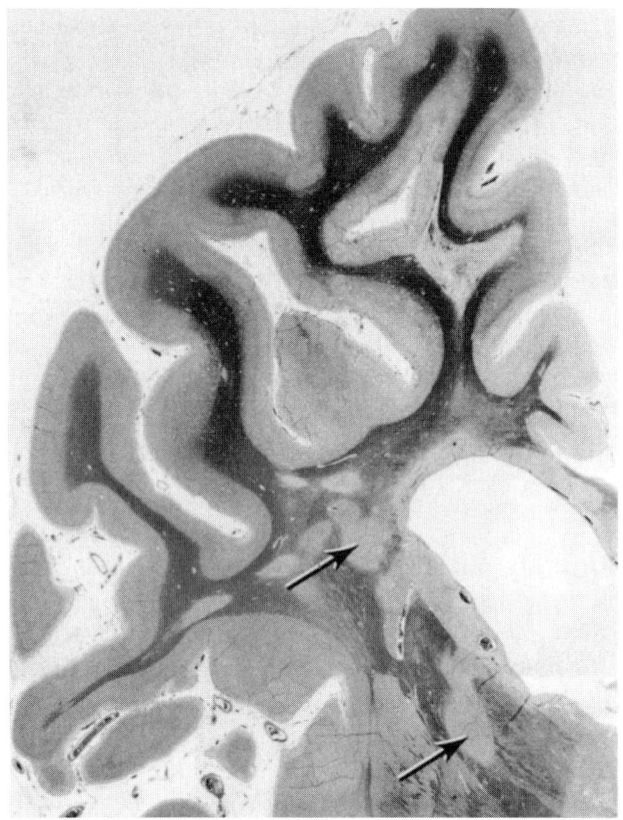

Figure 4 Higher magnification of multiple sclerotic plaques showing sharp line of demarcation between normal myelin and demyelinated area (*arrows*) (hematoxylin and eosin, luxol fast blue, × 1.7).

prominent in older lesions. The plaques of MS are commonly surrounded by dense rings of macrophages/reactive microglia that express the human leucocyte antigen-DR (HLA-DR) (23). These cells expressing the MHC class II glycoprotein are believed to play a pivotal role in presenting antigen to T-helper/inducer (CD4+) lymphocytes.

Apart from differences in the appearance of the plaques, which relate to the age of the lesion, there seems to be a continuous variation from the typical, relatively indolent lesions, to those which characterize the severe atypical clinical cases in which the tempo of the pathologic processes is accelerated. In the latter patients, the lesions tend to be more destructive, and then axis cylinders and even nerve cell bodies are destroyed. The cellular reaction is also more intense, with an extensive perivascular infiltration of lymphocytes and lesser numbers of plasma cells. Such rapidly progressive tumefactive demyelinating plaques (demyelinating pseudotumors) can clinically and radiographically mimic the features of a neoplasm including glioblastoma. The diagnosis is confirmed by the recognition of a dense macrophage infiltrate with preserved axons within the lesion. This is best demonstrated by an immunohistochemical stain for components of axons, such as neurofilament protein, and may help distinguish the lesion from an infarct, whereby the axons are typically destroyed. The macrophage population can be highlighted by a Ham56 immunostain. There is often reactive astrogliosis within and adjacent to the lesion, a feature which can be shown with a glial fibrillary acidic protein (GFAP) immunostain. LFB staining shows a paucity of myelin, some of which is seen within the cytoplasm of the macrophages. Other histological clues pointing to a reactive pathological process including demyelination are reactive astrocytes with dispersion of their chromosomes "granular mitoses," and large protoplasmic glial cells containing fragmented chromatin (Creutzfeldt cells).

The "plaques" of MS have been extensively investigated by transmission electron microscopy (TEM), and although many studies were concerned principally with descriptive morphology, others have disclosed structures resembling paramyxovirus nucleocapsids within some plaques (155,165,199,217), but as discussed elsewhere in this section, the significance of this observation remains unknown.

Thorough histopathologic studies of the optic nerve during the initial stages of their involvement in MS have not been reported, but are presumably identical to those elsewhere in the brain.

Variants of Multiple Sclerosis

Besides the classical form of MS (Charcot type) described above, other rare variants of the disease, in which more destructive lesions are generally found, are recognized in a younger age group.

Acute Multiple Sclerosis (Marburg Type)

Some patients die after an acute or subacute illness with lesions that are virtually all of recent onset and are necrotizing with a more florid inflammatory cellular reaction (148) than is customary in the Charcot type of the disease. As in the Schilder and Devic types of MS, this variant of the disease is common in younger patients and is often preceded by, or accompanied by, a febrile illness (148).

Neuromyelitis Optica (Devic Type)

The designation Devic disease refers to the combination of severe visual impairment and paraplegia occurring within several days or weeks of each other due to demyelinating lesions in the optic nerves and spinal cord (38,107,195). Most cases are believed to be examples of acute MS, but the same clinical picture can arise from other causes, such as acute disseminated encephalomyelitis. Patients with Devic disease seldom die as an immediate result of their illness and consequently knowledge about the histopathology of the more benign cases of Devic disease is sparse (159).

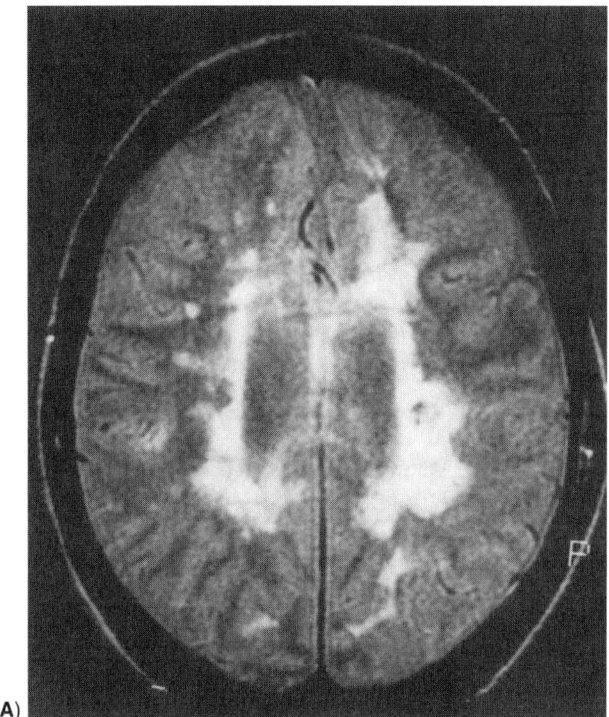

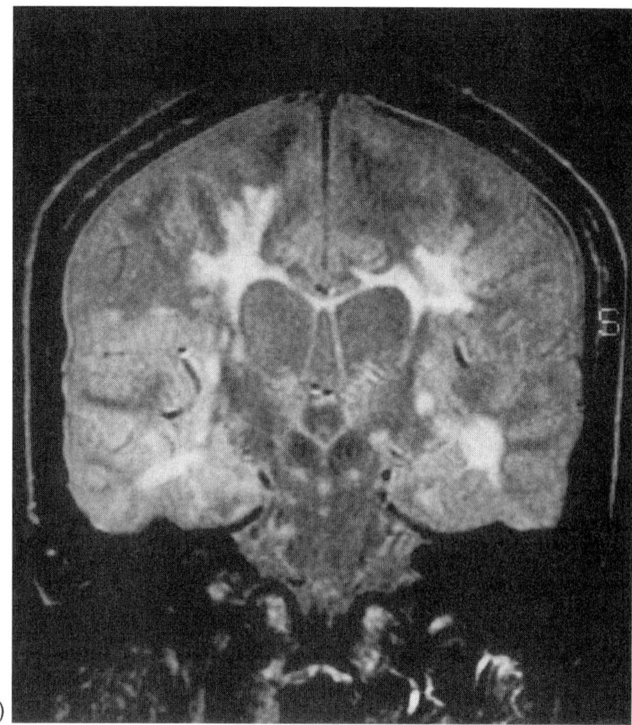

Figure 5 The plaques of multiple sclerosis appear white and are readily seen in the living patient with the aid of magnetic resonance imaging. (**A**) Horizontal section through head. (**B**) Coronal section. *Source*: Courtesy of Dr. O.B. Boyko.

Postmortem examinations in most lethal cases, however, have disclosed dispersed demyelinating lesions with attributes of acute MS, but frequently with considerable axonal degeneration. These lesions, which are of variable age, have a predisposition for the optic nerves and upper thoracic spinal cord, but may also involve other parts of the CNS, such as the brainstem and cerebral hemispheres. Necrosis is often a conspicuous feature of the lesions in the spinal cord and optic chiasm, and this is believed to occur as a consequence of ischemia secondary to the acute edema that develops in these sites that possess a limited ability to undergo rapid expansion because of their constraining coverings. The necrosis frequently leads to cavitation, especially in the spinal cord, but also sometimes in the optic chiasm. The extent of the gliosis reflects the intensity of the necrosis and duration of survival.

Although the lesions in milder cases may be indistinguishable from the "plaques" of acute MS, severe cases have massive areas of central demyelination with destruction of axons, and occasionally central liquefaction of the optic chiasm. Since tissue necrosis is not regarded as a feature of MS, some regard its presence as testimony of a different disease. However, the necrotic lesions in the optic nerve and spinal cord may be secondary to ischemia caused by severe edema, which sometimes accompanies acute lesions in MS. Indeed, the spinal cord is frequently explored surgically in Devic syndrome and found to be swollen. Apart from the necrotic and demyelinated portions of the optic nerves and spinal cord, the remainder of the CNS is often normal apart from Wallerian degeneration.

Neuromyelitis optica clinically resembles subacute myelo-optico-neuropathy which occurs in Japan and Latin America and which has been attributed to Entero-Vioform (clioquinol) (107). From the late 1950s until 1972 it is estimated that more than 10,000 individuals with subacute myelo-optico-neuropathy were diagnosed in Japan. A herpes virus related to avian infectious laryngotracheitis virus has been isolated from the feces and cerebrospinal fluid (CSF) of patients with subacute myelo-optico-neuropathy (89) and may be a causal agent of this entity. Neuromyelitis optica has been associated with pulmonary tuberculosis (11) raising the possibility that the disorder is a sequel to an immunological reaction.

Schilder Type

The Schilder type of MS has a more rapid course than the usual variety and a clinical picture dominated by progressive loss of intellectual functions due to extensive, usually confluent, areas of demyelinization in the cerebral hemispheres with or without small lesions elsewhere. In childhood the lesions are usually not associated with disseminated plaques, and the disease is typically characterized by an acute or subacute progressive course with mental disturbances, blindness and deafness. In acute cases, with large destructive lesions, there is often considerable cerebral edema, and a brain tumor or encephalitis is often suspected clinically. Should the affected tissue be biopsied, the pathologist may face a difficult diagnostic problem since the astrocytic proliferation may be prominent and some astrocytes may be enormous and multinucleated, suggestive of a glioma. When disseminated plaques are present, the age of onset and the clinical course are usually indistinguishable from the Charcot type of MS (discussed above), with extensive involvement of the cerebral white matter.

In the past the connotation Schilder disease (diffuse sclerosis) was applied to a heterogeneous group of idiopathic neurologic disorders primarily of childhood. Some Schilder cases probably included adrenoleucodystrophy, subacute sclerosing encephalitis, and other disorders with diffuse cerebral damage.

Concentric Sclerosis (Balo Type)

This rare pathological curiosity is characterized by laminated concentric zones of demyelination separated by narrow bands of more or less intact myelin. Most cases have occurred in the second and third decades of life and have been typified clinically by a rapid fulminant neurological illness (43).

Etiology and Pathogenesis

Ever since MS became recognized as an entity, this disease has challenged the minds of innumerable investigators and a single dominant mechanism for its pathogenesis has not yet emerged. Morphologic, epidemiologic, and immunologic observations on this disease have revealed information relevant to our understanding of the disease, but a similar disease is not known to occur naturally in animals, and a comparable condition has not been produced experimentally. A systemic infection has been hypothesized to cause the regulation of adhesion molecules on the vascular endothelium of the brain and spinal cord, allowing leukocytes to traverse blood vessel walls and enter the normally immunologically privileged CNS. Lymphocytes may then be able to trigger a cascade of events resulting in the formation of an acute inflammatory, demyelinating lesion, especially if they are programmed to recognize myelin antigen (64).

Morphologic Clues to the Pathogenesis

The basic morphologic lesion is the destruction of myelin within the CNS. This is followed by its phagocytosis by macrophages and subsequently by an astrocytic proliferation with a production of glial fibrils. The perivenous location of small multiple sclerotic "plaques" (55,60,61) as well as their frequent periventricular distribution, suggests a myelinolytic substance that diffuses from the blood or CSF or both. The existence of such a substance is underscored by the observation that sera from patients with MS can destroy myelin in tissue culture (22,164). A humoral immune process seems to be operative, since complement and immunoglobulins have been demonstrated in the active plaques (124,203), but whether cellular hypersensitivity plays a role in MS remains uncertain (15). Trypan blue, which does not normally cross the blood–brain barrier leaks from the cerebral veins in MS plaques following perfusions of the brain with this dye (30). The role of this breakdown in the blood–brain barrier in the genesis of the lesion also remains to be established, but a breach in the blood–brain barrier in a person who is genetically predisposed to the disease is generally believed to be the origin of the histological hallmark of the multiple sclerosis plaque.

Contribution of Epidemiology

Epidemiologic investigations indicate that the incidence of MS varies considerably in different geographic areas and that critical environmental factors influence the appearance of the disease. A high-frequency band occurs in the northern temperate zones of Europe and North America and in southern Australia and New Zealand, while MS is uncommon in Asia (110) and rare in the tropics (1). The disease is nonexistent, or extremely rare, among African blacks. Currently 2.5 million people are suspected of having MS worldwide and about half a million people are estimated to have MS in the United States. Women are affected slightly more often than men, and whites more often than African blacks. Other ethnic groups such as Inuits and Southeast Asians are less likely to acquire MS. It is noteworthy that MS preferentially affects people from relatively high socioeconomic backgrounds (111).

Studies of migrant populations suggest that the risk of an individual developing MS depends on where the individual lived during the first 15 to 20 years of life. Residence in high-risk regions during that age period retain a high incidence of MS (47,109). Thus, an emigrant from a high- to a low-risk area retains the high-risk or vice versa.

Genetic Aspects

Despite the lack a strong familial aggregation of MS much evidence suggests a genetic susceptibility to MS (141), including numerous documented familial cases (127), an increased prevalence of MS in affected families (183), and associations with immune response genes (13,92,142,200,221). Twin siblings, however, have not shown concordance rates compatible with a strong inherited predisposition (20,108). Genetic analyses have provided evidence that several genes are involved in the susceptibility to MS. These genes have been mapped to chromosome 1 (1q31–q32), chromosome 6 (6q21,6p21.3), and chromosome 16 (16p13). The identified genes are *PTPRC* (1q31–q32), which encodes protein tyrosine phosphatase receptor type C (also known as leukocyte common antigen) and CD24 (6q21). Certain major histocompatibility antigens are more frequent in patients with MS than in the population at large, but the specific histocompatibility genes that are found with an increased incidence in MS vary from country to country. In the Unites States and Europe, individuals with the antigens HLA-A3 and HLA-B7 have at least twice the risk of developing MS than individuals with other histocompatibility antigens (16,93,112,142). High-risk Northern European populations are associated with the HLA-DRB1*1501-DQB1*0602 haplotype.

Immunologic Aspects

Following extensive studies on the immune competence of patients with MS (5,91,121,143–145,165, 196,222) the following observations have been made: reduced T-cell responsiveness to mitogens, apparently linked to histocompatibility type (91,143,145); a reduction in circulating T cells with preservation of normal numbers of B cells (121,144,167); borderline suppressor T-cell activity in young, but not elderly patients with inactive MS and not in patients with recent exacerbations (5). The question remains unanswered whether the under-represented circulating population of T lymphocytes reflects the genetic endowment of patients with MS or an acquired loss of T cells. In patients with MS the lymphocyte reactivity to measles, parainfluenza, and vaccinia viruses does not differ significantly from controls until the subject becomes disabled. This suggests that the deficient cellular response to certain viruses is a consequence of the disease rather than a causal factor (196). Mutant T-cell clones isolated from the peripheral blood of MS patients have been found to proliferate in response to myelin basic protein (MBP), an antigen envisaged to partake in the induction of MS, even without prior exposure to this antigen (4). T cells that are reactive to MBP use the gene for the variable region of the T-cell receptor β (TCR Vβ) chain for the recognition of MBP. MBP has two immunodominant regions: residues MBP (84–102) and MBP (143–168). Individuals with MS have a higher frequency of T cells reactive with MBP (84–102) in their blood than do controls, and reactivity with MBP (84–102) is associated with the DR2 allele of the HLA region, while MBP (143–168) is associated with the DRwll allele (225). An analysis of the TCR Vβ genes used by T-cell lines from both MS and healthy individuals has disclosed that Vβ17 is selectively involved in the recognition of the immunodominant MBP (84–102). This finding is of potential value in the immunotherapy of MS as 60% of patients with MS are DR2+ (225).

Humoral immunity in MS has also attracted attention. The CSF immunoglobin G (IgG) is usually elevated (95,120,202) and the IgM is often elevated as well (221). The elevated immunoglobulin is oligoclonal in type and there is evidence for its synthesis within the CNS (120). That the antibody is formed locally in the CNS rather than from other sources points to the presence of antigenic stimulation within the neural tissue. Antibodies to myelin are present in serum of most patients and correlate with the active phases of the disease (124). Immunofluorescent studies have disclosed antimyelin antibodies, particularly of the IgG type, together with complement at the edges of demyelinated plaques (124).

One focus of research has centered on the role of CD4+ T cells and CD8+ T cells. Myelin-specific CD8+ T cells appear to be more abundant in patients with relapsing multiple sclerosis than in healthy persons. Also demonstrated within the CSF has been proliferation of B cells with increased mutations in B-cell receptors suggesting that a B-cell response to a specific antigen is occurring. The ability of myelin-specific T cells to cause inflammation in the CNS may be due to their cytokine-producing phenotype. Inflammatory immune or delayed hypersensitivity responses are primarily mediated by type 1 helper T cells (Th1) that produce gamma interferon (IFNγ). Myelin-reactive T cells from multiple sclerosis patients produce cytokines consistent with a Th1-mediated response whereas myelin-reactive T cells from healthy individuals are more likely to produce cytokines that characterize a type 2 helper T-cell mediated response (Th2). Several interleukins, including interleukin 12 (IL12), interleukin 17 (IL17), and interleukin 23 (IL23) have also been implicated in the regulation of T-cell responses that have potential relevance to multiple sclerosis (37).

Evidence for an Infectious Agent

An infectious agent has long been suspected, but nobody has isolated a pathogen that produces MS in experimental animals (156). Sabin and Messare (180) reported specific immunofluorescence for *Herpes simplex* in the tissues of several patients with MS and others have noted a slightly elevated titer of antimeasles antibodies in the serum and CSF in a high proportion of these patients (2,29,156) compared with control subjects. However, in contrast to SSPE (see Chapter 8), not all patients with MS have elevated levels of measles antibody. It is noteworthy that an antigenic similarity between measles virus and the most active constituent of brain extracts capable of inducing experimental allergic encephalomyelitis (encephalitogenic factor) of central myelin has been claimed (128). It seems unlikely that the measles virus is the causative agent of MS as its geographic distribution is difficult to reconcile with the worldwide presence of measles. Moreover, antibodies to various other common viruses, including herpes simplex, influenza, mumps, parainfluenza, poliomyelitis, and vaccinia are also often elevated in the serum and CSF in patients with MS (28,96,172). Structures resembling paramyxovirus nucleocapsids have been identified by TEM in mononuclear cells of plaques (155,165,199,217). However, viruses cannot be identified unequivocally by morphology alone and similar virus-like structures have been seen in a variety of unrelated conditions (113,155). More significantly, a parainfluenza type I virus, named 6/94, has been isolated by co-cultivation of brain tissue from two patients with MS (201).

Current Concept of Multiple Sclerosis

MS remains an elusive disorder, but the aforementioned epidemiologic, morphologic, genetic, and immunologic observations taken together are consistent with the hypothesis that MS has a genetic susceptibility. The causal agent is most likely a virus which is prevalent in some parts of the world and which usually causes trivial symptoms and a life-long immunity. Alternatively and rarely, perhaps because of a genetic susceptibility, an individual who seems unable to develop immunity to certain antigens and infectious agents develops MS. Some viral infections are characterized by long incubation periods, often many years preceding the overt disease. Since the recognition of such "slow viruses," a pathogen of this nature has been suspected in MS (60). A persistent (latent) virus disease analogous to SSPE (see Chapter 8) or an immunological disorder resulting from an infection akin to post-infective encephalomyelitis (191) both remain possible. The well established observation that persons who migrate from a region of high risk for MS to an area of low risk before the age of 15 years acquire the risk of their new home strongly suggests that exposure to the pathogen responsible for MS needs to occur before puberty.

ACUTE DISSEMINATED ENCEPHALOMYELITIS

Acute disseminated encephalomyelitis is characterized by an acute onset of multiple lesions throughout the CNS, including the optic nerve and other visual pathways. In contrast to MS the specific lesions are smaller (a few mm in diameter), but more extensive with a striking perivenous distribution in both gray and white matter (hence the older connotation of acute perivenous encephalomyelitis). There is an intense lymphocytic and plasma cell inflammatory response. The ultimate outcome is variable and, while sometimes fatal, a good recuperation may ensue.

Acute disseminated encephalomyelitis may follow a specific infection (particularly measles and vaccinia, but also smallpox, varicella, and influenza) (post-infectious encephalomyelitis) or vaccination (such as anti-rabies vaccination with emulsions of nervous tissue) (post-vaccinial encephalomyelitis). Sometimes the entity develops in the apparent absence of an antecedent vaccination or infection (spontaneous acute disseminated encephalomyelitis). An unusually fulminant variety of encephalomyelitis that affects mainly young men is typified by vessel wall necrosis, hemorrhage, and a prominent polymorphonuclear leukocytic infiltrate (acute hemorrhagic leukoencephalitis).

The human disease closely resembles experimental allergic encephalomyelitis induced by injecting foreign peripheral nerve tissue with Freund adjuvant (213). Guinea pigs sensitized with isogenic spinal cord emulsified with Freund adjuvant develop acute allergic optic neuritis with clinical features of "retrobulbar optic neuritis" and "neuroretinitis" and with histopathologic features of experimental acute disseminated encephalomyelitis (166). Such animals develop multiple foci of a mononuclear cell infiltrate in the retrobulbar portion of the optic nerve and chiasm with associated demyelination.

Leukodystrophies

A heterogeneous group of clinically distinct neurologic disorders is characterized by defective myelination of the CNS, a loss of sensory, motor, and intellectual functions and eventual death. These so-called leukodystrophies include metachromatic leukodystrophy, globoid (Krabbe) leukodystrophy (see Chapter 41), the adrenoleukodystrophies, Canavan disease, Pelizaeus–Merzbacher disease, Cockayne syndrome, and Alexander disease.

Adrenoleukodystrophies

The adrenoleukodystrophies are rare disorders characterized by mental and neurologic deterioration due to a diffuse paucity of myelin within the CNS and atrophic, hypofunctional adrenal glands (low plasma cortisol levels that do not increase after corticotropin administration). Very long-chain fatty acids (VLCFA) accumulate within various tissues, the serum and other body fluids because of their impaired oxidation (135,140). In the past many cases of adrenoleukodystrophy were designated Schilder disease (bronze Schilder disease).

Clinical Features

Bronzing of the skin and other clinical features of Addison disease may or may be evident (154) and adrenocortical disease may precede evidence of neurologic disease. Seven clinical variants of the X-linked adrenoleukodystrophy are recognized: childhood adrenoleukodystrophy (childhood cerebral form), adolescent adrenoleukodystrophy (adolescent cerebral form), adult adrenoleukodystrophy (adult cerebral form), adrenal insufficiency without neurologic disease, asymptomatic adrenoleukodystrophy, heterozygote adrenoleukodystrophy, and adrenomyeloneuropathy (139). In addition, there is an autosomal recessive neonatal adrenoleukodystrophy. The pathologic changes are comparable in these variants (73) and the biochemical alterations have similarities but are due to defects in different genes (*ABCD1, PEX1, PEX10, PEX13, PEX26*) involved in VLCFA metabolism. In childhood adrenoleukodystrophy, VLCFA acyl-CoA synthetase is defective (9). Progressive visual loss secondary to bilateral optic atrophy or involvement of other visual pathways develops early in the neonatal and childhood variants of the adrenoleukodystrophies and proceeds within months to no light perception.

Childhood Adrenoleukodystrophy

The childhood X-linked form of adrenoleukodystrophy is the commonest variant. Gaze nystagmus and sluggish pupillary responses may precede the cortical blindness and optic atrophy due to a severe loss of nerve fibers in the optic nerve head (41,224).

Adrenomyeloneuropathy

In the X-linked adrenomyeloneuropathy (MIM #300100) young adult males develop progressive spastic paraparesis and a distal symmetric polyneuropathy in addition to adrenal gland dysfunction (73). Individuals with this variant of adrenoleukodystrophy may have affected male kindred with the childhood variant and persons with childhood adrenoleukodystrophy and adrenomyeloneuropathy have both been mapped to the long arm of the X chromosome (Xq28) and are caused by a mutation in the same *ABCD1* gene, which encodes for an ATPase binding cassette protein (220). Moreover, the phenotypic difference between non-neonatal adrenoleukodystrophy and adrenomyeloneuropathy is not necessarily a consequence of allelic heterogeneity due to different mutations in the same gene. Some individuals with either adrenomyeloneuropathy or childhood adrenoleukodystrophy have had abnormal color vision, which is accounted for by genetic defects involving the contiguous *RCP* (red visual pigment) and *GCP* (green visual pigment) genes located in the same Xq28 part of the X-chromosome (9). In at least one family adrenomyeloneuropathy has been associated with cataracts (102).

Autosomal Neonatal Adrenoleukodystrophy

The neonatal variant of adrenoleukodystrophy (MIM #202370) affects both sexes and has an autosomal recessive mode of inheritance. Dolichocephaly, a prominent high forehead, epicanthal folds, broad nasal bridge, and low-set ears typify the external appearance of the head in neonatal adrenoleukodystrophy. Mental retardation is severe and seizures are common. Nystagmus and a pigmentary retinopathy are early manifestations of neonatal adrenoleukodystrophy (41,130). This disorder is caused by mutations in genes encoding the peroxisome receptor 1 (peroxin-1), namely *PEX1* (51) and other related genes, such as *PEX10* (peroxin-10), *PEX13* (peroxin-13), and *PEX26* (peroxin-26).

Histopathology

The white matter of the CNS contains confluent areas of active demyelination surrounding inflammatory zones that contain necrotic axons. This inflammatory reaction, which includes macrophages and reactive astrocytes, as well as T lymphocytes of the T4 and CD45R subsets, distinguishes the adrenoleukodystrophies from other leukodystrophies. B-lymphocytes and plasma cells are uncommon (153). Birefringent intracytoplasmic crystals accumulate within the brain, adrenal gland and other affected tissues. By TEM the crystals appear lamellar.

The eyes from several individuals with the childhood (41,224) and neonatal forms of adrenoleukodystrophy (41) have been studied by light microscopy late in the course of the disease. Extensive atrophy of the nerve fiber and ganglion cell layers of the retina and a diffuse optic atrophy with narrowing of the nerve fiber bundles, glial hypercellularity, and partial demyelination have been features. Marked axonal loss, numerous intracytoplasmic inclusions, including dense lipofuscin granules and macrophages have been prominent in affected regions. The optic atrophy appears to be secondary to CNS and optic nerve lesions (descending optic atrophy), as well to retinal neuronal destruction (ascending atrophy atrophy) (41). Swelling of the optic nerve head may occur probably as a sequel to elevated intracranial pressure (41). The photoreceptors degenerate and cells in the outer retina may contain pigment in a configuration reminiscent of retinitis pigmentosa (41). TEM has disclosed a marked decrease in myelin as well as axonal degeneration. Advanced demyelination of the optic chiasm with loss of oligondendroglia and an increased number of astrocytes and numerous macrophages accumulate. The typical intracytoplasmic inclusions that gather in the brain and other tissues, have not been identified in the optic nerve or optic chiasm, implying that the process in these parts of the visual pathway are involved secondarily rather than by the primary metabolic defect.

Metabolic Defect and Pathogenesis

At one time the adrenoleukodystrophies were thought to be a genetically determined lipid storage diseases caused by an error in membrane sterol metabolism (33,152), but they are now known to be due to an inherited deficiency of a peroxisomal enzyme known as VLCFA acyl-Co-A synthetase (lignoceroyl-CoA ligase). The deficiency results in defective beta oxidation of VLCFA, which accumulate largely in the brain and adrenal gland. These predominantly saturated VLCFA are toxic and account for the destruction of numerous cell types, including adrenocortical cells, the testicular interstitial cells of Leydig, and Schwann cells. An inherent myelin instability together with the cytotoxic effect of VLCFA on myelin and oligodendroglia are believed to cause myelin breakdown. The characteristic inflammatory response around areas of demyelination seems to be a natural response to demyelination, rather than the cause of it (153).

Pelizaeus–Merzbacher Disease

Pelizaeus–Merzbacher disease (MIM #312080) is a rare clinically heterogeneous X-linked recessive slowly progressive sudanophilic leukodystrophy with severe psychomotor retardation, dwarfism in childhood and premature aging. Neurological manifestations are secondary to a failure of oligodendrocyte differentiation and defective myelination due to point mutations in, or deletions of, the *PLP1* gene that encodes for the main integral protein of myelin (proteolipid protein 1) (52), which is found on the short arm of the X-chromosome (Xp22) (209). The mutated protein is misfolded and usually trapped in the endoplasmic reticulum during transportation to the cell surface, which eventually leads to oligodendrocyte cell death in persons with the severe phenotype (101). Ocular manifestations include demyelination and atrophy of optic nerve axons, loss of retinal ganglion cells and gliosis, "salt and pepper" retinopathy, anterior segment pigment dispersion, cataract, corneal ulceration and opacification, and pupillary aberrances (163). Death usually occurs in the second or third decade. Pelizaeus–Merzbacher disease is allelic with spastic paraplegia type 2 (88).

Apart from humans, mutations have been identified in the *PLP* gene in several animal models with X-chromosome linked disorders of myelin [jimpy mouse, msd-mouse, myelin-deficient (md) rat, and shaking pup] (218).

Cockayne Syndrome

Cockayne syndrome, is characterized by an onset in childhood of developmental and mental retardation leading to dwarfism, a distinctive facies with prognathism and bird-like features, mental retardation, loss of subcutaneous fat, partial deafness, and a photosensitive dermatitis. In common with Pelizaeus–Merzbacher disease premature aging is a feature and affected individuals usually also die within the second or third decade.

The ocular manifestations of this autosomal recessive condition, include cataracts, demyelination, and atrophy of optic nerve axons with gliosis, a degenerative retinopathy (with a loss of retinal ganglion cells and atrophy of the photoreceptors and outer nuclear layer), irregular hypo- and hyperpigmentation of the RPE (giving the retinal fundus a "salt and pepper" appearance on ophthalmoscopy), anterior segment pigment dispersion, ulceration and other abnormalities of the cornea, nystagmus, and an unresponsiveness of the pupils to mydriatics (27,39,82,116,147,175,228). Exposure and inadequate moistening of the corneal surface secondary to anhidrosis, failure of the Bell phenomenon (movement of eyes up and backward on forced closure), and loss of blinking are thought to be major reasons for the corneal lesions.

Cockayne syndrome shares some features with xeroderma pigmentosum including an increased sensitivity to ultraviolet (UV) light irradiation (184) and an abnormality in DNA repair. Two variants of Cockayne syndrome are recognized: Cockayne syndrome type A (MIM #216400) and Cockayne syndrome type B (MIM #133540), which are caused by mutations in the genes that encode for group 8 excision-repair cross-complementing protein (*ERCC8*) (81) and group 6 excision-repair cross-complementing protein (*ERCC6*) (208), respectively.

Canavan Disease

Canavan disease (MIM #271900) is a rare autosomal recessive lethal disorder of infancy characterized by a spongy state of the white matter in the brain and defective myelination. This condition, which is associated with elevated levels of N-acetylaspartic acid in the plasma and urine due to a deficiency of aspartoacylase is caused by a mutation in the *ASPA* gene that encodes for aspartoacyclase. Canavan disease is considered in Chapter 43.

Alexander Disease

A rare leukodystrophy (MIM 203450), which was first described in an infant by Alexander in 1949 (3), is characterized by megalocephaly, progressive mental retardation, a heavy brain, and an abundance of homogeneous eosinophilic carrot-shaped bodies. These so-called Rosenthal fibers are located in the white matter, including that of the optic nerve and visual pathways, especially around blood vessels. These structures contain chaperones αB-crystallin and HSP27 (see Chapter 36) as well as mutated GFAP, and brain tissue from patients with Alexander disease contain abundant phosphorylated αB-crystallin (129). Rosenthal fibers are sparse in the retrobulbar optic nerve and do not accumulate in Müller cells of the retina (205). Identical structures are sometimes conspicuous in optic nerve astrocytomas (see Chapter 63). Alexander disease has been subdivided into infantile, juvenile, and adult varieties depending upon the age of onset, the clinical manifestations, and the extent of the abnormalities (42,212). Numerous missense point mutations in GFAP have been identified in infantile, juvenile, and adult forms of Alexander disease (25,118) and they usually arise spontaneously during spermatogenesis (119). To date all GFAP mutations in Alexander disease have all been heterozygous indicating that the mutant protein is dominant over the normal one (48).

DISEASES OF NEURONS

Many diseases of the CNS involve distinct neuronal populations situated in different parts of the brain with specific characteristics (83).

Prion Diseases

The prion diseases are a group of lethal neurodegenerative spongiform encephalopathies that bridge the gap between disorders caused by infectious agents and genetic defects. The term prion was coined by Prusiner for a protein infectious agent (160). These unconventional agents are encoded by the *PRNP* gene on chromosome 20 (20pter–p12) and produce disease after a long latent period. In contrast to orthodox pathogens, prions lack nucleic acids and are impervious to maneuvers that alter or demolish nucleic acids. Prions have as yet not been shown to induce a detectable immune reaction, and they are able to resist physical and chemical inactivation (including ionizing and UV irradiation, formaldehyde, and chlorine dioxide) (66,194).

The prion diseases, can be infectious, sporadic, or genetic and include bovine spongiform encephalopathy (BSE) or "mad cow disease" of cattle, scrapie of sheep, and Creutzfeldt–Jakob disease (CJD), kuru, Gerstmann–Sträussler–Scheinker (GSS), disease and fatal familial insomnia (FFI) of humans. Some of these diseases are transmissible as autosomal dominant inherited disorders (194). The hallmark of all prion diseases is the aberrant metabolism that culminates in an accumulation of the prion protein. This results from the conversion of the normal cellular isoform protein (PrP) into the abnormal disease-causing isoform (PrPSc) (161,162,182). The manner by which prions replicate remains as mysterious as the infectious agents themselves. Infectious prions cause characteristic spongiform encephalopathies in which an abnormal folded protease resistant isoform of PrP known as PrPSc accumulates. As with other proteins that pass through the endoplasmic reticulum, the misfolded prion protein becomes transported back into the cytosol for degradation by the proteosome (see Chapter 36). Available evidence indicates that it is extremely neurotoxic. Sporadic prion disease occurs mainly in persons homozygous for a common PrP polymorphism at residue 129. Some inherited PrP mutations cause disease, not through an accumulation of PrPSc, but by the formation of a transmembrane form of PrP known as CtmPrP (80). Disease-specific mutations in the *PRNP* gene account for 15% of these diseases. Point and insertional mutations in *PRNP* vary in frequency between countries and the particular mutations are disease-specific and the age of onset relates to the mutation. The products of several other genes, such as *PRND*, which is downstream of *PRNP*, interact with Prp. It is noteworthy that a relative resistance to prion disease is conferred by a heterozygosity for a common polymorphism in *PRNP* (134) and that mice which do not express PrP are not susceptible to scrapie (188). For a comprehensive review of the genetics of the prion diseases see Mead (133).

Creutzfeldt–Jakob Disease

CJD (MIM #123400) is characterized by progressive dementia and other neurological manifestations and usually death within 6 months. Sporadic CJD (sCJD) accounts for 85% of all cases of human prion disease, and familial CJD (fCJD) accounts for 10% to 15% of cases. Variant CJD (vCJD), which is strongly linked to contaminated food obtained from cattle with BSE was first described in 1996 (219). It affects younger patients (average age 29 years as apposed to 65 years) and the duration of illness is relatively longer (mean of 14 months versus 4.5 months). The abnormal prion protein has been demonstrated in brains with CJD by immunohistochemical methods in association with synaptic structures, but the tissue processing needs special fixatives to yield positive results (99). The disorder is important to ophthalmologists not only because of visual field defects that frequently accompany the cerebral disease, but also because of the risk of person-to-person transmission by corneal grafting (57). Only 1.3 of the approximately 45,000 cornea donors in the United States each year are expected to have CJD, and most of the estimated risk is due to preclinical disease. Attention on donor screening criteria for cornea transplantation has resulted in the recognition of two possible cases of transmission of CJD through corneal transplant, one from Japan and one of from Germany (86,97). Despite the apparent transmission of CJD by keratoplasty in a human patient (57), the pathogen has not been identified in, or isolated from, human corneal tissue (31). It has, however, been detected in corneas of guinea pigs with experimental CJD (31). Histological studies of eyes from persons dying of CJD have disclosed either no abnormalities (173) or a questionable mild optic atrophy (115).

Scrapie

Scrapie, a naturally occurring spongiform encephalopathy of sheep and goats, is also caused by a prion. Dark retinal patches and spots have been observed ophthalmoscopically in affected sheep (12) and degenerative changes have been reported in the outer retina of hamsters following intracerebral inoculation of the scrapie agent (34,35,85).

Mitochondrial Encephalomyopathies

The so-called mitochondrial encephalomyopathies comprise several distinct syndromes caused by genetic disorders of mitochondrial DNA. They include Leigh syndrome, Alper syndrome, Kearns–Sayre syndrome, myoclonus epilepsy with "ragged-red fibers" (MERRF), and MELAS (mitochondrial myopathy, encephalopathy, lactic acidosis, strokelike episodes) (see Chapter 72) and Leber hereditary optic neuropathy (LHON) (see Chapter 35).

Subacute Necrotizing Encephalomyelopathy

General Remarks

Subacute necrotizing encephalomyelopathy (Leigh syndrome or disease, infantile Wernicke disease, MIM #256000) is a progressive, degenerative neurological condition that was first described by Leigh (114). It usually has an insidious onset and typically affects infants and children between the ages of 2 months and 6 years. The condition occasionally occurs in adults (17).

Clinical Features

The clinical features of Leigh syndrome vary considerably and include alterations in the state of consciousness, intention tremor, truncal ataxia, hypoactive tendon reflexes, a disordered central regulation of respiration, recurrent vomiting, difficulty in swallowing, failure to thrive, dysfunction of multiple cranial nerves secondary to necrosis of the nerve nuclei, progressive psychomotor retardation and deterioration, a non-specific generalized weakness, proximal hypotonia and paresis, bilateral pyramidal signs, and peripheral neuropathy.

Diagnostic imaging displays the lesions conspicuously in the living patient. The T2-weighted MRI (71,131,227) and computed tomography (CT) (71,131,197) display the images remarkably well. Bilateral symmetrically distributed low attenuation areas on CT that are suggestive of necrosis can be readily detected in the tectum of the midbrain, caudate nuclei, putamina, globus pallidi, and substantia nigra, but, in contrast to Wernicke encephalopathy, the mammillary bodies and red nuclei are spared. Ultrasonography is also useful in detecting early intracranial lesions in Leigh disease, because of the hyperechoic nature of the major lesions during the preclinical stage (227). The abnormal images, especially in the putamina, which appear to be invariably involved, are not only of diagnostic value to the clinician, but enable the evolution of the lesions within the brain to be documented serially.

Disordered skeletal and cardiac muscle function is conspicuous (see Chapter 72) and progressive general muscle weakness and hypotonia from infancy is followed by an inability to sit, stand, or walk. Respiratory difficulties commonly ensue and usually culminate in death after several weeks to 15 years.

Histopathology

The peripheral nerves have thin hypomyelinated sheaths. Numerous vacuoles account for characteristic spongy lesions in the central gray matter of the CNS, but white matter is also affected. The vacuolar abnormalities seem to form as a consequence of myelin splitting (98). Many tissues (including striated muscle, vascular smooth muscle, choroid plexus epithelia, ependymal cells, astrocytes, and some neurons) contain numerous abnormal mitochondria (without crystalline inclusions) which may be deformed and bizarre. The damaged areas may contain an increased number of astrocytes (reactive gliosis).

Other histopathologic abnormalities include intracytoplasmic ovoid to round proteinaceous inclusions that cross-react with antisera to tropomyosin (117) and the loss of immunohistochemically detectable cytochrome *c* oxidase subunits (137). Neuropathological features of Pelizaeus–Merzbacher disease have accompanied at least one case of subacute necrotizing encephalopathy (44).

Ophthalmic Manifestations

Abnormalities in the brain and extraocular muscles as well as optic atrophy account for the ophthalmologic manifestations (87,186). The tissue of few eyes have been studied after death and reported abnormalities include loss of retinal ganglion cells (especially in the macular area), thinning of the nerve fiber layer, and loss of myelin and axons, with some sparing of peripheral axonal bundles in the optic nerve (53,74,87). Retinal mitochondria manifest destruction of the cristae and accumulations of intramitochondrial electron-dense material.

The optic tracts and chiasm may also be demyelinated with axonal loss. Lesions of the optic nerves, brainstem, ocular innervation, and extraocular muscles account for abnormal visual evoked responses and other bilateral ophthalmic manifestations. The latter include strabismus, ocular motility disorders, optic nerve abnormalities, a diminished pupillary response to light, ptosis, external and internuclear ophthalmoplegia, diplopia, and episodic downward gaze with limitation of horizontal eye movement, wandering eye movements, and nystagmus (21).

Genetics

Although sometimes occurring sporadically this genetically heterogeneous disorder results from mutations in mitochondrial DNA as well as in many nuclear genes that are involved in energy metabolism. Some cases probably have an autosomal recessive mode of inheritance and parental consanguinity is common (21,87). An X-linked recessive variant is also recognized. The responsible mutations affect mitochondrial respiratory chain complexes I (mitochondrial encoded *MTND3*, *MTND5*, *MTND6*, and nuclear encoded *NDUFV1*, *NDUFS1*, *NDUFS3*, *NDUFS4*, *NDUFS7*, and *NDUFS8*), complex II (*SDHA*), complex III (*BCS1L*), complex IV (mitochondrial encoded *MTCO3* and nuclear encoded *COX10*, *COX15*, *SCO2*, *SURF1*), and complex V (*MTATP6*) (see Chapter 1). In addition mutations have been detected in genes that encode mitochondrial tRNA (*MTTV, MTTK, MTTW*, and *MTTL1*) and components of the pyruvate dehydrogenase complex (*DLD, PDHA1*).

This mitochondrial disorder of oxidative phosphorylation is characterized by markedly elevated blood and *CSF* lactate and pyruvate concentrations. An intravenous pyruvate loading test can aid in the diagnosis of mitochondrial (encephalo-) myopathies (211). These mutations result in defects in a variety of mitochondrial enzymes involved in the respiratory chain (enzyme complex I (65,171), enzyme complexes IV (8,49,100,122,136,137), a deficiency of the pyruvate dehydrogenase complex or NADH dehydrogenase (103,192), as well as from biotinidase deficiency with decreased carboxylase activities (propionyl CoA carboxylase, 3-methylcrotonyl-CoA carboxylase, pyruvate carboxylase) (14). An inhibitor of the conversion of thiamine pyrophosphate to thiamine triphosphate is present in the blood, urine, and CSF of some patients with Leigh disease (149–151). The enzymatic defects can be detected in assays of many tissues as well as cultured skin fibroblasts. Values of hepatic cytochrome *c* oxidase activity have varied immensely.

Pathogenesis

Potential causes of the metabolic defect in Leigh disease include a deficiency of cytochrome *c* oxidase due to mutations of either the nuclear (136) or the mitochondrial DNA encoding for different subunits of the enzyme, or large deletions of mtDNA. It is noteworthy that cytochrome *c* oxidase defects may accompany syndromes other than Leigh syndrome, presumably because of selective or more widespread involvement of specific organ systems. This delicate status of oxidative metabolism probably accounts for the apparent predisposition of individuals with Leigh syndrome to significant risks of general anesthesia (70).

Alzheimer Disease

Alzheimer disease (AD) is an extremely common disorder of aging that affects approximately four million people in the United States, and it is the most frequent neurodegenerative disorder. In other parts of the developed world where the population is aging, AD is also common and may be just as prevalent. The prevalence of AD is approximately 1 in 10,000 in patients who are 60 years old, but it affects more than one in three of those who are 85 years and older. AD can be classified into familial and sporadic forms. Most cases are sporadic, with 10% or less being inherited. Familial AD is rare and has an autosomal dominant mode of inheritance. It presents in patients <65 years old, and several different types are recognized. AD1 (MIM #104300) is caused by mutations in the *APP* gene on chromosome 21 (21q) that encodes for amyloid precursor protein. AD2 (MIM #104310) is associated with the APOE*4 allele on chromosome 19. AD3 (MIM #607822) is due to mutations in the *PSEN1* gene on chromosome 14 (14q) that encodes presenilin-1 and AD4 (MIM #606889) has mutations in *PSEN2*, the gene for presenilin-2 on chromosome 1 (1q31–q42).

Atrophy of the cerebral cortex affects particularly the frontal lobes (Fig. 6). Histologically, the characteristic lesions in AD are senile or neuritic plaques, and neurofibrillary tangles (Fig. 7). Pathogenic mechanisms responsible for these changes include amyloid-beta (Aβ) aggregation and deposition resulting in plaque development, and hyperphosphorylation of tau with formation of the tangles. Neurovascular dysfunction, oxidative stress, mitochondrial dysfunction, cell-cycle abnormalities, and inflammatory processes have also been implicated in the pathophysiology of the disease (19).

Although visual abnormalities are not a feature in the vast majority of cases, optic atrophy has been reported in some (84,181). In view of the rarity of

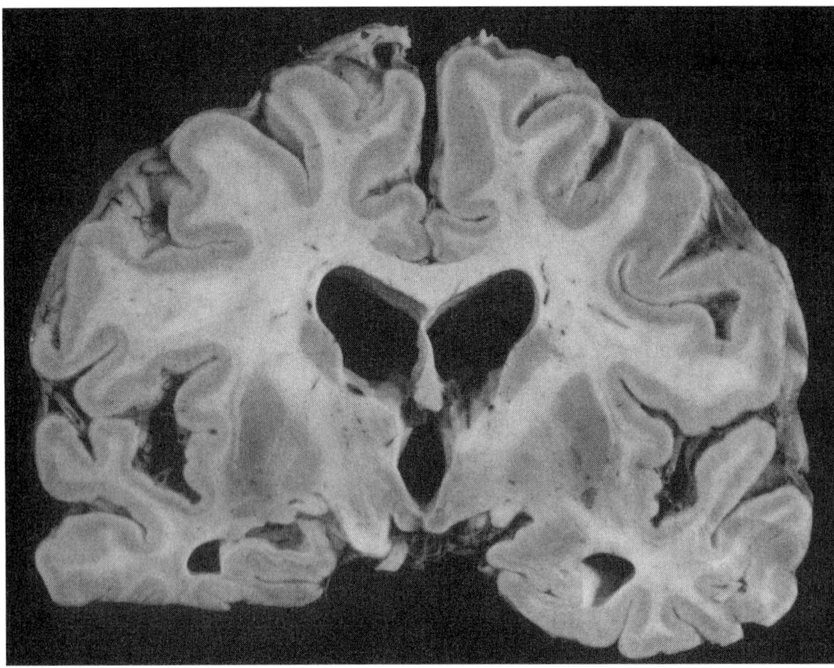

Figure 6 Coronal section of the brain showing ventricular dilatation (hydrocephalus ex-vacuo), gyral atrophy, and sulcal widening in a patient with Alzheimer disease.

conspicuous abnormalities in the optic nerve in AD, the question of whether the reported abnormalities in the optic nerve are a sequel to AD or a non-specific reaction to other common cerebral disorders associated with aging, such as arteriolar sclerosis, remains to be determined. Apoptosis, or programmed cell death (see Chapter 2), has been implicated in the mechanism resulting in the death of retinal ganglion cells. Apoptosis is initiated by the activation of specific proteases termed caspases, which have been shown to be activated in other chronic neurodegenerative diseases such as AD. The discovery that caspase-3 and caspase-8, which are thought to initiate apoptosis, are activated in retinal ganglion cells, has

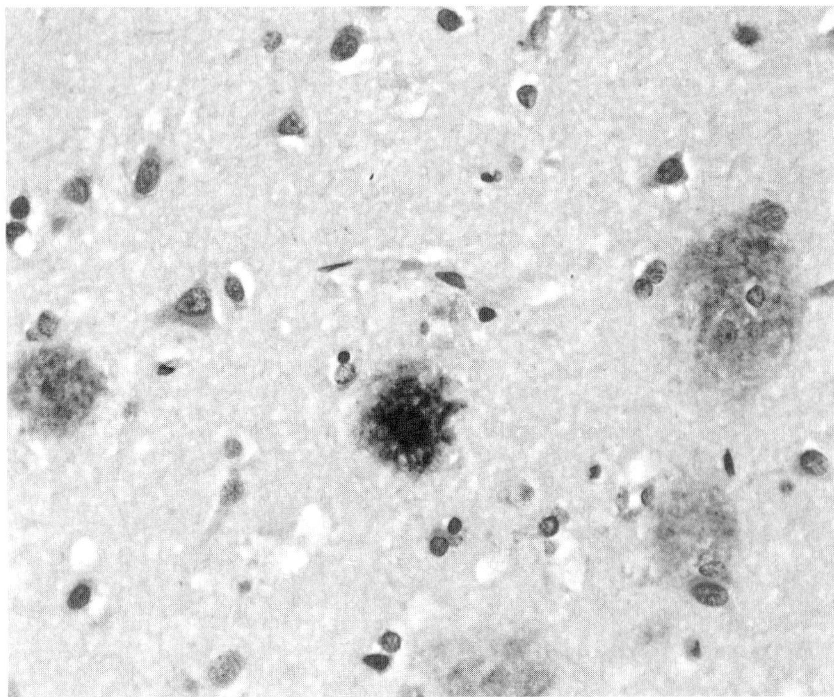

Figure 7 Neuritic plaques of Alzheimer disease with central amyloid cores (immunohistochemical stain for beta-amyloid precursor protein, $\times$ 46).

spawned the hypothesis that the neural degeneration associated with glaucoma mimics AD at the molecular level and that it results from cleavage of APPs to produce neurotoxic fragments including Aβ. Chronic caspase activity results in loss of the protective effect of amyloid precursor protein and the upregulation of toxic amyloid precursor protein fragments resulting in ganglion cell death (132).

Parkinson Disease

Parkinson disease (PD) is a common human neurodegenerative disorder affecting both sexes in all ethnic groups throughout the world (185). Its incidence increases with age and approximately 80% of cases occur in the seventh and eighth decades of life. Young-onset parkinsonism starts between the ages of 21 and 40 years, and is associated with the same pathologic changes as the much more common late-onset disease (169). Individuals with PD often exhibit a clinical appearance characterized by motor manifestations including resting tremor, rigidity, gait disturbance, and bradykinesia (170). Non-motor manifestations may include depression and cognitive dysfunction, including dementia in the late stages of the disease. Sleep, sensation, and perception modalities may also be disturbed (46).

PD is a disorder of the nigrostriatal dopaminergic system resulting from a depletion of dopamine in the striatum. Post-mortem examinations of brains afflicted by PD typically display a loss of pigmented dopaminergic neurons in the pars compacta of the substantia nigra (Fig. 8), and Lewy bodies (LBs) within the surviving neurons (Fig. 9). LBs are round or oval-shaped intracytoplasmic inclusion bodies with an eosinophilic hyaline core that is often surrounded by a clear zone or halo. Individual neurons may contain one or many LBs.

The major component of LBs appears to be α-synuclein (α-SYN), a presynaptic cytosolic protein widely expressed in the neuropil. Although the function of α-SYN is not completely understood, aggregation of α-SYN within neurons is thought to be toxic to the cells by disrupting normal cellular physiology and topography (190). Interactions involving protein aggregation, impaired protein degradation (dysfunction of the lysosome and proteosome systems), and mitochondrial dysfunction/oxidative stress appear to be some of the pathogenic mechanisms involved in PD (190).

Patients with PD may exhibit a wide variety of ophthalmological features, and the visual dysfunction has been considered to contribute to the parkinsonian disability through its influence on cognition and locomotion (210). Individuals with PD perform significantly worse than neurologically normal older adults in tests of vision and cognition, contrast sensitivity, visual speed of processing and attention, spatial and motor perception, visual and verbal memory, executive functions, depression, and motor function (18,210).

For reasons that are not apparent the most common ocular complaints suggest ocular surface irritation and include dry eyes and blepharitis. Impaired visual function has also been associated with decreased color discrimination (blue cone pathway) and retinal dopamine deficiency. Visual hallucinations, abnormal eyelid movements including reduced spontaneous blink, blepharospasm, and apraxia of eyelid opening, have also been documented. Abnormal eye movements in PD may relate to decreased adaptive modification of saccade

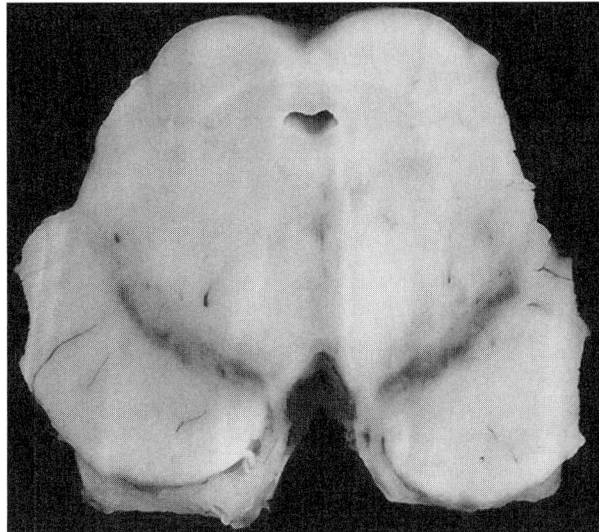
(A)

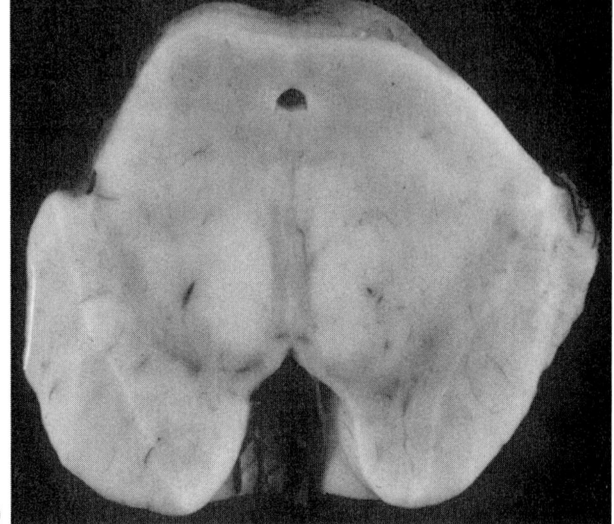
(B)

Figure 8 Sections of the midbrain (**A**) from a normal person and (**B**) from an individual with Parkinson disease (PD), (**B**) showing the markedly pale substantia nigra that is typical of PD.

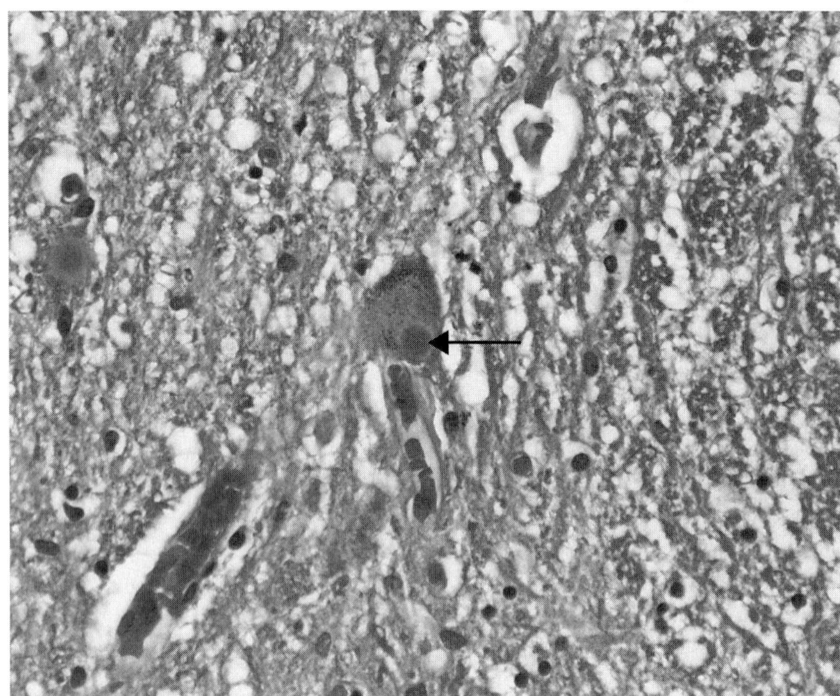

Figure 9 A Lewy body (*arrow*) is identified in a dopaminergic neuron within the substantia nigra in a patient with Parkinson disease (luxol fast blue, hematoxylin and eosin, ×46).

amplitudes, deficit of memory-guided saccades, ocular microtremor, and rapid eye movement sleep behavior disorder. Individuals who have undergone surgical pallidotomy therapy may acquire a contralateral homonymous hemianopia (18,46,168,198).

Apart from its role in motor function, dopamine is a major neurotransmitter and modulator in the retina of the neural adaptation to light (78,223). Dopaminergic neurons located at the border of the inner nuclear and inner plexiform layers of the retina synthesize and release dopamine. These neurons react to light and neuroactive chemicals by modifying dopamine production and release (223). In PD, some visual functions that are partially controlled by dopamine, including color vision, temporal sensitivity, and spatial contrast sensitivity are impaired (50,90). Observations obtained with optical coherence tomography (OCT) suggest that the inferotemporal area of the circumpapillary retinal nerve fiber layer becomes thinner than normal in patients with PD (90).

The pathogenesis of PD remains poorly understood, but environmental and genetic factors are suspected of being involved it its causation (185). Although most cases of PD arise sporadically, others are familial. Mutations in several genes involved in protein degradation and aggregation, including those which encode α-SYN (*PARK1*), ubiquitin E3 ligase parkin (*PARK2*), and ubiquitin C-terminal hydrolase L1 (*PARK5*), have been identified in families with PD (170).

Spinocerebellar Degenerations

The spinocerebellar degenerations (spinocerebellar ataxias) are a heterogeneous group of inherited neurodegenerative diseases that involve neurons in the cerebellum and brainstem and which cause nystagmus. One type (spinocerebellar ataxia type VII) (MIM #164500) also involves the retina causing a macular degeneration that eventually progresses into the peripheral retina. A fine sprinkling of pigment granules may be evident in the region of the macula. Other ophthalmological manifestations include a progressive external ophthalmoplegia which appears to have a supranuclear origin. Ptosis is not a feature. Spinocerebellar type VII results from a highly unstable trinucelotide (CAG) repeat in the *ATX7* gene on chromosome 3 (3p12–13) which encodes for the ataxin 7 protein (45,56).

OTHER

Idiopathic Intracranial Hypertension

Idiopathic intracranial hypertension (IIH) is the development of manifestations of increased intracranial pressure in the absence of a intracranial mass lesion This entity, which is also known as pseudotumor cerebri, predominantly affects obese women of child-bearing age, and other reported risk factors include vitamin A toxicity (see Chapter 49), adrenal insufficiency, Cushing disease, hypoparathyroidism, and hypothyroidism (215). Medications that have been implicated include corticosteroids, among others. Clinically, patients may present with non-specific symptoms of elevated intracranial pressure such as headache, pulsatile tinnitus, and horizontal diplopia. Additional studies that are useful in making the diagnosis include documentation of the opening CSF pressure from lumbar puncture, and the finding of compressed or slit-like ventricles on CT.

Visual loss is one of the major complications of IIH, and patients may exhibit papilledema with transient visual obscurations and progressive loss of peripheral vision in one or both eyes. Physical signs of acute papilledema include peripapillary flame hemorrhages, venous engorgement, and hard exudates. Chronic papilledema may result in peripapillary subretinal neovascularization, resulting in intraocular hemorrhage, and sudden visual loss. Chronic papilledema is also associated with telangiectatic blood vessels on the surface of the optic nerve head, optociliary shunt veins, and optic disc pallor (104,174,214,216).

Although IIH is a disorder of unknown cause, theories regarding its pathophysiology include resistance to CSF outflow at the arachnoid granulations, narrowing of the transverse dural venous sinus, and cerebral edema. However, the usual neurological and pathological findings of cerebral edema have not been documented in patients with IIH.

Therapeutic successes in lowering the intracranial pressure with medications such as carbonic anhydrase inhibitors or with lumboperitoneal shunting, ventriculoperitoneal, or ventriculoatrial shunting suggest that pressure elevations in the CSF are an important component of the disorder. Further support for this notion comes from the creation of fenestrations in the optic nerve sheath to permit the flow of CSF fluid directly into the orbital fat where it is absorbed into the venous circulation (69). For reasons that are not clear some patients with severe symptoms respond to a short course of high-dose corticosteroids.

Glaucoma

Over the years glaucoma has been regarded solely as a disease of the eye and the pathologic changes have been identified mainly in the anterior chamber angle, retina, and optic nerve head (see Chapters 20 and 21), but recently it has become recognized that the brain becomes involved in chronic glaucoma as a consequence of the trans-synaptic degeneration of the axons derived from the ganglion cells in the retina (75,76). This has been shown in experimental glaucoma in the monkey (229,230) and recently in a clinicopathological study of human glaucoma (77). Apart from optic atrophy the magnocellular and parvocellular layers of the lateral geniculate body undergo degenerative changes and these are accompanied by a loss of neurons in the visual cortex.

REFERENCES

1. Acheson ED. The epidemiology of multiple sclerosis. In: McAlpine D, Lumsden CE, Acheson ED, eds. Multiple Sclerosis: A Reappraisal. 2nd ed. Chapters 1 and 2. London: Churchill Livingstone, 1972:3–80.
2. Adams JM, Imagawa DT. Measles antibodies in multiple sclerosis. Proc Soc Exp Biol Med 1962; 111: 562–6.
3. Alexander WS. Progressive fibrinoid degeneration of fibrillary astrocytes associated with mental retardation in a hydrocephalic infant. Brain 1949; 72:373–81.
4. Allegretta M, Nicklas JA, Sriram S, Albertini RJ. T cells responsive to myelin basic protein in patients with multiple sclerosis. Science 1990; 247:718–21.
5. Antel JP, Weinrich M, Arnason BGW. Mitogen responsiveness and suppressive cell function in multiple sclerosis. Neurology 1978; 28:999–1003.
6. Archambeau PL, Hollenhorst RW, Rucker CW. Posterior uveitis as a manifestation of multiple sclerosis. Mayo Clin Proc 1965; 40:544–51.
7. Arnold AC, Pepose JS, Helper RS, Foos RY. Retinal periphlebitis and retinitis in multiple sclerosis. I. Pathologic characteristics. Ophthalmology 1984; 91: 255–62.
8. Arts WF, Scholte HR, Loonen MC, et al. Cytochrome c oxidase deficiency in subacute necrotizing encephalomyelopathy. J Neurol Sci 1987; 77:103–15.
9. Aubourg P, Feil R, Guidoux S, et al. The red-green visual pigment gene region in adrenoleukodystrophy. Am J Hum Genet 1990; 46:459–69.
10. Bamford CR, Ganley JP, Sibley WA, Laguna JF. Uveitis, perivenous sheathing and multiple sclerosis. Neurology 1978; 28:119–24.
11. Barbizet J, Degos J-D, Meyrignac C. Neuromyélite optique aiguë associée a une tuberculose pulmonaire aiguë. Rev Neurol (Paris) 1980; 136:303–9.
12. Barnett KC, Palmer AC. Retinopathy in sheep affected with natural scrapie. Res Vet Sci 1971; 12:383–5.
13. Batchelor JR, Compston A, McDonald WI. The significance of the association between HLA and multiple sclerosis. Br Med Bull 1978; 34:279–84.
14. Baumgartner ER, Suormala TM, Wick H, et al. Biotinidase deficiency: a cause of subacute necrotizing encephalomyelopathy (Leigh syndrome): report of a case with lethal outcome. Pediatr Res 1989; 26:260–6.
15. Behan PO, Behan WMH, Feldman RG, Kies MW. Cell-mediated hypersensitivity to neural antigens: occurrence in humans and non-human primates with neurological diseases. Arch Neurol Psychiat 1972; 27:145–52.
16. Bertrams J, Kuwert E. HL-A antigen frequencies in multiple sclerosis. Eur Neurol 1972; 7:74–8.
17. Bianco F, Floris R, Pozzessere G, Rizzo PA. Subacute necrotizing encephalomyelopathy (Leigh's disease): clinical correlations with computerized tomography in the diagnosis of the juvenile and adult forms. Acta Neurol Scand 1987; 75:214–7.
18. Biousse V, Skibell BC, Watts RL, et al. Ophthalmologic features of Parkinson's disease. Neurology 2004; 62:177–80.

19. Blennow K, de Leon MJ, Zetterberg H. Alzheimer's disease. Lancet 2006; 368:387–403.
20. Bobowick AR, Kurtzke JF, Brody JA, et al. Twin study of multiple sclerosis: an epidemiologic inquiry. Neurology 1978; 28:978–87.
21. Borit A. Leigh's necrotizing encephalomyelopathy: neuro-ophthalmological abnormalities. Arch Ophthalmol 1971; 85:438–42.
22. Bornstein MB. A tissue-culture approach to demyelinative disorders. Nat Cancer Inst Monogr 1963; 11:197–214.
23. Boyle EA, McGeer PL. Cellular immune response in multiple sclerosis plaques. Am J Pathol 1990; 137: 575–84.
24. Breger BC, Leopold IH. The incidence of uveitis in multiple sclerosis. Am J Ophthalmol 1966; 62:540–5.
25. Brenner M, Johnson AB, Boespflug-Tanguy O, et al. Mutations in GFAP, encoding glial fibrillary acidic protein, are associated with Alexander disease. Nat Genet 2001; 27:117–20.
26. Brockhurst RJ, Schepens CL, Okamura ID. Peripheral uveitis: clinical description, complications and differential diagnosis. Am J Ophthalmol 1960; 49:1257–66.
27. Brodrick JD, Dark AJ. Corneal dystrophy in Cockayne' s syndrome. Br J Ophthalmol 1973; 57:391–9.
28. Brody JA. Epidemiology of multiple sclerosis and a possible virus aetiology. Lancet 1972; 2:173–6.
29. Brody JA, Sever JL, Edgar A, McNew J. Measles antibody titers of multiple sclerosis patients and their siblings. Neurology 1972; 22:492–9.
30. Broman T. Supravital analysis of disorders in the cerebral vascular permeability. II. Two cases of multiple sclerosis. Acta Psychiat Neurol Scand Suppl 1947; 46:58–71.
31. Brown P. An epidemiologic critique of Creutzfeldt-Jakob disease. Epidemiol Rev 1980; 2:113–35.
32. Burde RM. Retrobulbar neuritis revisited. Am J Ophthalmol 1975; 79:695–7.
33. Burton BK, Nadler HL. Schilder's disease: abnormal cholesterol retention and accumulation in cultivated fibroblasts. Pediatr Res 1974; 8:170–5.
34. Buyukmichci N, Marsh RF, Albert DM, Zelinski K. Ocular effects of scrapie agent in hamsters: preliminary observations. Invest Ophthalmol Vis Sci 1977; 16:319–24.
35. Buyukmichci N, Rorvik M, Marsh FF. Replication of the scrapie agent in ocular neural tissues. Proc Natl Acad Sci USA 1980; 77:1169–71.
36. Charcot JM. Lectures on the Disease of the Nervous System, first series (translated by G. Sigerson), delivered 1868, lecture 6. London: The New Sydenham Society, 1877.
37. Charo IF, Ransohoff RM. The many roles of chemokines and chemokine receptors in inflammation. N Engl J Med 2006; 354:610–21.
38. Cloys DE, Netsky MG. Neuromyelitis optica. In: Vinken PJ, Bruyn GW, eds. Handbook of Clinical Neurology. Vol. 9, Chapter 14. Amstersdam: North Holland Publishing Co., 1970:426–36.
39. Cockayne EA. Dwarfism with retinal atrophy and deafness. Arch Dis Child 1936; 11:1–8.
40. Cohen MM, Lessel S, Wolf PA. A prospective study of the risk of developing multiple sclerosis in uncomplicated optic neuritis. Neurology 1979; 29:208–13.
41. Cohen SMZ, Green WR, De la Cruz ZC, et al. Ocular histopathologic studies of neonatal childhood adrenoleukodystrophy. Am J Ophthalmol 1983; 95:82–96.
42. Cole G, DeVilliers F, Proctor NSF, et al. Alexander's disease: case report including histopathological and electron microscopic features. J Neurol Neurosurg Psychiatr 1979; 42:619–24.
43. Courville CB. Concentric sclerosis. In: Vinken PJ, Bruyn GW, eds. Handbook of Clinical Neurology. Vol. 9. Amsterdam: North Holland Publishing Co., 1970:437–51.
44. Cruz-Sanchez FF, Cervos-Navarro J, Rossi ML, Lafuente JV. Pelizaeus–Merzbacher disease with thiamine deficiency or Leigh disease with extensive involvement of white matter? Case report. Clin Neurol Neurosurg 1989; 91:261–3.
45. David G, Abbas N, Stevanin G, et al. Cloning of the SCA7 gene reveals a highly unstable CAG repeat expansion. Nat Genet 1997; 17:65–70.
46. Davidsdottir S, Cronin-Golomb A, Lee A. Visual and spatial symptoms in Parkinson's disease. Vision Res 2005; 45:1285–96.
47. Dean G, Kurtzke JF. On the risk of multiple sclerosis according to age at immigration to South Africa. Br Med J 1971; 3:725–9.
48. Der Perng M, Su M, Wen S, et al. The Alexander disease-causing glial fibrillary acidic protein mutant, R416W, accumulates into Rosethal fibers by a pathway that involves filament aggregation and the association of αB-crystallin and HSP27. Am J Hum Genet 2006; 79:197–213.
49. DiMauro S, Servidei S, Zeviani M, et al. Cytochrome c oxidase deficiency in Leigh syndrome. Ann Neurol 1987; 22:498–506.
50. Djamgoz MB, Hankins MW, Hirano J, et al. Neurobiology of retinal dopamine in relation to degenerative states of the tissue. Vision Res 1997; 37:3509–29.
51. Dodt G, Braverman N, Wong C, et al. Mutations in the PTS1 receptor gene, PXR1, define omplementation group 2 of the peroxisome biogenesis disorders. Nat Genet 1995; 9:115–25.
52. Doll R, Natowicz MR, Schiffman R, Smith FI. Molecular diagnostics for myelin proteolipid protein gene mutations in Pelizaeus–Merzbacher disease. Am J Hum Genet 1992; 51:161–9.
53. Dooling EC, Richardson EP Jr. Ophthalmoplegia and Ondine's curse. Arch Ophthalmol 1977; 95:1790–3.
54. Donders PC. Eales' disease. Docum Ophthalmol 1958; 12: 1–105.
55. Dow RS, Berglund G. Vascular pattern of lesions of multiple sclerosis. Arch Neurol Psychiat 1942; 47:1–18.
56. Duenas AM, Goold R, Giunti P. Molecular pathogenesis os spinocerebellar ataxias. Brain 2006; 129: 1357–70.
57. Duffy P, Wolf J, Collins G, DeVoe AG, Streeten B, Cowen D. Possible person-to-person transmission of Creutzfeldt-Jakob disease. N Engl J Med 1974; 290:692.
58. Engell T, Jenson OA, Klinken L. Periphlebitis retinae in multiple sclerosis: a histopathological study of two cases. Acta Ophthalmol 1985; 63:83–8.
59. Esiri MM, Kennedy PGE. Viral diseases. In: Graham DI, Lantos PL, eds. Greenfield's Neuropathology. 6th ed. Vol. 1, Chapter 1. London: Arnold, 1997:3–50.
60. Field EJ. Slow virus infections of the nervous system. Int Rev Exp Path 1969; 8:129–239.
61. Fog T. The topographic distribution of plaques in the spinal cord in multiple sclerosis. Arch Neurol Psychiat 1950; 63:382–414.
62. Fog T. The topography of plaques in multiple sclerosis. Acta Neurol Scand 1965; 41(Suppl.15):1–161.
63. Frohman EM, Frohman TC, Zee DS, et al. The neuro-ophthalmology of multiple sclerosis. Lancet Neurol 2005; 4:111–21.

64. Frohman EM, Racke MK, Raine CS. Multiple sclerosis—the plaque and its pathogenesis. N Engl J Med 2006; 354: 942–55.
65. Fujii T, Ito M, Okuno T, et al. Complex I (reduced nicotinamide-adenine dinucleotide-coenzyme Q reductase) deficiency in two patients with probable Leigh syndrome. J Pediatr 1990; 116:84–7.
66. Gajdusek DC. Unconventional viruses and the origin and disappearance of Kuru. Science 1977; 197:943–60.
67. Gartner S. Optic neuropathy in multiple sclerosis: optic neuritis. Arch Ophthalmol 1953; 50:718–26.
68. Giles CL. Peripheral uveitis in patients with multiple sclerosis. Am J Ophthalmol 1970; 70:17–9.
69. Goh KY, Schatz NJ, Glaser JS. Optic nerve sheath fenestration for pseudotumor cerebri. Neuroophthalmol 1997; 17:86–91.
70. Grattan-Smith PJ, Shield LK, Hopkins IJ, Collins KJ. Acute respiratory failure precipitated by general anesthesia in Leigh's syndrome. J Child Neurol 1990; 5:137–41.
71. Greenberg SB, Faerber EN, Riviello JJ, et al. Subacute necrotizing encephalomyelopathy (Leigh disease): CT and MRI appearances. Pediatr Radiol 1990; 21:5–8.
72. Gregson NA. The molecular biology of myelin. In: Hallpike JF, Adams CWM, Tourtellotte WW, eds. Multiple Sclerosis: Pathology, Diagnosis and Management. Chapter 1. Baltimore: Williams and Wilkins, 1983:1–28.
73. Griffin JW, Goren E, Schaumburg H, et al. Adrenomyeloneuropathy: a probable variant of adrenoleukodystrophy. Neurology 1977; 27:1107–13.
74. Grover WD, Green WR, Pileggi AJ. Ocular findings in subacute necrotizing encephalomyelitis. Am J Ophthalmol 1970; 70:599–603.
75. Gupta N, Yücel YH. Glaucoma and the brain. J Glaucoma 2001; 109(Suppl. 5):S28–9.
76. Gupta N, Yücel YH. Brain changes in glaucoma. Eur J Ophthalmol 2003; 13:32–5.
77. Gupta N, Ang LC, Tilly LN, et al. Human glaucoma and neural degeneration in intracranial optic nerve, lateral geniculate nucleus, and viual cortex. Br J Ophthalmol 2006; 90:674–8.
78. Gustincich S, Contini M, Gariboldi M, et al. Gene discovery in genetically labeled single dopaminergic neurons of the retina. Proc Natl Acad Sci U S A 2004; 101:5069–74.
79. Haarr M. Periphlebitis retinae in association with multiple sclerosis. Acta Psychiatr Neurol Scand 1953; 28:175–90.
80. Hegde RS, Tremblay P, Groth D, et al. Transmissible and genetic prion diseases share a common pathway of neurodegenertaion. Nature 1999; 402:822–6.
81. Henning KA, Li L, Iyer N, et al. The Cockayne syndrome group A gene encodes a WD repeat protein that interacts with CSB protein and a subunit of RNA polymerase II TFIIH. Cell 1995; 82:555–64.
82. Hijikata F, Hirooka M, Ohno T. Cockayne's syndrome: a histopathological study of the ocular tissues. Rinsho Ganka 1969; 23:187–94.
83. Hinton DR, Henderson VW, Blanks JC, et al Monoclonal antibodies react with neuronal subpopulations in the human nervous system. J Comp Neurol 1988; 267: 398–408.
84. Hinton DR, Sadun A, Blanks JC, Miller CA. Optic nerve degeneration in Alzheimer's disease. N Engl J Med 1986; 315:485–7.
85. Hogan RN, Baringer JR, Prusiner SB. Progressive retinal degeneration in scrapie-infected hamsters. Lab Invest 1981; 44:34–42.
86. Hogan RN, Cavanagh HD. Transplantation of corneal tissue from donors with diseases of the central nervous system. Cornea 1995; 14:547–53.
87. Howard RO, Albert DM. Ocular manifestations of subacute necrotizing encephalomyelopathy (Leigh's disease). Am J Ophthalmol 1972; 74:386–93.
88. Inoue K. PLP1-related inherited dysmyelinating disorders: Pelizaeus–Merrzbacher diases and spastic paraplegia type 2. Neurogenetics 2004; 6:1–16.
89. Inoue YK. An avian-related new herpesvirus infection in man: subacute myelo-optico-neuropathy (SMON). Progr Med Virol 1975; 21:35–42.
90. Inzelberg R, Ramirez JA, Nisipeanu P, et al. Retinal nerve fiber layer thinning in Parkinson disease. Vision Res 2004; 44:2793–7.
91. Jensen MK. Lymphocyte transformation in multiple sclerosis. Acta Neurol Scand 1968; 44:200–6.
92. Jersild C, Hansen GS, Svejgaard A, Fog T, Thomsen M, Dupont B. Histocompatibility determinants in multiple sclerosis, with special reference to clinical course. Lancet 1973; 2:1221–5.
93. Jersild C, Svejgaard A, Fog T, Ammitzboll T. HL-A antigens and diseases: I. Multiple sclerosis. Tissue Antigens 1973; 3:243–50.
94. Johnson HC. Retinal venous sheathing in multiple sclerosis. Am J Ophthalmol 1946; 29:1150–1.
95. Kabat EA, Freedman DA, Murray JP, Knaub V. A study of a crystalline albumin, gamma globulin and total protein in the cerebrospinal fluid of 100 cases of multiple sclerosis and in other diseases. Am J Med Sci 1950; 219:55–64.
96. Kempe CH, Takabayashi K, Miyamato H, et al. Elevated cerebrospinal fluid antibodies in multiple sclerosis. Arch Neurol 1973; 28:278–97.
97. Kennedy RH, Hogan RN, Brown P, et al. Eye banking and screening for Creutzfeldt-Jakob disease. Arch Ophthalmol 2001; 119:721–6.
98. Kimura S, Kobayashi T, Amemiya F. Myelin splitting in the spongy lesion in Leigh encephalopathy. Pediatr Neurol 1991; 7:56–8.
99. Kitamoto T, Shin R-W, Doh-ura K, et al. Abnormal isoform of prion proteins accumulates in the synaptic structures of the central nervous system in patients with Creutzfelt-Jakob disease. Am J Pathol 1992; 140:1285–94.
100. Koga Y, Nonaka I, Nakao M, et al. Progressive cytochrome c oxidase deficiency in a case of Leigh's encephalomyelopathy. J Neurol Sci 1990; 95:63–76.
101. Koizume S, Takizawa S, Fujita K, et al. Aberrant trafficking of a proteolipid protein in a mild Pelizaeus–Merzbacher disease. Neuroscience 2006; 141:1861–9.
102. Komori T, Nagashima T, Hirose K, et al. Adrenomyeloneuropathy associated with congenital cataract: report of a family with MRI study (Japanese). Rinsho Shinkeigaku Clin Neurol 1988; 28:532–5.
103. Kretzschmar HA, DeArmond SJ, Koch TK, et al. Pyruvate dehydrogenase complex deficiency as a cause of subacute necrotizing encephalopathy (Leigh disease). Pediatrics 1987; 79:370–3.
104. Krogsaa B, Soelberg Sorensen P, Seedorff HH, et al. Ophthalmologic prognosis in benign intracranial hypertension. Acta Ophthalmol Suppl 1985; 173:62–4.
105. Kuhl W. Seltene "Begleit"-Bilder bei periphlebitis retinae. Acta Ophthalmol 1968; 46:1105–12.
106. Kurland LT, Beebe EW, Kurtzke JF, et al. Studies on the natural history of multiple sclerosis. 2. Optic neuritis as a prelude to multiple sclerosis. Acta Neurol Scand 1966; 42 (Suppl. 19):157–76.

107. Kuroiwa Y. Neuromyelitis optica (Devic's disease, Devic's syndrome). In: Vinken PJ, Bruyn GW, eds. Handbook of Clinical Neurology. Chapter 13, Vol. 47 (revised series). North Holland: Elsevier, 1985;397–408.
108. Kurtzke JF. Familial incidence and geography in multiple sclerosis. Acta Neurol Scand 1965; 41:127–39.
109. Kurtzke JF. On the time of onset in multiple sclerosis. Acta Neurol Scand 1965; 41:140–53.
110. Kurtzke JF. A reassessment of the distribution of multiple sclerosis: parts one and two. Acta Neurol Scand 1975; 51: 110–36, 137–57.
111. Kurtzke JF, Kurland LT. Multiple sclerosis in the epidemiology of neurologic disease. In: Baker AB, Baker LH, eds. Clinical Neurology. Vol. 3, Chapter 48. New York: Harper and Row, 1976:22–30.
112. Kuwert EK, Bertrams HJ. Genetic aspects of multiple sclerosis. In: ter Meulen V, Katz M, eds. Slow Virus Infections of the Central Nervous System. New York: Springer, 1975:186–99.
113. Lampert F, Lampert PW. Multiple sclerosis: morphologic evidence of intranuclear paramyxovirus or altered chromatin fibers. Arch Neurol 1975; 32:425–7.
114. Leigh D. Subacute necrotizing encephalopathy in an infant. J Neurol Neurosurg Psychiat 1951; 14: 216–21.
115. Lesser RL, Albert DM, Bobowick AR, O'Brien FH. Creutzfeldt-Jakob disease and optic atrophy. Am J Ophthalmol 1979; 87:317–21.
116. Levin PS, Green WR, Victor DI, MacLean AL. Histopathology of the eye in Cockayne's syndrome. Arch Ophthalmol 1983; 101:1093–7.
117. Lew EO, Rozdilsky B, Munoz DG, Perry G. A new type of neuronal cytoplasmic inclusion: histological, ultrastructural, and immunocytochemical studies. Acta Neuropathol 1989; 77:599–604.
118. Li R, Johnson AB, Salomons G, et al. Glial fibrillary acidic protein mutations in infantile, juvenile, and adult forms of Alexander disease. Ann Neurol 2005; 57:310–26.
119. Li R, Johnson AB, Salomons GS, et al. Propensity for paternal inheritance of de novo mutations in Alexander disease. Hum Genet 2006; 119:137–44.
120. Link H, Tibbling G. Principles of albumin and IgG analyses in neurological disorders. III. Evaluation of IgG synthesis within the central nervous system in multiple sclerosis. Scand J Clin Invest 1977; 37:397–401.
121. Lisak RP. Multiple sclerosis: evidence for immunopathogenesis. Neurology 1980; 39:99–105.
122. Lombes A, Nakase H, Tritschler HJ, et al. Biochemical and molecular analysis of cytochrome c oxidase deficiency in Leigh's syndrome. Neurology 1991; 41:491–8.
123. Lucarelli MJ, Pepose JS, Arnold AV, Foos RY. Immunopathologic features of retinal lesions in multiple sclerosis. Ophthalmology 1991; 98:1652–6.
124. Lumsden CE. The immunogenesis of the multiple sclerosis plaque. Brain Res 1971; 28:365–90.
125. McAlpine D. The benign form of multiple sclerosis. Brain 1961; 84:186–203.
126. McAlpine D. The benign form of multiple sclerosis: results of a long term study. Br Med J 1964; 2:1029–32.
127. McAlpine D, Lumsden CE, Acheson ED. Multiple Sclerosis: A Reappraisal. 2nd ed. Edinburgh and London: Livingstone, 1972.
128. McDermott JR, Field EJ, Caspary EA. Relation of measles virus to encephalitogenic factor, with reference to the aetiopathogenesis of multiple sclerosis. J Neurol Neurosurg Psychiat 1974; 37:282–7.
129. Mann E, McDermott MJ, Goldman J, et al. Phosphorylation of alpha-crystallin B in Alexander's disease brain. FEBS Lett 1991; 294:133–6.
130. Manz HJ, Schuelein M, McCullough DC, et al. New phenotype variant of adrenoleukodystrophy: pathologic, ultrastructural and biochemical study in two brothers. J Neurol Sci 1980; 45:245–60.
131. Martin JJ, Van de Vyver FL, Scholte HR, et al. Defect in succinate oxidation by isolated muscle mitochondria in a patient with symmetrical lesions in the basal ganglia. J Neurol Sci 1988; 84:189–200.
132. Mc Kinnon SJ. Glaucoma: ocular Alzheimer disease? Frontiers Biosci 2003; 8:s1140–56.
133. Mead S. Prion disease genetics. Eur J Hum Genet 2006; 14: 273–81.
134. Mead S, Stumpf MPH, Whitfield J, et al. Balancing selection at the prion protein gene consistent with prehistoric kurulike epidemics. Science 2003; 300:640–3.
135. Menkes JH, Corbo LM. Adrenoleukodystrophy: accumulation of cholesterol esters with very long-chain fatty acids. Neurology 1977; 27:928–32.
136. Miranda AF, Ishii S, DiMauro S, Shay JW. Cytochrome c oxidase deficiency in Leigh's syndrome: genetic evidence for a nuclear DNA-encoded mutation. Neurology 1989; 39:697–702.
137. Miyabayashi S, Ito T, Abukawa D, et al. Immunochemical study in three patients with cytochrome c oxidase deficiency presenting Leigh's encephalomyelopathy. J Inherit Metabol Dis 1987; 10:289–92.
138. Morse PH. Retinal venous sheathing and neovascularization in disseminated sclerosis. Ann Ophthalmol 1975; 7: 949–52.
139. Moser HW, Loes DJ, Melhem ER, et al. X-linked adrenoleukodystrophy: overview and prognosis as a function of age and brain magnetic resonance imaging abnormality: a study involving 372 patients. Neuropedriatics 2000; 31:227–39.
140. Moser HW, Moser AB, Frayer KK, et al. Adrenoleukodystrophy: increased plasma content of saturated very long-chain fatty acids. Neurology 1981; 31:1241–9.
141. Myrianthopoulos NC. Genetic aspects of multiple sclerosis. In: Vinken PJ, Bruyn GW, eds. Handbook of Clinical Neurology. Vol. 9. Amsterdam: North-Holland, 1970: 85–106.
142. Naito S, Namerow N, Mickey MR, Terasaki PI. Multiple sclerosis: association with HL-A3. Tissue Antigens 1972; 2:1–4.
143. Offner H, Konat G, Clausen J. Effects of phytohemagglutinin, basic protein and measles antigen on myo-(2-H3) inositol incorporation into phosphatidylinositol of lymphocytes from patients with multiple sclerosis. Acta Neurol Scand 1974; 50:791–800.
144. Oger JF, Arnason BGW, Wray SH, Kistler JP. A study of B and T cells in multiple sclerosis. Neurology 1975; 25:444–7.
145. Paty DW, Cousin HK, Stiller CR. HLA antigens and mitogen responsiveness in multiple sclerosis. Transplant Proc Suppl 1977; 19:187–9.
146. Paufique L, Étienne R. Un signe peu connu de la sclérose en plaque: la périphlébite des veines rétiniennes. Ann Oculist 1955; 188:701–7.
147. Pearce WG. Ocular and genetic features of Cockayne's syndrome. Can J Ophthalmol 1972; 7:435–43.
148. Peters G. Multiple Sklerose. In: Lubarsch O, Henke F, Rossle R, eds. Hundbuch der speziellen pathologischen Anatomie und Histologie. Vol. 13/2A. Berlin: Springer, 1958:519–602.

149. Pincus JH, Cooper JR, Itokawa Y, Gumbinas M. Subacute necrotizing encephalomyelopathy: effects of thiamine and thiamine propyl disulfide. Arch Neurol 1971; 24: 511–7.
150. Pincus JH, Cooper JR, Piros K, Turner V. Specificity of the urine inhibitor test for Leigh's disease. Neurology 1974; 19:885–90.
151. Pincus JH, Itokawa Y, Cooper JR. Enzyme-inhibiting factor in subacute necrotizing encephalomyelopathy. Neurology 1969; 19:841–5.
152. Powell H, Tindall R, Schultz P, et al. Adrenoleukodystrophy: electron microscopic findings. Arch Neurol 1975; 32:250–60.
153. Powers JM, Liu Y, Moser AB, Moser HW. The inflammatory myelinopathy of adreno-leukodystrophy: cells, effector molecules, and pathogenetic implications. J Neuropathol Exp Neurol 1992; 51:630–43.
154. Powers JM, Schaumburg HH. The adrenal cortex in adrenoleukodystrophy. Arch Pathol 1973; 96:304–10.
155. Prineas J. Pathology of the early lesion in multiple sclerosis. Hum Pathol 1975; 6:531–54.
156. Prineas JW. The neuropathology of multiple sc1erosis. In: Vinken PJ, Bruyn GW, eds. Handbook of Clinical Neurology. Chapter 8, Vol. 47 (revised series). Amsterdam: North Holland Publishing Co., 1985:213–57.
157. Prineas JW, Kwon EE, Goldenberg PZ, et al. Interaction of astrocytes and newly formed oligodendrocytes in resolving multiple sclerosis lesions. Lab Invest 1989; 61: 489–503.
158. Prineas JW, Kwon EE, Goldenberg PZ, et al. Multiple sclerosis: oligodendrocyte proliferation and differentiation in fresh lesions. Lab Invest 1989; 61:489–503.
159. Prineas JW, McDonald IW. Demyelinating diseases. In: Graham DI, Lantos PL, eds. Greenfield's Neuropathology. 6th ed. Vol. 2, Chapter 13. London: Arnold, 1997:813–81.
160. Prusiner SB. Novel proteinaceous infectious particles cause scrapie. Science 1982; 216:136–44.
161. Prusiner SB. Prion diseases and the BSE crisis. Science 1997; 278:245–51.
162. Prusiner SB. Shattuck Lecture–Neurodegenerative diseases and prions. N Engl J Med 2001; 344:1516–26.
163. Rahn EK, Yanoff M, Tucker S. Neuro-ocular considerations in the Pelizaeus–Merzbacher syndrome: a clinicopathologic study. Am J Ophthalmol 1968; 66:1143–51.
164. Raine CS, Hummelgard A, Swanson E, Bornstein MB. Multiple sclerosis: serum-induced demyelination in vitro. J Neurol Sci 1973; 20:127–48.
165. Raine CS, Powers JM, Suzuki I. Acute multiple sclerosis: confirmation of 'paramyxovirus-like' intranuclear inclusions. Arch Neurol 1974; 30:39–46.
166. Rao NA, Tso MOM, Zimmerman LE. Experimental allergic optic neuritis in guinea pigs: preliminary report. Invest Ophthalmol Vis Sci 1977; 16:338–42.
167. Reddy MM, Goh RO. B and T lymphocytes in man: III. B, T, and "null" lymphocytes in multiple sclerosis. Neurology 1976; 26:997–9.
168. Repka MX, Claro MC, Loupe DN, et al. Ocular motility in Parkinson's disease. J Pediatr Ophthalmol Strabismus 1996; 33:144–7.
169. Revesz T, Gray F, Scaravill F. Parkinson's disease. In: Duckett S, de la Torre JC, eds. Pathology of the Aging Nervous System. 2nd ed. New York: Oxford University Press, 2001:264–308.
170. Riess O, Kruger R, Schultz JB. Spectrum of pheotypes and genotypes in Parkinson's disease. J. Neurol 2002; 249 (Suppl. 3):III/15–III/20.
171. Robinson BH, De Meirleir L, Glerum M, et al. Clinical presentation of mitochondrial respiratory chain defects in NADH-coenzyme Q reductase and cytochrome oxidase: clues to pathogenesis of Leigh disease. J Pediatr 1987; 110: 216–22.
172. Ross CAC, Lenman JAR, Melville ID. Virus antibody levels in multiple sclerosis. Br Med J 1969; 3:512–3.
173. Roth AM, Keltner JL, Ellis WG, Martins-Green M. Virus-simulating structures in the optic nerve head in Creutzfeldt-Jakob disease. Am J Ophthalmol 1979; 87: 823–7.
174. Rowe FJ, Sarkies NJ. Assessment of visual function in idiopathic intracranial hypertension prospective study. Eye 1998; 12:111–8.
175. Rowlatt U. Cockayne's syndrome: report of case with necropsy findings. Acta Neuropathol (Berl.) 1969; 14: 52–61.
176. Rucker CW. Sheathing of the retinal veins in multiple sclerosis. Mayo Clin Proc 1944; 19:176–8.
177. Rucker CW. Sheathing of the retinal veins in multiple sclerosis. J Am Med Assoc 1945; 127:970–3.
178. Rucker CW. Retinopathy of multiple sclerosis. Trans Am Ophthalmol Soc 1947; 45:564–70.
179. Rucker CW. Sheathing of the retinal veins in multiple sclerosis. Mayo Clin Proc 1972; 47:335–40.
180. Sabin AB, Messare G. Fluorescent antibody technique in the study of fixed tissues from patients with encephalitis. In: Van Bogaert L, Radermecker J, Hozay J, Lowenthal A, eds. *Encephalitides: Proceedings of a Symposium on the Neuropathology, Electroencephalography and Biochemistry of Encephalitides Antwerp, 1959*. Amsterdam: Elsevier, 1961: 621–6.
181. Sadun AA, Borchert M, DeVita E, et al. Assessment of visual impairments in patients with Alzheimer's disease. Am J Ophthalmol 1987; 104:113–20.
182. Safar JG, Geschwind MD, Deering C, et al. Diagnosis of human prion disease. Proc Natl Acad Sci USA 2005; 102: 3501–6.
183. Schapira K, Poskanzer DC, Miller H. Familial and conjugal multiple sclerosis. Brain 1963; 86:315–32.
184. Schmickel RD, Chu EHY, Trosko JE, Chang CC. Cockayne syndrome: a cellular sensitivity to ultraviolet light. Pediatrics 1977; 60:135–9.
185. Schwartzman RJ, Alexander GM. The scientific basis of Parkinsonian syndromes. In: Duckett S, de la Torre JC, eds. *Pathology of the Aging Nervous System*, 2nd ed. New York: Oxford University Press, 2001:309–21.
186. Sedwick LA, Burde RM, Hodges FJ. Leigh's subacute nectrotizing encephalopathy presenting as spasmus nutants. Arch Ophthalmol 1984; 102:1046–8.
187. Shaw PJ, Smith NM, Ince PG, Bates D. Chronic periplebitis retinae in multiple sclerosis: a histopathological study. J Neurol Sci 1987; 77:147–52.
188. Shmerling D, Hegyi I, Fischer M, et al. Expression of amino-terminally truncated PrP in the mose leading to ataxia and specific cerebellar lesions. Cell 1998; 93: 203–14.
189. Shibasaki H, Okirhiro MM, Kuroiwa Y. Multiple sclerosis among Orientals and Caucasians in Hawaii: a reappraisal. Neurology 1978; 28:109–12.
190. Shults CW. Lewy bodies. Proc Natl Acad Sci U S A 2006; 103(6):1661–8.
191. Sibley WA, Foley JM. Infection and immunization in multiple sclerosis. Ann Acad Sci 1965; 122:457–68.
192. Siemes H, Goebel HH, Sengers RCA, et al. Subakute nekrotisierende Encephalomyelopathie Leigh infolge

verminderter Aktivatat des Pyruvat-Dehydrogenase-Komplexes. Monatsschr Kinderheilk 1987; 135:821–6.
193. Smith ME. The turnover of myelin proteins. Neurobiology 1972; 2:35–40.
194. Stahl N, Prusiner SB. Prions and prion proteins. FASEB J 1991; 5:2799–812.
195. Stansbury FC. Neuromyelitis optica (Dévic's disease). Arch Ophthalmol 1949; 42:292–335, 465–501.
196. Symington GR, Mackay IR. Cell-mediated immunity to measles virus in multiple sclerosis: correlation with disability. Neurology 1978; 28:109–12.
197. Taccone A, Di Rocco M, Fondelli P, Cottafava F. Leigh disease: value of CT in presymptomatic patients and variability of the lesions with time. J Comput Assist Tomogr 1989; 13:207–10.
198. Tamer C, Melek IM, Duman T, et al. Tear film tests in Parkinson's disease patients. Ophthalmology 2005; 112: 1795–800.
199. Tanaka R, Iwasaki Y, Koprowski A. Unusual intranuclear filament in multiple sclerosis brain. Lancet 1974; 1:1236–7.
200. Terasak PI, Park MS, Opelz GG, Ting A. Multiple sclerosis and high incidence of a B lymphocyte antigen. Science 1976; 193:1237–45.
201. Ter Meulen B, Koprowski H, Iwasaki Y, et al. Fusion of cultured multiple sclerosis brain cells: presence of nucleocapsids and virions and isolation of parainfluenza-type virus. Lancet 1972; 2:1–5.
202. Tourtellotte WW. Cerebrospinal fluid in multiple sclerosis. In: Vinken PJ, Bruyn GW, eds. Handbook of Clinical Neurology. Chapter 4, Vol. 47. Amsterdam: North Holland, 1985:79–130.
203. Tourtellotte WW. Cerebrospinal fluid immunoglobulins and the central nervous system as an immunological organ particularly in multiple sclerosis and subacute sclerosing panencephalitis. Res Publ Assoc Res Nerv Ment Dis 1971; 49:112–55.
204. Toussaint D, Perier O, Verstappen A, Bervoets S. Clinicopathological study of the visual pathways, eyes, and cerebral hemispheres in 32 cases of disseminated sclerosis. J Clin Neuro-Ophthalmol 1983; 63:211–20.
205. Towfighi J, Young R, Sassani J, Horoupian DS. Alexander's disease: further light-, and electron-microscopic observations. Acta Neuropathol 1983; 61:36–42.
206. Traub RG and Rucker CW. The relationship of retrobulbar neuritis to multiple sclerosis. Am J Ophthalmol 1954; 37: 494–7.
207. Treusch JV, Rucker CW. Incidence of changes in the retinal veins in multiple sclerosis. Proc Mayo Clin 1944; 19:253–4.
208. Troelstra A, van Gool J, de Wit J, et al. ERCC6, a member of a subfamily of putative helicases, is involved in Cockayne's syndrome and preferential repair of active genes. Cell 1992; 71:939–53.
209. Troffatter JA, Dlouhy SR, DeMeyer W, et al. Pelizaeus–Merzbacher disease: tight linkage to proteolipid protein gene exon variant. Proc Natl Acad Sci U S A 1989; 86:9427–30.
210. Uc EY, Rizzo M, Anderson SW, et al. Visual dysfunction in Parkinson disease without dementia. Neurology 2005; 65:907–1913.
211. van Erven PMM, Gabreëls FJ, Wevers RA, et al. Intravenous pyruvate loading test in Leigh syndrome. J Neurol Sci 1987; 77:217–27.
212. Vogel FS, Hallervorden J. Leukodystrophy with diffuse Rosenthal fiber formation. Acta Neuropathol 1962; 2:126–43.
213. Waksman BH, Adams RD. Allergic neuritis: an experimental disease of rabbits induced by the injection of peripheral nervous tissue and adjuvants. J Exp Med 1955; 102:231–5.
214. Wall M, George D. Visual loss in pseudotumor cerebri. Incidence and defects related to visual field strategy. Arch Neurol 1987; 44:170–5.
215. Wall M, George D. Idiopathic intracranial hypertension. A prospective study of 50 patients. Brain 1991; 114: 155–80.
216. Wall M, Hart WM Jr, Burde RM. Visual field defects in idiopathic intracranial hypertension (pseudotumor cerebri). Am J Ophthalmol 1983; 96:654–69.
217. Watanabe I, Okazaki H. Virus-like structure in multiple sclerosis. Lancet 1973; 2:569–70.
218. Weimbs T, Dick T, Stoffel W, Boltshauser E. A point mutation at the X-chromosomal proteolipid locus in Pelizaeus–Merzbacher disease leads to disruption of myelinogenesis. Biol Chem Hoppe-Seyler 1990; 371: 1175–83.
219. Will RG, Ironside JW, Zeildler M, et al. A new variant of Creutzfeldt-Jacob disease in the UK. Lancet 1996; 347: 921–5.
220. Willems PJ, Vits L, Wanders RJ, et al. Linkage of DNA markers at Xq28 to adrenoleukodystrophy and adrenomyeloneuropathy present within the same family. Arch Neurol 1990; 47:665–9.
221. Williams AC, Mingioli ES, McFarland HF, et al. Increased CSF IgM in multiple sclerosis. Neurology 1978; 28:996–8.
222. Winchester RJ, Ebers G, Fu SM, et al. B-cell alloantigen Ag 7a in multiple sclerosis. Lancet 1975; 2:814.
223. Witkovsky P. Dopamine and retinal fuction. Doc Ophtahlmol 2004; 108:17–40.
224. Wray SH, Cogan DG, Kuwabara T, et al. Adrenoleukodystrophy with disease of the eye and optic nerve. Am J Ophthalmol 1976; 82:480–5.
225. Wucherpfennig KW, Ota K, Endo N, et al. Shared human T cell receptor Vβ usage to immunodominant regions of myelin basic protein. Science 1990; 248:1016–9.
226. Wybar KC. The ocular manifestations of disseminated sclerosis. Proc R Soc Med 1952; 45:315–20.
227. Yamagata T, Yano S, Okabe I, et al. Ultrasonography and magnetic resonance imaging in Leigh disease. Pediatr Neurol 1990; 6:326–9.
228. Yamaguchi K, Okabe H, Tamai, M. Corneal perforation in a patient with Cockayne's syndrome. Cornea 1991; 10:79–80.
229. Yücel YH, Yang Q, Weinreb RN, et al. Atrophy of relay neurons in magno- and parvocellular layers in the lateral geniculate nucleus in experimental glaucoma. Invest Ophthalmol Vis Sci 2001; 42:3216–22.
230. Yücel YH, Yang Q, Weinreb RN, et al. Atrophy of relay neurons in mangnocellular and parvocellular layers in the LGN in glaucoma. Arch Ophthalmol 2000; 118: 378–84.

71

Amblyopia

Anne B. Fulton
Department of Ophthalmology, Children's Hospital, Boston, Massachusetts, U.S.A.

Suzanne P. McKee
Smith-Kettlewell Eye Research Institute, San Francisco, California, U.S.A.

Janine D. Mendola
Center for Advanced Imaging, West Virginia University School of Medicine, Morgantown, West Virginia, U.S.A.

Anne Moskowitz and Carolyn S. Wu
Department of Ophthalmology, Children's Hospital, Boston, Massachusetts, U.S.A.

INTRODUCTION

Animal experiments laid the groundwork for understanding plasticity of the immature visual system and the functional and structural consequences of abnormal visual experience during development. The results of this traditional work spawned studies of the pathobiology of human amblyopia using non-invasive psychophysical procedures (48) and magnetic resonance imaging (MRI) (11,50).

Amblyopia is defined as reduced visual acuity in the presence of optimal refractive correction and in the absence of ocular abnormalities or visual system disease sufficient to account for the acuity deficit (71,72). Typically, the visual deficit is monocular. In young patients with an immature visual system, amblyopia is an acute developmental disorder.

Amblyopia is a heterogeneous disorder with clinical categories that can be defined by ocular features that typically produce asymmetry of visual inputs from each eye to the brain. Thus, not only visual acuity, but also binocular vision is altered.

ORIGIN OF AMBLYOPIA

Human amblyopia originates with abnormal visual experience in infancy and childhood. This view is supported by clinical observations and investigations in animal models which demonstrate that anomalous visual inputs alter the structure and function of the developing brain. The plasticity, or responsiveness, of the immature visual system to extrinsic factors decreases as the visual system develops (13,14,35). Induced or naturally occurring extrinsic factors that predispose to amblyopia include ocular misalignment (strabismus), asymmetric optical focus in the two eyes (anisometropia), and deprivation of a clear retinal image. Age of application of the extrinsic factor is a crucial variable. The young ages during which visual inputs alter the brain are termed the critical, or sensitive, periods. Multiple critical periods (13,23) coincide with periods of normal development of multiple visual functions (5,19–21,45,47,58,73); selected functions are shown in Figures 1–3.

The developmental segregation of ocular dominance columns in the visual cortex (32) coincides with the onset of stereopsis (24). Classical studies described suppression and binocular competition (35,70) and provided the foundation for further investigations of plasticity in the developing brain. The effects of visual experience are now characterized in functionally discrete areas of the brain that are distinguished by different cell types, molecular expression patterns, microcircuitry, and connectivity that shape the brain's response to the sensory inputs (44).

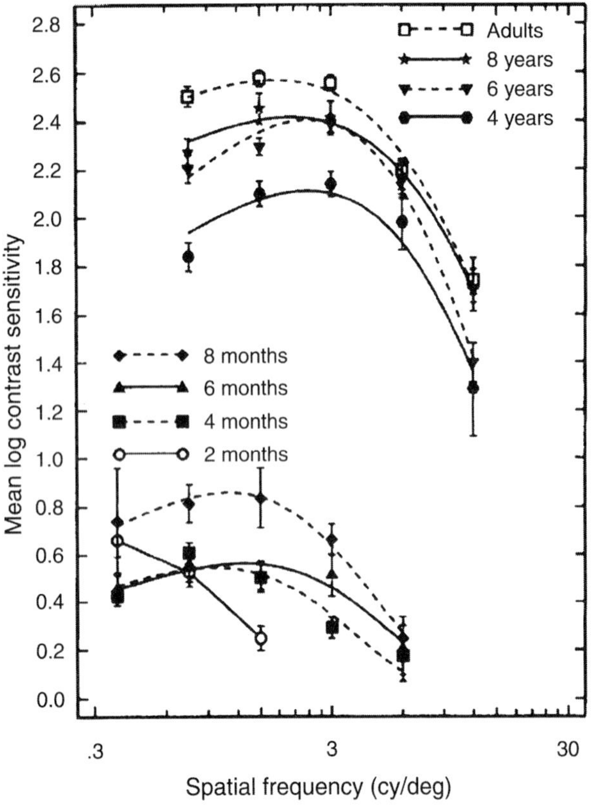

Figure 1 Mean contrast sensitivity, measured using psychophysical techniques, is shown as a function of spatial frequency for infants, children, and adults. Error bars represent ±1SEM. Peak sensitivity improved almost two log units from infancy to adulthood. Note that peak sensitivity has not reached adult levels at 4, 6, and 8 years, ages at which amblyopia is an acute disorder. *Source*: Adapted from Ref. 20.

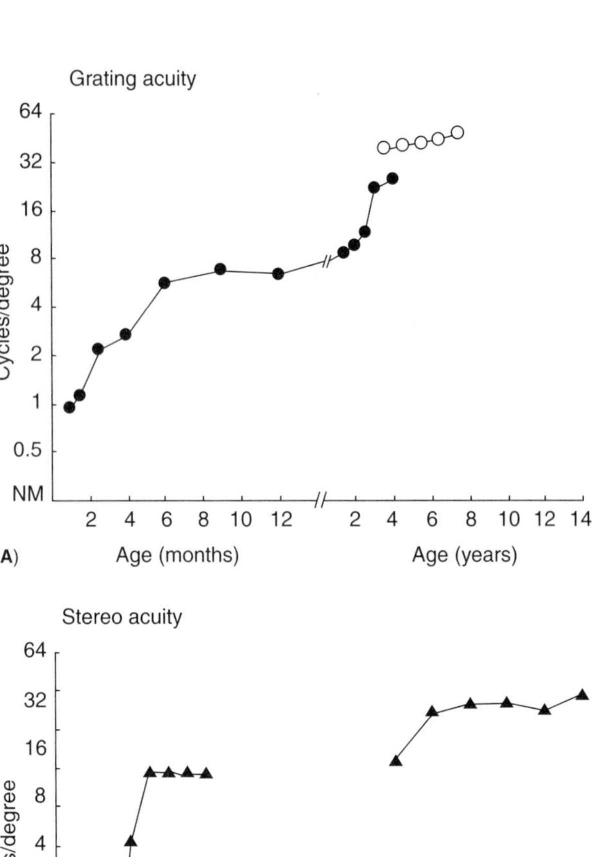

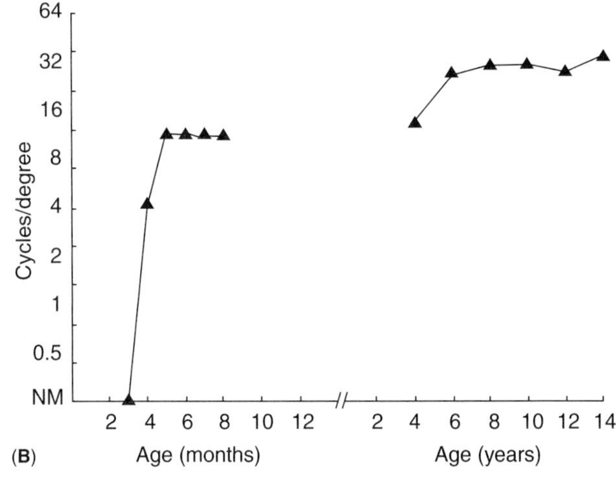

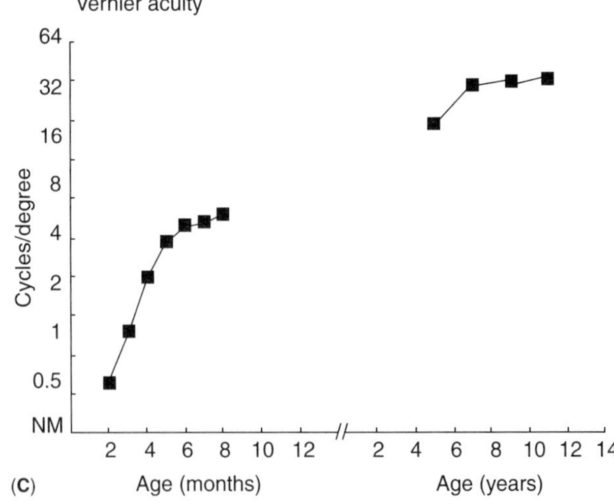

Figure 2 (**A**) Grating acuity as a function of age is replotted from Mayer et al. (infants) (45) and Gwiazda et al. (children) (19). (**B**) Stereo acuity as a function of age is replotted from Gwiazda et al. (19). (**C**) Vernier acuity as a function of age is replotted from Gwiazda et al. (19). Grating, stereo, and Vernier acuity develop rapidly during infancy, with continued slower development during childhood.

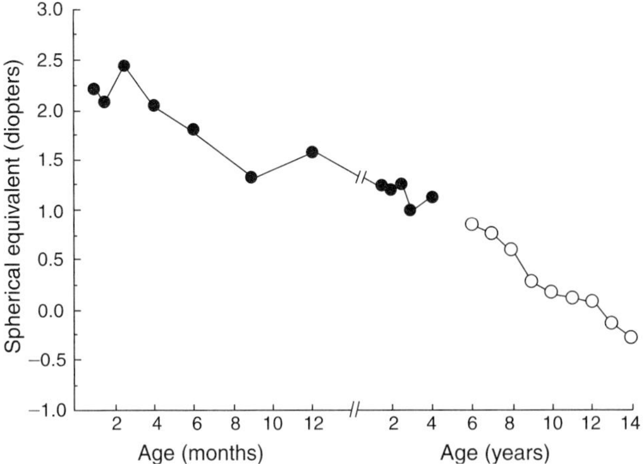

Figure 3 Development of refraction in normal subjects is replotted from Mayer et al. (1 month to 4 years; cycloplegic retinoscopy) (47) and Zadnik et al. (school-aged children; cycloplegic autorefraction) (73). Mean spherical equivalent is shown as a function of age. Hyperopia declined significantly with increasing age. Anisometropia, a recognized risk factor for amblyopia, is uncommon; anisometropia greater than 1 D occurred in only 1% of 514 normal subjects, aged 1 month to 4 years (47).

Clinically, the anomalous inputs are identified by an examination of the eyes. Strabismus, especially esotropia with a fixation preference, is the ophthalmic condition most often associated with amblyopia. Refractive error that is asymmetric between right and left eye at a young age, even if optically corrected, is also commonly associated with amblyopia. Deprivation of a clear retinal image, such as by a cataract, is the least frequent condition associated with amblyopia. A child with an immature visual system (Figs. 1–3), who has strabismus, anisometropia or deprivation of a clear retinal image, is at risk for amblyopia. Strabismus and anisometropia may coexist in the same patient, and strabismus is common in young patients who are deprived of a clear retinal image.

In contrast to immature subjects with acute amblyopia, adults and older children have been the subjects of much of the definitive work on the pathobiology of human amblyopia. In adults, amblyopia is a static condition. In further contrast to the acute clinical condition in which the ophthalmic practitioner concentrates on assessment of ocular features, investigators of adults and older children concentrate on an analysis of visual processes in the brain using noninvasive psychophysical and imaging procedures.

CLASSIFICATION OF AMBLYOPIA

Amblyopes are usually classified by the associated condition: anisometropia, strabismus, or deprivation. These conditions are thought to produce different patterns of visual deficits, and therefore, different types of amblyopia (68). However, amblyopia could be a simple abnormality that varies only in severity, but not in kind. To explore this issue, the early psychophysical studies measured contrast sensitivity and various types of acuity in small samples of anisometropic and strabismic amblyopes (8,26,43).

Despite the variety and rigor of the measurements, these small studies did not produce incontrovertible evidence for different types of amblyopia. For example, it has been frequently demonstrated that grating acuity, which is a simple measure of resolution, underestimates the deficit in the optotype acuity (the ability to identify letters) and Vernier acuity (the ability to detect an offset between two lines) of strabismics but not of anisometropes (18,41–43,46). That is, the ratio of optotype or Vernier acuity to grating acuity is different in strabismic and anisometropic amblyopes. In a study of 53 amblyopes, Birch and Swanson (7) found that the Vernier to grating ratio among moderate amblyopes was significantly different between strabismics and anisometropes. This difference, however, was not evident among the severe amblyopes in their sample. Birch and Swanson suggested that functional distinctions among different clinically defined groups depended on severity.

In the largest study to date, McKee et al. (48) recruited 427 adult abnormal subjects, who were currently amblyopic or who had risk factors for amblyopia during development. The study included the "at risk" subjects because the definition of amblyopia is based on an arbitrary visual acuity cutoff, e.g., 20/40, when in fact, it is likely that the deficiency in visual acuity is actually a continuum. A control group of 68 normal subjects was also recruited. The large sample size made it possible to group abnormal subjects into non-standard clinical categories (Table 1) to explore whether subtle differences in the associated conditions produced differences in visual function.

In addition to a standard measure of optotype acuity (the Bailey–Lovie LogMAR chart), McKee et al. (48) made precise psychophysical measurements of visual functions known to be abnormal in amblyopia—contrast sensitivity, grating acuity, Vernier acuity, and binocularity. Because the distribution of amblyopic measurements was skewed and, therefore, not amenable to standard statistical analysis that depend on the assumption of a normal distribution, McKee et al. analyzed their measurements by permutation analysis to assess whether there were significant differences among the clinically defined groups. These measurements were then transformed into *z*-scores, and factor analysis was used to assess the number of variables needed to account for the underlying functional losses. Two factors were

Table 1 Clinically Defined Categories of Abnormal Subjects in McKee et al. Amblyopia Study

Anisometropes (*N*= 84): a difference in interocular refractive error of ≥1D
Strabismics (*N*= 40): constant ocular deviation and no anisometropia
Strabismic-anisometropes (*N*= 101): constant ocular deviation and anisometropia
Inconstant strabismics (*N*= 24): intermittent ocular deviation
Inconstant strabismic-anisometropes (*N*= 44): intermittent ocular deviation and anisometropia
Former strabismics (*N*= 18): no ocular deviation, but history of surgery
Eccentric fixators (*N*= 35): non-centric monocular fixation, no ocular deviation
Deprivationals (*N*= 24): history of deprivation
Refractives (*N*= 27): refractive error ≥4D, but no anisometropia
Other abnormals (*N*= 30): history of patching, anisometropia, or oculomotor abnormality

Source: From Ref. 48.

sufficient—one related to contrast sensitivity, the other related to acuity.

Based on their statistical analysis, McKee et al. (48) concluded that amblyopia is a heterogeneous abnormality that is influenced by the associated condition. It cannot be characterized simply by the deficit in visual acuity. Figure 4 provides a succinct summary of the results on the weaker eye of the abnormal subjects. This figure shows the mean locations of the clinically defined sub-groups (Table 1) within the two-factor space; the *x*-axis of this space is the acuity factor and the *y*-axis is the contrast sensitivity factor. It can be considered a map of amblyopia, with the normal subjects in the east, the strabismics in the north, the anisometropes in the south, and the strabismic-anisometropes in the west.

FUNCTIONAL DIFFERENCES BETWEEN SUBTYPES OF AMBLYOPIA

The location of these groups reveals information about the functional differences among the various subtypes of amblyopia. It is no surprise that the normal subjects have far better acuity than any of the abnormal groups, but the location of the strabismic groups is unexpected. Their position above the normal subjects on the sensitivity axis indicates that their monocular contrast sensitivity is better than normal. Despite their superior contrast sensitivity, the acuity of strabismics is no better than the acuity of the anisometropic group with poor contrast sensitivity. It is noteworthy that the deprivational subjects are near the anisometropes, which suggests that mild-to-moderate deprivation produces deficits in acuity and contrast sensitivity similar to those produced by the blurred optical image in anisometropia. The strabismic-anisometropes and eccentric fixators (individuals with a fixed strabismus but such poor acuity that their eyes do not move under cover) have the poorest acuity. In examining the dispersion of the strabismic-anisometropic group, McKee et al. (48) noted that those with moderate acuity loss resemble the pure strabismics with their high contrast sensitivity, while those with poor acuity move toward the anisometropic group in sensitivity. The double-hit of strabismus and anisometropia leads to the poorest outcome.

The persistent blurred or degraded optical imagery associated with deprivation or anisometropia

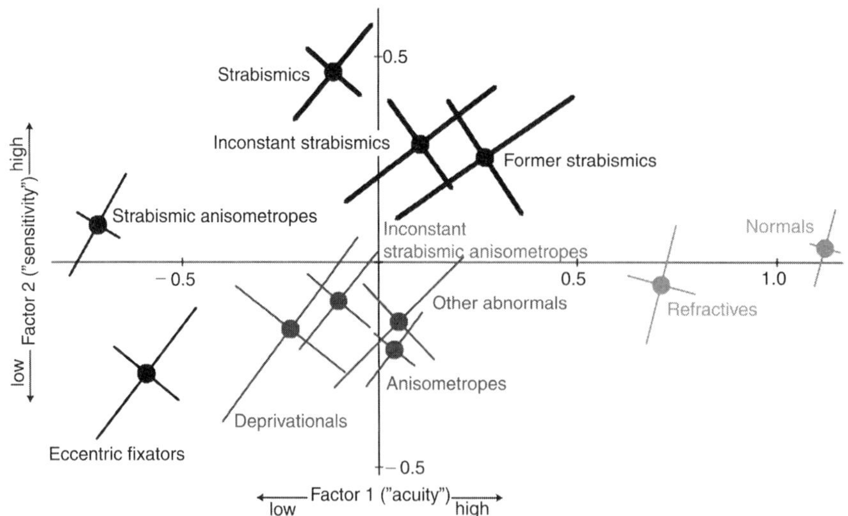

Figure 4 Mean locations of the 10 clinically defined categories and normal subjects in the two-factor space. The diagonal bars show ±1 SEM measured along the principal axes of the elliptical distributions. *Source*: Adapted from Ref. 48.

undoubtedly accounts for the abnormalities in visual function found in these groups—namely, the loss of fine detail in all acuity measures and poor contrast sensitivity. The puzzle is what accounts for the pattern of deficits associated with strabismus.

An important difference between strabismics and anisometropes is not shown in Figure 4. Strabismics generally have no binocular function, as measured by stereopsis or other measures that require cooperative interaction between the eyes. On the other hand, many anisometropes have some residual binocular function (28). McKee et al. (48) found that 64% of their anisometropic group passed their two tests of binocularity; indeed, 35% of the anisometropes, classified as amblyopic by a visual acuity worse than 20/40, passed both tests. To explore the effects of the loss of binocularity, McKee et al. classified all of their abnormal subjects as "binocular" if they passed both of their binocular tests, or "non-binocular" if they failed both tests; subjects failing one test were excluded from this analysis. The right side of Figure 5 shows optotype acuity plotted as a function of grating acuity for binocular (black dots) and non-binocular (gray dots) subjects; the left side shows Vernier acuity as a function of grating acuity for the same two groups. Two things are apparent in this figure. First, for mild-to-moderate losses in grating acuity (gray region on left of graphs), the loss in optotype and Vernier acuity is generally greater in the non-binocular group than in the binocular group. Thus, the numerous previous studies showing that grating acuity underestimates optotype and Vernier acuity in strabismic amblyopes probably reflect the lack of binocular function in strabismics. Second, once the loss in grating acuity exceeds 3 minutes of arc, almost all observers lack binocular function. So, the difference in the ratio of optotye to grating acuity between strabismic and anisometropic subjects disappears among severe amblyopes, as Birch and Swanson (7) found, because both the strabismics and the anisometropes lack binocular function.

NEURAL CIRCUITRY IN AMBLYOPIA

McKee et al. (48) speculated that the loss of binocularity in strabismic subjects produces a profound reorganization of neural circuitry that, in turn, leads to enhanced monocular sensitivity. It also leads to suppression of the image from one eye, since strabismics lack the neural machinery to combine the two retinal images into a single, fused percept. Very likely, the continuous suppression of one image accounts for the loss of pattern acuity associated with the identification of letters and Vernier offsets.

These observations regarding the differences between strabismic and anisometropic subtypes in terms of visual performance are important not only for the practicing clinician, but also because they may shed light on etiology, e.g., the degree to which amblyopia develops as a consequence or is a cause of strabismus/anisometropia. The fact that impairment in binocular functions may predict the pattern of monocular deficits suggests possible mechanisms of amblyopia, as described above (48). In particular, interocular suppression may be an important etiological factor in the progressive development of amblyopia (1,60). As previously discussed, Vernier acuity is more impaired in subjects with poor binocularity, such that deficits cannot be predicted by linearly scaling the grating acuity (Fig. 5). Vernier acuity is a hyperacuity, thought to depend on cortical

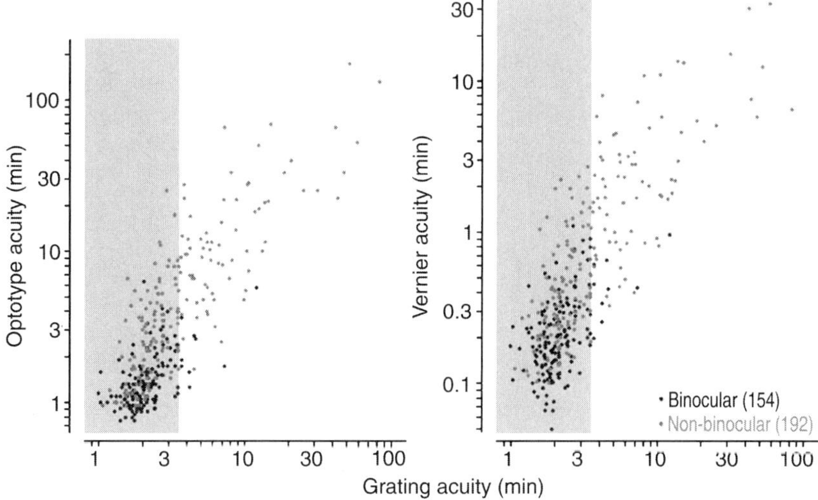

Figure 5 The graph on the left shows optotype acuity plotted against grating acuity; the graph on the right shows Vernier acuity plotted against grating acuity. At any given level of grating acuity, non-binocular observers ($N=192$; *gray dots*) generally show worse optotype and Vernier acuity than binocular observers ($N=154$; *black dots*). *Source*: Adapted from Ref. 48.

regions including and beyond the primary visual cortex. The hypothesis that Vernier acuity relies on neural pathways that overlap with binocular integration pathways is attractive (54,58,64). In addition, these functions show a similar developmental time course. Vernier acuity and binocular acuity approach adult levels by the end of the first decade (61,66). In contrast, grating acuity develops rapidly during infancy and then continues to develop more slowly, reaching adult levels at age 3 to 6 years (Fig. 2A) (19).

Many subjects with amblyopia show impairments on binocular tests. Categorization into binocular versus non-binocular groups is based on results of tests of stereopsis (1,48) and binocular motion integration (for low spatial frequencies) (1). The non-binocular group can be further characterized by performance on tests of interocular suppression, such as dichoptic contrast masking (1,22,40). The non-binocular group displays a strong asymmetry in interocular masking, whereas the binocular group shows little asymmetry (Fig. 6). For non-binocular subjects, a masking stimulus presented to the non-dominant (amblyopic) eye produces relatively little threshold elevation in the dominant eye. On the other hand, a masking stimulus presented to the dominant eye produces marked threshold elevation in the non-dominant eye.

These results encourage the idea that a history of interocular suppression distinguishes the non-binocular group and is an important etiological determination of their constellation of deficits. Even with monocular viewing, spatial localization abilities such as Vernier acuity may be particularly impaired because subjects without binocular vision suppress or "neglect" input from the amblyopic eye (57).

Maintaining residual binocularity is desirable in the treatment of subjects with amblyopia, regardless of clinical subtype, so treatment regimens should incorporate sufficient binocular vision. In the case of esotropia, early treatment results in better stereoacuity, and residual stereoacuity is associated with reduced risk of recurrence after surgery (6). Because stereopsis may improve during treatment along with visual acuity (38), regular testing of stereopsis is desirable and might be considered a separate factor in treatment optimization.

BRAIN IN AMBLYOPIA

Until recently, few techniques were available for assessing the structure or function of specific regions of the brain in patients with amblyopia. Psychophysical impairments in such patients have been interpreted to result from fewer neurons in primary visual cortex (15,33,56). While no significant change in thickness of retinal nerve fiber layer has been found in amblyopic eyes (3,10), significant shrinkage of cell size has been reported in the lateral geniculate nucleus in one strabismic subject (67). Only two patients with amblyopia, one due to strabismus and one due to anisometropia, have provided visual cortex for histological analysis. No change in the pattern of cytochrome oxidase ocular dominance staining was found in either subject (30,31). It is clear from invasive studies of animal models that abnormalities may be observed in primary visual cortex, the first level at which the separate inputs from the two eyes are combined. Both anatomical (16,25,29,65) and physiological (34,52,62) studies document the disadvantaged input from the weaker eye and lack of

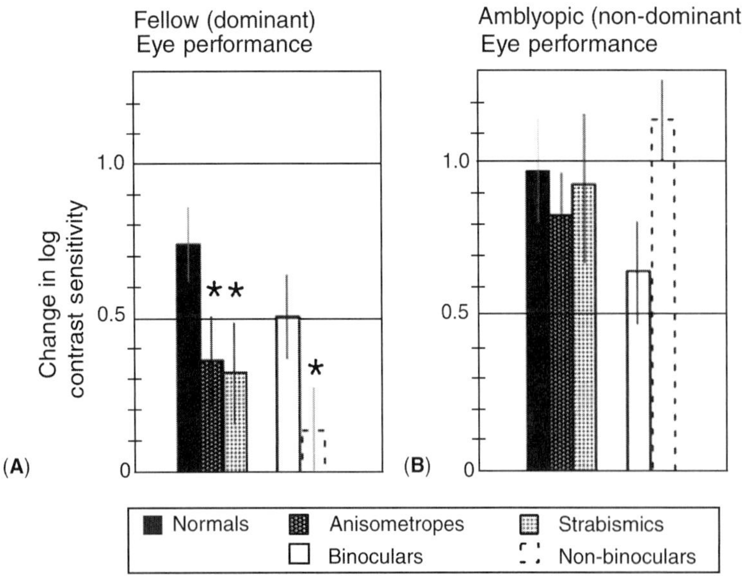

Figure 6 (**A**) Change in contrast sensitivity (in log units) of the fellow (dominant) eye due to dichoptic contrast masking by a 1 log unit supra-threshold 2 cpd grating presented to the amblyopic (non-dominant) eye (i.e., the ratio of contrast sensitivity with a homogeneous background to that with a 2 cpd background). Seven anisometropic, six strabismic, and seven control subjects were tested. Ordinate values indicate threshold elevation, i.e., interocular inhibition. Error bars indicate ±1SEM. Amblyopic groups show less inhibition of their fellow eye than normal subjects. Asterisks indicate groups performing significantly different from normal. (**B**) Change in contrast sensitivity of the amblyopic (non-dominant) eye due to the presence of a masking grating presented to the fellow (dominant) eye. Conventions are the same as for (**A**). *Source*: Adapted from Ref. 48.

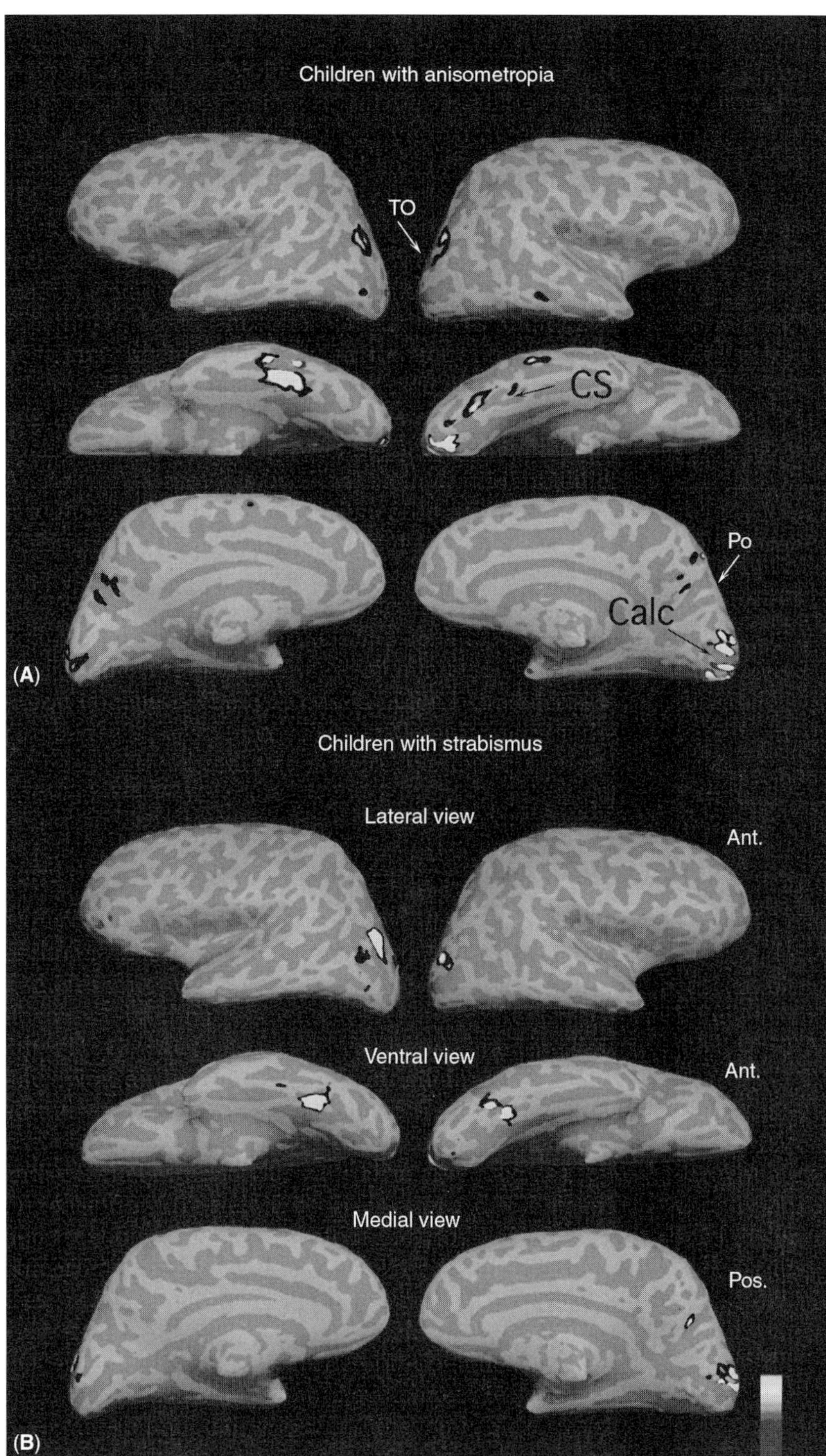

Figure 7 Localization of voxel-based morphology gray matter reductions in visual cortex in children with anisometropic and strabismic amblyopia compared to normal subjects. (**A**) Statistically significant gray matter volume reductions are shown for the anisometropic group. The changes are plotted on three inflated views of both hemispheres (*white regions surrounded by black*). From top to bottom row, the lateral, ventral, and medial views of the brain are shown. Left column shows left hemisphere, and right column shows right hemisphere. Cortical gyri and sulci are uniformly light and dark gray, respectively. The cortical surface of one normal child is used for the display. *Abbreviations*: TO, transverse occipital sulcus; CS, collateral sulcus; PO, parieto-occipital sulcus; Calc, calcarine sulcus. (**B**) The equivalent gray matter volume reductions are shown for the strabismic group. All conventions are the same as for (**A**). *Abbreviations*: Ant., anterior pole; Pos., posterior pole. *Source*: Adapted from Ref. 50.

binocular integration. Abnormalities have also been observed in extrastriate areas, in accordance with some behavioral evidence for "high-level" deficits (17,27,57) and with suggestions that the physiological abnormalities observed in primary visual cortex neurons do not fully account for behavioral loss in monkeys (35).

Recent morphological studies (50) indicate abnormalities of both gray and white matter in 7- to 12-year-old children with anisometropic or strabismic amblyopia. Group-based statistical analysis of anatomical MRI scans shows reductions in amount and intensity of gray matter in multiple regions. The scans were of a high resolution

(1.2 × 0.9 × 0.9 mm), optimized for contrast between gray and white matter and analysis was automated with voxel-based morphology (volumetric element-by-element comparison of the local concentration of gray matter) (2). This involved segmentation of the images into gray and white matter components, followed by combination of the brains of subjects with the same age group and diagnosis. Abnormalities were found in four cortical regions: para-calcarine, medial parietal-occipital junction, lateral parietal-occipital junction, and ventral temporal cortex (Fig. 7). In adult anisometropic and strabismic subjects (age 18–35 years), changes were similar but more restricted in the para-calcarine area; these results have been replicated in a separate study of strabismic adults (9).

Cortical fiber tracts may also be anomalous in amblyopia. It has been shown that inducing amblyopia in animal models causes an expansion of the zone of corpus callosum connections in the visual cortex (51,69). The corpus callosum has been recently examined using the non-invasive MRI technique diffusion tensor imaging (DTI) (49), which relies upon the ability to measure water diffusion within brain tissues that reflects the tissue structure at the microscopic level. Anisotropic diffusion is found in regions containing fibers and fiber tracts (37). DTI scans were obtained for a cohort of children similar to the one examined with voxel-based morphology (50) and compared to control children. The posterior corpus callosum showed reduced anisotropic diffusion in children with both anisometropic and strabismic amblyopia.

These morphological results are entirely consistent with the increasingly apparent role of higher-level cortex in the neurological account of amblyopia. There is growing evidence for extrastriate abnormalities in amblyopia from animal studies (12,35,36, 55,59,63) and from human neuroimaging (4,39,53). In fact, amblyopia may be considered to represent a functional deafferentation that increases at progressively higher stages of the visual pathway.

These morphological studies have not shown a large degree of difference between subjects with amblyopia associated with anisometropia versus strabismus. At this time, it is not possible to distinguish between the role of form deprivation versus lack of binocularity because all extant studies have focused on subjects who have both amblyopia and reduced binocularity. The extent to which such cortical changes represent the "cause" or the "result" of amblyopia remains to be defined. There could be eye-to-brain as well as brain-to-eye effects. Moreover, the degree to which these changes are genetically determined or experience-dependent is a central question for the future.

REFERENCES

1. Agrawal R, Conner IP, Odom JV, et al. Relating binocular and monocular vision in strabismic and anisometropic amblyopia. Arch Ophthalmol 2006; 124:844–50.
2. Ashburner J, Friston KJ. Voxel-based morphometry—the methods. Neuroimage 2000; 11:805–21.
3. Baddini-Caramelli C, Hatanaka M, Polati M, et al. Thickness of the retinal nerve fiber layer in amblyopic and normal eyes: a scanning laser polarimetry study. J AAPOS 2001; 5:82–4.
4. Barnes GR, Hess RF, Dumoulin SO, et al. The cortical deficit in humans with strabismic amblyopia. J Physiol 2001; 533:281–97.
5. Birch EE, Gwiazda J, Held R. Stereoacuity development for crossed and uncrossed disparities in human infants. Vision Res 1982; 22:507–13.
6. Birch EE, Stager DR, Sr, Berry P, Leffler J. Stereopsis and long-term stability of alignment in esotropia. J AAPOS 2004; 8:146–50.
7. Birch EE, Swanson WH. Hyperacuity deficits in anisometropic and strabismic amblyopes with known ages of onset. Vision Res 2000; 40:1035–40.
8. Bradley A, Freeman RD. Is reduced Vernier acuity in amblyopia due to position, contrast or fixation deficits? Vision Res 1985; 25:55–66.
9. Chan ST, Tang KW, Lam KC, et al. Neuroanatomy of adult strabismus: a Voxel-based morphometric analysis of magnetic resonance structural scans. Neuroimage 2004; 22:986–94.
10. Colen TP, de Faber JT, Lemij HG. Retinal nerve fiber layer thickness in human strabismic amblyopia. Binocul Vis Strabismus Q 2000; 15:141–6.
11. Conner IP, Sharma S, Lemieux SK, Mendola JD. Retinotopic organization in children measured with fMRI. J Vis 2004; 4:509–23.
12. Crewther DP, Crewther SG. Neural site of strabismic amblyopia in cats: spatial frequency deficit in primary cortical neurons. Exp Brain Res 1990; 79:615–22.
13. Daw NW. Critical periods and amblyopia. Arch Ophthalmol 1998; 116:502–05.
14. Daw NW. Mechanisms of plasticity in the visual cortex. The Friedenwald Lecture. Invest Ophthalmol Vis Sci 1994; 35:4168–79.
15. Demanins R, Wang YZ, Hess RF. The neural deficit in strabismic amblyopia: sampling considerations. Vision Res 1999; 39:3575–85.
16. Fenstemaker SB, Kiorpes L, Movshon JA. Effects of experimental strabismus on the architecture of macaque monkey striate cortex. J Comp Neurol 2001; 438:300–17.
17. Giaschi DE, Regan D, Kraft SP, Hong XH. Defective processing of motion-defined form in the fellow eye of patients with unilateral amblyopia. Invest Ophthalmol Vis Sci 1992; 33:2483–9.
18. Gstalder RJ, Green DG. Laser interferometric acuity in amblyopia. J Pediatr Ophthalmol 1971; 8:251–6.
19. Gwiazda J, Bauer J, Held R. From visual acuity to hyperacuity: a 10-year update. Can J Psychol 1989; 43:109–20.
20. Gwiazda J, Bauer J, Thom F, Held R. Development of spatial contrast sensitivity from infancy to adulthood: psychophysical data. Optom Vis Sci 1997; 74:785–89.
21. Gwiazda J, Scheiman M, Held R. Anisotropic resolution in children's vision. Vision Res 1984; 24:527–31.
22. Harrad RA, Hess RF. Binocular integration of contrast information in amblyopia. Vision Res 1992; 32:2135–50.
23. Harwerth RS, Smith EL 3rd, Crawford ML, von Noorden GK. Behavioral studies of the sensitive periods of

development of visual functions in monkeys. Behav Brain Res 1990; 41:179–98.
24. Held R. Two stages in the development of binocular vision and eye alignment. In: K. Simons, ed. Early Visual Development, Normal and Abnormal. London: Oxford Press; 1993:250–7.
25. Hendrickson AE, Movshon JA, Eggers HM, et al. Effects of early unilateral blur on the macaque's visual system. II. Anatomical observations. J Neurosci 1987; 7:1327–39.
26. Hess RF, Holliday IE. The spatial localization deficit in amblyopia. Vision Res 1992; 32:1319–39.
27. Hess RF, Wang YZ, Demanins R, et al. A deficit in strabismic amblyopia for global shape detection. Vision Res 1999; 39:901–14.
28. Holopigian K, Blake R, Greenwald MJ. Selective losses in binocular vision in anisometropic amblyopes. Vision Res 1986; 26:621–30.
29. Horton JC, Hocking DR, Kiorpes L. Pattern of ocular dominance columns and cytochrome oxidase activity in a macaque monkey with naturally occurring anisometropic amblyopia. Vis Neurosci 1997; 14:681–9.
30. Horton JC, Hocking DR. Pattern of ocular dominance columns in human striate cortex in strabismic amblyopia. Vis Neurosci 1996; 13:787–95.
31. Horton JC, Stryker MP. Amblyopia induced by anisometropia without shrinkage of ocular dominance columns in human striate cortex. Proc Natl Acad Sci USA 1993; 90: 5494–8.
32. Hubel DH, Wiesel TN. Receptive fields, binocular interaction and functional architecture in the cat's visual cortex. J Physiol 1962; 160:106–54.
33. Katz LM, Levi DM, Bedell HE. Central and peripheral contrast sensitivity in amblyopia with varying field size. Doc Ophthalmol 1984; 58:351–73.
34. Kiorpes L, Kiper DC, O'Keefe LP, et al. Neuronal correlates of amblyopia in the visual cortex of macaque monkeys with experimental strabismus and anisometropia. J Neurosci 1998; 18:6411–24.
35. Kiorpes L, McKee SP. Neural mechanisms underlying amblyopia. Curr Opin Neurobiol 1999; 9:480–6.
36. Kiorpes L, Walton PJ, O'Keefe LP, et al. Effects of early-onset artificial strabismus on pursuit eye movements and on neuronal responses in area MT of macaque monkeys. J Neurosci 1996; 16:6537–53.
37. Le Bihan D, Breton E, Lallemand D, et al. MR imaging of intravoxel incoherent motions: application to diffusion and perfusion in neurologic disorders. Radiology 1986; 161: 401–7.
38. Lee SY, Isenberg SJ. The relationship between stereopsis and visual acuity after occlusion therapy for amblyopia. Ophthalmology 2003; 110:2088–92.
39. Lerner Y, Pianka P, Azmon B, et al. Area-specific amblyopic effects in human occipitotemporal object representations. Neuron 2003; 40:1023–9.
40. Levi DM, Harwerth RS, Smith EL 3rd. Humans deprived of normal binocular vision have binocular interactions tuned to size and orientation. Science 1979; 206:852–4.
41. Levi DM, Klein S. Differences in Vernier discrimination for grating between strabismic and anisometropic amblyopes. Invest Ophthalmol Vis Sci 1982; 23:398–407.
42. Levi DM, Klein S. Hyperacuity and amblyopia. Nature 1982; 298:268–70.
43. Levi DM, Klein SA. Vernier acuity, crowding and amblyopia. Vision Res 1985; 25:979–91.
44. Majewska AK, Sur M. Plasticity and specificity of cortical processing networks. Trends Neurosci 2006; 29:323–9.
45. Mayer DL, Beiser AS, Warner AF, et al. Monocular acuity norms for the Teller Acuity Cards between ages one month and four years. Invest Ophthalmol Vis Sci 1995; 36:671–85.
46. Mayer DL, Fulton AB, Rodier D. Grating and recognition acuities of pediatric patients. Ophthalmology 1984; 91: 947–53.
47. Mayer DL, Hansen RM, Moore BD, et al. Cycloplegic refractions in healthy children aged 1 through 48 months. Arch Ophthalmol 2001; 119:1625–8.
48. McKee SP, Levi DM, Movshon JA. The pattern of visual deficits in amblyopia. J Vis 2003; 3:380–405.
49. Mendola J, Bahekar A, Conner I, et al. DTI shows white matter abnormalities in children with amblyopia. 11th International Conference on Functional Mapping of the Human Brain. Neuroimage 2005; 26:S46.
50. Mendola JD, Conner IP, Roy A, et al. Voxel-based analysis of MRI detects abnormal visual cortex in children and adults with amblyopia. Hum Brain Mapp 2005; 25: 222–36.
51. Milleret C, Houzel JC. Visual interhemispheric transfer to areas 17 and 18 in cats with convergent strabismus. Eur J Neurosci 2001; 13:137–52.
52. Movshon JA, Eggers HM, Gizzi MS, et al. Effects of early unilateral blur on the macaque's visual system. III. Physiological observations. J Neurosci 1987; 7: 1340–51.
53. Muckli L, Kohler A, Kriegeskorte N, Singer W. Primary visual cortex activity along the apparent-motion trace reflects illusory perception. PLoS Biol 2005; 3:e265.
54. Mussap AJ, Levi DM. Binocular processes in Vernier acuity. J Opt Soc Am A Opt Image Sci Vis 1995; 12: 225–33.
55. Schroder JH, Fries P, Roelfsema PR, et al. Ocular dominance in extrastriate cortex of strabismic amblyopic cats. Vision Res 2002; 42:29–39.
56. Sharma V, Levi DM, Coletta NJ. Sparse-sampling of gratings in the visual cortex of strabismic amblyopes. Vision Res 1999; 39:3526–36.
57. Sharma V, Levi DM, Klein SA. Undercounting features and missing features: evidence for a high-level deficit in strabismic amblyopia. Nat Neurosci 2000; 3:496–501.
58. Shimojo S, Birch EE, Gwiazda J, Held R. Development of Vernier acuity in infants. Vision Res 1984; 24:721–8.
59. Sireteanu R, Best J. Squint-induced modification of visual receptive fields in the lateral suprasylvian cortex of the cat: binocular interaction, vertical effect and anomalous correspondence. Eur J Neurosci 1992; 4:235–42.
60. Sireteanu R. Human amblyopia: consequence of chronic interocular suppression. Hum Neurobiol 1982; 1:31–3.
61. Skoczenski AM, Norcia AM. Late maturation of visual hyperacuity. Psychol Sci 2002; 13:537–41.
62. Smith EL 3rd, Chino YM, Ni J, et al. Residual binocular interactions in the striate cortex of monkeys reared with abnormal binocular vision. J Neurophysiol 1997; 78: 1353–62.
63. Thiele A, Bremmer F, Ilg UJ, Hoffmann KP. Visual responses of neurons from areas V1 and MT in a monkey with late onset strabismus: a case study. Vision Res 1997; 37:853–63.
64. Tsao DY, Vanduffel W, Sasaki Y, et al. Stereopsis activates V3A and caudal intraparietal areas in macaques and humans. Neuron 2003; 39:555–68.
65. Tychsen L, Burkhalter A. Nasotemporal asymmetries in V1: ocular dominance columns of infant, adult, and strabismic macaque monkeys. J Comp Neurol 1997; 388:32–46.

66. Tychsen L. Binocular Vision. In: W. Hart, ed. Adler's Physiology of the Eye: Clinical Applications. St. Louis, MO: Mosby Year Book; 1992:773–853.
67. von Noorden GK, Crawford ML. The lateral geniculate nucleus in human strabismic amblyopia. Invest Ophthalmol Vis Sci 1992; 33:2729–32.
68. von Noorden GK. Burian-von Noorden's Binocular Vision and Ocular Motility. 3 ed. St. Louis: CV Mosby, 1985.
69. Watroba L, Buser P, Milleret C. Impairment of binocular vision in the adult cat induces plastic changes in the callosal cortical map. Eur J Neurosci 2001; 14:1021–9.
70. Wiesel TN. Postnatal development of the visual cortex and the influence of environment. Nature 1982; 299: 583–91.
71. Wu C, Fulton AB. Amblyopia. In: Hunter DG, Mills MD, eds. Albert and Jacobiec's Principles and Practice of Ophthalmology. 3rd ed. New York: Elsevier, 2008.
72. Wu C, Hunter DG. Amblyopia: diagnostic and therapeutic options. Am J Ophthalmol 2006; 141:175–84.
73. Zadnik K, Manny RE, Yu JA, et al. Ocular component data in schoolchildren as a function of age and gender. Optom Vis Sci 2003; 80:226–36.

72

Muscular Disorders

Edward H. Bossen
Department of Pathology, Duke University, Durham, North Carolina, U.S.A.

INTRODUCTION

Most evaluations of muscle disease have been derived from the study of extremity muscles, which differ from extraocular muscles (EOMs). Before discussing muscle diseases that affect the eye, the structure of both extremity (limb) muscles and EOMs will be compared.

NORMAL LIMB MUSCLES

A skeletal muscle, such as the biceps, consists of bundles (fasciculi) of individual muscle fibers with connective tissue surrounding each fasciculus (perimysium), and individual muscle fibers (endomysium) (Fig. 1). The contractile element of the muscle fiber is the myofibril, which is composed of essentially parallel arrays of actin and myosin filaments. Skeletal muscle is called striated muscle because of its banded microscopic appearance due to the A (anisotropic), I (isotropic), and Z (Zwischenscheibe) bands. The I band, which is pale when stained with hematoxylin and eosin, contains the actin filaments (5–8 nm in diameter), which are anchored at the thin, dense, Z band. The dark A band contains the thicker (15 nm in diameter) myosin filaments as well as actin filaments, which slide between the myosin filaments during contraction. The basic contractile unit of skeletal muscle is the sarcomere, which extends from Z band to Z band (Fig. 2).

In addition to myofibrils, the muscle fibers contain mitochondria, which contribute energy, and other cytoplasmic components, including glycogen, ribosomes, and rare lysosomes. The sarcoplasmic reticulum is important in the release and uptake of calcium essential for muscle contraction and relaxation and transverse tubules aid in transmission of the action potential from the periphery to the interior of the cells (Fig. 3).

The concept of the motor unit—a neuron, its axon, and the muscle fibers it innervates—is important for understanding the histopathology of muscle disease. The muscle fibers contract when stimulated by the axon at a specialized portion of

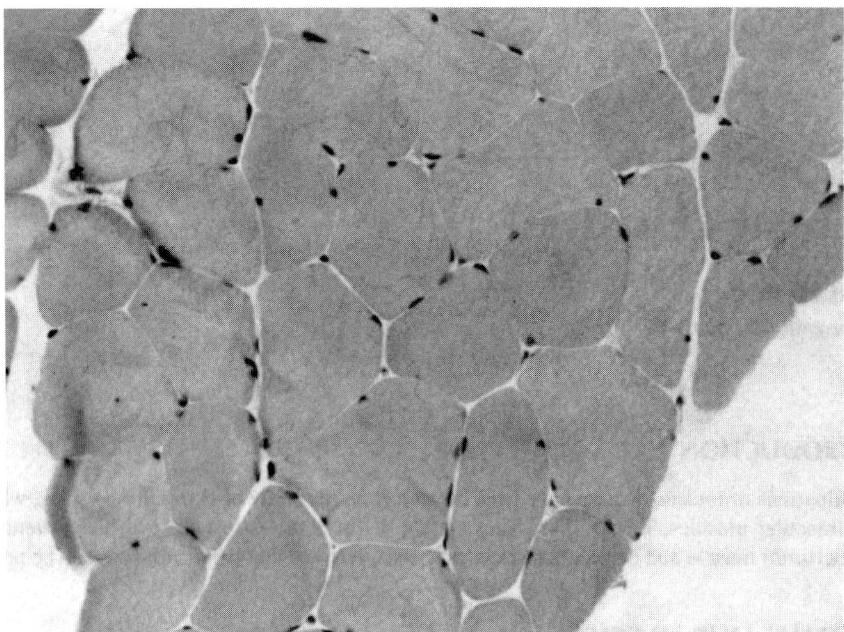

Figure 1 Normal muscle (hematoxylin and eosin, ×250).

the fiber, the motor end plate. The action potential travels along the surface of the muscle fiber and into the interior of the fibers via the transverse tubules. A portion of the sarcoplasmic reticulum, known as junctional sarcoplasmic reticulum, abuts the plasmalemma at the transverse tubule and the periphery of the fiber (7). Calcium bound within the junctional sarcoplasmic reticulum is released, by an unknown mechanism, by the action potential, allowing contraction. Relaxation occurs when calcium is taken up by the free sarcoplasmic reticulum, which lacks the granules of the junctional sarcoplasmic reticulum.

Reference should be made to specialized texts for more detailed information on the structure and physiology of muscle (16,53).

NORMAL EXTRAOCULAR MUSCLES

EOMs differ from limb muscles. The fibers are rounder, smaller (10–38 μm in diameter versus 40–60 μm) (41), have more internal nuclei, and there is more endomysial tissue than limb muscle. Variation in fiber size is normal for EOM fibers, with larger fibers tending to be in the center of muscles and smaller fibers at the periphery (Fig. 4). These features, normal in EOM, would be considered myopathic in limb muscle. Ringbinden (ringed fibers—see the section entitled Myotonic Dystrophy) can also be seen in normal EOM (23,192).

There have been several classifications of the type of EOMs. A commonly used older system

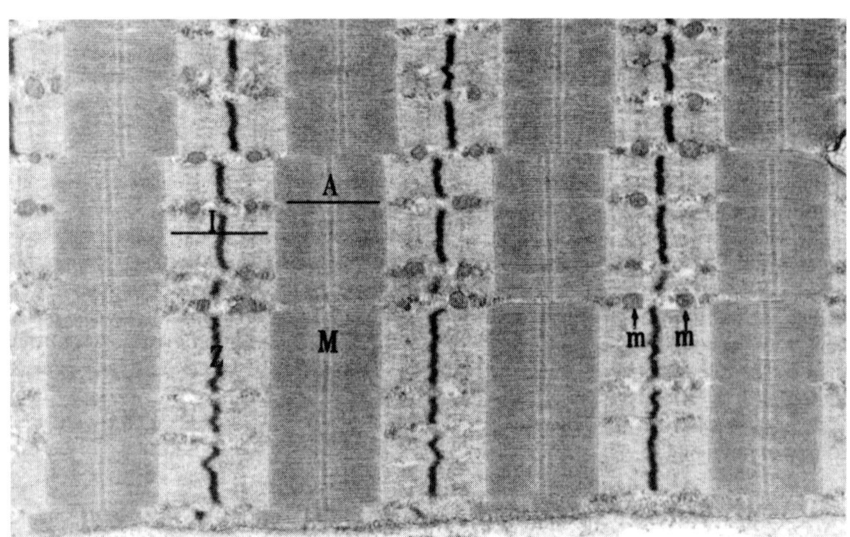

Figure 2 Apperance of normal striated muscle by transmission electron microscopy. *Abbreviations*: A, A band; I, I band; M, M line (middle of A band); m, mitochondria (×11,500).

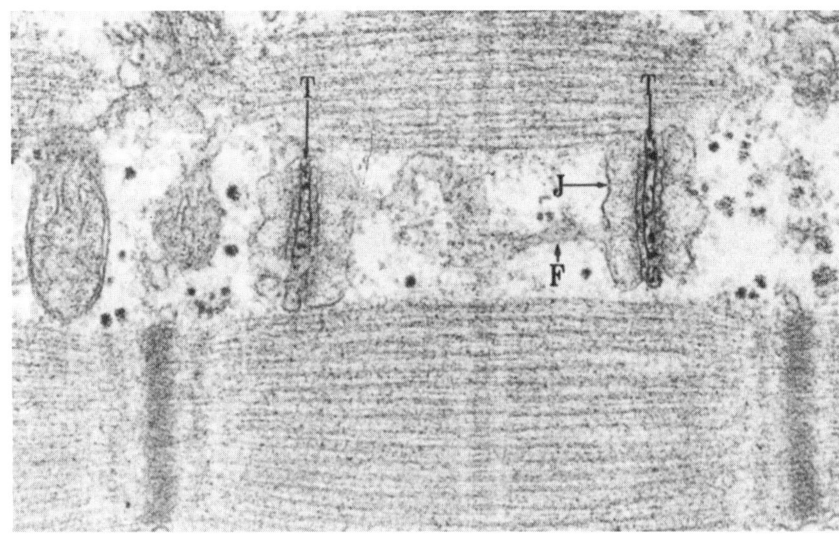

Figure 3 Normal striated muscle by transmission electron microscopy. *Abbreviations*: T, transverse tubular system; J, junctional sarcoplasmic reticulum; F, free sarcoplasmic reticulum (×45,500).

divided the EOMs into three principal fiber types: fine, granular, and coarse (Table 1). The fine and granular fibers are referred to as "Fibrillenstruktur" and the coarse as "Felderstructur" in the older literature (72,209). In the levator palpebrae superioris the three types are arranged randomly but in the oblique and rectus muscles peripheral (orbital), intermediate, and central (global) zones are discernible (41,72,208,267,279). In the levator palpebrae superioris 75% to 80% of the fibers are coarse with the remainder being granular. In the oblique and rectus muscles the peripheral and intermediate zones consist of 80% coarse and 20% fine fibers, whereas the granular fibers comprise 75% of the central zone, the remainder being composed of equal portions of fine and coarse fibers.

Histochemical staining of EOMs reveals that the fine fibers resemble limb muscle fiber type 1, although they have less succinic dehydrogenase and other oxidative enzyme activity. The granular fibers resemble type 2 limb muscle fibers, staining intensely for myosin adenosine triphosphatase and weakly for succinic dehydrogenase. The coarse fibers have properties of both type 1 and type 2 fibers, staining

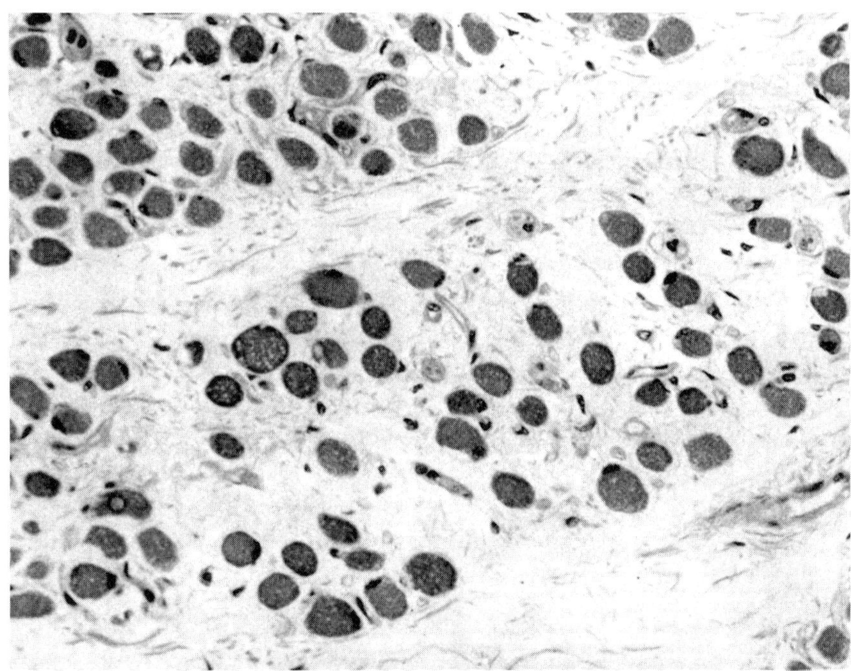

Figure 4 Normal extraocular muscle. Note the variation in fiber size, rounding of fibers, and abundant connective tissue. The fiber size is not directly comparable with illustrations of skeletal muscle since this is of fixed tissue and the skeletal muscle illustrations are of frozen tissue except as indicated (hematoxylin and eosin, ×260).

Table 1 Muscle Fiber Types: Limb Muscles

	Muscle type	
Attribute	**Type 1**	**Type 2**
Myosin adenosine triphosphatase stain	Pale	Dark
Succinic dehydrogenase stain	Dark	Pale
Mitochondria	More	Fewer
Twitch type	Slow	Fast

strongly for both myosin adenosine triphosphatase and succinic dehydrogenase (72,267).

EOM can also be divided into six subtypes. These are: orbital single innervated, orbital multiple innervated, global red single innervated, global intermediate single innervated, global pale single innervated, and global multiple innervated fibers (379). The fibers that are multiply innervated are those with en grappe endplates. These fibers do not develop an action potential and have slow, graded, tonic contractions in contrast to the action potential generated twitch contraction of limb muscle and the single innervated EOM (379).

The EOM fibers with en grappe neuromuscular junctions have multiple neuromuscular junctions and may be supplied by more than one nerve. The en grappe neuromuscular junctions lack the secondary junctional folds of singly innervated extremity endplates, which may be a factor in the susceptibility of these fibers to myasthenia gravis (34).

The importance of these studies of normal EOMs lies in the interpretation of myopathic as opposed to neurogenic changes in these muscles, the criteria for which were developed with respect to limb muscles. Do these rules also apply to EOMs? Drachman et al. (64) studied the EOMs of dogs following intracranial avulsion or crushing of the oculomotor nerve. They found the most striking changes 2 weeks to 1 month following denervation, with a gradual restoration of normal morphology thereafter. During the period of maximum change they noted infiltrates of inflammatory cells (predominantly lymphocytes), central nuclei in 20% of the fibers (normal in their study being 3–5%), fiber degeneration, myophagocytosis, basophilic fibers with plump vesicular nuclei (probably regenerating fibers), occasional fiber splitting, and increased connective tissue around individual fibers (endomysial fibrosis) and about muscle fasciculi (perimysial fibrosis). These findings would indicate a myopathy in limb muscle. The one feature these authors noted which was not typical of a myopathy was loss of nerve fibers in the denervated animals. Large groups of atrophic fibers (64,72,267) were not seen in experimental denervation of EOMs, presumably because the size of the motor unit is much smaller in these muscles compared to those of the limbs. However, Minoda (209) reports group atrophy in neurogenic EOM paralysis in humans.

Durston studied denervated EOM in baboons (72) with histochemical techniques and noted type grouping 6 months after denervation. The grouped fibers were predominantly of the fine type, which is most comparable to the principal fiber type involved in denervation of limb muscle (limb type 1 fibers).

Ringel et al. (267) did not find type grouping in their studies of EOM denervation in rhesus monkeys and had difficulty in establishing the diagnosis of denervation by the morphologic criteria used in limb muscle. Employing alpha-bungarotoxin they were able to demonstrate extrajunctional binding, a characteristic of experimental denervation in limb muscle. This phenomenon is not diagnostic of denervation; moreover, only a minority of fine and granular fibers gave a positive response, and none did after 12 weeks.

Another component of limb muscle is the muscle spindle. The muscle fibers of the spindle, referred to as intrafusal muscle fibers, are divided into "nuclear chain" and "nuclear bag" fibers. As in limb muscles, muscle spindles also occur in human EOM, but the muscle fibers of the spindle (intrafusal fibers) cannot be differentiated into nuclear chain or nuclear bag types.

When viewed by transmission electron microscopy (TEM) EOMs basically resemble limb skeletal muscle, but Z-band alterations, abnormal mitochondria, and leptomeres (zebra bodies) have been reported in otherwise normal EOMs (192). The proportion of cytoplasm containing mitochondria is greater in EOMS muscles than in limb muscles (41). Singly innervated orbital muscle fibers are the most oxidative (319).

Readers desiring more details of EOM structure and function are referred to reviews (41,279,281).

GENERAL CONCEPTS OF MUSCLE PATHOLOGY

Abnormalities of any of the components of the motor unit may lead to neuromuscular disease, of which there are two main categories: myopathies and neurogenic disorders. The characteristic histologic features of a myopathy, as defined in limb muscle, are: variation in fiber size, rounding of normally polygonal fibers, both hypertrophic and atrophic fibers, central nuclei in more than 3% of fibers, fiber regeneration and degeneration, myophagocytosis (macrophages within degenerating muscle fibers), endomysial fibrosis (increase in connective tissue around individual fibers), and fiber splitting (Fig. 5). Polymyositis, an inflammatory

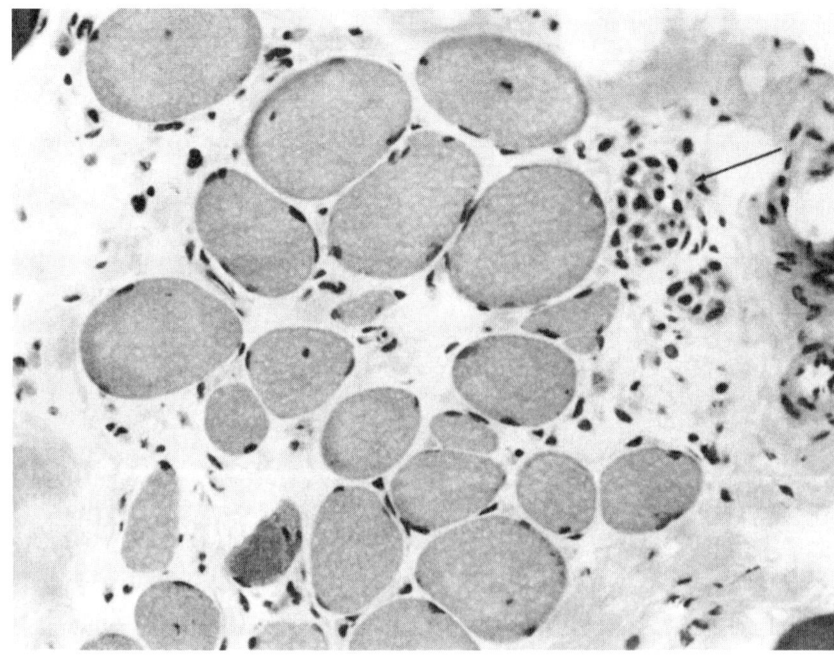

Figure 5 Myopathy. Note the rounded fibers, internal nuclei, increased connective tissue around fibers, and myophagocytosis (*arrow*) (hematoxylin and eosin, ×250).

myopathy, has an infiltrate of lymphocytes, plasma cells, and sometimes eosinophils in addition to the aforementioned features.

Neurogenic atrophy is characterized by group fiber atrophy with angulation of the atrophic fibers (Fig. 6). Central nuclei and endomysial fibrosis are not basic features of neurogenic atrophy but can be seen, together with degenerating, regenerating, and hypertrophic fibers, in long-standing denervation. This pattern is referred to as myopathic change secondary to chronic denervation.

Enzyme histochemistry is a considerable aid in the diagnosis of neuromuscular disorders, its usefulness being based on the fact that all muscle fibers do not have the same distribution of cytoplasmic components. For diagnostic purposes, human skeletal muscle fibers can be divided into two major groups: type 1 and type 2. In general, type 1 fibers are slow-twitch fibers with predominantly aerobic metabolism reflected by the presence of numerous mitochondria. Type 2 fibers are fast-twitch, mainly anaerobic, and have fewer mitochondria. Fiber characteristics are

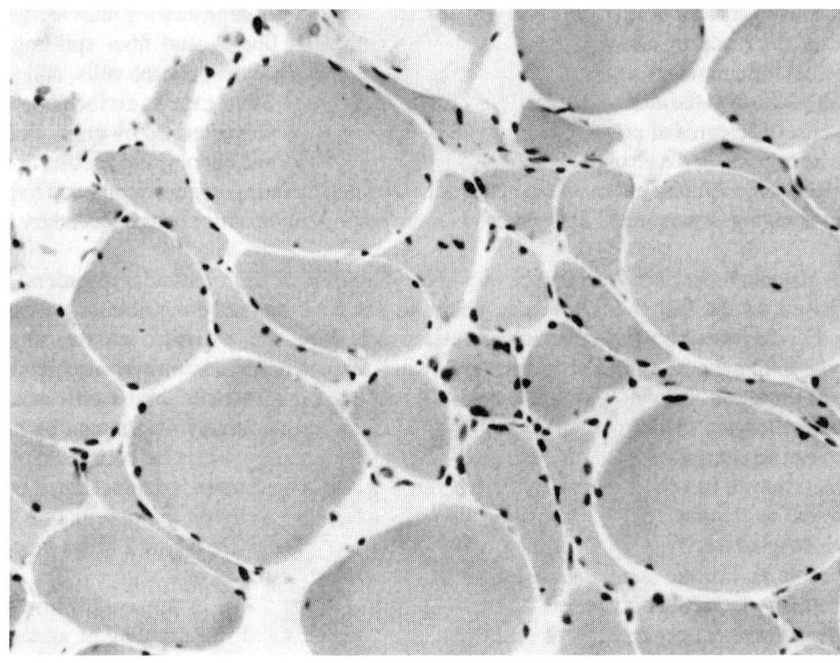

Figure 6 Neurogenic atrophy, group fiber atrophy (hematoxylin and eosin, ×250).

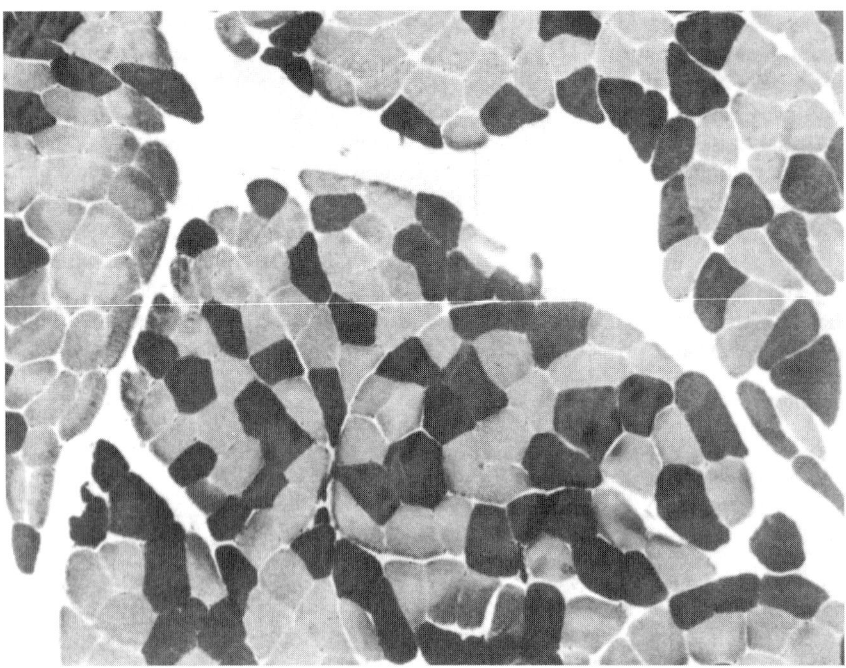

Figure 7 Normal muscle with myosin adenosine triphosphatase stain, illustrating the checkerboard pattern with pale type 1 and dark type 2 fibers (×110).

largely determined by neurogenic influence and can be altered by cross-innervation (67,272). In humans, muscles are composed of both type 1 and 2 fibers, arranged in a checkerboard pattern (Figs. 7 and 8). This pattern is demonstrated by a variety of histochemical techniques, but muscle fiber typing is based primarily on the distribution of myosin adenosine triphosphatase. Type 1 fibers stain poorly for this enzyme, whereas type 2 fibers stain intensely (Fig. 8; Table 2). Further subdivisions can be based on other staining procedures (69).

Histochemistry is particularly helpful in the diagnosis of denervation (Fig. 9). In denervating diseases, some fibers lose their nerve supply and atrophy, but others are reinnervated by sprouting from axons that supply adjacent muscle fibers. When this occurs, the reinnervated fibers assume the histochemical staining of the neighboring fibers normally supplied by that axon. This results in a pattern termed "fiber-type grouping" rather than the normal checkerboard pattern (Fig. 10). Such fibers may be of normal size and configuration and so fail to

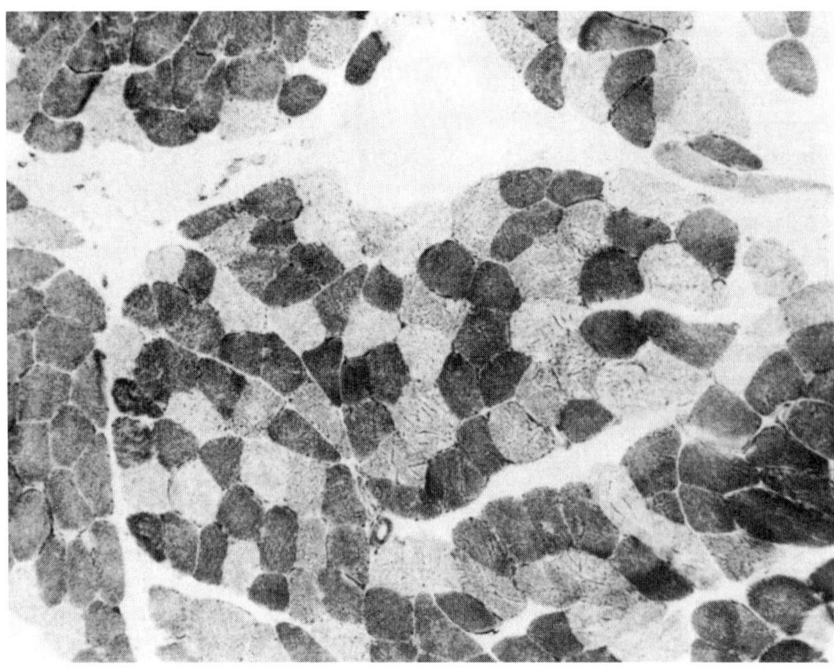

Figure 8 Normal muscle illustrating dark type 1 and pale type 2 fibers. Compare with Figure 7, which is the same field but slightly rotated (nicotinamide adenine dinucleotide tetrazolium reductase stain, ×100).

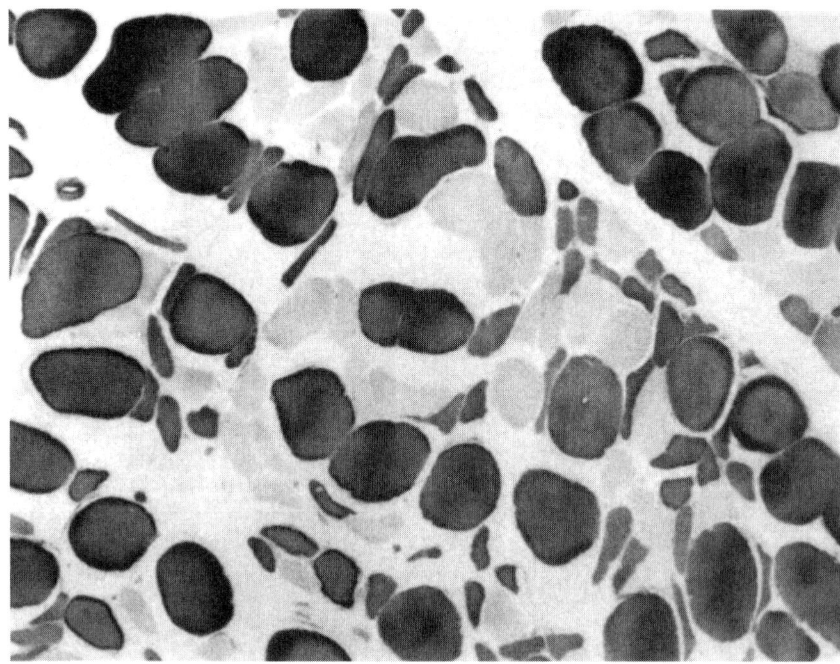

Figure 9 Denervation. Angulated, atrophic fibers that are both type 1 (*pale*) and type 2 (*dark*) are seen (myosin adenosine triphosphatase stain, $\times$100).

be recognized in the absence of histochemical enzyme staining. Eventually, the neuron or axon supplying this group of fibers may itself become involved in the disease process, resulting in the classic feature of denervation-group fiber atrophy (Fig. 6). In denervation, atrophic fibers are both type 1 and 2 (Fig. 9), whereas in disuse atrophy or steroid myopathy the atrophic fibers are type 2.

Another characteristic of denervation best seen with histochemical stains is that of the "target" fiber (Fig. 11). In denervation there is segmental central disruption of the myofibrils with loss of membranous structures, including mitochondria, in this central zone and aggregation of mitochondria at the periphery of the disrupted area. Staining of a cross section of muscle for nicotinamide-adenine dinucleotide tetrazolium reductase, which demonstrates mitochondria, reveals a central unstained zone (no mitochondria) surrounded by an intensely staining zone (aggregates of mitochondria), with the remainder of the fiber having normal staining characteristics. Not all denervated muscle manifests this change but, when it is seen, it is strongly suggestive of denervation.

Table 2 Muscle Fiber Types: Extraocular

	Muscle Type		
Attribute	**Coarse**	**Fine**	**Granular**
Myosin adenosine triphosphatase stain	Dark	Pale	Dark
Succinic dehydrogenase stain	Dark	Intermediate	Pale
	En grappe	En plaque	En plaque

Source: Modified from Durston JHJ. Histochemistry of primate extraocular muscles and the changes of denervation. Br J Ophthalmol 58:193, 1974.

NEUROMUSCULAR DISORDERS

Myasthenia Gravis

Clinical Features

Myasthenia gravis is a neuromuscular disorder characterized clinically by increasing weakness with repetitive muscle use, but improved by anticholinesterase drugs. Estimates of the incidence of myasthenia gravis range from 2 to 10 per 100,000, with 20% of the cases beginning in patients under 20 years old (298). It is most commonly a generalized disease, with 69% to 90% of the patients having EOM involvement, but in 13% to 14% of the cases there is only ptosis and/or ophthalmoplegia (120,190). Approximately one-half of patients with ocular myasthenia, defined as involvement only of the EOMs, levator palbebrae superioris, and orbicularis oculi muscles (74), will become generalized within 2 years (180). Ninety percent of individuals who present with pure ocular myasthenia, but who develop generalized myasthenia gravis, do so within 3 years of onset of their ocular diseases (74). Chinese have a higher frequency of pure ocular myasthenia (45).

The best diagnostic tool is the presence of serum anti-acetylcholine receptor (anti-ACR) antibodies, but

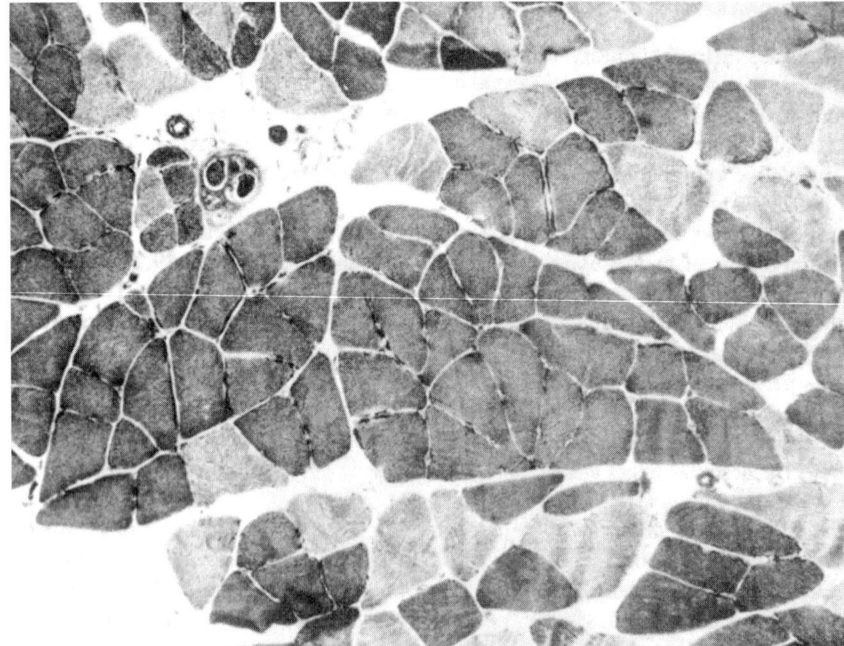

Figure 10 Denervation. The normal checkerboard pattern is lost, with almost entire fasciculi of one type, a change referred to as type grouping. In this instance the dark fibers are type 1 (nicotinamide adenine dinucleotide tetrazolium reductase stain, ×100).

approximately 10% or patients with clinical myasthenia lack these antibodies (178). Thirty to 50% of those with pure ocular myasthenia lack anti-ACR antibodies (155,249). Ten to 40% of those who are seronegative for ACR antibodies have anti-MuSK (muscle specific tyrosine kinase) antibodies. These patients are usually women who are difficult to treat and have bulbar symptoms (74,358). Patients with pure ocular myasthenia do not have MuSK antibodies (381). Patients who are seronegative for both ACR and MuSK tend to have mild disease (74).

In adults generalized myasthenia gravis affects females twice as often as males. The onset, usually between the ages of 20 and 35 years, may be gradual or sudden, and may be precipitated by an illness or emotional disturbance. The course is variable, with most deaths occurring during the first year and rarely after 10 years. In a large study in Italy, 4% of patients

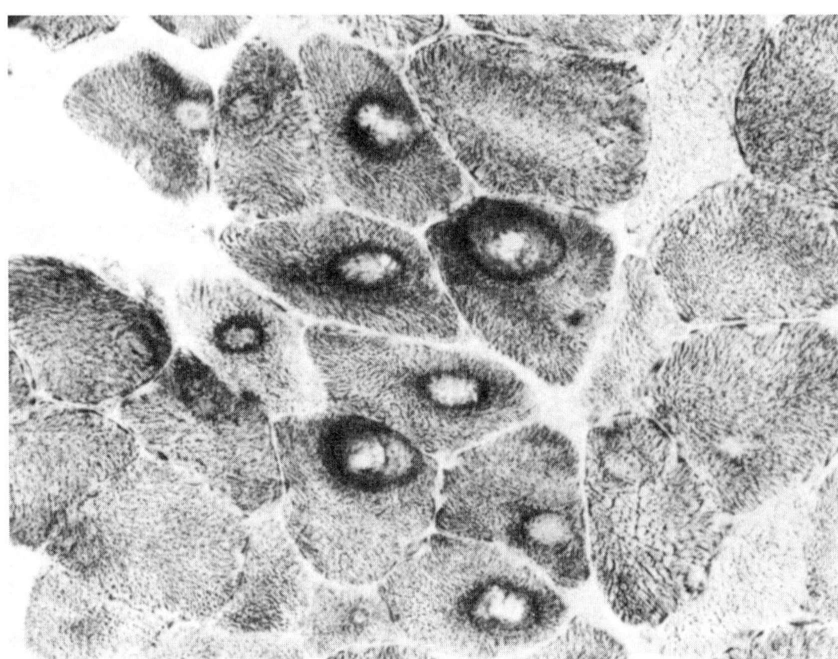

Figure 11 Denervation. The fibers in the middle of this micrograph contain a central pale zone surrounded by a dark rim. These are target fibers (nicotinamide adenine dinucleotide tetrazolium reductase stain, ×260).

died of myasthenia gravis (190). Although any muscle may be affected, the EOMs are most commonly involved, with the neck muscles being the next most frequently affected. Motor function of other cranial nerves may be affected, but sensory changes are uncommon (80).

Involvement of the EOMs is manifest by ptosis and external ophthalmoplegia, which may be alternating and recurrent (24,107,238). Pure ocular myasthenia is slightly more common in males, but the female to male ratio in patients under 20 years of age is 2:1. The EOMs might be particularly vulnerable because of a lower safety factor for neuromuscular transmission which is due to the rapidity of firing and the simplified endplates normally present in these muscles (229). The fetal isoforms of ACR present in the multiterminal fibers of EOMs may make the eye muscles more susceptible (150,229). Myasthenia gravis may be mistaken for progressive external ophthalmoplegia (35) or a focal lesion of the medial longitudinal fasciculus (114,204). Internal ophthalmoplegia, characterized by dilated unequal pupils which respond to anticholinesterase agents, is very rare (13,132).

Approximately 10% to 20% of cases of myasthenia gravis occur in association with other autoimmune diseases, including rheumatoid arthritis (1,238, 342), Sjögren syndrome (128), systemic lupus erythematosus (238,342), polymyositis (163), scleroderma (238,245), hyperthyroidism (238), and Hashimoto thyroiditis (237,342) (see Chapter 47). Patients over the age of 40 years are most likely to have other autoimmune diseases (49). Patients treated with D-penicillamine for rheumatoid arthritis (294) or Wilson disease (see Chapter 48) may also develop myasthenia gravis (195). From the standpoint of ophthalmologists the association with thyroid disease is particularly important, since both myasthenia gravis and hyperthyroidism affect the EOMs.

An inherited predisposition to myasthenia gravis may exist. Three to 5% of cases are familial. Studies on the association with human leukocyte antigens (HLA) (see Chapter 3) have shown an increased frequency of HLA8 (225). Pirskanen reported 72% of female myasthenics under 35 years old are HLA8-positive (controls 17.5%) (253). More than 70% of myasthenics with thymic hyperplasia are also HLA8-positive, whereas only 6% to 10% of those with thymoma are HLA8-positive (102). However, myasthenics with thymomas have a higher frequency of HLA2 and a lower incidence of HLA1 than do controls or myasthenics without thymoma. The myasthenic patients with thymoma generally possess antibodies to skeletal muscle striations, whereas only 11% of those without thymoma have these antibodies (234). Pure ocular myasthenia gravis does not correlate with specific HLAs (253). Fritze and colleagues (102) has suggested that there are two forms of adult myasthenia gravis: a form occurring in females under 40 years old with thymic hyperplasia and low-antimuscle antibody titers who are HLA8-positive, and non-HLA8-negative patients, usually males over 40 years of age, with thymomas and high-antimuscle antibody titers. The antibodies referred to here are those detected at muscle striations and not anti-ACRs, which will be discussed later. Compston and colleagues (49) found the highest anti-ACR antibody titers in patients with thymomas and the lowest in males over 40 years of age.

In myasthenia gravis electromyography discloses a diminished muscle action potential with repetitive nerve stimulation and reduced miniature end-plate potential amplitude. Miniature end-plate potentials are normal and produced by spontaneous release of small quantities of acetylcholine. Their amplitude is usually well below the threshold required to produce muscle contraction. The pharmacologic tests for myasthenia gravis include improvement with anticholinesterase drugs, such as edrophonium or neostigmine, and increased sensitivity to curare. EOMs may not respond to neostigmine but are curare-sensitive (35).

Morphologic Features

In myasthenia gravis morphologic abnormalities occur principally in skeletal muscle and the thymus. The muscle changes consist of a denervation pattern (234) with group fiber atrophy, angulated fibers, type grouping (Fig. 8), and focal infiltrates of lymphocytes ("lymphorrhages"). Maselli and colleagues (193) demonstrated monocytes or macrophages at the neuromuscular junction. In an analysis of 61 muscle biopsies from 46 myasthenics, Oosterhuis and Bethlem (234) found 17 examples of neurogenic atrophy and 26 of lymphorrhages. Nine of 17 patients with thymoma had lymphorrhages, but the denervation pattern did not correlate with the presence of thymoma. The question of denervation in myasthenia gravis is controversial despite morphologic evidence of its presence. Cöers and Telerman-Toppet point out that myasthenic patients characteristically have enlarged, elongated motor endings, whereas denervation is characterized by collateral branching of motor endings. However, they did find evidence of denervation in seven of 45 patients, all over 50-years old (46).

Seventy-five percent of myasthenic individuals have thymic abnormalities, either hyperplasia (85%) or a thymoma (15%) (223). Chinese have a higher incidence of thymoma, 13/27 patients in one study, approximately two to three times the level in Western countries (337). About one-half of patients with thymoma develop myasthenia gravis (74,273).

Ninety-five percent of patients between the ages of 20 and 30 with myasthenia gravis have thymic hyperplasia, which is defined as the presence of germinal centers in the thymus (225). Berrih-Aknin and colleagues (20) point out that germinal centers may also occur in the thymus in other autoimmune diseases. Thymectomy is advocated early in the course of the disease for young patients (99,288), who usually have thymic hyperplasia (thymoma is rare in persons under 20 years of age) (99,280). Following thymectomy, improvement is gradual, increasing from 10% to 12% remission in the first postoperative year to 30% to 37% in the fifth year, but eventually improvement occurs in 90% of those with thymic hyperplasia. The presence of germinal centers in the thymus may be of prognostic significance, and those patients who lack germinal centers or only have rare ones, improve more quickly than those with many germinal centers (110,242); but 10 years after thymectomy the improvement rate is equal regardless of the number of germinal centers (248). Moran and colleagues (215) found no correlation between numbers of germinal centers and clinical improvement, but they did find that the mean cross-sectional area, perimeter, and diameter of germinal centers were less in those who improved than in those who did not.

Patients with thymoma do not respond to thymectomy as do patients with thymic hyperplasia, with the first year remission and improvement rates being 6.5% and 18.8%, respectively. Patients who survive 2 years reportedly have a 33% remission rate if male and 13% if female (242). Thymectomy is not used for pure ocular myasthenia (111). Durelli et al. (71) found that patients who underwent thymectomy within 1 year after onset who did not require additional immunosuppressive therapy had a stable remission rate within 2 years of 44% versus 26% for other postthymectomy patients. They also found improved remission rates after trans-sternal extended thymectomy, but not after cervical thymectomy.

The thymus is a source of anti-ACR antibody production (104,290), with thymic plasma cells being a major producer (371). Thymectomy not only reduces a source of antibody, but it also removes a source of antigen, which maintains the autoimmune response (178). There is a steady decrease in anti-ACR antibody titers between 6 weeks and 1 year after thymectomy (168). The source may be thymic myoid cells or a source within the epithelial component of the thymus (20).

Myasthenic patients with thymoma also develop antibodies against titin, the third most common protein in skeletal muscle, and ryanodine receptors (273). These are discussed further in the next section.

Etiology and Pathogenesis

Initially myasthenia gravis was thought to be a presynaptic defect. Elmqvist and colleagues (73) demonstrated reduced miniature end-plate potential amplitude, which was interpreted as a difficulty in packaging acetylcholine. TEM, however, disclosed normal cholinergic vesicles, and a decreased surface area of the postsynaptic membrane with simplification of the postsynaptic area (specifically loss of secondary clefts), suggesting a postsynaptic defect (83). Ito and colleagues (143) demonstrated normal acetylcholine release and increased acetylcholine in intercostal muscle of myasthenic patients. Thornell and colleagues (343) suggested that degeneration of the postsynaptic folds with subsequent increased distance between pre- and postsynaptic areas may account for the diminished miniature end-plate potential and explain previous interpretations of a presynaptic defect.

The discovery that alpha-bungarotoxin in snake venom binds irreversibly to ACRs has enabled investigators to study these receptors, which are located principally on the terminal portions of the postsynaptic folds (82), where there are estimated to be 20,000 to 25,000 per sq. mm. (256). The number of receptors is markedly reduced in myasthenia gravis (11–30% of controls) (81) and correlates with the patient's clinical status and the amplitude of the miniature end-plate potential (82). Currently, myasthenia gravis is believed to result from antibodies to the ACR at the motor end plate. Anti-MuSK (muscle specific kinase) antibodies also act at the neuromuscular junction (338).

The anti-ACR antibody titer cannot be used to predict severity when comparing groups of patients, but the decline in titer in patients with transient infantile myasthenia gravis (157) or undergoing plasma exchange (224) correlates with the clinical improvement in particular patients. The lowest titers occur in pure ocular myasthenia gravis (179). The antibody to ACR does not correlate with a second type of antibody in myasthenia gravis, which is directed toward muscle striations (174), and the binding site of anti-ACRs is not the same as the bungarotoxin binding site, since the antibody only incompletely blocks toxin binding (158,179). Anti-ACR antibodies are polyclonal (349). Blocking, binding, and modulating antibodies exist (135), but destruction of the ACR-bearing membrane is main problem. The presence of fewer ACRs has been postulated as a reason for the increased susceptibility of the ocular muscles.

A key link in the chain of evidence for the role of immunoglobulin in myasthenia gravis was the demonstration of IgG and the third component of complement (C3) at the sites of ACRs in patients with myasthenia (77). Similar findings develop in experimental autoimmune myasthenia gravis, in which the amplitude of the miniature end-plate potential correlates with the length of the postsynaptic membrane containing IgG and C3 (283).

Experimental autoimmune myasthenia gravis induced in various mammals by injection of purified ACR from electric eels (285,335,343) is characterized morphologically by an inflammatory infiltrate at the end plate 7 to 11 days after injection. The postsynaptic region of the end plate degenerates but in most animals it gradually regenerates, although some suffer a relapse with severe degeneration as in the human disease (84).

Antibodies against ACR produce their effect by causing end-plate degeneration mediated by complement, accelerated degeneration of ACRs, or by blocking the ACR (11,66). Another reason postulated for the greater susceptibility of ocular muscles compared to limb muscles is the lower levels of decay accelerating factor (DAF), which inhibits complement deposition (379). The basic reason for the development of ACR antibodies remains unknown, but speculation centers on the concept that myasthenia gravis is an autoimmune disease (312) and the role of the thymus in myasthenia gravis and other autoimmune diseases (116). Autoantibodies, until recently were thought to be "forbidden," but increasingly sensitive tests have shown them to be normal (302). Why they increase to damaging levels in some individuals is not known. The antibodies are a T-cell mediated and major histocompatibility complex restricted process in humans (303). The antibodies probably develop in response to an endogenous source such as extrajunctional receptors in denervated muscle (370), thymic myoid cells (152,293) or the epithelial component of the thymus (50). The epithelial and myoid cells may arise from a primitive pericapillary desmin-positive mesenchymal cell in the medulla of the thymus (383). Alpha-bungarotoxin binds to thymic epithelial cells of myasthenic patients (86), suggesting the presence of ACRs. The presence of these cells has led to the belief that the changes in skeletal muscle are due to cross-reactivity between skeletal muscle and the thymic myoid cells. Indeed, Aharonov and colleagues (6) have demonstrated cross-reactivity between calf thymus and eel ACRs and thymuses from patients with myasthenia gravis have epitopes of the ACR (161).

Ninety percent of myasthenic patients have anti-thymic antibodies (136) and it is conceivable that a viral infection of the thymus affecting thymic myoid cells leads to the production of antibodies against these cells, with such antibodies cross-reacting with skeletal muscle. One theory postulates that exposure to viruses and bacteria leads to the formation of antibodies against ACRs because of shared epitopes between the organisms and the receptors or because of shared epitopes in the antibodies against the microorganisms and the ACR. Numerous microorganisms have been identified as possible culprits (62). Schwimmbeck and colleagues (304) demonstrated cross-reactivity between a subunit of ACRs and herpes simplex virus. Increased B cells and decreased T cells have also been noted in the thymus in myasthenia gravis (181), suggesting that decreased T suppressor cells permit the synthesis of autoantibodies. Anti-ACR production by the thymus, as well as T lymphocytes, has been shown (359), and the favorable therapeutic effect of thymectomy may result from the removal of sources of both antibody production and antigen.

Another theory suggests that any inflammatory process that affects the thymic medulla could allow peripheral CD4+ T cells to enter the thymus, encounter ACRs in the thymus, and then stimulate ACR reactive B cells to produce antibodies (177).

Thymomas do not have myoid cells but there is evidence that they have genomic loci with a very restricted nucleotide sequence similar to the ACR alpha subunit gene (112). Two types of antibodies other than anti-ACR antibodies are particularly associated with thymoma. These are anti-titin antibodies and anti-ryanodine receptor antibodies. The combination of anti-ryanodine receptor and anti-titin antibodies has a 95% sensitivity and specificity and 70% positive predictive value for thymoma (314).

Titin is located near the A band-I band junction. It keeps thick filaments in register and builds passive resistance to stretch. Antibody titers to titin correlate with myopathic findings in myasthenic patients. Ninety-five percent of myasthenics with thymoma have anti-titin antibodies, as do one-half of late onset myasthenics without thymoma (314).

The ryanodine receptor is important for calcium release by the sarcoplasmic reticulum and is located at the junctions of T-tubules, sarcolemma, and sarcoplasmic reticulum. Anti-ryanodine receptor antibodies inhibit calcium ion release. Although present in only 75% of myasthenics with thymoma, ryanodine receptor antibodies are more specific than anti-titin antibodies for thymoma and are more likely to be associated with aggressive, malignant thymomas. The combination of anti-ryanodine receptor and anti-titin antibodies has a 95% sensitivity and specificity and 70% positive predictive value for thymoma (314).

Childhood Forms of Myasthenia Gravis

Several forms of childhood myasthenia gravis are recognized (95):

Juvenile Myasthenia Gravis. Juvenile myasthenia gravis is similar to the adult disease, but with onset after the first year of life. Seventy-five percent of the cases involve children over 10 years of age. Complete spontaneous remissions occur in approximately 20% of patients, including almost all with symptoms restricted to EOMs and facial muscles.

Transitory Neonatal Myasthenia Gravis. Although all infants of mothers with myasthenia gravis have anti-ACR antibodies, only 12% of children born to myasthenic mothers develop a transitory myasthenic syndrome (222). This usually begins on the first day of life and persists for a few weeks, but sometimes for as long as 5 months. The level of anti-ACR antibodies correlates better with severity in the transitory infantile myasthenia gravis than in adult myasthenia gravis (90).

Toyka (346) demonstrated decreased miniature end-plate potential amplitude and fewer ACRs in mice after repeated injections with serum from myasthenic patients and identified the active fraction as IgG. This would explain infantile transient myasthenic gravis, since IgG can cross the placenta. In experimental autoimmune myasthenia gravis of neonatal rats (see below), anti-ACR is passed through milk (285).

Familial Limb-Girdle Myasthenia Gravis. Patients with familial limb-girdle myasthenia gravis are usually adolescents. They manifest an abrupt onset of symmetrical weakness of the proximal limb muscles without ocular involvement (146,200). Other apparently non-immune mediated forms of congenital myasthenia are recognized (85).

Congenital Myasthenia Gravis. Congenital myasthenia gravis also begins shortly after birth, but the mother is not a myasthenic, although the siblings may be, and EOM involvement is the predominant feature (109).

Familial Infantile Myasthenia Gravis. Infants with familial infantile myasthenia gravis have severe respiratory and feeding difficulties with little or no EOM involvement. The siblings, but not the mother, may have myasthenia gravis. Spontaneous remissions can occur, but apnea may reappear with infection (50,119).

Congenital Acetylcholinesterase Deficiency. The only patient reported with congenital acetylcholinesterase deficiency had small nerve terminals, reduced acetylcholine release, and reduced acetylcholinesterase in the muscle (81,317).

Slow-Channel Syndrome. There is involvement of the cervical, scapular, and finger extensor muscles as well as oculomotor weakness in slow-channel syndrome. There are degenerative changes at the neuromuscular junction. Engel (85) predicted that a mutation in the ACR hinders the closure of the ACR ion channel and the condition has now been show to be caused by different mutations in the genes that encode for the alpha (*CHRNA1*), beta (*CHRNB1*), delta (*CHRND*) and epsilon (*CHRNE*) subunits of ACR.

Myotonic Dystrophy

General Considerations

Myotonic dystrophy is divided into myotonic dystrophy type 1 (DM1, classic myotonic dystrophy, Steinert disease, MIM #160900) and myotonic dystrophy type 2 (DM2, proximal myotonic myopathy (PROMM), Ricker syndrome, MIM #602668).

The first descriptions of classic myotonic dystrophy, hereafter referred to as DM1, as a multisystem disorder are credited to Steinert in 1909 (323) and Batten and Gibb (347). Earlier descriptions of the skeletal muscle component considered DM1 to be atypical Thomsen disease or termed it myotonia atrophica (347). DM1 is said to have an incidence of 1 per 8000 (214). Northeastern Quebec has a carrier rate as high as 1/550 compared to 1/5000 to 1/50000 in other areas (378). The estimated prevalence in Italy of 69 to 90/1,000,000 population, makes it the most common neuromuscular disease in that country (217). Roses (276), based on his experience with large pedigrees, found that less than 20% of heterozygotes were clinically affected, indicating the prevalence of the gene is greatly underestimated. He believes it to be the most common dystrophy. Shaw and Harper (307) believe it to be the most common dystrophy in adults. The mean age at death is mid-fifties, usually from cardiac and respiratory complications (126).

DM2 is now the designation for cases previously described as PROMM. Proximal DM1 is considered a more general clinical term (263). DM2 is similar clinically to DM1, but lacks a congenital form that is part of the DM1 spectrum and mental retardation is not seen in young patients as it is in DM1. DM2 is generally less severe than DM1 with less atrophy and weakness. Proximal involvement is more common than in DM1. The frequency of DM2 is not clear, because detection requires genetic analysis. There is speculation that DM2 is as prevalent as DM1 in Germany (60), but accounts for <1% of myotonic dystrophy elsewhere (126).

The main difference between DM1 and DM2 is their underlying genetic abnormalities (see later).

Clinical Features

Ptosis, cataracts, facial weakness, cardiac conduction defects, atrophy of the distal limb musculature, mental impairment, and, in males, frontal baldness and testicular atrophy are the most common findings in DM1. Myotonia, which is prolonged contraction of muscle after stimulation or a delay in muscle relaxation after a strong contraction, is a key feature. An abnormal glucose tolerance and decreased IgG levels are present in some affected individuals (269). The phenotype varies considerably, some patients having any combination of the foregoing features, whereas others manifest no apparent clinical characteristics, and are only recognized by biochemical abnormalities or because they are obligate heterozygotes (275).

DM2 differs from DM1 clinically in that it is generally milder, and mental impairment is less. Other differences noted between DM1 and DM2 include normal deep tendon reflexes in DM2 versus hypoactive reflexes in DM1; pain is common in DM2, but not in DM1; and calf hypertrophy in some cases of DM2 which is not a feature of DM1 (202). Muscle atrophy is uncommon in DM2.

Congenital myotonic dystrophy is seen in DM1, but not in DM2. The affected parent is the mother. The chance of her offspring having myotonic dystrophy is high, 59% to 100%, depending on the size of the trinucleotide repeat (see section on Molecular Biology) and age under 30 (351). Megalocolon, constipation, or sprue-like symptoms may occur in childhood (176). Profound hypotonia, clubfeet, and cerebral abnormalities have been noted, and involvement of respiratory muscles may cause apnea in children and adults (31,39,41,44). Patients who survive infancy show facial diplegia and delay in motor development. With age, hypotonia decreases but myotonia becomes manifest (275). Cataracts are rare in childhood myotonic dystrophy. Lotz and Van der Meyden reported cataracts in a 27 year old with congenital myotonic dystrophy (183).

Morphologic Features

The morphologic features discussed are those of DM1. The findings in DM2 are generally similar but differences between the two forms will be indicated where appropriate.

Limb Muscle

The principal histologic findings in skeletal muscle are fiber atrophy, particularly of type 1 fibers (259), fiber hypertrophy, long chains of internal nuclei, ringed fibers (Ringbinden), and pale-staining peripheral portions of fibers (sarcoplasmic pads) (374) (Fig. 12). DM2 differs in that the atrophic fibers tend to be type 2, not type 1 as in DM1 (202).

Fiber differentiation may be poor in infants. With histochemical techniques oxidative enzymes are evident in the center of the muscle fiber but not at their periphery, resulting in a halo effect (Fig. 13) (94).

When Ringbinden are present, a fiber seen in cross section will have myofibrils running at oblique angles to other myofibrils, usually at the periphery but sometimes associated with a more peripheral sarcoplasmic pad (Figs. 12 and 14). Ringbinden have been described in numerous normal and abnormal muscles, including EOMs (23), and is probably a non-specific response to muscle fiber injury (148).

TEM studies have shown the sarcoplasmic pads to consist of disorganized cytoplasmic components, including myofibrils, sarcoplasmic reticulum, glycogen, lipids, and lysosomes (92,162,165, 220). Fiber degeneration and regeneration are occasionally seen, and endomysial fibrosis may be present in advanced cases. Ultrastructural abnormalities of the myofibrils in myotonic dystrophy have led some authors to suggest a defect in the synthesis of myofibrils (5). The sarcoplasmic reticulum, important in muscle contraction and relaxation, has been suspected of being important in myotonic dystrophy, but morphologic changes in it, such as dilatation and multiple terminal cisternae, are non-specific.

Intramuscular nerves exhibit extensive sprouting of subterminal axons, increase in end-plate size, and multiple end plates in single fibers (more than in denervation) (8,47). Denervation, however, has been reported in myotonic dystrophy (380).

In myotonic dystrophy the muscle fibers of the muscle spindles (intrafusal fibers) resemble those outside the muscle spindles (extrafusal fibers) (198), but the intrafusal fibers are considerably increased in number (>100: normal 5–14) (326,327,329). Histochemical stains disclose most of the intrafusal fibers in myotonic dystrophy to be type 1, instead of both type 1 and type 2 (130). This may indicate type grouping, a feature of the reinnervation phase of denervation, or it could result from an increased need for oxidative activity due to chronic overloading of the spindle by myotonia. Studies of motor innervation to the spindle have shown an increased number of motor axon sprouts (329), many of which do not appear to terminate on the simplified end plates. The question of whether the abnormal innervation leads to the splitting of intrafusal fibers or constitutes an attempt to innervate previously split fibers remains unanswered. Currently, the latter view is favored (198,326,327).

Ocular Muscles

EOM weakness is uncommon, occurring in only 7% of patients (183). There are, however, abnormalities of eye movements, which may involve central nervous system (CNS) abnormalities (126).

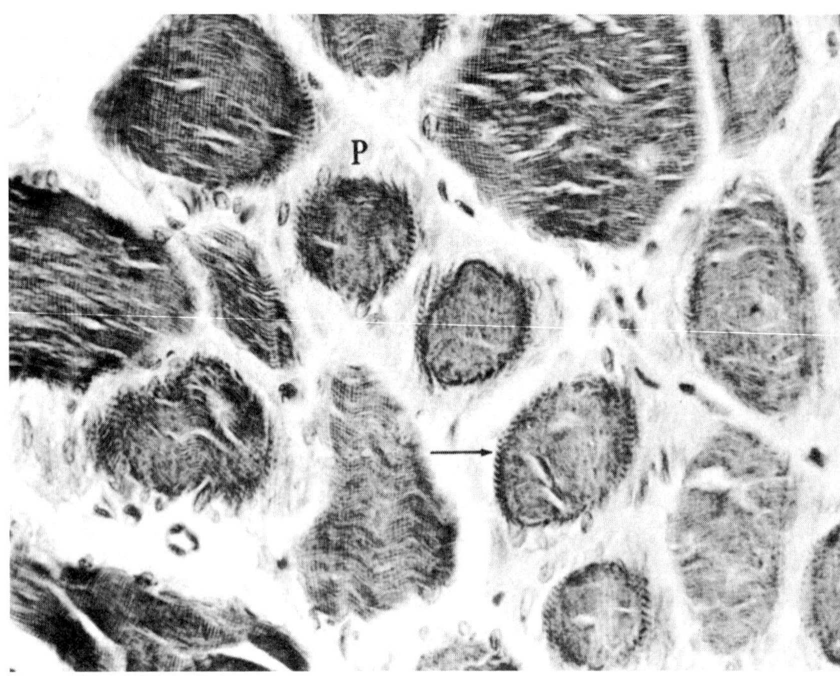

Figure 12 Myotonic dystrophy (adult). Several fibers contain Ringbinden (*arrow*) and sarcoplasmic pads (P) (hematoxylin and eosin, formalin fixed, ×415).

Histologic studies of the EOMs, including the levator palpebrae superioris, have shown various degrees of fiber atrophy and hypertrophy, centrally placed nuclei sometimes in chains, as well as increased connective tissue and fat (59,149,246,372).

Ultrastructural observations have included only non-specific changes, including disorganization and loss of myofibrils, clusters of sarcoplasmic reticulum and transverse tubules, and abnormal Z lines (170,171). Increased numbers of inner cristae of mitochondria with concentrically arranged cristae are sometimes noted (171). Similar alterations have been observed in the EOMs of rats fed diazacholesterol (239). Neuromuscular junctions are said to be normal except for a few synaptic vesicles and swollen mitochondria (170).

Non-Muscular Ocular Abnormalities

Ocular Hypotonia. Ocular hypotonia is common in myotonic dystrophy (261,305,367). Junge (149) found

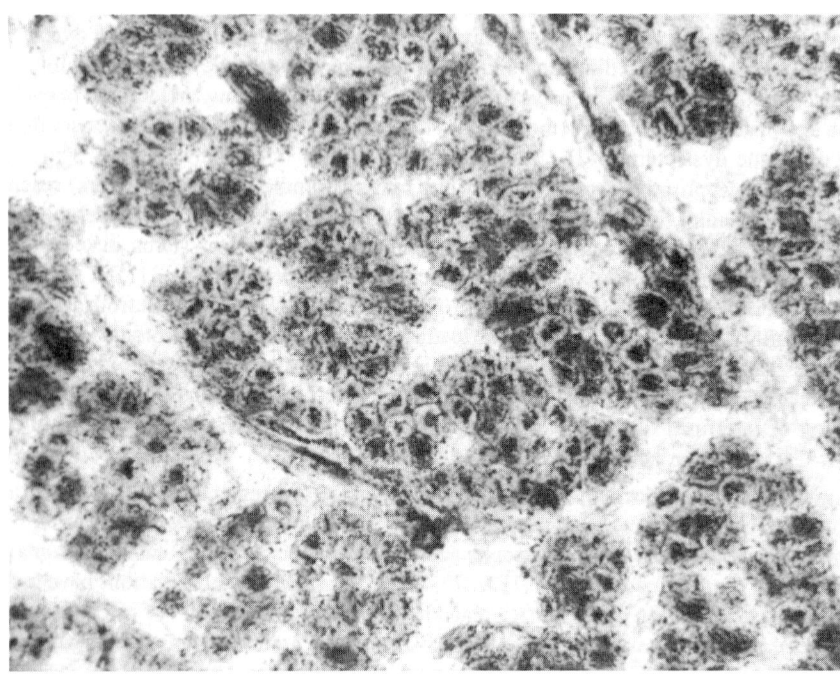

Figure 13 Myotonic dystrophy. This is muscle from a 1-day-old infant. Note the peripheral halo (nicotinamide adenine dinucleotide tetrazolium reductase, ×410).

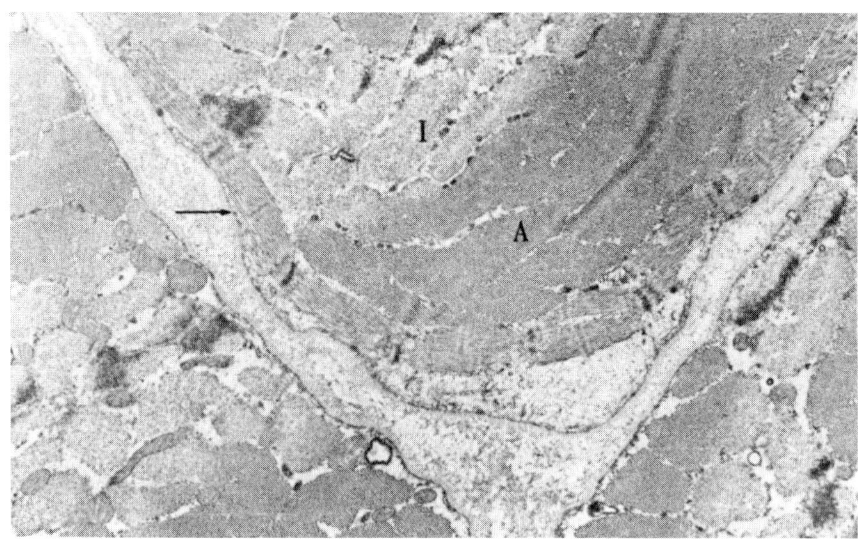

Figure 14 Myotonic dystrophy. Cross section of a muscle fiber with a longitudinally oriented myofibril (*arrow*) at the periphery (×11,600). *Abbreviations*: A, A band; I, I band.

the intraocular pressure (IOP) to be low in 84 of 101 eyes from 51 patients with myotonic dystrophy (control mean 16.3 mmHg; myotonic mean 8.8 mmHg), and in a few instances the IOP was lower than normal in asymptomatic blood relatives of myotonic patients. Junge speculated that the ocular hypotonia might in part be due to degeneration of the ciliary muscle, which has been described in myotonic dystrophy. Atrophy (205), hyaline degeneration, and vacuole formation in ciliary muscles have been reported several times (38,189,348), but the vacuolar change has also been found in individuals without myotonic dystrophy. Burns (38) reported a fibrotic sphincter pupillae and sparse muscle fibers in the dilator pupillae.

Cataracts. Opacities form in the lens in most adults with myotonic dystrophy, both DM1 and DM2 (126,129), but rarely in childhood. Younger patients with severe muscle disease may not have cataracts, whereas older individuals presenting with cataracts may have little or no muscle symptoms (126).

The clinical features of myotonic cataracts have been well characterized since the first report more than 50 years ago (153). They pass through three stages of development (70): (*i*) dust like irregularly shaped opacities intermingled with iridescent crystals of varying red and green hue appear in the anterior and posterior lens cortex just beneath the capsule (361); (*ii*) the opacities become more diffuse, increase in density, and assume a stellate shape (153); (*iii*) finally, vacuoles and lamellar separations develop (9,70).

There is some evidence that not all patients presenting with the characteristic lens abnormalities of myotonic dystrophy have the disorder, confirmed by genetic analysis (113). Histological studies have shown nucleated fibers in the vicinity of vacuoles and lacunae (348,365), which may contain crystalline material (289). The suggestion that lipids, particularly cholesterol, cause the iridescence of the lens in myotonic dystrophy (36) has not been confirmed histochemically. TEM studies (57,87) show the iridescent particles corresponded to vacuoles containing whorls of multilaminated membranes. Filaments (8–12 nm in diameter) appearing as hollow tubes on cross sections have also been described. They are also seen in the aging lens (57).

Decreased lenticular glutathione is associated with cataract formation while gamma-glutamyl transpeptidase, which aids in the catabolism of glutathione, has been found to be increased in the serum of patients with myotonic dystrophy (356). Horrobin and Morgan (133) suggested zinc could play a role in cataract development because zinc deficiency not only has some similarities to myotonic dystrophy, but also causes cataracts in trout (133) and in humans with acrodermatitis enteropathica (257).

Changes in the Iris and Ciliary body. The vasculature of the iris is said to be abnormal in myotonic dystrophy and to be characterized by a slow circulation, leakage, and peripupillary tufting (194,324). The myotonic patients with tufts described by Mason (194) were all latent diabetics and it should be noted that non-myotonic diabetics may also have tufts. Meyer and colleagues (205) described vacuolization of the pigmentary and non-pigmentary epithelium of the iris. Depigmentation of the ciliary processes has also been noted (129).

Retina. Retinal degeneration is common and degenerated photoreceptors, increased pigment cells, and cystic changes have been noted in tissue sections of the retina (134,189). Eighty-five percent of patients with myotonic dystrophy have abnormal electroretinograms (ERGs) (37,149). Patterned dystrophy and peripheral yellow flecks in the retina believed to be in the deep retinal pigment epithelium (RPE) or Bruch membrane (129), fundus scars (261), and abnormal visual evoked potentials (252) have been reported.

Cornea. Studies of the cornea in myotonic dystrophy have been few (88,149), and lesions seen have been attributed to disordered function of the eyelids or deficient tear secretion.

Heart

Cardiac abnormalities, principally electrocardiographic, occur in 68% of DM1 patients (96). Although conduction defects with the consequent possibility of sudden death (249) are the most common cardiac abnormality, the conduction system has rarely been evaluated completely (341). Fatty infiltration and fibrosis of the cardiac muscle are common (21,333,340,350).

Twenty percent of DM2 patients have conduction abnormalities and 7% develop a cardiomyopathy unrelated to ischemia (60).

Nervous System

Mental deficiency may be prominent (43,277,340) in DM1, but not in DM2. Neurofibrillary tangles are reported in both DM1 and DM2, as are Marinesco bodies (197). Loss of neurons in the brainstem nuclei, particularly in patients with sleep disturbance or hypoventilation, has been noted (126).

Neuronal and cytoplasmic inclusion bodies have been described in the thalamus (56). Although electromyographic studies suggest peripheral nerve involvement (199,213), morphologic changes are seldom seen in peripheral nerves (30,255) and these are not thought to be significant (126). A quantitative study of the spinal cord reported no decrease in the number of motor neurons (368).

Endocrine and Metabolic Dysfunction

Interest in the endocrine glands in myotonic dystrophy dates from 1917, when Naegeli (221) suggested that the primary defect resided in the endocrine glands. The most common pathologic change is testicular atrophy, but abnormal ovaries have also been reported (21). Plasma follicle stimulating and luteinizing hormones are increased, while testosterone is decreased, supporting the concept of a primary gonadal disorder rather than a pituitary defect (125,282). The pituitary gland is morphologically normal in three-quarters of cases (21), but non-specific changes may occur in the pituitary and other endocrine glands (275).

Diabetes mellitus is present in 7% of patients with DM1 (275), but abnormal glucose tolerance is present in 16% (126) and 23% with DM2 (60). Thyroid, parathyroid, and adrenal cortical function are not significantly affected (126).

The relationship between the ocular and the other manifestations of myotonic dystrophy is not clear. They do not seem to be related to defects in carbohydrate metabolism, although cataracts are more common in myotonics with diabetes mellitus (275,311). An abnormal lipid metabolism has been suspected in the evolution of the cataract, in part because hypocholesterolemic drugs can produce cataracts and myotonia (160,372). Thomas and Harper (339), however, failed to detect abnormalities of lipid composition in membranes of erythrocytes or cultured skin fibroblasts of patients with myotonic dystrophy.

Molecular Biology

DM1 is caused by an expansion of cytosine-thymine-guanine (CTG) trinucleotide repeats on human chromosome 19 (19q13.3), in the region of the *DMPK* gene (169). Whereas normal persons may have up to 50 of these repeats, myotonic patients can have thousands (214).

DM2 is associated with an expansion of a tetraplet cystine-cystine-thyme-guanine (CCTG) nucleotide repeat, in intron 1 of the *ZNF9* gene on chromosome 3 (3q21.3) (169).

How these gene alterations produce myotonic dystrophy has been the source of debate. The involvement of the *DMPK* gene in DM1 led to speculation that *DMPK* alterations led to the disease. Indeed, *DMPK* is reduced in congenital DM1 and myoblasts from these patients are defective in fusion and differentiation (18). However, DM1 and DM2, which are clinically broadly similar, are related to abnormalities of different genes, and *DMPK* is not affected in DM2.

Other proposed mechanisms for myotonic dystrophy are disruption of splicing and other functions by accumulation of the repeats in the nucleus, interference with adjacent genes, or some combination of these (263). Abnormal RNA is currently the favored mechanism (108).

The myotonia is thought to be due to abnormalities of the chloride channels (108,169). Other pre mRNA targets altered include cardiac troponin T and the insulin receptor (108), microtubule-associated tau, myotubularin-related protein, and *N*-methyl D-aspartate receptor 1 (197).

Progressive External Ophthalmoplegia

General Remarks

Von Graefe (363,364) is usually credited with the first clinical description of progressive external ophthalmoplegia, but Hutchinson (139) introduced the term "ophthalmoplegia externa" for what he thought was of syphilitic origin. The brain of one of Hutchinson's cases had changes in the oculomotor, trochlear, and abducent nerves and their nuclei (118). This led to the concept that external ophthalmoplegia was of nuclear origin (25), while Möbius (210) thought it was congenital and heredofamilial, a view bolstered by family studies (17).

Histologic studies (103,159,286,300,310) challenged the neurogenic nature of progressive external ophthalmoplegia by demonstrating normal oculomotor, trochlear and abducent nerve nuclei (300), and what were interpreted as myopathic changes (159). Involvement of muscles in the limbs, pharynx, larynx, face, and neck in some patients gave further support to progressive external ophthalmoplegia being a form of muscular dystrophy, hence the terms ocular myopathy, ocular dystrophy, and oculopharyngeal muscular dystrophy (147,219,268,336) terms which today would be applied differently, as discussed below.

The aforementioned histopathologic reports, however, did not end the controversy over the pathogenesis of progressive external ophthalmoplegia. Studies of experimental denervation in EOM (64) show that denervation of EOMs produces morphologic changes comparable to myopathies in limb muscle, thus invalidating previous conclusions on the origin of progressive external ophthalmoplegia based on the "myopathic" changes in EOMs.

Clinical Features

Ophthalmoplegia is frequently associated with and preceded by ptosis. Weakness of facial, neck, and limb muscles are common but may occur years after the onset of ophthalmoplegia (54). Paralysis of the EOMs clearly has many causes and classification of these disorders remains controversial. The primary abnormality may involve the oculomotor, trochlear, and abducent nerves, their nuclei or central connections in the cerebral cortex or midbrain, as well as the myoneural junction, or the EOMs themselves. The possible insults include trauma, toxins, degenerative disorders, infectious agents, metabolic disorders, and neoplasms. Ophthalmoplegia may be associated with other disease processes or injury (Table 3).

Only a few of the disorders associated with ophthalmoplegia will be discussed in this chapter, namely progressive external ophthalmoplegia related to mitochondrial dysfunction.

These disorders may present with isolated ophthalmoplegia with some progressing to involve the orbicularis oculi, other facial muscles, and sometimes limb muscles (descending ocular myopathy).

Table 3 Some Associations with Ophthalmoplegia

Clinical and laboratory findings (Refs.)
Ocular
Cataracts (247)
Optic atrophy (64)
Pigmentary retinopathy (64,233,274)
Proptosis (64,309)
Ear, nose, and throat
Hearing loss (64,155)
Dysphonia (64)
Nervous system
Absent tendon jerks (153)
Ataxia (54,64,153,274)
Abnormal electroencephalogram (64,155,230,233)
Cerebellar atrophy (153)
Elevated CSF protein (155,233,296)
Mental retardation (64,153,230,274)
Peripheral neuropathy (54)
Seizures (274)
Musculoskeletal
Dysarthria (153,230,274)
Dystonia (274)
Extremity weakness (54,64,155,274,309)
Facial weakness (54,64)
Myopathic electromyogram (155,233,315)
Myotonia (172)
Neck flexor weakness (42,54,233,309)
Short stature (153,155,156,296)
Cardiac
Abnormal electrocardiogram (heart block commonly) (58,155,296)
Gastrointestinal
Diarrhea (308,233)
Dysphagia (54,64,230,274)
Masticatory weakness (155)
Genital
Genital hypoplasia (156,186)
Associated disorders
Bassen-Kornzweig syndrome (274)
Dermatomyositis (325)
Diabetes mellitus (172)
Hypoparathyroidism (345)
Infantile spinal muscular atrophy (274)
Juvenile spinal muscular atrophy (2)
Marfan syndrome (121)
Möbius syndrome (159,210,211)
Primary biliary cirrhosis (264)
Syphilis (139)
Wernicke encephalopathy (360)
Associated physical and chemical agents
Drugs and toxins (coal gas, diphenylhydantoin, primadone) (235)
Trauma (306)

Some cases of progressive external ophthalmoplegia are associated with a pigmentary retinopathy, cardiomyopathy (usually with conduction defects and a propensity to sudden death), cerebellar disorders, deafness, short stature, and mental retardation. Onset is before the end of the second decade of life, and the CSF protein is elevated. These are referred to as examples of Kearns–Sayre (Kearns–Shy, Kearns Sayre–Daroff) syndrome (MIM #530000) (19,155).

Histopathology

Because there are relatively few detailed morphologic studies in individuals with external ophthalmoplegia and the uncertainty of many earlier studies, the histopathology of all cases will be discussed together except when stated otherwise. Readers interested in an extensive historical account should consult specific publications (54,156).

Extraocular Muscles and Levator Palpebrae Superioris

Variation in fiber size, fiber degeneration and/or atrophy (not fiber group atrophy), and increased fat and connective tissue are frequently observed in biopsies of EOMs in progressive external ophthalmoplegia (54,64,103,286,310). Ring fibers may occur (54), while intramuscular nerves at motor end plates are unremarkable (42).

TEM has disclosed loss of myofibrils, irregularities of the sarcoplasmic reticulum, and transverse tubular system in addition to an accumulation of mitochondria, many of which contain concentric cristae and crystalloids (42,296,382), and excess glycogen (292).

Skeletal Muscle

Skeletal muscle abnormalities have been interpreted as myopathic (268,274), but frequently the limb muscles are normal, or contain only rare atrophic or degenerated fibers in hematoxylin and eosin-stained microscopic sections (141,332). However, in many cases staining with a modified Gomori trichrome reveals abnormal fibers with accumulations of red staining material, particularly beneath the sarcolemma (141,216,332,345). The appellation "ragged-red fibers" has been applied to these abnormal fibers (233), which usually constitute fewer than 5% of the fibers (153), although 20% to 60% of the fibers may be of this type (140). The red-staining areas react positively with histochemical methods for oxidative enzymes (nicotinamide-adenine dinucleotide tetrazolium reductase; succinic dehydrogenase) (Fig. 15) and may also contain increased amounts of stainable glycogen and lipids. These abnormalities affect the type 1 fibers (based on myosin adenosine triphosphatase activity) much more frequently than type 2 fibers (42,141,153,216,230,315).

TEM of these abnormal zones reveals accumulations of unusual mitochondria (extremely large mitochondria with concentric cristae, distended with granular material, with and without electron dense bodies, and crystalloids) (Figs. 16 and 17). Lipid deposits and glycogen may be prominent in the mitochondrial aggregates (63), presumably secondary to defective mitochondrial metabolism. Other ultrastructural changes include non-specific Z-band streaming and myofibril degeneration.

Patients with progressive external ophthalmoplegia frequently have ragged-red fibers, but these are not specific for that condition. Rarely they are observed in hypothyroidism, glycogen storage disease type 2 (Pompe disease) (see Chapter 39), myotonic dystrophy, polymyositis, regenerating muscle, Luft disease (a hypermetabolic mitochondrial disease)

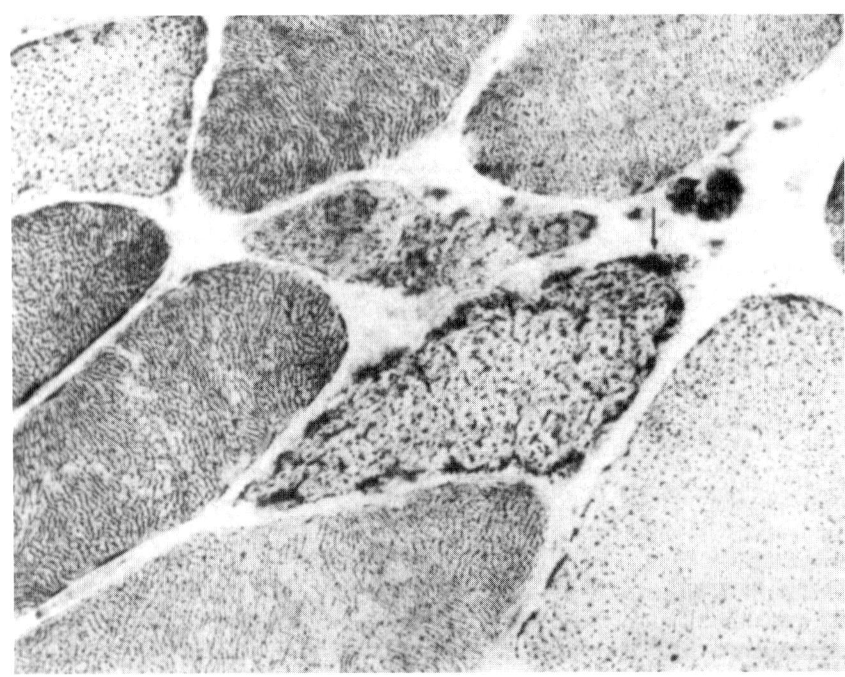

Figure 15 Progressive external ophthalmoplegia, with accumulation of dense material in a fiber (*arrow*) (nicotinamide adenine dinucleotide tetrazolium reductase stain, ×410).

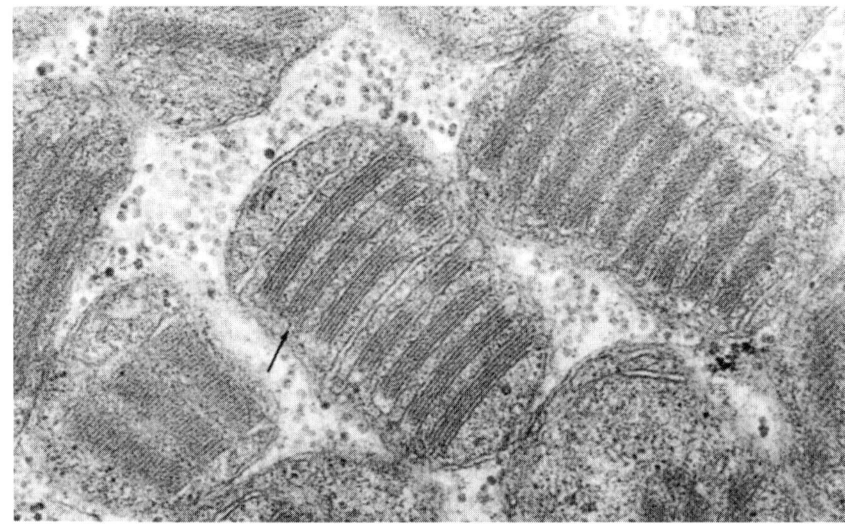

Figure 16 Progressive external ophthalmoplegia. Crystalline array (*arrow*) between cristae of mitochondria (×69,000).

(63,184), Leigh disease (55) (see Chapter 70), and other disorders.

Ragged-red fibers and their mitochondrial abnormalities, with and without ophthalmoplegia, are associated with loose coupling of oxidative phosphorylation (defective respiratory control and normal phosphorylative ability) (26,28,63,299). Some or a few ragged-red fibers are produced when uncouplers of oxidative-phosphorylation (2,4-dinitropbenocarbonylcyanide-*m*-chlorophenylhydrazine and oleic acid) are introduced into the hind limbs of rats (201). However, these mitochondrial inclusions are not identical to the crystalloids of human ragged-red fibers, perhaps because the human diseases are chronic. Korman and colleagues (166) suggest that the paracrystalline array most likely forms in the non-energized configuration of mitochondria (which presumably develops in the uncoupled state).

The significance of ragged-red fibers in progressive external ophthalmoplegia remains unclear, but their number does not appear to correlate with the muscle weakness. In Luft disease (MIM 251900) most mitochondria are abnormal, yet muscle weakness may be negligible (184). Moreover, usually fewer than 5% of mitochondria in the ragged-red fibers of progressive external ophthalmoplegia are morphologically abnormal.

Nervous System

Changes in the CNS are central to the question of whether the cause of progressive external ophthalmoplegia is neurogenic or myogenic. Unfortunately,

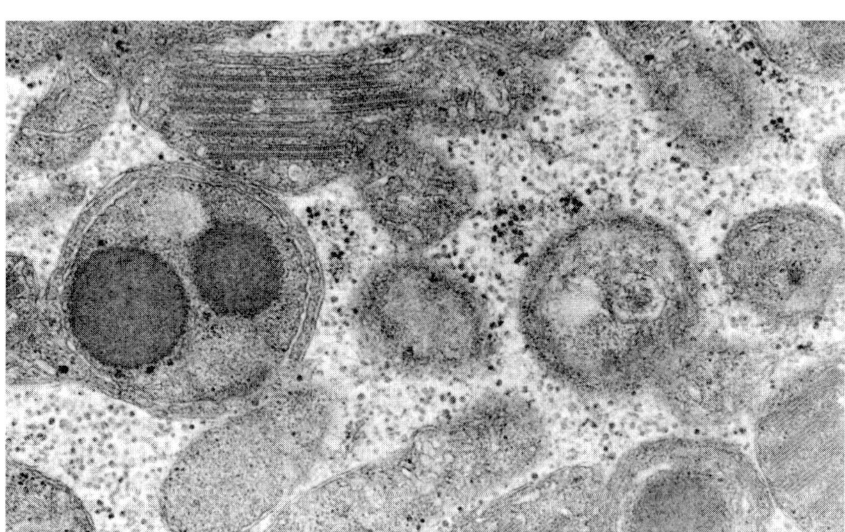

Figure 17 Progressive external ophthalmoplegia. Transmission electron micrograph showing crystalline arrays, electrondense material, and concentric cristae (×46,000).

available data do not provide a clear-cut answer. The nerves supplying the EOMs and their nuclei are described as normal by some authors (54,155) but abnormal by others (173,300). Croft and coworkers (54) reported neuronal loss and astrocytic hyperplasia in subthalamic nuclei and foci of neuronal degeneration with gliosis in the substantia nigra. Crystalloids in the mitochondria of Purkinje and granular cells of the cerebellum, loss of neurons and siderosis in the lateral portion of the substantia nigra and vestibular nuclei, and increased astrocytes in the substantia nigra have also been described (296), as has siderosis of the globus pallidus, vestibular nuclei, and substantia nigra (155).

The neurons of the oculomotor, trochlear, and abducent nerves are reported as being reduced in number (58,173), smaller and rounder with fewer dendrites than normal (300), and with abnormal variations in size and shape (173).

Vacuoles have been described in the brain (58,155) being so diffuse in one case (58) that spongiform encephalopathy was diagnosed. These alterations are of questionable significance because they are common artifacts.

A normal spinal cord has been reported in one case (48), but spinal cord and peripheral nerve abnormalities have been observed in others. Croft and colleagues (54) observed demyelination of the posterior columns, loss of ganglion cells, hypertrophied capsular cells of dorsal root ganglia, and nodules of cells with hyperchromatic nuclei and scant cytoplasm in the lower lumbar posterior roots, and loss of myelinated fibers in the peroneal nerve. A hypertrophic interstitial neuropathy has been documented (65). "Zebra" bodies similar to those seen in the mucopolysaccharidoses have been observed in Schwann cells of a peripheral nerve (117).

Other Tissues

A pigmentary retinopathy accompanies many of the same disorders as progressive external ophthalmoplegia (e.g., cardiac conduction defects, auditory disorders, cerebellar anomalies) (32,145). A loss of RPE may be associated with circinate atrophic areas in a pseudorosette pattern in Giemsa-stained flat retinal preparations (155,156).

Heart block is a common electrocardiographic abnormality, but the heart, including its conducting system, may be normal (58). Cardiac hypertrophy, subendocardial fibrosis, and a thickened epicardium have also been described (156).

Radiography and motility studies suggest that the smooth muscle in the lower esophagus is abnormal, but histologic abnormalities have not been reported (268).

In progressive external ophthalmoplegia the mitochondrial abnormalities are not restricted to muscle and have been noted in the liver (230) and sweat glands (153).

Etiology and Pathogenesis

Progressive external ophthalmoplegia may be considered as a mitochondrial disorder, but biochemical abnormalities are not always detected and they are not consistent. A detailed discussion of these mitochondrial disorders is beyond the scope of this chapter. Briefly, the mitochondrial disorders of muscle include the following major syndromes: Kearns–Sayre syndrome (MIM #530000), myoclonic epilepsy with red-ragged fibers (MERRF) (MIM #545000), mitochondrial myopathy, encephalopathy, lactic acidosis, and stroke-like episodes (MELAS) (MIM #540000), and mitochondrial neurogastrointestinal encephalopathy syndrome (MNGIE) (MIM #603041). Over 100 point mutations in mtDNA have been reported with varying clinical manifestations (320).

The metabolic pathways in the mitochondria involve: transport of metabolites, substrate utilization, the Krebs cycle, oxidative phosphorylation, and the respiratory chain. Mitochondrial DNA codes 13 respiratory chain subunits (320).

There is an interplay between the nucleus and mitochondria such that abnormalities of nuclear genes can cause mtDNA defects (254). For example, MNGIE is believed to be due to multiple mtDNA deletions, but in turn these are due to mutations in thymidine phosphorylase on chromosome 22 (22q13.32) (14).

The reverse can also be true, in that mitochondrial dysfunction prompts nuclear changes to overcome the metabolic deficiency (206).

Disorders of the respiratory chain of interest to ophthalmologists, including the Kearns–Sayre syndrome (associated with combined complexs I and III deficiencies) and Leber optic atrophy (associated with defects of complex I), are reported to manifest type atrophy in the muscle (291). The complexes are discussed in Chapter 1.

Harding and Holt (124) noted that in 40% of 71 cases of mitochondrial myopathy up to one-half of the mitochondrial DNA was deleted, and that all of these cases manifested progressive external ophthalmoplegia, but a specific biochemical deletion did not correlate with chronic external ophthalmoplegia. Twelve of 43 patients with chronic external ophthalmoplegia had no apparent deletion of mitochondrial DNA.

Morphology and biochemistry may be insufficient to diagnose and characterize cases of mitochondrial disorders (167). This has prompted advocacy of genetic classification (354).

Oculopharyngeal Muscular Dystrophy

Oculopharyngeal muscular dystrophy is inherited as an autosomal dominant trait and patients develop ptosis and dysphagia in their middle age. The condition is most common in French Canadians, but has been reported in several other ethnic groups (344). The carrier prevalence is 1:1000 in French Canadians, while the rate in the general French population is 1:100,000. The highest rate is in Bukhara Jews, 1:600 (91). It is rare in African Americans (278).

The genetic basis is a relatively short increase in a guanine-cytosine-guanine (GCG) nucleotide repeat from 6 to 7–13 in the poly(A) binding protein nuclear 1 gene, resulting in 12–17 alanines in the N-terminal domain instead of 10 alanines. A rare $(GCG)_7$ autosomal recessive form is reported (91). There are also combinations of a nucleotide repeat with guanine-cytosine-adenine (GCA) interspersions (270).

External ophthalmoplegia occurs, but is rarely complete (344). Progression to the facial muscles takes place, and, late in the disease, the proximal limb muscles may be involved. Distal muscle involvement has been reported in Japan (105) and in an elderly German, who was subsequently autopsied and found to have some anterior horn cell loss (295). Otherwise autopsy studies have not suggested a neurogenic origin (182). Cardiac abnormalities are unusual but a few cases with bundle branch block have been reported.

Abnormalities detected by skeletal muscle biopsy include variation in fiber size, fibrosis, increased muscle fibers with internal nuclei, and rarely, necrosis and inflammation. Angulated atrophic fibers may be seen, but this could be an aging change. Ragged-red fibers are not a feature of this disorder. Vacuoles with a basophilic edge (rimmed-vacuoles) may be seen in skeletal muscle (68). The key morphologic abnormality is the presence of intranuclear filaments (approximately 8 nm in diameter) (Fig. 18) which frequently palisade. These are considered unique for oculopharyngeal muscular dystrophy, but they need to be distinguished from intranuclear filaments found in other disorders, such as inclusion body myositis (Fig. 19) (51). The filaments in the latter disease are approximately 12–18 nm in diameter and occur in cytoplasmic vacuoles as well as within the nucleus. Interestingly, Fukuhara and colleagues (105) described a patient with oculopharyngeal muscular dystrophy and distal muscle weakness whose rimmed vacuoles contained filaments similar to those of inclusion body myositis.

The intranuclear filaments have been shown to contain polyadenylate binding protein 1 (PABN1), molecular chaperones, proteosome subunits, ubiquitin and poly (A)-mRNA (52).

Miscellaneous Disorders with External Ophthalmoplegia

Möbius Syndrome

The Möbius syndrome, also referred to as facial diplegia, congenital oculofacial paralysis, or infantile nuclear aplasia, is characterized by paralysis of lateral gaze and varying degrees of facial paresis (131,254,322,362). Clubfeet, micrognathia, absent portions of the extremities, peripheral neuropathy, hypogonadism, and other anomalies may also be present (4,131,232,271). Möbius (211,212) thought the disorder was degenerative; currently, some consider the basic defect to be in the CNS, whereas others believe that it involves the mesoderm, or mesoectoderm, and that the neurologic changes are secondary. The few documented morphologic studies (137,254,318) show abnormalities in the brainstem, such as diminished numbers of cell bodies in cranial nerves, particularly the abducent nerves. These findings thus support a primary defect in the CNS, as do electromyographic observations and a morphologically normal biopsied external rectus muscle (352). Proponents of a mesodermal origin of the disorder (89,265) argue that there is no obvious direct link between the neurologic and the musculoskeletal abnormalities. They contend that the decreased number of neurons in the brainstem is secondary to a defective development of mesodermal structures toward the end of the second fetal month (89). Pitner and colleagues (254) have performed a meticulous anatomical study of this disorder and, although they found abnormalities of the cerebellum, the cranial nerves and their nuclei were normal. These investigators reported extensive fatty and fibrous replacement of facial muscles and interpreted their findings as being due to a primary failure of muscle development. They suggested, however, that like arthrogryposis multiplex congenita, the Möbius syndrome may be produced by multiple factors. Interestingly, at least one patient with arthrogryposis also had the Möbius syndrome (322).

Genetic studies have identified several abnormalities. These include reciprocal translocations between chromosome 1 (1p34) and 13 (13q13), between chromosome 1 and 11:t(1;11)(p22;p13), and between chromosome 1 and 2:t(1;2)(p22.3;q21). A deletion of chromosome 13q12 has also been reported. Two other loci are found at chromosomes 3 (3q21–q22) and 10 (10q21.3–q22).

A study of a large Dutch pedigree suggests mutations of the *PLXND1* gene, a member of the plexin gene family, which is expressed in the nervous system and endothelium of developing blood vessels (353).

Arthrogryposis Multiplex Congenita

Arthrogryposis multiplex congenita (MIM 108110) is a syndrome characterized by fixation of multiple joints at birth. It may be caused by anything that decreases fetal movement, but most commonly is associated with neurogenic features. Reported associations include external ophthalmoplegia, a decreased corneal

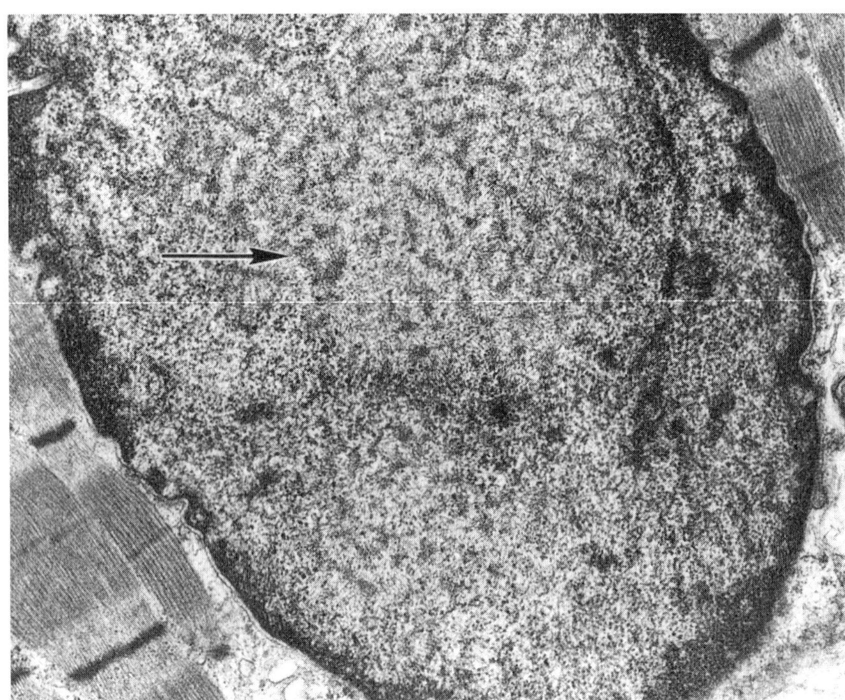

Figure 18 Short filaments (*arrow*) within the nucleus of a muscle cell of a patient with oculopharyngeal dystrophy (×16,000).

blinking reflex, deteriorated visual evoked responses (241), trichiasis of the upper eyelid (191), optic atrophy (100), as well as cataracts and glaucoma (330).

Distal arthrogryposis is defined as a family of disorders with dominant inheritance of congenital contractures of the distal extremities without abnormal muscle biopsies. Keratoconus, strabismus, astigmatism, and limited ocular motility are reported (15,284).

Centronuclear Myopathy

First reported by Spiro and colleagues (321), centronuclear myopathy (X-linked myotubular myopathy,

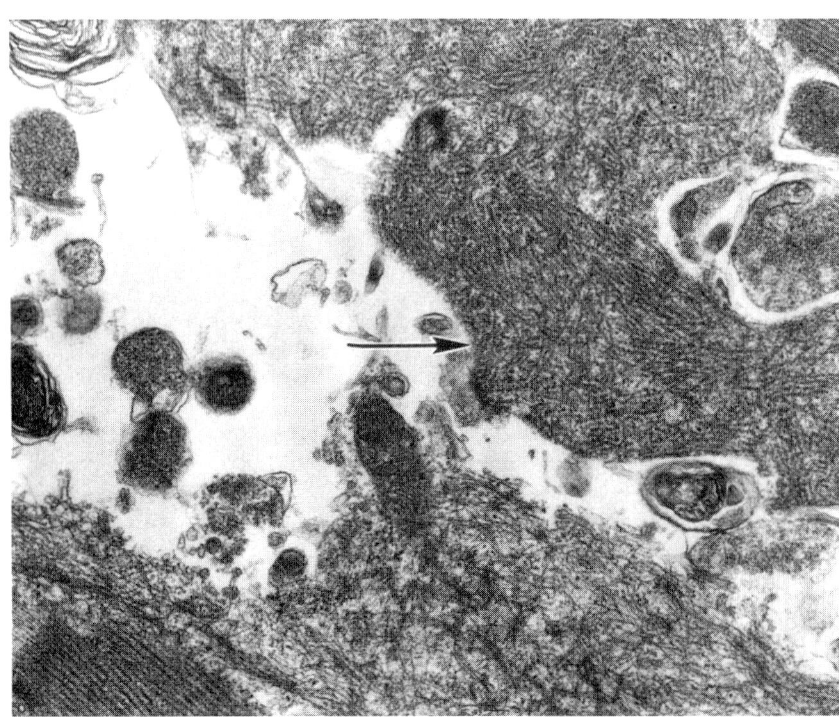

Figure 19 Intracytoplasmic filaments (approximately the size of myosin filaments) are present within the striated muscle of a patient with inclusion body myositis. Similar filaments may be found in nuclei. These filaments are approximately three times the diameter of those seen in oculopharygeal muscular dystrophy (×20,600).

MIM #310400) is named for its histologic appearance. In this disease most of striated muscle fibers have central nuclei, in contrast to normal muscle, in which fewer than 3% of the fibers have nuclei in this location. Because the muscle in this disorder resembles the myotubular phase of developing muscle, the term "myotubular myopathy" is sometimes used (22).

The condition is characterized by a non-progressive, or slowly progressive, weakness and wasting of many muscle groups and with ptosis and/or external ophthalmoplegia being present in over one-half the cases (22). Facial weakness is also common (22,236,244,297). Severe distal muscle deficits may also be evident (93). The age of onset is variable, although most patients are floppy infants (262,297). Ptosis is less frequent when the disease is diagnosed in adults, and the adult and childhood forms may be different diseases (115).

Histochemical stains disclose both types 1 and 2 fibers in limb muscles, although type 1 may predominate (244,258). When viewed with TEM, a zone devoid of myofibrils is evident adjacent to the centralized nuclei (236). The muscle differs from true embryonic fibers since this clear zone does not occupy the full length of the fiber and because fiber differentiation is present (258); hence, the term myotubular myopathy is misleading.

A case of centronuclear myopathy in a patient with Marfan syndrome, who also had "fingerprint" inclusions in his muscle biopsy, has been reported. The patient had bilateral ptosis, alternate divergent strabismus, myopia, bilateral cataracts, subluxed lenses, and reduced pupillary reflexes to convergence (144).

One form of centronuclear myopathy is X-linked myotubular myopathy. These patients are hypotonic at birth and commonly have ophthalmoplegia. Prognosis is poor in this disorder, which is caused by mutations in the *MTM1* gene located on the X chromosome (Xq28), which encodes myotubularin, a member of a family of proteins involved in cytoskeletal organization, cell signaling, and vesicle traffic. Nearly 200 mutations of the *MTM1* gene (251) are known.

There are several forms of autosomal centronuclear myopathies, both recessive and dominant. Ophthalmoparesis can be used to identify more severely affected early-onset autosomal dominant patients.

The genes for the autosomal forms of centronuclear myopathy have not yet been identified (251).

Multiminicore Disease

Multiminicore disease (multicore disease, MIM #117000) first described by Engel in 1966 (79), is a congenital, non-progressive myopathy characterized morphologically by multiple focal areas of myofibrillar degeneration in many striated muscle fibers. Sporadic as well as familial cases have been reported. A mitochondrial abnormality has been suggested to play a role in the pathogenesis of multiminicore diseases (78,98). The condition is genetically heterogeneous and caused by mutations of the *RYR1* gene on chromosome 19 (19q13.1) that encodes for the ryanodine receptor gene as well as mutations in *SEPN1*, the selenoprotein N gene on chromosome 1 (1p36–p35) (227).

The clinical presentation is variable, but includes proximal muscle weakness, Marfanoid features, weakness of the orbicularis oris (79), ptosis, and external ophthalmoplegia (78,142,328).

Congenital Ophthalmoplegia

A few cases of congenital ophthalmoplegia are associated with hypotonia (159), aminoaciduria (138), as well as syndromes, such as the Möbius syndrome.

Spinal Muscular Atrophy

External ophthalmoplegia has been reported in infantile spinal muscular atrophy (Werdnig–Hoffman disease, MIM #253300) (240,274), juvenile spinal muscular atrophy (Kugelberg–Welander syndrome, MIM #158600) (3), and in a Japanese family with progressive spinal muscular atrophy (196).

Celiac Disease

Sandyk and Brennan (287) reported a 12-year-old girl with celiac disease, who had diplopia due to medial rectus weakness. Treatment of her celiac disease eliminated the diplopia.

Other Neuromuscular Diseases Affecting the Eye

Muscle–Eye–Brain Disease, Walker–Warburg Syndrome, and Fukuyama Congenital Muscular Dystrophy

Muscle–eye–brain (MEB) disease (MIM #253280), Walker–Warburg syndrome (MIM #236670), and Fukuyama congenital muscular dystrophy (FCMD) (MIM #253800) are three autosomal recessive disorders that can manifest in varying degrees, abnormalities of skeletal muscle and brain. They have been grouped together as "cobblestone" lissencephalies but differ genetically.

There is overlap in the clinical findings, but the following serves as a diagnostic guide. MEB disease is primarily found in Finland. Brain abnormalities include mental retardation, cerebellar hypoplasia, hydrocephalus, pachygyria and a flat brainstem. Myoclonic jerks are also present. Ocular findings include congenital myopia and glaucoma, pallor of the optic disc and retinal hypoplasia. The children are hypotonic and have dystrophic changes within the muscle biopsy (377). MEB disease is caused by loss-of-function mutations to a gene on chromosome 1p32–34 which codes protein O-linked mannose beta 1, 2-*N*-acetylglucosaminyltransferase 1 (POMGnT1). The brain changes are more severe if the mutation occurs near the 5′ terminus rather than the 3′ terminus (334).

Fukuyama congenital muscular dystrophy is limited to Japan, where it is one of the commonest autosomal recessive disorders. The brain manifests polymicrogyria and the patients have severe mental retardation and seizures. The patients are hypotonic with weakness of facial as well as limb muscles (331). Ocular changes tend to be the mildest of the three diseases (355). Fukuyama congenital muscular dystrophy is the result of mutations to the *FCMD* gene on chromosome 9 (9q31) encoding fukutin. Fukutin is important for neuronal migration, muscle fiber integrity, and eye development (331). The disease is unusual in that most patients have a founder 3 kb retrotransposal element in the 3′ untranslated region of *FCMD* (334).

Walker–Warburg syndrome is worldwide in distribution. Lissencephaly, agenesis of the corpus collosum, cerebellar hypoplasia, dilatation of the fourth ventricle, fusion of the hemispheres, and occipital encephalocele are brain findings. Ocular abnormalities include cataract, microphthalmia, buphthalmos and persistent hyperplastic primary vitreous (PHPV) (355). Walker–Warburg syndrome has a heterogenous genetic makeup. Like Fukuyama congenital muscular atrophy some cases demonstrate abnormalities of the *FCMD* gene. Others have mutations in the *POMT1* gene on chromosome 9(9q34), or in the *FKRP* gene encoding fukutin-related protein gene. These only account for 20% of the cases (355).

All three disorders are linked by abnormalities in the glycosylation of alpha-dystroglycan (123,334), which is a component of the dystrophin glycoprotein complex (151). It is an important receptor for extracellular ligands in muscle, nerve and brain (207).

Dermatomyositis

Dermatomyositis is an inflammatory myopathy that also has skin abnormalities. Ocular abnormalities include retinopathy, optic atrophy (61,127,218), nystagmus (366), external ophthalmoplegia (243,325), incomplete eyelid closure (27), diplopia (228), and ocular myositis (164). The childhood form of dermatomyositis may have other systemic manifestations, such as gastrointestinal hemorrhages (12,175,373), presumably because of the vascular involvement (see Chapter 6).

Schwartz–Jampel Syndrome

The Schwartz–Jampel syndrome (MIM #255800) is characterized by blepharophimosis, dwarfism, skeletal and facial anomalies, and myotonia (2,101,301) and in most cases hypertrophied muscle (101). Normal (2) or scattered atrophic fibers (301) are seen by light microscopy, but TEM has disclosed intermyofibrillar vacuoles (2) and perinuclear lamellar dense bodies (203). Features of arthrogryposis multiplex congenita and the Schwartz-Jampel syndrome may be present in the same patient (97). Genetic studies have identified mutations in the *HSPG2* gene on chromosome 1 (1p36.1), which encodes perlecan, a heparan sulfate proteoglycan found in basement membranes (226) (see Chapter 40).

Duchenne Pseudohypertrophic Muscular Dystrophy

Duchenne pseudohypertrophic muscular dystrophy (MIM #310200), which is associated with a deficiency of the cytoskeletal protein dystrophin, is a sex-linked disorder which usually becomes symptomatic by the age of 3 to 5 years, progressing to death in the late teens. It is caused by a mutation in the *DMD* gene on the X-chromosome (Xp21.2). Impairment of eye movements is usually not apparent clinically, but has been demonstrated with the electrooculographic technique (185). Abnormal ERGs have been noted and dystrophin has been localized in the porcine retina (29). Deutan color blindness has been reported in some individuals with Duchenne muscular dystrophy as well as in Becker muscular dystrophy (MIM #300376), which is also caused by mutations in the *DMD* gene and Becker muscular dystrophy similar to Duchenne muscular dystrophy clinically but with a later onset and slower course (75,76,250).

Local Anesthetic Myopathy

Postoperative diplopia and ptosis have been described in some patients following exposure of the rectus muscles to local anesthetics (260). Some local anesthetics induce myotoxic effects experimentally in EOMs (40,231).

Marcus Gunn Syndrome

Marcus Gunn in 1883 (122) described a 15 year old with ptosis of the left eyelid which would involuntarily jerk upward while eating or speaking. Gunn found that the elevation of the levator palpebrae was produced by movement of the jaw to the right, which involves the action of the left external pterygoid muscle. Many theories have been proposed concerning this phenomenon, sometimes referred to as the "winking jaw" phenomenon (369). Lyness et al. (188) have studied the levator palpebrae superioris muscle and demonstrated neurogenic atrophy in the affected eyelid as well as in some clinically unaffected eyelids from the same patients. They postulate a pathologic process in the brainstem.

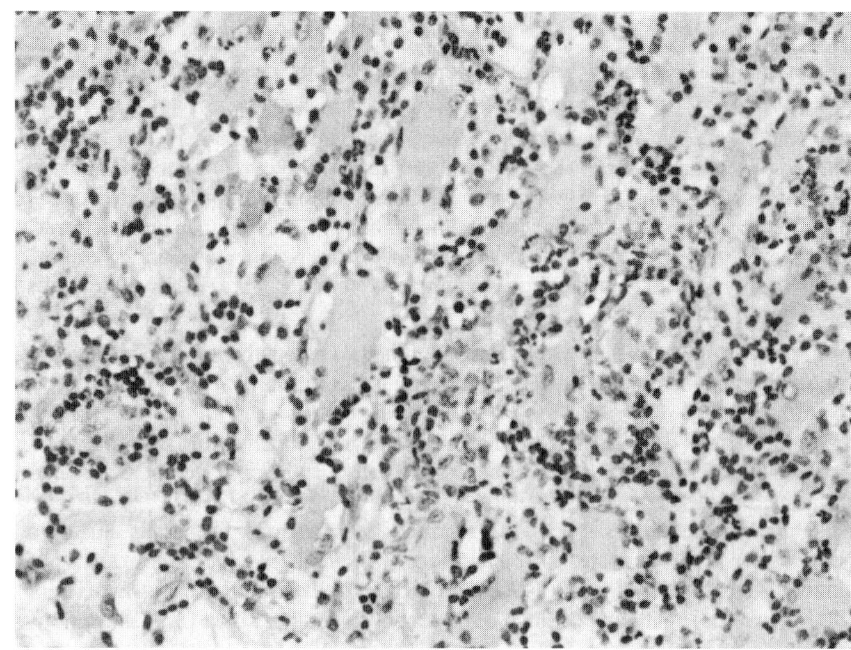

Figure 20 Ocular myositis. An infiltrate of mononuclear cells and neutrophils is associated with degenerating muscle fibers (hematoxylin and eosin, formalin fixed, ×285).

Other Disorders of Muscle

Desmin-Related Myofibrillar Myopathy

Desmin-related myofibrillar myopathy (DRM, MIM #601419) is a rare myopathy characterized by an accumulation of intrasarcoplasmic aggregates of desmin in association with other sarcoplasmic proteins. Affected individuals suffer from skeletal muscle weakness and cardiac abnormalities (conduction blocks, arrhythmias and restrictive heart failure). About a third of the cases are caused by a mutation in the *DES* gene that encodes for desmin. The disorder can also result from mutations in other genes, such the one for αB-crystallin (*CRYAB*) and cataracts (see Chapter 33) (357). Mice lacking the *Cryab* gene develop a myopathy in the absence of cataracts (33).

Other

The literature contains a report of four siblings with Coats disease, muscular dystrophy, mental retardation, and deafness (316).

Acute and chronic forms of ocular myositis (266,375) may present as proptosis, sometimes alternating from one orbit to the other (Fig. 20) (154).

A study of 21 individuals with gyrate atrophy of the choroid and retina (see Chapter 35) (313) disclosed type 2 fiber atrophy in all cases and tubular aggregates in 13 patients. Tubular aggregation in muscle is non-specific, but their frequency in gyrate atrophy is unusual.

Several reports document unspecified myopathies with visual impairment or ocular abnormalities (visual loss, cataracts, retinopathy, and corneal crystals), sometimes associated with anomalies in other tissues (10,106,186,376).

REFERENCES

1. Aarli JA, Milde EJ, Thunold S. Arthritis in myasthenia gravis. J Neurol Neurosurg Psychiat 1975; 38: 1048–1105.
2. Aberfeld DC, Namba T, Vye MV, Grob D. Chondrodystrophic myotonia: report of two cases, myotonia, dwarfism, diffuse bone disease, and unusual ocular and facial abnormalities. Arch Neurol 1970; 22: 455–62.
3. Aberfeld DC, Namba T. Progressive ophthalmoplegia in Kugelberg-Welander disease: report of a case. Arch Neurol 1969; 20:253–6.
4. Abid F, Hall R, Hudgson P, Weiser R. Moebius syndrome, peripheral neuropathy, and hypogonadotrophic hypogonadism. J Neurol Sci 1978; 35:309–15.
5. Adams RD, Rebeiz JJ. Histopathologie der myotonischen Erkrankungen. In Kuhn E. ed. Progressive Muskeldystrophie, Myotonie, Myasthenie, Berlin: Springer-Verlag, 1966:191–203.
6. Aharonov A, Tarrab-Hazdai R, Abramsky O, Fuchs S. Immunological relationship between acetylcholine receptor and thymus: a possible significance in myasthenia gravis. Proc Natl Acad Sci U S A 1975; 72:1456–9.
7. Alexander CB, Bossen EH. Peripheral couplings in human skeletal muscle. Lab Invest 1978; 39:17–20.
8. Allen DE, Johnson AG, Woolf AL. The intramuscular nerve endings in dystrophia myotonica: a biopsy study by vital staining and electron microscopy. J Anat 1969; 105:1–26.
9. Allen JH, Barer CG. Cataract of dystrophia myotonica. Arch Ophthalmol 1940; 24:867–84.
10. Arnold RW, Stickler GB, Bourne WM, Mellinger JF. Corneal crystals, myopathy and nephropathy: A new syndrome? J Ped. Ophthalmol Strabis 1987; 24:151–5.
11. Ashizawa T, Appel SH. Immunopathologic events at the endplate in myasthenia gravis. Springer Sem Immunopath 1985; 8:177–96.
12. Banker BQ, Victor M. Dermatomyositis systemic angiopathy of childhood. Medicine 1966; 45:261–89.

13. Baptista AG, Souza HS. Pupillary abnormalities in myasthenia gravis, report of a case. Neurology 1961; 11: 210–3.
14. Barboni P, Savini G, Plazzi G, Bellan M, Valentino ML, Zanini M, Montagna P, Hirano M, Carelli V. Ocular findings in mitochondrial neurogastrointestinal encephalomyopathy: a case report. Graefe's Arch Clin Exp Ophthalmol 2004; 242:878–80.
15. Beals RK, Weleber RG. Distal arthrogryposis 5: a dominant syndrome of peripheral contractures and ophthalmoplegia. Am J Med Genet 2004; 131A:67–70.
16. Beam KG, Horowicz P. Excitation–contraction coupling in skeletal muscle. In: Engel AG, Franzini-Armstrong C, eds. Myology, 3rd ed. Vol. 1. New York: McGraw-Hill, 2004: 257–80.
17. Beaumont WM. Family tendency to ophthalmoplegia externa. Trans Ophthalmol Soc UK 1900; 20:258–64.
18. Beffy P, Barsanti C, Del Carratore R, Simi S, Benedetti PA, Benzi L, Prelle A, Ciscto P. Expression and localization of myotonic dystrophy protein kinase in human skeletal muscle cells determined with a novel antibody: possible role of the protein in cytoskeleton rearrangements during differentiation. Cell Biol Internat 2005; 29:742–53.
19. Berenberg RA, Pellock JM, DiMauro S, Schotland DL, Bonilla E, Eastwood A, Hays A, Vicale CT, Behrens M, Chutorian A, Rowland LP. Lumping or splitting? "Ophthalmoplegia Plus" or Kearns-Sayre syndrome. Ann Neurol 1977; 1:37–54.
20. Berrih-Aknin S, Morel E, Raimond F, Safar D, Gaud C, Binet J P, Levasseur P, Bach JF. The role of the thymus in myasthenia gravis: immunohistological and immunological studies in 115 cases. Ann N Y Acad Sci 1987; 505:50–70.
21. Berthold H. Zur pathologischen Anatomie der Dystrophia myotonica Curschmann-Steinert. Dtsch Z Nervenheilkd 1958; 178:394–412.
22. Bethlem J, van Wijngaarden GK, Mumenthaler M, Meijer AEF. Centronuclear myopathy with type 1 fiber atrophy and "myotubes". Arch Neurol 1970; 23:70–3.
23. Bethlem J, van Wijngaarden GK. The incidence of ringed fibers and sarcoplasmic masses in normal and diseased muscle. J Neurol Neurosurg Psychiatry 1963; 26:326–32.
24. Bielschowsky A. Bietrag zur Kenntnis der rezidivierenden und alternierenden Ophthalmoplegia exterior. Albrecht von Graefes Arch Ophthalmol 1915; 90:433–51.
25. Birdsall, W.R. Progressive paralysis of the external ocular muscle, or ophthalmoplegia externa. J Nerv Ment Dis 1887; 14:65–77.
26. Black JT, Judge D, Demers L, Gordon S. Ragged-red fibers, a biochemical and morphological study. J Neurol Sci 1975; 26:479–88.
27. Bogousslavsky J, Perentes D, Regli F, Deruaz JP. Polymyositis with severe facial involvement. J Neurol Sci 1982; 228:277–81.
28. Bonilla E, Schotland DL, DiMauro S, Lee C-P. Luft's disease: an electron cytochemical study. J Ultrastruct Res 1977; 58:1–9.
29. Bordais A, Bolaños-Jimenez F, Fort P, Varela C, Sahel J-A, Picaud S, Rendon A. Molecular cloning and protein expression of Duchenne muscular dystrophy gene products in porcine retina. Neuromusc Disord 2005; 15:476–87.
30. Borenstein S, Noel P, Jacquy J, Flament-Durand J. Myotonic dystrophy with nerve hypertrophy: report of a case with electrophysiological and ultrastructural study of the sural nerve. J Neurol Sci 1977; 34:87–99.
31. Bossen EH, Shelburne JD, Verkauf BS. Respiratory muscle involvement in infantile myotonic dystrophy. Arch Pathol 1974; 97:250–2.
32. Botermans CHG. Primary retinal degeneration and its association with neurological diseases. In Vinken PJ, Bruyn GW eds. Handbook of Clinical Neurology, Neuroretinal Degeneration, Vol. 13, New York: American Elsevier, 1972:148–379.
33. Brady J P, Garland DL, Green DE, Tamm ER, Giblin FJ, Wawrousek EF. αB–crystallin in lens development and muscle integrity: a gene knockout approach. Invest Ophthalmol Vis Sci 2001; 42:2924–34.
34. Brandt DE, Leeson CR. Structural differences of fast and slow fibers in human extraocular muscle. Am J Ophthalmol 1966; 62:478–87.
35. Brust JC-M, List TA, Catalano LW, Lovelace R. Ocular myasthenia gravis mimicking progressive external ophthalmoplegia, rare case of myasthenia associated with peripheral neuropathy and spastic paraparesis. Neurology 1974; 24:755–60.
36. Bunge E. Der cholestesingehalt normaler und getrübter menschlicher Linsen. Albrecht von Graefes Arch Ophthalmol 1938; 139:50–61.
37. Burian HM, Burns CA. Ocular changes in myotonic dystrophy. Trans Am Ophthalmol Soc 1966; 64:250–73.
38. Burns CA. Ocular histopathology of myotonic dystrophy: a clinicopathologic case report. Am J Ophthalmol 1969; 68:416–22.
39. Cannon PJ. The heart and lungs in myotonic muscular dystrophy. Am J Med 1962; 32:765–75.
40. Carlson BM, Emerick S, Komorowski TE, Rainin EA, Shepard BM. Extraocular muscle regeneration in primates. Local anesthetic-induced lesions. Ophthalmology 1992; 99:582–9.
41. Carry MR, Ringel SP. Structure and histochemistry of human extraocular muscle. Bull Soc Belge Ophtalmol 1989; 237:303–19.
42. Castaigne P, Laplane D, Fardeau M, Dordain G, Autret A, Hirt L. Myopathie avec anomalies mitochondriales localisées aux fibres de type 1. Rev Neurol 1972; 126:81–96.
43. Caughey JE, Myrianthopoulos NC. Dystrophia Myotonica and Related Disorders. Springfield, IL: Charles C Thomas, 1963:119–23.
44. Caughey JE, Pachomov N. The diaphragm in dystrophia myotonica. J Neurol Neurosurg Psychiat 1956; 22:311–3.
45. Chiu HC, Vincent A, Newsom-Davis J, Hsieh KH, Hung TP. Myasthenia gravis: population differences by disease expression and acetylcholine receptor antibody titers between Chinese and Caucasians. Neurology 1987; 37:1854–7.
46. Coërs C, Telerman-Toppet N. Morphological and histochemical changes of motor units in myasthenia. Ann NY Acad Sci 1976; 274:6–19.
47. Coërs, C, Woolf AL. The Innervation of Muscle. Springfield, IL: Charles C Thomas, 1959:107–12.
48. Cogan DG, Kuwabara T, Richardson EPG. Pathology of abiotrophic ophthalmoplegia externa. Bull Johns Hopkins Hosp 1962; 111:42–56.
49. Compston DAS, Vincent A, Newsom-Davis J, Batchelor JR. Clinical, pathological, HLA antigen and immunological evidence for disease heterogeneity in myasthenia gravis. Brain 1980; 103:579–601.
50. Conomy JP, Levinsohn M, Fanaroff A. Familial infantile myasthenia gravis: a case of sudden death in young children. J Pediatr 1975; 87:428–30.
51. Coquet M, Vital C, Julian J. Presence of inclusion body myositis-like filaments in oculopharyngeal muscular dystrophy: ultrastructural study of 10 cases. Neuropathol Appl Neurobiol 1990; 16:393–400.

52. Corbeil-Girard L-P, Klein AF, Sasseville AM-J, Lavoie H, Dicaire M-J, Saint-Denis A, Pagé M, Duranceau A, Codère F, Bouchard J-P, Karpati G, Rouleau GA, Massie B, Langelier Y, Brais B. PABN1 overexpression leads to upregulation of genes encoding nuclear proteins that are sequestered in oculopharyngeal muscular dystrophy nuclear inclusions. Neurobiol Dis 2005; 18:551–67.
53. Craig RW, Padrón R. Molecular structure of the sarcomere. In: Engle AG, Franzini-Armstrong C, eds. Myology. 3rd ed. Vol. 1. New York: McGraw-Hill, 2004:129–66.
54. Croft PB, Cutting JC, Jewesbury ECO, Blackwood W, Mair WGP. Ocular myopathy progressive external ophthalmoplegia with neuropathic complications. Acta Neurol Scand 1977; 55:169–97.
55. Crosby TW, Chou SM. "Ragged-red" fibers in Leigh's disease. Neurology 1974; 24:49–54.
56. Culebras A, Feldman RG, Merk F. Cytoplasmic inclusion bodies within neurons of the thalamus in myotonic dystrophy: a light and electron microscopic study. J Neurol Sci 1973; 19:319–29.
57. Dark AJ, Streeten BW. Ultrastructural study of cataract in myotonia dystrophica. Am J Ophthalmol 1977; 84:666–74.
58. Daroff RB, Solitare GB, Pincus JH, Glaser GH. Spongiform encephalopathy with chronic progressive external ophthalmoplegia. Neurology 1966; 16:161–9.
59. Davidson SI. The eye in dystrophia myotonica, with a report on electromyography of the extra-ocular muscles. Br J Ophthalmol 1961; 45:183–96.
60. Day JW, Ricker K, Jacobsen JF, Rasmussen LJ, Dick KA, Kress W, Schneider C, Koch MC, Beilman GJ, Harrison AR, Dalton JC, Ranum, LPW. Myotonic dystrophy type 2. Molecular, diagnostic and clinical spectrum. Neurology 2003; 60:657–64.
61. DeVries S. Retinopathy in dermatomyositis. Arch Ophthalmol 1951; 46:432–5.
62. Dieperink ME, Stefansson K. Molecular mimicry and microorganisms: a role in the pathogenesis of myasthenia gravis. Curr Topics Microbiol Immunol 1989; 145:57–65.
63. DiMauro S, Schotland DL, Bonilla E, Lee C-P, Gambetti P, Rowland LP. Progressive ophthalmoplegia, glycogen storage, and abnormal mitochondria. Arch Neurol 1973; 29:170–9.
64. Drachman DA, Wetzel N, Wasserman M, Naito H. Experimental denervation of ocular muscles, a critique of the concept of "ocular myopathy". Arch Neurol 1969; 21:170–83.
65. Drachman DA. Ophthalmoplegia plus: the neurodegenerative disorders associated with progressive external ophthalmoplegia. Arch Neurol 1968; 18:654–74.
66. Drachman DB, De Silva S, Ramsay D, Pestronk A. Humoral pathogenesis of myasthenia gravis. Ann N Y Acad Sci 1987; 505:90–105.
67. Dubowitz V. Cross-innervated mammalian skeletal muscles: histochemical physiological and biochemical observations. J Physiol 1967; 193:481–96.
68. Dubowitz V. Muscle Biopsy. A Practical Approach, 2nd ed. Philadelphia: Bailliere Tindall, 1985:398–404.
69. Dubowitz V. Muscle Biopsy: A Modern Approach. 2nd ed. Philadelphia: W. B. Saunders, 1985:28–30.
70. Duke-Elder S. Diseases of the Lens and Vitreous; Glaucoma and Hypotony: System of Ophthalmology, Vol. 1. London: Kimpton, 1969:183–9.
71. Durelli L, Maggi G, Casadio C, Ferri R, Rendine S, Bergamini L. Actuarial analysis of the occurrence of remissions following thymectomy for myasthenia gravis in 400 patients. J Neurol Neurosurg Psychiat 1991; 54: 406–11.
72. Durston JHJ. Histochemistry of primate extraocular muscles and the changes of denervation. Br J Ophthalmol 1974; 58:193–216.
73. Elmqvist D, Hofmann WW, Kugelberg J, Quastel DMJ. An electrophysiological investigation of neuromuscular transmission in myasthenia gravis. J Physiol 1964; 174: 417–34.
74. Elrod RD, Weinberg DA. Ocular myasthenia gravis. Ophthalmol Clin N Am 2004; 17:275–309.
75. Emery AEH, Smith CAB, Sanger R. The linkage relations of the loci for benign Becker type X-borne muscular dystrophy, colour blindness and the Xg blood groups. Ann Hum Genet 1969; 32:261–9.
76. Emery AEH. Genetic linkage between the loci for colour blindness and Duchenne type muscular dystrophy. J Med Genet 1966; 3:92–5.
77. Engel A, Lambert EH, Howard FM, Jr. Immune complexes IgG and C3 and the motor end-plate in myasthenia gravis. Mayo Clin Proc 1977; 52:267–80.
78. Engel AG, Gomez MR, Groover RV. Multicore disease: a recently recognized congenital myopathy associated with multifocal degeneration of muscle fibers. Mayo Clin Proc 1971; 46:666–681.
79. Engel AG, Gomez MR. Congenital myopathy associated with multifocal degeneration of muscle fibers. Trans Am Neurol Assoc 1966; 91:222–3.
80. Engel AG, Hohlfeld R. Acquired Autoimmune Myasthenia Gravis. In: Engel AG, Franzini-Armstrong C, eds. Myology. 3rd ed. Vol. 1. New York: McGraw-Hill, 2004:1755–90.
81. Engel AG, Lambert EH, Gomez MR. A new myasthenic syndrome with end-plate acetylcholinesterase deficiency, small nerve terminals, and reduced acetylcholine release. Ann Neurol 1977; 1:315–30.
82. Engel AG, Lindstrom JM, Lambert EH, Lennon VA. Ultrastructural localization of the acetylcholine receptor in myasthenia gravis and in its experimental autoimmune model. Neurology 1977; 27:307–15.
83. Engel AG, Santa T. Histometric analysis of the ultrastructure of the neuromuscular junction in myasthenia gravis and in the myasthenic syndrome. Ann NY Acad Sci 1971; 183:46–63.
84. Engel AG, Tsujihata M, Lindstrom JM, Lennon VA. The motor end plate in myasthenia gravis and in experimental autoimmune myasthenia gravis: a quantitative ultrastructural study. Ann NY Acad Sci 1976; 274:60–79.
85. Engel AG. Congenital disorders of neuromuscular transmission. Sem Neurol 1990; 10:12–26.
86. Engel WK, Trotter JL, McFarlin DF, McIntosh CL. Thymic epithelial cells contain acetylcholine receptor. Lancet 1977; 1:1310–1.
87. Eshaghian J, March WF, Goossens W, Rafferty NS. Ultrastructure of cataract in myotonic dystrophy. Invest Ophthalmol VisSci 1978; 17:289–93.
88. Eustace P. Corneal lesions in myotonic dystrophy. Br J Ophthalmol 1969; 53:633–7.
89. Evans PR. Nuclear agenesis, Möbius' syndrome: the congenital facial diplegia syndrome. Arch Dis Child 1955; 30:237–43.
90. Eymard B, Vernet-der Garabedian B, Berrih-Aknin S, Pannier C, Bach J-F, Morel E. Anti-acetylcholine receptor antibodies in neonatal myasthenia gravis: heterogeneity and pathogenic significance. J Autoimmun 1991; 4:185–95.
91. Fan X, Rouleau GA. Progress in understanding the pathogenesis of oculopharyngeal muscular dystrophy. Can J Neurol Sci 2003; 30:8–14.

92. Fardeau M, Lapresle I, Milhaud M. Contribution à l'étude des lèsions élémentaires du muscle squelettique: ultrastructure des masses sarcoplasmiques latérales (observées dans un cas de dystrophie myotonique). C R Soc Biol Paris 1965; 159:15–7.
93. Fardeau M. Some orthodox or non-orthodox considerations on congenital myopathies. EEG 1987; 39 (Suppl): 85–90.
94. Farkas E, Tome FMS, Fardeau M, Arsenio-Nunes ML, Dreyfus P, Diebler MF. Histochemical and ultrastructural study of muscle biopsies in 3 cases of dystrophia myotonica in the newborn child. J Neurol Sci 1974; 21:273–88.
95. Fenichel GM. Clinical syndromes of myasthenia in infancy and childhood, a review. Arch Neurol 1978; 35: 97–103.
96. Fisch C. The heart in myotonica atrophia. Am Heart J 1951; 41:525–38.
97. Fitch N, Karpati G, Pinsky L. Congenital blepharophimosis, joint contractures, and muscular hypotonia. Neurology 1971; 21:1214–20.
98. Fitzsimons RB, Tyer HDD. A study of a myopathy presenting as idiopathic scoliosis: multicore disease or mitochondrial myopathy. J Neurol Sci 1980; 46:33–48.
99. Fonkalsrud EW, Herrmann C, Jr, Mulder DG. Thymectomy for myasthenia gravis in children. J Pediatr Surg 1970; 5:157–65.
100. Fowler M. Case of arthrogryposis multiplex congenita with lesions in the nervous system. Arch Dis Child 1959; 34:505–10.
101. Fowler WM Jr, Layzer RB, Taylor RG, Eberle ED, Sims GE, Munsat TL, Philippart M, Wilson BW. The Schwartz-Jampel syndrome. J Neurol Sci 1974; 22:127–46.
102. Fritze D, Herrmann C, Jr, Naeim F, Smith GS, Zeller E, Walford RL. The biologic significance of HL-A antigen markers in myasthenia gravis. Ann NY Acad Sci 1976; 274:440–50.
103. Fuchs E. Ueber isolirte doppelseitige Ptosis. Albrecht von Graefes Arch Ophthalmol 1890; 36:234–59.
104. Fujii Y, Hashimoto J, Mondeu Y, Ito T, Nakahase K, Kawashima Y. Specific activation of lymphocytes against acetylcholine receptor in the thymus in myasthenia gravis. J Immunol 1986; 136:887–91.
105. Fukuhara N, Kumamato T, Tsubaki T, Mayuzumi T, Nitta H. Oculopharyngeal muscular dystrophy and distal myopathy: intrafamilial difference in the onset and distribution of muscular involvement. Acta Neurol Scand 1982; 65:458–67.
106. Furukawa T, Takagi A, Nakao K, Sugita H, Tsukagoshi H, Tsubaki T. Hereditary muscular atrophy with ataxia retinitis pigmentosa, and diabetes mellitus, a clinical report of a family. Neurology 1968; 18:942–7.
107. Garcin R, Fardeau M, Godet-Guillain M. A clinical and pathological study of a case of alternating and recurrent external ophthalmoplegia with amyotrophy of the limbs observed for forty-five years: discussion of the relationship of this condition with myasthenia gravis. Brain 1965; 88:739–52.
108. Gatchel JR, Zoghbi HY. Diseases of unstable repeat expansion: mechanisms and common principles. Nature Rev Genet 2005; 6:743–51.
109. Gath I, Kayan A, Leegaard J, Sjaastad, O. Myasthenia congenita: electromyographic findings. Acta Neurol Scand 1970; 46:323–30.
110. Genkins G, Papatestas AE, Horowitz SH, Kornfeld P. Studies in myasthenia gravis: early thymectomy, electrophysiologic, and pathologic correlations. Am J Med 1975; 58:517–24.
111. Genkins GL, Kornfeld P, Papatestas AE, Bender AN, Matta RJ. Clinical experience in more than 2000 patients with myasthenia gravis. Ann N Y Acad Sci 1987; 505:500–16.
112. Geuder KI, Marx A, Witzemann V, Schalke B, Kirchner T, Müller-Hermelink HK. Genomic organization and lack of transcription of the nicotinic acetylcholine receptor subunit genes in myasthenia gravis-associated thymoma. Lab Invest 1992; 66:452–8.
113. Giordano M, Comoli AM, DeAngelis MS, Mutani R, Sebastiani F, Richiardi PM. Reassessment of the specificity of lens opacity in myotonic dystrophy. Ophthal Res 1996; 28:224–9.
114. Glaser JS. Myasthenic pseudo-internuclear ophthalmoplegia. Arch Ophthalmol 1966; 75:363–6.
115. Goebel HH, Meinck HM, Reinecke M, Schimrigk K, Mielke U. Centronuclear myopathy with special consideration of the adult form. Eur Neurol 1984; 23:425–34.
116. Goldstein AL, Thurman GB, Cohen GH, Rossio JL. The endocrine thymus: potential role for thymosin in the treatment of autoimmune disease. Ann N Y Acad Sci 1976; 274:390–401.
117. Gonatas NK. A generalized disorder of nervous system, skeletal muscle, and heart resembling Refsum's disease and Hurler's syndrome. Part II. Ultrastructure. Am J Med 1967; 42:169–78.
118. Gowers WR. A Manual of Diseases of the Nervous System. 2nd ed., Philadelphia: Blakiston, 1897:196–7.
119. Greer M, Schotland M. Myasthenia gravis in the newborn. Pediatrics 1960; 26:101–08.
120. Grob D, Arsura EL, Brunner NG, Namba T. The course of myasthenia gravis and therapies affecting outcome. Ann N Y Acad Sci 1987; 505:472–99.
121. Gross MLP, Teoh R, Legg NJ, Pallis C. Ocular myopathy and Marfan's syndrome. J Neurol Sci 1980; 46:105–12.
122. Gunn M. Congenital ptosis with peculiar associated movements of the affected lid. Trans Ophthalmol Soc UK 1883; 3:283–7.
123. Haliloglu G, Gross C, Senbil N, Talim B, Hehr U, Uyanik G, Winkler J, Topaloglu H. Clinical spectrum of muscle-eye-brain disease: from the typical presentation to severe autistic features. Acta Myol 2004; 23:137–9.
124. Harding AE, Holt IJ. Mitochondrial myopathies. Br Med Bull 1989; 45:760–71.
125. Harper P, Penny R, Roley TP, Jr, Migeon CJ, Blizzard RM. Gonadal function in males with myotonic dystrophy. J Clin Endocrinol Metab 1972; 35:852–6.
126. Harper PS. Myotonic Dystrophy, 3rd ed. New York: Saunders, 2001.
127. Harrison SM, Frenkel M, Grossman BJ, Matalon R. Retinopathy in childhood dermatomyositis. Am J Ophthalmol 1973; 76:786–90.
128. Havard CWH. Progress in myasthenia gravis. Br Med J 1977:1008–11.
129. Hayasaka S, Kiyosawa M, Katsumata S, Honda M, Takase S, Mizuno K. Ciliary and retinal changes in myotonic dystrophy. Arch Ophthalmol 1984; 102:88–93,.
130. Heene R. Histological and histochemical findings in muscle spindles in dystrophia myotonica. J Neurol Sci 1973; 18:369–72.
131. Henderson JL. The congenital facial diplegia syndrome: clinical features, pathology, and aetiology. Brain 1939; 62: 381–403.
132. Herishanu Y, Lavy S. Internal "ophthalmoplegia" in myasthenia gravis. Ophthalmologica 1971; 163:302–5.
133. Horrobin DF, Morgan RO. Myotonic dystrophy: a disease caused by functional zinc deficiency due to an abnormal zinc-binding ligand? Med Hypoth 1980; 6:375–88.

134. Houber JP, Babel J. Les lésions uvéo-rétiniennes de la dystrophie myotonique. Ann Ocul 1970; 203:1067–76.
135. Howard FM Jr, Lennon VA, Finley J, Matsumoto J, Elveback LR. Clinical correlations of antibodies that bind, block, or modulate human acetylcholine receptors in myasthenia gravis. Ann NY Acad Sci 1987; 505:526–38.
136. Huang S-OW, Rose JW, Mayer RF. Assessment of cellular and humoral immunity of myasthenics. J Neurol Neurosurg Psychiat 1977; 40:1053–9.
137. Huebner O. Cited in Henderson (1939) (131).
138. Hurwitz LJ, Carson NAJ, Allen IV, Chopra JS. Congenital ophthalmoplegia, floppy baby syndrome, myopathy, and aminoaciduria. J Neurol Neurosurg Psychiat 1969; 32: 495–508.
139. Hutchinson J. On ophthalmoplegia externa or symmetrical immobility (partial) of the eyes, with ptosis. Med Chir Trans Lond 1879; 62:307–29.
140. Hyman BN, Patten BM, Dodson RF. Mitochondrial abnormalities in progressive external ophthalmoplegia. Am J Ophthalmol 1977; 83:362–71.
141. Iannaccone ST, Griggs RC, Markesbery WR, Joynt RJ. Familial progressive external ophthalmoplegia and ragged-red fibers. Neurology 1974; 24:1033–8.
142. Isaacs H, Badenhorst M. Multicore disease. South Afr Med J 1980; 57:543–6.
143. Ito Y, Miledi R, Molenaar PC, Vincent A, Polak RL, van Elder M, Davis JN. Acetylcholine in human muscle. Proc R Soc Lond [Biol] 1976; 192:475–80.
144. Jadro-Santel D, Grcevic N, Dogan S, Franjic J, Benc H. Centronuclear myopathy with type I fibre hypotrophy and fingerprint inclusions associated with Marfan's syndrome. J Neurol Sci 1980; 45:43–56.
145. Jeger BV, Fred HL, Butler RB, Carnes WH. Occurrence of retinal pigmentation, ophthalmoplegia, ataxia, deafness and heart block: report of a case, with findings at autopsy. Am J Med 1960; 29:888–93.
146. Johns TR, Campa JF, Crowley WJ. Familial myasthenic myopathy. Neurology 1971; 21:449.
147. Johnson CC, Kuwabara T. Oculopharyngeal muscular dystrophy. Am J Ophthalmol 1974; 77:872–9.
148. Jonecko A. Die Ringbinden als eine allgemeine unspezifische Reaktion der quergestreiften Muskulatur. Experientia 1962; 18:166–7.
149. Junge J. Ocular changes in dystrophia myotonica, paramyotonia, and myotonia congenita. Doc Ophthalmol 1966; 21:1–115.
150. Kaminski HJ, Maas E, Spiegel P, Ruff RL. Why are eye muscles frequently involved in myasthenia gravis. Neurology 1990; 40:1663–9.
151. Kano H, Kobayashi K, Herrmann R, Tachikawa M, Manya H, Nishino I, Nonaka I, Straub V, Talim B, Voit T, Topaloglu H, Endo T, Yoshikawa H, Toda T. Deficiency of alpha dystroglycan in Muscle–Eye–Brain disease. Biochem Biophy Res Commun 2002; 291:1283–6.
152. Kao I, Drachman DB. Thymic muscle cells bear acetylcholine receptors: possible relation to myasthenia gravis. Science 1977; 195:74–5.
153. Karpati G, Carpenter S, Larbrisseau A, Lafontaine R. The Kearns-Shy syndrome, a multisystem disease with mitochondrial abnormality demonstrated in skeletal muscle and skin. J Neurol Sci 1973; 19:133–51.
154. Keane JR. Alternating proptosis, a case report of acute orbital myositis defined by the computerized tomographic scan. Arch Neurol 1977; 34:642–64.
155. Kearns TP, Sayre GP. Retinitis pigmentosa, external ophthalmoplegia and complete heart block, unusual syndrome with histologic study in one of two cases. Arch Ophthalmol 1958; 60:280–9.
156. Kearns TP. External ophthalmoplegia, pigmentary degeneration of the retina, and cardiomyopathy: a newly recognized syndrome. Trans Am Ophthalmol Soc 1965; 63:559–625.
157. Keesey J, Lindstrom J, Cokely H, Herrmann C, Jr. Antiacetylcholine receptor antibody in neonatal myasthenia gravis. N Engl J Med 1977; 296:55.
158. Keesey J, Shaikh I, Wolfgram F, Chao L-P. Studies on the ability of acetylcholine receptors to bind alpha-bungarotoxin after exposure to myasthenic serum. Ann NY Acad Sci 1976; 274:244–53.
159. Kiloh LG, Nevin S. Progressive dystrophy of the external ocular muscles (ocular myopathy). Brain 1951; 74:115–43.
160. Kirby TJ, Achoc RWP, Perry HO, Winkelmann RK. Cataract formation after triparanol therapy. Arch Ophthalmol 1962; 68:486–9.
161. Kirchner T, Tzartos S, Hoppe F, Schalko B, Wekerle H, Müller-Hermelink HK. Pathogenesis of myasthenia gravis, acetylcholine receptor-related antigenic determinants in tumor-free thymuses and thymic epithelial tumors. Am J Pathol 1988; 130:268–80.
162. Kito S, Yamamoto M, Fujimori N, Itoga E, Kosaka K. Studies on myotonic dystrophy. Part I. Ultrastructural lesions of the muscle and the nerve in myotonic dystrophy. In Takulas B, ed. Basic Research in Myology. Amsterdam: Excerpta Medica, 1973:651–73.
163. Klein JJ, Gottlieb AJ, Mones RJ, Appel SH, Osserman KE. Thymoma and polymyositis: onset of myasthenia gravis after thymectomy: report of two cases. Arch Intern Med 1964; 113:142–52.
164. Kokotis P, Theodossiadis P, Bouros C, Sfikakis PP. Bilateral ocular myositis as a late complication of dermatomyositis. J Rheumatol 2005; 32:379–81.
165. Korenyi-Both A, Lapis K, Gallai M, Szobor A. Fine structural alterations of muscle fibers in diseases accompanied by myotonia. Beitr Pathol 1975; 156:241–56.
166. Korman EF, Harris RA, Williams CH, Wakabayashi T, Green DE, Valdivia E. Paracrystalline arrays in mitochondria. Bioenergetics 1970; 1:387–404.
167. Kornblum C, Kunz WS, Klockgether T, Roggenkamper P, Schroder R. Diagnostic value of mitochondrial DNA analysis in chronic progressive external ophthalmoplegia (CPEO). Klin Monatsbl Augenheilkd 2004; 221:1057–61.
168. Kuks JBM, Oosterhuis HJGH, Limburg PC, The TH. Antiacetylcholine receptor antibodies decrease after thymectomy in patients with myasthenia gravis. Clinical Correlations. J Autoimmun 1991; 4:197–211.
169. Kurihara T. New classification and treatment for myotonic disorders. Internal Med 2005; 44:1027–32.
170. Kuwabara T, Lessell S. Electron microscopic study of extraocular muscles in myotonic dystrophy. Am J Ophthalmol 1976; 82:303–9.
171. Lagoutte F, Coquet M, Vital C. Étude ultrastructurale de la musculature oculaire dans deux cas familiaux de maladie de Steinert. Arch Ophtalmol Paris 1976; 36:565–74.
172. Lakin M, Locke S. Progressive ocular myopathy with ovarian insufficiency and diabetes mellitus: report of a case. Diabetes 1961; 10:228–31.
173. Langdon HM, Cadwalader WB. Chronic progressive external ophthalmoplegia: report of a case with necropsy. Brain 1928; 51:321–33.
174. Lefvert AK, Matell G. Antibodies against human cholinergic receptor proteins in patients with myasthenia gravis: studies during immunosuppressive treatment. Acta Med Scand 1977; 20:181–2.

175. Lell ME, Swerdlow ML. Dermatomyositis of childhood. Pediatr Ann 1977; 6:203–212.
176. Lenard HG, Goebel HH, Weigel W. Smooth muscle involvement in congenital myotonic dystrophy. Neuropediatr 1977; 8:42–52.
177. Levinson AI, Song D, Gaulton G, Zheng Y. The intrathymic pathogenesis of myasthenia gravis. Clin Dev Immunol 2004; 11:215–20.
178. Lindstrom J, Shelton D, Fujii Y. Myasthenia gravis. Adv Immunol 1988; 42:233–84.
179. Lindstrom JM, Seybold ME, Lennon VA, Whittingham S, Duane DD. Antibody to acetylcholine receptor in myasthenia gravis. Neurology 1976; 26:1054–9.
180. Linton DM, Philcox D. Myasthenia gravis. Disease-a-Month 1990; 36:595–637.
181. Lisak RP, Abdou NI, Zweiman B, Zmijewski C, Penn A. Aspects of lymphocyte function in myasthenia gravis. Ann NY Acad Sci 1976; 274:402–10.
182. Little BW, Perl DP. Oculopharyngeal muscular dystrophy: an autopsied case from the French-Canadian kindred. J Neurol Sci 1982; 53:145–58.
183. Lotz BP, Van der Meyden CH. Myotonic dystrophy. Part II. A clinical study of 96 patients. S Afr Med J 1985; 67: 815–7.
184. Luft R, Ikkos D, Palmierl G, Ernster L, Afzelius B. A case of severe hypermetabolism of non-thyroid origin with a defect in maintenance of mitochondrial respiratory control: a correlated clinical, biochemical, and morphological study. J Clin Invest 1962; 41:1776–804.
185. Lui F, Fonda S, Merlini L, Corazza R. Saccadic eye movements are impaired in Duchenne muscular dystrophy. Doc Ophthalmol 2001; 103:219–28.
186. Lundberg PO. Hereditary myopathy, oligophrenia, cataract, skeletal abnormalities, and hypergonadotrophic hypgonadism: a new syndrome. Eur Neurol 1973; 10: 261–80.
187. Lundberg PO. Ocular myopathy with hypogonadism. Acta Neurol Scand 1962; 38:142–55.
188. Lyness RW, Collin JRO, Alexander RA, Garner A. Histological appearances of the levator palpebrae superioris muscle in the Marcus Gunn phenomenon. Br J Ophthalmol 1988; 72:104–9.
189. Manschot WA. Histological findings in a case of dystrophia myotonica. Ophthalmologica 1968; 155:294–6.
190. Mantegazza R, Beghi E, Pareyson D, Antozzi C, Peluchetti D, Sghirlanzoni A, Cosi V, Lombardi M, Piccolo G, Tonali P, Evoli A, Ricci E, Batocchi A P, Angelini C, Micaglio GF, Marconi G, Tailuti R, Bergamini Durelli L, Cornelio F. A multicentre follow-up study of 1152 patients with myasthenia gravis in Italy. J Neurol 1990; 237:339–44.
191. Margolis S, Luginbeuhl B. Eye abnormalities associated with arthrogryposis multiplex congenita. J Ped Ophthalmol 1975; 12:57–60.
192. Martinez AI, Hay S, McNeer KW. Extraocular muscles, light microscopy, and ultrastructural features. Acta Neuropathol 1976; 34:237–53.
193. Maselli RA, Richman DP, Wollmann RL. Inflammation at the neuromuscular junction in myasthenia gravis. Neurology 1991; 41:1497–504.
194. Mason GI. Iris neovascular tufts: relationship to rubeosis, insulin, and hypotony. Arch Ophthalmol 1979; 97:2346–2.
195. Masters CL, Dawkins RL, Zilko PJ, Simpson JA, Leedman RJ, Lindstrom, J. Penicillamine-associated myasthenia gravis, antiacetylcholine receptor, and antistriational antibodies. Am J Med 1977; 63:689–94.
196. Matsunaga M, Inokuchi T, Ohnishi A, Kuroiwa Y. Oculopharyngeal involvement in familial neurogenic muscular atrophy. J Neurol Neurosurg Psychiat 1973; 36:104–111.
197. Maurage CA, Budd MM, Ruchoux, P.V, Kalimo H, Krahe R, Delacourte A, Sergeant N. Similar brain tau pathology in DM2/PROMM and DM1/Steinert disease. Neurology 2005; 65:1636–8.
198. Maynard JA, Cooper RR, Ionaescu VV. An ultrastructure investigation of intrafusal muscle fibers in myotonic dystrophy. Virchows Arch [A] Pathol Anat Histopathol 1977; 373:1–13.
199. McComas AJ, Campbell MJ, Sica REP. Electrophysiological study of dystrophia myotonica. J Neurol Neurosurg Psychiat 1971; 34:132–9.
200. McQuillen MP. Familial limb-girdle myasthenia. Brain 1966; 89:121–65.
201. Melmed C, Karpati G, Carpenter S. Experimental mitochondrial myopathy produced in vivo uncoupling of oxidative phosphorylation. J Neurol Sci 1975; 26: 305–318.
202. Meola G, Moxley RT III. Myotonic dystrophy type 2 and related myotonic disorders. J Neurol 2004; 251: 1173–82.
203. Mereu TR, Porter IH, Hug G. Myotonia, shortness of stature, and hip dysplasia, Schwartz-Jampel syndrome. Am J Dis Child 1969; 117:470–8.
204. Metz HS. Myasthenia gravis presenting as internuclear ophthalmoplegia. J Pediatr Ophthalmol 1977; 14:23–4.
205. Meyer E, Navon D, Auslender L, Zonis S. Myotonic dystrophy: pathological study of the eyes. Ophthalmologica (Basel) 1980; 181:215–20.
206. Miceli MV, Jazwinski SM. Common and cell-type specific responses of human cells to mitochondrial dysfunction. Exp Cell Res 2005; 302:270–80.
207. Michele DE, Barresi R, Kanagawa M, Saito F, Cohn RD, Satz JS, Dollar J, Nishino I, Kelley RI, Somer H, Straub V, Mathews KD, Moore SA, Campbell KP. Post-translational disruption of dystroglycan-ligand interactions in congenital muscular dystrophies. Nature 2002; 418:417–22.
208. Miller JE. Cellular organization of rhesus extraocular muscle. Invest Ophthalmol 1967; 6:18–39.
209. Minoda K. Histochemical and electron microscopic studies of extraocular muscles. Part IV. Fine structure or neuropathic extraocular muscles. Acta Soc Ophthalmol Jpn 1971; 75:1184–95.
210. Möbius PJ Über periodische oculomotoriuslahmung. Dtsch Z Nervenheilk 1900; 17:294–305.
211. Möbius PJ. Über infantilen Kernschwund. Muench Med Wochenschr 1892; 39:17–21, 41–3, 55–8.
212. Möbius PJ. Ueber angeborenedoppelseitige Abducens-Facialis-Lähmung. Muench Med Wochenschr 1888; 35: 91–4.
213. Mongia SK, Lundervold A. Electrophysiological abnormalities in cases of dystrophia myotonica. Eur Neurol 1975; 13:360–76.
214. Mooers BHM, Logan JS, Berglund JA. The structural basis of myotonic dystrophy from the crystal structure of CUG repeats. Proc Natl Acad Sci U S A 2005; 102:16626–31.
215. Moran CA, Suster S, Jagirdar J. Morphometric analysis of germinal centers in nonthymomatous patients with myasthenia gravis. Arch Path Lab Med 1990; 114: 689–91.
216. Morgan-Hughes JA, Cooper JM, Schapira AHV, Hayes DJ, Clark JB. The mitochondrial myopathies: defects of the mitochondrial respiratory chain and

oxidative phosphorylation system. EEG (Suppl.) 1987; 39:103–14.
217. Mostacciuolo ML, Barujani G, Armani M, Danieli GA, Angelini C. Genetic epidemiology of myotonic dystrophy. Genet Epidemiol 1987; 4:289–98.
218. Munro S. Fundus appearances in a case of acute dermatomyositis. Br J Ophthalmol 1959; 43:548–58.
219. Murphy SF, Drachman DB. The oculopharyngeal syndrome. J Am Med Assoc 1968; 203:1003–8.
220. Mussini ID, Mauro S, Angelini C. Early ultrastructural and biochemical changes in muscle in dystrophia myotonica. J Neurol Sci 1970; 10:585–604.
221. Naegeli W. Über Myotonica atrophica, speziell über die Symptome und die Pathogenese der Krankheit nach 22 eigenen Fällen. Muench Med Wochenschr 1917; 64: 1631–2.
222. Namba T, Brown SB, Grob D. Neonatal myasthenia gravis: report of two cases and review of the literature. Pediatrics 1970; 45:488–504.
223. Namba T, Nakata Y, Grob D. The role of humoral and cellular immune factors in neuromuscular block in myasthenia gravis. Ann N Y Acad Sci 1976; 274:493–515.
224. Newsom-Davis J, Pinching AJ, Vincent A, Wilson SG. Function of circulating antibody to acetylcholine receptor in myasthenia gravis: investigation by plasma exchange. Neurology 1978; 28:266–72.
225. Newsom-Davis J, Willcox N, Schluep M, Harcourt G, Vincent A, Mossman S, Wray D, Burges J. Immunological heterogeneity and cellular mechanisms in myasthenia. Ann NY Acad Sci 1987; 505:12–38.
226. Nicole S, Topaloglu H, Fontaine B. 102nd ENMC international workshop on Schwartz-Jampel syndrome, 14–16 December 2001, Naarden, The Netherlands. Neuromusc Disord 2003; 13:347–51.
227. North K. Congenital myopathies. In Engel AG, Franzini-Armstrong C. Myology, 3rd ed. Vol. 2. New York: McGraw-Hill, 2004:1473–1533.
228. O'Leary PA, Waisman M. Dermatomyositis: a study of forty cases. Arch Dermatol Syphilol 1940; 41:1001–19.
229. Oda K. Motor innervation and acetylcholine receptor distribution of human extraocular muscle fibres. J Neurol Sci 1986; 74:125–33.
230. Okamura K, Santa T, Nage K, Omae T. Congenital oculoskeletal myopathy with abnormal muscle and liver mitochondria. J NeurolSci 1976; 27:79–91.
231. Oklund S, Komorowski TE, Carlson BM. Ultrastructure of mepivacaine-induced damage and regeneration in rat extraocular muscle. Invest Ophthamol Vis Sci 1989; 20: 1643–51.
232. Olsen WK, Bardin CW, Walsh O, Engel WK. Moebius syndrome:lower motor neuron involvement and hypogonadotrophic hypogonadism. Neurology 1970; 20: 1002–8.
233. Olson W, Engel WK, Walsh GO, Einaugler R. Oculocraniosomatic neuromuscular disease with "ragged-red" fibers. Arch Neurol 1972; 26:193–211.
234. Oosterhuis H, Bethlem J. Neurogenic muscle involvement in myasthenia gravis, a clinical and histopathological study. J Neurol Neurosurg Psychiat 1973; 36:224–54.
235. Orth DN, Almeida H, Walsh FB, Henda M. Ophthalmoplegia resulting from diphenylhydantoin and primidone intoxication: report of four cases. J Am Med Assoc 1967; 201:225–7.
236. Ortiz deZarate JC, Maruffo A. The descending ocular myopathy of early childhood: myotubular or centronuclear myopathy. Eur Neurol 1970; 3:1–12.
237. Osher RH, Smith JL. Ocular myasthenia gravis and Hashimoto's thyroiditis. Am J Ophthalmol 1975; 79: 1038–43.
238. Osserman KE, Genkins G. Studies in myasthenia gravis: review of a twenty year experience in over 1200 patients. Mt Sinai J Med N Y 1971; 38:497–537.
239. Pachter BR, Eberstein A, Breinin GM. Electromyographic and electron microscopic findings in the central extraocular muscles of the myotonic rat. Exp Neurol 1977; 57: 971–83.
240. Pachter BR, Pearson J, Davidowitz J, Reuben R, Boal D, Carr R, Breinin GM. Congenital total external ophthalmoplegia associated with infantile spinal muscular atrophy: fine structure of extraocular muscle. Invest Ophthalmol 1976; 15:320–24.
241. Paez JH, Tuulonen A, Yarom R, Arad H, Zelikovitch A, Ben Ezra D. Ocular findings in arthrogryposis multiplex congenita. J Ped Ophthalmol Strabis 1982; 19:75–9.
242. Papatestas AE, Genkins G, Horowitz SH, Kornfeld P. Thymectomy in myasthenia gravis: pathologic, clinical, and electrophysiologic correlations. Ann N Y Acad Sci 1976; 274:555–73.
243. Pearson CM. Polymyositis. Ann Rev Med 1966; 17:63–82.
244. PeBenito R, Sher JH, Cracco JB. Centronuclear myopathy: clinical and pathologic features. Clin Pediatr 1978; 17: 259–65.
245. Peck SM, Osserman KE, Weiner LB, Lefkovits A, Osserman RS. Studies in bullous diseases: immunofluorescent serologic tests. N Engl J Med 1968; 279:951–8.
246. Pendefunda G, Cernea P, Dobrescu G. Manifestarile oculare in miotonia atrofica Steinert. Oftalmol. 1964; 8: 219–24.
247. Pepin B, Mikol J, Goldstein B, Aron JJ, Lebuisson DA. Familial mitochondrial myopathy with cataract. J Neurol Sci 1980; 45:191–203.
248. Perlo VP, Arnason B, Poskanzer D, Castleman B, Schwab RS, Osserman KE, Papatestis A, Alpert L, Kark A. The role of thymectomy in the treatment of myasthenia gravis. Ann NY Acad Sci 1971; 183:308–17.
249. Petkovich NJ, Dunn M, Reed W. Myotonia dystrophica with A-V dissociation and Stokes-Adams attacks. Am Heart J 1964; 68:391–6.
250. Philip U, Walton JN, Smith CAB. Colour blindness and the Duchenne-type muscular dystrophy. Ann Hum Genet 1956; 21:155–8.
251. Pierson CR, Tomzak K, Agrawal P, Moghadaszadeh B, Beggs AH. X-linked myotubular and centronuclear myopathies. J Neuropathol Exp Neurol 2005; 64:555–64.
252. Pinto F, Amantini A, de Scisciolo G, Scaioli V, Frosini R, Pizzi A, Marconi G. Electrophysiological studies of the visual system in myotonic dystrophy. Acta Neurol Scand 1987; 76:351–8.
253. Pirskanen R. On the significance of HL-A and LD antigens in myasthenia gravis. Ann NY Acad Sci 1976; 274:451–60.
254. Pitner SE, Edwards JE, McCormick WF. Observations on the pathology of the Moebius syndrome. J Neurol Neurosurg Psychiat 1965; 28:362–74.
255. Pollock M, Dyck PJ. Peripheral nerve morphometry in myotonic dystrophy. Arch Neurol 1976; 33:33–9.
256. Porter CW, Barnard, E.A. Ultrastructural studies on the acetylcholine receptor at motor end plates of normal and pathologic muscles. Ann NY Acad Sci 1976; 274:85–107.
257. Racz P, Kovacs B, Varga L, Ujlaki E, Zombai E, Karbuczky S. Bilateral cataract in acrodermatitis enteropathica. J Pediat Ophthalmol Strabis 1979; 16:180–2.

258. Radu H, Killyen I, Ionescu V, Radu A. Myotubular centronuclear neuro-myopathy. I. Clinical, genetical, and morphological studies. Eur Neurol 1977; 15:285–300.
259. Radu H, Pendefunda G, Blucher G, Radu A, Darko Z, Godri I. Comparative and correlative study of the myotonias. In: Walton JN, Canal N, Scarlato G, eds. Amsterdam: Excerpta Medica, 1970:332–6.
260. Rainin EA, Carlson BM. Postoperative diplopia and ptosis: a clinical hypothesis based on the myotoxicity of local anesthetics. Arch Ophthamol 1985; 103:1337–9.
261. Raitta C, Karli P. Ocular findings in myotonic dystrophy. Ann Ophthalmol 1982; 14:646–50.
262. Raju TNK, Vidyasagar D, Reyes MG, Chokroverty S. Centronuclear myopathy in the newborn period causing severe respiratory distress. Pediat. 1977; 59:29–34.
263. Ranum LPW, Day JW. Myotonic dystrophy: RNA pathogenesis comes into focus. Am J Hum Genet 2004; 74:793–804.
264. Remacle J-P Pellissier J-F, Chamlian A, Benkoël L, Aubert L, Monges H. Progressive ophthalmoplegia associated with asymptomatic primary biliary cirrhosis. Hum Pathol 1980; 11(Suppl.):540–8.
265. Richards RN. The Möbius syndrome. J Bone Joint Surg 1953; 35A:37–444.
266. Ricker K, Pohlenz S. Ocular myositis and neuromyositis. Eur Neurol 1968; 1:41–9.
267. Ringel SP, Engel WK, Bender AN, Peters ND, Yee RD. Histochemistry and acetylcholine receptor distribution in normal and denervated monkey extraocular muscle. Neurology 1978; 28:55–63.
268. Roberts AH, Bamforth J. The pharynx and esophagus in ocular muscular dystrophy. Neurology 1968; 18:645–52.
269. Roberts DF, Bradley WG. Immunoglobulin levels in dystrophia myotonica. J Med Genet 1977; 14:16–9.
270. Robinson DO, Hammans SR, Read SP, Sillibourne J. Oculopharyngeal muscular dystrophy (OPMD): analysis of the PABN1 gene expansion sequence in 86 patients reveals 13 different expansion types and further evidence for unequal recombination as the mutational mechanism. Human Genet 2005; 116:267–71.
271. Rogers EL, Hitch GF, Jr, Gray I. Möbius syndrome and limb abnormalities. J Pediatr Ophthalmol 1977; 14:134–8.
272. Romanul FCA, van der Meulen JP. Slow and fast muscles after cross-innervation, enzymatic, and physiological changes. Arch Neurol 1967; 17:387–402.
273. Romi F, Gilhus NE, Aarli JA. Myasthenia gravis: clinical, immunological, and therapeutic advances. Acta Neurol Scand 2005; 111:134–41.
274. Rosenberg RN, Schotland DL, Lovelace RE, Rowland LP. Progressive ophthalmoplegia. Arch Neurol 1968; 19: 362–76.
275. Roses AD, Harper PS, Bossen EH. Myotonic muscular dystrophy. In: Vinken PJ, Bruyn FW, eds. Handbook of Clinical Neurology, Vol. 40, Part 1. New York: American Elsevier, 1979:485–532.
276. Roses AD. Myotonic muscular dystrophy: from clinical description to molecular genetics. Arch Intern Med 1985; 145:1487–9.
277. Rosman NP, Kakulas BA Mental deficiency associated with muscular dystrophy: a neuropathological study. Brain 1966; 89:769–88.
278. Rubin FH, Cross SA. Oculopharyngeal dystrophy. Arch Int Med 1981; 141:1103.
279. Ruff R, Kaminski H, Maas E, Spiegel P. Ocular muscles: physiology and structure-function correlations. Bull Soc Belge Ophthalmol 1989; 237:321–52.
280. Ryniewicz B, Badurska B. Follow-up study of myasthenic children after thymectomy. J Neurol 1977; 217:133–8.
281. Sadeh M. Extraocular muscles. In: Engel AG, Franzini-Armstrong C, eds. Myology. 3rd ed. Vol. 1. New York: McGraw-Hill, 2004:119–27.
282. Sagel J, Distiller LA, Morley JE, Isaacs H. Myotonia dystrophica: studies on gonadal function using luteinizing hormone-releasing hormone LRH. J Clin Endocrinol Metab 1975; 40:lll0–3.
283. Sahashi K, Engel AG, Lindstrom JM, Lambert EH, Lennon WA. Ultrastructural localization of immune complexes IgG and C3 at the end-plate in experimental autoimmune myasthenia gravis. J Neuropathol Exp Neurol 1978; 37:212–23.
284. Sahni J, Kaye SB, Fryer A, Hiscott P, Bucknall RC. Distal arthrogryposis Type IIB: unreported ophthalmic findings. Am J Med Genet 2004; 127A:35–9.
285. Sanders DB, Cobb EE, Winfield JB. Neonatal experimental autoimmune myasthenia gravis. Muscle Nerve 1978; 1: 146–50.
286. Sandifer PH. Chronic progressive ophthalmoplegia of myopathic origin. J Neurol Neurosurg Psychiat 1946; 9: 81–3.
287. Sandyk R, Brennan MJW. Isolated ocular myopathy and celiac disease in childhood. Neurology 1983; 33:792.
288. Sarnat HB, McGarry JD, Lewis JE. Effective treatment of infantile myasthenia gravis by combined prednisone and thymectomy. Neurology 1977; 27:550–3.
289. Sautter H. Myotonie und cataracta myotonica. Albrecht von Graefes Arch Ophthalmol 1941; 143:1–26.
290. Scadding GK, Vincent A, Newsom-Davis, J, Henry K. Acetylcholine receptor antibody synthesis by thymic lymphocytes: correlation with thymic histology. Neurology 1981; 31:935–43.
291. Scarlato G, Pellegrini, G, Veicsteinas A. Morphologic and metabolic studies in a case of oculo-cranio-somatic neuromuscular disease. J Neuropathol Exp Neurol 1978; 37:1–12.
292. Scelsi R, Marchetti C, Faggi L, Sandrini G, Rocchelli B. An ocular myopathy with glycogen storage and abnormal mitochondria in muscle fibers: histochemical and ultrastructural findings. Eur Neurol 1981; 20:440–4.
293. Schluep M, Willco N, Vincent A, Dhoot GK, Newsom-Davis J. Acetylcholine receptors in human thymic myoid cells in an immunohistological study. Ann Neurol 1987; 22:212–22.
294. Schmidt D, Kommerell G. Okuläre myasthenie durch D-penicillamin-Behandlung Klin Msbl Augenheilkd 1976; 168:409–13.
295. Schmitt HP, Krause K-H. An autopsy study of a familial oculopharyngeal muscular dystrophy OPMD with distal spread and neurogenic involvement. Muscle Nerve 1981; 4:296–305.
296. Schneck L, Adachi M, Briet P, Wolintz A, Volk BW. Ophthalmoplegia plus with morphological and chemical studies of cerebellar and muscle tissue. J Neurol Sci 1973; 19:37–44.
297. Schochet SS Jr, Zellweger H, Ionasescu V, McCormick WF. Centronuclear myopathy: disease entity or a syndrome? Light and electron-microscopic study of two cases and review of the literature. J Neurol Sci 1972; 16:215–28.
298. Schönbeck S, Chrestal S, Hohlfeld R. Myasthenia gravis: prototype of the antireceptor diseases. Int Rev Neurobiol 1990; 32:175–200.
299. Schotland DL, DiMauro S, Bonilla E, Scarpa A, Lee C-P. Neuromuscular disorder associated with a defect in

mitochondrial energy supply. Arch Neurol 1976; 33: 475–9.

300. Schwartz G-A, Liu C-N. Chronic progressive external ophthalmoplegia, a clinical and neuropathologic report. Arch Neurol Psychiat 1954; 71:31–53.
301. Schwartz O, Jampel RS. Congenital blepharophimosis associated with a unique generalized myopathy. Arch Ophthalmol 1962; 68:82–7.
302. Schwartz R. Some speculations on the origins of autoantibodies. Ann NY Acad Sci 1987; 505:8–11.
303. Schwartz RH. T-lymphocyte recognition of antigen in association with gene products of the major histocompatibility complex. Ann Rev Immunol 1985; 3:237–61.
304. Schwimmbeck PL, Dyrberg T, Drachman DB, Oldstone MBA. Molecular mimicry and myasthenia gravis: an autoantigenic site of the acetylcholine receptor alpha-subunit that has biologic activity and reacts immunochemically with Herpes simplex virus. J Clin Invest 1989; 89:1174–9.
305. Segal BS. The retinopathy of dystrophia myotonia Steinert. Metab Pediat Ophthalmol 1986; 9:585–8.
306. Senita GR, Fisher ER. Progressive dystrophic external ophthalmoplegia following trauma. Arch Ophthalmol 1958; 60:422–6.
307. Shaw DJ, Harper PS. Myotonic dystrophy: developments in molecular genetics. Br Med Bull 1989; 45:745–55.
308. Shy GM, Gonatas NK. Human myopathy with giant abnormal mitochondria. Science 1964; 145:493–6.
309. Shy GM, Silberberg DH, Appel SH, Mishkin M M, Godfrey E H. A generalized disorder of nervous system, skeletal muscle, and heart resembling Refsum's disease and Hurler's syndrome. I. Clinical, pathologic, and biochemical characteristics. Am J Med 1967; 42:163–8.
310. Silex P. Progressive paralysis of the levator. Arch Ophthalmol 1899; 28:430.
311. Simon KA. Diabetes and lens changes in myotonic dystrophy. Arch Ophthalmol 1962; 67:312–5.
312. Simpson JA, Behan PO, Dick HM. Studies on the nature of autoimmunity in myasthenia gravis: evidence for an immunodeficiency type. Ann N Y Acad Sci 1976; 274: 382–9.
313. Sipila I, Simell O, Rapola J, Sainio K, Tuuteri L. Gyrate atrophy of the choroid and retina with hyperornithinemia: tubular aggregates and type 2 fiber atrophy in muscle. Neurology 1979; 29:996–1005.
314. Skeie GO, Romi F, Aarli JA, Bentsen PT, Gilhus NK. Pathogenesis of myositis and myasthenia associated with titin and ryanodine receptor antibodies. Ann N Y Acad Sci 2003; 998:343–50.
315. Slaiman WR, Doyle D, Johnson RH, Jennett S. Myopathy with mitochondrial inclusion bodies: histological and metabolic studies. J Neurol Neurosurg Psychiat 1974; 37: 1236–46.
316. Small RG. Coats' disease and muscular dystrophy. Trans Am Acad Ophthalmol Otolaryngol 1968; 72: 225–31.
317. Smit LME, Veldman H, Jennekens FGI, Molenaar PC, Oen BS. A congenital myasthenic disorder with paucity of secondary synaptic clefts: deficiency and altered distribution of acetylcholine receptors. Ann NY Acad Sci 1987; 505:346–56.
318. Spatz H, Ullrich O. Klinischer und anatomischer Beitrag zu den angeborenen Beweglichkeits-defekten in Hirnnervenbereich. Z Kinderheilkd 1931; 51:579–97.
319. Spencer RF, McNeer K.W. Morphology of the extraocular muscles in relation to the clinical manifestation of strabismus. In: Lennerstrand G, von Noorden GK, Campos EC, eds. Strabismus and Amblyopia. Experimental Basis for Advances in Clinical Management. New York: Plenum Press, 1988:37–41.
320. Spinazzola A, Carrara F, Mora M, Zeviani M. Mitochondrial myopathy and ophthalmoplegia in a sporadic patient with the 5698 G>A mitochondrial DNA mutation. Neuromuscul Disord 2004; 14:815–7.
321. Spiro AJ, Shy GM, Gonatas NK. Myotubular myopathy. Arch Neurol 1966; 14:1–14.
322. Sprofkin BE, Hillman JW. Moebius's syndrome-congenital oculofacial paralysis. Neurology 1956; 6:50–4.
323. Steinert H. Über das Klinische und anatomische Bild des Muskelschwunds der Myotoniker. Dtsch Z Nervenheilkd 1909; 37:59–104.
324. Stern LZ, Cross HE, Crebo AR. Abnormal iris vasculature in myotonic dystrophy. Arch Neurol 1978; 35:224–7.
325. Susac JO, Garcia-Mullin R, Glaser JS. Ophthalmoplegia in dermatomyositis. Neurology 1973; 23:305–10.
326. Swash M, Fox KP. Abnormal intrafusal muscle fibers in myotonic dystrophy: a study using serial sections. J Neurol Neurosurg Psychiat 1975; 38:91–9.
327. Swash M, Fox KP. The fine structure of the spindle abnormality in myotonic dystrophy. Neuropathol Appl Neurobiol 1975; 1:171–87.
328. Swash M, Schwartz MS. Familial multicore disease with focal loss of cross-striations and ophthalmoplegia. J Neurol Sci 1981; 52:1–10.
329. Swash M. The morphology and innervation of the muscle fibers in dystrophia myotonica. Brain 1972; 95: 357–68.
330. Swinyard CA, Mayer V. Multiple congenital contractures. Public health considerations of arthrogryposis multiplex congenita. J Am Med Assoc 1963; 183:23–27.
331. Takeda S, Kondo M, Sasaki J, Kurahashi H, Kano H, Arai K, Misaki K, Fukui T, Kobayashi K, Tachikawa M, Imamura M, Nakamura Y, Shimizue T, Murakami T, Sunada Y, Fujikado T, Matsumrua K, Terashima T, Toda T. Fukutin is required for maintenance of muscle integrity, cortical histiogenesis and normal eye development. Hum Mol Genet 2003; 12:1449–59.
332. Tamuna K, Santa T, Kuroiwa Y. Familial oculocranioskeletal neuromuscular disease with abnormal muscle mitochondria. Brain 1974; 97:665–72.
333. Tanaka N, Nanaka H, Takeda M, Niimura T, Kanehisa T, Terashi S. Cardiomyopathy in myotonic dystrophy: a light and electron microscopic study of the myocardium. Jap Heart J 1973; 14:202–12.
334. Taniguchi K, Kobayashi K, Saito K, Yamanouchi H, Ohnuma A, Hayashi YK, Manya H, Jin DK, Lee M, Parano E, Falsaperia R, Pavone P, Van Coster R, Talim B, Steinbrecher A, Straub V, Nishino I, Topaloglu H, Voit T, Endo T, Toda T. Worldwide distribution and broader clinical spectrum of muscle-eye-brain disease. Hum Mol Genet 2003; 12:527–34.
335. Tarrab-Hazdai R, Aharonov A, Silman I, Fuchs S, Abramsky O. Experimental autoimmune myasthenia induced in monkeys by purified acetylcholine receptor. Nature 1975; 256:128–30.
336. Taylor EW. Progressive vagus-glossopharyngeal paralysis with ptosis: a contribution to the group of family diseases. J Nerv Ment Dis 1915; 42:129–39.
337. Teoh R, McGuire L, Wong K, Chin D. Increased incidence of thymoma in Chinese myasthenia gravis: possible relationship with Epstein-Barr virus. Acta Neurol Scand 1989; 80:221–5.
338. Thanvi BR, Lo TCN. Update on myasthenia gravis. Postgrad Med J 2004; 80:690–700.

339. Thomas NST, Harper PS. Myotonic dystrophy: studies on the lipid composition and metabolism of erythrocytes and skin fibroblasts. Clin Chim Acta 1978; 83:13–23.
340. Thomasen E. Myotonia. In Thomsen's Disease, Paramyotonia Dystrophia Myotonica. A Clinical and Heredobiologic Investigation. Copenhagen: Munksgaard, 1948:121–124, 128–132.
341. Thomson AMP. Dystrophia cordis myotonica studied by serial histology of the pacemaker and conducting system. J Pathol Bacteriol 1968; 96:285–95.
342. Thoriacius S, Aarli JA, Riise T, Matre R, Johnsen HJ. Associated disorders in myasthenia gravis: autoimmune diseases and their relation to thymectomy. Acta Neurol Scand 1989; 80:290–5.
343. Thornell LE, Sjöstrom M, Mattson CH, Heilbronn E. Morphological observations on motor end-plates in rabbits with experimental myasthenia. J Neurol Sci 1976; 29:389–410.
344. Tome FMS, Fardeau M. Ocular myopathies. In Myology, Vol. 2. Engel AG, Banker BQ eds. New York: McGraw-Hill, 1986:1327–47.
345. Toppet M, Telerman-Toppet N, Szliwowski HB, Vainsel M, Coers C. Oculocraniosomatic neuromuscular disease with hypoparathyroidism. Am J Dis Child 1977; 131:437–41.
346. Toyka KV, Drachman DB, Griffin DE, Pestronk A, Winkelstein JA, Fischbeck JH Jr, Kao I. Myasthenia, gravis: study of humoral immune mechanisms by passive transfer to mice. N Engl J Med 1977; 296:125–31.
347. Tramonte JJ, Burns Ted M. Myotonic dystrophy. Arch Neurol. 2005; 62:1316–9.
348. Trelles JP, Gutierrez C, Aranibar A, Palomino L. Estudio anatomoclínico de la enfermedad de Steinert. Riv Neuro-Psiquiat 1956; 19:139–204.
349. Tzartos SJ, Seybold ME, Lindstrom JM. Specificities of antibodies to acetylcholine receptors in sera from myasthenia gravis patients measured by monoclonal antibodies. Proc Natl Acad Sci U S A 1982; 79:188–92.
350. Uemura N, Tanaka H, Niimura T, Hashiguchi H, Yoshimura M, Terushi S, Kenehisa, T. Electrophysiological and histological abnormalities of the heart in myotonic dystrophy. Am Heart J 1973; 96:616–24.
351. Upadhyay K, Thomson A, Luckas MJM. Congenital Myotonic Dystrophy. A case report. Fetal Diag Therapy 2005; 20:512–4.
352. Van Allen MW, Blodi FC. Neurologic aspects of the Möbius syndrome. Neurology 1960; 10:249–59.
353. van der Zwaag B, Verzijl HTFM, Wichers KH, Beltran-Valero de Bernabe, D, Brunner HG, van Bokhoven H, Padberg GW. Sequence analysis of the PLEXIN-D1 gene in Möbius syndrome patients. Ped Neurol 2004; 31:114–8.
354. Van Goethem G, Martin JJ, Van Broeckhoven C. Progressive external ophthalmoplegia characterized by multiple deletions of mitochondrial DNA: unraveling the pathogenesis of human mitochondrial DNA instability and the limitation of a genetic classification. Neuromuscul Med 2003; 3:129–46.
355. Van Reeuwijk J, Brunner HG, van Bokhoven H. Glyc-O-genetics of Walker-Warburg syndrome. Clin Genet 2004; 67: 189–281.
356. Vassilopoulos D, Alevizos B, Spengos M. Cataract and y-glutamyl cycle in myotonic dystrophy. Ophthalmologica 1976; 174:167–9.
357. Vicart P, Caron A, Guicheney P, Li Z, Prévost M-C, Faure A, Chateau D, Chapon F, Tomé F, Dupret J-P, Paulin D, Fardeau M. A missense mutation in the αB-crystallin chaperone gene causes a desmin-related myopathy. Nat Genet 1998; 20:92–95.
358. Vincent A, Rothwell P. Myasthenia gravis. Autoimmunity 2004; 37:317–9.
359. Vincent A, Thomas HC, Scadding GK, Newsom-Davis J. *In vitro* synthesis of anti-acetylcholine receptor antibody by thymic lymphocytes in myasthenia gravis. Lancet 1978; 1:305–7.
360. Vogel R M, Lee RV. Bilateral ptosis in Wernicke's disease. Neurology 1967; 17:85–6.
361. Vogt A. Die Cataract bei myotonischer Dystrophie. Schweiz Med Wochenschr 1921; 51:669–74.
362. Von Graefe A. Diagnostic der Augen muskellähmungen, §42 In Graefe A, Saemisch T eds. Handbuch der gesammten Augenheilkunde, Vol. 6, Engelmann: Leipzig, 1880:59–61.
363. Von Graefe A. Notizen vermischten lnhalts. Arch Ophthalmol 1856; 2:299–329.
364. Von Graefe A. VI. Verhandlungen ärzlicher Gesellschaften. Berl Klin Wochenschr 1868; 5:126–7.
365. Vos TA. 25 years dystrophia myotonica (D.M.). Ophthalmologica 1961; 141:37–44.
366. Wagner E. Fall einer seltnen Muskel krankheit. Arch Heilk Lpz 1863; 4:282–3.
367. Walker SP, Brubaker RF, Magataki S. Hypotony and aqueous humor dynamics in myotonic dystrophy. Invest Ophthalmol VisSci 1982; 22:744–51.
368. Walton JN, Irving D, Tomlinson BE. Spinal cord limb motor neurons in dystrophia myotonica. J Neurol Sci 1977; 34:199–211.
369. Wartenberg R. Winking-jaw phenomenon. Arch Neurol Psychiat 1948; 59:734–53.
370. Weinberg CB, Hall ZW. Antibodies from patients with myasthenia gravis recognize determinants unique to extrajunctional acetylcholine receptors. Proc Natl Acad Sci USA 1979; 76:504–8.
371. Willcox HNA, Newsom-Davis J, Calder LR Cell types required for anti-acetylcholine receptor antibody synthesis by cultured thymocytes and blood lymphocytes in myasthenia gravis. Clin Exp Immunol 1984; 58:97–106.
372. Winer N, Klachko DM, Baer RD, Langley PL, Burns TW. Myotonic response induced by inhibitors of cholesterol biosynthesis. Science 1966; 153:312–3.
373. Winfield J. Juvenile dermatomyositis with complications. Proc R Soc Med 1977; 70:548–51.
374. Wohlfart G. Dystrophia myotonica and myotonica congenita, histopathologic studies with special reference to changes in the muscles. J Neuropathol Exp Neurol 1951; 10:109–24.
375. Wolter JR, Hoy JE, Schmidt DM. Chronic orbital myositis, its diagnostic difficulties and pathology. Am J Ophthalmol 1966; 62:292–8.
376. Yong SL, Lowry RB, Jan JE. Syndrome of myopathy, short stature, seizures, retinitis pigmentosa, and cleft lip. Birth Defect 1977; 13:210–5.
377. Yoshida A, Kobayashi K, Manya H, Taniguchi K, Kano H, Mizuno M, Inazu T, Mitsuhashi H, Takahshi S, Takeuchi M, Herrmann R, Straub V, Talim B, Voit T, Topaloglu H, Toda T, Endo T. Muscular dystrophy and neuronal migration disorder caused by mutations in a glycosyltransferase, POMGnT1. DevelopCell 2001; 1: 717–24.
378. Yotova V, Labuday D, Zietkiewicz E, Gehl D, Lovell A, Lefebvre J-F, Bourgeois S, Lemieux-Blanchard É, Labuda M, Vézina H, Houde L, Tremblay M, Toupance B, Heyer E,

Hudson TJ, Laberge C. Anatomy of a founder effect: myotonic dystrophy in Northeastern Quebec. Hum Genet 2005; 117:177–87
379. Yu Wai Man CY, Chinnery PF, Griffiths PG. Extraocular muscles have fundamentally distinct properties that make them selectively vulnerable to certain disorders. Neuromuscul Dis 2005; 15:17–23.
380. Zacks S. The Motor Endplate. Huntington, N.Y.: Krieger, 1973:363–366.
381. Zhou L, McConville J, Chaudhry V, Adams R, Skolasky RL, Vincent A, Drachman DB. Clinical comparison of muscle-specific tyrosine kinase (MuSK) antibody-positive and –negative myasthenic patients. Muscle Nerve 2004; 30:55–60.
382. Zintz R, Villiger W. Elektronmikroskopische befunde bei 3 Fällen von chronisch progressive okulärer Muskeldystrophie. Ophthalmologica 1967; 153:439–59.
383. Zoltowska A. Myoid and epithelial cell differentiation in myasthenic thymuses. Thymus 1991; 17:237–48.

Abbreviations

when used as a prefix with a Mendelian Inheritance in Man (MIM number) it indicates a descriptive entry and not a unique locus

+ when used as a prefix with a Mendelian Inheritance in Man (MIM number) it indicates that the entry contains a description of known sequence and a phenotype

% when used as a prefix with a Mendelian Inheritance in Man (MIM number) it indicates that the entry describes a confirmed mendelian phenotype or phenotypic locus for which the underlying molecular basis is not known

***** when used as a prefix with a Mendelian Inheritance in Man (MIM number) it indicates a gene of known sequence

αβ T-cell a subset of T cells with a distinct T cell receptor on their surface with one α cahin and one β

γδ T-cell a subset of T cells with a distinct T cell receptor on their surface with one γ chain and one δ

α-MSH α-melanocyte-stimulating hormone

α-SYN α-synuclein

A adenine and anisotropic

Aβ amyloid beta

A2B5 a type 2 astrocyte precursor marker

A2E a vitamin A-based fluorophore in lipofuscin

A3AR the gene for adenosine receptor A3

AA amyloid protein A, apparent anisotrophy

AANF atrial natriuric factor

AApoAI apolipoprotein AI derived amyloid

AApoAII apolipoprotein AII derived amyloid

AApoAIV apolipoprotein AIV derived amyloid

AASS a gene on chromosome 7 (7q31.3) that codes for α-aminoadipic semialdehyde synthase

AASV ANCA-associated vasculitides

AAV adeno-associated virus

Aβ Aβ protein precursor

Aβ_2M β_2-microglobulin derived protein

ABCA4 the ATP-binding cassette transporter retinal gene on chromosome 1 (1p22.1–p21) (also known as *ABCR*, *RP19*, and *STGD1*)

Abca4 the murine ATP-binding cassette transporter retinal gene

ABCA7 adenosine triphoshate binding cassette protein A7

ABCC6 a gene on chromosome 16 (16p13.1) that causes pseudoxanthoma elasticum when mutated

ABCD1 the gene for ATP-binding cassette subfamily D member 1 on the X chromosome (Xq28)

ABCG5 the ATP-binding cassette subfamily G member 5 gene on chromosome 2 (2p21)

ABCG8 a ATP-binding cassette subfamily G member 8 gene on chromosome 2 (2p21)

ABCR ATP-binding cassette transporter

ABCR the ATP-binding cassette gene on chromosome 1 (1p21–p13) (also known as *ABCA4*, *RP19*, and *STGD1*)

AC anterior chamber

ACA anticentromere antibody

ACAID anterior chamber associated immune deviation

ACal calcitonin derived amyloid

ACE angiotensin-converting enzyme

ACE gene for angiotensin-converting enzyme on chromosome 17 (17q23)

ACL **A**cromegaloid features, **C**utis verticis gyrata and **L**eukoma syndrome

ACR acetylcholine receptor and American College of Rheumatology

ACTA1 the α-actin sketetal muscle gene on chromosome 1 (1q42.1)

ACTA2 the α-2 actin smooth muscle gene on chromosome 10 (10q22–q24)

ACTB the β-actin gene on chromosome 7 (7p22–p12)

ACTC the α-actin cardiac muscle gene on chromosome 15 (15q14) (also known as *ACTC1)*

ACTG1 the γ-1 actin gene on chromosome 17 (17q25.3)

ACTG2 the γ-2 actin gene on chromosome 2 (2p13.1)

ACTH adrenocorticotrophin

ACys cystatin C derived amyloid

AD autosomal dominant, Alzheimer disease

AD1 an autosomal dominant familial type of Alzheimer disease

AD2 a type of Alzheimer disease associated with the APOE*4 allele on chromosome 19

AD3 a type of Alzheimer disease caused by *PSEN1* mutations

AD4 a type of Alzheimer disease caused by *PSEN2* mutations

Ad5E1 early region 1 of human adenovirus type 5

Ad5E1A early region 1A of human adenovirus type 5

ADAID anterior chamber associated immune deviation

ADAMTS10 the gene on chromosome 19 (19p13.3–p13.2) that codes for a disintegrin-like and metalloproteinase with thrombospondin type 1 motif

ADC apparent diffusion coefficient

ADCC antibody-dependent cell mediated cytotoxicity

adCOD autosomal dominant cone dystrophy

adCORD autosomal dominant cone-rod dystrophy

adCSNB autosomal dominant congenital stationary night blindness

ADEN acute disseminated epidermal necrosis

ADH aldehyde dehydrogenase

ADM2 adrenomodulin 2; also known as intermedin

adMD autosomal dominant macular dystrophy

ADOA autosomal dominant optic atrophy

ADP adenosine diphosphate

ADR adverse drug reaction
adRP autosomal dominant retinitis pigmentosa
ADTB3A the gene on chromosome 5 (5q14.1) that causes Hermansky–Pudlak syndrome type 2 when mutated (also known as *HPS1* and *AP3B1)*
ADVIRC **A**utosomal **D**ominant **Vi**treo **R**etino **C**horoidopathy
AEC ankyloblepharon-ectodermal dysplasia-cleft lip/palate
AEF amyloid enhancing factor
AEI/AE3 a pancytokeratin antibody
aFGF acidic fibroblast growth factor
AFib fibrinogen α-chain derived amyloid
AGA the aspartlglycosaminidase gene on chromosome 4 (4q32–q33)
AGC1 the aggregan gene on chromosome 15 (15q26.1)
AGE advanced glycation end-product
AGel gelsolin derived amyloid
AgKS antigenic keratan sulfate
AGL the glycogen debranching enzyme gene on chromosome 1 (1p21)
AGRN the tenascin gene on chromosome 1 (1pter–p32)
AH gamma globulin heavy chain derived amyloid
AHC acute hemorrhagic conjunctivitis
AIAPP islet amyloid polypeptide derived amyloid
AIDS acquired immune deficiency syndrome
AIF apoptosis inducing factor
AIMP2B intergral membrane protein derived amyloid
AIns insulin derived amyloid
AIPL1 the arylhydrocarbon-interacting receptor protein-like 1 gene on chromosome 17 (17p13.1) (also known as *LCA4*)
AKC acute keratoconjunctivitis
AKAP2 the gene for A-kinase anchor protein 2 on chromosome 9 (9q31–q33)
AKAP2 A-kinase anchor protein 2
AKer kerato-epithelin (transforming growth factor beta induced protein) derived amyloid
AKT a protein kinase product of an oncogene
AKT1 an oncogene on chromosome 14 (14q32.3)
AL amyloid protein L (amyloid light chain protein)
Ala alanine
ALac lactoferrin derived amyloid
ALCL anaplastic large cell lymphoma
ALDH aldehyde dehydrogenase
ALDH1A1 aldehyde dehydrogenase family 1 , subfamily A, member 1
ALDH3A1 aldehyde dehydrogenase family 3 , subfamily A, member 1
ALDOA the fructose 1,6-biphosphate aldolase A gene on chromosome 16 (16q22–q24)
ALK anterior lamellar keratectomy
ALL acute lymphoblastic leukemia
ALSG aplasia of the lacrimal and salivary glands
ALV avian leukosis virus
ALys lysozyme derived amyloid
AMD age-related macular degeneration
AMed medin amyloid (lactadherin derived amyloid)
AMP adenosine monophosphate
AMS ablepharon–macrostomia syndrome
An adult nucleus of crystalline lens
ANA antinuclear antibodies
ANCA anti-neutrophil cytoplasmic antibody
ANCL adult neuronal ceroid-lipofuscinosis
ANG1 angiopoetin-1
ANG2 angiopoetin-2
Ank the mouse gene for progressive ankylosis
ANKH a gene on chromosome 5 (5q15.2–p14.1) that is a homolog of the murine *Ank* gene
ANS 8-anilino-l-naphthalenesulfonate
ANT adenine translocator, adenosine nucleotide translocator (also known as ADP/ATP translocator)
Anti-CCP anti-cyclic citrullinated peptide
Anti-La an antibody to SS-B
Anti-Ro an antibody to SS-A
ANVOs abortive neovascular outgrowths
Anx1 annexin 1
AP amyloid p-component
AP sites apurinic/pyrimidinic sites
Apaf-1 apoptotic protease activating factor 1
AP3B1 the gene on chromosome 5 (5q14.1) that causes Hermansky–Pudlak syndrome type 2 when mutated (also known as *HPS2* and *ADTB3A)*
APC antigen presenting cell; adenomatous polyposis coli; and the encoded product of the *APC* gene
APC the gene responsible for adenomatous polyposis coli
APECED **A**utoimmune, **P**oly**E**ndocrinopathy, **C**andidiasis, and **E**ctodermal dystrophy
aPL anti-phospholipid
APO1 cell surface death receptor 2 (also known as CD95)
APO2 death receptor 4 (DR4) (also known as tumor necrosis factor related apoptosis-inducing ligand receptor 1[TRAILR1])
APO2L tumor necrosis factor-related apoptosis inducing ligand (TRAIL)
APO3 death receptor 3 (DR3) (also known as LARD, TRAMP and WSL1)
apoA apolipoprotein A
APOA1 the gene for apolipoprotein AI on chromosome 11 (11q23)
APOA2 the gene for apolipoprotein AII on chromosome 1 (1q21–q23)
APOA4 the gene for apolipoprotein AIV on chromosome 11 (11q23)
apoB apolipoprotein B
APOB the gene for apolipoprotein B on chromosome 2 (2p24–p23)
APOD the gene for apolipoprotein D on chromosome 3 (3q26.2–qter)
apoE apolipoprotein E
APOE the gene for apolipoprotein E on chromosome 19 (19q13.2)
APP a amyloid precursor protein gene on chromosome 21 (21q)
APro prolactin derived amyloid
APrP prion protein derived amyloid
APS antiphospholipid syndrome
APUD cells **A**mine **P**recursor **U**ptake and **D**ecarboxylation cells
AqH aqueous humor
AQP aquaporin
AQP0 aquaporin 0

AR autosomal recessive or aldose reductase
ARA American Rheumatism Association (a former name for the American College of Rheumatology)
ARAT retinal acyltransferase
arCOD autosomal recessive cone dystrophy
arCORD autosomal recessive cone-rod dystrophy
AREDS age-related eye disease study
AREDSII age-related eye disease study II
Arf the murine gene for a protein that stabilizes p53
ARF cyclin-dependent kinase inhibitor 2A (also known as p14)
Arg arginine
ARIX a homolog of the Drosophila aristaless homeobox gene on chromosome 11 (11q13.3–q13.4)
arLCA autosomal recessive Leber congenital amaurosis
ARN acute retinal necrosis
arRP autosomal recessive retinitis pigmentosa
ARS Axenfeld–Rieger syndrome
ARSA the arylsulfatase A gene on chromosome 22 (22q13.31)
ARSB the arylsulfatase B gene on chromosome 5 (5q11–q13)
AS ankylosing spondylitis
ASA the reduced form of ascorbic acid and arylsulfatase A
ASAH the ceramidase gene on chromosome 8 (8p22–p21.3)
ASD anterior segment dysgenesis
Ash a murine gene that is expressed in retinal progenitor cells
ASM acid sphingomyelinase
ASMD anterior segment mesenchymal dysgenesis
Asn asparagine
Asp aspartate
ASPA the aspartocyclase gene on chromosome 17 (17pter–p13)
ASPN the asporin gene on chromosome 9 (9q21.3–q22)
AT ataxia telangiectasia
Ath3 a murine gene that is expressed in retinal progenitor cells
Ath5 a murine gene that is expressed in retinal progenitor cells
ATM the gene on chromosome 11 (11q22.3) that causes ataxia-telangiectasia when mutated
ATP adenosine triphosphate
ATP7A a copper transport P-type adenosine triphosphatase gene on the X chromosome (Xq13)
ATP7B a copper transport P-type adenosine triphosphatase gene on chromosome 13 (13q14.3)
ATPase adenosine triphosphatase
ATTR transthyretin derived amyloid
ATV acute transforming viruses
AUG the codon for methionine
AVM arteriovenous malformation

B2M the β_2-microglobulin gene on chromosome 15 (15q21–q22)
b-HLH-Zip a family of transcription factors that bind to DNA as dimers
β2GP1 β2 glycoprotein 1
βTG β-thromboglobulin
B7 family a group of immunoadjuvant molecules
BAD/Bad BCL2 antagonist of cell death
BAER brainstem evoked response
BALT bronchus associated lymphoid tissue
Bax BCL2-associated X protein
Bak BCL2 antagonist killer 1, also known as BAK1, BCL2L7
BAK benzalkonium chloride
BB an airgun with a smooth bore barrel
BCC basal cell carcinoma
B cell B lymphocyte
BCD Bietti crystalline dystrophy
BCG Bacillus Calmette-Guérin
BCL-1 cyclin D1 (also known as PRAD1)
Bcl-2 an anti-apoptotic factor (also known as B-cell lymphoma 27
Bcl-3 oncogene B-cell lymphoma 3 (formerly Bcl-4)
Bcl-XL a regulator of apoptosis found in mitochondrial membranes
Bcl-w a member of the bcl-2 family
BCL2 the Bcl-2 gene on chromosome 18 (18q21.3)
BCNU bis (chloroethyl) -1-nitrosourea
BCOR the BCL6 corepressor gene on the X chromosome (Xp11.4)
BCR/ABL a fusion gene at the breakpoint cluster region on chromosome 22 (22q11.27)
BCS brittle cornea syndrome
BCSH a gene that codes a component of the mitochondrial respiratory chain complex III
BD Behçet disease
BDNF brain-derived neurotrophic factor
BDUMP bilateral diffuse uveal melanocytic proliferation
BE receptors binding apo-E lipoprotein
BED Bornholm eye disease
bFGF basic fibroblast growth factor (also known as FGF2)
BFP biologic false-positive
BGN the biglycan gene on the X chromosome (Xq28)
BH domains a fragment of the Rho family (RhoGAPS) with guanosine triphoshate hydrolase activity
bHLH basic helix–loop–helix
bHLHZip basic-helix–loop/leucine zipper
Bid/BID BH3-interacting domain death agonist
BIGH3 a former abbreviation for the *TGFBI* gene
BIM/Bim a portion of the Bcl-2 family produced by the *BIM* gene
BIR baculoviral inhibitor of apoptosis (IAP) repeats
BIR2 the second domain of baculoviral inhibitor of apoptosis repeat
BIR3 the third domain of baculoviral inhibitor of apoptosis repeat
BKV a human polyomavirus
BLD basal laminar deposit (basal linear deposit)
BLOC1S3 the gene on chromosome 19 (19q13) that causes Hermansky–Pudlak syndrome type 8 when mutated
bp base pairs
BMI body mass index
BMPR1A the gene for bone morphogenetic protein receptor type IA on chromosome 10 (10q22.3)
BMPR2 the bone morphogenetic protein receptor type II gene on chromosome 2 (2q33)
BMT bone marrow transplantation

Bok a BCL2 related protein involved in apoptosis
BP benzo(a)pyrene, blood pressure
BPAG1 bullous pemphigoid antigen 1
BPES blepharophimosis-ptosis-epicanthus inversus syndrome
BRCA1 breast cancer 1 gene on chromosome 17 (17q21)
BRCA1 the growth inhibitory factor secreted by breast epithelium that is encoded by the *BRCA1* gene
BRCA2 breast cancer 2 gene on chromosome 13 (13q12.3)
Brn3b a murine gene for a transcription factor needed for retinal ganglion cell differentiation
Brn3b a murine transcription factor needed for retinal ganglion cell differentiation
BRUCE baculoviral inhibitor of apoptosis (BIR) repeat containing ubiquitin-conjugating enzyme
BSA bovine serum albumin
BSE bovine spongioform encephalopathy (also known as "mad cow disease")
bZIP basic region leucine zipper

c crystalline lens cortex
C cytosine
C1 first component of complement
C1q q subfraction of first component of complement
C1r r subfraction of first component of complement
C1s s subfraction of first component of complement
C2 second component of complement
C2a a fragment of second component of complement
C2b b fragment of second component of complement
C3 third component of complement
C3a a fragment of third component of complement
C3b b fragment of third component of complement
C3d d fragment of third component of complement
C4 fourth component of complement
C4b b fragment of fourth component of complement
C4S chondroitin-4-sulfate
C5 fifth component of complement
C5a a fragment of fifth component of complement
C5b b fragment of fifth component of complement
C5b67 complex of C5b with C6 and C7
C6 sixth component of complement
C6S chondroitin-6-sulfate
C7 seventh component of complement
C8 eighth component of complement
C9 ninth component of complement
Ca^{2+} calcium ions
Ca^{2+}-stimulated ATPase calcium stimulated adenosine triphosphatase
CA cytosine-adenine dinucleotide
CA15.3 cancer antigen 15.3 (an ocofetal antigen)
CA4 the carbonic anhydrase IV gene on chromosome 17 (17q23.2) (also known as *RP17*)
CACNA1F the calcium channel-voltge dependent alpha-IF subunit on the X chromosome (Xp11.23) (also known as *CSNB2*)
CaGC calgranulin C
CAK chronic actinic keratopathy
CALCA the (pro)calcitonin gene on chromosome 11 (11p15.2–p15)
CALLA common acute lymphoblastic antigen
CALT conjunctiva associated lymphoid tissue
CAM 5.2 an antibody that recognizes low molecular weight cytokeratin
CAMAK **C**ataract, **M**icrocephaly, **A**rthrogryposis and **K**yphosis
CAMFAK **C**ataract, **M**icrocephaly, **F**ailure to thrive, **A**rthrogryposis and **K**yphosis
cAMP cyclic adenosine monophosphate
CAM cell adhesion molecule
CAM5.2 a pancytokeratin antibody
cANCA cytoplasmic staining anti-neutrophil cytoplasmic antibody
Cap capsule
CAR cancer-associated retinopathy
CARD caspase recruitment domain
CASR a gene on chromosome 3 (3q13.3–q21) that codes for an extracellular calcium-sensing receptor
CATT cytosine-adenine-thymine-thymine
CBH cutaneous basophil hypersensitivity
CBS the cystathionine beta-synthase gene on chromosome 21 (21q22.3)
CCP cyclic citrullinated peptide
CCR2 the chemokine CC motif receptor 2 gene on chromosome 3 (3p21)
CCR3 the chemokine CC motif receptor 3
CCR4 the chemokine CC motif receptor 4
CCR5 the chemokine CC motif receptor 5 gene on chromosome 3 (3p21)
CCRG cooperative cataract research group
CCS Churg Strauss syndrome
CD cluster of differentiation antigen
CD4 marker for helper T lymphocytes
CD8 marker for suppressor T lymphocytes
CD11b receptor for C3bi (also known as CR3, Mac-1 antigen)
CD11c receptor for C3bi and C3dg (also known as CR4)
CD14 monocyte differentiation antigen (also known as myeloid cell-specific leucine-rich glycoprotein)
CD18 a leucocyte cell adhesion molecule (also known as integrin-beta 2)
CD19 CD19 B lymphocyte antigen
CD19 the gene on chromosome 16(16p11.2) for the CD19 B lymphocyte antigen
Cd21 receptor for C3d (also known as CR2)
CD25 interleukin 2 receptor alpha (also known as TAC antigen)
CD26 a T-cell activation antigen (also known as adenosine deaminase complexing protein 2)
CD31 platelet-endothelial cell adhesion molecule 1; a vascular emdothelial cell marker
CD34 hematopoietic progenitor cell antigen; a vascular emdothelial cell marker
CD35 receptor for C3b (also known as CR1)
CD36 leukocyte differentiation antigen
CD40 an immunoadjuvant molecule
CD46 membrane cofactor protein; the measles virus receptor

CD55 decay-accelerating factor for complement (also known as Cromer blood group)
CD59 protectin (also known as human leukocyte antigen MIC11)
CD62 also known as GMP-140 and granule membrane protein
CD68 a macrophage antigen (also known as macrosialin)
CD80 an immunoadjuvant molecule
CD86 an immunoadjuvant molecule
CD91 low density lipoprotein receptor-related protein 1 (also known as apolipoprotein receptor)
CD95 FAS (also known as aopotosis antigen 1 and FAS antigen)
CD99 surface antigen MIC2
CD117 stem cell factor receptor (also known as c-kit)
CDB corneal dystrophy of Bowman layer and the superficial stroma
CDC Centers for Disease Control and Prevention
Cdc27 cell division cycle 27 homolog
CDH11 the cadherin 11 gene on chromosome on 17 (17q21–q22.1))
CDH23 the cadherin 23 gene on chromosome on 10 (10q22)
Cdk cyclin-dependent kinase
CDK climatic droplet keratopathy
CDK4 cyclin-dependent kinase 4
CDKN2A the cyclin-dependent kinase inhibitor 2A gene on chromosome 9 (9p21)
cDNA complimentary deoxyribonucleic acid
CDP cytidine diphosphate
CEA carcinoembryonic antigen
CERKL the ceramide kinase-like protein gene on chromosome 2 (2q31.3) (also known as *RP26*)
CETP cholesterol ester transfer protein
CEV cell-associated virus
CF complement fixation
CFEOM congenital fibrosis of the extraocular muscles
CFEOM1 congenital fibrosis of the extraocular muscles type 1
CFEOM2 congenital fibrosis of the extraocular muscles type 2
CFH complement factor H
CFH the gene for complement factor H on chromosome 1 (1q32)
CG cytosine-guanine dinucleotide
cGMP cyclic guanosine monophosphate
CGRP calcitonin gene-related peptide
CHARGE association coloboma, heart defects, choanal atresia, mental retardation, genitourinary defects, and ear anomalies
CHED congenital hereditary endothelial dystrophy
CHED1 congenital hereditary endothelial dystrophy type 1
CHED2 congenital hereditary endothelial dystrophy type 2
CHIP 28 aquaporin 1 (also known as aquaporin-CHIP)
CHM choroideremia
CHRNA1 the gene for the α subunit of the acetylcholine receptor on chromosome 2 (2q24–q32)
CHRNB1 the gene for the β subunit of the acetylcholine receptor on chromosome 17 (17p12–p11)
CHRND the gene for the δ subunit of the acetylcholine receptor chromosome 2 (2q33–q34)
CHRND1 the gene for the δ subunit of the acetylcholine receptor on chromosome 2 (2q33–q34)
CHRNE the gene for the ε subunit of the acetylcholine receptor on chromosome 17 (17p13–p12)
CHRNE1 the gene for the ε subunit of the acetylcholine receptor on chromosome 17 (17p13–p12)
CHRPE congenital hypertrophy of the retinal pigment epithelium
CHS1 the gene on chromosome 1 (1q34) that causes Chédiak–Higashi syndrome when mutated
CHST5 the carbohydrate sulfotransferase 5 gene on chromosome 16 (16q22)
CHST6 the carbohydrate sulfotransferase 6 gene on chromosome 16 (16q22)
CHX10 a gene that is abundantly expressed in the retina (also known as the homeobox 10 gene)
C-Fos a proto-oncogene involved in cellular proliferation
c-IAP2 an inhibitor of apoptosis
CIAS1 the gene on chromosome 1 (1q44) that is mutated in familial cold hypersensitivity and the Muckel–Wells syndrome
c-Jun a proto-oncogene
CIN conjunctival intraepithelial neoplasm
CI-MPR cation-independent mannose-phosphate receptor
CJD Creutzfeldt-Jakob disease
Ckd4 cyclin-dependent kinases 4
CLDN19 the claudin 12gene on chromosome 1 (1p34.2)
CLL chronic lymphocytic leukemia
CLN ceroid lipofuscinosis, neuronal
CLN1 ceroid lipofuscinosis, neuronal type 1 (also known as infantile neuronal ceroid lipofuscinosis)
CLN1 the palmitoyl-protein thioesterase-1 gene on chromosome 1 (1p32)
CLN2 ceroid lipofuscinosis, neuronal type 2 (also known as late infantile neuronal ceroid lipofuscinosis)
CLN2 the gene on chromosome 11 (11p15.5) that is responsible for ceroid lipofuscinosis, neuronal type 2
CLN3 ceroid lipofuscinosis, neuronal type 3; also known as juvenile neuronal ceroid lipofuscinosis
CLN3 the gene on chromosome 16 (16p12.1) that is responsible for ceroid lipofuscinosis, neuronal type 3
CLN4 ceroid lipofuscinosis, neuronal type 4 (also known as adult neuronal ceroid lipofuscinosis)
CLN5 ceroid lipofuscinosis, neuronal type 5 (also known as variant late infantile neuronal ceroid lipofuscinosis)
CLN5 the gene on chromosme 13 (13q21.1–q32) that is responsible for ceroid lipofuscinosis, neuronal type 5
CLN6 ceroid lipofuscinosis, neuronal type 6 (also known as variant late infantile neuronal ceroid lipofuscinosis)
CLN6 the gene on chromosome 15 (15q21–q23) that is responsible for ceroid lipofuscinosis, neuronal type 6
CLN7 ceroid lipofuscinosis, neuronal type 7
CLN8 ceroid lipofuscinosis, neuronal type 8 (also known as Turkish variant late infantile neuronal ceroid lipofuscinosis)
CLN8 the gene on chromosome 8 (8pter–p22) that is responsible for ceroid lipofuscinosis, neuronal type 8
CLN9 ceroid lipofuscinosis, neuronal type 9

CLU gene for clusterin on chromosome 8 (8p21–p12)
cm centimeter
cM centimorgan
CME cystoid macular edema
CMV cytomegalovirus
CNBr cyanogen bromide
CNCG the gene on chromosome 4 (4p12) that codes for the alpha subunit of the rod cyclic guanosine monophosphate-gated channel (also known as *CNGA1 and CNCG1*)
CNCG1 the gene on chromosome 4 (4p12) that codes for the alpha subunit of the rod cyclic guanosine monophosphate-gated channel (also known as *CNCG and CNGA1*)
CNGA cyclic nucleotide-gated channel
CNGA1 the gene on chromosome 4 (4p12) that codes for the alpha subunit of the rod cyclic guanosine monophosphate-gated channel (also known as *CNCG and CNCG1*)
CNGA3 the cyclic nucleotide-gated channel alpha-3 gene on chromosome 2 (2q11.2)
CNGB3 the cyclic nucleotide-gated channel beta-3 gene on chromosome 8 (8q21–q22)
CNS central nervous system
CNV choroidal neovascularization
CO2 carbon dioxide
CoA coenzyme A
CO-Ag a cornea associated antigen (also known as corneal calgranulin C)
COI a mitochondrial DNA cytochrome c oxidase subunit I gene of respiratory Complex IV (also known as *MTCO1*)
COII a mitochondrial DNA cytochrome c oxidase subunit II gene of respiratory Complex IV (also known as *MTCO2*)
COIII a mitochondrial DNA cytochrome c oxidase subunit III gene of respiratory Complex IV (also known as *MTCO3*)
COD cone dystrophy
COD1 the gene on the X chromosome (Xp11.4) for retinitis pigmentosa guanosine triphosphate hydrolase regulator (also known as *RP3, CORDX and RPGR*)
COD2 a locus for cone dystrophy on the X chromosome (Xq27)
COD3 the gene for guanylate cyclase activator 1A on chromosome 6 (6p21.1) (also known as *GUCA1A* and *GCAP1*)
COD4 a locus for cone and cone-rod dystrophy on the X chromosome(Xq11–q13.1)
COG Children's Oncology Group
COL1A1 the collagen type 1 alpha-1 gene on chromosome 17 (17q21.31–q22)
COL2A1 the collagen type II alpha-1 polypeptide gene on chromosome 7 (7q22.1)
COL3A1 the collagen type III alpha-1 polypeptide gene on chromosome 2 (2q31)
COL4A1 the collagen type IV alpha-1 polypeptide gene on chromosome 13 (13q34)
COL4A2 the collagen type IV alpha-2 polypeptide gene on chromosome 13 (13q34)
COL4A3 the collagen type IV alpha-3 polypeptide gene on chromosome 2 (2q36–q37)
COL4A4 the collagen type IV alpha-4 polypeptide gene on chromosome 2 (2q36–q37)
COL4A5 the collagen type IV alpha-5 polypeptide gene on the X chromosome(Xp22.3)
COL4A6 the collagen type IV alpha-6 polypeptide gene on the X chromosome(Xp22.3)
Col5a1 the murine collagen type V alpha-1 polypeptide gene
COL5A1 the collagen type V alpha-1 polypeptide gene on chromosome 9 (9q34.2–q34.3)
COL5A2 the collagen type V alpha-2 polypeptide gene on chromosome 2 (2q31)
COL5A3 the collagen type V alpha-3 polypeptide gene on chromosome 19 (19p13.2)
COL6A1 the collagen type VI alpha-1 polypeptide gene on chromosome 21(21q22.3)
COL6A2 the collagen type VI alpha-2 polypeptide gene on chromosome 21(21q22.3)
COL6A3 the collagen type VI alpha-3 polypeptide gene on chromosome 2 (2q37)
COL7A1 the collagen type VII alpha-1 polypeptide gene on chromosome 3 (3p21.3)
COL8A1 the collagen type VIII alpha-1 polypeptide gene on chromosome 3 (3q12–q13)
COL8A2 the collagen type VIII alpha-2 polypeptide gene on chromosome 1 (1p34.3–p32.3)
Col8a1 the murine collagen type 8 alpha-1 polypeptide gene
Col8a2 the murine gene for collagen type 8 alpha-2 polypeptide
COL9A1 the collagen type IX alpha-1 polypeptide gene on chromosome 6 (6q13)
COL9A2 the collagen type IX alpha-2 polypeptide gene on chromosome 1 (1p33–p32.2)
COL10A1 the collagen type X alpha-1 polypeptide gene on chromosome 6 (6q21–q22.3)
COL11A1 a collagen type XI alpha-1 polypeptide gene on chromosome 1 (1p21)
COL11A2 a collagen type XI alpha-2 polypeptide gene on chromosome 6 (6p21.3)
COL12A1 a collagen type XII alpha-1 polypeptide gene on chromosome 6 (6q12–q13)
COL13A1 the collagen type XIII alpha-1 polypeptide human gene on chromosome 10 (10q22)
COL14A1 a collagen type XIV alpha-1 polypeptide gene on chromosome 8 (8q23)
COL15A1 a collagen type XV alpha-1 polypeptide gene on chromosome 9 (9q21–q22)
COL16A1 a collagen type XVI alpha-1 polypeptide gene on chromosome 1 (1p34)
COL17A1 a collagen type XVII alpha-1 polypeptide gene on chromosome 10 (10q24.3)
COL18A1 a collagen type XVIII alpha-1 polypeptide gene on chromosome 21 (21q22.3)
COL19A1 a collagen type XIX alpha-1 polypeptide gene on chromosome 6 (6q12–q14)
COL20A1 a collagen type XX alpha-1 polypeptide gene on chromosome 20 (20q13.33)

COL21A1 a collagen type XXI alpha-1 polypeptide gene on chromosome 6 (6p12.3–11.2)
COL22A1 a collagen type XXII alpha-1 polypeptide gene on chromosome 8 (8q24.3)
COL23A1 a collagen type XXIII alpha-1 polypeptide gene on chromosome 5 (5q35)
COL24A1 the collagen type XXIV alpha-1 polypeptide gene on chromosome 1 (1p22.3)
COL25A1 a collagen type XXV alpha-1 polypeptide gene on chromosome 4 (4q25)
COL26A1 the collagen type XXVI alpha-1 polypeptide gene on chromosome 7 (7q22.1)
COL27A1 the collagen type XXVII alpha-1 polypeptide gene on chromosome 9 (9q32)
COL28A1 the collagen type XXVIII alpha-1 polypeptide gene on chromosome 7 (7p21.3)
COMP cartilage oligomeric matrix protein
COMS Collaborative Ocular Melanoma Study
ConA concanavalin-A
CORD cone-rod dystrophy
CORD2 the gene on chromosome 19 (19q13.3) that codes for cone-rod otx photoreceptor homeobox transcription factor (also known as *CRX*)
CORD4 a locus for cone-rod dystrophy on chromosome 17 (17q)
CORD6 the retinal-specific guanylate cyclase gene on chromosome 17 (17p13.1) (also known as *LCA1, GUCY2D, and RETGC1*)
CORD7 autosomal dominant cone-rod dystrophy
CORD8 a locus for cone-rod dystrophy on chromosome 1 (1q12–q24)
CORD9 a locus for cone-rod dystrophy on chromosome 8 (8p11)
CORDX the retinitis pigmentosa guanosine triphosphate hydrolase regulator gene on the X chromosome (Xp11.4) (also known as *RP3, RPGR and COD1*)
CORDX2 a locus for cone-rod dystrophy on the X chromosome (Xq27–28)
CORDX3 a locus for cone-rod dystrophy on the X chromosome (Xp11–q13)
CoQ Coenzyme Q also known as ubiquinone
COX10 a nuclear gene on chromosome 17 (17p12–p11.2) that codes a component of the mitochondrial respiratory chain complex IV
COX15 a nuclear gene on chromosome 10 (10q24) that codes a component of the mitochondrial respiratory chain complex IV
CP cicatricial pemphigoid
CP49 an early name for phkinin in the lens
CP115 an early name for filensin; also known as cytoskeletal protein 115 kD
CPE ciliary pigmented epithelium; cyopathic effect
CpG cytosine phosphate guanine dinucleotide
C/PL cholesterol phospholipid ratio
CR1 receptor for C3b (also known as CD35)
CR2 receptor for C3d (also known as CD21)
CR3 receptor for C3bi (also known as CD11b)
CR4 receptor for C3bi and C3dg (also known as CD11c)
CRALBP cellular retinaldehyde-binding protein
CRALBP the cellular retinaldehyde-binding protein gene on chromosome 15 (15q26) (also known as *RLBP1*)
CRB1 a gene on chromosome 1 (1q31–q32.1) that codes for a homolog of Drosophila Crumbs 1 (also known as *RP12*)
CRB(II) intestinal intracytoplasmic retinol-binding protein
CRBP cellular retinol-binding protein; also known as retinol-binding protein 1 (RBP1)
CRBP2 cellular retinol-binding protein 2
CREBBP a gene on chromosome 16 (16p13.3) that codes for a transcription factor for a cAMP-response element binding protein
CREST syndrome calcinosis, Raynaud phenomenon, esophageal dysmotility, sclerodactyly, and telangiectasia syndrome
CRP C-reactive protein
CRP the gene for C-reactive protein
Crry complement receptor related protein
CRS congenital rubella syndrome
C-Rel a member of the Rel/NFκB family of transcription factors
CRX the gene on chromosome 19 (19q13.3) that codes for cone-rod otx photoreceptor homeobox transcription factor (also known as *CORD2*)
CRYAA the alpha-A crystallin gene on chromosome 21 (21q22.3)
CRYAB the B-crystallin gene on chromosome 11 (11q22.1–q23.2)
Cryab the murine gene for αB-crystallin
CRYBB1 the beta-B1 crystallin gene on chromosome 22 (22q11.2–q12.1)
CRYBB2 the gene for βB2-crystallin on chromosome 22 (22q11.2)
CRYBB3 the gene for βB3-crystallin on chromosome 22 (22q11.2)
CRYGC the gene for γC-crystallin on chromosome 2 (2q33–q35)
CRYGD the gene for γD-crystallin on chromosome 2 (2q33–q35)
CRYGS the gene for γS-crystallin on chromosome 3 (3q25–qter)
CS chondroitin sulfate
CSF cerebrospinal fluid
CSNB congenital stationary night blindness
CSNB the calcium channel-voltge dependent alpha-IF subunit on the X chromosome (Xp11.23) (also known as *CACNA1F*)
CSNB1 the nyctalopin gene on the X chromosome (Xp11.4) (also known as *NYX*)
CSNB3 the rod cyclic guanosine monophosphate phosphodiesterase beta subunit gene on chromosome 4 (4p16.3) (also known as *PDE6B*)
CSPG2 the versican gene on chromosome 5 (5q13–q14)
CSPG6 the bamacan gene on chromosome 10 (10q25)
CSS Churg–Strauss syndrome
CST3 the cystatin C gene on chromosome 20 (20p11.2)
CT computed tomography
CTG a cytosine-thymine-guanine trinucleotide
CTAP connective tissue activating protein
CTGF connective tissue growth factor
CTH ceramide trihexoside
CTL cytotoxic T lymphocyte
CTLA4 cytotoxic T lymphocyte-associated antigen 4 (also known as CD152)

CTNS a cystine transporter gene on chromosome 17(17p)
CtmPrP a transmembrane form of prion protein
CTRP5 a collagen–like member of the C1q/tumor necrosis factor superfamily gene on chromosome 11 (11q23.3)
CTRP5 a collagen–like member of the C1q/tumor necrosis factor superfamily
CXCL12 chemokine CXC motif ligand 12 (also known as stromal cell-derived factor 1 (SDF-1)
CXCR2 chemokine (C-X-R) receptor 2 (also known as beta interleukin 8 receptor)
CXCR4 chemokine (C-X-R) receptor 4
Cu2+ cupric ions
CU18 an antibody that recognizes breast carcinoma associated antigen 225
CVD cardiovascular disease
CVS chorionic villous sample
cw cataract webbed (a mutant deer mouse)
Cyclin A2 a cyclin encoded by a gene on chromosome 4 (4q27)
Cyclin B1 a cyclin encoded by a gene on chromosome 5 (5q12)
Cyclin C a cyclin encoded by a gene on chromosome 6 (6q21)
Cyclin E2 a cyclin that controls the initiation of DNA synthesis
Cyclin G1 a cyclin encoded by a gene on chromosome 5 (5q32–q34)
Cyclin T2 a cyclin encoded by a gene on chromosome 2 (2p14–q21.3)
CYP1B1 the cytochrome p450 subfamily 1 polypeptide 1 gene on chromosome 2 (2p22–p21)
CYP4V2 the cytochrome p450 family 4 subfamily V polypeptide 2 gene on chromosome 4 (4q35.1)
CYP27A1 the sterol 27-hydroxylase (also known as cytochrome p450 subfamily XXVIIA polypeptide 1 gene on chromosome 2 (2q33–qter)

1D one-dimensional
1D SDS-PAGE one-dimensional sodium dodecyl sulfate-polyacrylamide gel electrophoresis
2D DIGE two-dimensional difference gel electrophoresis
2D PAGE two-dimensional polyacrylamide gel electrophoresis
3D three dimensional
5D4 an anti-keratan sulfate antibody
D diopter
D2-40 a lymphatic-endothelial marker recognizing podoplanin
Da Dalton
DAF decay-accelerating factor
DAG diaminoglycol
DBS dried blood spot
DC dendritic cell
DCC the "delete in colon cancer" gene on chromosome 18 (18q21.3)
DCN the biglycan gene on chromosome 12(12q13.2)
DCR1 decoy receptor 1 (also known as TRAIL3, tumor necrosis factor related apoptosis-inducing ligand receptor 3 [TRAILR3], death receptor 3 [DR3], and TRAIL receptor without an intracellular domain [TRID], and tumor necrosis factor receptor superfamily member 10C [TNFRSF10C])
DcR2 tumor necrosis factor-related apoptosis inducing ligand 4 (TRAIL4)
DcR3 tumor necrosis factor-related apoptosis inducing ligand (TRAIL) (also known as APO2L)
Dct a murine gene involved in melanin production
DED death effector domains
DES the desmin gene on chromosome 2 (2q35)
DESK Descemet stripping endothelial keratoplasty
DG diacylglycerol
DH delayed hypersensitivity
DHA dehydroascorbic acid
DHEAS dehydroepiandrosterone sulfate
DHICA 5,6-dihydroxyindole-2-carboxylic acid
DHRD Doyne honeycomb retinal dystrophy
DHS dehydroascorbic acid
Diablo direct IAP-binding protein with low PI; also known as second mitochodria-derived activator of caspase (SMAC)
DIDMOAD diabetes insipidus, diabetes mellitus, optic atrophy, and deafness
DIF direct immunofluorescence
DLBCL diffuse large B cell lymphoma
DLD a gene that codes for a component of the pyruvate dehydrogenase complex
DLEK deep lamellar endothelial keratoplasty
dLGN dorsal lateral geniculate nucleus
DLN draining lymph node
DM1 myotonic dystrophy type 1 (also known as classic myotonic dystrophy)
DM2 myotonic dystrophy type 2 (also known as proximal myotonic dystrophy)
DMD the dystrophin gene on the X chromosome (Xp21.2) that causes Duchenne muscular dystrophy when mutated
DMN dimethylnitrosamine
DMPK the dystrophia myotonica protein kinase gene on chromosome 19 (19q13.3)
DMS dimethylsulfate
DNA deoxyribonucleic acid
DNMT3B DNA methyltransferase 3B
DR1 death receptor 1 (also known as TNFR1 and CD120a)
DR2 death receptor 2
DR3 death receptor 3 (also known as lymphocyte-associated receptor of death [LARD],TRAMP, WSL1 decoy receptor 1 [DCR1]; TRAIL3, tumor necrosis factor related apoptosis-inducing ligand receptor 3 [TRAILR3], TRAIL receptor without an intracellular domain [TRID], and tumor necrosis factor receptor superfamily member 25 [TNFRSF25])
DR4 death receptor 4 (also known as tumor necrosis factor - related apoptosis-inducing ligand receptor 4 [TRAILR4], DCR2, TRUNDD, and decoy receptor 2)
DR5 death receptor 5 (also known tumor necrosis factor receptor superfamily, member 10B [TNFR10B], tumor necrosis factor-related apoptosis-inducing ligand receptor 2 [TRAIL2], KILLER and TRICK2)

DR6 death receptor 6 (also known as tumor necrosis factor receptor superfamily member 21, osteoprotegenin [OPG], osteoclastogenesis inhibitory factor, and interleukin 1-beta convertase)
DRM desmin-related myofibillar myopathy
DRP-1 dynanim- related protein 1
DS dermatan sulfate
DS PG dermatan sulfate proteoglycan
dsDNA double stranded DNA
DsrNA-RT single standed desoxyribonucleic acid-reverse transcriptase
DSPG3 the epiphycan gene on chromosome 12 (12q21)
dsRNA double stranded RNA
DTI diffusion tensor imaging
DTH delayed type hypersensitivity
DTNBP1 the gene on chromosome 6 (6p22.3) that causes Hermansky–Pudlak syndrome type 7 when mutated
DTT dithiothreitol
dUTP 2′-deoxyuridine 5′-triphosphate

E1A an adenovirus oncoprotein
E1B a gene in adenovirus
E2F a transcription factor that binds to the retinoblastoma gene (*RB1*)
E6 a gene in papillomaviruses
E7 a gene in papillomaviruses
EAF2 a component of the ELL-mediated RNA polymerase II elongation factor
EAU experimental autoimmune uveitis
EB elementary body
EBV Epstein-Barr virus
EC vascular endothelial cell
ECD1 an autoantigen with extracellular domains in Sjögren syndrome
ECF-A eosinophilic chemotactic factor of anaphylaxis
ECG electrocardiograph
ECM extracellular matrix
ECM1 the extracellular matrix protein 1 gene on chromosome 1 (1q21)
ECM2 the extracellular matrix protein 2 gene on chromosome 9 (9q21.3–q22)
ECP eosinophil cationic protein
ECS extracellular space
EDAR ectodysplasin A receptor
EDRF endothelial dependendent relaxation factor
EDS Ehlers–Danlos syndrome
EDS1 Ehlers–Danlos syndrome type 1
EDTA ethylenediaminetetraacetic acid
EDN eosinophil derived neurotoxin
EDN1 gene for endothelin 1 on chromosome 6 (6p24–p23)
EDN1 endothelin 1
EDNRA endothelin receptor type A
EDNRA a gene for endothelin receptor type A on chromosome 4 (4q31.2)
EDNRB a gene for endothelin receptor type B on chromosome 13 (13q22)
EDNRB endothelin receptor type B
EEC syndrome ectodactyly, ectodermal dysplasia, and cleft lip/palate syndrome
EEG electroencephalography; electroencephalograph; electroencephalogram
EEP EDTA-extractable protein
EETs epoxyeicosatrienoic acid
EEV extracellular enveloped virus
EFEMP1 the fibulin 3 gene on chromosome 2 (2p16) (also known as FBLN3)
EFTF eye field transcription factor
e.g. for example
EGF epidermal growth factor
EGFR the gene for epidermal growth factor receptor on chromosome 7 (7p12.3–p12.1)
EIA enzyme-linked immunoassay
EJ-ras an oncogene
EKC epidemic keratoconjunctivitis
EKG electrocardiogram
EKH4 monoclonal antikeratin antibody predominantly expressed in basal epithelial cells
EKH5 monoclonal antikeratin antibody predominantly expressed in eccrine secretory part of structures
EKH6 monoclonal antikeratin antibody predominantly expressed in normal eccrine and ductal structures
ELAM-1 endothelial leukocyte adhesion molecule-1
ELISA enzyme-linked immunosorbent assay
ENA extractable nuclear antigen
ELN the elastin gene on chromosome 7 (7q11.2)
ELOVL4 elongation of very long chain fatty acids-like 4
ELOVL4 the elongation of very long chain fatty acids-like 4 gene on chromosome 6 (6q14)
EM erythema multiforme; electron microscopy
EMA epithelial membrane antigen
EMG electromyograph
EMT epithelial-mesenchymal transition
Endo endothelial cells
ENOS the β-enolase gene on chromosome 17 (17pter–p12)
ENPP2 the ectonucleotide pyrophosphatase/phosphodiesterase gene on chromosome 8 (8q24.1)
en embryonic nucleus of crystalline lens
env a gene in Rous sarcoma virus
Eo eosinophils
EOG electro-oculography
EOM extraocular muscle
ep epithelium
EP300 a gene on chromosome 22 (22q13) that codes for a histone acetyltransferase (p300) that regulates transcription
Epi epithelial cells
EPMR epilepsy with mental retardation (also known as neuronal ceroid lipofuscinosis type 8)
EPR electron spin resonance
ER endoplasmic reticulum
Erb-B an oncogene
ERCC1 group 1 excision-repair cross-complemeting protein
ERCC6 group 6 excision-repair cross-complemeting protein
ERCC8 group 8 excision-repair cross-complemeting protein
ERG electroretinogram
ERK extracellular signal-regulated kinase (a subgroup of mitogen activated protein kinases, MAPKs)

ERM epiretinal membrane
ERP early receptor potential
ERT enzyme replacement therapy
ESAF endothelial cell angiogenesis factor
ESCB enhanced S-cone syndrome
ESCS a gene on chromosome 15 (15q23) that codes for nuclear receptor subfamily 2, group E, member 3 (also known as *NR2E3* and *PNR*)
ESI electrospray ionization
ESI-LC-MS/MS electrospray ionization liquid chromatography tandem mass spectrometry
ESR erythrocyte sedimentation rate
EST expressed tags
EVR1 exudative vitreoretinopathy type 1
EVR2 exudative vitreoretinopathy type 2
EVR3 exudative vitreoretinopathy type 3
EVR4 exudative vitreoretinopathy type 4

5-Fu 5-fluoruracil
F6H8 perfluorohexyloctane
FA fluorescein angiography
Fab fragment antigen binding
Factor VIII an essential blood clotting factor; a vascular cell marker
FACS fluorescence activated cell sorter
FAD flavin adenine dinucleotide
FADD Fas-assciated death domain
FADH2 reduced flavin adenine dinucleotide
FAH the fumarylacetoacetate hydrolase gene on chromosome 15 (15q23–q25)
FAP familial amyloid polyneuropathy, familial adenomatous polyposis
FAS/Fas apoptosis antigen 1 (APO1) (also known as CD95, cell surface death receptor 2, and FAS antigen)
FASL/Fasl Fas ligand
Fb fibroblasts
FBLN3 the fibulin 3 gene on chromosome 2 (2p16) (also known as *EFEMP1*)
FBLN5 the fibulin 5 gene on chromosome 14 (4q32.1)
FBLN6 the fibulin 6 gene on chromosome 1 (1q24–q25)
FBN1 the fibrillin-1 gene on chromosome 15 (15q21.1)
FBN2 the fibrillin-2 gene on chromosome 5 (5q23–q31)
FBN3 the fibrillin-3 gene on chromosome 19 (19p13.3–p13.2)
Fc constant fragment of immunoglobulin; crystallizable fragment of immunoglobulin
FCD Fuchs corneal dystrophy
fCJD familial Creutzfelt-Jakob disease
FCMD Fukuyama congenital muscular dystrophy
FCMD the fukudin gene on chromosome 9(9q31)
FD fleck corneal dystrophy
Fe^{2+} ferrous ions
Fe^{3+} ferric ions
FEVR familial exudative vitreoretinopathy
FFA fundus fluorescein angiogram
FFI fatal familial insomnia
FMM fundus flavimaculatus
FGA the fibrinogen α-chain gene on chromosome 4 (4q28)
FGF fibroblast growth factor
FGF1 the fibroblast growth factor 1 (acidic fiboblast growth factor) gene on chromosome 5 (5q31)
FGF2 fibroblast growth factor 2 (also known as basic fibroblast growth factor [bFGF])
FGF2 the gene for fibroblast growth factor 2 (basic fibroblast gowth factor) on chromosome 4 (4q25–q27)
Fgf2 the murine gene for fibroblast growth factor 2 (basic fibroblast gowth factor)
FGF8 fibroblast growth factor 8
FGF8 the gene for fibroblast growth factor 8 on chromosome 10 (10q24)
FGF9 fibroblast growth factor 9
FGF9 the gene for fibroblast growth factor 9 on chromosome 13 (13q11–q12)
Fgf10 the murine gene for fibroblast growth factor 10
FGF10 the gene for fibroblast growth factor 10 on chromosome 5 (5p13–p12)
FGFR1 fibroblast growth factor receptor 1
FH familial hypercholesterolemia
FHI Fuchs heterochromic iridocyclitis
FIP-2 an adenoviral protein
FIS1 homolog of *S. cerevisiae*, also known as tetratricipeptide repeat domain 11
FISH fluorescent in situ hybridization
FKH7 the former term for forkhead box C1 transcription factor now known as FOXC1
FKH7 a former term for the gene on chromosome 6 (6p25) that codes for forkhead box C1 transcription factor; now known as *FOXC1*
FKRP4 the fukutin-related protein gene on chromosome 19 (19q13.3)
FLAIR fluid attenuated inversion recovery
FLICE caspase 8 apoptosis-related cysteine protease
FLIP FLICE inhibitory protein
$FLIP_L$ FLICE-like inhibitory protein long-form
$FLIP_S$ FLICE-like inhibitory protein short-form
Flk1 vascular endothelial growth factor receptor 2
Flt-1 fms-like tyrosine kinase-1
FLNA the actin-binding protein filamin A
FMN flavin mononucleotide
FMOD the fibromodulin gene on chromosome 1 (1q32.1)
fn fetal nucleus of the crystalline lens
FN1 the fibronectin gene on chromosome 2 (2q31)
FOXC1 the forkhead box C1 transcription factor gene on chromosome 6 (6p25) (formerly known as *FKHL7*)
Foxc1 the murine forkhead box C1 gene that codes for transcription factor
FOXC1 the forkhead box C1 gene on chromosome 6 (6p25)
Foxc2 the murine forkhead box C2 gene that codes for transcription factor
FOXC2 the forkhead box C2 gene on chromosome 16 (16q24.3)
Foxd1 a transcription factor
FOXE3 the gene for forkhead box E3 on chromosome 1 (1p32)
FOXL2 the forkhead transcription factor
FOXL2 the forkhead transcription factor FOXL2 gene on chromosome 3 (3q23)
FOXP1 the glutamine-rich factor 1 gene on chromosome 3 (3p14.1)

FRAS1 the gene on chromosome 4 (4q) that is responsible for Fraser syndrome
FREM2 the FRAS1-related extracellular matrix protein 2 gene on chromosome 13 (13q13.3)
FSCN2 the retinal fascin homolog 2 actin binding protein gene on chromosome 17 (17q25) (also known as *RP30*)
Fuc fucose
FUCA1 the α-L-fucosidase gene on chromosome 1 (1p34)
FZD4 the gene on chromosome 11 (11q14–q21) that codes a homolog of Drosophila frizzled 4 a member of the"frizzled" gene family
FZD6 the gene coding a homolog of Drosophila frizzled 6 a member of the"frizzled" gene family

g gram
G guanine
G protein a glycoprotein on the surface of rhabdoviruses
G-protein a guanine nucleotide binding protein
G0 the resting phase of the cell cycle
G1 the presynthetic phase of the cell cycle
G2 the phase in the cell cycle between the S and M phases
G3P glyceraldehyde 3-phosphate
G3PD glyceraldehyde 3-phosphate dehydrogenase
G6P glucose-6-phosphate
G6PC the glucose-6-phosphatase gene on chromosome 17 (17q21)
G6PD glucose 6-phosphate dehydrogenase
G6PT1 the glucose 6 phosphate transporter 1 gene on chromosome 11 (11q23)
GA geographic atrophy and gyrate atrophy
GA733-1 a former name for the *TACSTD2* gene on chromosome 1 (1P32)
GAA an acid α-glucosidase gene on chromosome 17 (17q25.2–q25.3)
GABA gamma aminobutyric acid
Gadd45 the gene product of the growth arrest and DNA damage–inducible gene (GADD45A)
GADD153 a DNA repair protein
GADD153 a DNA repair protein gene on chromosome 12 (12q13.1–q13.2)
gag a gene in Rous sarcoma virus
GAG glycosaminglycan; codon for glutamic acid
GAGs glycosaminoglycans
Gal galactose
Gal6ST galactose-6-sulfotransferase
GALC galactosylceramidase
GALC the galactosylceramidase gene on chromosome 14 (14q31)
GalCer galactosylceramide
GalNAc N-acetylgalactosamine
GALNS the galactose 6-sulfatase gene on chromosome 16 (16q24.3)
GALT gut associated lymphoid tissue
GAPO growth retardation, alopecia, pseudoanodontia and optic atrophy syndrome
GAS6 growth arrest-specific 6
GB3 globotriaosylyceramide
GBA the glucocerebrosidase gene on chromosome 1 (1q21)
GBC globotribosyl ceramide
GBE1 the glycogen branching enzyme gene on chromosome 3 (3p12)
GBM glomerular basement membrane
GCA giant cell arteritis and a guanine-cytosine-adenine trinucleotide
GCAP guanylate cyclase activation protein
GCAP1 an isoform of a calcium-binding protein involved in the replenishment of cyclic guanosine monophosphate in rods and cones (also kown as GUCA1A)
GCAP1 the gene for guanylate cyclase activator 1A on chromosome 6 (6p21.1) (also known as *GUCA1A* and *COD3*)
GCAP2 an isoform of a calcium-binding protein involved in the replenishment of cyclic guanosine monophosphate in rods and cones (also known as GUCA1B)
GCAP2 the gene for guanylate cyclase activator 1B on chromosome 6 (6p21.1) (also known as *GUCA1B*)
GCAP3 an isoform of calcium-binding protein involved in the replenishment of cyclic guanosine monophosphate in rods and cones (also known as GUCA1C)
GCD granular corneal dystrophy
GCG a guanine-cytosine-guanine trinucleotide
GCP the gene for green visual pigment on the X chromosome (Xq28)
GD Gaucher disease
GDLD gelatinous drop-like corneal dystrophy
GDP guanosine diphosphate
GFAP glial fibrillary acidic protein
GH growth hormone
GHMP an enzyme superfamily that includes galactokinase, homoserine kinase, mevalonate kinase and phosphomevonate kinase
GIT gastrointestinal tract
GJ gap junction
GJA8 the gap junction protein alpha-8 gene on chromosome 1 (1q21.1)
GJB2 the gap junction protein beta-2 (connexin 26) gene on chromosome 13 (13q11–q12)
GLA the α-galactosidase A gene on the X chromosome (Xq22–24)
Glb1 the murine gene that codes β-galactosidase
GLB1 β-galactosidase
GLB1 the acid β-galactosidase gene on chromosome 3 (3p21.33)
Glc glucose
GLC3A the locus for primary congenital glaucoma type 3 on chromosome 2 (2p21–2p25), where there are homozygous mutations in the cytochrome P4501B1 gene (*CYP1B1*)
GLI glioma associated oncogene
GLRX the glutaredoxin gene on chromosome 5 (5q14)
Glu glutamate
GluCer glucosylceramide
GLUT1 the glucose transporter 1 gene on chromosome 1 (1p35–p31.3)
Gly glycine
GlyNAc6St N-acetylglucosamine 6-O-sulfotransferase
GM2A the GM_2-activator protein gene on chromosome 5 (5q31.3–q33.1)

GM-CSF granulocyte-macrophage colony stimulating factor
GMP-140 granule membrane protein
GNA the *N*-acetylglucosamine 6-sulfatase gene on chromosome 12 (12q14)
GNAS the guanine nucleotide-binding protein, alpha-stimulating activity polypeptide 1 gene on chromosome 20 (20q13.2)
GNAS1 the guanine nucleotide-binding protein, alpha-stimulating activity polypeptide 1 gene on chromosome 20 (20q13.2)
GNAT1 the guanine nucleotide-binding protein alpha-transducing activity polypeptide 1 gene on chromosome 3 (3p21)
GNAT2 the guanine nucleotide-binding protein alpha-transducing activity polypeptide 2 gene on chromosome 1 (1p13.1)
GNPTAB the N-acetylglucosamine-1-phosphotransferase gene on chromosome 12 (12q23.3)
GNPTG the gene on chromosome 16 (16q) for the gamma subunit of N-acetylglucosamine-1-phosphotransferase
gp75 a differentiation antigen of melanocytes
GP100 a melanocyte protein (also known as melanocyte protein 17)
GPC1 the glypican 1 gene on chromosome 2 (2q35–q37)
GPC2 the glypican 2 gene on chromosome 7 (7q22.1)
GPC3 the glypican 3 gene on the X chromosome (Xq26)
GPC4 the glypican 4 gene on the X chromosome (Xq26)
GPC5 the glypican 5 gene on chromosome 13 (13q32)
GPC6 the glypican 6 gene on chromosome 13 (13q32)
GPCR G-protein coupled receptor
Gpr2a a murine gene on chromosome 16
GRIPs glypican-related integral membrane proteoglycans
GRK1 the rhodopsin kinase gene on chromosome 13 (13q34) (also known as *RHOK*)
GRM6 the metabotropic glutamate receptor 6 gene on chromosome 5 (5q35.3)
GRO (MGSA) a cytokine
GRODS granular osmiophilic deposits
GSD glycogen storage diseases
GSH glutathione reduced form
GSL glycosphingolipids
GSN the gelsolin gene on chromosome 9 (9q34)
GSS Gerstmann–Stäussler-Scheinker disease
GSSG oxidized glutathione
GST glutathione S-transferase
GST 5.6 an isoenzyme of glutathione S-transferase
GST 7.4 an isoenzyme of glutathione S-transferase
GSTM1 the glutathione S-transferase mu 1(mGST-1) gene on chromosome 1 (1p13.3)
GSTP1 the gene for glutathione S-transferase pi 1 on chromosome 11 (1q13)
GSTT1 glutathione S-transferase theta 1
GSTT1 the gene for glutathione S-transferase theta 1 (GST-T1) on chromosome 22 (22q11.2)
GTM3 a transformed/immortalized trabecular meshwork cell strain
GTP guanosine triphosphate
GTPase guanosine triphosphate hydrolase
GUCA1A an isoform of a calcium-binding protein involved in the replenishment of cyclic guanosine monophosphate in rods and cones (also kown as GCAP1)
GUCA1A the gene for guanylate cyclase activator 1A on chromosome 6 (6p21.1) (also known as *COD3* and *GCAP1*)
GUCA1B an isoform of a calcium-binding protein involved in the replenishment of cyclic guanosine monophosphate in rods and cones (also known as GCAP2)
GUCA1C an isoform of calcium-binding protein involved in the replenishment of cyclic guanosine monophosphate in rods and cones (also known as GCAP3)
GUG codon for valine
GUSB the β-D-glucuronidase gene on chromosome 7 (7q21.11)
GUCY2D retinal guanylate cyclase-1 (also known as RetGC1)
GUCY2D the retinal-specific guanylate cyclase gene on chromosome 17 (17p13.1) (also known as *CORD6*, *LCA1*, and *RETGC1*)
GVF Goldmann visual field
Gy grey ($1GY=100rad=J/kg=m^2/s^2$)
GYS2 the glycogen synthase gene on chromosome 12 (12p12.3)

5-HT 5-hydroxytryptamine
5-HETE 5-hydroxyeicosatetraenoic acid
12-HETE 12-hydroxyeicosatetraenoic acid
12(R)-HETE 12(R)-hydroxyeicosatetraenoic acid
15-HETE 15-hydroxyeicosatetraenoic acid
H heparin
H_2O_2 hydrogen peroxide
HA hyaluronic acid (also known as hyaluran)
HAMP a gene on chromosome 19 (19q13) that causes hemochromatosis when mutated
HAV hepatitis A virus
HbA adult hemoglobin
HbC hemoglobin C
HB-EGF heparin-binding epidermal growth factor-like growth factor
HbF fetal hemoglobin
HBID hereditary benign intraepithelial dyskeratosis
HBO hyperbaric oxygen
HbS hemoglobin S (sickle cell hemoglobin)
HbSC hemoglobin SC
HBV hepatitis B virus
HBVcAg hepatitis B virus core antigen
HBVsAg hepatitis B virus surface antigen
HCV hepatitis C virus
HD homeodomain
HDL high density lipoprotein
HBV hepatitis B virus
HBVsAg hepatitis B virus surface antigen
HCS hyperferritinemia-cataract syndrome
HDM2 double minute gene (also known as MDM2)
HDM2 the double minute 2 gene, also known as *MDM2*
HDV hepatitis D virus
HEP high-energy phosphates

Hes1 a murine gene that is expressed in retinal progenitor cells
HESX1 a gene on chromosome 3 (3p21.2–p21.1) known as the homeobox gene expressed in ES cells and as the Rathke pouch homeobox gene
HETEs hydroxyeicosatetraenoic acids
HEXA the α-subunit of β-hexosaminidase gene on chromosome 15 (15q23–q24)
HEXA an isoform of β-hexosaminidase consisting of an α- and β-subunit
HEXB the β-subunit of β-hexosaminidase gene on the chromosome 5 (5q13)
HEXB an isoform of β-hexosaminidase consisting of two β-subunits
HFE a gene on chromosome 6 (6p) that causes hemochromatosis when mutated
HFMD hand-foot and mouth disease
Hg mercury
HGF hepatocyte growth factor
HGF the gene for hepatocyte growth factor on chromosome 7 (7q21.1)
HGD the homogentisate 1,2-dioxygenase gene on chromosome 3 (3q21–q23)
HGSNAT the acetyl-CoA-glucosamine *N*-acetyltransferase gene on chromosome 8 (8p11.1)
HHV8 human herpes virus 8
HI hemagglutination inhibition
HIF hypoxia-inducible factor
HIF the hypoxia-inducible transcription factor-1 gene on chromosome 14 (14q21–q24)
HIF$_\alpha$ hypoxia–inducible factor alpha
His histidine
HIV human immunodeficiency virus
HDL high density lipoprotein
HDL-1 high density lipoprotein fraction 1
HDL-2 high density lipoprotein fraction 2
HDL-3 high density lipoprotein fraction 3
HEP high energy phosphates
HGD the homogentisate 1,2 dioxygenase gene on chromosome 3 (3q21–q23)
HHV-6 human herpes virus 6
HHV-8 human herpes virus 8
HK hexokinase
HLA human leukocyte antigen
HLA-A11 haplotype of human leukocyte antigen (HLA)
HLA-B40 haplotype of human leukocyte antigen (HLA)
HLA-B51 haplotype of human leukocyte antigen (HLA)
HLA-B87 haplotype of human leukocyte antigen (HLA)
HLA-DR class II histocompatibility antigen
HLA-DR2 haplotype of class II histocompatibility antigen
HLA-DR4/DRW53 haplotype of class II histocompatibility antigen
HLA-DR15 haplotype of class II histocompatibility antigen
HLA-DR17 haplotype of class II histocompatibility antigen
HLA-DR51 haplotype of class II histocompatibility antigen
HLA-DRB1 haplotype of class II histocompatibility antigen
HLE human lens epithelium
HLOD hierachical level of detail; heterogeneity likelihood of the odds (lod) score
HMB45 antibody that reacts with a neuraminidase sensitive oligosaccharide side chain of a glycoconjungate in immature melanosomes
HMB50 antibody that recognizes a different epitope on the same antigen in melanoctes as HMB45
HMG hydroxymethylglutaryl
HMW kininogen high molecular weight kininogen
HNK-1 human natural killer-1; a marker for the astrocyte type 1 precursor
HPETEs hydroperoxyeicosatetraenoic acids
HPF high power field
HPLC high pressure liquid chromatography
HPS1 the gene on chromosome 10 (10q23.1) that causes Hermansky–Pudlak syndrome type 1 when mutated
HPS2 the gene on chromosome 5 (5q14.1) that causes Hermansky–Pudlak syndrome type 2 when mutated (also known as *ADTB3A* and *AP3B1*)
HPS3 the gene on chromosome 3 (3q24) that causes Hermansky–Pudlak syndrome type 3 when mutated
HPS4 the gene on chromosome 22 (22q11.2–q12.2) that causes Hermansky–Pudlak syndrome type 4 when mutated
HPS5 the gene on chromosome 11 (11p15–p13) that causes Hermansky–Pudlak syndrome type 5 when mutated
HPS6 the gene on chromosome 10 (10q24.32) that causes Hermansky–Pudlak syndrome type 6 when mutated
HPV human papilloma virus
HPV16 human papilloma virus type 16
hr hour
HRP horseradish peroxidase
HRPT2 hyperparathyroidism-2
HRPT2 the gene on chromosome 1 (1q25–q31) responsible for hyperparathyroidism-2
HS heparan sulfate
HSF4 the gene for heat shock transcription factor-4 on chromosome 16 (16q22.12)
HSK herpetic stromal keratitis
HSP heat shock protein
HSP27 heat shock protein 27
HSP40 heat shock protein 40
HSP60 heat shock protein 60
HSPB1 the heat shock protein 27 gene on chromosome 7 (7q11.23)
HSPD1 the heat shock protein 60 gene on chromosome 2 (2q33.1)
HSPF1 the heat shock protein 40 gene on chromosome 19 (19p13.2)
HSPG2 the perlecan gene on chromosome 1 (1p36.1)
HSV herpes simplex virus
HSV-1 herpes simplex virus type 1
HSV-2 herpes simplex virus type 2
HTGL hepatic triglyceride lipase
HTLV-1 human T cell leukemia virus 1
HTLV-2 human T cell leukemia virus 2
HtrA2 HtrA serine peptidase 2 (also known as serine proteinase 25)
HUMARA human androgen-receptor gene on the X chromosome (Xq11.2–q12)
HV-B herpes virus B
HYAL1 the hylauronidase gene on chromosome 3 (3p21.3–p21.2)

I isotropic
IAP inhibitor of apoptosis
IAPP the islet amyloid polypeptide gene on chromosome 12 (12p12.3–p12.1)
IBD identity by descent
ICA internal carotid artery
ICAM intercellular adhesion molecule
ICAM-1 intercellular adhesion molecule-1
ICAM-2 intercellular adhesion molecule-2
ICAM-3 intercellular adhesion molecule-3
ICE syndrome the irido-corneal-endothelial syndrome that includes iris nevus syndrome, Chandler syndrome, and essential iris atrophy
ICZ inner collagenous zone
ID3 A transcription factor inhibitor of DNA binding 3
IDL intermediate density lipoproteins
IDO indoleamine pyrrole 2,3 dioxygenase
IDS the iduronate-2 sulfatase gene on the X chromosome (Xq28)
IDUA the α-L-iduronidase gene on chromosome 4 (4p16.3)
IEF isoelectric focusing
IEV intracelluar enveloped virus
IF immunofluorescence
IFA indirect fluorescent antibody (also immunofluoresecent antibody)
IFκ B nuclear factor of kappa light chain enhancer in B cells inhibitor
IFN interferon
IFNα interferon alpha
IFNβ interferon beta
IFNγ interferon gamma
Ig immunoglobulin
IgA immunoglobulin A
IgD immunoglobulin D
IgE immunoglobulin E
IGF insulin-like growth factor
IGF1 insulin like growth factor 1
IGF2 insulin like growth factor 2
IgG immunoglobulin G
IgG_1 a subgroup of immunoglobulin G
IgG_2 a subgroup of immunoglobulin G
IgG_3 a subgroup of immunoglobulin G
IgG_4 a subgroup of immunoglobulin G
IgGκ immunoglobulin G kappa
IGHD the immunoglobulin delta heavy chain gene on chromosome 14 (14q32.33)
IGHE the immunoglobulin epsilon heavy chain gene on chromosome 14 (14q32.33)
IGHG1 the gamma immunoglobulin heavy chain gene on chromosome 14 (14q32.33)
IGHM the immunoglobulin mu heavy chain gene on chromosome 14(14q32.33)
IGLJ the gene for immunoglobulin κ or λ light chain on chromosome 22 (22q11.2)
IgM immunoglobulin M
IHA indirect hemagglutination
IIH idiopathic intracranial hypertension (also known as pseudotumor cerebri)
IIRC International Intraocular Retinoblastoma Classification
iNOS inducible nitric oxide synthase
IL interleukin
IL1 interleukin 1
IL1α interleukin 1 alpha
IL1β interleukin 1 beta
IL2 interleukin 2
IL2 the interleukin 2 gene on chromosome 4 (4q26–q27)
IL3 interleukin 3
IL4 interleukin 4
IL5 interleukin 5
IL6 interleukin 6
IL7 interleukin 7
IL8 interleukin 8
IL9 interleukin 9
IL10 interleukin 10
IL12 interleukin 12
IL18 interleukin 18
IL1A the interleukin 1 alpha gene on chromosome 2 (2q14)
IL1B the interleukin 1 beta gene on chromosome 2 (2q14)
IL1RN the interleukin 1 receptor antagonist gene on chromosome 2 (2q14.2)
IL2R interleukin 2 receptor
IL18 the interleukin 18 gene on chromosome 11 (11q22.2–q22.3)
IL8RB IL 8 receptor beta gene on chromosome 2 (2q35)
Ile isoleucine
ILGF2 insulin-like growth factor 2
ILL inner limiting lamina of retina
ILM inner limiting membrane of retina
IMPDH1 the inosine monophosphate dehydrogenase 1 gene on chromosome 7 (7q32.1) (also known as *RP10*)
IMV intracellular mature virus
INCL infantile neuronal ceroid-lipofuscinosis
iNOS inducible nitric acid oxide synthase
INS the insulin gene on chromosome 11 (11p15.5)
$InsP_3$ inositol 1,4,5-triphosphate
IOL prosthetic intraocular lens
IOP intraocular pressure
IPCV idiopathic polypoidal choroidal vasculopathy
IP1 inositol phosphate
IP2 inositol biphosphate
IP3 inositol triphosphate
IPE iris pigmented epithelium
IPM interphotoreceptor matrix
IRBP interphotoreceptor cell-binding protein (also known as interstitial retinol-binding protein)
IRE iron-responsive element
IRMA intraretinal microvascular abnormality
IRP iron regulatory protein
ISCOM immunostimulatory complexes
ISSD infantile sialic acid storage disease
ISSVA Internatioanl Society for the Study of Vascular Anomalies
ITM2B the integral membrane protein 2B gene on chromosome 13 (13q14)

JA juvenile rheumatoid arthritis
j-Bid a cleavage product of BH3-interacting domain death agonist (BID)
JCT juxtacanalicular connective tissue

JCV a human polyomavirus
JIA juvenile idiopathic arthritis
JNCL juvenile neuronal ceroid-lipofuscinosis
JOAG juvenile open angle glaucoma
JNK c-Jun N-terminal protein kinase
JNKK1 mitogen-activated protein kinase 4 (also known as MAP2K4)

K^+ potassium ion
K cell killer T lymphocyte
kb kilobase
KC keratoconus
KCS keratoconjunctivitis sicca
KD Kawasaki disease
kDa kilodalton
Ker keratinocyte
KERA the keratocan gene on chromosome 12 (12q22)
Ki-67 a marker for cell cycle proliferation (also known as Mib-1)
KID **K**eratitis, **I**chthyosis, **D**eafness syndrome
KIF21A the kinesin family member 21A gene on chromosome 12 (12q12)
KGF keratocyte growth factor
Ki-ras a family of retrovirus-associaited DNA sequences (ras) originally isolated from Kirsten murine sarcoma virus
KLHL7 an antigen that elicits autoantibodies in Sjögren syndrome
KLHL12 an antigen that elicits autoantibodies in Sjögren syndrome
KM Michaelis constant
KP keratic precipitate
KRT3 the cytokeratin 3 gene on chromosome 12 (12q13)
KRT12 the cytokeratin 12 gene on chromosome 17 (17q12)
KS keratan sulfate; Kaposi sarcoma
KS-I corneal keratan sulfate
KS-II cartilaginous keratan sulfate
KS-IIA cartilaginous keratan sulfate containing α-(1,3)-fucose and α-(2,6)-linked *N*-acetyl-neuraminic acid residues
KS-IIB cartilaginous keratan sulfate lacking α-(1,3)-fucose and α-(2,6)-linked *N*-acetyl-neuraminic acid residues
KSHV Kaposi sarcoma associated herpesvirus
KSPG keratan sulfate proteoglycan

L lutein
L cone red cone
LADD syndrome lacrimo-auriculo-dento-digital syndrome
LAK lymphokine activated killer cell
LAMP lysosome associated membrane protein
LANA latency-associated nuclear antigen
LAR a transmembrane phosphotyrosine phosphatase
LARD lymphocyte-associated receptor of death (also known as death receptor 3 [DR3])
LASER light amplication by stimulated emission of radiation
LASIK laser assisted *in situ* keratomileusis
LATs latency-associated transcripts
LBL lymphobastic B cell lymphoma
LC liquid chromatography
LCA leukocyte common antigen and Leber congenital amaurosis
LCA1 the retinal-specific guanylate cyclase gene on chromosome 17 (17p13.1) (also known as *CORD6, GUCY2D, and RETGC1*)
LCA2 the retinal pigment epithelium-specific 65 kDa protein gene on chromosome 1 (1p31) (also known as *RPE65* and *RP20*)
LCA3 a locus for Leber congenital amaurosis on chromosome 14 (14q23.3)
LCA4 the arylyhydrocarbon-interacting receptor protein-like 1 gene on chromosome 17 (17p13.1) (also known as *AIPl1*)
LCA5 a locus for Leber congenital amaurosis on chromosome 6 (6q14.1)
LCA6 the RPGR-interating protein 1 gene on chromosome 14 (14q11) (also known as *RPGRIP1*)
LCA9 a locus for Leber congenital amaurosis on chromosome 1 (1p36)
LCAT lecithin-cholesterol-acyltransferase
LCAT the lecithin-cholesterol-acyltransferase gene on chromosome 16 (16q22.1)
LCD lattice corneal dystrophy
LC-MS/MS liquid chromatography–mass spectrometry/mass spectrometry
LD linkage disequilibrium
LD syndrome lymphadema-trichiasis syndrome
LDH lactic dehydrogenase
LDH the lactate dehydrogenase gene on chromosome 11 (11p15.4)
LDL low density lipoprotein
LE lupus erythematosus
LEC CAMs lectin-epithelial growth factor-complement binding adhesion molecules
LECAM-1 lectin-EGF-complement adhesion molecule
LEF lymphoid enhancer-binding factor
LEMNDS a gene on chromosome 12 (12q14) that causes the Buschke–Ollendorff syndrome when mutated
Lens1 a murine gene involved in the induction of the lens placode
LEOPARD multiple lentigines, electrocardiographic conduction abnormalities, ocular hypertelorism, pulmonary stenosis, abnormal genitalia, retardation of growth, sensorineural deafness
Leu leucine
LeY Lewis Y antigen
LFA-1 synonym for CD18
LFB luxol fast blue
LGL large granular lymphocytes
L-GPs lactosaminoglycan-glycoproteins
LGV lymphogranuloma venereum
LHON Leber hereditary optic neuropathy
Lhx2 a murine eye field transcription factor
LI labelling index
LINCL late infantile neuronal ceroid-lipofuscinosis
LIPA an acid lipase gene on chromosome 10 (10q24–q25)
LMW low molecular weight

LMX1B a gene on chromosome 9 (9q34.1) that causes nail patella syndrome when mutated
LMYC an oncogene on chromosome 1 (1p32) with homology to a small region of bothMYC and NMYC (also known as MYCL1)
LN lymph node
LOCS lens opacities case-control classification system
LOCS III lens opacity classification system III
LOD logarithm of the odds
lop a mutant mouse with lens opacities
LORD late-onset retinal degeneration
LOX-1 lectin like oxidized low-density lipoprotein receptor-1
LOXL1 the gene for lysyl oxidase-like 1 on chromosome 15 (15q22)
LPL lipoprotein lipase
LPS lipopolysaccharide
LRAT lecithin retinol acyltransferase
LRAT the lecithin retinol acyltransferase gene on chromosome 4 (4q31.1)
LRN laboratory response network
LRP5 low density lipoprotein receptor-related protein 5
LRP5 the low density lipoprotein receptor-related Protein 5 on chromosome 11 (11q13.4)
LRR leucine-rich repeat
LSC long-space collagen
LSD lysosomal storage disease
LTB_4 leukotriene B_4
LTBP1 the latent TGFβ binding protein 1 gene on chromosome 2 (2p12–q22)
LTBP2 the latent TGFβ binding protein 2 gene on Chromosome 14 (14q24)
LTBP-1 latent TGFβ binding protein 1
LTBP-2 latent TGFβ binding protein 2
LTC_4 leukotriene C_4 (previously known as SRS-A)
LTD_4 leukotriene D_4
LTE_4 leukotriene E_4
LTF the lactoferrin gene on chromosome 3 (3q21–q23)
LTR long terminal repeat, log-transformed refraction
LUM the lumican gene on chromosome 12 (12q21.3–q22)
Lys lysine
LYVE-1 lymphatic vessel endothelial receptor 1
LYZ the gene for lysozyme

4MUGS 4-methylumbelliferyl-*N*-acetylglucosamine-6-sufate
5mc 5-methylcytosine
7MG methylation of guanine on nitrogen in the 7th position
m meter
M molar; also the phase of mitosis in the cell cycle
M1S1 a former name for the *TACSD2* gene on chromosome 1 (1p32)
M-cell a special epithelial cell in the gut
Mab monoclonal antibody
Mab21L1 a murine gene for a homologue of *C. elegans* cell fate-determinng protein mab21 that is expressed in the retina
MAC membrane attack complex
MadCAM1 mucosal addressin cell adhesion molecule
MAF the gene for v-maf avian musculoaponeurotic fibrosarcoma oncogene homolog on chromosome 16 (16q22–q23)
Maf a murine gene that codes for a transcription factor involved in the regulation of crystalline lens induction and development
MAGE melanoma antigen gene
MAGE-3 melanoma-specific antigen 3
MAGP-1 microfibril- associated glycoprotein
MALDI matrix-assisted laser desorption ionization
MALDI-TOF MS matrix-assisted laser desorption ionization-time of flight mass spectrometry
MALT mucosa associated lymphoid tissue
Man mannose
MAN2B1 the α-mannosidase class 2B1-gene on chromosome 19 (19cen–q12)
MANBA the β-mannosidase gene on chromosome 4 (4q22–q25)
Man-6-P mannose 6-phosphate
MAP mitogen-activated protein
MAP2K mitogen-activated protein kinase kinase
MAP3K mitogen-activated protein kinase kinase kinase
MAPK mitogen-activated protein kinase
MAPK14 the gene for mitogen-activated protein kinase p38
MART-1 melanoma antigen recognized by T cells (also known as Melan-A)
MAS McCune–Albright syndrome
Mash1 a murine gene involved in retinal differentiation
Math3 a murine gene involved in retinal development
Math5 a murine gene involved in retinal development
MATP a membrane-associated transporter protein gene on chromosome 5 (5p13.3)
MBP major basic protein (product of eosinophils); myelin basic protein
MBL mannose-binding lectin
MBP myelin basic protein
MC mast cells
MCAF macrophage/monocyte chemotactic and activating factor
MCB membranous cytoplasmic body
MCD macular corneal dystrophy
mcg microgram; same as μg
MCL mantle cell lymphoma
MCL1 a gene on chromosome 1 (1q21) originally isolated from the ML-1 myeloid leukemia cell line
MCOLN1 the mucolipin 1 gene on chromosome 19 (19p13.3–p13.2)
M cone green cone
MCOPS5 microphthlamia syndromic 5
MCP metacarpophalangeal
MCP-1 monocyte chemotactic protein-1
Md myelin-deficient
MD macular dystrophy
MDA malondialdehyde
MDP muramyl dipeptide
MDPF 2-methoxy-2,4-diphenyl-3(2*H*)-furanone
MDM2 double minute 2 gene on chromosome 12 (12q14.3–q15) (also known as *HDM2*)
MEB Muscle-Eye-Brain

MECD Meesmann corneal dystrophy
MEI metastatic efficiency index
MEFV the Mediterranean fever gene on chromosome 16 (16p13)
MEK MARK/ERK kinase
MEL-14 lymphocyte homimg receptor in mice
Melan-A melanoma antigen recognized by T cells (also known as MART-1)
MELAS myoclonic epilepsy, lactic acidosis, and stroke-like episodes
MEN multiple endocrine neoplasia
MEN1 the gene on chromosome 11 (11q13) that is responsible for multiple endocrine neoplasia syndrome type 1A
MEN2A multiple endocrine neoplasia syndrome type 2A
MEN2B multiple endocrine neoplasia syndrome type 2B
MER A novel tyrosine kinase
MERRF myoclonic epilepsy with red ragged fibers
MERTK the MER tyrosine kinase proto-oncogene on chromosome 2 (2q14.1)
MFG–E8 milk-fat-globule-EGF-factor 8
MFGE8 the lactadherin gene on chromosome 15 (15q25)
MFN1 mitofusin 1
MFN2 mitofusin 2
MFRP the membrane-type frizzled-related protein gene on chromosome 11 (11q23.3)
MFRP membrane-type frizzled-related protein
Mg magnesium
Mg^{2+} magnesium ions
MGSA (GRO) a cytokine
mGST-1 glutathione S-transferase mu
MHC major histocompatibility complex
MIA melanoma inhibitory activity
Mib-1 a marker for cell cycle proliferation; also known as Ki-67
MICA the major histocompatibility complex class 1 chain related gene A on chromosome 6 (6p21.3)
MIF macrophage migration inhibitory factor
MIP major intrinsic protein of lens (also known as MP26 and aquaporin-0)
MIP the MIP (aquaporin-0) gene on chromosome 12 (12q13)
MITF microphthalmia transcription factor
Mitf the murine gene that codes for microphthalmia transcription factor
MitfA a major isoform of microphthalmia transcription factor found in the retinal pigment epithelium
MitfD a major isoform of microphthalmia transcription factor found in the retinal pigment epithelium
MitfH a major isoform of microphthalmia transcription factor found in the retinal pigment epithelium
Mkk7 mitogen-activated protein kinase 7 (also known as MAP2K7)
ML-I mucolipidosis I
ML-II mucolipidosis II
ML-III mucolipidosis III
ML-IV mucolipidosis IV
MLB multilamellar body
MLCRD syndrome microcephaly-lymphedema-chorioretinal dysplasia syndrome
MLD metachromatic leukodystrophy
MLGAPC mucin-like glycoprotein associated with photoreceptor cells
MLH1 a DNA repair protein
MLS mucolipidosis
mm millimeter
mM millimolar
MMACHC the gene on chromosome 1 (1p34.1) that causes homocystinemia and methylmalonic aciduria when mutated
MMP matrix metalloproteinase [Zn(2+)-binding endopeptidase] and mitochondrial permeability
MMP-1 matrix metalloproteinase 1 (also known as collagenase)
MMP-2 matrix metalloproteinase 2 (also known as gelatinase, collagenase type IV, collagenase type IV A, and gelatinase A)
MMP-3 matrix metalloproteinase 3 (also known as stromelysin)
MMP-7 matrix metalloproteinase 7
MMP-9 matrix metalloproteinase 9
MMP-14 matrix metalloproteinase 14 (also known as MTI-MMP)
MMP1 the matrix metalloproteinase 1 gene on chromosome 11 (11q22–q23)
MMP2 matrix metalloproteinase 2 gene on chromosome 16 (16q13)
MMP3 matrix metalloproteinase 3 gene on chromosome 11 (11q23)
MMP9 matrix metalloproteinase 9 gene on chromosome 20 (20q11.2–q13.1)
Mn manganese
MNGIE mitochondrial neurogastointestinal encephalopathy syndrome
Mn^{2+} manganese ion
MØ macrophages/monocytes
MOCS1 the molybdenum cofactor synthesis 1 gene on chromosome 6 (6p21.3)
MOCS2 the molybdopterin synthase gene on chromosome 5 (5q11)
MOMP major outer membrane protein
MP macular pigment
MPA microscopic polyangiitis
MP17 a lens membrane protein with calmodulin binding properties
MP20 a lens plasma membrane protein
MP22 a truncated product MP70
MP26 the highly conserved major intrinsic protein of the crystalline lens (also known as aquaporin 0)
MP38 a cleavage product of MP70
MP64 a lens plasma membrane protein
MP70 an outer cortical lens fiber protein now known as connexin 50
MPO myeloperoxidase
MPR a mannose-6-phosphate receptor in the Golgi membranes
MPNST malignant peripheral nerve sheath tumor
MPS mucopolysaccharidosis
MPS I mucopolysaccharidosis type I
MPS IH mucopolysaccharidosis type IH (Hurler syndrome)
MPS IS mucopolysaccharidosis type IS (Scheie syndrome)

MPS IH/S mucopolysaccharidosis type IH/S
MPS II mucopolysaccharidosis type II (Hunter syndrome)
MPS III mucopolysaccharidosis type III (Sanfillipo syndrome)
MPS IIIA mucopolysaccharidosis type IIIA (Sanfillipo syndrome type A)
MPS IIIB mucopolysaccharidosis type IIIB (Sanfillipo syndrome type B)
MPS IIIC mucopolysaccharidosis type IIIC (Sanfillipo syndrome type C)
MPS IIID mucopolysaccharidosis type IIID (Sanfillipo syndrome type D)
MPS IV mucopolysaccharidosis type IV (Morquio syndrome)
MPS IVA mucopolysaccharidosis type IVA (Morquio syndrome type A)
MPS IVB mucopolysaccharidosis type IVB (Morquio syndrome type B)
MPS V mucopolysaccharidosis type V (former term for mucopolysaccharidosis type IS)
MPS VI mucopolysaccharidosis type VI (Maroteaux–Lamy syndrome)
NPS VII mucopolysaccharidosis type VII (Sly syndrome)
MPS VIII mucopolysaccharidosis type VIII (an entity that is no longer recognized)
MPS IX mucopolysaccharidosis type IX (Natowicz disease)
M_r molecular radius/relative molecular mass
MRCS syndrome microcornea, rod-dystrophy, cataract and posterior staphyloma syndrome
MRI magnetic resonance imaging
mRNA messenger ribonucleic acid
MRS magnetic resonance spectroscopy
MS multiple sclerosis
MSA muscle specific actin
MSD multiple sulfatase deficiency
m/sec meters/second
MSH2 aberrant mismatched repair gene
MTCO1 a mitochondrial DNA cytochrome c oxidase subunit I gene of respiratory complex IV (also known as *COI*)
MTCO2 a mitochondrial DNA cytochrome c oxidase subunit II gene of respiratory complex IV (also known as *COII*)
MTCO3 a mitochondrial DNA cytochrome c oxidase subunit III gene of respiratory complex IV (also known as *COIII*)
MTATP6 a gene that codes a component of the mitochondrial respiratory chain complex V
MtDNA mitochondrial DNA
MTHFR 5,10-methlenetetrahydrofolate reductase
MTHFR the gene for 5,10 methylenetetrahydrofolate reductase on chromosome 1 (1p36.3)
MTM1 the myotubularin gene on the X chromosome (Xq28)
MTI-MMP matrix metalloproteinase 14 (also known as MMP14)
MTND1 the subunit 1 of the mitochondrial DNA that codes for nicotinamide adenine dinucleotide dehydrogenase (complex I of the mitochondrial respiratory chain)
MTND2 the subunit 2 of the mitochondrial DNA that codes for nicotinamide adenine dinucleotide dehydrogenase (complex I of the mitochondrial respiratory chain)
MTND3 the subunit 3 of the mitochondrial DNA that codes for nicotinamide adenine dinucleotide dehydrogenase (complex I of the mitochondrial respiratory chain)
MTND4 the subunit 4 of the mitochondrial DNA that codes for nicotinamide adenine dinucleotide dehydrogenase (complex I of the mitochondrial respiratory chain)
MTND5 the subunit 5 of the mitochondrial DNA that codes for nicotinamide adenine dinucleotide dehydrogenase (complex I of the mitochondrial respiratory chain)
MTND6 the subunit 6 of the mitochondrial DNA that codes for nicotinamide adenine dinucleotide dehydrogenase (complex I of the mitochondrial respiratory chain)
MTND7 the subunit 7 of the mitochondrial DNA that codes for nicotinamide adenine dinucleotide dehydrogenase (complex I of the mitochondrial respiratory chain)
MTTK the gene that codes mitochondrial tRNA lysine from mitochondrial nucleotides 8295–8364
MTTL1 the gene that codes mitochondrial tRNA leucine from mitochondrial nucleotides 3230–3304
MTTV the gene that codes mitochondrial tRNA valine from mitochondrial nucleotides 1602–1670
MTTW the gene that codes mitochondrial tRNA tryptophan from mitochondrial nucleotides 5512–5576
mTOR mammalian target of rapamycin. It is a serine/threonine protein kinase
MudPIT multidimensional protein identification technology
MuSK muscle specific kinase
MVD microvascular density
MW molecular weight
MYC an oncogene on chromosome 8 (8q24.12–q24.13)
MYOC the myocilin gene on chromosome 1 (1q21-31)
MYO7A the myosin VIIa gene on chromosome 11 (11q13)
MYP a locus for myopia
MYP1 a locus for myopia on the X chromosome (Xq28)
MYP2 a locus for myopia on chromosome 18 (18p11.31)
MYP3 a locus for myopia on chromosome 12 (12q21–23)
MYP4 a locus for myopia on chromosome 7 (7q36)
MYP5 a locus for a myopia on chromosome 17 (17q21–23)
m/z mass-to-charge ratio where m is the mass and z is the charge)
MZL marginal zone lymphoma

Na^+ sodium ion
NA nucleic acid
NAA N-acetyl aspartic acid
NAAT nucleic acid amplification test
Na^+, K^+-ATPase sodium-potassium adenosine triphosphatase

NaCl sodium chloride
NAD^+ nicotinamide adenine dinucleotide (oxidized form)
NADH nicotinamide adenine dinucleotide (reduced form)
$NADP^+$ nicotinamide adenine dinucleotide phosphate (oxidized form)
NADPH nicotinamide adenine dinucleotide phosphate (reduced form)
NAGA the α-*N*-acetylgalactosaminidase gene on chromosome 22 (22q11)
NAGLU the α-N-acetylglucosaminidase gene on chromosome 17 (17q21)
NAION non-arteritic anterior ischemic optic neuropathy
NAIP neuronal apoptosis inhibiting protein
NARP neurogenic muscle weakness, ataxia and retinitis pigmentosa
NB84 a marker of neuroblastoma
NBCCS nevoid basal cell carcinoma syndrome
NB-DGJ N-butyldeoxygalactonojirimycin
NC nucleocapsid
N-CAM neural cell adhesion molecule
NCL neuronal ceroid-lipofuscinosis
ND Norrie disease
nDNA nuclear DNA
NDP the norrin gene on the X-chromosome (Xp11.4)
NDUFS1 a nuclear gene on chromosome 2 (2q33–q34) that codes a component of the mitochondrial respiratory chain complex I
NDUFS3 a nuclear gene on chromosome 11 (11p11.11) that codes a component of the mitochondrial respiratory chain complex I
NDUFS4 a nuclear gene on chromosome 5 (5q11.1) that codes a component of the mitochondrial respiratory chain complex I
NDUFS7 a nuclear gene on chromosome 19 (19p13) that codes a component of the mitochondrial respiratory chain complex
NDUFS8 a nuclear gene on chromosome 11 (11q13) that codes a component of the mitochondrial respiratory chain complex I
NDUFV1 a nuclear gene on chromosome 11 (11q13) that codes a component of the mitochondrial respiratory chain complex I
NDV Newcastle disease virus
Nd:YAG neodymium-doped yttrium aluminum garnett laser
NEDD8
NEU1 the neuraminidase 1 gene on chromosome 6 (6p21.3)
NeuroD a murine gene that is expressed in retinal progenitor cells
NF neurofilaments
NF1 neurofibromatosis type 1
NF1 the gene responsible for neurofibromatosis type 1
NF2 neurofibromatosis type 2
NF2 the gene for neurofibromatosis type 2 on chromosome 22 (22q12.2)
NFκB nuclear factor of kappa light chain gene enhancer in B cells
NFκB1 nuclear factor kappa-B subunit 1
NFκB2 nuclear factor kappa-B subunit 2
N-FKyn 3-hydroxykynurenine
NGF nerve growth factor
NGFR nerve growth factor receptor
Ngn2 a murine gene that is expressed in retinal progenitor cells
NH_4OH ammonia hydroxide
NHL non-Hodgkin lymphoma
NHS the gene on the X-chromosome (Xp22.13) that is responsible for Nance–Horan syndrome
NICH non-involuting cogenital hemangioma
NIH National Institutes of Health
NK cell natural killer cell
nm nanometer
NMYC an oncogene on chromosome 2 (2p24.1) that homologous with the *MYC* oncogene that was amplified in neuroblastoma cell line (also known as *MYCN*)
NMDA N-methyl-D-aspartate
NMR nuclear magnetic resonance
NO nitric oxide
NOEV N-acyl beta-valienamine
nop nuclear opacification (a mutant mouse)
NOS1 the gene for nitric oxide synthase on chromosome 12 (12q24.2–q24.31)
NPC1 a lipid trafficking protein gene on chromosome 18 (18q11–q12)
NPC2 the gene on chromosome 14 (14q24.3) that is responsible for Niemann-Pick disease type C2
NPCE nonpigmented ciliary epithelium
NPD Niemann-Pick disease
NP-A Niemann-Pick disease type A
NP-B Niemann-Pick disease type B
NP-C1 Niemann-Pick disease type C1; formerly designated Niemann-Pick disease type D
NP-C2 Niemann-Pick disease type C2
NP-D Niemann-Pick disease type D
NPL non-parametric linkage
NPPA the atrial natriuretic factor gene on chromosome 1 (1p36.2)
NPS nail patella syndrome
NR2E3 the nuclear receptor subfamily 2, group E, member 3 gene on chromosome 15 (15q23) (also known as *ESCS* and *PNR*)
NRAMP1 the natural resistance-associated macrophage protein 1 gene on chromosome 2 (2q35)
NRAMP2 the natural resistance-associated macrophage protein 2 gene on chromosome 12 (12q13)
NRL the neural retina leucine zipper gene on chromosome 14 (14q11.2) (also known as *RP27*)
NSAIDs non-steroidal anti-inflammatory drugs
NSC nuclear sclerotic cataract
NSE neuron specific enolase
NTF3 neurotrophin 3
NTF4 neurotrophin 4
NTF5 neurotrophin 5
NYX the nyctalopin gene on the X chromosome (Xp11.4) (also known as *CSNB1*)

3-OH Kyn N-formylkynurenine
O_2 oxygen radical also known as superoxide anion
O^4MT methylation of thymine on oxygen in 4th position
O^6MG methylation of guanine on oxygen in 6th position

OA ocular albinism
OAT L-ornithine:2-oxoacid aminotranferase
OCA oculocutaneous albinism
OCA1 oculocutaneous albinism type 1
OCA1A oculocutaneous albinism type 1A
OCA1B oculocutaneous albinism type IB
OCA2 oculocutaneous albinism type 2
OCA2 the gene on chromosome 15 (15q11.2–q12) that causes oculocutaneous albinism type 2 when mutated
OCA3 oculocutaneous albinism type 3
OCA4 oculocutaneous albinism type 4
Ocl-2 protoncogene which inhibits apoptosis
OCP ocular cicatricial pemphigoid
OCRL1 a gene on the X chromosome (Xq26.1) that codes for phosphatidylinositol 4,5-bisphosphate 5-phosphatase in the trans Golgi network
OCSS oculocraniosomatic syndromes
OCT optical coherent tomography
OCZ outer collagenous zone
ODFR oxygen-derived free radicals
OGN the osteoglycin gene on chromosome 9 (9q21.3–q22)
OH• hydroxyl radical
OI osteogenesis imperfecta
OLM outer limiting membrane of retina; also ocular larva migrans
OMD the osteomodulin gene on chromosome 9 (9q22)
Omi HTRA serine peptidase 2; also known as HTRA2 and serine protease 25
OMIM Online Mendelian Inheritance in Man
OMNTI oral melanotic neuroectodermal tumor of infancy
OMP1 the gene for MOMP
Omp1 a single copy gene on the *C. trachamatis* chromosome
OPA1 optic atrophy 1
OPA4 optic atrophy 4
OPA5 optic atrophy 5
OPG osteoprotegerin (also known as death receptor 6 (DR6), tumor necrosis factor receptor superfamily member 21, osteoclastogenesis inhibitory factor, and interleukin 1-beta convertase)
OPMD oculopharyngeal muscular dystrophy
OPN1LW an opsin 1 red cone pigment gene on the X chromosome (Xq28)
OPN1MW an opsin 1 green cone pigment gene on the X chromosome (Xq27)
OPTC the opticin gene on chromosome 1 (1q32.1)
OPTN the optoneurin gene on chromosome 10 (10p15–p14)
ORF open reading frame
ORF15 open eading frame 15
ORF73 protein encoded by Kaposi sarcoma associated herpes virus (KSHV)
Otx the family of murine genes that code for orthodenticle-related transcription factors
OTX2 the gene on chromosome 14 (14q21–q22) that is the homolog of the Drosophila orthodentide gene
Otx2 a murine eye field transcription factor that is the homolog of the *Drosophila* orthodentide gene
OVA ovalbumin
OXYS oxidation sensitive

6PGD 6-phosphogluconate dehydrogenase
P platelets, probability, short arm of a chromosome
P16 cyclin-dependent kinase inhibitor 2A (also known as CDKN2A and INK4)
p21 cyclin-dependent kinase inhibitor 1A (also known as CDKN1A)
p27 cyclin-dependent kinase inhibitor 1B (also known as CDKN1B)
P30/32^{MIC2} a cell surface antigen that reacts with antibodies against CD99 (surface antigen MIC2)
p50 nuclear factor kappa-B subunit 1 (also known as transcription factor NFKB1)
p52 repressor of the inhibitor of protein kinase 52-KDa
P53 the protein product of the *TP53* gene on chromosome 17 (17p13.1)
P63 the protein product of the *TP73L* gene on chromosome 3 (3q27)
P65 Golgi peripheral membrane protein P65 (also known as Golgi reassembly stacking protein 1)
PA polyarteritis nodosa
PABN1 polyadenylate-binding nuclear protein 1
PABN1 polyadenylate-binding nuclear protein 1 gene
PACAP pituitary adenylate cyclase-activating protein
PACG primary angle closure glaucoma
PAF platelet activating factor
PADGEM platelet activation-dependent granule external membrane protein
PAGE polyacrylamide gel electrophoresis
PAM primary acquired melanosis
PAMP pathogen–associated molecular pattern
pANCA perinuclear staining anti-neutrophil cytoplasmic antibody
PAP1 the PIM1-kinase associated protein 1 gene on chromosome 7 (7p14.3) (also known as *PIM1* and *RP9*)
PARK1 the α-SYN gene on chromosome 4 (4q21)
PARK2 the ubiquitin E3 ligase gene on chromosome 6 (6q25.2–q27)
PARK3 the ubiquitin C-terminal hydrolase L1 gene on chromosome 2 (2p13)
PARP poly (ADP-ribose) polymerase
PAS periodic acid Schiff
PAX2 the paired box gene 2 on chromosome 10 (10q24)
Pax2 the murine gene for paired box-2
PAX6 the gene for paired box-6 on chromosome 11 (11p13)
Pax6 the murine gene for paired box-6
PC phosphatidylcholine
PCDH15 the protocadherin-15 gene on chromosome 10 (10q21)
PCF pharyngeal conjunctival fever
PCG primary congenital glaucoma
PCR polymerase chain reaction
PCTH1 a gene on chromosome 9 (9q22.3)that codes for a transmembrane protein that suppresses TGFβ and Wnt families of signally proteins
PD polyol dehydrogenase, pseudoefficiency and Parkinson disease
PDCD1 the programmed cell death 1 gene on chromosome 2 (2q37.3)
PDE phosphodiesterase

PDE6A the rod cyclic guanosine monophosphate phosphodiesterase alpha subunit gene on chromosome 5 (5q33.1)
PDE6B the rod cyclic guanosine monophosphate phosphodiesterase beta subunit gene on chromosome 4 (4p16.3) (also known as *CSNB3*)
PDGF platelet derived growth factor
PDHA1 a gene on the X chromosome (Xp22.2–p22.1) that codes for a component of the pyruvate dehydrogenase complex
PDR proliferative diabetic retinopathy
PDS pigment dispersion syndrome
PDZ domain a structural domain of 80-90 amino acids that is found in certain signaling proteins
PE phosphatidylethanolamine
PEDF pigment epithelium-derived growth factor
PET positron emission tomography
PEX pseudoexfoliation syndrome
PEX1 the peroxisome biogenesis factor 1 (peroxin-1) gene on chromosome 7 (7q21–q22)
PEX10 the peroxisome biogenesis factor 10 (peroxin-10) gene on chromosome 1 (1p36.32)
PEX13 the peroxisome biogenesis factor 13 (peroxin-13) gene on chromosome 2 (2p15)
PEX26 the peroxisome biogenesis factor 26 (peroxin-26) gene on chromosome 22 (22q11.21)
PF-4 platelet factor 4
PFKM the muscle phosphofructokinase gene on chromosome 12(12q13.3)
PFV persistent fetal vasculature
PG proteoglycan; prostaglandin, pigmentary glaucoma
PGAM2 the muscle phosphoglycerate mutase gene on chromosome 7 (7p13–p12.3)
PGD_2 prostaglandin D2
PGE_2 prostaglandin E2
PGF placenta growth factor
PGF_2 prostaglandin F2
PGG_2 prostaglandin G2
PGH_2 prostaglandin H2
PGI_2 prostacyclin
PGP 9.5 ubiquitin carboxyl-terminal esterase L1
pH a measure of the of the acidity of a solution in terms of the hydrogen ions
PHA phytohemaglutinin
Phako phacoemulsification
PHKA1 the muscle isoform of the α-subunit of phosphorylase kinase gene on the X chromosome (Xq13)
PHKA2 the α-subunit of phosphorylase kinase gene on the X chromosome (Xp22.2–p22.1)
PHKB the β-subunit of liver and muscle phosphorylase kinase gene on chromosome 16 (16q12–q13)
PHKG2 the gene on the chromosome 16 (16q11–p12) that codes for the testis/liver isoform of the γ-subunit of phosphorylase kinase
PHLDA1 the gene on chromosome 12 (12q15) for pleckstrin homology-like domain Family A member 1 (also known as T cell death–associated gene 51)
PHPV persistent hyperplastic primary vitreous
Pi inorganic phosphate
PI phosphatidylinositol
pI isoelectric point
PI3K phosphoinositide-3 kinase
PIK3R3 phosphatidylinositol 3 kinase
PIM1 the PIM1-kinase associated protein 1 gene on chromosome 7 (7p14.3) (also known as *PAP1 and RP9*)
PIP proximal interphalangeal
PIP_2 phosphatidylinositol 4, 5-bisphosphate
PIP5K3 the phosphatiditylinositol-3-phosphate 5 kinase type III gene on chromosome 2 (2q35)
PITC phenylisothiocyanate
PITX2 the paired-like homeodomain transcription factor 2
PITX2 the paired-like homeodomain transcription factor 2 gene on chromosome 4 (4q25–q26)
Pitx2 the murine paired-like homeodomain transcription factor 2 gene
PITX3 the paired-like homeodomain transcription factor 3
PITX3 the paired-like homeodomain transcription factor 3 gene on chromosome 10 (10q25)
PLOD the lysyl hydroxylase gene on chromosome 1 (1p36.3–36.2)
PLP1 the main integral protein of myelin (proteolipid protein 1) gene on the X chromosome (Xq22)
PLXND1 the plexin D1 gene on chromosome 3 (3q21.3)
PM plasma membrane
PMMA polymethylmethacrylate
PML progressive multifocal leukoencephalopathy
PMN polymorphonuclear leukocyte/polymorphonuclear neutrophils
PMR polymyalgia rheumatica
PN polyarteritis nodosa
PNET primitive neuroectodermal tumor
PNR photoreceptor cell-specific nuclear receptor
PNR a gene on chromosome 15 (15q23) that codes for nuclear receptor subfamily 2, group E, member 3 (also known as *NR2E3* and *ESCS*)
PNS peripheral nervous system
POAG primary open angle glaucoma
Pol a gene of Rous sarcoma virus
POLA Pathologies Ocularies Liees a l'Age
POMGnT1 protein O-linked mannose beta 1,2-N-acetylglucosaminyltransferase 1
POMT1 the protein O-mannosyltransferase gene on chromosome 9 (9q34.1)
PORN progressive outer retinal necrosis
POU the gene for POU proteins (a family of proteins that are transcription factors with a bipartite DNA binding domain (POU domain); named after three mammalian transripton factors (Pit-1, Oct-1/Oct-2, and Unc-86)
PPAR peroxisome proliferator-activated receptor
PPCD posterior polymorphous corneal dystrophy
PPCRA pigmented paravenous chorioretinal atrophy
PPD purified protein derivative of tuberculin
PPGB the cathepsin protective protein gene on chromosome 20 (20q13.1)
PPP pentose phosphate pathway
PPP2CA the protein phosphatase 2A gene on chromosome 5 (5q23–q31)
PPRPE recessive retinitis pigmentosa with para-arteriolar preservation of the retinal pigment epithelium
PPT1 palmitoyl-protein thioesterase 1

PRAD1 parathyroid adenomatosis 1 (also known as cyclin D1 and BCL-1)
pRb retinoblastoma gene product
PRELP a small interstitial proteoglycan with proline arginine-rich end leucine rich repeats
PRELP the gene on chromosome 1 (1q32) that codes for the proteoglycans known as PRELP
pre-mRNA precursor messenger mRNA
PRG1 the serglycin gene on chromosome 10 (10q22.1)
PRKAR1A the protein kinase cAMP-dependent regulatory type 1 alpha gene on chromosome 17 (17q23–q24)
PRL the prolactin gene on chromosome 6 (6p22.2–p21.3)
PRNP the gene for prions on chromosome 20 (20pter–p12)
PROMM proximal myotonic myopathy
ProMMP-2 promatrix metalloproteinase-2
Prox1 the prospero-related homeobox 1 murine gene that codes for a transcription factor that is involved in the regulation of crystalline lens induction and development
PrP the normal cellular isoform of prion protein
PrP^c wildtype prion protein
PRPF3 a gene for human homolog of yeast pre-mRNA splicing factor 3 on chromosome 1 (1q21.2) (also known as *RP18*)
PRPF8 a gene for the human homolog of yeast pre-mRNA splicing factor C8 on chromosome 17 (17p13.3) (also known as *RP13*)
PRPF31 a gene for human homolog of yeast pre-mRNA splicing factor 31 on chromosome 19 (19q13.42) (also known as *RP11*)
PRPH2 the peripherin 2 gene on chromosome 6 (6p21.1–cen) (also known as *RDS* and *RP7*)
PrP^{sc} mutated prion protein (also known as PrPSC)
PrPSC mutated prion protein (also known as PrP^{SC})
PrPSc the abnormal disease-causing isoform of prion protein
PRR pattern recognition receptor
PSAP the saposin sulfatide activator gene on chromosome 10 (10q22.1)
PSC posterior subcapsular cataract
PSEN1 the presenilin-1 gene on chromosome 14 (14q)
PSEN2 the presenilin-2 gene on chromosome 1 (1q31–q42)
PSH proteinthiol
pSS primary Sjögren syndrome
PSH protein thiol
PTC phenylthiocarbamoyl
PTCH the human homolog of the *Drosophila* patch gene on chromosome 22 (23–q31)
PtdSer phosphatidylserine
PTEN a phosphatase and tensin homolog gene on chromosome 10 (10q23.31) that is mutated in Cowden syndrome
PTH phenylthiohydantoin; parathyroid hormone
PTLD post-transplant lymphoproliferative disease
PTMs post-translational modifications
PTP permeability transition pore
PTPN22 protein tyrosine phosphatase non-receptor 22
PTPRC protein kinase phosphatase receptor type C gene on chromosome 1(1q31–q32)
PU phacoantigenic uveitis
PUFA polyunsaturated fatty acid
PUK peripheral ulcerative keratitits
PVD posterior vitreous detachment
pVHLD the von Hippel-Lindau disease protein
PVR proliferative vitreoretinopathy
PYGL the liver phosphorylase gene on chromosome 14 (14q21–q22)
PYGM the muscle phosphorylase gene on chromosome 11 (11q13)
^{31}P-NMR phosphorous 31-nuclear magnetic resonance

q long arm of a chromosome
QTL quantitative trait locus

R rad
RA rheumatoid arthritis
Rab a family of small guanosine triphosphate (GTP)-binding proteins within the Ras superfamily that regulates vescicular trafficking pathways
RAB3A a protein that regulates synaptic vesicle exocytosis
RAB8A a Ras-associated protein
RAD51 a gene on chromosome 15 (15q15.1) that codes a homolog of *S. cerevisiae* RAD51
RAG1 recombination activating gene 1 on chromosome 11 (11p13)
RAG2 recombination activating gene 2 on chromosome 11 (11p13)
RANTES a cytokine (**R**egulated on **A**ctivation, **N**ormal **T** **E**xpressed and **S**ecreted)
RAR retinoic acid receptor
RARE retinoic acid-response element
Ras retrovirus-associated DNA sequences originally isolated from murine sarcoma virus; the Ras superfamily of small guanosine triphosphate (GTP)-binding proteins regulates vescicular trafficking pathways and includes the Rab family
^{86}Rb rubidium 86
Rb retinoblastoma
RB reticulate body
RB1 the retinoblastoma gene on chromosome 13 (13q14)
RBC red blood cell
RBP retinol binding protein
RBP1 retinol-binding protein 1 (also known as cellular retinol-binding protein [CRBP])
RCP the gene for red visual pigment on the X chromosome (Xq28)
RCS Royal College of Surgeons
RD retinal detachment
RDH1 the 11-*cis* retinol dehydrogenase 5 gene on chromosome 12 (12q13–q14) (also known as *RDH5*)
RDH5 retinol dehydrogenase 5
RDH5 the 11-*cis* retinol dehydrogenase 5 gene on chromosome 12 (12q13–q14) (also known as *RDH1*)
RDH12 retinol dehydrogenase 12
RDH12 the retinol dehydrogenase 12 gene on chromosome 14 (14q24.1)
rDNA ribosomal deoxyribonucleic acid
RDS the peripherin 2 gene on chromosome 6 (6p21.1–cen) (also known as *PRPH2* and *RP7*)

RDH5 the 11-*cis* retinol dehydrogenase 5 gene on chromosome 12 (12q13–q14) (also known as *RDH1)*

REAL classification Revised European American Lymphoma Classification

RECQL2 the recq protein-like 2 gene on chromosome 8 (8p12–p11.2)

RELA the A homolog of V-REL avian reticuloendotheliosis viral oncogene on chromosome 11 (11q12–q13)

RELB the B homolog of V-REL avian reticuloendotheliosis viral oncogene on chromosome 19 (19q13.32)

REP-1 Rab excort protein 1

REP-2 Rab excort protein 2

RER rough endoplasmic reticulum

RET the rearranged during transfection proto-oncogene on chromosome 10 (10q11.2)

RetGC1 retinal guanylate cyclase-1 (also known as GUCY2D)

RETGC1 the retinal-specific guanylate cyclase gene on chromosome 17 (17p13.1) (also known as *CORD6, GUCY2D*, and *LCA1*)

RF rheumatoid factor

RGC reinal ganglion cell

RGD an integrin-binding motif (ArgGlyAsp)

RGR retinal pigment epithelium-retinal G-protein coupled receptor

RGR the retinal pigment epithelium-retinal G-protein Coupled receptor gene on chromosome 10 (10q23.1)

Rho a family of small guanosine triphosphate (GTP) binding proteins

RHO the rhodopsin gene on chromosome 3 (3q21–q24) (also known as *RP4*)

RHOK the rhodopsin kinase gene on chromosome 13 (13q34) (also known as *GRK1*)

RICH rapidly involuting congenital hemangioma

RIM a protein involved in the regulation of glutamate release at the ribbon synapse of photoreceptors

RIMS1 protein regulating synaptic membrane exocytosis 1 gene on chromosome 6 (6q12–q13)

RK radial keratotomy

RLBP1 the cellular retinaldehyde-binding protein gene on chromosome 15 (15q26) (also known as *CRALBP*)

RNFLI retinal nerve fiber layer infarct (also known as "cotton wool" spot)

Ro Sjögren syndrome related antigen

ROBO3 a gene on chromosome 11 (11q23–q25) that codes a homolog of *Drosophila* roundabout 3

ROI reactive oxygen intermediates

ROM1 the rod outer segment protein 1 gene on chromosome 11 (11q13)

ROP retinopathy of prematurity

ROS reactive oxygen species

RP retinitis pigmentosa, refractive power, and relapsing polychondritis

RP1 the oxygen-regulated photoceptor protein 1 gene on chromosome 8(8q12.1)

RP3 the gene on the X chromosome (Xp11.4) for retinitis pigmentosa guanosine triphosphate hydrolase regulator (also known as *RPGR, CORDX* and *COD1*)

RP4 the rhodopsin gene on chromosome 3 (3q21–q24) (also known as *RHO*)

RP7 the peripherin 2 gene on chromosome 6 (6p21.1–cen) (also known as *RDS* and *PRPH2)*

RP9 the PIM1-kinase associated protein 1 gene on chromosome 7 (7p14.3) (also known as *PAP1 and PIM1*)

RP10 the inosine monophosphate dehydrogenase 1 gene on chromosome 7 (7q32.1) (also known as *IMPDH1*)

RP11 a gene on chromosome 19 (19q13.42) that codes for human homolog of yeast pre-mRNA splicing factor 31 (also known as *PRPF31*)

RP12 a gene on chromosome 1 (1q31–q32.1) that codes for a homolog of *Drosophila* Crumbs 1 (also known as *CRB1*)

RP13 a gene on chromosome 17 (17p13.3) that codes for human homolog of yeast pre-mRNA splicing factor C8 (also known as *PRPF8*)

RP14 the tubby–like protein 1 gene on chromosome 6 (6p21.3) (also known as *TULP1*)

RP17 the gene for carbonic anhydrase IV on chromosome 17 (17q23.2) (also known as *CA4*)

RP18 a gene on chromosome 1 (1q21.2) that codes for human homolog of yeast pre-mRNA splicing factor 3 (also known as *PRPF3*)

RP19 the ATP-binding cassette transporter retinal gene on chromosome 1 (1p21–p13) (also known as *ABCA4, ABCR*, and *STGD1*)

RP20 a gene on chromosome 1 (1p31) that codes for retinal pigment epithelium-specific 65 kDa protein (also known as *RPE65* and *LCA2*)

RP22 a locus for retinitis pigmentosa on chromosome 16 (16p12.3–p12.1)

RP25 a locus for retinitis pigmentosa on chromosome 6 (6cen–q15)

RP26 the gene for ceramide kinase-like protein on chromosome 2 (2q31.3) (also known as *CERKL*)

RP27 a gene on chromosome 14 (14q11.2) that codes for neural retina leucine zipper (also known as *NRL*)

RP28 a locus for retinitis pigmentosa on chromosome 2 (2p16–p11)

RP29 a locus for retinitis pigmentosa on chromosome 4 (4q32–q34)

RP30 the gene on chromosome 17 (17q25) that codes for retinal fascin homolog 2 actin bindig protein (also known as *FSCN2*)

RP31 a locus for retinitis pigmentosa on chromosome 9 (9p22–p13)

RP32 a locus for retinitis pigmentosa on chromosome 1 (1p34.3–p13.3)

RPE retinal pigment epithelium

RPE65 retinal pigment epithelium-specific 65 kDa protein

RPE65 a gene on chromosome 1 (1p31) that codes for retinal pigment epithelium-specific 65 kDa protein (also known as *LCA2* and *RP20*)

RPED retinal pigment epithelium detachment

RPGR the gene on the X chromosome (Xp11.4) for retinitis pigmentosa guanosine triphosphate hydrolase regulator (also known as *RP3, CORDX* and *COD1*)

RPGR-ORF15 a highly repetitive purine-region in the open reading frame 15 of the *RRGR* gene

RPGRIP1 the RPGR-interating protein 1 gene on chromosome 14 (14q11.2) (also known as *LCA6*)

RRD rhegmatogenous retinal detachment
RS Reiter syndrome
RS1 the retinoschism gene on the X chromosome (Xp22.2–p22.1)
RSV Rous sarcoma virus
RT-PCR reverse transcription-polymerase chain reaction
RVFV rift valley fever virus
RX the retina and anterior neural fold homeobox gene on chromosome 18 (18q21.3) (also known as *RAX*)
Rx1 a murine eye field transcription factor
RYR1 the ryanodine receptor 1 gene on chromosome 19 (19q13.1)

^{35}S sulfur isotope 35
S sulfur and the phase of synthesis in the cell cycle
S-antigen arrestin
S100 a calcium binding protein
SAA serum amyloid protein A
SAA1 the serum amyloid A1 gene on chromosome 11 (11p15.1)
SAA1 serum amyloid A1
SAA2 the serum amyloid A2 gene on chromosome 11 (11p15.1)
SAA2 serum amyloid A2
SAA3 the serum amyloid A3 gene on chromosome 11 (11p15.1–p14))
SAA3 serum amyloid A3
SAA4 the serum amyloid A4 gene on chromosome 11 (11p15.1)
SAA4 serum amyloid A4
SAAL an acute phase reactant protein; a precursor of SAA
SAC seasonal allergic conjunctivitis
SAG the arrestin gene on chromosome 2 (2q37.1)
SAGE serial analysis of gene expression
SALT skin associated lymphoid tissue
SAM senescence accelerated mouse; also sterile alpha motif
SANS the sans gene on chromosome 17 (17q24)
SAP serum amyloid protein
SAP-A saposin A
SAP-B saposin B
SAP-C saposin C
SAP-D saposin D
SAPK stress-activated protein kinase
SARA2 a gene on chromosome 5 (5q31.10 that causes chylomicron retention disease when mutated
SAT1 the spermidine/spermine N(1)-acetyltransferase-1 gene on the X chromosome (Xp22.1)
SBF2 a gene on chromosome 17 (17q11.2) that causes Charcot-Marie Tooth disease type 4 when mutated
SCC squamous cell carcinoma
S cone blue cone
SCD Schnyder corneal dystrophy
SCID severe combined immune deficiency
sCJD sporadic Creutzfelt-Jakob disease
SC02 a nuclear gene on chromosome 22 (22q13) that codes for a component of the mitochondrial respiratory chain complex IV
SDC1 the syndecan 1 gene on chromosome 2 (2p24.1)
SDC2 the syndecan 2 gene on chromosome 8 (8q22–q24)
SDC3 the syndecan 3 gene on chromosome 1 (1p32)
SDC4 the syndecan 4 gene on chromosome 20 (20q12–q13)
SDF-1 stromal cell-derived factor 1 (also known as chemokine CXC motif ligand 12)
SDHA a gene on chromosome 5 (5p15) that codes a component of the mitochondrial respiratory chain complex II
SDS sodium dodecyl sulfate
SDS-PAGE sodium dodecyl sulfate-polyacrylamide gel electrophoresis
Se selenium
sec second
SED spondyloepiphyseal dysplasia with dwarfism
SEER **S**urveillance, **E**pidemiology, and **E**nd **R**esults
SEGA subependymal giant cell astrocytoma
SELDI-TOF surface-enhanced laser desorption ionization time-of flight
SEM scanning electron microscopy and standard error of the mean
SEMA4A semaphorin 4A (also known as SEMAB)
SEMA4A the semaphorin 4A gene on chromosome 1 (1q22) (also known as *SEMAB*)
SEMAB the semaphorin 4A gene on chromosome 1 (1q22) (also known as *SEMA4A*)
SEN subependymal nodules
SEPN1 the selenoprotein N gene on chromosome 1 (1p36–p35)
Ser serine
SFAs semifluorinated alkanes
SFD Sorsby fundus dystrophy
SGSH the heparan *N*-sulfatase gene on chromosome 17 (17q25.3)
SH sulfhydryl group
SH3BP2 SH3 domain-binding protein 2
SHH the sonic hedgehog gene on chromosome 7 (7q36)
Shh the murine sonic hedgehog gene
sHSPs small heat shock proteins
SIAT9 the sialyltransferase-9 gene on chromosome 2 (2p11.2)
sICAM-1 soluble form of ICAM-1
SIgA sectory component of immunoglobulin A
sIL-2r soluble interleukin 2 receptor
SILAC stable isotope labelling with amino acids in cell culture
Sip1 a murine gene that codes a transcription factor that is involved in crystalline lens induction and develpment
Six3 a murine eye field transcription factor that is the homolog of the Drosophila sine oculis homeobox 3 gene
SIX5 the gene for sine oculis-5 on chromosome 19 (19q13.3)
SIX6 a gene on chromosome 14 (14q23) that is the homolog of the Drosophila sine oculis homeobox 6 gene
Six6 a murine eye field transcription factor that is the homolog of the Drosophila sine oculis homeobox 6 gene
SJS Stevens Johnson syndrome
Ski a murine proto-oncogene
SLC4A11 the sodium borate cotransporter gene on chromosome 20 (20p13–p12)

SLC39A4 a gene on chromosome 8 (8q24.3) that controls zinc absorption from the intestine
SLC40A1 a gene on chromosome 2 (2q32) that causes hemochromatosis when mutated
SLC1745 a gene on chromosome 6 (6q14–q15)that codes for a transporter of sialic acid into the lysosome
SLE systemic lupus erythematosus
SLEB2 a locus for systemic lupus erythematosus susceptibility on chromosome 2 (2q37)
SLIPS syndecan-like integral membrane proteoglycans
SLL small lymphocytic lymphoma
SLRR a superfamily of small proteoglycans containing tandem arrays of leucine-rich repeats
SLS segment long spacing
Smac/SMAC second mitochondria-derived activator of caspases
SMADs a group of related intracellular proteins critical for transmitting to the nucleus signals from TGFβ
SMPD1 a sphingomyelinase gene on chromosome 11 (11p15.4–p15.1)
SNAILs a family of zinc finger transcription factors first identified in *Drosophila*
SNAP-25 a protein involved in the regulation of acetylcholine release
SNP single nucleotide polymorphism
SO sympathetic ophthalmia
SOC53 suppressor of cytokine signaling
SOD superoxide dismutase
SOD2 the manganese superoxide dismutase gene on chromosome 6 (6q25.3)
SOX1 the Sry-box 1 gene on chromosome 13 (13q34)
Sox1 the murine Sry-box 1 gene
SOX2 the Sry-box 2 gene on chromosome 3 (3q26.3–q27)
Sox2 the murine Sry-box 2 gene
SOX3 the Sry-box 3 gene on the X chromosome 3 (Xq26.3)
Sox3 the murine Sry-box 3 gene
SOX9 SRY-Box 9 the product of the SRY-related HMG-box gene 9
sp. species
SPARC secreted protein, acidic, cysteine-rich (also known as osteonectin)
SPK superficial punctate keratitis
SRBC sheep red blood cell
Src a gene in Rous sarcoma virus
SRP signal recognition particle
SRS-A slow reacting substance of anaphylaxis (currently known as leukotreine C_4)
SRT substrate reduction therapy
SS Sjögren syndrome
SS-A an antigen to Sjögren syndrome
SS-B an antigen to Sjögren syndrome
SSc systemic sclerosis
SSCP single-stranded conformational polymorphism
ssDNA single standed deoxyribonucleic acid
SSH suppression subtraction hybridization
SSPE subacute sclerosing panencephalitis
ssRNA-RT single standed ribonucleic acid-reverse transcriptase
sSS secondary Sjögren syndrome
ST sulfotransferase
STGD Stargardt disease
STGD1 Stargardt disease type 1
STGD1 the ATP-binding cassette transporter retinal gene on chromosome 1 (1p21–p13) (also known as RP19, *ABCA4*, and *ABCR*)
STGD2 Stargardt disease type 3
STGD3 Stargardt disease type 3
STS serologic test for syphilis
STS a gene for steroid sulfatase on the X chromosome (Xp22.32)
SUMF1 the gene on the chromosome 3 (3p26) that codes for a sulfatase that acts on all substates
SUOX the sulfite oxidase gene on chromosome 12
SubRPE subretinal pigment epithelium
SURF1 a nuclear gene on chromosome 9 (9q34) that codes a component of the mitochondrial respiratory chain complex IV
SV systemic vasculidides
SV40 simian virus 40
SWS Sturge–Weber syndrome
SYPRO™ a registered tradename of Molecular Probes

T thymine
T1-weighted image a magnetic resonance image using short TE and TR times; it has greater signal intensity from fat containing tissues
T2-weighted image a magnetic resonance image made with a sequence with long TR and TE to show contrast in tissues with varying T2 relaxation times; water gives a strong signal
T3 triiodothyronine
T4 thyroxine
TA Takayasu arteritis
TACSTD2 the current name for the gene on chromosome 1 (1p32) that was formerly called *M1S1*, *TROP2*, and *GA733-1*
TALL1 tumor necrosis factor and Apo1-related leukocyte-expressed ligand 1 (also known as tumor necrosis factor ligand, member 13B [TNFSF13B] and B cell activating factor, and zTNF4)
TAP transporter associated with antigen processing
TAT the tyrosine aminotransferase gene on chromosome 16 (16q22.1–q22.3)
TATA thymine-adenine-thymine-adenine
TBA thiobarbituric acid
TBD Thiel-Behnke corneal dystrophy
tBid truncated Bid
Tc phase separation temperature
Tc cytotoxic T-cell
TCA tricarboxylic acid cycle (also known as Krebs cycle and citric acid cycle)
T cell T lymphocyte
TCF8 a transcription factor 8 gene on chromosome 10 (10p11.2)
TCR T-cell receptor
TCR Vβ variable region of the T-cell receptor β chain
TdT terminal deoxynucleotidyl transferase
TDT transmission disequilibrium test
TEK gene encoding endothelial cell-specific tyrosine kinase receptor
TEM transmission electron microscopy

TEN toxic epidermal necrolysis
TEWL transepithelial water loss
TFR2 a gene on chromosome 7 (7q22) that causes hemochromatosis when mutated
TG thymine-guanine dinucleotide
TGase transglutaminase
TG2 tissue transglutaminase
TG3 epidermal transglutaminase
TGF transforming growth factor
TGFα transforming growth factor α
TGFβ transforming growth factor β
TGFB the transforming growth factor β1 gene on chromosome 19 (19q13.1), also known as *TGFB1*
TGFβ1 transforming growth factor β1
TGFB1 the transforming growth factor β1 gene on chromosome 19 (19q13.1)
TGFβ2 transforming growth factor β2
TGFBI the transforming growth factor beta induced gene on chromosome 5 (5q31)
TGFBIp transforming growth factor beta induced protein
TGFBR2 the TGFβ receptor 2 gene on chromosome 3 (3p22)
TGIF the transforming growth factor beta-induced factor gene on chromosome 18 (18p11.3)
TGM2 the transglutaminase-2 gene on chromosome 20 (20q11.2–q12)
Th helper T cell
Th0 precursors of other helper T cells
Th1 helper T cell type 1 that is involved in cell-mediated immunity (also known as Th1-cell)
Th2 helper T cell type 2 that stimulates antibody production by B-cells (also known as Th2-cell)
Thr threonine
Thy-1 a major cell surface protein of T lymphocytes
TIGR an former term for the *MYOC* gene on chromosome 1 (1q21–31) that codes for myocilin
TIL tumor infiltrating lymphocytes
TIMP tissue inhibitor of metalloproteinase
TIMP1 the tissue inhibitor of metalloproteinase 1 gene on the X chromosome (Xp11.3–p11.23)
TIMP2 the tissue inhibitor of metalloproteinase 2 gene on chromosome 17 (17q25)
TIMP3 the tissue inhibitor of metalloproteinase 3 gene on chromosome 22 (22q12.1–q13.2)
TIMP1 tissue inhibitor of metalloproteinase 1
TIMP2 tissue inhibitor of metalloproteinase 2
TIMP3 tissue inhibitor of metalloproteinase 3
tk thymine kinase
TKT transketolase
Tll the murine paired box-6 gene
TLR Toll-like receptor
TM trabecular meshwork
TMS triple-membrane structure
TNC the tenascin C gene on chromosome 9 (9q33)
TNF tumor necrosis factor
TNF the tumor necrosis factor gene on chromosome 6 (6p21.3)
TNFα tumor necrosis factor α
TNFβ tumor necrosis factor β
TNR the tenascin R gene on chromosome 1 (1q24)
TNFR tumor necrosis factor receptor
TNFR1 tumor necrosis factor receptor 1 (also known as tumor necrosis factor receptor superfamily member 1A, death receptor 1 and CD120a)
TNFR2 tumor necrosis factor receptor 2 (also known as CD120b)
TNFRSF1A tumor necrosis factor receptor superfamily, member 1A
TNFRSF1B tumor necross factor receptor superfamily, member 1B
TNFRSF12 tumor necrosis factor receptor superfamily member 12 (also known as death receptor 3 [DR3], lymphocyte-associated receptor of death [LARD], TRAMP, and WSL1)
TNFR25 tumor necrosis factor receptor 1
TNFSF13B tumor necrosis factor ligand, member 13B (also known as B cell activating factor, TALL1 and zTNF4)
TNM tumor-nodes-metastases
TP53 the tumor protein p53 gene on chromosome 17 (17p13.1)
TP73L the gene on chromosome 3 (3q27) that codes for tumor protein p73-like (also known as tumor protein p63)
TPA 12-O-tetradecanoylphobol-13-acetate
TPO thyroid peroxidase
TRADD tumor necrosis factor receptor associated death domain
TRAF1 tumor necrosis factor receptor associated factor 1
TRAR2 tumor necrosis factor receptor associated factor 2
TRAIL tumor necrosis factor-related apoptosis inducing ligand (also known as APO2L)
TRAIL3 tumor necrosis factor-related apoptosis inducing ligand 3 (also known as DCR1)
TRAIL4 tumor necrosis factor-related apoptosis inducing ligand 4 (also known as DCR2)
TRAILR1 Tumor necrosis factor (TNF)-related apoptosis-inducing ligand receptor 1 (also known as death receptor 4 [DR4] and APO2)
TRAILR2 Tumor necrosis factor (TNF)-related apoptosis-inducing ligand receptor 2 (also known as death receptor 5 [DR5], KILLER and TRICK2)
TRAILR3 Tumor necrosis factor (TNF)-related apoptosis-inducing ligand receptor 3 (also known as death receptor 3 [DR3], tumor nerosis factor receptor superfamily member 10C [TNFRSF10C], decoy receptor 1 [DCR1] and TRAIL receptor without an intracellular domain [TRID])
TRAILR4 Tumor necrosis factor (TNF)-related apoptosis-inducing ligand receptor 4
TRAP150 the thyroid hormone receptor associated protein 3 gene on chromosome 1 (1p34.3)
TRB trilateral retinobastoma
Treg regulatory T-cells
TRH thyrotropin releasing hormone
TRIC trachoma and inclusion conjunctivitis
TRICK 2 death receptor 5 (DR5) also known as tumor necrosis factor-related apoptosis-inducing ligand receptor 2 [TRAIL2] and KILLER)
TRKA tyrosine kinase receptor A
TRKB tyrosine kinase receptor B
TRKC tyrosine kinase receptor C

TROP2 a former name for the *TACSTD2* gene on chromosome 1 (1p32–p31)
TRP1 a tyrosinase-related protein enzyme that catalyzes DHICA polymerization
TRP1 the tyrosinase-related protein 1 gene on chromosome 9 (9q23)
TRYP-1 enzyme that catalyzes the polymerization of 5,6-dihydroxyindole-2-carboxylic acid
tRNA transfer RNA
Ts suppressor T-cell
TSC tuberous sclerosis complex
TSC1 a gene for tuberous sclerosis complex on chromosome 9 (9q34)
TSC2 a gene for tuberous sclerosis complex on chromosome 16 (16p13.3)
TSD Tay-Sachs disease
TSH thyroid stimulating hormone
TSTA tumor-specific transplantation antigens
TTF-1 thyroid transcription factor 1
TTP1 tripeptidyl peptidase 1
TTP1 the tripeptidyl peptidase 1 gene on chromosome 8 (8q13.1–q13.3)
TTR the transthyretin gene on chromosome 18 (18q11.2–q12.1)
TTT transpupillary thermotherapy
Try a murine gene involved in melanin production
TUCAN tumor-up-regulated caspase recruitment domain (CARD)-containing antagonist
TULP1 Tubby–like protein 1
TULP1 the tubby–like protein 1 gene on chromosome 6 (6p21.3) (also known as *RP14*)
TUNEL terminal deoxynucleotidyl transferase (TdT) mediated 2′-deoxyuridine 5′-triphosphate (dUTP) nick-end labelling
Tyr tyrosine
TYR the tyrosinase gene on chromosome 11 (11q14-21)
Tyrp1 a murine gene involved in melanin production
TWIST a transcription factor
TXA_2 thromboxane A_2

U uracil
UBE2A the ubiquitin conjugating enzyme E2A gene on the X chromosome (Xq24–q25)
UBE2B the ubiquitin conjugating enzyme E2B gene on chromosome 5 (5q23–q31)
UBIAD1 a gene on chromosome 1 (1p34–1p36) that encodes a potential prenyltransferase
UDP uridine diphosphate
UGH uveitis-glaucoma-hyphema
U.K. United Kingdom
UNC119 the retinal gene 4 on chromosome 17 (17q11.2)
UNICEF Unted Nations International Children's Emergency Fund
UP ubiquinated proteins
UPS ubiquitin-proteasome system
US$ US dollars
U.S. United States
USH syndrome Usher syndrome
USH1 a type of Usher syndrome that has been mapped to chromosome 14 (14q32)
USH1B a type of Usher syndrome due to a mutation in the *MYO7A* gene
USH1C a type of Usher syndrome due to a mutation in the *USH1C* gene
USH1C the harmonin gene on chromosome 11 (11p15)
USH1D a type of Usher syndrome due to a mutation in the *CDH23* gene
USH1E a type of Usher syndrome that has been mapped to chromosome 21 (21q21)
USH1F a type of Usher syndrome due to a mutation in the *PCDH15* gene
USH1G a type of Usher syndrome due to a mutation in the *SANS* gene
USH2 a type of Usher syndrome
USH2A a type of Usher syndrome due to a mutation in the *USH2A* gene
USH2A the usherin gene on chromosome 1 (1q41)
USH2B a type of Usher syndrome that has been mapped to chromosome 3 (3p24)
USH2C a type of Usher syndrome due to a mutation in the *VLGR1* gene
USH3 a type of Usher syndrome
USH3A a type of Usher syndrome due to a mutation in the *USH3A* gene
USH3A a clarin-1 gene on chromosome 3 (3q21–25)
USP6 ubiquitin-specific protease 6
USP6 the ubiquitin-specific protease 6 gene on chromosome 17 (17p13)
UV ultraviolet
UVA ultraviolet A (100–290 nm)
UVA1 ultraviolet A1 (340–400 nm)
UVA2 ultraviolet A2 (320–340 nm)
UVB ultraviolet B (290–320 nm)

−ve negative
+ve positive
VDAC voltage-dependent anion channel
Val valine
Vax1 a murine ventral anterior homeobox gene
Vax2 a murine ventral anterior homeobox gene
VCAM-1 vascular cell adhesion molecule-1
vCJD variant Creutzfeldt-Jakob disease
VDAC voltage dependent anion channel (also known as porin)
VDR the vitamin D receptor gene on chromosome 12 (12q–q14)
VEGF vascular endothelial growth factor
$VEGF_{120}$ an isoform of vascular endothelial growth factor with 120 amino acids
$VEGF_{145}$ a human isoform of vascular endothelial growth factor with 145 amino acids
$VEGF_{165}$ a human isoform of vascular endothelial growth factor with 165 amino acids
$VEGF_{164}$ a murine isoform of vascular endothelial growth factor with 165 amino acids

$VEGF_{188}$ a murine isoform of vascular endothelial growth factor with 189 amino acids
$VEGF_{189}$ a human isoform of vascular endothelial growth factor with 189 amino acids
$VEGF_{206}$ a human isoform of vascular endothelial growth factor with 206 amino acids
VEGF-A vascular endothelial growth factor A
VEGF-B vascular endothelial growth factor B
VEGF-C vascular endothelial growth factor C
VEGF-D vascular endothelial growth factor D
VEGF-E vascular endothelial growth factor E
VEGFR1 vascular endothelial growth factor receptor 1
VEGFR2 vascular endothelial growth factor receptor 2
VEGFR3 vascular endothelial growth factor receptor 3
VEP visual evoked potential
VER visual evoked response
VHL von Hippel-Lindau protein
VHL the gene on chromosome 3 (3p25–26) that causes von Hippel-Lindau disease when mutated
VHLD von Hippel-Lindau disease
VIP vasoactive intestinal peptide
VIPR vasoactive intestinal peptide receptor
vJNCL variant juvenile neuronal ceroid lipofuscinosis
VKC vernal keratoconjunctivitis
VKH Vogt–Koyanagi–Hirada syndrome or disease
VLCFA very long chain fatty acid
VLDL very low density lipoproteins
VLGR1 the very large G-protein coupled receptor 1 gene on chromosome 5 (5q14)
vLINCL variant late infantile onset neuronal ceroid lipofuscinosis
VLM visceral larva migrans
VMD2 the bestrophin gene on chromosome 11 (11q13)
VSX1 the visual system homeobox gene 1 on chromosome 20 (20p11.2)
VSV vesicular stomatitis virus
VTNS the gene on chromosome 17 (17p13) that codes for a transporter of cystine
VWF von Willebrand factor
VZV varicella zoster virus

WAGR syndrome Wilms tumor-aniridia-genitourinary anomalies-mental retardation syndrome
WD repeat-containing protein 36
WDR36 a gene on chromosome 5 (5q22.1) that causes primary open glaucoma when mutated
WEE1 the Wee1 tyrosine kinase gene on chromosome 11 (11p15.3–p15.1)
WG Wegener granulomatosis
WHO World Health Organization
WNTs a family of highly conserved developmental control genes involved in signaling pathways that were first identified in *Drosophila*
Wnt4 a murine developmental control gene involved in signaling pathways that were first identified in *Drosophila*
WRD-36 an unusual extracellular matrix protein
WT1 a gene on chromosome 11 (11p13) for a zinc finger DNA–binding protein
WTV weak transforming viruses

XIAP X-linked inhibitor of apoptosis protein
XLRP X linked recessive retinitis pigmentosa
XLRS X-linked retinoschisis
XP xeroderma pigmentosum
XR x-linked recessive
xRP X-linked recessive retinitis pigmentosa

Z zeaxanthin and Zwischenscheibe
Z band a perpendicularly arranged band in striated muscle
ZIP a family of metal ion transporters
Zip4 the protein product of the *SLC39A4* gene
zTNF4 tumor necrosis factor ligand, member 13B (also known as B cell activating factor [TNFSF13B])
ZNF9 the zinc finger protein 9 gene on chromosome 3 (3q21.3)

Index

Note: Page numbers followed by F indicate figures; page numbers followed by T indicate tables.